Cardiological Society of India

CARDIOLOGY

UPDATE 2024

Cardiological Society of India

CARDIOLOGY

UPDATE 2024

Volume 2

Editor-in-Chief

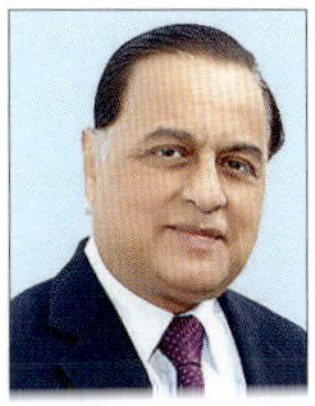

Sanjay Tyagi

MD(Medicine) DM(Cardiology) FAMS FICP FCSI FICA FRCP(Edinburgh) FSCAI FESC FACC(USA)
Dr BC Roy National Awardee
Senior Consultant, Academic Advisor (HOD) and Clinical Director Cardiology
Apollo Hospitals, Northern Region, New Delhi, India
President-Elect, Cardiological Society of India
Secretary General (India), International College of Cardiology (USA)
National Coordinator, Cardiology and Interventional Cardiology, National Board of Examination

Formerly

Director General Health Services, Govt of India
Dean, Maulana Azad Medical College, New Delhi
Director, Professor and HOD Cardiology
GB Pant Institute of Postgraduate Medical Education and Research

Co-Editors

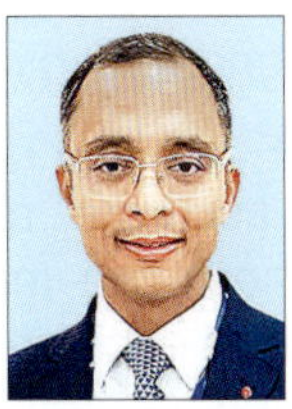

Mohit D Gupta MD DM FAMS FACC(USA)
Director–Professor, Department of Cardiology
GB Pant Institute of Postgraduate Medical Education and Research
New Delhi, India

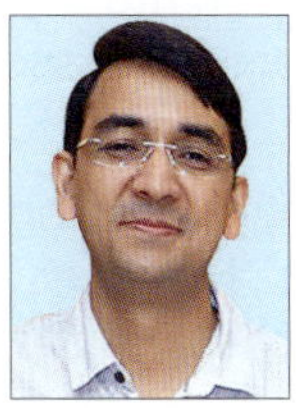

Saurabh Kumar Gupta MD DM
Professor, Department of Cardiology
All India Institute of Medical Sciences
New Delhi, India

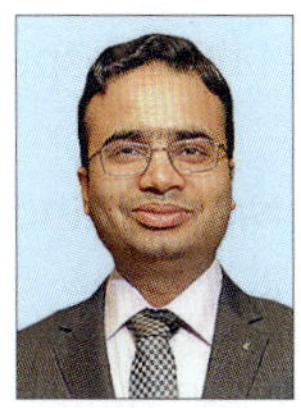

Ankit Bansal MD DM(Cardiology)
Professor, Department of Cardiology
GB Pant Institute of Postgraduate Medical Education and Research
New Delhi, India

Foreword

M Khalilullah

JAYPEE

JAYPEE BROTHERS MEDICAL PUBLISHERS
The Health Sciences Publisher
New Delhi | London

JAYPEE **Jaypee Brothers Medical Publishers (P) Ltd**

Headquarters
EMCA House
23/23-B, Ansari Road, Daryaganj
New Delhi 110 002, India
Landline: +91-11-23272143, +91-11-23272703
+91-11-23282021, +91-11-23245672
E-mail: jaypee@jaypeebrothers.com

Corporate Office
Jaypee Brothers Medical Publishers (P) Ltd.
4838/24, Ansari Road, Daryaganj
New Delhi 110 002, India
Phone: +91-11-43574357
Fax: +91-11-43574314
E-mail: jaypee@jaypeebrothers.com

Overseas Office
JP Medical Ltd.
83, Victoria Street, London
SW1H 0HW (UK)
Phone: +44-20 3170 8910
Fax: +44(0)20 3008 6180
E-mail: info@jpmedpub.com

Website: www.jaypeebrothers.com
Website: www.jaypeedigital.com

Inquiries for bulk sales may be solicited at: jaypee@jaypeebrothers.com

CSI Cardiology Update 2024 (Volume 2) / Sanjay Tyagi

First Edition: **2025**

ISBN: 978-93-6616-795-4

Printed at: Samrat Offset Pvt. Ltd.

DEDICATION

We dedicate this book to our parents and teachers for their inspiration, unwavering support, guidance and making us believe that we can overcome any challenges.

We are indebted to wives and children for their encouragement and most importantly sparing us the invaluable time required for this arduous task.

We owe our deepest gratitude to our patients for their trust and being part of our journey.

Contributors

Editor-in-Chief

Sanjay Tyagi MD(Medicine) DM(Cardiology) FAMS FICP FCSI FICA FRCP(Edinburgh) FSCAI FESC FACC(USA)
Dr BC Roy National Awardee
Senior Consultant, Academic Advisor (HOD) and Clinical Director Cardiology
Apollo Hospitals, Northern Region, New Delhi, India
President-Elect, Cardiological Society of India
Secretary General (India), International College of Cardiology (USA)
National Coordinator, Cardiology and Interventional Cardiology, National Board of Examination

Formerly
Director General Health Services, Govt of India
Dean, Maulana Azad Medical College, New Delhi
Director, Professor and HOD Cardiology
GB Pant Institute of Postgraduate Medical Education and Research

Co-Editors

Mohit D Gupta MD DM FAMS FACC(USA)
Director–Professor
Department of Cardiology
GB Pant Institute of Postgraduate Medical Education and Research
New Delhi, India

Saurabh Kumar Gupta MD DM
Professor
Department of Cardiology
All India Institute of Medical Sciences
New Delhi, India

Ankit Bansal MD DM(Cardiology)
Professor
Department of Cardiology
GB Pant Institute of Postgraduate Medical Education and Research
New Delhi, India

Contributing Authors

Aarya A Naik MBBS
PGY1 MD (Medicine)
University of Tennessee Medical Center
Memphis, Tennessee, USA

Abhilasha MD
Senior Resident
SRM Medical College
SRM Institute of Science and Technology
Chennai, Tamil Nadu, India

Abhinav Aggarwal MD(Medicine) DNB(Medicine)
Senior Resident
Department of Cardiology
VMMC and Safdarjung Hospital
New Delhi, India

Abhinay Tibdewal MD DNB DM FSCAI
Consultant Interventional Cardiologist
Medica Superspeciality Hospital
Kolkata, West Bengal, India

Abhishek Chaturvedi MD
Interventional Cardiology Fellow
Georgetown University MedStar
Washington Hospital Center
Washington DC, USA
International Fellow
Center for Chronic Disease Control (CCDC)
New Delhi, India

Lt Col (Dr) Abhishek Mallick MD(Pediatrics) DNB(Pediatrics) DM(Pediatric Cardiology)
Senior Resident
Department of Cardiology
Advanced Cardiac Center
Postgraduate Institute for Medical Education and Research
Chandigarh, India

Abhishek Garg MD DM
Resident, Department of Cardiology
Dayanand Medical College and Hospital
Unit-Hero DMC Heart Institute
Ludhiana, Punjab, India

Abhishek Goyal MD DM
Professor
Department of Cardiology
Dayanand Medical College and Hospital
Unit-Hero DMC Heart Institute
Ludhiana, Punjab, India

Abhishek Kumawat MD
3rd Year (DM)
ABVIMS and DR RML Hospital
New Delhi, India

Abraham Oomman MD DM(Cardiology)
Senior Consultant Interventional Cardiologist
Apollo Main Hospital
Chennai, Tamil Nadu, India

Abraham Paul MD DM(Cardiology)
Consultant, Aster Medcity
Kochi, Kerala, India

Achukatla Kumar Pharm D
Senior Research Consultant
Apollo Hospitals
Indore, Madhya Pradesh, India

AD Arun Mohan MD DrNB(Cardiology)
Resident, Meenakshi Hospital
Thanjavur, Tamil Nadu, India

Aditi A Naik MBBS
3rd Year
NHL Medical College and VS Hospital
Ahmedabad, Gujarat, India

Aditya Kapoor MD DM
Professor and Head
Department of Cardiology
Sanjay Gandhi Postgraduate Institute of Medical Sciences
Lucknow, Uttar Pradesh, India

Advait Akash MD DM(Cardiology)
Cardiologist
Heart Hospital
Patna, Bihar, India

Aftab Khan MD(Medicine) DM(Cardiology) DNB(Cardiology)
Consultant Interventional Cardiologist
Department of Cardiology
Director, Electrophysiology Services
Apollo Multispeciality Hospitals
Kolkata, West Bengal, India

Aishwarya Gaur DNB(General Medicine)
Resident
Department of Medicine
ESIC Model Hospital
Jaipur, Rajasthan, India

Aishwarya Vyas MD DM
Resident
Department of Cardiology
SMS Medical College
Jaipur, Rajasthan, India

Ajay Bahl FRCP DM
Professor
Postgraduate Institute of Medical Education and Research
Chandigarh, India

Ajay Kumar Sinha MD PhD FRCP(Edinburgh) FACC FESC FCSI FICC FAPSCC
Director
Department of Clinical Cardiology and Research
Jai Prabha Medanta Superspecialty Hospital
Patna, Bihar, India

Ajay M Naik MD DM DNB FACC FHRS
Cardiac Electrophysiologist
Marengo CIMS Hospital
Ahmedabad, Gujarat, India

Ajay S Chaurasia MD DM(Cardiology)
Professor and Head
Department of Cardiology
Topiwala National Medical College and BYL
Nair Charitable Hospital
Mumbai, Maharashtra, India

Ajit Desai MD DM(Cardiology) DNB(Cardiology) FACC
Additional Director
Department of Cardiology
Jaslok Hospital
Mumbai, Maharashtra, India

Ajit D Pai BA MPH
Data Scientist
Cardiovascular Specialists of Redlands and Inland Empire
Redlands, CA, USA

Ajit Kumar Valaparambil MD DM
Senior Consultant
Kerala Institute of Medical Science
Former Dean and Head
Department of Cardiology
Sree Chitra Tirunal Institute
Thiruvananthapuram, Kerala, India

Ajit S Mullasari MD DM
Chairman and Head
Department of Cardiology
Institute of Cardio Vascular Diseases
The Madras Medical Mission Hospital
Professor of Practice
Indian Institute of Technology – Madras
Chennai, Tamil Nadu, India

A Kader Sahib MD DrNB MRCP(London)
Consultant Cardiologist
Apollo Hospitals
Trichy, Tamil Nadu, India

Akash Gopi MD DNB(Cardiology)
Cardiologist
Fortis Hospitals
Bengaluru, Karnataka, India

Akash Shah MD(Medicine)
3rd Year DM Cardiology Resident
Bombay Hospital
Mumbai, Maharashtra, India

Akhilesh Kumar MD(Medicine) DrNB(Cardiology)
Senior Resident
Fortis Escort Heart Institute
New Delhi, India

AK Pancholia MD FACC FESC FCSI FISH FIMSA MAMS
Head
Department of Medicine, Clinical and Preventive Cardiology
Arihant Hospital
Indore, Madhya Pradesh, India
BC Roy and Charak Awardee of MPIMA

Amal Khan MD MNAMS DM
Former Professor
Department of Cardiology
WBMES
Visiting Consultant
Manipal Hospital, Salt Lake
Kolkata, West Bengal, India

Amartya Khan MD(Anesthesiology) DrNB
Critical Care Medicine Trainee
RN Tagore International Institute of Cardiac Sciences
Kolkata, West Bengal, India

Amitabha Chattopadhyay DCH DNB
Fellowship in Pediatric Cardiology (Australia)
Chief Pediatric Cardiologist and Clinical Lead Eastern India
Department of Pediatric Cardiology
Narayana Superspeciality Hospital
Howrah, West Bengal, India

Amit Aggarwal DNB MNAMS FIACM FICP
Senior Specialist
Department of Medicine
ABVIMS and Dr RML Hospital
New Delhi, India

Amit Garg MD(Radiodiagnosis)
Senior Consultant
Department of Imaging
Fortis Escort Heart Institute
New Delhi, India

Amit Malviya MD DM
Additional Professor
Department of Cardiology
NEIGRIHMS
Shillong, Meghalaya, India

Amit Mittal MD DM(Cardiology)
Senior Consultant
Department of Cardiology
Indraprastha Apollo Hospital
New Delhi, India

A Muruganathan MD
Chairman
Shristi AG Hospital
Tirupur, Tamilnadu, India
Director Elect – API Physicians Research Foundation

(Col) Anil Dhall Sena Medal MD(Medicine) DM(Cardiology) FACC FESC FAHA FRCP(Edinburgh) FSCAI FHRS FCSI
Professor and Head
Department of Cardiology
Janakpuri Super Speciality Hospital
New Delhi, India

Anil Sharma MD DM(Cardiology) FAPSC FSCAI FACC
Professor and Head
Department of Cardiology
Bombay Hospital
Mumbai, Maharashtra, India

Anil Sivadasan Radha MD DNB(Pediatrics) DNB(Cardiology) EPGB
Senior Consultant Interventional Pediatric Cardiologist
Lisie Hospital
Kochi, Kerala, India

Animesh Mishra MD DM
Senior Professor and Head
Department of Cardiology
NEIGRIHMS
Shillong, Meghalaya, India

Anindya Mukherjee MD DM
Senior Clinical Fellow
Adult Congenital Heart Disease
Bristol Heart Institute
United Kingdom

Anirban Das MD DM
Senior Resident
Burdwan Medical College
Burdwan, West Bengal, India

Anish Bhargav MD DM
Senior Resident and EP Fellow
JIPMER
Puducherry, India

Anish Keepanasseril MD(Obstetrics and Gynecology) DNB(Obstetrics and Gynecology) MNAMS MRCPI(Obgyn) MSc Epidemiology(LSHTM, UK)
Professor, Department of Obstetrics and Gynecology, JIPMER
Puducherry, India

Anish Kumar Khan DM(Cardiology) MD(Pulmonary Medicine) FCCP(USA) DAA(CMC Vellore) EDARM(HERMES)
Consultant Interventional Cardiologist and Pulmonologist
Visiting Consultant
Manipal Hospital, Salt Lake
Kolkata, West Bengal, India

Anita Saxena MD DM FACC
Vice Chancellor
Pt BD Sharma University of Health Sciences
Rohtak, Haryana, India

Ankit Bansal DM(Cardiology)
Professor
Department of Cardiology
GB Pant Institute of Postgraduate Medical Education and Research
New Delhi, India

Ankit Garg MS FNB
Assistant Professor
Department of Pediatric Cardiology
Pediatric Super-Specialty Wing
Amrita Institute of Medical Sciences
Faridabad, Haryana, India

Ankit Kumar Sahu MD DM
Associate Professor
Department of Cardiology
Sanjay Gandhi Postgraduate Institute of Medical Sciences
Lucknow, Uttar Pradesh, India

Ankur Handa MD DM
Senior Resident
Department of Cardiology
Cardiothoracic Sciences Centre
All India Institute of Medical Sciences
New Delhi, India

Anne Princy Steaphen MD DM
Assistant Professor
Department of Cardiology
Tamil Nadu Government Multi Super Speciality Hospital
Chennai, Tamil Nadu, India

AN Patnaik MD DM DNB FACC
Senior Consultant Cardiologist
Star Hospitals
Hyderabad, Telangana, India

Anuja Gadre MD DM(Cardiology)
Senior Resident
Department of Cardiology
Postgraduate Institute of Medical Education and Research
Chandigarh, India

Anuj Gupta MBBS
Student, All India Institute of Medical Sciences, Bhopal
Bhopal, Madhya Pradesh, India

Anupam Srivastava MD(Medicine)
Senior Resident
Department of Cardiology
Assam Medical College and Hospital
Dibrugarh, Assam, India

Anushree Kumbhalkar MD DM(Cardiology)
Senior Resident
Department of Cardiology
All India Institute of Medical Sciences, Nagpur
Nagpur, Maharashtra, India

Archit Dahiya MD(Medicine) DM(Cardiology)
Senior Interventional Cardiologist
Holy Heart Hospital
Rohtak, Haryana, India

Arif Mustaqueem MD(Medicine) DNB(Cardiology)
Associate Director
Department of Cardiology
Max Super Specialty Hospital
Saket, New Delhi, India

Arijit Ghosh MD DM
In-charge Cath Lab
Manipal Hospital
Kolkata, West Bengal, India

Arijit Kumar Ghosh MD DM FACC FESC FSCAI FAPSIC FAPVS FICC FCSI
Professor and Head
Department of Cardiology
All India Institute of Medical Sciences, Nagpur
Nagpur, Maharashtra, India

Arjun Mali MD DM(Cardiology)
Assistant Professor
Department of Cardiology
Topiwala National Medical College and BYL
Nair Charitable Hospital
Mumbai, Maharashtra, India

Arpita Katheria MD
Assistant Professor
Department of Cardiology
Sanjay Gandhi Postgraduate Institute of Medical Sciences
Lucknow, Uttar Pradesh, India

Arun Arul David MD
DrNB Cardiology Registrar
Department of Cardiology
Apollo Speciality Hospital, Vanagaram
Chennai, Tamil Nadu, India

Arun Mohanty MD DM FESC FACC
Professor
Sir Ganga Ram Hospital
New Delhi, India

Arup Dasbiswas MD DM(Cardiology) FCSI FICC FIAE FIAMS FICP FSCAI(USA) FACC(USA) FESC(Europe) FAPVS(Asia)
Emeritus Professor (Cardiology)
PKG Medical College and Hospital
Ex-Director, ICVS, IPGMER
Ex-Professor and Head
Department of Cardiology
IPGMER and SSKM Hospital
Kolkata, West Bengal, India

Arvind Kumar Jaiswal MD DM
Consultant Cardiologist
Shekhar Hospital
Lucknow, Uttar Pradesh, India

Arvind Kumar MD DM(Cardiology) FESC FICC FACC
Senior Consultant Cardiologist
Jeevak Heart Hospital
Patna, Bihar, India

Arya Subhadra DNB DM DrNB
Consultant Cardiology
St Gregorios Medical Mission Hospital
Parumala, Kerala, India

Aseem Basha MD
Assistant Professor
Department of Cardiology
All India Institute of Medical Sciences
New Delhi, India

Asha Moorthy MD DM FCCP FIACM FICP FIMSA FICC
Professor and Head
Department of Cardiology
Saveetha Medical College
Chennai, Tamil Nadu, India

Asharam Panda MD DM
Assistant Professor
Department of Cardiology
Dreams University and Health Sciences and Padmini Care Hospital
Cuttack, Odisha, India

Ashish Deshpande MD DM(Cardiology) FACC
Consultant Interventional Cardiologist
Department of Cardiology
Oriion Citicare Superspeciality Hospital
Ex-Professor and Head, MGM Medical College and Hospital
Aurangabad, Maharashtra, India

Ashish Jai Kishan MD(Medicine) DNB(Cardiology)
Senior Consultant
Fortis Escort Heart Institute
New Delhi, India

Ashish Kumar Jain MD DNB(Cardiology)
Associate Consultant Cardiologist
Sir Ganga Ram Hospital
New Delhi, India

Ashish Kumar Jha MD DM(Cardiology) FACC FSCAI
Cardiologist, Heart Hospital
Patna, Bihar, India

Ashish Kumar MD DM
Associate Consultant
Division of Interventional Cardiology
Medanta Heart Institute
Medanta – The Medicity
Gurugram, Haryana, India

Ashmit Bhardwaj MBBS
Medical Student
University of Leeds
Leeds, United Kingdom

Ashok Seth FRCP FACC MSCAI FAPSIC DSc
Chairman
Fortis Escorts Heart Institute
New Delhi, India

Ashwani Mehta DM(Cardiology)
Senior Consultant Cardiologist
Sir Ganga Ram Hospital
New Delhi, India

Ashwin Mahesh MD
Cardiovascular Disease Fellow
University of Pittsburgh Medical Center (UPMC)
Harrisburg, PA, USA

A Sreenivas Kumar MD DM FACC
Senior Consultant Cardiologist and Director
Department of Cardiology and Clinical Research
Apollo Hospital, Jubilee Hills
Hyderabad, Telangana, India

Atul Mathur MD(Medicine) DM(Cardiology)
Chairman and Head
Department of Cardiology
Fortis Escort Heart Institute
New Delhi, India

Avani Jain MD
Medical Officer
DNS Hospital
Indore, Madhya Pradesh, India

Avinash Mani MD DM(Cardiology)
Consultant
Department of Cardiology
Fortis Escorts Heart Institute
New Delhi, India

Avishkar Agrawal MD
Senior Resident
Department of Cardiology
All India Institute of Medical Sciences
New Delhi, India

Awadesh Kumar Sharma MD DM
Associate Professor
LPS Institute of Cardiology
Kanpur, Uttar Pradesh, India

Ayush Malhotra MD(Medicine) DrNB(Cardiology)
Specialist Grade
Department of Cardiology
Janakpuri Super Speciality Hospital
New Delhi, India

Ayush Shukla MD DM FAPSIC FSCAI
Assistant Professor
Department of Cardiology
King George's Medical University
Lucknow, Uttar Pradesh, India

Babu Reddy MD DM
Associate Professor
Department of Cardiology
Sri Jayadeva Institute of Cardiovascular Sciences and Research
Bengaluru, Karnataka, India

Balachander Jayaraman MD DM
Professor (Retired)
JIPMER
Puducherry, India

Balbir Singh MD DM
Chairman Cardiac Sciences
Max Hospital
Saket, New Delhi, India

Barun Kumar DM(Cardiology)
Additional Professor
Department of Cardiology
All India Institute of Medical Sciences, Rishikesh
Rishikesh, Uttarakhand, India

BC Srinivas MD DM(Cardiology)
Former Professor and Head
Department of Cardiology
Sri Jayadeva Institute of Cardiovascular Sciences and Research
Bengaluru, Karnataka, India

BG Vinodkumar MD
Junior Registrar
Billroth Hospital
Chennai, Tamil Nadu, India

Bhanu Duggal DM(Cardiology)
Professor and Head
Department of Cardiology
All India Institute of Medical Sciences, Rishikesh
Rishikesh, Uttarakhand, India

Bharat Dalvi MD DM
Consultant Cardiologist
Sir HN Reliance Hospital and Glenmark Cardiac Centre
Mumbai, Maharsahtra, India

Bhavuk Jaiswal MD(Medicine) DNB(Medicine) DM(Cardiology)
Associate Consultant
Fortis Escort Heart Institute
New Delhi, India

Bhushan Shah MD DNB(Cardiology)
Assistant Professor
Department of Cardiology
All India Institute of Medical Sciences, Bhopal
Bhopal, Madhya Pradesh, India

Bhushan Tile DM(Cardiology)
Senior Resident
ABVIMS and Dr RML Hospital
New Delhi, India

B Hygriv Rao MD DM FACC FESC
Director
Division of Pacing and Electrophysiology
KIMS Group of Hospitals
Hyderabad, Telangana, India

Bidyut Roy MD(Medicine) DM(Cariology)
Senior Resident
Department of Cardiology
IPGMER
Kolkata, West Bengal, India

Biraja Prasad Beura MD
Senior Resident Cardiology
MKCG Medical College
Berhampur, Odisha, India

Biswajit Majumder MD DM FACC FESC FSCAI FCSI FICP FAPSIC
Professor and Head
Department of Cardiology
RG Kar Medical College and Hospital
Kolkata, West Bengal, India

Biyanka Jaltotage MBBS(Hons) MSc
Cardiologist, Fiona Stanley Hospital
Perth, Western Australia, Australia

Blessvin Jino MD DM FNB
Consultant Interventional Cardiologist
Meditrina Hospital
Kollam, Kerala, India

BR Mishra MD DM FCSI FIAE FICC
Senior Consultant Cardiologist
Max Diagnostic
Cuttack, Odisha, India

B Shukti MBBS Dip GO MSc Medicine(Cardiology)(UK) FHEA(UK)
Senior Lecturer University/FE College
Senior Trust Doctor
United Kingdom

BS Yadav MD DM(Cardiology) FCSI FACC FSCAI
Professor and Head
Department of Cardiology
LN Medical College
Former Professor and Head
Department of Cardiology
Gandhi Medical College
Bhopal, Madhya Pradesh, India

Chandan Kumar Das MD(Medicine) DNB(Cardiology)
Super Specialist (Cardiology)
JLN Hospital and Research Center
Bhilai, Chhatisgarh, India

Chandra Bhan Meena MD DM FACC FSCAI FESC MHRS MAPHRS
Senior Professor
Department of Cardiology
SMS Medical College
Jaipur, Rajasthan, India

Chhabi Satpathy MD DM FACC FSCAI FESC FCSI FICC FIAE
Professor and Head
Division of Cardiology
MKCG Medical College
Berhampur, Odisha, India

CM Nagesh MD DM
Professor
Department of Cardiology
Sri Jayadeva Institute of Cardiovascular Sciences and Research
Bengaluru, Karnataka, India

C Rohit Swaminathan MD DM
DM Resident
Department of Cardiology
Amrita Institute of Medical Sciences
Kochi, Kerala, India

C Venkata S Ram MD MACP FACC FASH
Director
Apollo Institute for Blood Pressure Management
Apollo Group of Hospitals
Hyderabad, Telangana, India
Professor of Internal Medicine
University of Texas Southwestern Medical Center
Dallas, TX, USA

D Anuradha MD DNB
Junior Consultant Cardiologist
Apollo Hospitals Health City
Visakhapatnam, Andhra Pradesh, India

Dayasagar Rao V DM(Cardiology) FRCP(Canada) FRCP(Edinburgh)
Consultant Cardiologist
KIMS Hospital
Secunderabad, Telangana, India

Debabrata Biswas DNB(Medicine)
Postdoctoral Trainee
Department of Cardiology
NH-RTIICS
Kolkata, West Bengal, India

Debabrata Roy MD DM(Cardiology) FACC FESC FSCAI FAHA
Senior Consultant Interventional Cardiologist and Academic Co-ordinator
NH-RTIICS
Kolkata, West Bengal, India

Debasish Mohapatra MD(General Medicine) DM
Interventional Cardiologist
BM Birla Heart Hospital
Kolkata, West Bengal, India

Debayan Sarkar MBBS
Junior Specialist Doctor
University Hospitals
Biringham, United Kingdom

Debdatta Bhattacharyya MD MRCP CCST(Cardiology, UK)
Senior Consultant and Chief of Cath-lab
NH-RTIICS
Kolkata, West Bengal, India

Deepanjan Bhattacharya MD DM
Assistant Professor
Department of Cardiology
All India Institute of Medical Sciences, Kalyani
Kalyani, West Bengal, India

Deepa S Kumar MD DM(Cardiology) PDF(Pediatric Cardiology)
Additional Professor
Department of Cardiology
Sree Chitra Tirunal Institute for Medical Sciences and Technology
Thiruvananthapuram, Kerala, India

Deepthi Kodati MD DM FESC
Consultant Cardiologist
Trust Health Care
Durgabai Deshmukh Hospital
Hyderabad, Telangana, India

Deepti Chopra DTCD MD MAMS ACME FAIMER(2nd year)
Professor and Head
Department of Pharmacology
All India Institute of Medical Sciences, Bilaspur
Bilaspur, Himachal Pradesh, India

Devanu Ghosh Roy MD DM
Senior Consultant
Department of Cardiology
Peerless Hospital and BK Roy Research Centre
Kolkata, West Bengal, India

Dev B Pahlajani DNB(Medicine) DNB(Cardiology) FSCAI
Head
Department of Cardiology
Breach Candy Hospital
Mumbai, Maharashtra, India

Devesh Kumar DM(Cardiology)
Assistant Professor
Department of Cardiology
VMMC and Safdarjung Hospital
New Delhi, India

Dhananjay Kumar MD
Additional Director
Fortis Escorts Heart Institute
New Delhi, India

Dharmendra Jain DM
Professor
Department of Cardiology
Institute of Medical Sciences
Banaras Hindu University
Varanasi, Uttar Pradesh, India

Dhiman Kahali MD Dip(Cardiology) DM(Cardiology)
Senior Consultant and Director
BM Birla Heart Research Centre
Kolkata, West Bengal, India

Dibya Kumar Baruah MD DM FACC FSCAI FAPSC FCSI
Senior Consultant and Director
Catheterization Laboratory
Apollo Hospital, Health City
Visakhapatnam, Andhra Pradesh, India

Dilip Kumar MD DM FACC FRCP(Glasgow) FSCAI FESC FICC FHRS FHFA Certified Cardiac Device Specialist(CCDS, HRS, USA)
Director – Cardiac Cath Lab Services
Senior Consultant Interventional Cardiologist and Electrophysiologist
Chief Academic Co-ordinator
Medica Institute of Cardiac Science
Kolkata, West Bengal, India

Dipankar Das MD DM FAPSIC
Head
Department of Cardiology
Hayat Super Speciality Hospital
Guwahati, Assam, India

Dipankar Ghosh Dastidar DCH MD(Medicine) DM(Cardiology) FACC FESC FCSI FICP FSCAI
Associate Professor and Head
Department of Cardiology
Burdwan Medical College
Burdwan, West Bengal, India

Disha Shetty MD DM
Assistant Professor
Department of Cardiology
Sri Jayadeva Institute of Cardiovascular Sciences and Research
Bengaluru, Karnataka, India

Dixit Goyal MD DM(Cardiology)
Assistant Professor
GB Pant Institute of Postgraduate Medical Education and Research
New Delhi, India

Dorairaj Prabhakaran MD DM(Cardiology) MSc FRCP FNASc FNA DSc(Honoris Causa)
Executive Director
Centre for Chronic Disease Control (CCDC)
Distinguished Professor – Public Health Foundation of India (PHFI)
New Delhi, India

DP Sinha MD DM FSCAI FJCS
Head
Department of Cardiology
ILS Hospital
Dum Dum, West Bengal, India

Ferooz Ahmad Banday MD(Medicine) DM(Cardiology)
Resident
Department of Cardiology
IPGMER
Kolkata, West Bengal, India

Ganesan Karthikeyan MD DM
Professor
Department of Cardiology
All India Institute of Medical Sciences
New Delhi, India

Gaurav Singhal DM(Cardiology)
Head
Department of Cardiology
ESIC Model Hospital
Jaipur, Rajasthan, India

Gaurav Tripathi MD DM FSCAI
Consultant and Head
Department of Cardiology
Suyash Hospital
Raipur, Chattisgarh, India

Gautam Sharma MD DM
Professor
Department of Cardiology
Professor-In-Charge
Centre for Integrative Medicine and Research
All India Institute of Medical Sciences
New Delhi, India

Gautam Singal MD DNB
Associate Professor
Department of Cardiology
Dayanand Medical College and Hospital
Unit-Hero DMC Heart Institute
Ludhiana, Punjab, India

Ghanshyam Sharma MD(Medicine)
Associate Professor
Department of Medicine
RD Gardi Medical College
Ujjain, Madhya Pradesh, India

Girish Dwivedi MD DM MRCP(UK) PhD(UK) FRACP FASE FESC FCSANZ FSCCT
Professor and Senior Cardiologist
Department of Cardiology
Fiona Stanley Hospital
Harry Perkins Institute of Medical Research
School of Medicine
The University of Western Australia
Perth, Western Australia, Australia

Girish MP MD DM
Professor
Department of Cardiology
GB Pant Hospital
New Delhi, India

Gopalakrishnan A DM
Additional Professor
Sree Chitra Tirunal Institute
Thiruvananthapuram, Kerala, India

Gopal Chandra Ghosh DM(Cardiology) FACC FESC
Consultant Cardiologist
GitaRam Hospital and RN Thakur Hospital
Berhampore, West Bengal, India

Gourav Bhattacharya MD DM(Cardiology)
Senior Resident
Department of Cardiology
Burdwan Medical College and Hospital
Burdwan, West Bengal, India

Goutam Datta MD DNB DM MRCP(UK) FESC FSCAI
Professor
IPGMER
Kolkata, West Bengal, India

G Ravi Kiran MD MRCP DM
Assistant Professor
Department of Cardiology
Nizamabad Medical College
Interventional Cardiologist
Medicover Hospital
Nizamabad, Telangana, India

Gurpreet S Wander MD DM FACC FAMS
Principal and Professor
Department of Cardiology
Dayanand Medical College and Hospital
Unit-Hero DMC Heart Institute
Ludhiana, Punjab, India

G Venkateshwara Reddy MD DM
Head
Department of Cardiology
Star Pinnacle Heart Centre
Visakhapatnam, Andhra Pradesh, India

Haresh Mehta MD(Medicine) DNB(Cardiology) FACC FESC FSCAI
Director – Interventional and Structural Cardiology,
SL Raheja – Fortis Hospital
Mumbai, Maharashtra, India

Harikrishnan S DM FACC FRCP FAMS
Professor and Head
Department of Cardiology
Sree Chitra Tirunal Institute for Medical Sciences and Technology
Thiruvananthapuram, Kerala, India

Harinder K Bali MD DM
Chairman Cardiac Sciences
Livasa Hospital
Mohali, Punjab, India

Harshit Khare MD DM(Cardiology)
Assistant Professor
Department of Cardiology
Sanjay Gandhi Postgraduate Institute of Medical Sciences
Lucknow, Uttar Pradesh, India

Harsh Wardhan MD(Medicine) DM(Cardiology)
Principal–Director, Cardiac Sciences
Supreme Hospital
Faridabad, Haryana, India

Hemant Kumar Satpathy MD
Maternal-Fetal- Medicine (MFN) Specialist
Methodist Women's Hospital
Omaha, NE, USA

Hem Chandra Kalita MD(Medicine) DM(Cardiology)
Professor
Department of Cardiology
Assam Medical College and Hospital
Dibrugarh, Assam, India

Hetan C Shah MD DNB(Cardiology) FACC FESC FSCAI
Professor
Department of Cardiology
Seth GS Medical College and KEM Hospital
Mumbai, Maharashtra, India

Himanshu Dabral MD DM
Director
Division of Interventional Cardiology
Medanta Heart Institute
Medanta – The Medicity
Gurugram, Haryana, India

Himanshu Jindal MD(General Medicine) DNB(Cardiology)
Resident
Max Super Speciality Hospital
Patparganj, New Delhi, India

HK Chopra MD DM FRCP FACC FISC FISCU FASE FCSI FIAE FIMSA
Senior Consultant Cardiologist
Medanta Moolchand Heart Institute
Chairman
CME Moolchand Medcity
New Delhi, India
Past President – National CSI

Ilayaraja U MD DM
Cardiologist
Billroth Hospital
Chennai, Tamil Nadu, India

I Sathyamurthy MD DM FACC FRCP DSc(Honoris Causa)
Senior Interventional Cardiologist
Department of Cardiology
Apollo Main Hospitals
Chennai, Tamil Nadu, India

Jacob Jose MD DM(Cardiology) FACC FASE FCCP MS
Consultant Cardiologist
Naruvi Hospitals
Vellore, Tamil Nadu, India

Jagdish Chander Mohan MD DM
Interventional Cardiologist
Department of Cardiology
Institute of Heart and Vascular Diseases
Jaipur Golden Hospital
Rohini, Delhi, India

Jaideep C Menon DM(Cardiology) MPH
Professor
Adult Cardiology and Public Health
Amrita Institute of Medical Sciences and Research Center
Amrita Vishwa Vidyapeetham
Kochi, Kerala, India

Jaideep Dey MD(General Medicine) DNB(Cardiology)
Associate Director
Department of Cardiology
BLK-Max Super Specialty Hospital
New Delhi, India

Jaishankar Krishnamoorthy MD DM FIAMS
Director and Clinical Lead of Cardiology and Electrophysiology
Director – Cath Lab Services
Medway Heart Institute
Chennai, Tamil Nadu, India

Jamal Yusuf MD DM(Cardiology) FSCAI FESC FNAMS
Director–Professor
GB Pant Institute of Postgraduate Medical Education and Research
New Delhi, India

Jayagopal PB MD DM DNB FACC FICC FCSI FESC FSCAI FRCP(E)
Director, Head and Senior Interventional Cardiologist
Lakshmi Hospital
Palakkad, Kerala, India

Jayranganath M MD DM(Cardiology)
Professor and Head
Sri Jay Deva Institute of Cardiovascular Science and Research
Bengaluru, Karnataka, India

Jenu Rose Jose E MD DNB DM(Cardiology) PDF(Pediatric Cardiology)
Consultant Pediatric Cardiologist
Lisie Hospital
Kochi, Kerala, India

Jesu Krupa MD DM(Cardiology)
Faculty
Department of Cardiology
Christian Medical College
Vellore, Tamil Nadu, India

John Jose E MD DM Fellowship in Interventional Cardiology
Professor and Head
Department of Cardiology Unit-2
Cardiac Valve and Structural Heart Disease
Christian Medical College Hospital
Vellore, Tamil Nadu, India

Joyal J Kandathil MD DM
Consultant Cardiology
St Gregorios Medical Mission Hospital
Parumala, Kerala, India

Joy M Thomas MD DM
Senior Consultant
Interventional Cardiology and Cardiac Electrophysiology
Department of Cardiology
Apollo Speciality Hospital, Vanagaram
Chennai, Tamil Nadu, India

JPS Sawhney DM FESC FACC FRCP
Chairperson
Department of Cardiology
Dharma Vira Heart Center
Sir Ganga Ram Hospital
New Delhi, India

JS Thomas Xavier Paulsingh DM FNB(Interventional Cardiology)
Associate Consultant and Interventional Cardiologist
Meenakshi Mission Hospital and Research Centre
Madurai, Tamil Nadu, India

Juan Lu BSc MPE PhD
AI Scientist
Harry Perkins Institute of Medical Research
School of Medicine
The University of Western Australia
Perth, Western Australia, Australia

Juhi Singh MD DNB(Medicine)
Senior Resident
Department of Cardiology
Sir Ganga Ram Hospital
New Delhi, India

Justin Paul Gnanaraj MD DNB(Medicine) DM DNB(Cardiology) FACC FESC FSCAI
Professor
Institute of Cardiology
Madras Medical College
Chennai, Tamil Nadu, India

Kabir Sethi MD DM
Department of Structural Heart Interventions
University Hospital of Mainz
Germany

Kajal Ganguly MD DM FACC
Consultant Interventional Cardiologist
Manipal Hospital
Kolkata, West Bengal, India

Kamal K Sethi MD DM FACC FHRS FCSI FISE
Director
Department of Cardiology
Chairman and Managing Director
Delhi Heart and Lung Institute
New Delhi, India

Kanika Kukreja MD(Medicine)
Senior Resident (Academic)
Department of Cardiology
All India Institute of Medical Sciences, Rishikesh
Rishikesh, Uttarakhand, India

Karthikeyan R MD
Senior Resident
ABVIMS and Dr RML Hospital
New Delhi, India

Kartik Pandurang Jadhav MD DM
Interventional Cardiologist
Department of Cardiology
Apollo Hospital
Hyderabad, Telangana, India

K Arun Kumar MD DM
Research Scholar
Department of Cardiology
Institute of Medical Sciences
Banaras Hindu University
Varanasi, Uttar Pradesh, India

Kaushik Manna MD(General Medicine) DM(Cardiology)
Consultant Interventional Cardiologist
NH-RTIICS
Kolkata, West Bengal, India

Kavita Tyagi MS DNB(Anatomy) DNB(Medicine) DNB(Cardiology) FNB(Interventional Cardiology)
Consultant Cardiologist
Sir Ganga Ram Hospital
New Delhi, India

Kayan Siodia MD FACC FSCAI
Interventional Cardiologist
Breach Candy Hospital
Mumbai, Maharashtra, India

Kiran Gaur MSc PhD
Associate Professor and Head
Department of Statistics, Mathematics and Computer Science
Government SKN Agriculture University
Jaipur, Rajasthan, India

KK Talwar MD DM FAMS FNA FACC DSc(Honoris Causa)
Chairman – Heart Institute
PSRI Hospital
New Delhi, India

KN Srinivasan MD DNB(Cardiology) FCSI FESC FSCAI
Senior Interventional Cardiologist
Department of Cardiology
Apollo Main Hospitals
Chennai, Tamil Nadu, India

Kranthi Kumar Gedala MD(General Medicine)
Senior Resident in Adult Cardiology
Amrita Institute of Medical Sciences and Research Center
Amrita Vishwa Vidyapeetham
Kochi, Kerala, India

Krishnamoorthy KM DM DNB
Professor
Sree Chitra Tirunal Institute
Thiruvananthapuram, Kerala, India

K Sivaprasad MD DM DNB FESC FSCAI
Professor and Head
Department of Cardiology
Government Medical College
Thiruvananthapuram, Kerala, India

Kumar Himanshu MD DM
Assistant Professor
LPS Institute of Cardiology
Kanpur, Uttar Pradesh, India

Lakshmi Durga Kumaraguruparan MD(Pediatrics) DNB(Pediatrics) DM
Resident
Department of Cardiology
Sri Ramachandra Institute of Higher Education and Research
Chennai, Tamil Nadu, India

Lekha Adik Pathak MD(Medicine) DM(Cardiology) FRCP(Edinburgh)
Director and Head
Department of Cardiology
Nanavati Max Super Speciality Hospital
Mumbai, Maharashtra, India

Louie Fischer MD DM MRCP(UK) FRCP(Edinburgh) FACC FSCAI FESC
Professor and Chief Interventional Cardiologist
MOSC Medical College Hospital
Kochi, Kerala, India

Maddury Jyotsna MD DM FACC FESC FICC
Professor and Head (Retired)
Department of Cardiology
Nizam's Institute of Medical Sciences
Hyderabad, Telangana, India

Madhu Shukla MBBS PhD
Head of Noninvasive Cardiology
Department of Cardiology
Institute of Heart and Vascular Diseases, Jaipur Golden Hospital
Rohini, New Delhi, India

Madhu Sreedharan MD DM MRCP(UK) FRCP FACC
Director
NIMS Heart Foundation
Thiruvananthapuram, Kerala, India

Madhuvanthi Rajendran DCH DNB
Registrar in Cardiology
Kovai Medical Centre Hospital
Coimbatore, Tamil Nadu, India

Mahendra Chouhan DNB(Medicine) DrNB
Senior Resident
Department of Cardiology
Janakpuri Super Speciality Hospital
New Delhi, India

Mahesh Nalin Kumar MD DrNB FACC FESC
Head and Senior Consultant Cardiology
St Gregorios Medical Mission Hospital
Parumala, Kerala, India

Mainak Mandal MBBS
Postgraduate Trainee
Department of General Medicine
KPC Medical College
Kolkata, West Bengal, India

Mainak Mukhopadhyay MD MRCP DM FESC CCDS
Consultant Interventional Cardiologist
Manipal Hospital
Kolkata, West Bengal, India

Manish Bansal MD DNB(Cardiology)
Senior Director Clinical and Preventive Cardiology
Medanta – The Medicity
Gurugram, Haryana, India

Manish Narang PhD MPharm
Director Medical Affairs
Asia Pacific and Japan
Abott Vascular
New Delhi, India

Manjira Sinha PhD
Senior Scientist
TCS Research
Kolkata, West Bengal, India

Manju Bhargav BR MD
Senior Resident
Department of Cardiology
Government Medical College
Thiruvananthapuram, Kerala, India

Manoj Kumar Agarwala MD(PGI) DM(PGI) FACC
Consultant Cardiologist
Department of Cardiology
Apollo Hospital, Jubilee Hills
Hyderabad, Telangana, India

Manojkumar Rohit MD DM(Cardiology) MNAMS
Professor
Department of Cardiology
Postgraduate Institute of Medical Education and Research
Chandigarh, India

Manoranjan Mandal MD Dip Card DM
Professor and Head
Department of Cardiology
NRS Medical College
Kolkata, West Bengal, India

Manu Gupta MBBS
Resident
Department of Medicine
PCMS and RC
Bhopal, Madhya Pradesh, India

Manu R MD DM
Senior Interventional Cardiologist
Meditrina Hospital
Kollam, Kerala, India

Mayank Shami MD
Senior Resident
Department of Cardiology
MAMC and GIPMER
New Delhi, India

Meenakshi Kadiyala MD(General Medicine) DM(Cardiology)
Professor and Head
Department of Cardiology
Saveetha Medical College
Chennai, Tamil Nadu, India

Meenu Nair MD DM
Resident
Department of Cardiology
Amrita Institute of Medical Sciences
Kochi, Kerala, India

Milind Kharche MD DM(Cardiology) FACC FESC FSCAI
Chief Interventional Cardiologist
Care CIIGMA Hospital
Aurangabad, Maharashtra, India

Milind Phadke MD DM
Additional Professor
Lokmanya Tilak Municipal Medical College and General Hospital
Mumbai, Maharashtra, India

Mohit D Gupta MD DM FAMS FACC(USA)
Director–Professor
Department of Cardiology
GB Pant Institute of Postgraduate Medical Education and Research
New Delhi, India

Mohit M Bhagwati DNB(Cardiology) FSCAI MNAMS
Incharge
Acute Cardiac Care and Heart Failure Clinic
Consultant
Department of Cardiology
Holy Family Hospital
New Delhi, India

Mohsin Raj Mantoo MD DM
Post-DM Senior Resident
Department of Cardiology
All India Institute of Medical Sciences
New Delhi, India

Mona Bhatia MD FRCR(UK) FSCMR(USA) FSCCT(USA)
Principal–Director and Head
Department of Imaging
Fortis Escort Heart Institute
New Delhi, India

Monika Bhandari MD DM FACC FESC FSCAI APSIC
Additional Professor
Department of Cardiology
King George's Medical University
Lucknow, Uttar Pradesh, India

Monika Jain MD
Final Year Resident Doctor
Department of Medicine
RD Gardi Medical College
Ujjain, Madhya Pradesh, India

Monika P Jawanjal MD DM
Assistant Professor
Department of Cardiology
Kasturba Medical College, Manipal
Manipal, Karnataka, India

MPS Chawla MD FACP FRCP FICP FIACM FISC FIMSA
Senior Professor and Former Head
Department of Medicine
ABVIMS and Dr RML Hospital
New Delhi, India

Mrinal Kanti Das MD DM FICP FICC FCSI FACC FESC
Consultant Cardiologist
CK Birla Hospitals (BMB/CMRI)
Kolkata, West Bengal, India

M Shanmathi MBBS
Duty Medical Officer
Meenakshi Hospital
Thanjavur, Tamil Nadu, India

MS Prashant MD
Resident
Department of Cardiology
Apollo Hospital
Hyderabad, Telangana, India

MS Ravi MD DM(Cardiology)
Former Director
Department of Cardiology
Madras Medical College and Rajiv Ghandhi Government General Hospital
Chennai, Tamil Nadu, India

Mukesh Goel MS MCh(CTVS)
Senior Consultant
Indraprastha Apollo Hospital
New Delhi, India

Mukund Prabhu MD DM PDF(Electrophysiology)
Associate Professor, Department of Cardiology (EP Division)
Kasturba Medical College, Manipal
Manipal, Karnataka, India

Muralidharan TR MD DM
Professor and Director
Institute of Cardiac Sciences
SRM GLOBAL Hospitals
SRM Institute of Science and Technology
Chennai, Tamil Nadu, India

Nadeem Akhtar MD
Senior Resident
Department of Cardiology
SP Medical College and HRMC Centre
Bikaner, Rajasthan, India

Nagaraj Desai MD DM(Cardiology) FACC
Director
Namana Medical Centre
Bengaluru, Karnataka, India

Nagendra Boopathy Senguttuvan MD DM FACC FSCAI Fellowship in Interventional Cardiology and Structural heart disease Interventions(USA)
Professor
Clinical Lead – Structural Heart Diseases Interventions
Department of Cardiology
Sri Ramachandra Institute of Higher Education and Research
Chennai, Tamil Nadu, India

Nakul Sinha MD DM
Chairman – Cardiology
Max Hospital
Former Professor and Head
Department of Cardiology
Sanjay Gandhi Postgraduate Institute of Medical Sciences
Lucknow, Uttar Pradesh, India

Nandhakumar Vasu MD DNB(Cardiology) FNB(Interventional Cardiology)
Senior Consultant
Department of Cardiology
Institute of Cardio Vascular Diseases
The Madras Medical Mission Hospital
Chennai, Tamil Nadu, India

Narra Lavanya MD(General Medicine) DrNB(Cardiology)
Consultant Interventional Cardiologist
KIMS Hospitals
Hyderabad, Telangana, India

Navanil Biswas MD(General Medicine) DrNB(Cardiology)
Consultant Interventional Cardiologist
Apollo Multispeciality Hospital
Kolkata, West Bengal, India

Navdeep Singh Sidhu MD DM FAPSIC FACC
Assistant Professor
Department of Cardiology
All India Institute of Medical Sciences, Bilaspur
Bilaspur, Himachal Pradesh, India

Naved Aslam MD DM
Professor
Department of Cardiology
Dayanand Medical College and Hospital
Unit-Hero DMC Heart Institute
Ludhiana, Punjab, India

Navjyot Kaur MD DNB MRCP DM
Assistant Professor
Department of Cardiology
Command Hospital (Air Force)
Bengaluru, Karnataka, India

Neeraj Awasthy MD FNB(Pediatric Cardiology)
Director
Department of Pediatric and Congenital Heart Disease
Fortis Escorts Heart Institute
New Delhi, India

Nikhil Borikar MD DM(Cardiology)
Associate Professor
Department of Cardiology
Topiwala National Medical College and BYL
Nair Charitable Hospital
Mumbai, Maharashtra, India

Nilesh Giri MD(Medicine) DM(Cardiology)
Resident
Department of Cardiology
IPGMER
Kolkata, West Bengal, India

Nirat Beohar MD FACC FSCAI
Professor of Medicine
Columbia University Medical Center
Director, Cardiac Catheterization Laboratory, Structural Heart Disease and Interventional Cardiology Fellowship
Columbia University Division of Cardiology
Mount Sinai Medical Center
Miami Beach, FL, USA

Nirmal Ghati MD DM
Assistant Professor
Department of Cardiology
Cardiothoracic Sciences Centre
All India Institute of Medical Sciences
New Delhi, India

Nishad Chitnis MD MRCP DNB
Consultant Cardiologist
Heart Care Clinic
Karveer Cardiac Centre
Kolhapur, Maharashtra, India

Nitin K Kabra MD DM FACC
Professor and Head
Department of Cardiology
Gandhi Medical College Hospital
Secunderabad, Telangana, India

Nitish Prasad MD DrNB
Consultant Cardiologist
Apollo Hospitals
Bhubaneswar, Odisha, India

NK Mohanty MD DM
Professor
Department of Cardiology
SCB Medical College
Cuttack, Odisha, India

NN Khanna MD DM FRCP(London Glasgow, Edinburgh) FACC FSCAI FESC FAPSIC FCCP FEISI FICC FCSI
Senior Consultant Cardiologist
Indraprastha Apollo Hospital
New Delhi, India
Advisor – Apollo Group of Hospitals in India

OP Yadava MS DNB
CEO and Chief Cardiac Surgeon
National Heart Institute
New Delhi, India

Oruganti Sai Satish MD DM(Fellowship in EP and Pacing)
Senior Professor and Head Unit 1
Department of Cardiology
Nizams Institute of Medical Sciences
Hyderabad, Telangana, India

Padma Madhab Bisoi MD(General Medicine)
Postdoctoral Trainee
BM Birla Heart Hospital
Kolkata, West Bengal, India

Panchanan Sahoo MD(Medicine) DM(Cardiology) FACC FESC FICC FISE
Professor, Senior Consultant and Electrophysiologist
Department of Cardiology
Kalinga Institute of Medical Sciences
Bhubaneswar, Odisha, India

Pankaj Harkut MD DM(Cardiology) FACC FESC
Consultant Interventional Cardiologist
Swasthyam Superspeciality Hospital
Nagpur, Maharashtra, India

Pankaj Kashyap MD DM(Cardiology)
Assistant Professor
Department of Cardiology
Topiwala National Medical College and BYL Nair Charitable Hospital
Mumbai, Maharashtra, India

Pankaj Manoria MD DM FACC FESC
Director
Manoria Heart and Critical Care Hospital
Bhopal, Madhya Pradesh, India

Parag Barwad MD DM FESC FSCAI CEPS-AC
Additional Professor
Department of Cardiology
Postgraduate Institute of Medical Education and Research
Chandigarh, India

Parayaru Kottayil Asokan MD DM FRCP FCSI FACC FESC FSCAI FICC
Chief Consultant Interventional Cardiologist
Department of Cardiology
Fathima Hospital
Kozhikode, Kerala, India

Paul V George MD DM
Senior Professor
Department of Cardiology Unit-2
Christian Medical College Hospital
Vellore, Tamil Nadu, India

Pawan Sharma MD(General Medicine) DM(Cardiology)
Senior Interventional Cardiologist
Associate Director and Unit-Head Cardiology
Max Superspeciality Hospital
Patparganj, New Delhi, India

P Chakradhar MD DM
Consultant Cardiologist
Apollo Hospitals Health City
Visakhapatnam, Andhra Pradesh, India

P Chandrasekhar MD DM FACC
Head and Professor
Department of Cardiology
Kurnool Medical College
Kurnool, Andhra Pradesh, India

PC Manoria MD DM FACC FESC FCAPSC
Director, Manoria Heart and Critical Care Hospital
Bhopal, Madhya Pradesh, India

PC Rath MD DM FICC FESC FACC FRCP(London) FRCP(Edinburgh)
Senior Consultant Cardiologist and Head
Department of Cardiology
Apollo Hospital, Jubilee Hills
Hyderabad, Telangana
Apollo Hospital
Bhubaneshwar, Odisha, India

Pintu Nahata MD DM(Cardiology) FACC FSCAI FESC FCI
Senior Professor and Head
Department of Cardiology
SP Medical College and HRMC Centre
Bikaner, Rajasthan, India

Pooja Sharma Gupta MBBS
Resident
Department of Dermatology
PCMS and RC
Bhopal, Madhya Pradesh, India

Prabahakar Koregol MD DM(Cardiology) FSCAI
Senior Consultant Cardiologist
Department of Cardiology
Fortis Hospitals and Namana Medical Centre
Bengaluru, Karnataka, India

Pradeep Kumar Mustepally MD DNB
Consultant Cardiologist
Apollo Hospital, Jubilee Hills
Hyderabad, Telangana, India

Pradyumna Kumar Singh MD
Senior Resident
Department of Cardiology
ABVIMS and Dr RML Hospital
New Delhi, India

Prakas Chandra Mondal MD MRCP(UK, Ireland) MRRCPS(Glasgow) DM(Cardilogy) DNB(Cardiology) FACC(USA)
Consultant Interventional Cardiologist and Head
Department of Cardiology
Apolo Multispeciality Hospital
Kolkata, West Bengal, India

Prasant Kr Sahoo MD DM FRCP FACC FSCAI FESC FAPSIC FCSI FICC
Director – Interventional Cardiology
Apollo Hospitals
Bhubaneswar, Odisha, India
Chairman CSI-NIC 2024-25

Prashant Bobhate MD(Pediatrics) FNB(Pediatrics Cardiology) FPVRi Fellowship in Pulmonary Hypertension(Canada)
Consultant Pediatric Cardiologist
Childrens Heart Center
Kokilaben Dhirubai Ambani Hospital
Mumbai, Maharashtra, India

Prashant Moorthy MD(FRCR)
Assistant Professor
Saveetha Medical College
Chennai, Tamil Nadu, India

Prashant Panda MD DM
Associate Professor
Department of Cardiology
Postgraduate Institute of Medical Education and Research
Chandigarh, India

Prasit Maity DNB
Consultant
Department of Imaging
Fortis Escort Heart Institute
New Delhi, India

Prathap Kumar N MD DM FIC
Chief Interventional Cardiologist
Meditrina Hospital
Kollam, Kerala, India

Pratishtha Mehra PhD
Senior Research Associate
Department of Cardiology
GB Pant Institute of Postgraduate Medical Education and Research
New Delhi, India

Praveen Arumugam MD
Senior Resident
Department of Cardiology
Cardiothoracic Sciences Centre
All India Institute of Medical Sciences
New Delhi, India

Pravin K Goel MD DM FACC FSCAI
Director – Interventional Cardiology
Medanta Heart Institute
Lucknow, Uttar Pradesh, India

Preetam Krishnamurthy MD DM PDF CCDS
Assistant Professor and Consultant Electrophysiologist
Sri Ramachandra Institute for Higher Education and Research
Chennai, Tamil Nadu, India

Preethi Caleb Harris MD DCH
Senior Resident
Department of Cardiology
NEIGRIHMS
Shillong, Meghalaya, India

Preeti Gupta MD(Internal Medicine) DrNB(Cardiology) FACC FESC FSCAI FICC FCSI
Professor
Department of Cardiology
VMMC and Safdarjung Hospital
New Delhi, India

Preetish Rath PhD
Candidate (Computer Science)
Tufts University, Medford
Massachusetts, USA

Priya Jagia MD DNB
Professor and Head
Department of Cardiovascular Imaging and Endovascular Interventions
Cardiothoracic Sciences Centre
All India Institute of Medical Sciences
New Delhi, India

PS Banerjee MD DM(Cardiology) FACC
Chief Interventional Cardiologist
Manipal Hospital
Former Head
Department of Cardiology
Medical College
Kolkata, West Bengal, India
Past President – Cardiological Society of India

Puneet Rastogii MD DM
Professor and Head
Department of Cardiology
GR Medical College
Gwalior, Madhya Pradesh, India

Punitha Lakxmi Ramesh MD
Senior Resident
Department of Cardiology
Sree Chitra Tirunal Institute for Medical Sciences and Technology
Thiruvananthapuram, Kerala, India

Purneshwar Pandey MD DM(Interventional Cardiology)
Consultant
Department of Cardiology
Fortis Hospital
Vasant Kunj, New Delhi, India

Purushotham Reddy Ramireddy Gari MD
Resident in Cardiology
Nizams Institute of Medical Sciences
Hyderabad, Telangana, India

Raghav R Nagpal MD
Consultant – Interventional and Structural Cardiology
SL Raheja – Fortis Hospital
Mumbai, Maharashtra, India

Rahul Nijhawan DM(Cardiology) PDF(Electrophysiology)
Assistant Professor
Department of Cardiology
GB Pant Institute of Postgraduate Medical Education and Research
New Delhi, India

Raja J Selvaraj MD DNB PDF EP
Professor
JIPMER
Puducherry, India

Rajeev Agarwal MD DM
Consultant Cardiologist
Jaswant Rai Speciality Hospital
Meerut, Uttar Pradesh, India

Rajeev Garg MD(Medicine) Dip Card(NIMS) DNB(Cardiology) MNAMS FSCAI FESC FACC Diplomate National Board
Senior Consultant Interventional Cardiologist
Aware Gleneagles Global Hospital
Hyderabad, Telangana, India

Rajeev Gupta MD PhD
Chair Preventive Cardiology and Medicine
Eternal Heart Care Centre and Research Institute
Jaipur, Rajasthan, India

Rajeev Gupta MD DM(Cardiology)
Professor and Head
Department of Cardiology
Gandhi Medical College
Bhopal, Madhya Pradesh, India

Rajendra Kumar Jain MD DM FACC DIU(Paris)
Founder and Director
KIMS Group of Hospitals
Hyderabad, Telangana, India

Rajesh Sharma MD DM
Associate Professor
Department of Cardiology
Indira Gandhi Medical College and Hospital
Shimla, Himachal Pradesh, India

Rajesh Thachathodiyil MD DM FACC
Head
Department of Cardiology
Amrita Institute of Medical Sciences
Kochi, Kerala, India

Rajesh Vijayvergiya MD DM FSCAI FACC FESC FISES
Professor
Department of Cardiology
Advanced Cardiac Centre
Postgraduate Institute of Medical Education and Research
Chandigarh, India

Rajiv C MD DM(Cardiology)
Senior Consultant
Aster Medcity
Kochi, Kerala, India

Rajiv Passey DNB(Medicine) DM(Cardiology) MNAMS FICP FESC
Senior Consultant Interventional Cardiologist
Co-Director Cath Lab and In-charge CCU
Dharma Vira Heart Centre
Sir Ganga Ram Hospital
New Delhi, India

Rajneesh Jain MD DM
Senior Consultant
Director – Cathlab and Vice Chairperson
Sir Ganga Ram Hospital
New Delhi, India

Rajneesh Kapoor MD DNB FACC
Chairman
Division of Interventional Cardiology
Medanta Heart Institute
Medanta – The Medicity
Gurugram, Haryana, India

Rajpal Prajapati DM
Associate Professor
Department of Cardiology
Institute of Medical Sciences
Banaras Hindu University
Varanasi, Uttar Pradesh, India

Rakesh Maurya MD DM
Consultant Cradiologist
Jaswant Rai Speciality Hospital
Meerut, Uttar Pradesh, India

Rakesh Yadav MD DM
Professor
Department of Cardiology
All India Institute of Medical Sciences
New Delhi, India

Ramakrishna J MD DM
Consultant Cardiologist
Apollo Hospital, Jubilee Hills
Hyderabad, Telangana, India

Ramdas G Pai MD FACC FRCP(Edinburgh)
Professor
California University of Science and Medicine
Colton, CA, USA

Ranjit K Nath MD DM FACC FSCAI FESC FCSI
Director–Professor and Head
Department of Cardiology
ABVIMS and Dr RML Hospital
New Delhi, India

Rathindra Nath Karmakar MD DM
Consultant
Department of Cardiology
Narayana Multispeciality Hospital
Kolkata, West Bengal, India

Ratul Ghosh MD
Resident
Department of Cardiology
RG Kar Medical College and Hospital
Kolkata, West Bengal, India

Ravikishore Amancharla MD DM FACC
Head and Senior Consultant
Cardiologist and Electrophysiologist
Health City
Cayman Islands

Ravikumar Rathnagiri MD DM FESC
Senior Consultant and Clinical Lead
Institute of Heart and Lung Transplant
MGM Healthcare
Chennai, Tamil Nadu, India

Ravi R Kasliwal MD DM(Cardiology)
Chairman Clinical and Preventive Cardiology
Medanta – The Medicity
Gurugram, Haryana, India

Ravi Vishnu Prasad MD(Medicine) DM(Cardiology)
Professor and Head
Department of Cardiology
Indira Gandhi Institute of Medical Sciences (IGIMS)
Patna, Bihar, India

Rishika Mehta MD(Pediatrics) DrNB(Pediatric Cardiology)
Pediatric Cardiologist
Department of Pediatric Cardiology
Narayana Superspeciality Hospital
Howrah, West Bengal, India

Rishi Sethi MD DM FACC FESC FRCP(Edinburgh, London) FSCAI FAPSIC FAMS FCSI FISC
Professor, Department of Cardiology
King George's Medical University
Lucknow, Uttar Pradesh, India

Rohan Naik MD
Assistant Professor
Department of Medicine
West Virginia University Heart and Vascular Institute
Morgantown, West Virginia, USA

Ronak Sheth MD FNB(Pediatric Cardiology)
Consultant Pediatric Cardiologist
Fortis Hospital
Mumbai, Maharashtra, India

Ronak V Ruparelia DNB(Medicine) DNB(Cardiology)
Interventional Cardiologist
Bankers Super Speciality Hospital
Vadodara, Gujarat, India

Roopa Salwan MD DM
Senior Director
Myocardial Infarction Program
Senior Consultant
Cardiology and Interventional Cardiology
Max Super Speciality Hospital
Saket, New Delhi, India

Roshan Rao MD DM FACC FESC FSCAI
Senior Interventional Cardiologist and Head
Department of Cardiology
Apollo Hospitals
Indore, Madhya Pradesh, India

R Rameshwar MD(General Medicine)
PG in DM(Cardiology)
Saveetha Medical College
Chennai, Tamil Nadu, India

Ruchi Sharma MD MD
Resident
ESIC Hospital
Faridabad, Haryana, India

Rufus Demel X MD DNB(Cardiology) FNB(Interventional Cardiology)
Chief Consultant Cardiologist
Devaki Heart Center
Madurai, Tamil Nadu, India

Rupendra Nath Saha MD
Senior Resident (Academic)
Department of Cardiology
All India Institute of Medical Sciences, Rishikesh
Rishikesh, Uttarakhand, India

Sabyasachi Pandey MD(Pediatrics) DM(Pediatric Cardiology)
Resident
Sri Jay Deva Institute of Cardiovascular Science and Research
Bengaluru, Karnataka, India

Sachin Maggo MD
Senior Resident
Department of Cardiology
Indira Gandhi Medical College and Hospital
Shimla, Himachal Pradesh, India

Sachin Raiya MD(Radiodiagnosis)
Department of Imaging
Fortis Escort Heart Institute
New Delhi, India

Safal MD DM
Professor
Department of Cardiology
MAMC and GIPMER
New Delhi, India

Sajan Narayanan MD(Internal Medicine) DM(Cardiology) FESC
Senior Consultant and Interventional Cardiologist
Little Flower Hospital and Research Institute
Kochi, Kerala, India

Sakshi Sachdeva MD DM
Assistant Professor – Pediatric Cardiology
ABVIMS and Dr RML Hospital
New Delhi, India

Sameer Shrivastava MD(General Medicine) DM(Cardiology)
Principal–Director and Chief of Noninvasive Cardiology
Max Super Specialty Hospital
Saket, New Delhi, India

Samshad Alam MD(Medicine) DM(Cardiology)
Associate Directror
Jai Prabha Medanta Superspecialty Hospital
Patna, Bihar, India

Samuel Jebavaram MD DNB
Senior Registrar, Billroth Hospital
Chennai, Tamil Nadu, India

Sandeep Kamat MD DM(Cardiology)
Assistant Professor
Department of Cardiology
Topiwala National Medical College and BYL
Nair Charitable Hospital
Mumbai, Maharashtra, India

Sandeep Seth DM(Cardiology)
Professor
Department of Cardiology
All India Institute of Medical Sciences
New Delhi, India

Sandeep Singh MD DM
Professor
Department of Cardiology
All India Institute of Medical Sciences
New Delhi, India

Sandipta Ray MD DM
Consultant Interventional Cardiologist
Manipal Hospital
Kolkata, West Bengal, India

Sangeeta Dhir MDS(Periodontology) Fellow(Implantology)
Consultant Dentistry and Clinical Research
Max Hospital
Saket, New Delhi, India

Sanjay Mehrotra MD DM
Consultant and Interventional Cardiologist
NH Institute of Cardiac Sciences
Bengaluru, Karnataka, India

Sanjay Tyagi MD(Medicine) DM(Cardiology) FAMS FICP FCSI FICA FRCP(Edinburgh) FSCAI FESC FACC(USA)
Dr BC Roy National Awardee
Senior Consultant, Academic Advisor (HOD) and Clinical Director Cardiology
Apollo Hospitals, Northern Region, New Delhi, India
President-Elect, Cardiological Society of India
Secretary General (India), International College of Cardiology (USA)
National Coordinator, Cardiology and Interventional Cardiology, National Board of Examination
Formerly
Director General Health Services, Govt of India
Dean, Maulana Azad Medical College, New Delhi
Director, Professor and HOD Cardiology
GB Pant Institute of Postgraduate Medical Education and Research

Sanjeev Asotra MD DM
Professor
Department of Cardiology
Indira Gandhi Medical College and Hospital
Shimla, Himachal Pradesh, India

Sanjeev Hanumantacharya Naganur MD(Pediatrics) DM(Cardiology) FICC FSCAI FPICS
Associate Professor
Department of Cardiology
Advanced Cardiac Center
Postgraduate Institute for Medical Education and Research
Chandigarh, India

Sanjeev Kathuria DM(Cardiology)
Professor
Department of Cardiology
GB Pant Institute of Postgraduate Medical Education and Research
New Delhi, India

Sanjeev Kumar MS MCh(Cardiothoracic and Vascular Surgery)
Professor and Head
Department of Cardiothoracic and Vascular Surgery (CTVS)
All India Institute of Medical Sciences, Patna
Patna, Bihar, India

Sankar Chandra Mandal MD(Medicine) DM(Cardiology) FACC(USA) FSCI FESC
Professor
Department of Cardiology
IPGMER
Kolkata, West Bengal, India

Sarita Rao MD DM FACC FSCAI
Senior Interventional Cardiologist and Director, Cath Lab
Apollo Hospitals
Indore, Madhya Pradesh, India

Saroj Mandal MD(Medicine) DM(Cardiology) FRCP(Edinburgh) FRCP(Glasgow) FACC(USA) FSCAI(USA) FESC(EURO)
Professor
Department of Cardiology
Institute of Cardiovascular Sciences
IPGMER
Kolkata, West Bengal, India

Sarumathi Thangavel MD FACC
Consultant Cardiologist
Lakshmi Hospital
Chennai, Tamil Nadu, India

Sateesh Reddy DNB(General Medicine) DM(Cardiology)
Senior Resident
Kalinga Institute of Medical Sciences
Bhubaneswar, Odisha, India

Satish K Parashar MD FACC
Senior Consultant Cardiologist and Director
Non-Invasive Cardiac Laboratory
Heart Centre
New Delhi, India

Satish Kumar MD(Pediatrics)
Senior Resident
Childrens Heart Center
Kokilaben Dhirubai Ambani Hospital
Mumbai, Maharashtra, India

Satya Sahitya Mandava MD DM
Senior Resident
Postgraduate Institute of Medical Education and Research
Chandigarh, India

Satya S Mandava MD DM
Fellow, Department of Cardiology
Advanced Cardiac Centre
Postgraduate Institute of Medical Education and Research
Chandigarh, India

Satyavan Sharma MD DM(Cardiology) MNAMS(Cardiology)
Honorary Consultant Cardiologist
Department of Cardiology
Bombay Hospital
Mumbai, Maharashtra, India

Satyavir Yadav MD DM
Associate Professor
Department of Cardiology
All India Institute of Medical Sciences
New Delhi, India

Satyendra Tewari MD DM(Cardiology) FACC FSCAI FCAPSC FESC FCSI FICC
Professor
Department of Cardiology
Sanjay Gandhi Postgraduate Institute of Medical Sciences
Lucknow, Uttar Pradesh, India

Saumitra Ray MD FRCP FESC FACC FSCAI FCSI FICP
Consultant
Woodlands Hospital
Kolkata, West Bengal, India

Saurabh Bhardwaj MD DrNB(Cardiology)
Junior Consultant Cardiologist
Indraprastha Apollo Hospitals
Sarita Vihar, New Delhi

Saurabh Dhumale MD DrNB(Cardiology)
Consultant Interventional Cardiologist
NH-RTIICS
Kolkata, West Bengal, India

Saurabh Kumar Gupta MD DM
Professor
Department of Cardiology
All India Institute of Medical Sciences
New Delhi, India

Saurav Mishra MD DM
Consultant – Interventional Cardiology
Medanta Heart Institute
Lucknow, Uttar Pradesh, India

Seenu Prasanth A MD(General Medicine) DM(Cardiology)
Senior Resident
Department of Cardiology
All India Institute of Medical Sciences, Nagpur
Nagpur, Maharashtra, India

Shabbir Ali Shaik MD DM FNB
Fellow Interventional Cardiologist
Department of Cardiology
Apollo Hospital, Jubilee Hills
Hyderabad, Telangana, India

Sharad Chandra DM FACC FESC FSCAI FAPSIC FCSI
Professor
Department of Cardiology
King George's Medical University
Lucknow, Uttar Pradesh, India

Shibba Takkar Chhabra MD DM
Professor
Department of Cardiology
Hero DMC Heart Institute
Dayanand Medical College and Hospital
Ludhiana, Punjab, India

Shinjan Patra MD(Internal Medicine) DM(Endocrinology)
Assistant Professor and Consultant Endocrinologist
Department of Endocrinology and Metabolism
All India Institute of Medical Sciences, Nagpur
Nagpur, Maharashtra, India

Shirisha Reddy Kommareddy MD DM
Consultant Cardiologist
KIMS Hospital
Hyderabad, Telangana, India

Shitij Chaudhary MD
Senior Resident
Department of Cardiology
All India Institute of Medical Sciences
New Delhi, India

Shivangi Tiwari MD
Final Year Resident Doctor
Department of Medicine
RD Gardi Medical College
Ujjain, Madhya Pradesh, India

Shivani Rao MD DM
Associate Professor
Department of Cardiology
ABVIMS and Dr RML Hospital
New Delhi, India

Shreyak P Kadu MD DM(Cardiology)
Assistant Professor
Department of Cardiology
Topiwala National Medical College and BYL
Nair Charitable Hospital
Mumbai, Maharashtra, India

Shreya Rani MBBS
Medical Officer
Jai Prabha Medanta Superspecialty Hospital
Patna, Bihar, India

Shridhar Dwivedi MD PhD FAMS FRCP(UK) FIACS(Canada)
Senior Consultant Cardiologist and Head, Academics
National Heart Institute
New Delhi, India

Shubhanshu Pal MD(Medicine)
Postdoctoral Trainee (3rd year)
Institute of Cardiovascular Sciences
IPGMER
Kolkata, West Bengal, India

Shyam Prasad Sahoo MBBS
Student
SRM Medical College
Chennai, Tamil Nadu, India

Siddhartha Pandey MD DM
Senior Resident
Department of Cardiology
SCB Medical College
Cuttack, Odisha, India

Sidhartha Chattopadhyay MRCP(1&2, UK)
Registrar
Department of Cardiology
Ruby General Hospital Limited
Kolkata, West Bengal, India

Sivashanmuganathan Velu MD DM
Consultant Cardiologist
Medway Heart Institute
Chennai, Tamil Nadu, India

Sivasubramanian Ramakrishnan MD DM
Professor
Department of Cardiology
All India Institute of Medical Sciences
New Delhi, India

SK Dwivedi MD DM FACC FESC FSCAI
Professor and Head
Department of Cardiology
King George's Medical University
Lucknow, Uttar Pradesh, India

Smit Shrivastava MD PGDHHM DM(Cardiology) FACC FSCAI FESC FICP FIMSA FICN FISE
Professor and Head
Advance Cardiac Institute
Pt JNM Medical College and Dr BRAM Hospital
Raipur, Chhattisgarh, India

S Murugarajan MD DM
Senior Assistant Professor
Department of Cardiology
National Centre of Ageing
Madras Medical College
Chennai, Tamil Nadu, India

Sneha Garg MD DM
Associate Consultant
Department of Cardiology
Max Hospital
Saket, New Delhi, India

Snehal Kulkarni MD DrNB FACC
Director – Pediatric Cardiac Sciences
Fortis Healthcare
Mumbai, Maharashtra, India

SN Routray MD DM FACC FESC FSCAI
Professor
Department of Cardiology
SCB Medical College
Cuttack, Odisha, India

Somnath Maji MD
Resident
Department of Cardiology
RG Kar Medical College and Hospital
Kolkata, West Bengal, India

Somnath Mukhopadhay MD DM(Cardiology) FESC
Consultant
Nightingale Hospital
Kolkata, West Bengal, India

Sonal Jain MD DrNB(Cardiology)
Resident
Sir Ganga Ram Hospital
New Delhi, India

Soormpally Vijay MD DM
Fellow in Electrophysiology
Department of Cardiac Electrophysiology, AIG Hospital
Hyderabad, Telangana, India

Soumik Ghosh DM
Associate Professor
Department of Cardiology
Institute of Medical Sciences
Banaras Hindu University
Varanasi, Uttar Pradesh, India

Soumya Patnaik MD
Assistant Professor
Department of Cardiology
University of Texas
Houston, Texas, USA

S Radhakrishnan MD DM
Professor and Head
Department of Pediatric Cardiology
Pediatric Super-Specialty Wing
Amrita Institute of Medical Sciences
Faridabad, Haryana, India

S Ramesh MD DM FACC FSCAI FESC
Professor and Senior Consultant
Sri Ramachandra Insitute of Higher Education and Research
Chennai, Tamil Nadu, India

SR Sharath Shanmugam MD(General Medicine)
PG in DM(Cardiology)
Sri Ramachandra Medical College
Chennai, Tamil Nadu, India

Sreelal Thazhathu Veettil MD DM
Resident, Department of Cardiovascular Imaging and Endovascular Interventions
Cardiothoracic Sciences Centre
All India Institute of Medical Sciences
New Delhi, India

Sridhar Kasturi MD DM FACC FESC FSCAI FICC
Head
Department of Cardiology and Cardiothoracic Surgery
KIMS – Sunshine Hospitals, Begumpet
Secunderabad, Telangana, India

Srina Ray MBBS
Senior House Officer
Scunthorpe General Hospital
United Kingdom

Srinivas Rao Maddury MD DM
Senior Interventional Cardiologist and Head
Department of Cardiology
Apollo Hospital
Hyderabad, Telangana, India

Sriram Easwaran MD DM
Assistant Professor
Lokmanya Tilak Municipal Medical College and General Hospital
Mumbai, Maharashtra, India

S Selvamani DNB(Cardiology)
Senior Consultant and Interventional Cardiologist
Meenakshi Mission Hospital and Research Centre
Madurai, Tamil Nadu, India

S Shanmugasundaram MD DM
Cardiologist
Department of Cardiology
Billroth Hospital
Chennai, Tamil Nadu, India

SS Iyengar DM(Cardiology) FRCP(Edinburg)
Consultant Cardiologist
Manipal Hospital
Bengaluru, Karnataka, India

SS Mishra MD FAIMS MCAM DoCM FCCP FIAE FICC FCSI
Professor and Director
SOA University, Bhubaneswar
Professor and Director
Dreams Health Sciences and Padmini Care Hospital
Director, Med 'n' Heart Clinic
Cuttack, Odisha, India

Subhasis Roy Chowdhury MD DM FSCAI
In-charge Cath Lab
Manipal Hospital
Kolkata, West Bengal, India

Subrahmanya Murti V MD DM
Senior Specialist Cardiology
Aster CMI Hospital
Bengaluru, Karnataka, India

Subrat Kumar Muduli DM(Cardiology)
Associate Professor
Department of Cardiology
GB Pant Institute of Postgraduate Medical Education and Research
New Delhi, India

Subroto Mandal MD DM DC FACC FICC FCPCI FSCAI
Professor and Head
Department of Cardiology
Director, Cath Lab
Ubuntu Heart and Super Specialty Hospital
Bhopal, Madhya Pradesh, India

Sudeep Verma MD FNB(Pediatric Cardiology)
Consultant
Department of Pediatric Cardiology
Krishna Institute of Medical Sciences (KIMS)
Secunderabad, Telangana, India

Sudeshna Jana MTech
Researcher
TCS Research
Kolkata, West Bengal, India

Sudhir Chandra Sinha MD DM FACC
Senior Consultant Cardiologist
Star Pinnacle Heart Centre
Visakhapatnam, Andhra Pradesh, India

Sudipta Mondal MD DM
Postdoctoral Fellow in Electrophysiology
Sree Chitra Tirunal Institute (SCTIMST)
Thiruvananthapuram, Kerala, India

Sujatha Vipperla MD DM FIC FSCAI
Consultant Cardiologist
Indus Hospitals
Visakhapatnam, Andhra Pradesh, India

Sulabh Chandrakar MD DM FSCAI
Director and Consultant Cardiologist
Prathmesh Hospital
Raipur, Chattisgarh, India

Suman Bhandari MD DM FACC FESC FSCAI FIMSA
Director
Department of Cardiology
Fortis Escorts Heart Institute
New Delhi, India

Sunandan Sikdar MD DM FACC
Consultant
Department of Cardiology
Narayana Multispeciality Hospital
Kolkata, West Bengal, India

Sundaram Chandrashekhar MD DM
Assistant Professor
Department of Cardiology
Trichy SRM College
Tiruchirappalli, Tamil Nadu, India

Sunil Kumar S MD DM(Cardiology) FESC FSCAI
Professor and Head
Department of Cardiology
JSS Medical College and Hospital
Mysuru, Karnataka, India

Sunita Kumbhalkar MD(Medicine) DNB(Cardiology)
Professor and Head
Department of General Medicine
All India Institute of Medical Sciences, Nagpur
Nagpur, Maharashtra, India

Supraja Moorthy MD DNB(FRCR)
Assistant Professor
Saveetha Medical College
Puducherry, India

Sura Kishore Mishra MD DM(Cardiology)
Professor and Head
Department of Cardiology
SCB Medical College
Cuttack, Odisha, India

Suvro Banerjee MD FRCP(London) FRCP(Edinburgh) FICC FCSI FSCAI FACC FESC
Senior Consultant
Department of Cardiology
Apollo Multispeciality Hospital
Kolkata, West Bengal, India

Suyash Tripathi DM
Associate Professor
Department of Cardiology
Institute of Medical Sciences
Banaras Hindu University
Varanasi, Uttar Pradesh, India

Tamagna Ghosh MD DM(Cardiology)
Assistant Professor
Department of Cardiology
Seth GS Medical College
KEM Hospital
Mumbai, Maharashtra, India

Tanmay Mukhopadhyay MD DM(Cardiology) FESC FSCAI
Associate Professor
Department of Cardiology
Burdwan Medical College and Hospital
Burdwan, West Bengal, India

Tanmoy Majee MD DM(Cardiology)
Consultant
Department of Cardiology
Ruby General Hospital Limited
Kolkata, West Bengal, India

Tanuja Makhani MD
Senior Resident
Department of Cardiology
Postgraduate Institute of Medical Education and Research
Chandigarh, India

Tarun Kumar MD DM FSCAI FACC
Professor
Department of Cardiology
ABVIMS and DR RML Hospital
New Delhi, India

T Govindan Unni MD DM(Cardiology)
Professor and Head
Department of Cardiology
Jubilee Mission Medical College and Research Institute
Thrissur, Kerala, India

Tharun David Varghese M MD DM
Consultant Interventional Cardiologist
MOSC Medical College Hospital
Kochi, Kerala, India

Thomas Alexander MD DM
Head, Department of Cardiology
Kovai Medical Centre Hospital
Coimbatore, Tamil Nadu, India

Tiny Nair MD DM FACC FRCP
Head, Department of Cardiology
PRS Hospital
Thiruvananthapuram, Kerala, India

Tirthankar Dasgupta PhD
Senior Scientist
TCS Research
Kolkata, West Bengal, India

Tom Devasia MD DM FACC FSCAI FESC PGDD MBA
Professor and Unit-Head
Department of Cardiology
Kasturba Medical College, Manipal
Manipal, Karnataka, India

Trinath Kumar Mishra MD DM FCSI FACC
Professor
Department of Cardiology
MKCG Medical College
Berhampur, Odisha, India

Umesh K Pandey DM
Associate Professor
Department of Cardiology
Institute of Medical Sciences
Banaras Hindu University
Varanasi, Uttar Pradesh, India

Umesh Tripathi MD DM
Assistant Professor
Department of Cardiology
King George's Medical University
Lucknow, Uttar Pradesh, India

Umeshwar Pandey MD DM
Professor and Head
LPS Institute of Cardiology
Kanpur, Uttar Pradesh, India

Upendra Kaul MD DM FCSI FSCAI FAPSIC FACC FAMS
Awarded Padmashiri and
Dr BC Roy Award
Chairman – Cardiology and
Dean- Academics and Research
Batra Hospital and Medical Research Center
New Delhi, India

Vaibhav Shukla MD DM
Senior Interventional Cardiologist
Apollo Hospitals
Indore, Madhya Pradesh, India

Valakkada J DM
Associate Professor
Sree Chitra Tirunal Institute
Thiruvananthapuram, Kerala, India

Vardhini Vijaykumar BDS MDS
Medical Advisor
Hyderabad, Telangana, India

Vibhav Sharma MD DM
Assistant Professor
Department of Cardiology
Amrita Institute of Medical Sciences
Faridabad, Haryana, India

Vidyut Jain MD FRCP(UK) FSCAI FESC FACC
Consultant Cardiologist
Choithram Hospital and Research Center
Indore, Madhya Pradesh, India

Vijaya Kumar Varada MD DM(Cardiology)
Post DM Senior Resident
Department of Cardiology
All India Institute of Medical Sciences, Rishikesh
Rishikesh, Uttarakhand, India

Vijay Bang MD DM FCSI FESC FSCAI FACC
Senior Interventional Cardiologist
Lilavati Hospital and Research Center
Honorable Professor and Head
Grant Medical College and
Sir JJ Group of Hospitals (Former)
Mumbai, Maharashtra, India

Vijay Garg MD FIAE FICP FCSI FICA(USA) FISE FACC(USA) FACP(USA) FIMSA FISC FESC(Europe)
Professor, Department of Medicine
RD Gardi Medical College
Ujjain, Madhya Pradesh, India

Vijay Kumar Chopra MD DM FESC FHFA FCSI
Senior Cardiologist
Max Super Speciality Hospital
Saket, New Delhi, India

Vijay Kumar MD DM
Associate Professor
Department of Cardiology
Sri Jayadeva Institute of
Cardiovascular Sciences and Research
Bengaluru, Karnataka, India

Vijay Kumar MD DNB(Cardiology)
Director
Department of Cardiology
Fortis Escorts Heart Institute
New Delhi, India

Vimal Mehta MD DNB(Medicine) DM(Cardiology) FESC FACC
Director–Professor
Department of Cardiology
Head of Unit-III
GB Pant Institute of Postgraduate
Medical Education and Research
New Delhi, India

Vinayaga Pandian DNB DrNB FSCAI
Consultant Cardiologist
Health City
Cayman Islands

Vinayak Agrawal MD DM
Senior Director and Head
Clinical Cardiology and Cardiac Imaging
Fortis Memorial Research Institute (FMRI)
Gurugram, Haryana, India

Vinit Kumar MD DM(Cardiology) FESC FSCAI FAPSIC
Cardiologist
Department of Cardiology
Heart Hospital
Patna, Bihar, India

Vinod Sharma MD DM(Cardiology) FRCP(London) FACC MBA(Healthcare Administration)
Vice-CEO and Head
Department of Cardiology Services
National Heart Institute
East of Kailash, New Delhi, India

Vinutha Rajesh MD FACC
Assistant Professor
Loma Linda University School of Medicine
Loma Linda, CA, USA

Vipin Kumar MD DM(Cardiology) FACC FSCAI
Senior Consultant Cardiologist
Ruban Memorial Hospital
Patna, Bihar, India

Vishal Batra MD DM
Professor
Department of Cardiology
GB Pant Institute of Postgraduate Medical Education and Research
New Delhi, India

Vishal Gavali MD(General Medicine)
Senior Registrar
Department of Cardiology
Jaslok Hospital
Mumbai, Maharashtra, India

Vishal Rastogi MD DM(Cardiology)
Director
Department of Cardiology
Fortis Escorts Heart Institute
New Delhi, India

Viveka Kumar MD DM FACC FSCAI FCSI
Director
Department of Cardiology
Max Hospital
Saket, New Delhi, India

Vivekanand S Gajapati MD DM
Consultant Cardiologist
SDM Narayana Heart Centre
Dharwad, Karnataka, India

Vivek BS MD DM
Senior Consultant
Director – Clinical Cardiology and Non-Invasive Imaging
Sir Ganga Ram Hospital
New Delhi, India

Vivek Chaturvedi MD DM FACC
Senior Consultant Cardiologist and Head
Department of Cardiology
Amrita Insitute for Medical Sciences and Research
Faridabad, Haryana, India

Vivek Kumar MD DM(Cardiology)
Senior Consultant
Department of Cardiology
Indraprastha Apollo Hospital
New Delhi, India

Vivek Narasimha V DNB(General Medicine) DrNB(Cardiology)
Fellow in Cardiology
KIMS Hospital
Secunderabad, Telangana, India

Vivudh Pratap Singh MD DM(Cardiology)
Senior Consultant – Interventional Cardiology
Fortis Escorts Heart Institute
New Delhi, India

Vinay Kumar Bahl MD DM(Cardiology)
Director – Cardiac Sciences
MS Ramaiah Medical College
Bengaluru, Karnataka, India

Yash Lokhandwala MD DM
Visiting Faculty
LTMG Hospital
Mumbai, Maharashtra, India

Yash Paul Sharma MD DM
Professor and Head
Department of Cardiology
Postgraduate Institute of Medical Education and Research
Chandigarh, India

Foreword

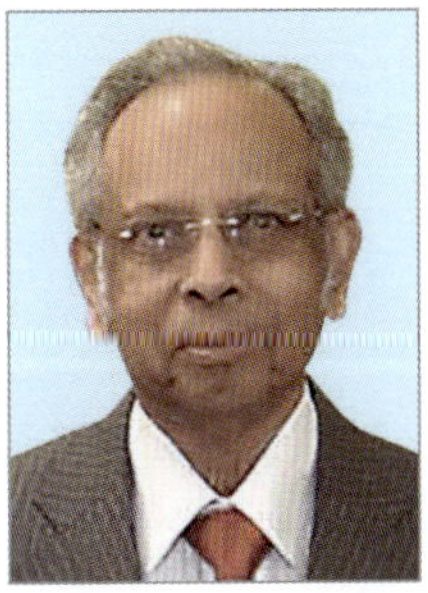

M Khalilullah
Padam Shree, Padam Bhushan, Dr BC Roy Awardee
Director and Senior Consultant Cardiologist
The Heart Centre, New Delhi, India
Former President, Cardiological Society of India
Director, GB Pant Institute of Postgraduate Medical Education and Research
New Delhi, India

It is with immense pride and respect for our profession that I introduce the *"CSI Cardiology Update 2024"*, an authoritative guide to the latest advancements and research in cardiovascular medicine, presented by the Cardiological Society of India. This annual volume, unveiled at the National Conference, reflects our continued commitment to elevating cardiology practice and enriching the knowledge of clinicians who dedicate themselves to the care of heart patients around the world.

The chapters in this edition are authored by some of the finest minds in cardiovascular medicine and interventional cardiology, each bringing a wealth of experience and insight into critical areas of our field. Their collective contributions span a remarkable range of topics, addressing everything from preventive strategies, advanced diagnostic approaches, medical management to innovative interventions. Together, they provide an invaluable resource for specialists, physicians, and fellows at all levels, seeking to keep pace with the rapid developments in cardiology and refine their approach to patient care.

As we stand at the forefront of cardiovascular healthcare, facing both the promise of new technologies and the persistent challenge of widespread cardiovascular disease, this book serves as a reminder of our shared mission: To improve the health and lives of those we serve. The knowledge contained in these pages is a testament to the dedication, expertise, and collaborative spirit that define our fraternity of cardiologists.

I extend my deepest gratitude to each contributor and to the editorial team for their hard work in bringing this volume to fruition. It is my hope that this update will not only inform but also inspire our readers to continue striving for excellence in their practice. May the insights found here empower you to make a meaningful difference in the lives of your patients and in the broader landscape of cardiovascular care.

Preface

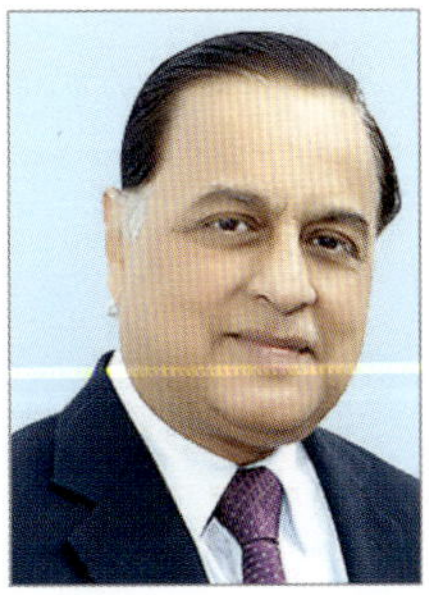

Sanjay Tyagi MD(Medicine) DM(Cardiology) FAMS FICP FCSI FICA FRCP(Edinburgh) FSCAI FESC FACC(USA)
Dr BC Roy National Awardee
Senior Consultant, Academic Advisor (HOD) and Clinical Director Cardiology
Apollo Hospitals, Northern Region, New Delhi, India
President-Elect, Cardiological Society of India
Secretary General (India), International College of Cardiology (USA)
National Coordinator, Cardiology and Interventional Cardiology, National Board of Examination
Formerly
Director General Health Services, Govt of India
Dean, Maulana Azad Medical College, New Delhi
Director, Professor and HOD Cardiology
GB Pant Institute of Postgraduate Medical Education and Research

A very warm greetings from the Cardiological Society of India (CSI).

It is an honor and a privilege to present the "*Cardiology Update 2024*" on behalf of CSI. It is a thoughtfully curated collection of the latest advances, research insights, and clinical practices in cardiovascular medicine. This edition, launched in conjunction with the Annual National Conference of the CSI, serves as a testament to the remarkable progress in our field and the relentless pursuit of excellence by cardiologists worldwide.

The updated book, largest till date, is divided into two volumes. It has been edited into 21 sections and 226 chapters written by eminent national and international authors. The chapters in this volume represent the contributions of distinguished experts, each a leader in their respective domain of cardiovascular care and research. This book addresses a wide spectrum of topics, from state-of-the-art interventional procedures and diagnostic innovations to the evolving paradigms in preventive cardiology, artificial intelligence, and complex disease management. Every chapter is crafted to ensure relevance and applicability to practicing cardiologists, merging latest in evidence-based research with real-world clinical insight.

Our aim is to provide cardiologists with a comprehensive, latest resource that enhances their clinical practice and supports them in delivering optimal care. With cardiovascular diseases remaining a leading cause of morbidity and mortality globally, the need for shared knowledge and refined clinical approaches is more critical than ever. It is our hope that this book will become an essential reference for clinicians, researchers, and healthcare providers dedicated to advancing cardiovascular science and patient outcomes.

I am deeply grateful to the galaxy of reputed national and international faculty for their expertise, commitment, and dedication to this project. Their work is the cornerstone of this book, reflecting the highest standards in cardiovascular medicine. I would also like to extend my appreciation to the CSI Scientific Committee and Executive Committee, especially Dr PC Rath, Dr Debabrata Roy, and Dr DP Sinha, whose support and organization were invaluable in bringing this publication to fruition. I would like to express my gratitude to my colleagues, Professor Jamal Yusuf, Professor Girish MP, Professor Vishal Batra, and Dr Subrat Kumar Muduli for their support. I would also like to place on record my sincere gratitude for Jaypee Brothers Medical Publishers, specially Ms Nedup for working tirelessly with the authors and compiling this book.

I dedicate this Update to my teachers, parents, patients, students, and family—wife Dr Mamta, son Dr Dhruv, and daughter Dr Swati—for being eternally supportive and encouraging throughout my journey.

May "*CSI Cardiology Update 2024*" inspire you, deepen your knowledge, and empower your practice as we all work toward a future of healthier hearts and lives.

Contents

VOLUME 1

SECTION 1: GENERAL CARDIOLOGY

SECTION 2: ECHOCARDIOGRAPHY/IMAGING

SECTION 3: ARTIFICIAL INTELLIGENCE IN CARDIOLOGY

SECTION 4: DYSLIPIDEMIA MANAGEMENT

SECTION 5: HYPERTENSION

SECTION 6: HEART FAILURE

SECTION 8: CARDIO-OBSTETRICS

SECTION 9: CONGENITAL HEART DISEASE

SECTION 10: VALVULAR HEART DISEASE/MISCELLANEOUS

SECTION 11: PULMONARY VASCULAR DISEASE

VOLUME 2

SECTION 12: CHRONIC CORONARY SYNDROMES

SECTION 13: ACUTE CORONARY SYNDROME

SECTION 14: CORONARY INTERVENTION

SECTION 15: STRUCTURAL INTERVENTION

SECTION 16: MECHANICAL CIRCULATORY SUPPORT

SECTION 17: VASCULAR INTERVENTIONS

SECTION 21: PREVENTIVE CARDIOLOGY

Scan the QR code to access references of all the chapters.

SECTION 12

Chronic Coronary Syndromes

Section Outline

CHAPTER

113

Latest Guidelines in Management of Stable Angina

Jamal Yusuf, Dixit Goyal

ABSTRACT

Chronic coronary syndromes (CCS) are the most common manifestation of ischemic heart disease, affecting almost half of the coronary artery disease (CAD) patients. The pathogenesis of stable angina is complex and often, albeit not always, involves flow-limiting epicardial coronary artery stenoses but also involves nonobstructive causes like coronary spasm and microvascular dysfunction. Proper risk stratification and selecting appropriate testing is important. Rational treatment requires a multifaceted and tailored approach for every individual combining lifestyle changes, aggressive management of modifiable risk factors, pharmacological therapy, and myocardial revascularization when appropriate.

Keywords: Coronary artery disease (CAD), chronic coronary disease (CCD), chronic coronary syndrome (CCS), microvascular dysfunction

INTRODUCTION

Coronary artery disease (CAD) is a leading cause of mortality worldwide and encompasses a wide spectrum of syndromes that occur due to an imbalance between myocardial oxygen demand and supply. The underlying pathological process is atherosclerotic plaque accumulation in the epicardial arteries, whether obstructive or nonobstructive. 2019 ESC guidelines have recommended the use of the term chronic coronary syndrome (CCS) instead of stable angina looking at the progressive nature of the disease and 2024 guidelines continued to use the same.[1,2] However, 2023 AHA guidelines, used the term chronic coronary disease (CCD).[3] Patients can have varied presentations ranging from long, stable periods to acute presentations due to an acute atherothrombotic event caused by plaque rupture or erosion. There is also a firm belief that epicardial stenosis is the leading cause of angina and ischemia. However, multiple RCTs failed to show any mortality benefit with revascularization in most stable CAD patients.[4] Thus, focusing unduly on epicardial coronary obstruction leads to overlooking of many other pathological mechanisms like epicardial or microvascular coronary vasospasm, coronary microvascular dysfunction (CMD), and derangements of myocardial energy or metabolism.[5] This chapter explores the comprehensive management strategies in the patients of CCS based on the latest guidelines and evidence.

CLASSIFICATION

Chronic coronary syndromes are a range of clinical presentations or syndromes that arise due to structural and/or functional alterations related to chronic diseases of the coronary arteries and/or microcirculation and 2024 ESC guidelines divided it into five frequently encountered scenarios **(Fig. 1)**:[2]

EVALUATION, DIAGNOSIS, AND RISK STRATIFICATION

Recent 2024 ESC guidelines have advised a four-step evaluation in a suspected case of CCS **(Fig. 2)**.[2]

Step 1: Initial Evaluation (General Clinical Examination)

The first step is a general clinical evaluation, focusing primarily on the signs and symptoms of CCS and ruling out acute coronary syndrome (ACS) and other noncardiac causes. Although chest pain is the cardinal symptom, merely 10–15% of patients present with typical angina.[6] Current guidelines focus on the detailed description of symptoms instead of using the terms typical or atypical chest pain.[2] The initial clinical evaluation requires recording a 12-lead

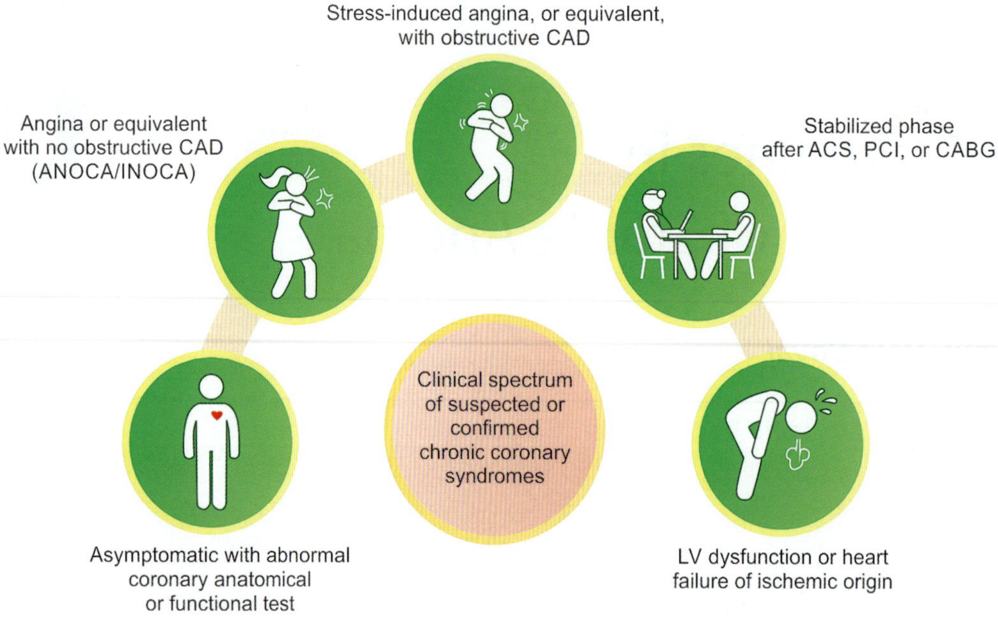

FIG. 1: Classification of CCS patients.[2]

resting electrocardiogram (ECG), basic blood tests, and in selected individuals, chest X-ray imaging and pulmonary function testing. Physical examination is important to assess the presence of anemia, hypertension, valvular heart disease, hypertrophic cardiomyopathy, or arrhythmias. It is also recommended to obtain the body mass index (BMI) and search for evidence of noncoronary vascular disease, which may be asymptomatic [includes palpation of peripheral pulses, auscultation of carotid and femoral arteries, as well as assessment of the ankle-brachial index (ABI)], and other signs of comorbid conditions such as thyroid disease, renal disease, or diabetes.

Step 2: Further Evaluation (Assess Clinical Likelihood of Obstructive Coronary Artery Disease)

The diagnosis of CCS is determined by assessing the individual's symptoms, considering the influence of age, gender, risk factors, and existing comorbidities on the probability of CCS, and selecting the most suitable diagnostic test to confirm the suspected condition. Earlier models used to estimate the likelihood of obstructive CAD, such as the Diamond-Forrester approach and the pretest probability model (2019 ESC), tended to overestimate the presence of obstructive CAD. 2024 ESC guidelines recommend the use of the risk-factor-weighted clinical likelihood (RF-CL) model which includes sex, age, angina symptoms, and the number of risk factors **(Fig. 3)**.[2] It classifies patients into 5 groups: Very low (≤5%), low (>5–15%), moderate (>15–50%), high (>50–85%), and very high (>85%) clinical likelihood of obstructive CAD. The RF-CL model classifies three times more individuals as having a very low (≤5%) likelihood of obstructive CAD compared to the ESC pretest probability (ESC-PTP) model, with 38% versus 12%, respectively.[7] It is advised to incorporate additional clinical information, such as peripheral artery examination, resting ECG, resting echocardiography, and evidence of vascular calcifications from prior imaging tests, to refine the estimate provided by the RF-CL model. Further noninvasive and invasive anatomical or functional testing is based on the percentage of likelihood.

Step 3: Confirming the Diagnosis (Selecting Appropriate Testing)

The step 3 is detailed in **Figures 4 and 5, and Table 1**.

The SCOT-HEART trial showed a modest but significant reduction in the combined endpoint of cardiovascular death or nonfatal myocardial infarction (MI), decreasing from 3.9 to 2.3% over a 5-year follow-up period in patients who underwent coronary computed tomography angiography (CCTA) in addition to routine testing (such as exercise ECG).[8] A network meta-analysis of randomized trials indicated that diagnostic testing with CCTA was associated with similar clinical outcomes compared to functional imaging in patients with suspected stable CAD.[9] In patients without significant obstructive disease on invasive coronary angiography (ICA) or CCTA, functional testing using noninvasive methods such as PET-CT myocardial blood flow (MBF), cardiac MRI, SPECT, or invasive techniques like FFR, iFR, IMR, and CFR should be performed to evaluate the functional significance of the lesion and to assess for microvascular dysfunction.

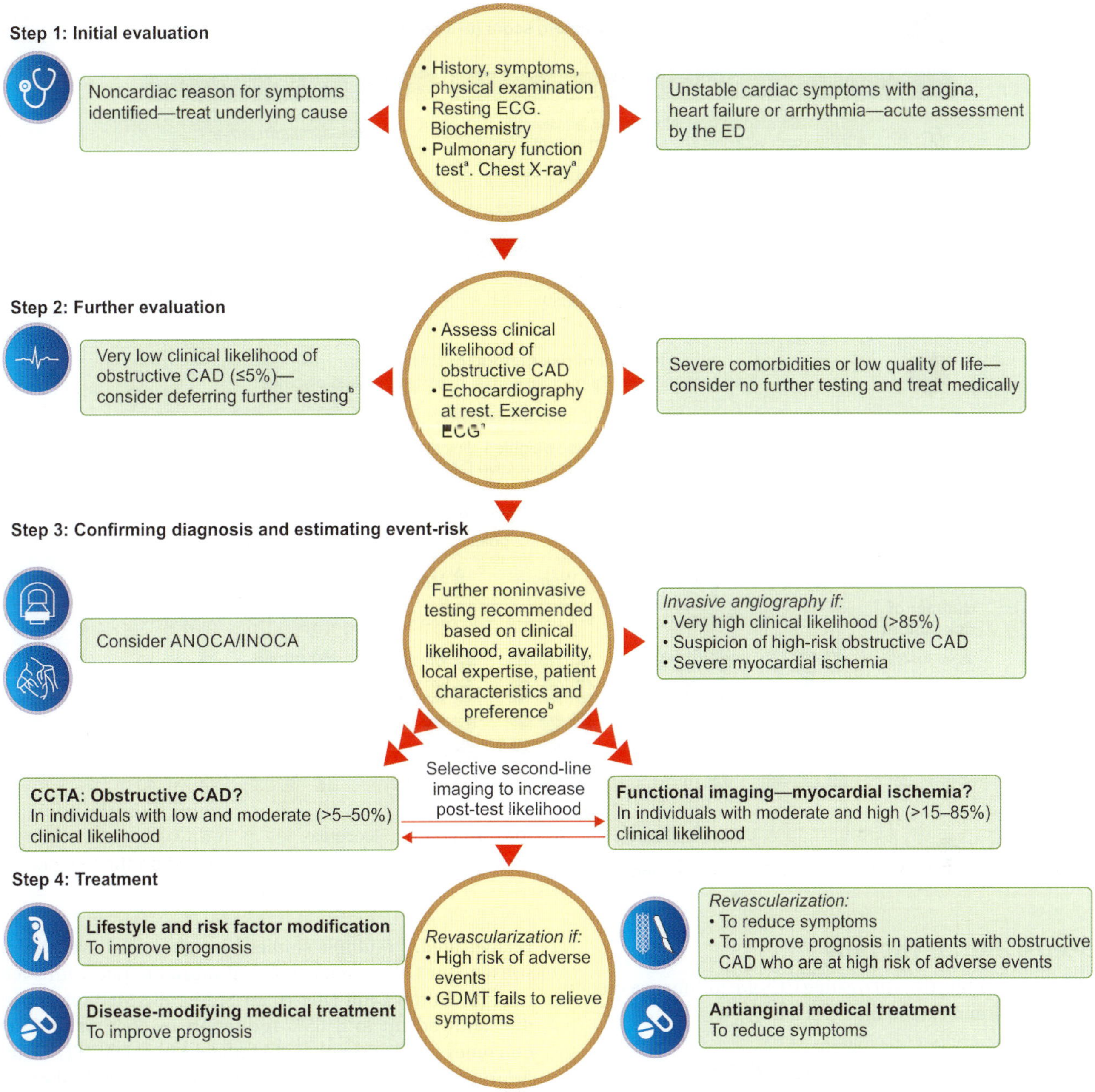

[a]In selected patients.

[b]Consider also coronary spasm or microvascular dysfunction.

FIG. 2: Four-step evaluation in a suspected case of CCS.

It is recommended that all patients with newly diagnosed obstructive CAD or myocardial ischemia undergo an assessment for adverse event risk to identify those at high risk of poor outcomes, who may benefit from revascularization beyond symptom management. According to data from large registries and historical randomized controlled trials (RCTs), high event risk is defined as a cardiac mortality rate of over 3% per year, intermediate risk as between 1% and 3% per year, and low risk as <1% per year.[10] The clinician should incorporate all available information, including noninvasive, invasive, or both, cardiovascular diagnostic testing results, and use validated risk scores **(Table 2)**. In individuals at high risk of adverse events, regardless of symptoms, ICA is recommended, supplemented by coronary pressure measurements (such as FFR or iFR) when appropriate. The goal is to refine risk stratification and enhance symptoms and cardiovascular outcomes through revascularization.

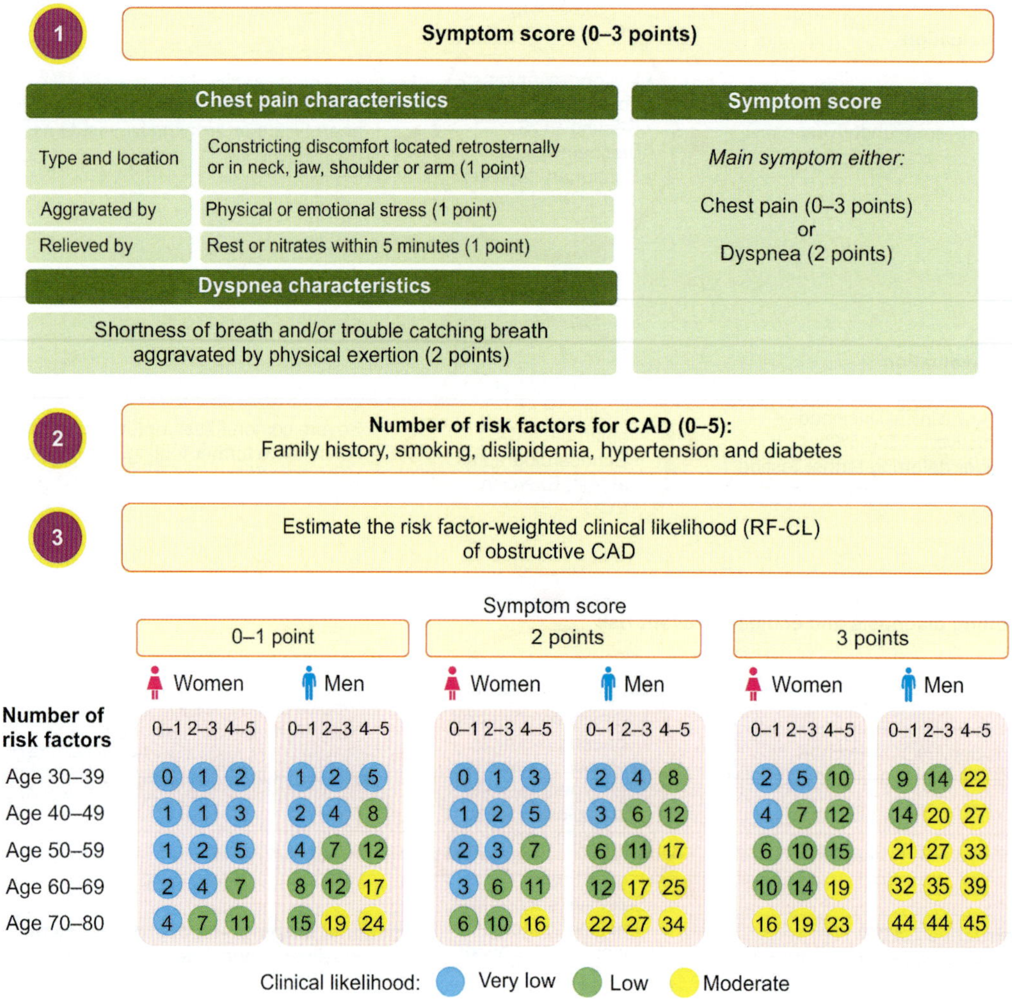

FIG. 3: Risk factor-weighted clinical likelihood model.[2]

Step 4: Initial Therapy

The primary objectives of treating CCS are to enhance quality of life (QoL) and extend life expectancy.

MANAGEMENT STRATEGIES GUIDELINE-DIRECTED MEDICAL TREATMENT

Guidelines recommend shared decision-making and a multidisciplinary team-based approach to improve health outcomes, facilitate modification of ASCVD risk factors, and improve health service utilization.[2]

Lifestyle Management

Healthy dietary choices are well known to improve the management of CVD risk factors. A Mediterranean dietary pattern high in fruit, vegetables, legumes, fiber, polyunsaturated fats, nuts, and fish, avoiding or limiting refined carbohydrates, red meat, dairy, and saturated fat, is advocated.[11] Multiple studies have shown a lower risk of subsequent CVD events and total mortality rate with such diet.[12,13] In the Lyon Diet Heart Study, the Mediterranean diet showed up to a 65% reduction in composite CVD outcomes (cardiac death and nonfatal MI).[14] DASH (Dietary Approaches to Stop Hypertension)-Sodium study showed that sodium reduction may improve biomarkers of cardiac injury, inflammation, and cardiac strain **(Table 3)**.[15] Smoking is a well-established risk factor, and e-cigarettes are often marketed as a less harmful alternative; however, emerging evidence suggests potential adverse effects on cardiovascular health.[16]

Pharmacotherapy

Antianginals: Beta-blockers, nondihydropyridine calcium channel blockers (CCBs), and ivabradine decrease myocardial oxygen demand (via decreasing contractility, heart rate, or both) while nitrates and CCBs increase arterial oxygenated blood supply via vasodilatory actions. The latest 2024 ESC guidelines emphasize that medical therapy for

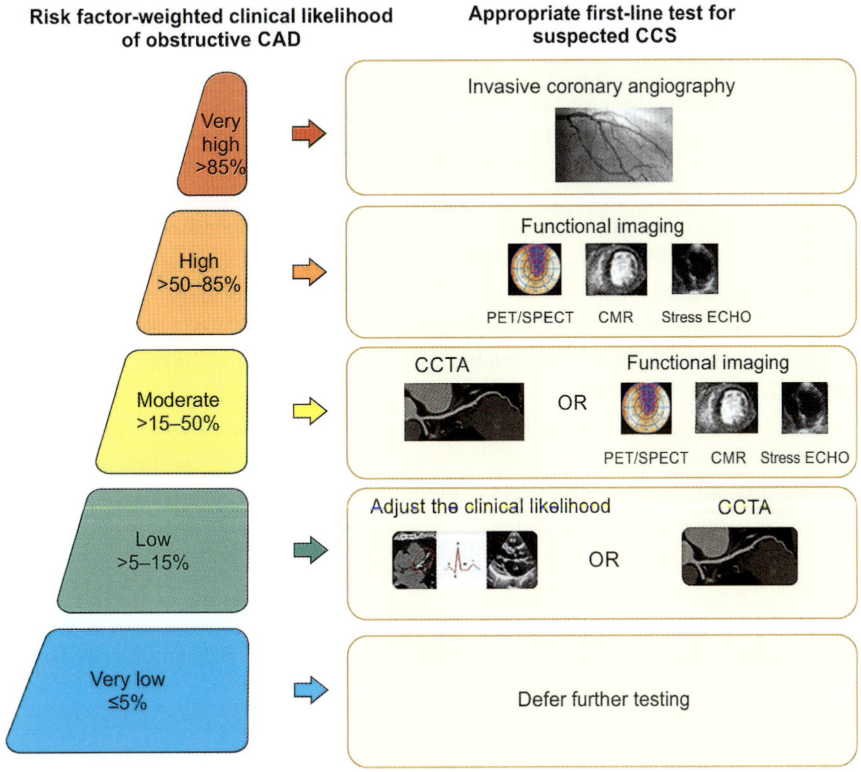

FIG. 4: Recommended initial testing for individuals showing symptoms of suspected chronic coronary syndrome.[2]

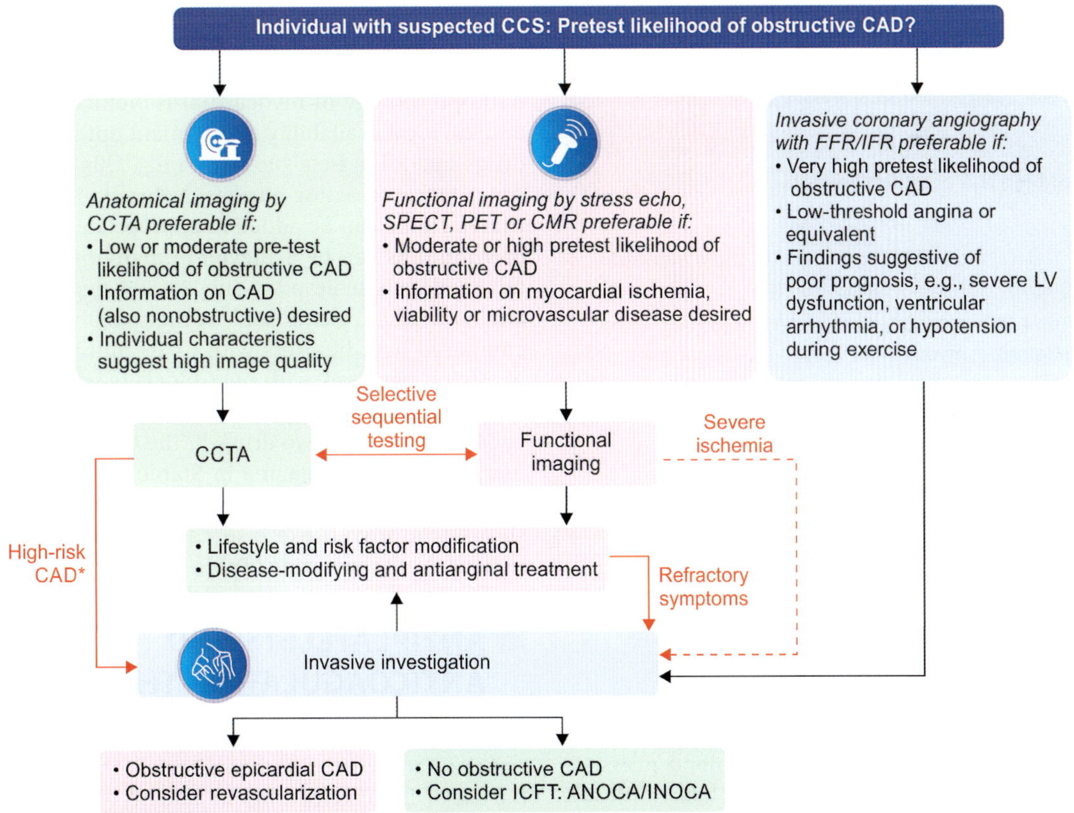

*High-risk CAD—obstructive CAD at high risk of adverse events by CCTA: ≥50% stenosis of the left main stem; three-vessel disease with severe stenoses (≥70% diameter stenosis); single- or two-vessel disease including the proximal LAD with severe stenoses.

FIG. 5: Choosing appropriate testing in suspected patients with CCS.[2]

TABLE 1: Recommendations for testing in patients with CCS.[2]

Recommendations for selection of test	COR	LOE
It is advised to choose the initial noninvasive diagnostic test by considering the pretest likelihood of obstructive coronary artery disease (CAD), relevant patient factors that may impact test performance, as well as local expertise and test availability	1	C
For symptomatic patients with a clinical assessment indicating a pretest likelihood of obstructive CAD greater than 5%, it is recommended to use coronary computed tomography angiography (CCTA) or noninvasive functional imaging for myocardial ischemia as the initial diagnostic test	1	B
Exercise ECG is recommended for patients where the results will influence the diagnostic or management strategy, helping to assess exercise tolerance, symptoms, arrhythmias, blood pressure response, and event risk	1	C
In individuals with a low (>5–15%) pretest likelihood of obstructive CAD, an exercise ECG may be considered to identify patients in whom further testing can be deferred	2b	C
Coronary CCTA is recommended as the preferred diagnostic method for ruling out obstructive CAD in individuals with a low-to-moderate pretest likelihood (>5–50%)	1	B
CCTA is recommended in individuals with low or moderate (>5–50%) pretest likelihood of obstructive CAD if functional imaging for myocardial ischemia is not diagnostic	1	B
Functional imaging for myocardial ischemia is recommended if CCTA has shown CAD of uncertain functional significance or is not diagnostic	1	B
Invasive coronary angiography with the availability of invasive functional assessments is recommended to confirm or exclude the diagnosis of obstructive CAD or ANOCA/INOCA in individuals with an uncertain diagnosis on noninvasive testing	1	B
Invasive coronary angiography is recommended to diagnose obstructive CAD in individuals with a very high (>85%) clinical likelihood of disease, severe symptoms refractory to guideline-directed medical therapy, angina at a low level of exercise, and/or high event risk	1	C
In individuals with de novo symptoms highly suggestive of obstructive CAD that occur at a low level of exercise, ICA with a view toward revascularization is recommended as first diagnostic test after clinical assessment by a cardiologist	1	C

TABLE 2: Features associated with high risk of adverse events.

Definition of high risk of adverse events	
Exercise ECG	Duke treadmill score <–10
Stress echocardiography	≥3 of 16 segments with stress-induced hypokinesia or akinesia
Stress SPECT or PET perfusion imaging	Area of ischemia ≥10% of the LV myocardium
Stress CMR	≥2 of 16 segments with stress perfusion defects or ≥3 dobutamine-induced dysfunctional segments
CCTA	Left main disease with ≥50% stenosis, three-vessel disease with ≥70 stenosis, or two-vessel disease with ≥70% stenosis, including the proximal LAD or one-vessel disease of the proximal LAD with ≥70% stenosis and FFR-CT ≤0.8

symptom management in CCS should be personalized based on each patient's hemodynamic profile (blood pressure and heart rate), comorbidities (especially heart failure), concurrent medications with potential drug interactions, and patient's preferences.[2] It should also consider the underlying pathophysiology of myocardial ischemia in each patient and the local availability of treatment options. The first-line drugs including beta-blockers and CCBs and second-line drugs like long-acting nitrates, ivabradine, ranolazine, and trimetazidine can be added in appropriate settings. Control of symptoms can be achieved in many patients; however, full freedom is achieved in only 40–50% depending upon the angina frequency at onset.[17] A meta-analysis of 72 studies compared beta-blockers with CCBs found fewer episodes of angina per week with beta-blockers with lower rates of drug discontinuation and no difference in the rate of death or MI between the two drugs.[18] The CARISA (Combination Assessment of Ranolazine in Stable Angina) trial and the ERICA (Efficacy of Ranolazine in Chronic Angina) trial showed improved exercise capacity with lesser angina episodes with ranolazine **(Table 4 and Fig. 6)**.[19,20]

ANTIPLATELETS AND ANTICOAGULATION THERAPIES

Platelet activation and aggregation are the drivers for symptomatic coronary thrombosis, forming the basis for the use of antiplatelet drugs in patients with CCS in view of a favorable balance between the prevention of ischemic events and increased risk of bleeding **(Table 5 and Fig. 7)**.

TABLE 3: Lifestyle changes recommended in patients with CCD.[2]

Lifestyle changes	LOE	COR
Diet emphasizing vegetables, fruits, legumes, nuts, whole grains, and lean protein is recommended to reduce the risk of CVD events	B-R	1
Reducing the percentage of calories from saturated fat (<6% of total calories) and replacing with dietary monounsaturated and polyunsaturated fat, complex carbohydrates, and dietary fiber	B-NR	2a
Minimization of sodium (<2.3 g/day, optimally <1.5 g/day) and minimization of processed meats (e.g., cured bacon and hot dogs)	B-NR	2a
Limiting refined carbohydrates (e.g., containing <25% whole grain by weight, including refined cold ready-to-eat breakfast cereal, white bread, and white rice) and sugar-sweetened beverages (e.g., soft drinks, energy drinks, and fruit drinks with added sugars)	B-NR	2a
Intake of trans fat should be avoided because trans fat is associated with increased morbidity and mortality rates	B-NR	3: harm
Use of nonprescription or dietary supplements, including omega-3 fatty acid, vitamins C, D, E, beta-carotene, and calcium, is not beneficial to reduce the risk of acute CVD events	B-NR	3: no benefit
Patients with CCD who regularly smoke tobacco should be advised to quit at every visit	A	1
Behavioral interventions are recommended to maximize cessation rates in combination with pharmacotherapy, including bupropion, varenicline, or combination long- and short-acting nicotine replacement therapy (NRT)	A	1
Limit alcohol intake (≤1 drink/day for women and ≤2 drinks/day for men) to reduce cardiovascular and all-cause death	B-NR	2a
An exercise regimen is recommended, including ≥150 minutes/week of moderate-intensity aerobic activities or ≥75 minutes/week of higher-intensity aerobic activities to improve functional capacity and QOL, and to reduce hospital admission and mortality rates	A	1

TABLE 4: Antianginal therapies.[2]

Recommendations for antianginal drugs	COR	LOE
Short-acting nitrates are recommended for immediate relief of angina	1	B
Initial treatment with beta-blockers and/or CCBs to control heart rate and symptoms is recommended for most patients with CCS	1	B
If anginal symptoms are not successfully controlled by initial treatment with a beta-blocker or a CCB alone, the combination of a beta-blocker and a DHP-CCB should be considered, unless contraindicated	2a	B
Long-acting nitrates or ranolazine should be considered as add-on therapy in patients with inadequate control of symptoms while on treatment with beta-blockers and or CCBs, or as part of initial treatment in properly selected patients	2a	B
Ivabradine should be considered as add-on antianginal therapy in patients with left ventricular systolic dysfunction (LVEF <40%) and inadequate control of symptoms, or as part of initial treatment in properly selected patients	2a	B
Nicorandil or trimetazidine may be considered as add-on therapy in patients with inadequate control of symptoms while on treatment with beta-blockers and or CCBs, or as part of initial treatment in properly selected patients	2b	B
Ivabradine is not recommended as add-on therapy in patients with CCS, LVEF >40%, and no clinical heart failure	3	B

Low-dose aspirin (75–100 mg once daily) is the traditional drug of choice in CCS patients regardless of prior MI. Meta-analysis of secondary prevention trials showed reduced combined risk of nonfatal MI, nonfatal ischemic stroke, or death from vascular causes [from 8.2 to 6.7% per year ($p < 0.0001$)], with relative risk (RR) reductions of 31%, 22%, and 9%, respectively with aspirin.[21] Recently, clopidogrel has been approved as an effective alternative to aspirin monotherapy for long-term secondary prevention in CCS patients based on a patient-level meta-analysis involving 24,325 patients (including recent ACS, post-CABG, or initial CCS patients) randomized to either aspirin monotherapy (12,147 patients) or P2Y12 inhibitor monotherapy [clopidogrel in 7,545 (62.0%), ticagrelor in 4,633 (38.0%)] and followed for 6–36 months. P2Y12 inhibitors reduced the combined ischemic outcome of cardiovascular death, MI, and stroke compared with aspirin (in doses of 100 or 325 mg daily), mainly through the reduction of infarction. The risk of major bleeding was similar, whereas GI bleeding and hemorrhagic stroke occurred less frequently with a P2Y12 inhibitor.[22]

A default dual antiplatelet therapy (DAPT) duration of 6 months is recommended after percutaneous coronary intervention (PCI) in CCS patients, however, in patients at high bleeding risk, a shorter duration of DAPT (1–3 months)

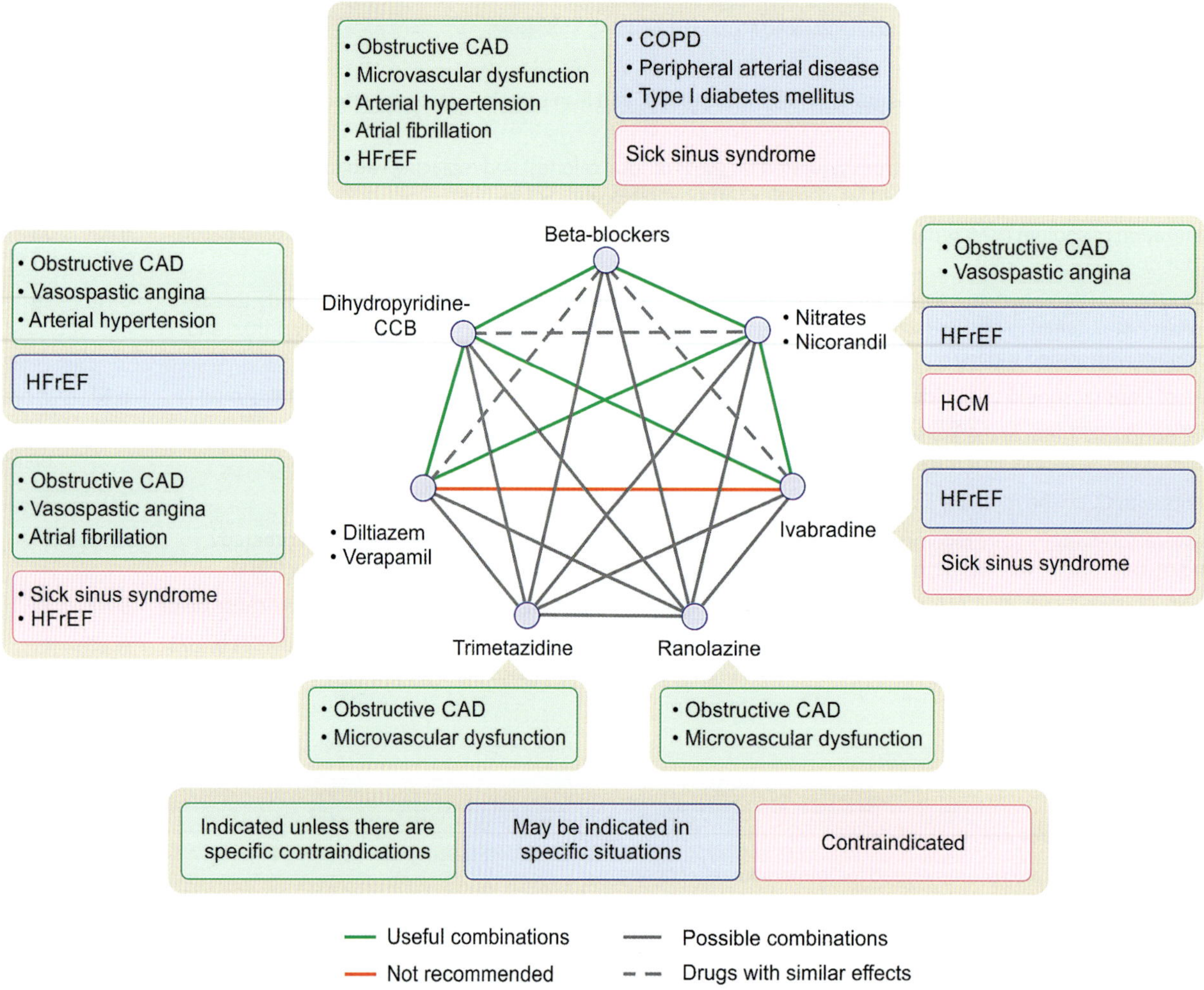

FIG. 6: Possible combinations of antianginal drugs.

TABLE 5: Recommendations for antiplatelet and anticoagulation therapies.[2]

Recommendations for antiplatelets and antithrombotic agents in CCS	COR	LOE
In CCS patients with a prior MI or remote PCI, aspirin 75–100 mg daily is recommended lifelong after an initial period of DAPT	1	A
In CCS patients with a prior MI or remote PCI, clopidogrel 75 mg daily is recommended as a safe and effective alternative to aspirin monotherapy	1	A
In CCS patients with no indication for oral anticoagulation, DAPT consisting of aspirin 75–100 mg and clopidogrel 75 mg daily for up to 6 months is recommended as the default antithrombotic strategy after PCI- stenting	1	A
In patients at high bleeding risk but not at high ischemic risk, it is recommended to discontinue DAPT 1–3 months after PCI and to continue with single antiplatelet therapy	1	A
Stopping DAPT after 1–3 months from PCI-stenting may be considered in patients who are not at high bleeding risk nor at high risk of ischemic events	2b	B
In CCS patients undergoing high-thrombotic risk stenting (e.g, complex left main stem, two-stent bifurcation, suboptimal stenting result, prior stent thrombosis, previously known CYP2C19 *2/*3 polymorphisms), prasugrel or ticagrelor (in addition to aspirin) may be considered instead of clopidogrel, for the first month, and up to 3–6 months	2b	C
After uncomplicated PCI in CCS patients with concomitant indication for OAC: • Early cessation of aspirin (≤1 week); • Followed by continuation of OAC and clopidogrel: ○ Up to 6 months in patients not at high ischemic risk or ○ Up to 12 months in patients at high ischemic risk; • Followed by OAC alone is recommended.	1	A

*Variants of genotype.

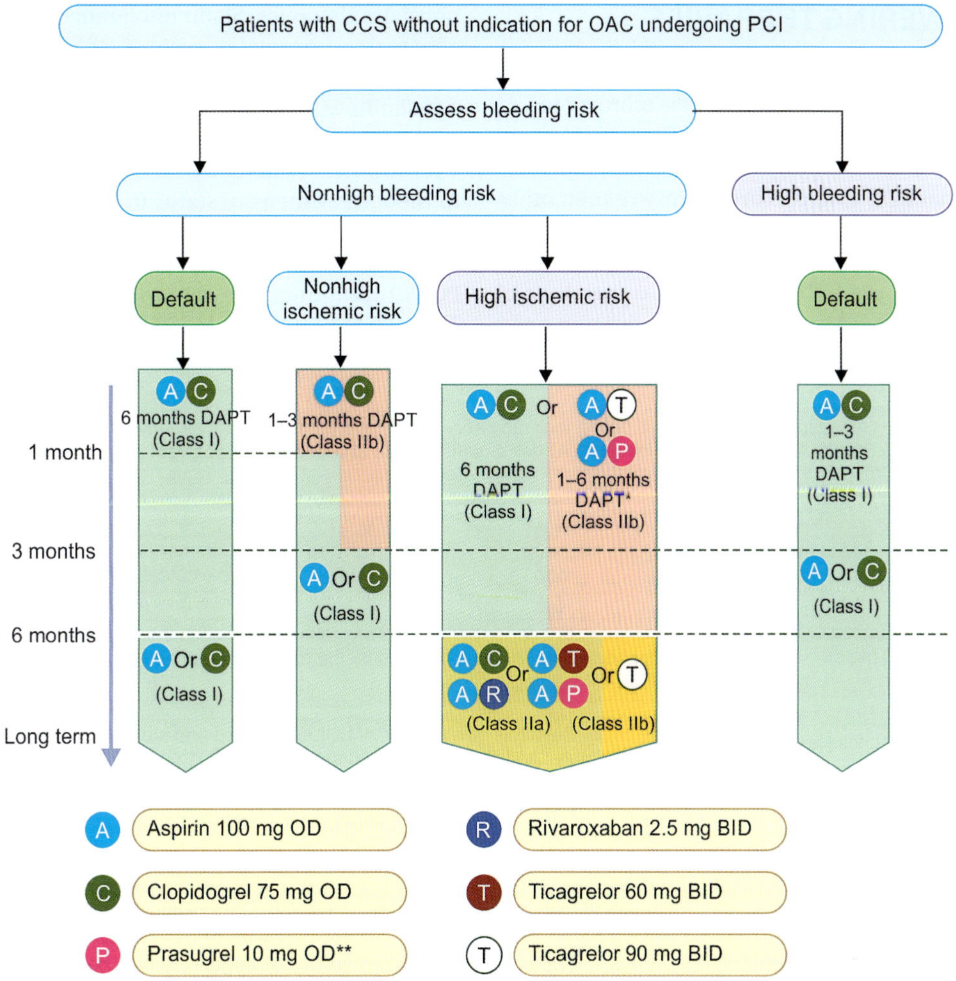

*In CCS patients undergoing high-thrombotic risk stenting (e.g., complex left main stem, 2-stent bifurcation, suboptimal stenting result, prior stent thrombosis, previously known CYP2C19 polymorphisms), prasugrel or ticagrelor (in addition to aspirin) may be considered instead of clopidogrel for the first month, and up to 3–6 months.

**Prasugrel 5 mg o.d. for patients aged ≥75 years or with a body weight.

FIG. 7: Recommended duration of antiplatelet therapies.[2]

can be beneficial. The MASTER-DAPT trial (Management of High Bleeding Risk Patients Post Bioresorbable Polymer Coated Stent Implantation with an Abbreviated versus Standard DAPT Regimen) involved 4,579 patients who underwent PCI, with about 50% having CCS. These high bleeding risk (HBR) patients were randomized, after 1 month of uneventful DAPT to either discontinue DAPT immediately or continue for at least 2 more months. After 335 days, the trial showed that early DAPT discontinuation was noninferior to the standard DAPT duration regarding ischemic events, while it significantly reduces major and clinically relevant nonmajor bleeding.[23] A meta-analysis revealed that an abbreviated DAPT regimen of 1-3 months led to reductions in both major bleeding and ischemic events, as well as cardiovascular mortality, compared to standard DAPT, regardless of whether patients presented with CCS or ACS.[24] In patients with high ischemic risk without HBR, there are three strategies to intensify antithrombotic therapy to reduce ischemic events, though with an increased risk of bleeding: (i) Continue DAPT with aspirin and clopidogrel, or aspirin and prasugrel post-PCI, as supported by the DAPT Study;[25] (ii) add ticagrelor to aspirin in post-MI patients, based on findings from the PEGASUS-TIMI 54 trial;[26] or (iii) in CCS patients, add very low-dose rivaroxaban to aspirin, as demonstrated in the COMPASS trial.[27] The findings from five RCTs and a meta-analysis have demonstrated that double antithrombotic therapy, as opposed to triple therapy, significantly reduces major or clinically relevant nonmajor bleeding without notably increasing ischemic events in patients with atrial fibrillation undergoing PCI.[28-33] This evidence supports the recommendation of using double antithrombotic therapy (oral anticoagulant plus a P2Y12 receptor inhibitor, primarily clopidogrel) after a 1-4 weeks period of triple therapy in CCS patients with atrial fibrillation undergoing PCI.

LIPID-LOWERING THERAPIES

Despite having lower LDL-C levels, Indians develop ASCVD a decade earlier than Western population.[34] According to LAI guidelines, patients with established ASVCD come into very high risk or extreme risk category A or B, and the guidelines recommended that LDL-C targets are aggressive than other guidelines **(Flowchart 1)**.[35] Reduction of 1 mmol/L (38.7 mg/dL) in LDL-C leads to 21% reduction in the risk of major vascular events over 5 years.[36] Statins are the cornerstone of therapy **(Table 6)**.[37] However, statins intolerance and need for additional LDL-C lowering stress upon the need of other nonstatin therapies. Statin intolerance is defined as adverse effects that improve or resolve with dose modification or discontinuation of statin therapy and require a trial of at least two statins with one at the lowest approved daily dose.[38]

In IMPROVE-IT (Improved Reduction of Outcomes; Vytorin Efficacy International Trial), the addition of ezetimibe to moderate-intensity statin therapy among patients with ACS resulted in a significant ASCVD risk reduction.[39] The FOURIER (Further Cardiovascular Outcomes Research with PCSK9 Inhibition Subjects with Elevated Risk) trial[40] and The ODYSSEY OUTCOMES (Evaluation of Cardiovascular Outcomes after an Acute Coronary Syndrome during

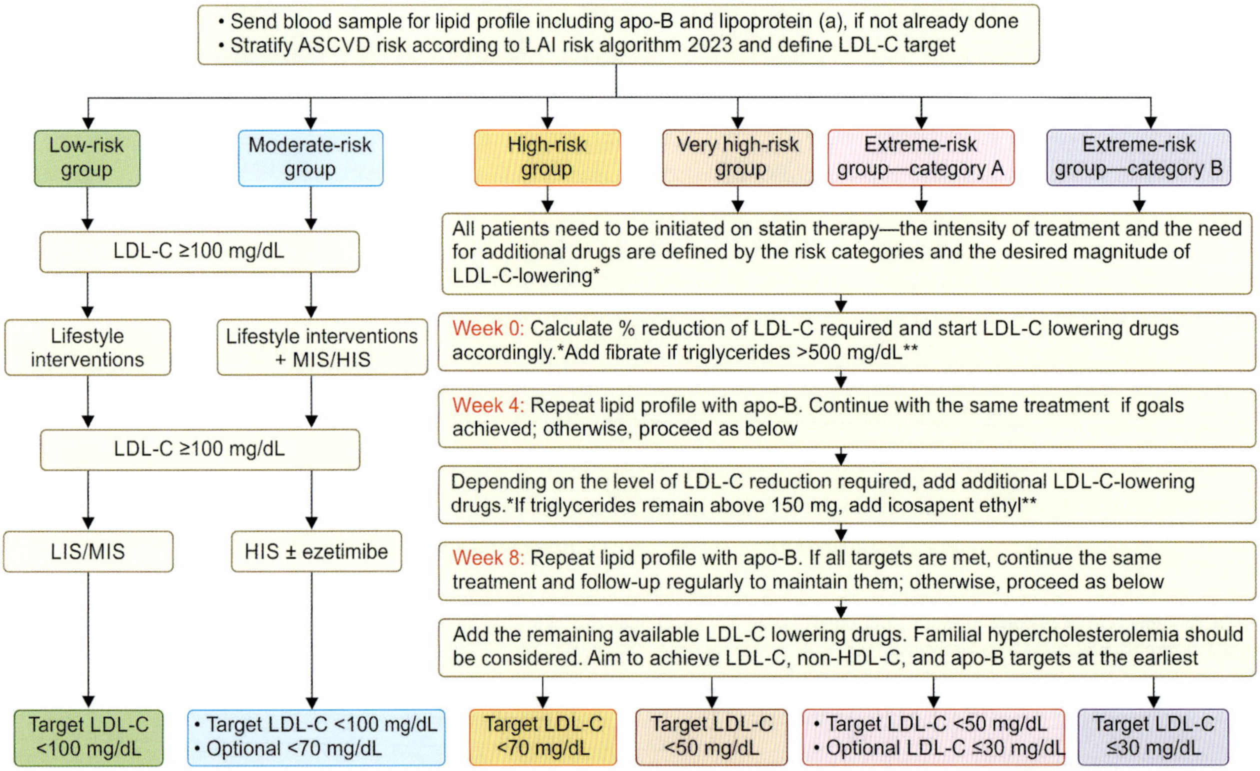

*To reduce LDL-C by 30%, start with MIS; to reduce it by 50%, start with HIS; and to reduce it by 65%, start with HIS + ezetimibe. Add bile acid sequestrant or bempedoic acid if an additional LDL-C reduction of 20% is required; if the additional LDL-C reduction is >20%, consider proprotein convertase subtilisin/kexin type 9 inhibitors.

**Look for and treat secondary causes of hypertriglyceridemia.

FLOWCHART 1: Lipid management.[35]

TABLE 6: Different strengths of statin therapies.[3]

	High intensity	Moderate intensity	Low intensity
LDL-C lowering	≥50%	30–49%	<30%
Statins	• Atorvastatin (40 and 80 mg) • Rosuvastatin (20 and 40 mg)	• Atorvastatin(10 and 20 mg) • Rosuvastatin (5 and 10 mg) • Simvastatin (20–40 mg)	Simvastatin (10 mg)
		• Pravastatin (40 and 80 mg) • Lovastatin (40 and 80 mg) • Fluvastatin XL (80 mg) • Fluvastatin (40 mg BID) • Pitavastatin (1–4 mg)	• Pravastatin (10–20 mg) • Lovastatin (20 mg) • Fluvastatin (20–40 mg)

Treatment with Alirocumab) trial[41] evaluated evolocumab and alirocumab, respectively and showed ~15% reduction in cardiovascular events with 60% reduction in LDL-C levels with both drugs. Bempedoic acid is an ATP citrate lyase inhibitor and reduces LDL-C by approximately 35% in combination with ezetimibe. In a pooled analysis of four randomized trials, LDL-C levels were significantly reduced with bempedoic acid in patients with ASCVD or heterozygous FH or both, and in statin-intolerant group.[42] Recently, CLEAR OUTCOMES trial showed significant LDL-C reductions and lower risk of MACE with bempedoic acid among statin-intolerant patients.[43] Inclisiran is a small interfering RNA that reduces synthesis of PCSK9 and LDL-C by ~ 50%.[44] However, due to limited evidence and cost issues other therapies should be preferred first. LAI recommends that at first, risk stratification of the patient should be done, and LDL-C target should be defined accordingly. To reduce LDL-C by 30%, start with moderate-intensity statin; to reduce it by 50%, start with high-intensity statin (HIS); and to reduce it by 65%, start with HIS+ ezetimibe. Add bile acid sequestrant or bempedoic acid if an additional LDL-C reduction of 20% is required; if the additional LDL-C reduction required is >20%, consider PCSK9 inhibitors.[35]

However, AHA 2023 guidelines have divided the patients with CCD into two groups: Not at very high risk and very high-risk group. Very high-risk and high-risk groups are shown in **Box 1** and should be managed accordingly **(Flowchart 2)**.

BOX 1 Very high-risk and high-risk groups according to AHA 2023.[3]

Definition of very high risk:
- History of multiple major ASCVD events

OR
- One major ASCVD event AND ≥2 high-risk conditions

Major ASCVD events:
- Recent ACS (within the past 12 months)
- History of MI (other than recent ACS events listed above)
- History of ischemic stroke
- Symptomatic peripheral artery disease (history of claudication with ABI < 0.85, or previous revascularization or amputation)

High-risk conditions:
- Age ≥ 65 years
- Familial hypercholesterolemia
- History of previous coronary artery bypass graft surgery or percutaneous coronary intervention outside of the major ASCVD event(s)
- Diabetes
- Hypertension
- Chronic kidney disease (eGFR, 15–59 mL/min/1.73 m^2)
- Current tobacco smoking
- Persistently elevated LDL-C ≥ 100 mg/dL despite maximally tolerated statin therapy and ezetimibe
- History of congestive heart failure

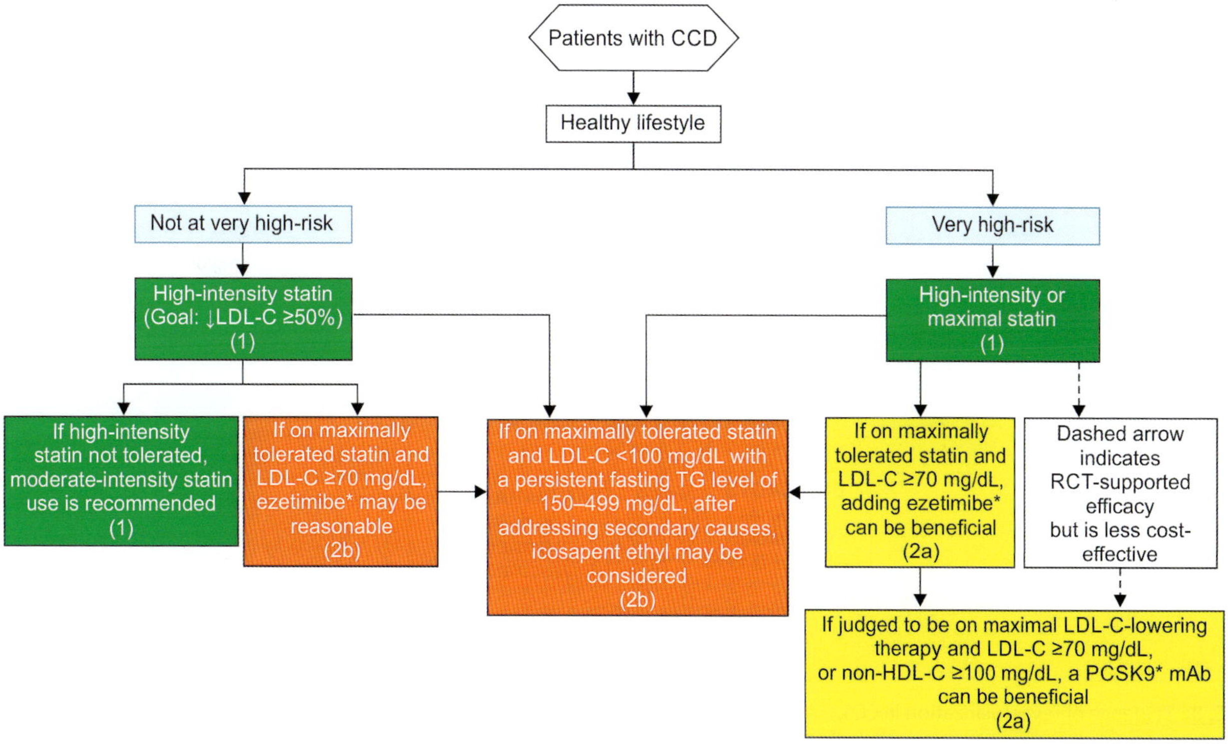

*Only when ezetimibe and PCSK9 mAb are deemed insufficient or not tolerated should bempedoic acid or inclisiran (in place of PCSK9 mAb) be considered to reduce LDL-C levels further.

FLOWCHART 2: Lipid-lowering therapies in CCD patients.[3]

ROLE OF COLCHICINE

Inflammation has a key role in atherosclerotic diseases, but the trials targeting these have shown mixed results. The COLCOT trial was the first trial to show efficacy of colchicine for secondary prevention in patients of ACS.[45] whereas the LoDoCo2 (Colchicine Reduces Risk of Major Cardiovascular Events in CCD) trial showed a reduced risk of recurrent cardiovascular events in patients taking colchicine 0.5 mg daily compared with placebo among patients with clinically stable ASCVD.[46] Recently a meta-analysis in patients with atherosclerotic CAD showed significantly lower MI, stroke, and unstable angina-driven revascularization with no significant difference for cardiovascular death, all-cause mortality, or GI events. In patients with CCS and atherosclerotic CAD, low-dose colchicine (0.5 mg daily) should be considered as a strategy to lower the risk of MI, stroke, and the need for revascularization and has a class 2a recommendation.[47] However, it has a narrow therapeutic index, which can lead to serious or toxic adverse effects and it is metabolized by cytochrome P450 3A4 and p-glycoprotein, making it prone to drug-drug interactions. Therefore, monitoring for adverse effects is of supreme importance.

Revascularization

This has always been a topic of debate as there is no strong evidence to support the effect of revascularization on all-cause mortality **(Fig. 8)**.

Three major RCTs including COURAGE (Clinical Outcomes Utilizing Revascularization and Aggressive Drug Evaluation), ISCHEMIA (International Study of Comparative Health Effectiveness with Medical and Invasive Approaches), and BARI-2D (Bypass Angioplasty Revascularization Investigation 2 Diabetes) showed no reduction in MACE with routine cardiovascular revascularization.[4,48,49] The COURAGE trial included patients with stabilized CCS class IV angina and at least a 70% stenosis in at least 1 coronary artery with evidence of ischemia, reported no difference in all-cause death or nonfatal MI between PCI and OMT over 15 years of follow-up.[4] In a secondary analysis of the COURAGE trial limited to 60% of patients with stress perfusion imaging and coronary angiography information available, there was no interaction between therapeutic strategy and either severity of ischemia or coronary anatomy.[50] The BARI-2D trial randomized patients with type 2 diabetes and CCD (at least 70% stenosis of a major coronary artery and angina or at least 50% stenosis of a major coronary artery with a positive stress test) to revascularization or GDMT and reported no difference in survival.[49] The ISCHEMIA trial included patients with stable ischemic heart disease with moderate-to-severe ischemia on noninvasive testing. Patients having >50% LM stenosis, LVEF <35%, NYHA III-IV heart failure, and refractory angina to drugs were excluded. Patients were randomized to routine invasive therapy (2,588) versus medial therapy (2,591). At 3.3 years, the primary outcome of cardiovascular death, MI, resuscitated cardiac arrest, or

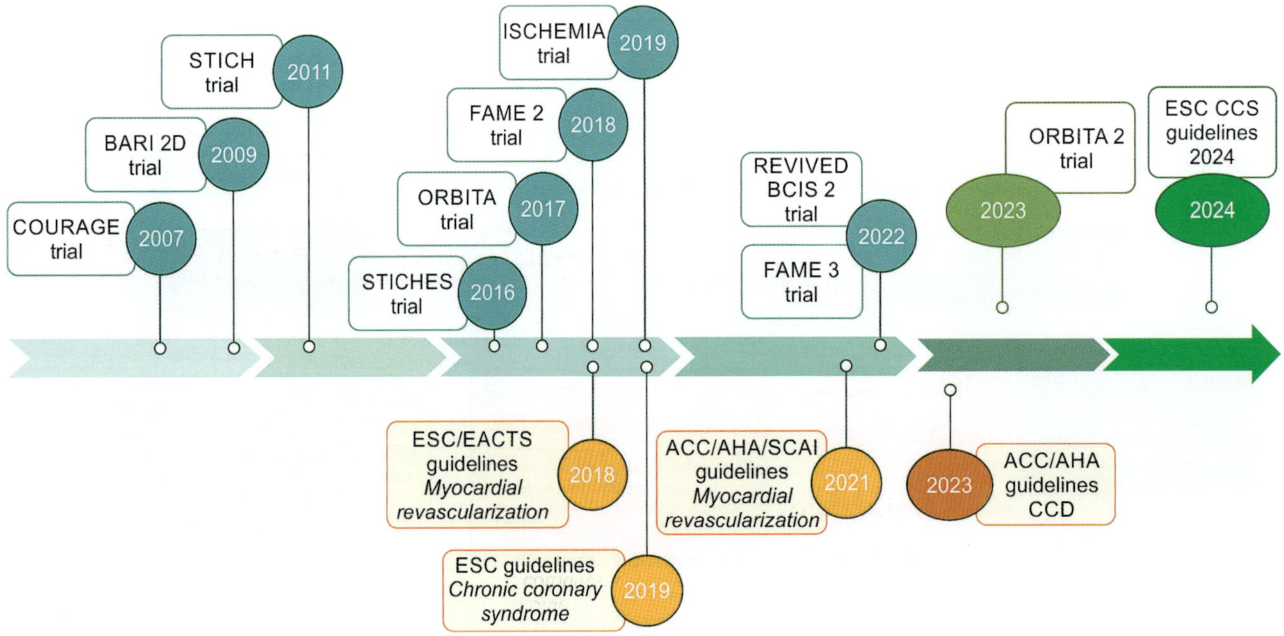

FIG. 8: Evidence of revascularization in CCS.

hospitalization for HF or unstable angina (USA) did not differ in two groups. However, there was a modest improvement in angina at 3 months, especially among those with daily/weekly angina, which persisted up to 36 months.[48] Also, at a longer follow-up of 7 years, a reduction in cardiovascular mortality with revascularization was observed. Moreover, in the ISCHEMIA trial, the incidence of procedural type 4a or type 5 MIs was increased with revascularization (20.1% of all MIs in the trial), but the incidence of late MI [spontaneous MI (type 1)], demand-induced MI (type 2), or MIs associated with stent thrombosis (type 4b) or with restenosis (4c) was reduced. A spontaneous MI was associated with a 2.4-fold increased hazard for all-cause death and a 3.4-fold increased hazard for cardiovascular mortality compared with no MI, whereas a procedural MI was not associated with all-cause or cardiovascular death.[51] A recent meta analysis confirmed a reduction in spontaneous MI with revascularization, but also noted an increase in procedural MI, with no improvement for MI overall with revascularization. However, revascularization reduced unstable angina (particularly among contemporary stent era trials) and unplanned revascularization in this and other meta-analyses.[52,53] The major limitations of these older trials were high cross-over rates, older generation stents, shorter follow-ups, and low angiographic complexities. Most recently, the ORBITA-2 (Sham-controlled Trial of Percutaneous Coronary Intervention for the Relief of Stable Angina) trial also found that PCI in CCS patients with stable angina (on little or no antianginal therapy) resulted in significantly less anginal symptoms when compared to placebo.[54] In the STICH trial, patients with ischemic cardiomyopathy and reduced ejection fraction of ≤35% showed improved survival at 10 years with CABG plus OMT in comparison to OMT alone.[55] In contrast, the REVIVED-BCIS2 trial found that PCI in CCS patients with ejection fraction ≤35%, did not yield improvement in survival when compared to OMT alone.[56] The STICH and REVIVED-BCIS2 trials differ in several key aspects. Patients in the REVIVED-BCIS2 trial were, on average, 10 years older than those in the STICH trial, had a lower incidence of prior MI (50% vs. 78%), and were more likely to be free of angina at baseline (67% vs. 36%). REVIVED-BCIS2 also included fewer patients with three-vessel disease (38% vs. 60%). Additionally, REVIVED-BCIS2 patients received more contemporary heart failure treatments and were more often treated with ICD or CRT devices (21%/53% vs. 2%/19%). The follow-up period in REVIVED-BCIS2 was also shorter than in STICH, which may have influenced the lack of survival benefit from PCI in the trial. Three large, RCTs have evaluated the clinical benefit of intracoronary imaging during complex PCI namely RENOVATE-COMPLEX PCI, OCTOBER, ILUMIEN IV.[57-59] FAME 2 trial showed improved MACE over 5 years when FFR guided revascularization (FFR ≤ 0.80) was done in intermediate stenosis **(Table 7)**.[60]

TABLE 7: Recommendations for revascularization.[2]

Recommendations for revascularization	COR	LOE
In CCS patients with LVEF >35%, myocardial revascularization is recommended, in addition to guideline-directed medical therapy for patients with functionally significant left main stem stenosis to improve survival	1	A
In CCS patients with LVEF >35%, myocardial revascularization is recommended, in addition to guideline-directed medical therapy, for patients with functionally significant three-vessel disease to improve long-term survival and to reduce long-term cardiovascular mortality and the risk of spontaneous myocardial infarction	1	A
In CCS patients with LVEF >35%, myocardial revascularization is recommended, in addition to guideline-directed medical therapy, for patients with functionally significant single-or two-vessel disease involving the proximal LAD, to reduce long-term cardiovascular mortality and the risk of spontaneous myocardial infarction	1	B
In surgically eligible CCS patients with multivessel CAD and LVEF ≤35%, myocardial revascularization with CABG is recommended over medical therapy alone to improve long-term survival	1	B
In selected CCS patients with functionally significant MVD and LVEF ≤35% who are at high surgical risk or not operable, PCI may be considered as an alternative to CABG	2b	B
In CCS patients with persistent angina or anginal equivalent, despite guideline-directed medical treatment, myocardial revascularization of functionally significant obstructive CAD is recommended to improve symptoms	1	A
Intracoronary imaging guidance by IVUS or OCT is recommended when performing PCI on anatomically complex lesions, in particular left main stem, true bifurcations, and long lesions	1	A
Intracoronary pressure measurement (FFR or iFR) or computation (QFR) is recommended to guide lesion selection for intervention in patients with multivessel disease	1	A

Angina/Ischemia with Nonobstructive Coronary Arteries

Although revascularization of epicardial stenosis provides symptomatic relief and better QoL, recent data shows that 20–30% of the patients present with recurrence of angina within 1 year and almost 40% of the patient within 3 years of successful PCI.[61]

Furthermore, repeat angiography in these patients often do not reveal any in-stent restenosis or residual obstruction, making it very important to consider nonobstructive causes of angina.[62] According to SCOT-Heart trail, four out of every five patients of suspected stable CAD had no significant epicardial stenosis.[63] Similarly, according to 2019 ESC guidelines, among patients with typical angina in the most common age range for detecting stable CAD (50–59 years), 68% of men and 87% of women did not have obstructive coronary stenosis[1] and the CorMicA (Coronary Microvascular Angina) trial revealed that approximately 45% of patients presenting with angina or ischemia did not have CAD at angiography.[64] In ischemia with nonobstructive coronary arteries (INOCA), the reasons for myocardial oxygen supply-demand mismatch could be coronary microvascular dysfunction (CMD), coronary vasospasm, or both. Microvascular angina is the clinical manifestation of CMD, and vasospastic angina is the clinical manifestation of myocardial ischemia caused by dynamic epicardial coronary obstruction due to a vasomotor disorder. In patients having angina without obstructive stenosis, subsequent testing should include stress perfusion imaging, PET, CMR, and/or invasive coronary angiography with functional testing using acetylcholine testing for spasm, coronary flow reserve, and microvascular resistance for CMD, to guide targeted pharmacologic treatment.[65] The evaluation and management of these different conditions are shown in **Flowchart 3** and **Table 8**.

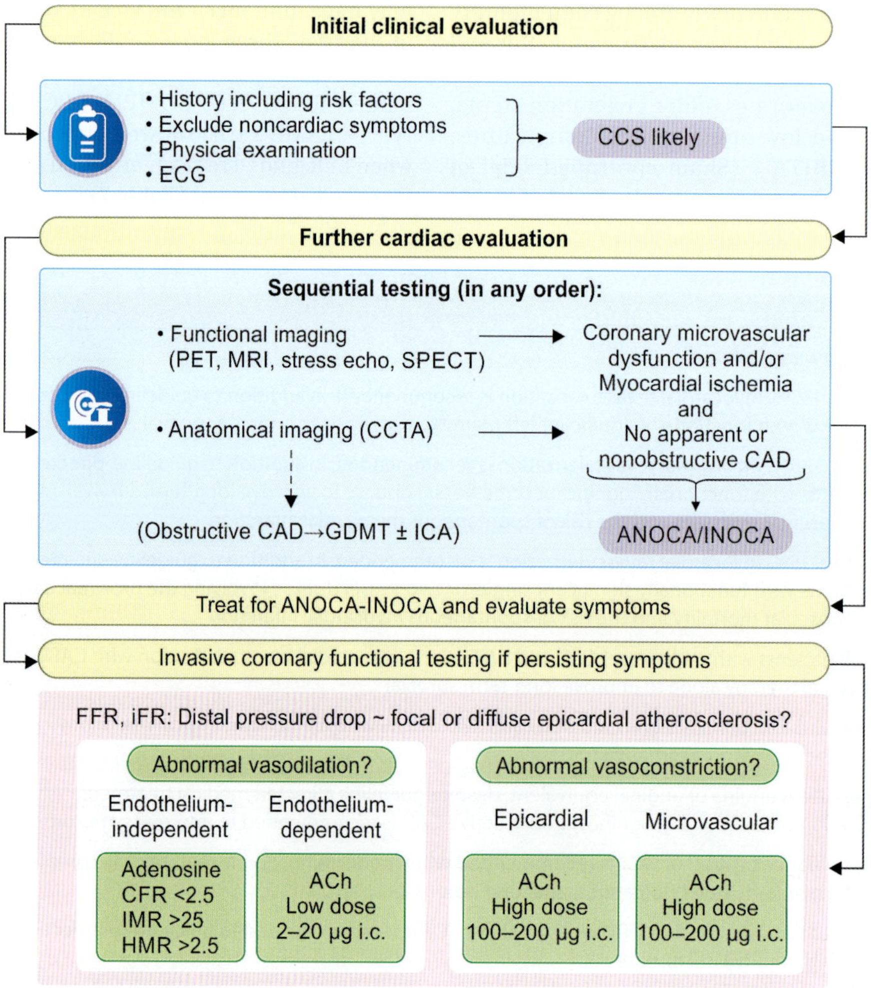

FLOWCHART 3: Evaluation of ANOCA/INOCA.[2]

TABLE 8: Management of ANOCA/INOCA.[3]

Endotype	Mechanism	Disorder of coronary artery function	Linked pharmacotherapy
Microvascular angina (nonobstructive CAD and proven CMD)	• ↑ Microvascular resistance • ↓ Coronary vasorelaxation • ↓ Microvasodilator capacity • Microvascular spasm	*IMR ≥25:* • IMR is a quantitative method for specifically assessing microvascular function-independent resting hemodynamics • IMR is distal coronary pressure* transmit time (average time for 3 saline bolus runs at hyperemia) *CFR by thermodilution < 2.0:* This reflects the inability to increase coronary flow above 2 times the resting flow *Resistive reserve ratio 2.0:* • This reflects the vasodilator capacity of the microcirculation to change from baseline to hyperemia (resistance at rest divided by resistance at hyperemia) • Angina during acetylcholine infusion or bolus with typical ischemic ST-segment changes and epicardial coronary constriction <90% reduction in epicardial coronary artery diameter represents inappropriate susceptibility microvascular constriction	*Baseline therapy:* • Consider aspirin, statin, and ACEi therapy in all patients. Sublingual nitroglycerin as needed • Smoking cessation and lifestyle changes *Antianginal Rx:* • *First line:* Beta-blocker (e.g., carvedilol 6.25 mg BID uptitrated) • *Second line:* CCB substituted [non DHP (e.g., verapamil 40 mg BID titrated)] where beta blockers are not tolerated or ineffective • *Third line:* Add in therapy: ○ CCB-DHP (e.g., amlodipine)-only for those on beta-blockers ○ Nicorandil* (5 mg BID, uptitrated) ○ Ranolazine (375 mg BID, uptitrated)
Vasospastic angina	Epicardial spasm	Epicardial coronary artery spasm is defined as reduction in coronary diameter >90% after intracoronary acetylcholine in comparison with baseline resting condition after intracoronary glyceryl trinitrate (nitroglycerin) administration in any epicardial coronary artery segment together with symptoms and ST-segment deviation on the ECG	*Baseline therapy:* • If atherosclerosis or endothelial impairment, aspirin and statin should be considered; Sublingual nitroglycerin as needed • Smoking cessation and lifestyle changes *Antianginal Rx:* • *First line:* CCB (e.g., verapamil 40 mg BID uptitrated) • *Second line:* Add long-acting nitrate (e.g., isosorbide monotitrate 10 mg BID) • *Third line:* Change nitrate to nicorandil (e.g., nicorandil 5 mg BID)
Mixed MVA/VSA	CMD and epicardial vasospasm	*Epicardial spasm plus any abnormality of:* • Microvascular resistance • Coronary vasorelaxation • Microvasodilator capacity	*Baseline therapy:* Consider aspirin, statin and ACEi therapy in all patients; sublingual nitroglycerin as needed

*Distal pressure multiplied by transit time.

CONCLUSION

Time has come for a paradigm shift in management of CCS patients. Once considered a disease of epicardial stenosis only, nowadays it is very important to consider CCS as an obstructive as well as a nonobstructive disease. Patients with INOCA should be thoroughly investigated using noninvasive or invasive functional testing for vasospastic disorders or CMD rather than labeling them as noncardiac pain. Lifestyle measures and GDMT continued to be underutilized, hence, procedural and pharmacologic interventions should not be considered as competing treatments but rather as complementary and additive therapeutic approaches, and the best-tailored approach for everyone should be followed to achieve optimal clinical outcomes and symptom relief **(Flowchart 4)**.

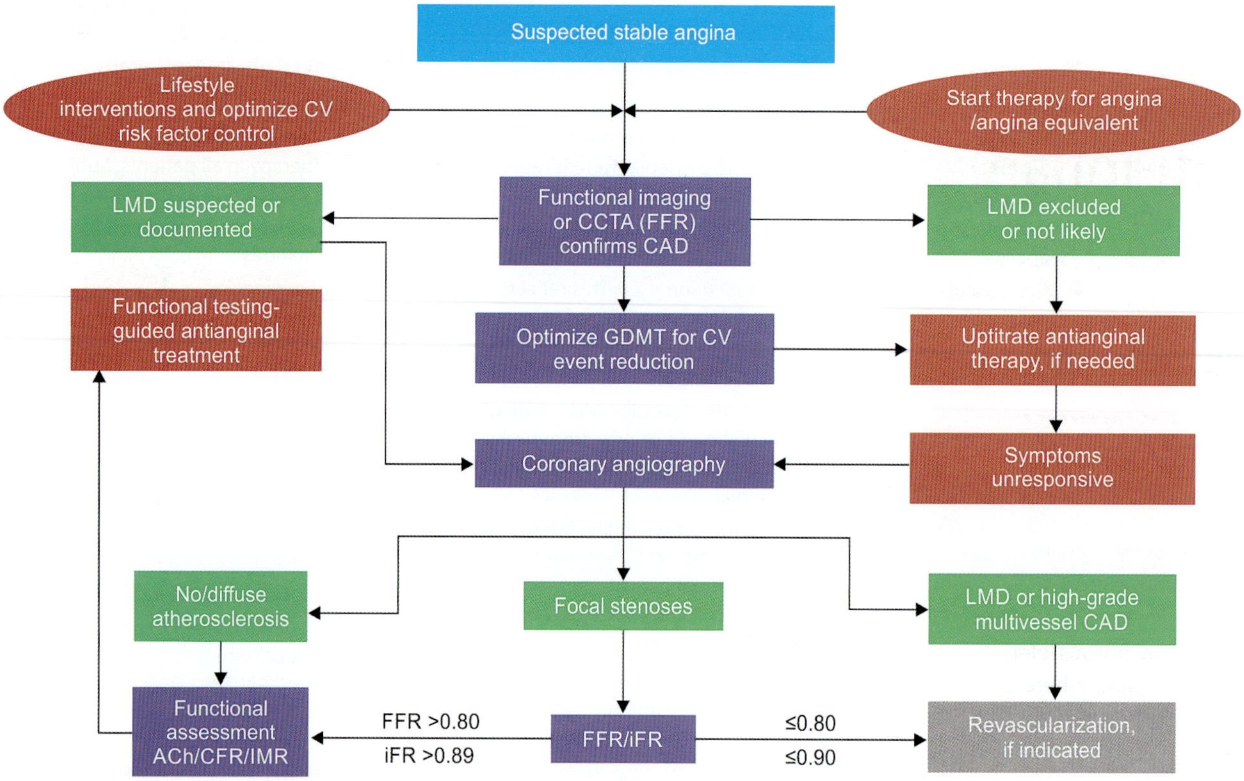

FLOWCHART 4: Management algorithm for suspected CCS patients.[66]

ONLINE REFERENCES

Please scan the QR code provided at the end of the table of contents for References of this chapter.

CHAPTER 114

Anti-inflammatory Drugs to Inhibit Atherosclerosis: Old and New

SS Mishra, BR Mishra, Asharam Panda

ABSTRACT

Atherosclerosis is an inflammatory disease of blood vessels that begins with the accumulation of lipids, inflammatory cells, and fibrous elements within the inner layers of arteries. This process that begins in utero is driven by chronic inflammation, where endothelial dysfunction plays a pivotal role. Looking at this pathophysiological mechanism, anti-inflammatory drugs appear a rational approach in its therapeutic strategy. After optimal medical therapy and control of traditional risk factors like diabetes, hypertension, and dyslipidemia, significant residual inflammatory risk for atherosclerosis persists. Commonly used agents include nonsteroidal anti-inflammatory drugs (NSAIDs), corticosteroids, and disease-modifying antirheumatic drugs (DMARDs) that have been used successfully to manage symptoms of inflammation in various conditions. However, their utility in atherosclerosis is limited due to potential adverse effects on the gastrointestinal tract and cardiovascular system, particularly in high-risk patients. Emerging biological therapies, such as monoclonal antibodies against cytokines or cell surface receptors, offer targeted approaches with reduced systemic side effects. Novel anti-inflammatory strategies involving colchicine, methotrexate, and monoclonal antibodies targeting inflammatory cytokines have emerged as a promising therapeutic option in the treatment of atherosclerosis. Molecules such as canakinumab, tocilizumab, and Janus kinase (JAK) inhibitors such as tofacitinib have shown promise to be used in atherosclerotic vascular disease.

Keywords: Inflammation, atherosclerosis, anti-inflammatory drugs, colchicine, monoclonal antibody

INTRODUCTION

Atherosclerosis is a chronic inflammatory disease characterized by the buildup of plaques within arterial walls and remains a leading cause of cardiovascular morbidity and mortality worldwide. This condition which begins in utero manifests few decades after leading to various atherosclerotic cardiovascular diseases (ASCVDs), including coronary artery disease (CAD), stroke, and peripheral artery disease (PAD), collectively accounting for a significant burden of morbidity and mortality worldwide.[1] While traditional therapies have focused on reducing cholesterol levels to prevent plaque formation which significantly improved mortality and morbidity, emerging research suggests that targeting inflammation within the arterial wall could offer additional benefit and hold promise to reduce the residual risk in managing atherosclerosis.[2] To address the issue, inflammatory markers have been identified and targeted for therapy.

ATHEROSCLEROSIS AND INFLAMMATION

Atherosclerosis begins with damage to the endothelial lining of arteries, which can be triggered by factors such as hypertension, dyslipidemia, smoking, diabetes mellitus, and environmental pollution. This damage allows low-density lipoprotein (LDL) cholesterol to infiltrate the arterial wall.[3] Once inside, LDL undergoes oxidation and is engulfed by macrophages, forming foam cells that initiate the formation of fatty streaks. Over time, these fatty streaks accumulate in smooth muscle cells, collagen, and other substances like cytokines and growth factors resulting in plaque formation that protrudes into the arterial lumen, restricting blood flow.[4]

The inflammatory cascade in atherosclerosis involves various cytokines, chemokines, and adhesion molecules that promote the recruitment and activation of immune cells.[5] Key inflammatory pathways include the NF-κB pathway, which regulates the expression of proinflammatory genes,

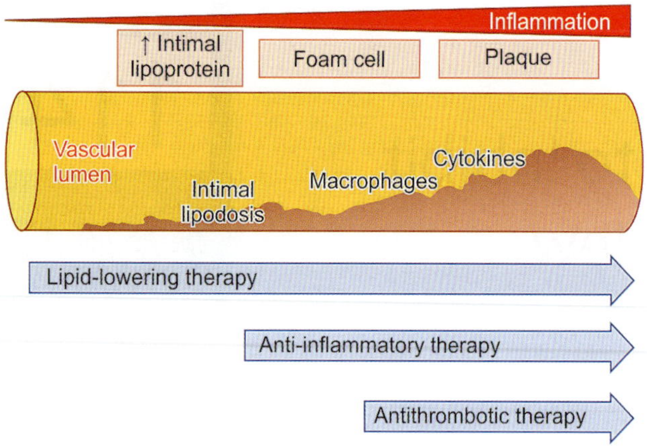

FIG. 1: Schematic presentation of role of inflammation in initiation and progression of atherosclerosis and role of therapeutic intervention.

and the inflammasome pathway, involved in the maturation of proinflammatory cytokines like interleukin-1β (IL-1β) **(Fig. 1)**.[6]

Cyclooxygenase (COX) enzymes, specifically COX-1 and COX-2, also play a distinct role in inflammation and cardiovascular health, influencing the progression of atherosclerosis. COX-1 is expressed in most tissues which are involved in maintaining normal physiological functions such as platelet aggregation, renal function, and gastric mucosal integrity.[7] In the context of atherosclerosis, COX-1-derived thromboxane A2 (TXA2) promotes platelet aggregation and vasoconstriction, contributing to the formation of thrombi and plaque. Inhibition of COX-1 by nonselective NSAIDs like aspirin reduces TXA2 synthesis, thereby preventing thrombosis and potentially stabilizing atherosclerotic plaques. COX-2 is induced by proinflammatory cytokines and growth factors; it is primarily associated with inflammation and pain response.[8] In atherosclerosis, COX-2 expression is upregulated within atherosclerotic lesions and endothelial cells under inflammatory conditions. COX-2-derived prostaglandins, particularly prostacyclin (PGI2), exert vasodilatory and antiplatelet effects, promoting vascular homeostasis.[9] Excessive COX-2 activity can lead to increased production of proinflammatory mediators and matrix metalloproteinases (MMPs), which contribute to plaque instability and rupture.[10]

TRADITIONAL ANTI-INFLAMMATORY THERAPIES

Anti-inflammatory therapy encompasses a diverse range of treatments aimed at reducing inflammation in various disease contexts. By targeting inflammatory pathways and mediators, these therapies mitigate tissue damage, alleviate symptoms, and improve overall patient outcome. Commonly used agents include nonsteroidal anti-inflammatory drugs (NSAIDs), corticosteroids, and disease-modifying antirheumatic drugs (DMARDs), each tailored to specific conditions such as arthritis, autoimmune diseases, and chronic inflammatory conditions. Historically, NSAIDs have been used to manage symptoms of inflammation in various conditions, including arthritis. However, their utility in atherosclerosis is limited due to potential adverse effects on the gastrointestinal tract and cardiovascular system, particularly in high-risk patients.[11]

COX-1 inhibitors such as aspirin irreversibly inhibit COX-1-mediated TXA2 synthesis in platelets, thereby reducing thrombotic events and potentially stabilizing atherosclerotic plaques. Low-dose aspirin is widely prescribed for secondary prevention of cardiovascular events in patients with atherosclerosis. In contrast, COX-2 inhibitors such as celecoxib were developed to minimize gastrointestinal side effects associated with nonselective NSAIDs. However, concerns arose regarding their cardiovascular safety due to COX-2's role in maintaining vascular homeostasis. Studies have suggested that COX-2 inhibitors may increase cardiovascular risk by disrupting the balance between vasodilatory prostaglandins and prothrombotic mediators. There is no benefit of COX-2 inhibitors in reducing the residual risk of ASCVD. Their use should be carefully weighed against potential cardiovascular risks, highlighting the need for personalized treatment strategies based on patient risk profiles and underlying inflammatory conditions.[12]

EMERGING THERAPEUTIC APPROACHES

Emerging biological therapies, such as monoclonal antibodies against cytokines or cell surface receptors, offer targeted approaches with reduced systemic side effects. The evolving landscape of anti-inflammatory therapy underscores its pivotal role in modern medicine, continually advancing to address the complexities of inflammatory diseases and enhance patient's quality of life. Novel anti-inflammatory strategies specifically targeting pathways are implicated in atherosclerosis.[13]

Colchicine

Colchicine, traditionally used for the treatment of gout and other inflammatory conditions, has garnered attention for its potential role in atherosclerosis management. Recent studies, including the landmark COLCOT (COLchicine Cardiovascular Outcomes Trial), have investigated colchicine's effects on cardiovascular outcomes in patients with recent myocardial infarction. In COLCOT, out of 4,745 patients, a total of 2,366 patients were given colchicine.[14] In a follow-up of average of 22.6 months, 5.5% treated with colchicine reached the primary endpoint compared with 7.1% treated with placebo with a hazard ratio of 0.77 and a confidence interval of 95%. Colchicine is believed to exert its anti-inflammatory effects by inhibiting microtubule polymerization and disrupting the function of inflammatory cells, particularly neutrophils and macrophages involved in plaque formation and destabilization.[14] By reducing inflammation within the arterial wall, colchicine may help stabilize atherosclerotic plaques, thereby potentially lowering the risk of cardiovascular events such as heart attacks and strokes. Ongoing research continues to explore colchicine's efficacy, safety profile, and optimal dosing strategies in the context of atherosclerosis, underscoring its potential as a promising adjunctive therapy in cardiovascular disease management.[15]

Methotrexate

Methotrexate, a well-known immunosuppressant and antirheumatic drug, has shown promise in the management of atherosclerosis due to its anti-inflammatory properties. Atherosclerosis is characterized by chronic inflammation of the arterial walls, leading to the development of plaques that can restrict blood flow and result in cardiovascular events.[16] Methotrexate works by inhibiting the enzyme dihydrofolate reductase, thereby reducing the proliferation of inflammatory cells and the production of proinflammatory cytokines. Clinical studies have suggested that methotrexate can reduce the levels of C-reactive protein (CRP), a marker of inflammation, and potentially slow the progression of atherosclerotic plaque formation. Although primarily used for conditions like rheumatoid arthritis and certain cancers, methotrexate's role in cardiovascular disease represents an exciting area of research, aiming to utilize this drug to improve outcomes for patients with atherosclerosis.[17]

BIOLOGICAL THERAPIES

Monoclonal antibodies targeting inflammatory cytokines have emerged as a promising therapeutic approach in the treatment of atherosclerosis. Atherosclerosis is driven by chronic inflammation within the arterial walls, where proinflammatory cytokines such as IL-1β, tumor necrosis factor-alpha (TNF-α), and interleukin-6 (IL-6) play pivotal roles in the progression of plaque formation and stabilization.[12] Monoclonal antibodies designed to neutralize these cytokines can significantly reduce inflammatory responses, thereby stabilizing plaques and preventing cardiovascular events. For instance, canakinumab, an IL-1β inhibitor, has demonstrated a reduction in cardiovascular events in clinical trials, highlighting the potential of this strategy.[6] By specifically targeting these key inflammatory mediators, monoclonal antibodies offer a targeted approach that can complement traditional lipid-lowering therapies, addressing both the lipid and the inflammatory components of atherosclerosis. This therapeutic innovation represents a significant advancement in the quest to reduce the burden of cardiovascular disease through precision medicine.[8]

Monoclonal antibodies targeting specific inflammatory cytokines, such as IL-1β (e.g., canakinumab) and IL-6 (e.g., tocilizumab), are under investigation for their potential to mitigate atherosclerosis progression.[9]

Canakinumab

Canakinumab, a monoclonal antibody targeting IL-1β, has shown significant potential in the treatment of atherosclerosis by addressing the underlying inflammation that contributes to the disease. IL-1β is a proinflammatory cytokine involved in the development and progression of atherosclerotic plaques.[10] By neutralizing IL-1β, canakinumab effectively reduces systemic inflammation, as evidenced by lowered levels of CRP, > 2 mg/L, a marker of inflammation. The CANTOS (Canakinumab Anti-inflammatory Thrombosis Outcomes Study) trial demonstrated that canakinumab significantly reduced the risk of recurrent cardiovascular events in patients with a history of myocardial infarction and elevated CRP levels, independent of lipid levels. The trial included more than 10,000 patients comparing 50, 150, and 300 mg canakinumab given subcutaneously 3 monthly with placebo for a primary endpoint of nonfatal myocardial infarction, nonfatal stroke, or cardiovascular death. A dose of 150 mg showed a statistically significant lower rate of primary endpoints compared to placebo.[18]

This finding underscores the crucial role of inflammation in atherosclerosis and highlights the potential of canakinumab to provide cardiovascular benefits beyond traditional lipid-lowering therapies. Canakinumab's success in clinical trials has paved the way for a new therapeutic approach targeting inflammation in the prevention and management of ASCVD.[19]

Tocilizumab

Tocilizumab, an anti-IL-6 receptor monoclonal antibody, has been investigated for its potential role in treating atherosclerosis by targeting the inflammatory processes central to the disease. IL-6 is a cytokine that promotes inflammation and is implicated in the development and progression of atherosclerotic plaques. By inhibiting the IL-6 receptor, tocilizumab can reduce the inflammatory cascade that exacerbates atherosclerosis. Clinical studies have shown that tocilizumab can decrease systemic inflammation, as evidenced by reduced levels of CRP and other inflammatory markers.[20] While primarily used in the treatment of rheumatoid arthritis and other inflammatory conditions, tocilizumab has shown promise in improving vascular function and reducing arterial stiffness, which are key factors in atherosclerosis progression. Ongoing research aims to further elucidate the cardiovascular benefits of tocilizumab, potentially offering a novel anti-inflammatory therapeutic strategy for reducing the burden of ASCVD.[21]

Janus Kinase Inhibitors

Drugs like tofacitinib, originally developed for rheumatoid arthritis, inhibit Janus kinase (JAK) pathways involved in inflammatory signaling and are being explored for their cardiovascular benefits.[22]

Tofacitinib, a JAK inhibitor, is being explored for its potential role in atherosclerosis due to its ability to modulate inflammatory pathways. JAK enzymes are critical in the signaling pathways of various proinflammatory cytokines, such as IL-6 and interferon-gamma (IFN-γ), which are involved in the pathogenesis of atherosclerosis. By inhibiting these enzymes, tofacitinib can reduce the activity of these cytokines, thereby dampening the inflammatory response that contributes to the formation and progression of atherosclerotic plaques. While tofacitinib is primarily used to treat autoimmune conditions like rheumatoid arthritis and psoriasis, its impact on vascular inflammation and immune cell activity makes it a promising candidate for atherosclerosis research. Preliminary studies suggest that tofacitinib can lower levels of inflammatory markers and improve endothelial function, potentially translating into reduced cardiovascular risk. Further clinical trials are needed to confirm its efficacy and safety in the context of cardiovascular disease, but tofacitinib represents a novel therapeutic avenue targeting inflammation in atherosclerosis.[23]

CHALLENGES AND FUTURE DIRECTIONS

While the concept of targeting inflammation to inhibit atherosclerosis is promising, several challenges remain. These include the need for further understanding of specific inflammatory pathways involved in plaque development, the identification of patients who would benefit most from anti-inflammatory therapy, and the management of potential side effects associated with long-term use of these medications. Future research and trial to establish the role of newer drugs in atherosclerosis management hold promise in reducing the burden of atherosclerosis in protecting blood vessels and different organs.[24]

CONCLUSION

Atherosclerosis remains a major health challenge globally, necessitating comprehensive strategies for prevention, early detection, and management. Advances in understanding its pathophysiology and the development of targeted therapies continue to shape clinical practice. Current research emphasizes the importance of inflammation in the genesis and sustenance of atherosclerosis and role of anti-inflammatory drugs helping in mitigating the burden of atherosclerosis and improving outcomes for affected individuals. Clinical markers of inflammation such as CRP and IL-6 are widely available that can be used as a screening modality.

The paradigm of using anti-inflammatory drugs to inhibit atherosclerosis represents a significant shift in the concept of cardiovascular medicine, from traditional NSAIDs to novel biological agents and targeted therapies. Ongoing research continues to explore how these treatments can complement existing strategies aimed at reducing cardiovascular risk. Ongoing research continues to explore our understanding of the inflammatory process and how these treatments can supplement the existing ones. By harnessing the power of inflammation modulation, healthcare providers may one day offer patients a new frontier in the prevention and management of atherosclerosis-related cardiovascular outcome.

ONLINE REFERENCES

Please scan the QR code provided at the end of the table of contents for References of this chapter.

CHAPTER

115

Latest Guidelines on Management of Chronic Coronary Disease (Syndromes)

Nagaraj Desai, Prabahakar Koregol, Akash Gopi, Sunil Kumar S

ABSTRACT

Chronic coronary disease (CCD) is a heterogeneous entity. Huge population, both symptomatic and asymptomatic, requires a patient-centric care enrolling him in clinical decision-making process, considering his social determinants of health. A comprehensive clinical evaluation of cardiovascular health, comorbid conditions, and risk factors to tailor the management of a patient is recommended. Pretest probability of CCD for a test may assist in economizing the care. Judicious and appropriate use of technologies to risk stratify, given the choices available, is recommended. The patients' preferences, costs, and technical expertise available may need to be accounted for. The clinical care has to be a team-based approach. The nonpharmacological therapies, for instance tobacco abstinence, require continuous vigilance for a better and reasonable success. Several pharmacological agents, sometimes in combination, are used for symptom relief, improvement of quality of life, and prognosis not only of cardiac issues but also of comorbidities and risk factors influencing the clinical outcomes. Guideline-directed medical therapies to optimize clinical status are recommended. In the drugs arena, new recommendations for the use of SGLT-2 inhibitors, GLP-1 agonists, conservative use of beta-blockers, including their discontinuation in some, have been made based on emerging evidence. Coronary revascularization, when offered, should consider the coronary anatomy, procedural risks, and short as well as long-term clinical outcomes. While it is welcomed, analysis of costs of care and value requires to be understood through the prism of demography of one's clinical practice. Prudence is suggested.

Keywords: Chronic coronary disease, chronic coronary syndromes, clinical practice guidelines

INTRODUCTION

Coronary artery disease (CAD) is a condition characterized by varying degrees (obstructive/nonobstructive) of luminal narrowing of the epicardial arteries initially starting as an atheromatous plaque. The growth of this plaque may be focal or diffuse and involve several segments of coronary tree. The timeframe over which the growth occurs is variable and dynamic. Importantly, the mechanisms of coronary luminal compromise may be several for instance, insidious growth of the plaques over years. It may cause symptoms, however, not always. Indeed, a large majority may remain asymptomatic, requiring several approaches to diagnose for instance, coronary imaging.

A term, chronic coronary syndromes (CCS), has been used in the 2019 European guidelines replacing the term stable angina.[1] Under this broad and overarching understanding, a patient may be symptomatic to a varying degree, or asymptomatic. On the other hand, a rapidly evolving thrombotic process at a focal site triggered by a plaque erosion or rupture with or without preexisting underlying lesion causing coronary luminal obstruction to a varying degree is called acute coronary syndromes (ACS). In a systematic review of clinical practice guidelines and consensus statements on chronic coronary syndrome, Jing et al. published in 2023, culling a total 10,699 citations according to Appraisal of Guidelines for research and Evaluation II instrument.[2] The authors evaluated 14 clinical practice guidelines and four consensus statements, each offering specific recommendations for CCS. The authors concluded that the published CCS guidelines varied in scope, quality, and recommendations; here is a need for a multidisciplinary approach to forge the broad-based, higher-quality evidence-based guidelines to enhance the efficacy and clinical outcomes for patients with CCS. In the same year, i.e., 2023, the multisociety ACC/AHA guidelines, using the term chronic coronary disease (CCD) to describe CCS, has published with some new features.[3] —Use of terms "disease" or "syndrome" to describe the entity, though strictly, not interchangeable, may be considered acceptable for a broader appreciation of the subject. In this brief chapter, for the consistency, the term CCD has been used.

What is new?

Besides the name itself, several new features find their place, for instance, costs versus value in care. The 2023 ACC/AHA guidelines makes nine specific recommendations on the use of several approaches including drugs (lipid management, SGLT-2 inhibitors, GLP-1 receptor agonists) and revascularization. The guidelines also have come up with newer recommendations on the use of beta-blockers. While considering the cost-benefit analysis, important caveat is being applicable to the specific geography—American. It may not be universally applicable, to be more specific, to Indian clinical practice, which may have its own several challenges. This underscores the importance of developing a country-specific clinical guidelines and continuous evaluation of its implementation and review as the landscape of clinical practice evolves with various therapies becoming more affordable.

POPULATION OF CHRONIC CORONARY DISEASE

Several clinical phenotypes may be considered and brought under the umbrella of CCD:[1,3]

- Patients with ACS post discharge after therapies and stabilized
- Patients with left ventricular dysfunction with known/suspected CAD
- Patients of stable angina medically managed with or without imaging test
- Patients with coronary vasospasm or microvascular angina
- Individuals with a positive screening test such as coronary CT angiography and considered as CAD

ICEBERG PHENOMENON AND CORONARY ARTERY DISEASE

There is a huge population, several times more than diagnosed CCD, which remains asymptomatic, undiscovered because it is untested and could be harboring CAD. This population, with or without risk factors, is counseled for the primary prevention of cardiovascular diseases.[4]

DIAGNOSIS

One of the most common clinical presentations of CCD is chest pain. At the initial presentation, a firm clinical diagnosis is the first step. In the evaluation, diagnosis and risk stratification are important components. The pretest probability of diagnosis of CAD should be considered in a given patient. This approach is clinically useful to prudently use resources. The ACC/AHA guidelines on approach to the chest pain, published in the year 2021, are useful in classifying the chest pain as typical angina, atypical angina, and noncardiac pain.[5] These guidelines discourages using the term atypical. It is important to appreciate that the anginal symptoms may be described by a patient variably and not necessarily limited to the chest. A detailed clinical evaluation including the physical limitations posed by anginal symptom for a given patient interfering with the quality of life, general health status, and comorbid conditions should be part of the evaluation.

LABORATORY EVALUATION

The guidelines recommend,[1,2] if there is an opportunity to do so, intensifying guideline-directed therapy (GDMT) and defer testing for ischemia.[3] In patients with CCD, change in symptoms or functional capacity that persists despite GDMT, imaging modalities such as PET/SPECT MRI, CMR imaging or stress ECHO are recommended. Using noninvasive tests to assess the severity of ischemia, estimate the future risks of adverse prognosis, has limitations because of several practical reasons though they are considered class I. Being capital-intensive, not widely available, expensive, and suboptimum availability of trained personnel, use of several noninvasive imaging techniques need to be judiciously considered. However, an exercise treadmill test is considered useful (and, also more widely available), but not without limitations. In those with frequent angina or severe stress-induced ischemia, invasive coronary angiogram (ICA) or noninvasive coronary computed tomography angiography (CCTA) could be considered. When revascularization is considered, assessment of functional significance of a coronary lesion at the time of angiography is recommended unless it is >90% diameter stenosis. The noninvasive evaluation of functional significance of a coronary lesion is now available and intuitively useful, but with no recommendation.

SALIENT FEATURES OF MANAGEMENT: GUIDELINES ON CCD

Team-based Care

The American guidelines recommend a "team-based" approach, involving professionals not only clinicians, a physician, including a subspecialist (or a superspecialist as we call them in India) and a nurse to optimize the care but also to include, for instance, experts in rehabilitation, diet, and, pharmacy, psychology, and social workers. Also, importantly, to enroll the patient in to his care—shared decision-making and, supporting the patient by providing education on continuous basis. The guidelines have discussed this topic extensively. It also advocates considering several aspects including socioeconomic determinants and several other related issues of health while planning risk assessment, testing, and treatment impacting the clinical decisions.

It should be that appreciated that an Indian physician delivers care, in many instances, in a restrictive "solo" practice setting. And, he wears multiple hats taking up several roles. Time being at a premium, given the patient load per physician this could play a dampener necessitating relooking in to the solutions for an effective, efficient , and economical care in his practice geography. An overarching approach to deliver committed care of cardiovascular diseases along with its several "mates" such as hypertension, diabetes may be a way forward in resource-restricted practice landscapes. Nevertheless, it's desirable to deliver a comprehensive care for a better clinical care experience for a patient.

With the burgeoning population suffering from CAD, especially CCD that requires to be managed and the complexities of care including the costs involved, a guideline/ or a consensus statement for the Indian care provider is not only desirable, but cannot be overemphasized.

Nonpharmacological Methods

The guidelines recommend healthy dietary habits and exercise for all diagnosed with CCD.[3,6]

Studies across diverse populations support the health benefits of a higher intake of whole grains and fiber, with lower intake of saturated fat, sodium, refined carbohydrates, and sweetened beverages. Healthy dietary choices combined with caloric reduction will support weight loss goals and improve cardiometabolic health for overweight and obese patients. In contrast, nonprescription nutrition or dietary supplements have insufficient evidence to support their use to reduce the risk of acute CVD events.[4,5]

The guidelines recommend patients to be physically active achieved through various forms of activities specifically reducing sitting time and engage in aerobic and resistance exercises. A structured cardiac rehabilitation program is recommended for the eligible patients with high risk to optimize the clinical outcomes. Those who require supervision to sail them through smoothly in to a chronic phase may have stable angina, recent myocardial infarction, or heart failure, etc.[3-5]

Tobacco use should be assessed and advised against the same. It should be reinforced at every visit. Behavioral or even pharmacological approach is recommended for those who are identified to benefit. Use of nicotine E-cigarettes, though may be successful for smoking cessation when compared to nicotine replacement therapy, their long-term effects may lead to dependence. At present, in the absence of long-term safety data, sustained use of the E-cigarettes are not recommended as the first-line therapy.[3]

Several substances including alcohol, cocaine, amphetamines, opioids, marijuana can adversely affect the cardiovascular system. In fact, the recent studies suggest that no safe level of alcohol use is acceptable and that previously observed cardioprotective effects of light-to-moderate alcohol use are likely confounded by other lifestyle and sociodemographic factors.[7]

Mental health has a major role in overall cardiovascular health and well-being in patients with CCD. But, despite being a modifiable prognostic risk factor for CCD outcomes, the screening, evaluation and management of the same is not addressed sufficiently. Nearly one out of five or even more may have concomitant mental health conditions necessitating care.

Importantly, potentially underpinning the bidirectional relationship between mental health and CCD is the resulting influence on health behaviors such as adherence to the care not only of several components of CCD but also of risk factors such as hypertension, diabetes, and dyslipidemias. A patient of CCD may benefit from several approaches such as psychotherapy and drugs. Studies have suggested that this approach has resulted reduction in recurrent cardiovascular events and mortality rate in patients with CCD.[8]

Pharmacotherapy: A Bird's Eye View

The aims of pharmacological management of CCD patients are to reduce angina, exercise-induced ischemia, improve quality of life, and to prevent cardiovascular events.

In the pharmacotherapies arena, the 2023 ACC/AHA guidelines have revisited the previous recommendation on use of certain class of drugs. For instance, class of drugs used in the management of diabetes mellitus such as SGLT-2 inhibitors, GLP-1 analogs in certain categories of patients even without diabetes.

It also recommends discontinuation of beta-blockers unless the patient had a myocardial infarction in the last 1 year, or has left ventricular dysfunction or another primary indication for its use.

Management of Angina

The therapies for angina work through two mechanisms—either by reducing myocardial oxygen demand or by improving myocardial blood supply.[9] While drugs such as beta-blockers, nondihydropyridine CCBs and ivabradine reduce myocardial oxygen demand, nitrates, dihydropyridine CCBs increase blood supply. Ranolazine and trimetazidine work at the cellular levels. The latter find no mention in the American guidelines while the European mentions it.[1,3]

The results of a network meta-analysis of 46 studies and 71 treatment comparisons supported the initial combination of a beta-blocker and a CCB.[10] The same meta-analysis suggested that several second-line add-on anti-ischemic drugs (long-acting nitrates, ranolazine, trimetazidine, and to a lesser extent, ivabradine) may prove beneficial in combination with a beta-blocker or a CCB as first-line therapy while no data were available for nicorandil.

The overriding goal is to maximize relief of symptoms while choosing therapy that will not exacerbate comorbidities, will not have important interactions with concomitant medications, and will be well tolerated. Control of symptoms may be achieved by most patients, but full freedom from angina is only achieved in 40–50%, depending on anginal frequency at the onset of treatment.[11]

Management of Risk Factors

The optimum control of risk factors such as high blood pressure, diabetes, and others is an integral part of the wholesome management of CCD.

Management of Lipids

Lipid goals, especially of LDL cholesterol, has witnessed continuous downward trend, buoyed by the several recent trials demonstrating efficacy and safety.[1,3]

For the control of lipids, the statins remain the drugs of first choice. Such patients require high-intensity dose of statins (restricted to atorvastatin and rosuvastatin). Those who are intolerant at least moderate-intensity doses are recommended. The list of nonstatin group of drugs is growing that includes ezetimibe, PCSK9 (proprotein convertase subtilisin/kexin type) inhibitors, inclisiran, and bempodoic acid. These nonstatin drugs are typically used in certain groups of patients like those who require more intense control of lipids (in combination), or considered in patients who are diagnosed statin intolerant. Importantly, some of them are very useful in genetically inherited dyslipidemias. The downside of these new medications in clinical practice is the cost involved over long term. The landscape of their use in a larger number of patients is likely to change with time. Also, for drugs such as inclisiran, the long-term cardiovascular outcome data is still awaited, although a recent patient level meta-analysis showed a favorable trend.[12]

Management of Blood Pressure

All guidelines on hypertension emphasize good control of hypertension to improve the prognosis, though the ESC and ACC/AHA may differ in some ways. More than one drug, and in combination, may be necessary to control. An ultimate goal of 130/80 mm Hg, without any new clinical issues, is recommended by all guidelines. The ISH guidelines take a pragmatic route for the global audience. [13-15]

Management of Diabetes

The management of diabetes has been witnessing a tectonic shift with the newer drugs such as GLP-1 agonists and SGLT-2 inhibitors being recommended in appropriate patients as an initial strategy as in patients with high cardiovascular risks, CKD, and heart failure. With wider availability of many of these drugs, their routine is likely to improve exponentially in the coming years.

However, all guidelines underscore individualizing the goals while providing clinical care and protecting a patient from potential risks of complications from medications.[16,17]

Use of Antiplatelets

Recently, the use of dual antiplatelet therapies after an episode of acute coronary syndrome, especially after a percutaneous intervention, has been evaluated, especially for a shorter duration for their efficacy and safety. And, the guidelines recommend considering the same in individuals in whom the risk of bleeding outweigh the ischemic risk. The use of validated risk scores to address bleeding risk can be useful in choice and duration of antiplatelet therapy. The more frequently used risk calculators are PRECISE DAPT (Predicting Bleeding Complications in Patients Undergoing Stent Implantation and Subsequent Dual Antiplatelet Therapy), DAPT, and PARIS (Patterns of Non-Adherence to Antiplatelet Regimen in Stented Patients) risk scores. Some patients may require additional DOACS. At present, it is concluded that the concurrent use of DOACS in the presence of atherosclerotic disease with or without AF is modest.[1,3,18]

Management of Comorbid Conditions

Patients of CCD who have comorbid conditions (e.g., CKD) are at a significantly elevated risk of developing symptomatic HF and recurrent cardiovascular events. Appropriate management of these conditions includes control of diabetes and blood pressure to the goals to decrease MACE in high-risk patients. Use of RAAS inhibitors is recommended. SGLT-2 inhibitors have also been shown to provide renal protection. It should be noted that the patients on RAAS inhibitors therapy require close follow-up after medication initiation and titration, including assessment of adherence, blood pressure control, laboratory testing, and evaluation for potential adverse effects. ARBs should be used as an alternative for patients who are ACE intolerant. Drugs such as ARNI are recommended in preference to other RAAS agents.

Sodium-glucose cotransporter-2 inhibitors are recommended in the presence of HF with or without diabetes and in both reduced as well as preserved rejection fraction. Also, beta-blockers and mineralocorticoid receptor antagonists (MRA) are recommended in optimum doses forming four pillars of therapy for the patients of heart failure with reduced ejection fraction.[1,3,19]

Inflammation and Coronary Artery Disease

Inflammation is a key component in the development of atherosclerosis.[3,20] The residual cardiovascular risks, despite the therapies, may be because of underlying chronic inflammation. Using select anti-inflammatory agents may have a role in improving cardiovascular outcomes. However, studies evaluating agents, thus, so far have shown mixed results. This calls for a conservative approach in the routine use of drugs such as colchicine.[1,3]

Revascularization in Chronic Coronary Disease

Coronary revascularization and its methods, as a strategy to improve clinical status of a patient with CCD beyond medical therapy, has been a matter of some "not so friendly" debate. A systematic review and a meta-analysis by Panuccio et al., and Laukkanen et al., respectively, concluded that the benefits of revascularization accrue on a longer-term follow-up and personalized approach based up on the clinical characteristics and lesion complexities may be more beneficial.[21,22] However, in the recent times, it has become a subject of clinical controversy. It's reflected in the recent American guidelines.[3] It finally resulted in cardiac surgeons not only withdrawing from the writing committee, but also not endorsing the same. Further, their society issued a critic, commenting that "it is misguiding," and has maintained that CABG should be recommended to improve survival as previously recommended. The 2021 American guidelines downgraded class of indication from 1 to IIB for CABG in three-vessel disease with normal LVEF. This was based on fact that after 70s and 80s BIG CABG trials, there has been no evidence to suggest CABG improved survival and proved in ISCHEMIA trial as well. The 2023 guidelines on chronic coronary disease gave class I recommendation for CABG to improve survival in patients with left main stenosis or three-vessel disease with severe LV dysfunction (LVEF < 35%). And in others, it gave class IIA indication for CABG, not to improve survival but to lower risk of cardiovascular events such as spontaneous MI, unplanned urgent revascularization, and cardiac death.

Chronic Coronary Disease with Angina with No Options of Revascularization

Refractory angina represents a small but important segment of the CCD population.[3] Patients are identified by three major features: (1) Uncontrolled angina (or equivalent symptoms) despite intensive medical therapy, (2) objective evidence ischemia, and (3) no option for coronary revascularization.[22] Typically, symptoms produce major lifestyle limitations, functional status limitations, and disabilities. Presently, there are no class I recommendation for its management. Enhanced external counterpulsation, which is FDA approved, has a weak support of a single randomized trial and used less often.[23] The direct transmyocardial laser revascularization has been studied in several RCTs and is FDA approved. However, presently, no recommendation is made after a thorough review.[24]

Chelating Agents

The use of chelation therapy such as intravenous infusions of disodium EDTA though prevalent since several decades, the data to support its use is not strong, and it is not FDA approved in the management of CCD. The results of TACT2 also did not show any role of routine chelation therapy, irrespective of diabetic status after a myocardial infarction.[25]

Vaccinations to Prevent Infections

Preventing infections such as influenza, pneumococcal using vaccinations has been shown to be useful in reducing cardiovascular events and costs.[26] Biological underpinnings of increase in events may be many and include proinflammatory mediators, sympathetic nervous stimulation, and coagulation cascade activation resulting alteration in a vulnerable plaque.[27] Promoting vaccination against such infections may be the best defense.

Management of Other Components

The emerging evidence suggests a manmade technology is proving to be a menacing in the form of microparticles arising out of widespread use of plastics. Data is provocative. Societal level intervention may reduce vascular diseases in general and also coronary disease.[28]

Ambient air pollution is being increasingly implicated in the development of atherosclerosis. Its control to mitigate the vascular diseases in general require societal and governmental interventions for the benefit of cohort of CCD.[29,30]

Follow-up Care

It should focus on the issues such as cardiac symptoms, quality of life, compliance to the care including use of medications, control of risk factors, and management of coexisting comorbidities. However, routine periodic anatomic or ischemic testing without a change in clinical or functional status is not recommended for risk stratification or to guide therapeutic decision-making in patients with CCD.[1,2] For comparison, sometimes, it may be occasionally useful to obtain a basic 12-lead ECG on a periodic basis.

CONCLUSION

The population of CAD is very huge, a majority comprising patients with various clinical phenotypes of CCD. Care of patients with CCD requires a multifaceted comprehensive, team-based approach. Integrating several strategies including pharmacological and nonpharmacological approaches on continuous basis are recommended to optimize clinical outcomes. Firm diagnosis and therapies to mitigate angina to improve quality of life should be considered. Newer approaches on the use of medications such as beta-blockers, considering shorter duration of dual antiplatelets therapies, optimizing statins, and novel therapies such as SGLT-2 inhibitors, GLP-1 agonists have been recommended. The nonpharmacological approaches including lifestyle modifications, optimum control of cardiovascular risk factors, and management of comorbid conditions should be addressed. Coronary revascularization, both percutaneous and surgical approaches, is useful in an appropriate case. The availability of technology, technical expertise and skills, affordable medications, costs and value, social determinants of health of a patient and his enrolment in to his care to enhance the compliance are some important drivers of the change and its widespread adaptation in the communities. The landscape of the management of CCD may be expected to evolve even further with refinements in our understanding of the disease and therapeutics.

ONLINE REFERENCES

Please scan the QR code provided at the end of the table of contents for References of this chapter.

CHAPTER 116

Management of Coronary Ectasia and Coronary Aneurysms: Current Concepts

P Chandrasekhar, G Ravi Kiran

ABSTRACT

Coronary artery aneurysms (CAA) or ectasias (CAE) are dilatations of arterial segments that commonly affect the right coronary artery. Microvascular dysfunction causes angina even in the absence of obstructive CAD. Genetics, inflammation, local wall injury, and hemodynamic factors are associated with CAE/CAA development. Stasis and endothelial dysfunction contribute to the development of local thrombus and atherosclerosis. Management is less evidence-based with intense control of cardiovascular risk factors, statins, ACE inhibitors when appropriate, and the avoidance of nitrates being considered in all. PCI in coronary vessels with CAE/CAA is usually associated with suboptimal results and higher target vessel/lesion revascularization. Aspirin is recommended for all patients with CAE and addition of warfarin should be individualized based on clinical and angiographic factors. For CAA, surgery is the main therapy except for small CAA, which can be treated percutaneously.

Keywords: Coronary artery, ectasia, aneurysms, coronary artery disease

INTRODUCTION

Bougon first described the abnormal dilation of coronary arteries in 1812. Since then, many studies have brought forth a deeper understanding of this entity. Two different phenotypes are suggested: Coronary artery aneurysm (CAA) and coronary artery ectasia (CAE) with arbitrary criteria being used to differentiate them; a focal dilation of coronary segments of at least 1.5 times the adjacent normal segment is described as CAA, whereas the CAE is defined as a dilation that is diffuse (exceeds one-third the length of the coronary vessel).[1]

Data from pooled analysis suggest a mean prevalence of ectasia/aneurysm being 3% (mean age 55 years)/1.65% (mean age 62 years). Isolated CAE is very rare with an angiographic frequency of 0.1–0.3%.[2,3] A large Indian study suggests a prevalence of 4%.[4] Common epidemiological features noted across many studies among patients with CAE/CAA include: (1) Majority are male and are seen dominantly in the right coronary artery with left main coronary artery being least commonly involved. Proximal parts of the coronary arteries are most commonly affected. (2) The etiology is atherosclerosis in around 50% of CAE/CAA patients. The incidence has been shown to be lower in Asia than in North America and Europe.

MORPHOLOGY AND ETIOLOGY

Topographically (Markis et al.) CAE is divided into four types: Diffuse ectasia of 2 or 3 vessels is classified as type I, diffuse ectasia in one vessel and focal dilatation in another vessel as type II, diffuse ectasia of one vessel only and focal aneurysm as types III and IV, respectively. Pseudoaneurysms are dilatations of the vessel, with single or double layers of the vessel wall, because of disruption of the media and external elastic membrane. In contrast, a true arterial aneurysm is three layered and may be saccular (when the longitudinal diameter is less than the transverse diameter) or fusiform. When a CAA is very large in size, it is defined as a giant CAA (GCAA); however, there is no clear consensus on the cutoff that must be used to define GCAA: Diameters >20, >40, or >50 mm, or quadruple the reference vessel diameter, have all been proposed as cutoffs by different authors. In the case of Kawasaki disease (KD), it was proposed to define CAA as giant if its diameter is >8 cm **(Figs. 1 and 2)**.

The etiology of CAE/CAA is atherosclerosis in 50% of cases and approximately 30% of CAE/CAA cases are associated with vasculitis, including KD, Takayasu arteritis, and connective tissue diseases such as Ehlers–Danlos and Marfan's syndrome. The remainder are congenital, idiopathic, infectious, or iatrogenic. In particular, congenital CAE/CAA has been documented with other cardiovascular abnormalities, including bicuspid aortic valve, aortic aneurysms, pulmonary stenosis, and ventricular septal defects.[5-8]

Three CAA subsets need special attention:

1. *Aortocoronary saphenous vein graft aneurysms (SVGAs):*[10,11] They commonly present very late following bypass surgery (more than two-thirds presents >10 years after CABG) as large aneurysms that usually progress over time and thus presenting with mechanical complications or rupture occasionally. Intimal calcification is the most common risk factor, followed by infection for development of SVGA after CABG.

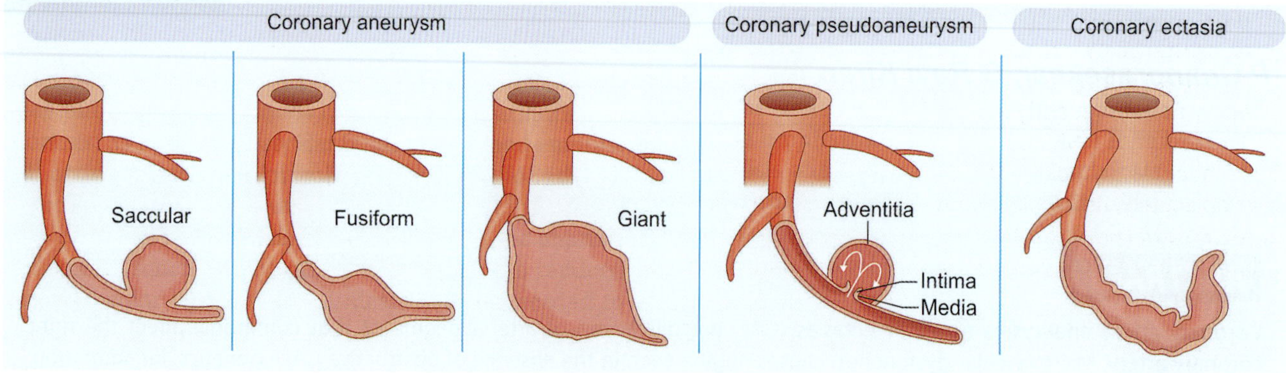

FIG. 1: Morphology of coronary artery ectasia (CAE) and coronary artery aneurysm (CAA).[9]

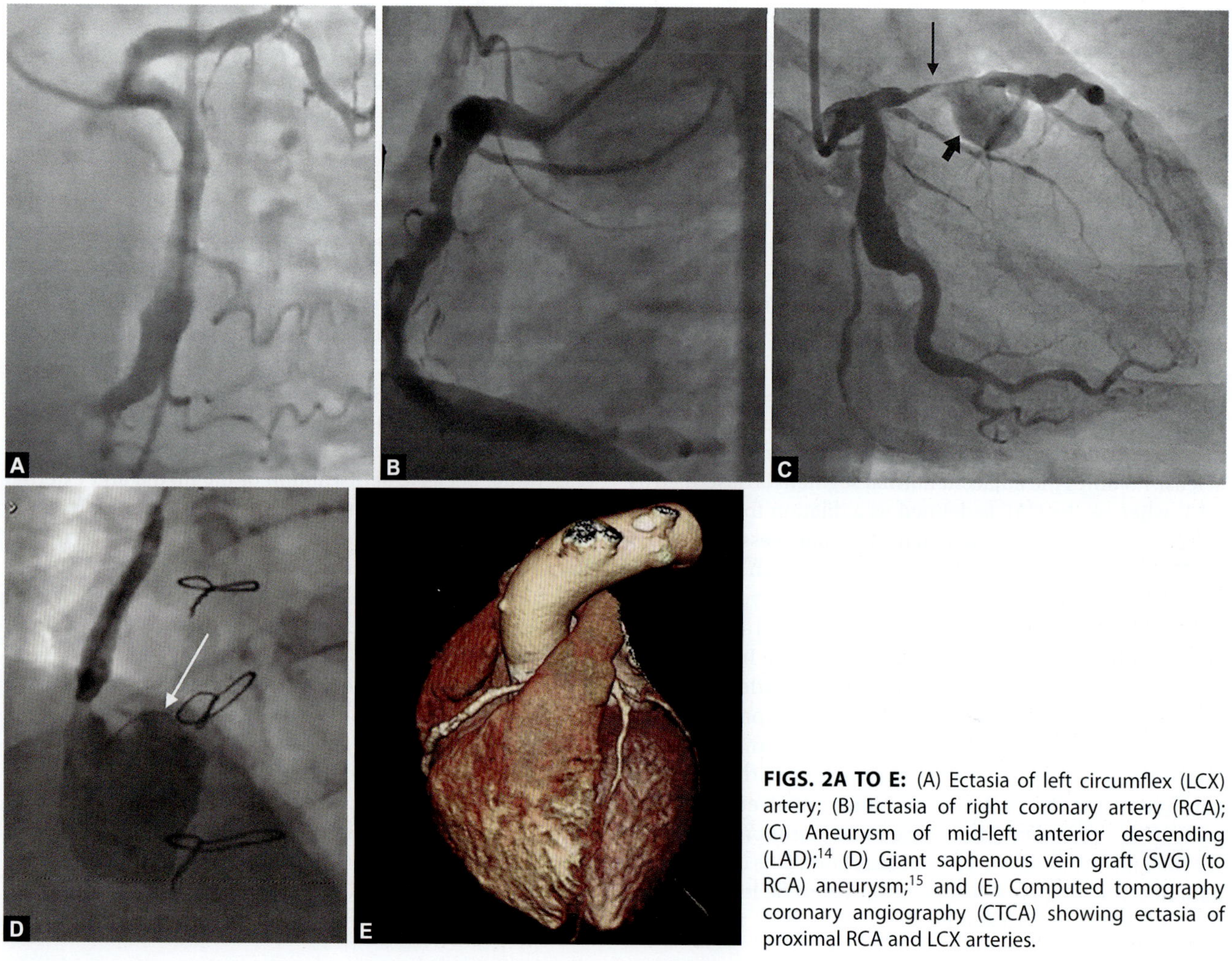

FIGS. 2A TO E: (A) Ectasia of left circumflex (LCX) artery; (B) Ectasia of right coronary artery (RCA); (C) Aneurysm of mid-left anterior descending (LAD);[14] (D) Giant saphenous vein graft (SVG) (to RCA) aneurysm;[15] and (E) Computed tomography coronary angiography (CTCA) showing ectasia of proximal RCA and LCX arteries.

2. *Mycotic aneurysms:*[12] They disproportionately involve young (*mean age:* 55 years) males (85%) and the responsible organism was either *Staphylococcus aureus* or *Streptococcus* in 75% of cases. They are often large with frequent presence of thick walls and thrombus (90%). Associated abnormal appearance of pericardium with either pericardial fluid, thickening, or loculation is common (80%).
3. *Iatrogenic CAA [Drug-eluting stent induced coronary aneurysm (DESCA)]:*[13] They have a pooled incidence of around 0.6% (in clinical trials) to 2% (in clinical registries) during the 6–9 months follow-up period and occur more frequently in type B2/C and CTO lesions.

The DES type (SES or PES or EES) did not show any significance. As per Aoki et al. DESCA is of three types: *Type I:* Develop acutely, usually <1 month, and is due to the arterial injury; *Type II:* Develop subacutely, usually within a year and is due to the arterial response to DES, namely inflammatory and nonproliferative effect; *Type III:* Infectious mycotic DESCA. One-third of patients present with ACS, and as per registry data, the development of CAA is not statistically associated with increased MACE.

CLINICAL PRESENTATION AND NATURAL HISTORY

Majority of CAAs/CAE are clinically silent and are only detected incidentally. However, clinical symptoms can develop due to the presence of concomitant obstructive CAD (resulting in angina) or formation of local thrombosis (causing ACS) or rarely due to rupture/mechanical compression of adjacent structures. Interestingly, myocardial ischemia (thus causing angina) due to microvascular dysfunction can be seen even in the absence of significant coronary stenosis. There are no significant changes in ectatic extent or coronary blood flow in either follow-up group of 1–5 years and 5–16 years, but there is a significant progression of coronary atherosclerotic changes during this period (thus the two diseases also have different progression rates, and CAE might present before CAD and is more likely to be an underlying risk factor for CAD progression). In contrast, studies have shown that at least 15–20% of aneurysms progress over a period of 5–7 years of follow-up, and the degree of baseline CAD severity is associated with the progression of CAA size.[16,17]

CAE/CAA has been associated with a 3–5-fold increase in the risk of major cardiac events, including cardiac death and myocardial infarction (MI) at 3–4 year follow-up. The reported incidence of CAE/CAA-associated events, such as thrombosis, distal embolization, rupture, and vasospasm, varies from 0.2 to 5%.[18] In a meta-analysis, CAE patients with STEMI had higher rates of PCI failure and no-reflow (in part due to high thrombus burden); however, MACE, mortality, reinfarction, target vessel revascularization during follow-up were comparable.[19] However, higher grades of CAE (Markis types I and II), multivessel CAE, and diffuse CAE were associated with reduced long-term survival and higher MACE compared to patients without CAE in many observational studies.[20,21]

PATHOGENESIS

A literature review[3,22-25] suggests the following factors contribute to CAE/CAA development:

- *Individual genetic susceptibility:* Genetic factors such as angiotensin-converting enzyme (ACE) DD genotype polymorphism, abnormal lipoprotein metabolism associated with familial hypercholesterolemia, potassium voltage-gated channel subfamily H member 1 (*KCNH1*) mutation, and autophagy related 16 like 1 (*ATG16L1*) gene mutations have all been linked to the development of CAE/CAA.
- *Inflammation:* The majority of newer studies imply that inflammation is an integral link in CAE/CAA pathogenesis and also inflammation may be more pronounced in patients suffering from CAE/CAA than CAD. Inflammatory mediators cause an exaggerated activity of metalloproteinases (MMP) and proteolysis of the extracellular matrix (ECM) weakens the vessel architecture and thus predisposing to the progressive dilatation of the artery. Elevated homocysteine levels, hyperinsulinemia, *Chlamydia pneumoniae* infection, smoking, and cocaine use may induce MMP activity in the arterial wall thus predisposing to vessel dilatation.
- *Hemodynamic factors:* Bench studies have shown that CAE can be caused by the pressure irregularities that are seen in arteries associated with significant coronary stenosis. It has also been proposed that high blood flow velocity causes endothelial damage and poststenotic vasodilation because of higher shear stress at the stenosis level.
- *Others:* Local wall injury following intracoronary manipulation (angioplasty, stenting, and brachytherapy) has been shown to provoke the formation of CAA. Due to their frequent association with CAD, CAE/CAA are generally believed to represent an exaggerated form of expansive vascular remodeling in response to atherosclerotic plaque growth. Loss of ECM integrity due to certain vasculitic and connective tissue diseases also predisposes to CAA/CAE development due to the abnormal architecture of the elastic lamina and media. Rarely, postinfectious CAAs have been seen and are due to the result of direct wall invasion or immune complex deposition. The abnormal vessel dilatation of CAE/CAA is associated with turbulent coronary flow, resulting in endothelial dysfunction, which in turn leads to the development of thrombosis and atherosclerotic plaques. In fact, in an OCT study, plaques occurred in nearly all CAE segments, of which >50% had high-risk features.
- *Risk factors:* Male sex, obesity, high triglyceride, and LDL/HDL ratio are all risk factors for CAE. Diabetes mellitus shows an inverse correlation with CAE and the effect of hypertension (HTN) on CAE is complex. When the vessel

was in normal condition, HTN was not very effective in increasing the chance of CAE and only increased the CAE chance by 3%, but when the vessel is ectatic, HTN is associated with the progression of CAE.

MANAGEMENT

General Principles

To date, there is no consensus regarding the optimal therapeutic strategy for CAE/CAA. All of the available studies have limitations such as nonrandomization, the absence of a control group, or a small number of patients (i.e., only case series). So, the management of CAA/CAE is individualized and depends mainly on the clinical presentation (incidentally discovered or symptomatic), characteristics of CAA/CAE (location, size/length, and etiology) and finally the patient profile (risk factors and comorbidities).

Coronary angiography is the invasive gold standard tool to assess the anatomic features of CAA/CAE, while coronary CT is the alternative noninvasive technique of choice for the follow-up. Intracoronary imaging (IVUS mainly) is extremely helpful; it helps to distinguish between true- and pseudo-aneurysm, accurately size the CAA, and/or any adjacent stenoses, and allow proper stent sizing if PCI is planned.

First, Intense control of cardiovascular risk factors is suggested in all patients with CAA/CAE regardless of the presence of concomitant obstructive CAD. Given the role of atherosclerosis and inflammation in their pathogenesis, statins (inhibits MMP) and ACE-inhibitors have been proposed as possible therapeutic options due to their pleiotropic effects on the endothelium. Hence, statins should be given to all patients, and among the patients with CAE/CAA and HTN, ACE inhibitors should be the first choice. Although, clinical data supporting this is scarce.

In addition, few studies have concluded that trimetazidine and ranolazine reduce the exercise-induced myocardial ischemia in patients with CAA/CAE. Nitrates should be avoided in patients with CAE/CAA because of their promotion of flow disturbances and exacerbation of myocardial ischemia.[26-28] The role of β-blockers and calcium channel blockers need to be properly defined as the data is limiting and conflicting.

Outcome data on PCIs in patients with CAA/CAE is limited (particularly if asymptomatic). In general,[29] PCI of an aneurysmal/ectatic culprit vessel in the setting of acute MI is associated with lower procedural success, higher incidence of no-reflow and distal embolization with higher rates of definite stent thrombosis, target vessel revascularization, and MI during follow-up, but the impact on overall mortality is controversial.

Management of Coronary Artery Ectasia

Meta-analytic data suggested that the patients with CAE had a significantly higher mean platelet volume than healthy individuals, indicating that platelet thrombotic effects may play a role in the genesis of CAE[30] suggesting a beneficial role of antiplatelet therapy. In fact, the prevalence of MI in patients with CAE who received aspirin was significantly lower than in patients with CAE who did not received antiplatelet treatment.[31] Hence, aspirin is routinely suggested. Limited evidence based on observational data[32] and a systematic review of data[33,34] suggests that antiplatelets (SAPT/DAPT) applied in combination with warfarin provided more efficient protection against major adverse cardiac events in CAE patients, and triple therapy with DOACs may be inferior to warfarin-based therapy.

Based on available evidence, it may be suggested that:

- *CAE with no ACS:* In patients with nonobstructive CAD and CAE, aspirin should be used and CAE patients with significant CAD might be better treated with DAPT (aspirin-clopidogrel). The additional benefit of anticoagulation for every patient with CAE is doubtful. Warfarin can be added to SAPT/DAPT for high-grade or diffuse CAE (warfarin should be in the target therapeutic range of 2.0–2.5 for at least >60% of the time) or when there is sluggish flow (TIMI I/II flow), particularly if bleeding risk is low. In a retrospective study, DAPT and SAPT + warfarin were associated with similar efficacy in the prevention of the ACS.[35]
- *CAE with ACS:* Due to the higher associated thrombus burden, PCI in CAE is frequently aided by thrombectomy, glycoprotein IIb/IIIa inhibitors and the use of intracoronary imaging is recommended. As coronary events are mainly arterial thrombotic event, DAPT is mandatory with aspirin and ticagrelor being suggested as better therapy with the addition of warfarin in patients with recurrent events even on DAPT.[36] However, upfront triple therapy with aspirin, clopidogrel, and warfarin can also be considered, though there is no comparative data. After the PCI with the latest generation DES, DAPT (aspirin + clopidogrel) with warfarin for at least 6 months may be suggested. In a typical patient, 1 year after PCI, SAPT + warfarin may be a balanced choice.

Management of Coronary Artery Aneurysms

Among patients with KD the use of IVIG along with glucocorticoids is associated with a reduced incidence of CAA.[37] Aspirin is indicated in Kawasaki patients with documented coronary aneurysms, and the addition of prophylactic anticoagulation is suggested in KD patients with giant aneurysms.[38,39] Dedicated studies are necessary to definitively establish which is the best medical therapy (anti-platelet, anticoagulant, or combined therapy) and when and how CAA should be considered for endovascular or surgical interventions. Despite the risk of thrombus formation and distal embolization described earlier, few retrospective studies conclude that the anticoagulation strategy is unbeneficial by showing a similar rate of thrombotic events in patients with and without CAA.[29] But one large piece of data from CAAR registry has shown that oral anticoagulant therapy (OAT) decreases the composite endpoint of UA, MI, and aneurysm thrombosis in patients with CAA, despite a nonsignificant higher risk of bleeding.[40]

Though the CAAR study found no major differences when comparing CABG versus PCI, suggesting the efficacy and safety of PCI in patients with CAAs, surgery remains the first line of therapy or even the only option in these patients. The indications in general[9] are: (1) Concomitant severe CAD or valve disease; (2) CAAs near the bifurcation of large branches or in the left main, (3) If they are multiple or giant (>20 mm or >4-fold dilation) or when they are infected; (4) Have mechanical complications such as fistula formation, compression of adjacent cardiac, or vascular structures; (5) Aortocoronary SVGAs (if >10 mm).

Surgical treatments include reconstruction, aneurysm resection or exclusion, ligation with concomitant CABG, patching, or hybrid repair. In view of the fact that the standard therapeutic surgical strategies for CCAs are not well established because of the scarcity of high-quality evidence, the tailored strategy for each patient should be employed. However, data suggests that the most common procedure is to bypass CAA and exclusion does not appear to offer any advantage over isolated revascularization (except in selected cases).[41] PCI is a relatively new therapeutic option that is considered when the clinical and/or anatomical risk is high.[29,40] To reduce the risks of stent thrombosis and stent displacement, proper sizing of the CAAs, IVUS guidance, micromesh stents, self-apposing stents, and additional short-term anticoagulation should be taken into account.

- Small-sized (<10 mm in diameter) CAA or pseudo-aneurysms can be treated with covered stent exclusion (if CAA is not involving a major side branch) or by balloon or stent-assisted coil embolization (if CAA involve a major side branch).
- In patients with large or rapidly expanding SVGAs or in those causing symptomatic external compression, percutaneous closure with Amplatzer occluders or coil embolization with or without PCI of the native grafted vessel is a feasible alternative to surgery.

CONCLUSION

- *Core point 1:* CAE/CAA are seen in 3–4/1–2% of angiographic studies, mainly in the proximal RCA. CAE may be high or low grades. CAA may be saccular or fusiform. Genetics, inflammation (activation of MMP), local wall injury (iatrogenic, infective, and immune complex mediated), and hemodynamic factors are associated with CAE/CAA development. With time, CAE usually does not progress, whereas CAA may be progressive and is associated with baseline CAD severity. Local thrombosis, shunt formation, and rupture may be seen thus contributing to higher MACE seen with CAE/CAA.
- *Core point 2:* CTCA is useful for follow-up, and intravascular imaging during PCI is advantageous. Intense control of risk factors, statins, ACEi and the avoidance of nitrates should be considered in all with a possible role for trimetazidine and ranolazine in chronic angina patients. Warfarin remains the anticoagulant of choice. PCI in coronary vessels with CAE/CAA is usually associated with higher target vessel/lesion revascularization.
- *Core point 3:* Aspirin is recommended for all CAE patients and clopidogrel is added in the presence of obstructive CAD. The addition of warfarin (*INR:* 2–2.5) to SAPT/DAPT should be individualized. All KD Patients with multivessel CAA, CAA *z*-score ≥10 or giant CAA should receive additional warfarin. For CAA, surgery is the therapy of choice, except for small CAA, which can be treated percutaneously or with aspirin (warfarin added if small CAAs are multiple or when patients deny any intervention).

ACKNOWLEDGMENTS

Authors would like to thank Dr Johann Christopher, MD, DrNB sir, Care hospital, Hyderabad for providing the CTCA image.

ONLINE REFERENCES

Please scan the QR code provided at the end of the table of contents for References of this chapter.

CHAPTER

117

Cardiac Syndrome X

Hetan C Shah, Tamagna Ghosh

ABSTRACT

Cardiac syndrome X (CSX), or angina with no flow-limiting stenosis on coronary angiogram, has been accepted as a condition with an excellent prognosis despite variable symptomatic improvement. Recent data show that patients with CSX with endothelial dysfunction have an increased risk for future adverse cardiovascular events. Current hypotheses of CSX pathophysiology emphasize a vascular endothelium dysfunction with reduced nitric oxide bioavailability leads to microvascular ischemia. Diagnosing microvascular ischemia involves multimodality testing using clinical history, electrocardiogram, stress testing, and imaging modalities like computed tomography (CT), CMR, and positron emission tomography (PET) scan and invasive modalities like Doppler wire measurement of coronary flow reserve and vasoreactivity testing. Treatments that target improving endothelial function such as statins, angiotensin-converting enzyme inhibitors, estrogen, and lifestyle modification are current standard in management for CSX. The goal of this chapter is to provide information for diagnosis, risk stratification, and therapy for the population with CSX. This group of patients benefits from treatment and timely diagnosis and is not as benign as previously considered.

Keywords: Cardiac syndrome X, coronary artery disease, major adverse cardiovascular events, coronary microvascular dysfunction, myocardial blood flow reserve, positron emission tomography, single-photon emission computed tomography, index of myocardial resistance, coronary flow reserve

INTRODUCTION

Syndrome X term was first used by Kemp in 1973[1] to define patients with angina like chest pain with normal or near-normal epicardial coronaries in angiography. This entity is now better known as "cardiac syndrome X" (CSX) and needs to be differentiated from "metabolic syndrome X." The latter is characterized by obesity, hypertension, dyslipidemia, and insulin resistance.

Cardiac syndrome X has multiple etiologies,[2] and its pathophysiology is based on (1) endothelial dysfunction, (2) microvascular spasm, and (3) abnormal pain sensitivity.[3] Patients in this group have impaired coronary flow reserve (CFR) and raised intramyocardial resistance due to abnormal endothelium-induced vasoreactivity. Microvascular dysfunction is caused by proinflammatory cytokines released from diseased endothelium. Autonomic imbalance is present in this group of patients leading to decreased pain threshold and hypersensitivity to changes in heart rate and contractility.[4] Coronary angiography is usually normal but may reveal atheromatous plaques on intravascular imaging.[5] Major risk factors and notable associations have been found in women who have impaired CFR. Others are age, hypertension, smoking history, elevated heart rate, and low HDL.

Studies have thrown light on the prognosis of patients with CSX, which is usually better than of those with obstructive coronary artery disease (CAD).[2] Recent studies have shown adverse cardiovascular outcomes in patients with CSX.[6] CSX has largely been replaced by coronary microvascular angina nowadays.

DEFINITION

Kanar and Sunbul have proposed the following definition of CSX:[7]

- Typical stable angina, exclusively or predominantly induced by effort
- Findings on workup compatible with myocardial ischemia/coronary microvascular dysfunction (CMVD)

- Angiography findings of normal or near-normal coronary arteries
- No other specific cardiac disease is present (e.g., variant angina, cardiomyopathy, and valvular disease).

RISK FACTORS

Cardiac syndrome X is likely more common in patients with the following:

- Hypertension
- Hypercholesterolemia
- Smoking
- Glucose intolerance
- Diabetes
- Female sex
- Estrogen deficiency

PATHOPHYSIOLOGY (FIG. 1)

The mechanism involved in pathology of CSX includes the following:

- Endothelial dysfunction
- Myocardial ischemia
- Insulin resistance
- Dysautonomia
- Increased cardiac sensitivity
- Estrogen deficiency

The *principal mechanism* is endothelial dysfunction, leading to microvascular ischemia.[8] The endothelium lines the vascular lumen and regulates blood flow mainly by regulating levels of nitric oxide. Dysfunctional endothelium leads to vasoconstriction with decrease in release of anti-inflammatory and antithrombogenic factors and reduced availability of nitric oxide.[9] There is a decreased level of nitric oxide and increased vasoconstrictor agent like endothelin-1 levels in these patients.[10] Cardiac MRI has demonstrated decrease in subendocardial blood flow with adenosine infusion.[8] Endothelial dysfunction cannot be demonstrated by invasive angiography alone and needs both invasive and noninvasive measures like nuclear imaging and CMR to demonstrate lack of normal vasodilatory reserve and increased intramyocardial resistance **(Fig. 2)**.[11,12]

EPIDEMIOLOGY

Approximately 20–30% of patients undergoing coronary angiography for evaluation of angina-like chest pain have nonobstructive CAD.[13] CSX is more common in women than in men.[14]

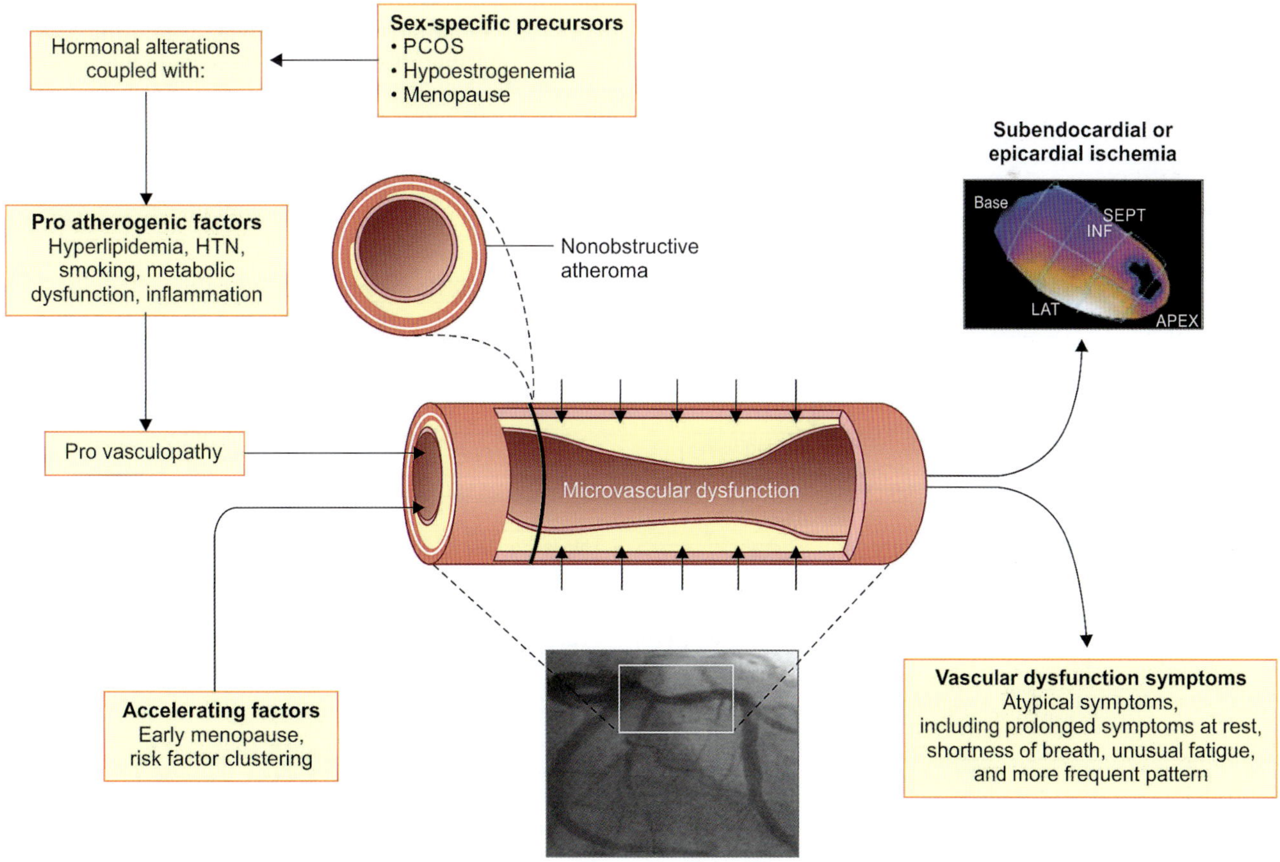

FIG. 1: Etiopathogenesis of cardiac syndrome X.

Source: Adapted from Arthur HM, Campbell P, Harvey PJ, et al. Women, cardiac syndrome X, and microvascular heart disease. Can J Cardiol. 2012;28 (2 Suppl):S42-9.

Cardiac syndrome X frequently occurs more in perimenopausal and postmenopausal women, which has a link with estrogen deficiency being a contributory reason.[15]

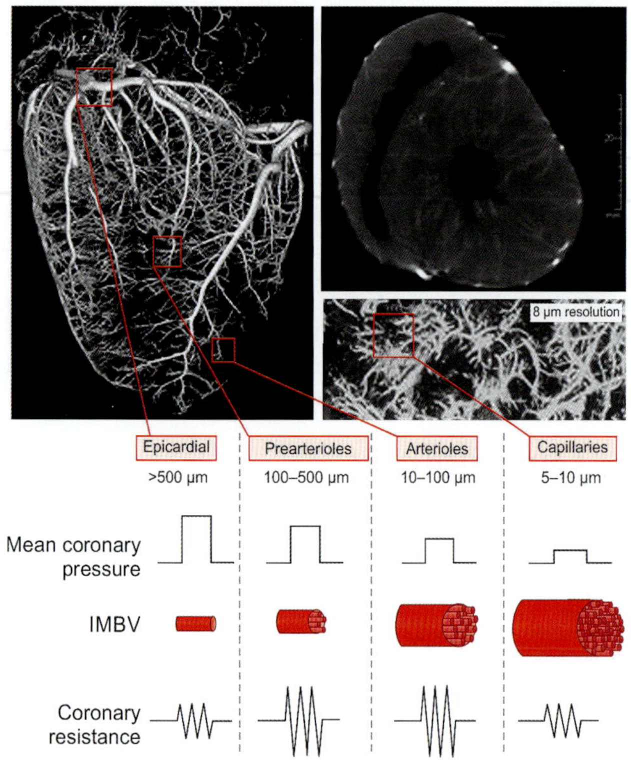

FIG. 2: Resistance vessels in myocardium are primarily the prearterioles and arterioles (10–500 μm).

EVALUATION

Cardiac syndrome X symptoms may range from typical or atypical chest pain to dyspnea often associated with exertion. These patients do not respond with conventional therapy like nitrates.[16]

There is proof of ischemia with ST-segment depression, abnormal stress imaging studies, and raised cardiac biomarker levels. Clinically, patients may or may not have changes on ECG or other noninvasive tests during chest pain episodes.

Diagnosis depends primarily on demonstrating endothelial dysfunction using nuclear imaging like single-photon emission computed tomography (SPECT) or cardiac MRI using dipyridamole or adenosine infusion.[8] The *gold standard* is to measure CFR using Doppler guidewire invasively in catheterization laboratory. Normal CFR is 2.5–3 times of baseline. CFR value of <2 signifies poor reserve due to endothelial dysfunction. Noninvasive measures of endothelial dysfunction like brachial artery reactivity[17] and peripheral artery tonometry[18] have been on par with invasive tests **(Flowchart 1)**.

Echocardiography

The first imaging modality for any patient with chest pain is a transthoracic echocardiography, which is essential to look for wall motion abnormalities, valvular abnormalities, or any other contributory cause for chest pain. In this modality, coronary blood flow (CBF) velocity is found to be enhanced during stress with opacification of the myocardium through microbubbles during myocardial contrast echocardiography.

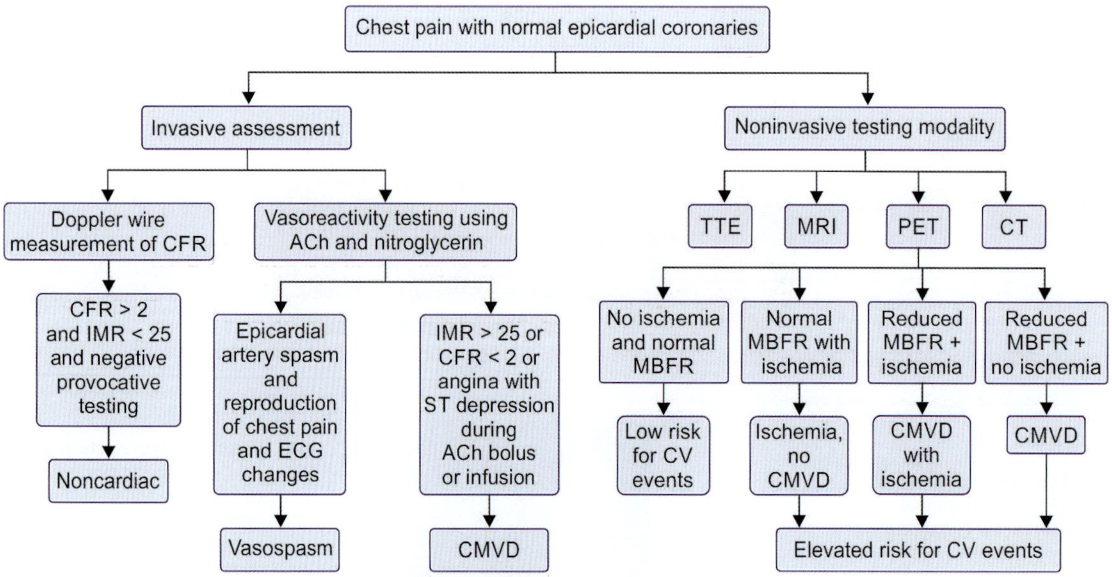

FLOWCHART 1: Diagnostic algorithm for chest pain with normal coronaries.
(IMR: index of myocardial resistance)

Vogel et al. also demonstrated the usefulness of echocardiography in determining myocardial blood flow. It has now been replaced by nuclear imaging and cardiac MRI due to better sensitivity in these tests.

Cardiac Magnetic Resonance Imaging

Cardiac MRI with gadolinium contrast helps in studying myocardial blood flow at rest and stress. Myocardial perfusion reserve index was compared with coronary reactivity testing. Thomson et al. evaluated 118 patients from the Women's Ischemia Syndrome Evaluation (WISE)-Coronary Vascular Dysfunction (CVD) study with 1.5-T CMRI using first-pass gadolinium perfusion imaging and adenosine. Results obtained from the study demonstrated that a threshold myocardial perfusion reserve index of 1.84 was predictive of CMVD with a sensitivity of 73% and specificity of 74% **(Figs. 3A and B)**.

Positron Emission Tomography

Positron emission tomography (PET) has been an important modality in assessing CFR. Through dynamic PET, myocardial blood flood, which helps to determine CFR, can be evaluated at rest and with stress. CBF has been shown to be a useful tool in evaluating CMVD even in patients with normal PET.

Using PET, we can calculate index of intramyocardial resistance, which gives a quantitative index for endothelial dysfunction.

Computed Tomography

With the use of computed tomography (CT) in assessing CMVD, one of the main reported advantages is the ability to assess anatomy and functionality in one study. Risk factors include radiation and renal affection due to contrast. Other concerns include poor estimation of myocardial blood flow. Grover et al., in their study of 30 patients with microvascular angina, demonstrated a lower mean total coronary lumen volume and mean myocardial mass compared to patients who were without angina.

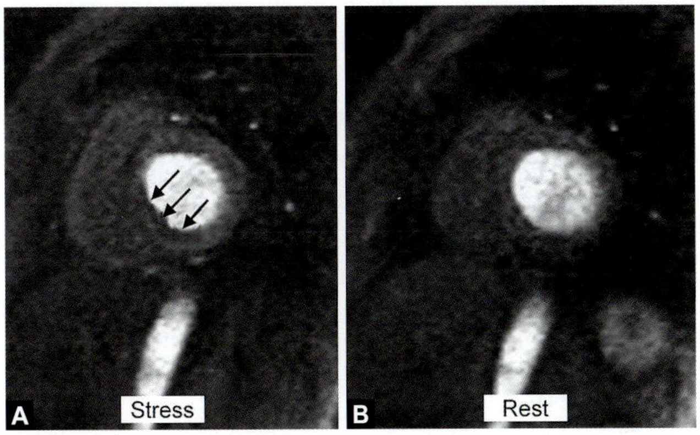

FIGS. 3A AND B: CMR showing stress-induced ischemia in CSX patient.

Vasoreactivity Testing

Coronary vasomotor tone regulation in patients with microvascular dysfunction involves several pathways. A >50% increase in CBF above baseline in response to acetylcholine and a CFR ratio of >2.5 in response to adenosine can be considered normal.[19] A decreased response to acetylcholine with a normal response to adenosine indicates endothelium-dependent disease. No response to nitroglycerin suggests nonendothelium-dependent dysfunction of epicardial arteries **(Table 1 and Fig. 4)**.

MANAGEMENT

Cardiac syndrome X is a diagnosis of exclusion in patients presenting with chest pain. Traditional treatment with agents like beta blockers and nitrates is not very effective in CSX. Studies undertaken have shown that less than half of these patients respond to nitrates.[19] Beta blockers and calcium channel blockers have been used in a small number of these patients. Verapamil and nifedipine have been shown to decrease anginal episodes and number of sublingual nitroglycerin tablets required.[20] Pain modulation by targeting nociceptor pathway using imipramine is a Class IIb recommendation by American College of Cardiology guidelines for treatment of CSX who do not respond to risk factor reduction, beta blockers, CCB, or nitrates.[21]

NEWER THERAPIES

Pharmacological Agents

- *Statin* therapy has been shown to be beneficial for primary prevention of CAD with dyslipidemia and also for secondary prevention in established CAD patients. Statins are known to decrease inflammation and C-reactive protein levels, and improve endothelial function.[22] In a large retrospective study by Wen-Hao Luo et al. based in China, statins decreased major adverse cardiovascular events (MACE) in microvascular dysfunction patients with a history of smoking and hypertension with or

TABLE 1: Coronary reactivity testing for microvascular dysfunction.

	Adenosine	Acetylcholine	Nitroglycerin
Microvascular	Nonendothelium dependent	Endothelium dependent	X
Epicardial	X	Endothelial dependent	Nonendothelium dependent

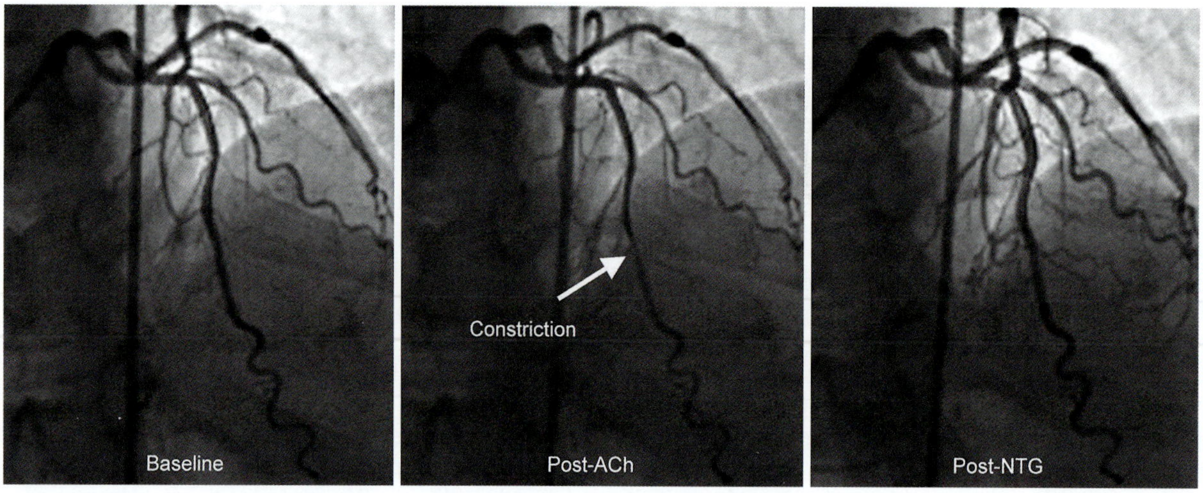

FIG. 4: Coronary blood flow in response to acetylcholine and nitroglycerin infusion.

without diabetes.[23] A small study of 40 patients with CSX showed improvement in endothelial function, exercise duration, and time to 1-mm ST depression on treadmill test in patients treated with pravastatin irrespective of cholesterol levels.[24] Simvastatin has shown to improve brachial artery reactivity time and time to ST depression on exercise testing in CSX patients.[25]

- *Angiotensin-converting enzyme inhibitors* are useful in preventing adverse events in patients at a high risk of obstructive CAD. This involves improvement in endothelial function. Chen et al. showed that CFR and exercise duration improved in CSX population after 8 weeks of enalapril therapy.[26] Pizzi et al. demonstrated a decrease in oxidative stress and improvement in endothelial function and quality of life in patients with CSX after using ramipril with atorvastatin.[27]
- Newer agents like *transdermal estrogen therapy* were shown to decrease frequency of angina episodes by approximately 50%, possibly by modifying endothelium-dependent vasodilatation and/or pain perception.[28]
- *L-Arginine* was shown to improve angina in some small studies. It also improved quality of life and blood pressure in the hypertensive group with microvascular angina.[29] Long-chain omega-3 fatty acids have been studied and observations show that they reverse stress test findings in patients with CSX after 4 months of therapy in one study.[30]
- *Gliflozins* have also hypothesized to be a possible treatment modality through modulation of vascular endothelial cell activation, especially in patients with HFpEF, where microvascular dysfunction is believed to be an underlying cause.[31]
- *Nicorandil* is an antianginal drug called *N*-(2-hydroxyethyl) nicotinamide nitrate, which has more than ATP. The mechanism of myocardial protection may be related to the opening of ATP-sensitive potassium channel, decreasing the production of excessive oxygen free radicals during myocardial ischemia, improving the antioxidant capacity of myocardium, and inhibiting the apoptosis and inflammation.[32] Nicorandil has been used in the treatment of microvascular angina, but there is a lack of high-quality randomized controlled trials on the clinical effectiveness.

Lifestyle Modification

Exercise improves mortality in overall population[33] and has shown to improve exercise capacity and decrease angina in the CSX group (26 patients) in one study.[34] Smoking cessation has an important role in modifying endothelial dysfunction.[35] Weight loss also has shown to improve endothelial function.[36] Evidence suggests Mediterranean diet is instrumental in preventing cardiovascular disease.[37]

GUIDELINE RECOMMENDATION BY AMERICAN HEART ASSOCIATION IN MANAGEMENT OF CSX

Recommendation from ACC for CSX management are given in **Box 1**.

STUDIES

- SWEDEHEART registry enrolled 9,138 patients with nonobstructive CAD for studying treatment with statins, ACE inhibitors/ARBs, beta blockers, and dual antiplatelets and MACE (composite of all-cause mortality or hospitalization for reinfarction, heart failure, or stroke). At a median follow-up of 4.1 years, there was a significantly lower event rate with statins (HR 0.77) and ACE inhibitors (HR 0.82) and a trend toward a lower

BOX 1 Recommendation from ACC for CSX management.

Class I:

- Reassurance and medical therapy with nitrates, beta blockers, and calcium channel blockers alone or in combination (LOE: B)
- Risk factor reduction (LOE: C)

Class II:

- Intravascular imaging to rule out any vulnerable plaque (LOE: B)
- If no ECG is available during chest pain episode and coronary spasm cannot be ruled out, then angiography with provocative testing with methylergonovine, acetylcholine, or methacholine (LOE: C)
- Hormone replacement therapy in postmenopausal women unless there is a contraindication (LOE: C)
- Imipramine for continued pain despite class I measures (LOE: C)

Class III:

- Medical therapy with nitrates, beta blockers, calcium channel blockers for patients with noncardiac chest pain is not recommended (LOE: C)

event rate with beta blockers (HR 0.86). Dual antiplatelets were not associated with a lower event rate[38] (HR 0.90; CI 0.74–1.08).

- MINOCA-BAT, a registry-based randomized, open label, multicenter trial with 2:2 factorial design, showed that oral beta blockers and ACE inhibitors reduced composite of death of any cause, readmission due to MI, ischemic stroke, or heart failure in patients with nonobstructive CAD after discharge with no previous signs of heart failure and ejection fraction of >40%.[39]
- StartMed-MINOCA[40] is an ongoing clinical trial, which will study whether an early risk stratification by CMVD (defined by index of microvascular resistance ≥25) associated with cardioprotective mineralocorticoid antagonist therapy with eplerenone could reduce the levels of N-terminal pro-brain natriuretic peptide (NT-proBNP) as a marker of damage in nonobstructive CAD patients.
- PROMISE clinical trial[41] which is ongoing will evaluate whether a "precision medicine approach" defined as a comprehensive diagnostic workup associated with consequent tailored pharmacological treatment of underlying etiology, compared to standard of care, may improve prognosis and quality of life in these patients.
- The Women's Ischemic Syndrome Evaluation study (WISE study), the largest and most thoroughly investigated cohort of middle-aged women with CSX, showed that 5-year annualized event rates for cardiovascular events were 16.0% in women with nonobstructive CAD and 7.9% in women with normal coronary arteries.[42]
- Women's Ischemia Trial to Reduce Events in Nonobstructive CAD (WARRIOR) trial suggested that resolvins, a class of omega-3 fatty acid-derived lipid mediators that reduce inflammation, play a role in CSX, and women with CMVD may not produce adequate quantities of resolvins to curb inflammation.[43]

CONCLUSION

Cardiac syndrome X is a challenging diagnosis with heterogenous etiologies. The population at a higher risk are postmenopausal women. These patients are often underdiagnosed and go untreated at times. There is growing evidence that this group of patients is at risk of future adverse cardiovascular events and needs to be treated. Prognosis is confounding and with variable results in terms of all-cause mortality, in-hospital mortality, and noncardiac deaths.[44] There is an unmet need for evidence to guide diagnosis and treatment of CMVD.

ONLINE REFERENCES

Please scan the QR code provided at the end of the table of contents for References of this chapter.

CHAPTER

118

Coronary Vasospasm: Update

Kranthi Kumar Gedala, Jaideep C Menon

ABSTRACT

Coronary vasospasm or coronary artery spasm (CAS) is a transient, abrupt narrowing of the coronary arteries, which can lead to myocardial ischemia, angina, and, in some cases, myocardial infarction. Despite advances in understanding its pathophysiology, diagnosis, and management, CAS remains a significant clinical challenge. This chapter reviews the latest insights into the mechanisms, diagnostic criteria, and treatment strategies for CAS, incorporating findings from recent guidelines and studies.

Keywords: Coronary artery spasm, vasospastic angina, myocardial ischemia, INOCA, MINOCA, coronary microvascular spasm

INTRODUCTION

Coronary artery spasm (CAS), also known as vasospastic angina, is characterized by temporary constriction of the coronary arteries, leading to reduced blood flow to the myocardium. It can manifest as chest pain and is often associated with ST-segment elevation on electrocardiograms (ECGs), mimicking acute coronary syndrome. While traditionally considered a benign condition, recent studies have highlighted its potential to cause serious cardiac events, including myocardial infarction and sudden cardiac death.[1] About one half of patients with INOCA and one-third of patients with MINOCA are found to have CAS.[2] This chapter aims to provide a comprehensive overview of CAS, drawing from recent guidelines and research findings.

PATHOPHYSIOLOGY

The pathophysiology of CAS involves complex interactions between endothelial dysfunction, smooth muscle hyperreactivity, and autonomic nervous system imbalances. Endothelial dysfunction reduces the production of nitric oxide, a key vasodilator, and increases endothelin-1, a potent vasoconstrictor.[3] Smooth muscle hyperreactivity in the coronary arteries leads to exaggerated responses to vasoconstrictive stimuli. Additionally, autonomic nervous system imbalances, particularly an increase in parasympathetic activity, can precipitate spasm.

Recent insights have also highlighted the role of inflammation and oxidative stress in the development of CAS. Inflammatory markers such as C-reactive protein (CRP) and interleukin-6 (IL-6) are elevated in patients with CAS, suggesting an inflammatory component to the disease.[1] Oxidative stress, resulting from an imbalance between reactive oxygen species (ROS) and antioxidant defenses, can further exacerbate endothelial dysfunction and smooth muscle hyperreactivity.

Further elucidating the mechanisms, research has identified genetic factors that may predispose individuals to CAS. Polymorphisms in genes related to endothelial function, such as the endothelial nitric oxide synthase (eNOS) gene, have been associated with increased susceptibility to vasospasm. Additionally, epigenetic modifications, which do not alter the DNA sequence but affect gene expression, have been implicated in the pathogenesis of CAS.

DIAGNOSTIC CRITERIA

The diagnostic criteria for CAS have been standardized by the Coronary Vasomotion Disorders International Study Group (COVADIS) to improve the consistency and accuracy of diagnosis. According to the COVADIS criteria, CAS is diagnosed based on the following:

- *Clinical symptoms*: Episodes of angina, particularly at rest and often in the early morning, lasting for a few minutes.

- *ECG changes*: Transient ST-segment elevation or depression during angina episodes.
- *Response to vasodilators*: Relief of symptoms and normalization of ECG changes with administration of nitrates or calcium channel blockers (CCBs).
- *Coronary angiography*: Demonstration of CAS, defined as >90% transient constriction of a coronary artery, induced by provocation tests (e.g., acetylcholine or ergonovine).[3]

CLINICAL PRESENTATION

Patients with CAS typically present with angina, which may occur at rest or during physical activity. The pain is often described as a pressure or tightness in the chest and can radiate to the arms, neck, or jaw. Unlike typical exertional angina, CAS-related angina often occurs at rest, particularly in the early morning hours, and is of a shorter duration.

In some cases, CAS can lead to more severe complications such as myocardial infarction, arrhythmias, or sudden cardiac death. These severe outcomes are more likely in patients with underlying atherosclerosis or other cardiovascular risk factors.[1]

EPIDEMIOLOGY

The prevalence of CAS varies widely depending on the population studied and the diagnostic criteria used. It is more common in East Asian populations, particularly in Japan, where it is a leading cause of myocardial infarction in young individuals. In Western populations, CAS is less common but still a significant cause of angina and myocardial ischemia.[4]

Risk factors for CAS include smoking, hyperlipidemia, hypertension, and a history of other vasospastic disorders such as Raynaud's phenomenon or migraine headaches. Acute emotional stress, physical exertion, exposure to cold temperatures, and certain medications (e.g., cocaine, sumatriptan) can provoke coronary artery vasospasm. Genetic factors may also play a role, as suggested by familial clustering of cases.

Smoking is particularly detrimental, as it exacerbates endothelial dysfunction and increases the propensity for CAS. Nicotine and other components of cigarette smoke can trigger vasoconstriction and enhance smooth muscle hyperreactivity. Therefore, smoking cessation is a critical component of managing patients with CAS.

DIAGNOSTIC TECHNIQUES

Noninvasive Testing

Noninvasive tests such as ECG, echocardiography, and stress testing can provide valuable information in the initial evaluation of patients with suspected CAS. During an angina episode, ECG may show transient ST-segment elevation or depression, which normalizes after symptom resolution. Holter monitoring can detect transient ischemic changes and correlate them with symptoms.

Stress testing, particularly with imaging modalities such as stress echocardiography or myocardial perfusion imaging, can help identify areas of reversible ischemia. However, stress testing may be less sensitive for CAS than for atherosclerotic coronary artery disease, as spasm is often triggered by rest or low-level exertion rather than peak exercise.

Invasive Testing

Coronary angiography with provocation testing remains the gold standard for diagnosing CAS. During angiography, vasospasm can be provoked using agents such as acetylcholine or ergonovine, which induce endothelial dysfunction and smooth muscle contraction. A positive test is defined by the reproduction of symptoms, transient ST-segment changes, and >90% constriction of a coronary artery.[3]

Intravascular ultrasound (IVUS) and optical coherence tomography (OCT) can provide additional insights into the structural characteristics of the coronary arteries, including the presence of atherosclerotic plaques, which may coexist with CAS.

Advanced imaging techniques, such as cardiac magnetic resonance imaging (MRI) and positron emission tomography (PET), are being increasingly utilized to assess myocardial perfusion and viability in patients with CAS. These modalities offer high-resolution images and can detect subtle changes in myocardial blood flow, improving the accuracy of CAS diagnosis.

CORONARY MICROVASCULAR SPASM

Coronary microvascular spasm, a related condition, involves the small coronary arteries and arterioles rather than the large epicardial coronary arteries. This condition can cause myocardial ischemia and angina similar to CAS but is often more challenging to diagnose due to the smaller size of the vessels involved.[2]

Patients with coronary microvascular spasm may present with angina at rest or during exertion, and traditional angiography may not reveal significant epicardial coronary artery stenosis.[5] Provocation tests, such as the administration of acetylcholine or hyperventilation, can induce microvascular spasm and help in diagnosing this condition. Noninvasive imaging techniques, such as stress cardiac MRI and PET, can also assess microvascular function and identify ischemia due to microvascular spasm.

MANAGEMENT

The management of CAS involves both pharmacological and nonpharmacological approaches aimed at preventing and relieving angina episodes, as well as reducing the risk of serious complications.

Pharmacological Therapy

Calcium Channel Blockers

Calcium channel blockers are the mainstay of treatment for CAS. They inhibit the influx of calcium ions into vascular smooth muscle cells, leading to vasodilation and reduced smooth muscle contractility.[4] Both dihydropyridine CCBs (e.g., amlodipine and nifedipine) and nondihydropyridine CCBs (e.g., verapamil, diltiazem) are effective in preventing and relieving CAS.

Nitrates

Nitrates, such as nitroglycerin, provide rapid relief of angina symptoms by causing vasodilation of the coronary arteries. Long-acting nitrates (e.g., isosorbide mononitrate) can be used for prophylaxis, but their use is limited by the development of tolerance.

Other Medications

Other medications that may be used in the management of CAS include:

- *Beta-blockers*: Although traditionally contraindicated due to concerns about unopposed alpha-adrenergic activity, some beta-blockers (e.g., nebivolol) with vasodilatory properties may be beneficial.
- *Statins*: Statins have anti-inflammatory and plaque-stabilizing effects and may reduce the frequency of vasospastic episodes.
- *Rho-kinase inhibitors*: These agents, which inhibit smooth muscle contraction, are being investigated for their potential to prevent CAS.[4]

Antiplatelet agents, such as aspirin, may be considered in patients with coexisting atherosclerosis to reduce the risk of thrombotic events. However, their role in isolated CAS remains unclear and should be individualized based on the patient's risk profile.

Nonpharmacological Therapy

Lifestyle modifications are essential in managing CAS. Patients are advised to avoid triggers that can precipitate spasm, such as smoking, cold exposure, and excessive stress. Regular physical activity, a healthy diet, and weight management are also recommended to improve overall cardiovascular health. Stress management techniques, such as mindfulness, yoga, and counseling, can help reduce the autonomic imbalances that contribute to CAS.

Refractory Cases

In patients with refractory CAS, despite optimal medical therapy, additional interventions may be considered. These include:

- *Coronary stenting*: In cases where spasm is localized to a discrete atherosclerotic lesion, stenting may provide relief.
- *Sympathectomy*: Surgical or chemical sympathectomy, which reduces sympathetic nervous system activity, has been used in severe refractory cases.[4]
- *Implantable cardioverter-defibrillator (ICD)*: In patients with a high risk of sudden cardiac death due to life-threatening arrhythmias triggered by CAS, an ICD may be warranted.

PROGNOSIS

The prognosis of CAS varies depending on the presence of underlying atherosclerosis and other cardiovascular risk factors. In patients with isolated CAS and no significant coronary artery disease, the long-term prognosis is generally favorable with appropriate treatment. However, in patients with coexisting atherosclerosis, the risk of adverse cardiovascular events, including myocardial infarction and sudden cardiac death, is higher.[1]

The long-term management of CAS involves regular follow-up to monitor the efficacy of treatment, adherence to lifestyle modifications, and surveillance for potential complications. Patient education is crucial in empowering individuals to recognize symptoms early and seek prompt medical attention.

RECENT GUIDELINES AND FUTURE DIRECTIONS

The 2023 guidelines from the Japanese Circulation Society, Japanese Association of Cardiovascular Intervention and Therapeutics, and Japanese College of Cardiology provide updated recommendations for the diagnosis and treatment of CAS. These guidelines emphasize the importance of early diagnosis and aggressive management to prevent complications.[4]

Emerging research is focusing on the molecular mechanisms underlying CAS, including the role of genetic factors, endothelial progenitor cells, and novel biomarkers. Advances in imaging techniques, such as cardiac MRI and PET, are also enhancing our ability to diagnose and monitor CAS.[1]

POTENTIAL AREAS FOR FUTURE RESEARCH

Several areas warrant further investigation to improve the understanding and management of CAS.

Genetic and Molecular Mechanisms

- *Genetic predisposition*: Studies exploring genetic polymorphisms and their association with CAS susceptibility can provide insights into the hereditary aspects of the disorder. Identifying genetic markers may help in risk stratification and personalized treatment approaches.

- *Molecular pathways*: Research into the specific molecular pathways involved in endothelial dysfunction, smooth muscle hyperreactivity, and inflammation can uncover novel therapeutic targets. The role of microRNAs and other noncoding RNAs in the regulation of these pathways is an emerging area of interest.

Biomarkers

Biomarkers for diagnosis and prognosis: The identification of reliable biomarkers for CAS could enhance diagnostic accuracy and prognostic assessment. Biomarkers related to endothelial function, inflammation, and oxidative stress are potential candidates. For instance, circulating levels of endothelin-1, nitric oxide metabolites, and inflammatory cytokines may serve as indicators of disease activity and treatment response.

Advanced Imaging Techniques

- *High-resolution imaging*: The development of advanced imaging techniques with higher resolution and greater sensitivity can improve the detection of subtle coronary artery changes and myocardial perfusion abnormalities associated with CAS. These technologies could facilitate early diagnosis, better monitoring of disease progression, and evaluation of therapeutic efficacy.
- *Functional imaging*: Functional imaging modalities, such as PET and MRI, can assess myocardial blood flow and metabolism, providing comprehensive information about the physiological impact of CAS on the myocardium.

Novel Therapeutics

- *Targeted therapies*: The development of targeted therapies aimed at specific molecular mechanisms involved in CAS, such as Rho-kinase inhibitors, offers promise for more effective treatment options. These agents could directly modulate smooth muscle contractility and endothelial function, reducing the frequency and severity of vasospastic episodes.
- *Combination therapies*: Investigating the efficacy of combination therapies, involving multiple classes of medications (e.g., CCBs, nitrates, statins), may optimize treatment outcomes. Combination regimens could address the multifactorial nature of CAS by targeting different pathophysiological pathways simultaneously.

CONCLUSION

Coronary artery spasm is a significant cause of myocardial ischemia and angina, with potential for serious cardiac events. Advances in our understanding of its pathophysiology, diagnosis, and management have improved outcomes for many patients. However, further research is needed to fully elucidate the mechanisms underlying CAS and to develop more effective and personalized treatment strategies.

The implementation of standardized diagnostic criteria and the adoption of evidence-based guidelines are critical steps in ensuring consistent and accurate diagnosis and management of CAS. Emerging insights into genetic and molecular mechanisms, novel biomarkers, advanced imaging techniques, and targeted therapies hold promise for further advancements in the field.

Clinicians must remain vigilant in recognizing CAS, particularly in patients presenting with atypical angina or those with a history of vasospastic disorders. Early diagnosis and aggressive management, including pharmacological therapy, lifestyle modifications, and, in refractory cases, interventional procedures, are essential to prevent complications and improve patient outcomes.

As our understanding of CAS continues to evolve, ongoing research and collaboration among healthcare professionals, researchers, and patients will be key to achieving better diagnostic, therapeutic, and prognostic outcomes in this complex and challenging condition.

ONLINE REFERENCES

Please scan the QR code provided at the end of the table of contents for References of this chapter.

CHAPTER

119

Nonobstructive Coronary Artery Disease: MINOCA and INOCA

Devanu Ghosh Roy, Deepanjan Bhattacharya

ABSTRACT

Physicians often encounter patients with evidence of angina but nonobstructive lesions on coronary angiography. These patients comprise the groups of ischemia with nonobstructive coronary artery disease (INOCA) and myocardial infarction with nonobstructive coronary artery disease (MINOCA). The term open artery ischemia (OAI) has also been proposed.

They require comprehensive stepwise evaluation of coronary physiology to understand the underlying pathophysiology.

Although therapy for these patients lies in the gray zone, trials and studies are underway to identify potential treatment strategies.

Keywords: Ischemia, myocardial infarction, coronary physiology

INTRODUCTION

Nonobstructive coronary artery disease (CAD) is atherosclerotic plaque that would not be expected to obstruct blood flow or result in anginal symptoms, accounting for 10–25% of patients undergoing coronary angiography. Significant CAD is defined as ≥70% obstruction for non-left main disease and ≥50% for left main disease.

Ischemia with nonobstructive coronary artery disease (INOCA) is defined as angiographic evidence of ischemia with nonobstructive lesions on coronary angiography.[1]

Myocardial infarction with nonobstructive coronary artery disease (MINOCA) is defined by clinical documentation of an acute myocardial infarction via an ischemic mechanism and the angiographic demonstration of nonobstructive coronary arteries.

The ESC proposed the diagnostic criteria for MINOCA in 2017,[2] which include:

- Positive ischemic cardiac biomarkers and corroborative clinical evidence of infarction (clinical symptoms, ECG ST-segment changes, LBBB or pathological Q waves, and loss of myocardial viability)
- Nonobstructive coronary arteries on angiography (no stenosis > 50% in an infarct-related artery)
- Nonclinically overt specific cause for acute presentation requiring further diagnostic evaluation

INOCA

The prevalence of INOCA is slowly increasing over years, with more than half of the patients being women.[3] It is significantly associated with an increased risk of major adverse cardiovascular events (MACE), stroke, and heart failure with preserved ejection fraction (HFpEF). Older age, hypertension, diabetes mellitus, and smoking further increase the risk of adverse outcomes.

Prevalence of INOCA among patients undergoing angiography is around 13%. The patients tend to be younger than those with obstructive CAD, with less comorbidities, with female preponderance.[4]

Patients with INOCA have a poorer quality of life as compared to those with stable CAD in terms of physical limitation, time missed from work, and angina frequency.

The Women's Ischemia Syndrome Evaluation (WISE) study estimated that at least 3–4 million women and men in the United States with signs and symptoms suggestive of ischemia have INOCA, with an estimated 10-year mortality of 13% (4.6 times higher than age-matched cohort).[5,6]

MINOCA

Patients with MINOCA account for 6% of all patients with myocardial infarction, with a striking female preponderance

(M:F ratio 1:1.8). They tend to be a decade younger than those with obstructive CAD and have less prevalence of dyslipidemia (21% vs. 32%).

Predominantly, the mode of presentation is NSTEMI, and the 1-year mortality is about 3.4%.[7]

Supply-demand mismatch (type 2 MI) is the most common cause of MINOCA, followed by plaque rupture, plaque erosion, microvascular dysfunction, vasospasm, thrombus, calcific nodule, and spontaneous coronary artery dissection (SCAD).

MECHANISM OF INOCA/MINOCA

Coronary microvascular dysfunction (CMD) accounts for the majority of cases of MINOCA/INOCA. It can be isolated endothelial dysfunction, smooth muscle dysfunction, or both.[8]

Heightened coronary vasoreactivity occurs in about 25% of patients, which can be in the epicardial coronaries or coronary microcirculation.

Abnormal thrombophilia screen is seen in as many as 19% of patients,[9] which include factor V Leiden, prothrombin variant G20210A, factor XII deficiency, and protein C and S deficiencies. Important acquired hypercoagulable states that may predispose to MINOCA include collagen vascular disorders, systemic vasculitis, systemic lupus, antiphospholipid syndrome, polycythemia vera, thrombocythemia, and the use of anabolic steroids or estrogens/progestins.

EVALUATION OF INOCA/MINOCA

Noninvasive

- *Cardiac MRI (CMR)* is a useful tool not only to rule out other causes of myocardial injury but also to assess myocardial perfusion and ventricular perfusion. The study by Pasupathy et al. showed that among all patients with suspected MINOCA, CMR was able to diagnose myocarditis in 33%, Takotsubo syndrome in 18%, and other cardiomyopathies in 12%, while 24% of patients had evidence of myocardial infarction.[10] Ischemic injury typically appears along vascular territory as myocardial edema or fibrosis affecting the subendocardial or transmural myocardium on T2 and LGE sequences.[9]
- *Coronary computed tomographic angiography (CCTA)* can be used to rule out obstructive CAD, as well as identify high-risk plaque features, evidence of inflammation, and SCAD.
- *Coronary flow reserve (CFR)* can be measured using transthoracic echocardiogram or measuring myocardial blood flow using PET or myocardial perfusion using CMR. CFR is defined as the ratio of coronary blood flow during maximum hyperemia to rest. CFR < 2 suggests microvascular dysfunction.[11]
- *Myocardial blood flow reserve (MBFR)* can be measured using PET scan. It is the ratio of myocardial blood flow during peak hyperemia to rest. Normal value is >2.3, while values < 1.5 indicate CMD.

Invasive

- *Intracoronary imaging* using optical coherence tomography (OCT) or intravascular ultrasound (IVUS) helps to evaluate lesions which were not evident on conventional angiography. It helps visualize plaque rupture, plaque erosion, calcific nodule, and SCAD **(Figs. 1A to C)**.
- *CFR* can be measured invasively using intracoronary Doppler wire. Average peak velocities are measured at baseline (APVb) and after maximal hyperemia (APVh) with adenosine (140 µg/kg intravenous, 30–60 µg/kg intracoronary for left coronary artery, and 20–30 µg/kg intracoronary for right coronary artery). Normal value is 3–5, while value <2 suggests microvascular dysfunction. Thermodilution can be used for measuring CFR, where it is equal to the ratio of meant transit time at hyperemia to rest (CFR = T_{mn} at hyperemia/T_{mn} at rest).[12]

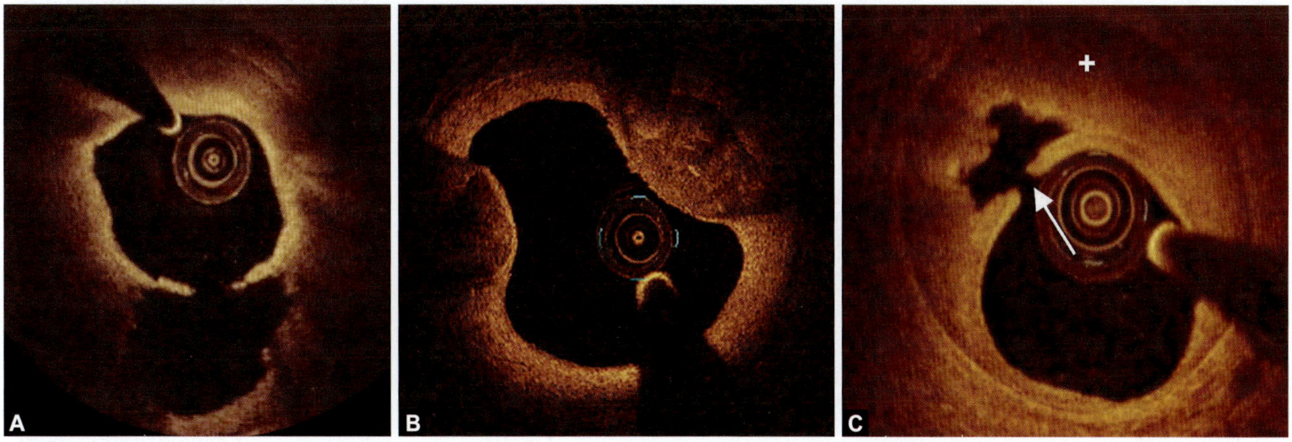

FIGS. 1A TO C: Coronary optical coherence tomography (OCT) showing (A) plaque rupture, (B) calcific nodule, and (C) SCAD.

- *Provocative coronary testing for coronary vasospasm* can be done using intracoronary acetylcholine. The dose is 20–100 μg for the left coronary artery and 20–50 μg for the right coronary artery, given over 20 seconds. Intravenous infusion of acetylcholine (0.36–3.6 μg over 2 minutes) is another option. A positive test is denoted by >90% coronary artery constriction with angina and/or new-onset ECG changes (ST depression/elevation > 0.1 mV or negative U waves). More than half of the patients with MINOCA demonstrate a positive provocation test.[13,14]
- *Index of microcirculatory resistance (IMR)* is considered as the gold standard for CMD. It is measured by the thermodilution technique, where mean transit time (T_{mn}) and distal coronary pressure (P_d) are measured, and IMR is calculated as the product of T_{mn} and P_d (IMR = $T_{mn} \times P_d$). Value > 25 is suggestive of CMD.[15]

The approaches to a patient with suspected INOCA and MINOCA are summarized in **Flowcharts 1 and 2**, respectively.

MANAGEMENT

Secondary prevention of MINOCA is similar to that of obstructive CAD and includes antiplatelets and high-intensity statins, along with lifestyle measures and cardiac rehabilitation.[16] Use of dual antiplatelets in patients with plaque rupture or erosion is controversial as there are insufficient data regarding the same.[17]

In those with documented coronary vasospasm, nitrates (both short and long acting) as well as calcium channel blockers (both dihydropyridine and nondihydropyridine) are beneficial. Cilostazol and nicorandil are also helpful in relieving vasospasm. Although low-dose aspirin is beneficial as it inhibits thromboxane synthesis, high doses can inhibit prostacyclin synthesis, thereby aggravating vasospasm.

The EDIT-CMD trial evaluated the role of diltiazem in patients with INOCA.[18] Patients with presence of vasospasm (after intracoronary acetylcholine provocation) and/or microvascular dysfunction (CFR < 2.0 or IMR ≥ 25) were randomized to receive oral diltiazem up to 360 mg/day or placebo. After 6 weeks, there was no significant improvement in CFR or IMR, but there was significant reduction of coronary vasospasm. There was also no significant improvement of quality of life or angina index.

Although data are scarce about the efficacy of drugs in CMD, β-blockers, ranolazine, dipyridamole, and long-term L-arginine therapy have shown some degree of benefit.

Around 70% of cases of SCAD show spontaneous resolution with conservative management. Intervention is indicated in patients with left main dissection, ongoing or

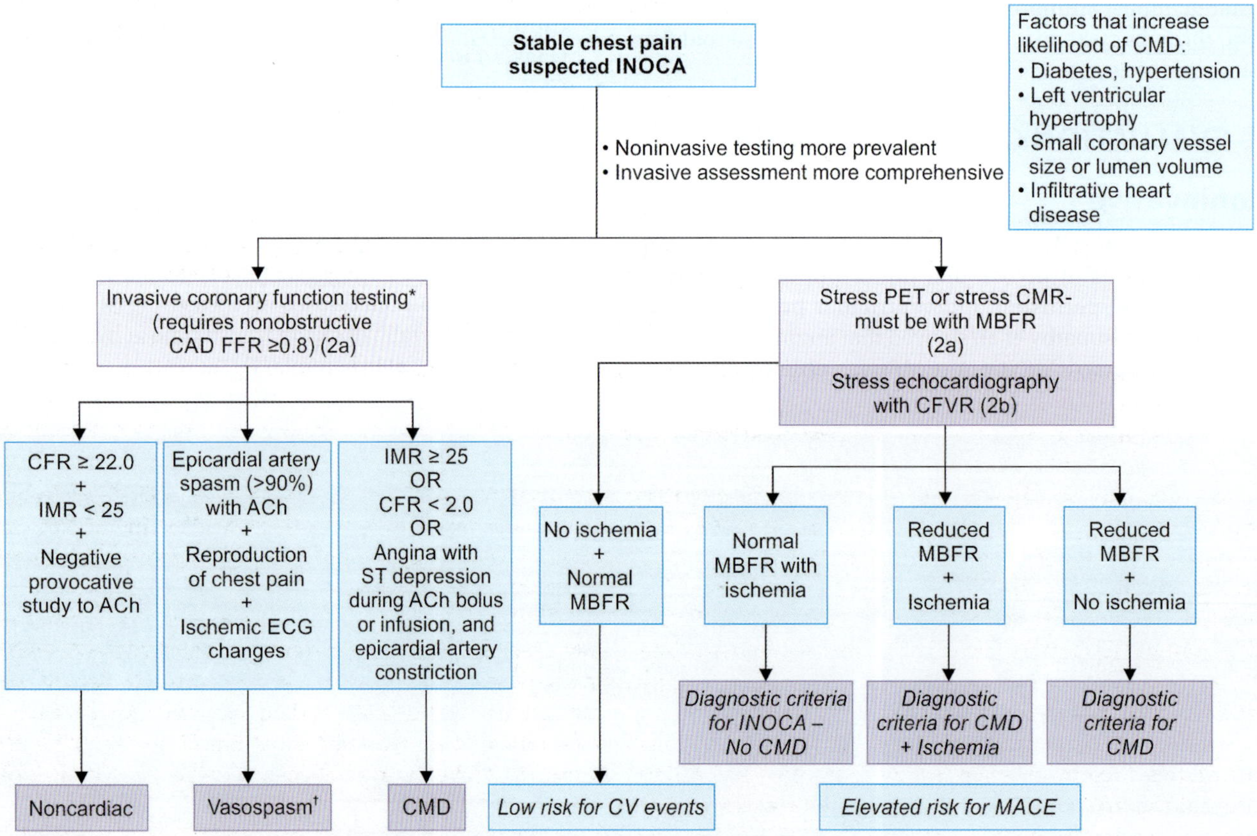

*Includes CFR, IMR and testing for provocation for vasospasm.

†Vasospasm indicated by >90% coronary artery constriction with angina and/or new onset ECG changes (ST depression/elevation >0.1 mm or negative U waves).

FLOWCHART 1: Approach to a patient with INOCA.

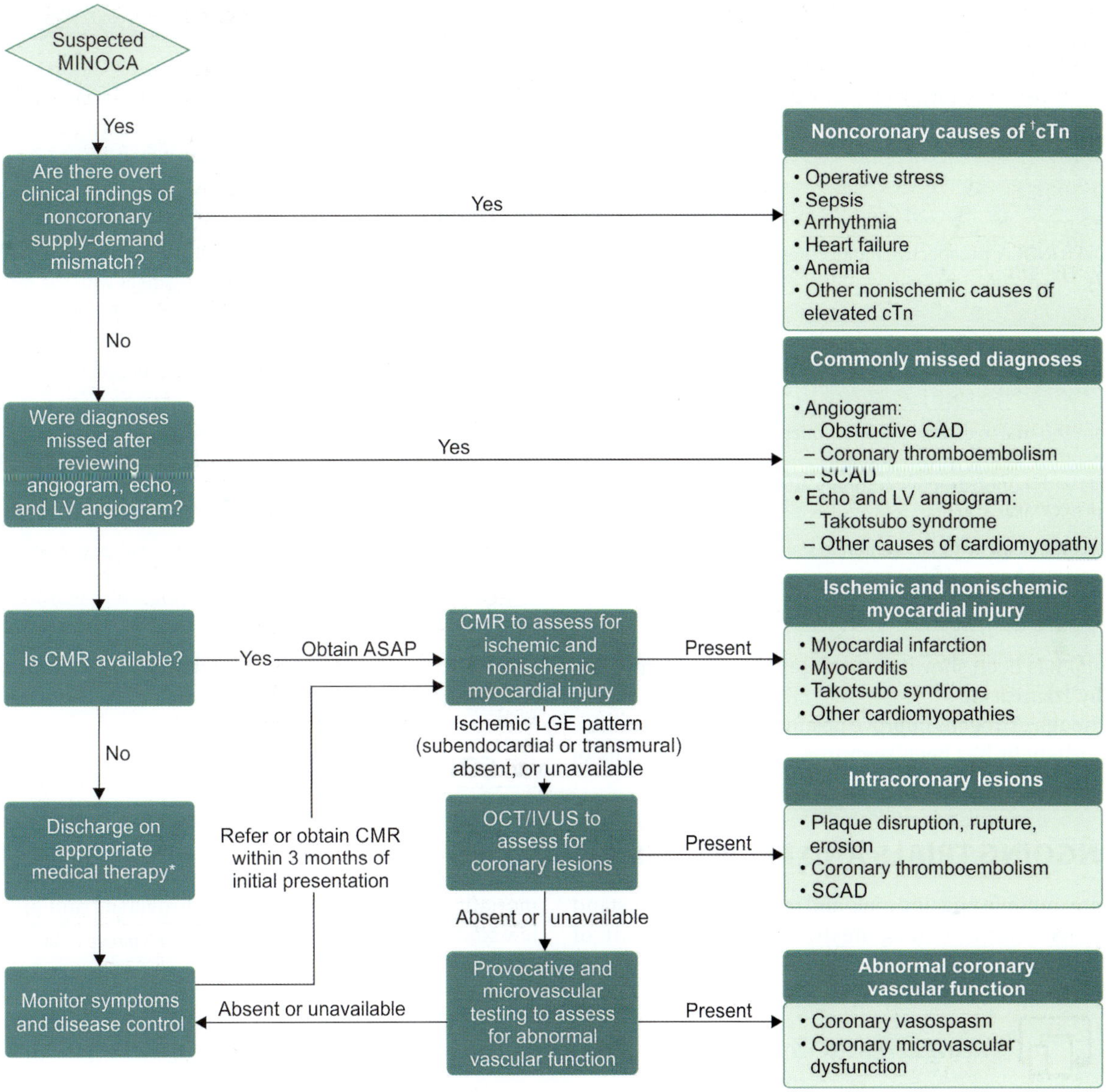

*Includes antiplatelets, high intensity statins, beta-blockers, ranolazine.
†Elevated cardiac troponin.

FLOWCHART 2: Approach to a patient with MINOCA.

recurrent angina, ventricular arrhythmias, and cardiogenic shock. Percutaneous coronary intervention (PCI) is considered for isolated left main SCAD, while coronary artery bypass graft, however, should be reserved for stable patients with high-risk clinical features and either an ostial left anterior descending (LAD) artery lesion or ≥2 proximal lesions when PCI is not feasible or there is left main dissection involving the LAD or left circumflex artery.[19,20]

The CorMica trial randomized patients with non-obstructive CAD to invasive testing followed by stratified medical therapy versus standard care.[21] Invasive testing included guidewire-based assessment of CFR, IMR, and fractional flow reserve, followed by vasoreactivity testing with acetylcholine. 73.5% of the patients were female with a median age of 61 years. Invasive testing led to a diagnosis of microvascular dysfunction in 51.7%, coronary vasospasm in 16.6%, and mixed disease in 20.5%. Stratified medical therapy in these patients significantly improved quality of life as well as angina index.

Angiotensin-converting enzyme (ACE) inhibitors attenuate sympathetic coronary vasoconstriction, reduce oxidative stress, and increase CFR through bradykinin-mediated, nitric oxide-dependent pathways. A meta-analysis by Abouzid et al. showed that ACE inhibitors significantly improve CFR but have no effect on angina episodes or blood pressure.[22]

Tricyclic antidepressants reduce the degree of nociception and can reduce angina episodes. Evidence for use of beta-blockers in heterogenous; nebivolol, with its vasodilatory effects, has shown efficacy. Intracoronary

TABLE 1: Summary of major trials and registries of MINOCA and INOCA.

Trial/registry	Purpose
Ischemia in patients with nonobstructive disease (INOCA) in Italy, INOCA-IT multicenter registry	Aims to enroll 200 consecutive patients with suspected chronic INOCA at clinically indicated coronary angiography in three Italian centers, for: • Investigating the prevalence of INOCA in women versus that in men • Stratification of patients into different INOCA endotypes • Implementing a stratified therapy
DISCOVER INOCA, prospective multicenter registry	Identify specific phenotypes of INOCA with both an anatomic evaluation (coronary angiography and intravascular imaging) and physiological assessment with the Abbott Coroventis CoroFlow Cardiovascular System, and to determine long-term outcomes
Women's Ischemia Trial to Reduce Events in Nonobstructive CAD (WARRIOR)	Prospective, randomized, open-blind multisite trial that will evaluate an intensive statin/ ACE-I (or ARB)/aspirin treatment strategy (IMT) versus primary prevention risk factor therapy treatment strategy (UC) in patients with INOCA
Randomized trial to examine a differential therapeutic response in symptomatic patients with nonobstructive coronary artery disease (EXAMINE-CAD)	Prospective, randomized, double-blind, placebo-controlled, crossover trial investigating the efficacy of bisoprolol and diltiazem therapy in symptomatic patients with INOCA
Precision Medicine with Zibotentan in Microvascular Angina (PRIZE) trial	Randomized, double-blind, placebo-controlled trial examining the efficacy of zibotentan in patients with microvascular angina

nebivolol has been shown to increase CFR significantly in a study by Togni et al.[23]

Although estrogens improve postmenopausal symptoms, no clear benefit has been seen in improving symptoms of ischemia.

ONGOING TRIALS AND REGISTRIES[24]

There are multiple ongoing trials and registries to understand the epidemiology, pathogenesis, and management of MINOCA and INOCA, few of which are summarized in **Table 1**.

CONCLUSION

INOCA and MINOCA are quite common in today's world and require comprehensive evaluation with stepwise testing. Although it is associated with an increased risk of mortality, therapy still remains controversial and limited to few studies.

ONLINE REFERENCES

Please scan the QR code provided at the end of the table of contents for References of this chapter.

acute and long-term phases of treatment. For over a decade, dual antiplatelet therapy (DAPT) with aspirin and clopidogrel has been considered the standard of care in the setting of ACS and PCI. However, a considerable number of adverse ischemic events continue to occur with this DAPT regimen, which has led to the development of newer and more potent antiplatelet agents.

- Aspirin acts to inhibit COX enzyme and thus attenuates production of PGs and TXA2.
- The ADP receptor antagonist binds the $P2Y_{12}$-receptor to prevent ADP-induced platelet activation.
- GPIIb/IIIa inhibitors impair platelet adhesion by preventing the formation of fibrinogen bridges between platelets.

Clopidogrel is a prodrug, which, after intestinal absorption, undergoes metabolization in the liver through a double oxidation process mediated by several cytochrome P450 (CYP) isoforms to finally generate an active metabolite that inhibits platelet activation and aggregation processes through irreversible blockade of the $P2Y_{12}$-receptor **(Fig. 2)**. Approximately 85% of clopidogrel is hydrolyzed prehepatically by esterases into an inactive. compound, thus, only 15% is available for hepatic metabolism. Prasugrel, like clopidogrel, is also an oral prodrug with a similar intestinal absorption process. However, in contrast to clopidogrel, esterases are part of prasugrel's activation pathway, and prasugrel is oxidized more efficiently to its active metabolite via a single CYP-dependent step. Direct-acting antiplatelet agents (cangrelor, ticagrelor, and cilostazol) have reversible effects and do not require hepatic metabolism for achieving pharmacodynamic activity. Ticagrelor and cilostazol are orally administered, and after intestinal absorption, inhibit platelet activation by direct blockade of the $P2Y_{12}$-receptor and PDE-III, respectively. Cangrelor is intravenously administered, and directly inhibits the $P2Y_{12}$-receptor, bypassing intestinal absorption. Genetic polymorphisms of target proteins/enzymes (intestine, liver, and platelet membrane) modulating clopidogrel-mediated platelet inhibition do not affect the pharmacodynamic activity of prasugrel, cilostazol, ticagrelor, and cangrelor, which ultimately inhibit platelet activation and aggregation processes by modulating intraplatelet levels of cAMP and VASP-P. **Table 1** shows comparison of pharmacokinetics of different antiplatelet drugs.

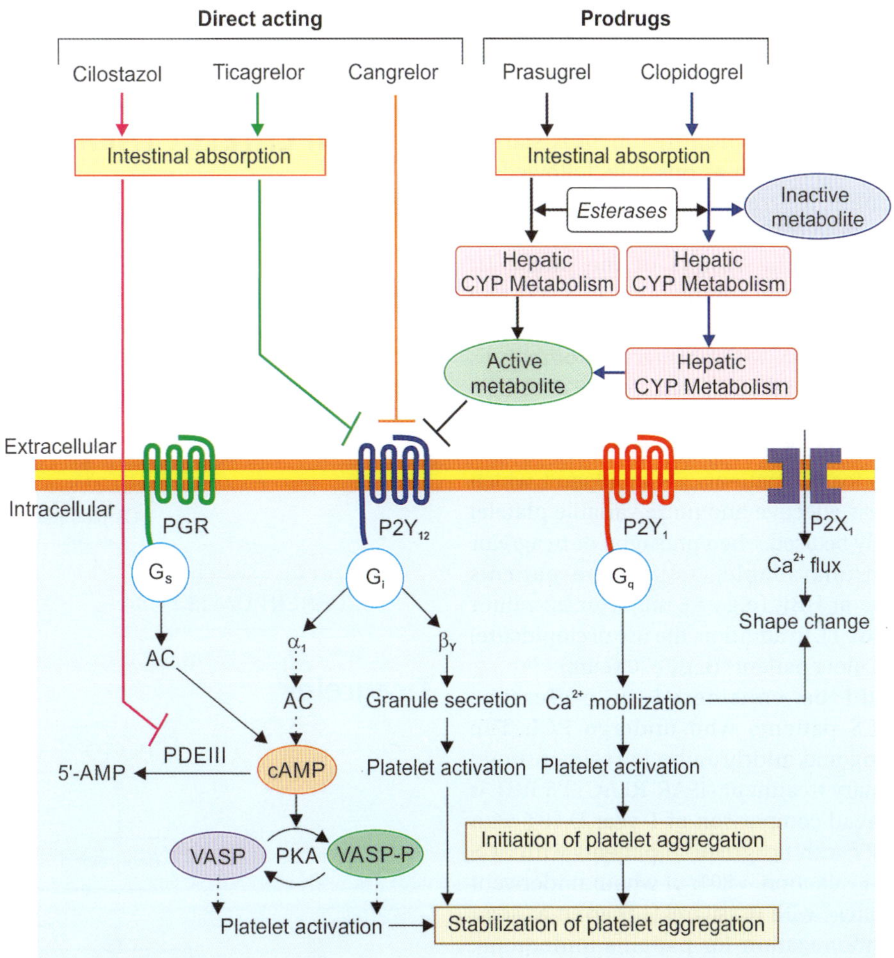

FIG. 2: Schematic of different therapeutic options for inhibition of platelet $P2Y_{12}$-receptor.

TABLE 1: Comparison of pharmacokinetics of different antiplatelet drugs.

	Clopidogrel	Prasugrel	Ticagrelor	Cangrelor
Chemical class	Thienopyridine	Thienopyridine	Cyclopentyl-triazolo-pyrimidine	Adenosine triphosphate analog
Administration route	Oral	Oral	Oral	Intravenous
Standard dosing:				
• Loading dose	300 or 600 mg	60 mg	180 mg	30 µg/kg bolus
• Maintenance dose	1 × 75 mg or 1 × 150 mg	1 × 10 mg or 1 × 5 mg	2 × 90 mg	4 µg/kg/min infusion
Prodrug	Yes	Yes	No	No
$P2Y_{12}$-receptor binding	Irreversible	Irreversible	Reversible	Reversible
Onset of antiplatelet effect	2–6 hours	30 minutes	30 minutes	2 minutes
Offset of antiplatelet effect	3–10 days	5–10 days	3–4 days	1–2 hours
Recommended withdrawal before surgery	5 days	7 days	5 days	1 hour

ANTIPLATELETS COMPARISON

The choice of antiplatelet regimen should take the bleeding risk of the patient into account. Factors associated with an elevated bleeding risk have been detailed by the Academic Research Consortium on high bleeding risk (ARC-HBR) presence of one major or two minor ARC-HBR risk factors indicates HBR. Of note, the presence of multiple major risk factors is associated with a progressive increase in the bleeding risk. Aspirin treatment is started with a loading dose (LD) as soon as possible, followed by maintenance treatment. Current evidence supports an aspirin maintenance dose (MD) of 75–100 mg once a day (OD) **Table 2**. Based on the results of the phase III PLATelet inhibition and patient outcomes (PLATO) and TRial to assess improvement in therapeutic outcomes by optimizing platelet InhibitioN with prasugrel thrombolysis in myocardial infarction 38 (TRITON-TIMI 38) studies, DAPT including aspirin and a potent $P2Y_{12}$-receptor inhibitor (prasugrel or ticagrelor) is recommended as the default DAPT strategy for ACS patients.[7,8] Clopidogrel, which is characterized by less effective and more variable platelet inhibition, should only be used when prasugrel or ticagrelor are contraindicated/unavailable, or in some patients considered otherwise at HBR (e.g., ≥1 major or ≥2 minor ARC-HBR criteria) **(Box 1)**. In addition, the use of clopidogrel may be considered in older patients (e.g., ≥70 years).

Prasugrel should be considered in preference to ticagrelor for ACS patients who undergo PCI. The intracoronary stenting and antithrombotic regimen rapid early action for coronary treatment (ISAR-REACT) 5 RCT is the largest head-to-head comparison of 1-year DAPT with prasugrel versus DAPT with ticagrelor in patients with ACS planned for invasive evaluation, >80% of whom underwent PCI.[9] A treatment strategy with prasugrel (LD given as soon as possible after randomization for patients undergoing primary PCI and after delineation of coronary anatomy for patients presenting with NSTE-ACS versus ticagrelor (LD given as soon as possible after randomization in all cases) significantly reduced the composite endpoint of death, MI, or stroke (6.9% vs. 9.3%, $p = 0.006$) without any increase in bleeding complications (4.8% vs. 5.4%, $p = 0.46$). Limitations of this study include an open-label design and limited data on medically managed or CABG-treated patients.

LANDMARK EFFICACY TRIALS ON ANTIPLATELET THERAPIES

Aspirin

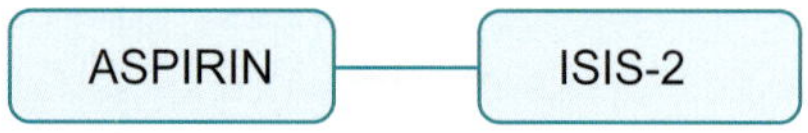

Clopidogrel

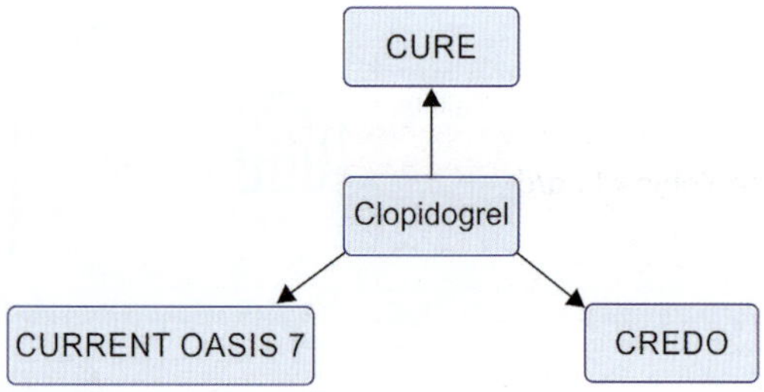

Ticagrelor

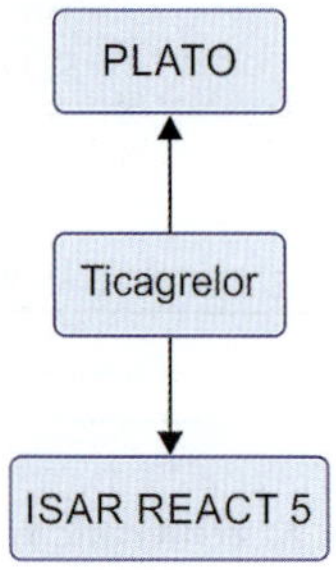

TABLE 2: Antiplatelet drug doses.

Antiplatelet drugs	
Aspirin	LD of 150–300 mg orally or 75–250 mg IV if oral ingestion is not possible, followed by oral MD of 75–100 mg OD; no specific dose adjustment in CKD patients
$P2Y_{12}$-receptor inhibitors (oral or IV)	
Clopidogrel	• LD of 300–600 mg orally, followed by an MD of 75 mg OD; no specific dose adjustment in CKD patients • *Fibrinolysis:* At the time of fibrinolysis an initial dose of 300 mg (75 mg for patients older than 75 years of age)
Prasugrel	LD of 60 mg orally, followed by an MD of 10 mg OD. In patients with body weight <60 kg. An MD of 5 mg OD is recommended. In patients aged ≥75 years, prasugrel should be used with caution, but an MD of 5 mg OD should be used if treatment is deemed necessary. No specific dose adjustment in CKD patients. Prior stroke is a contraindication for prasugrel
Ticagrelor	LD of 180 mg orally, followed by an MD of 90 mg BID; no specific dose adjustment in CKD patients
Cangrelor	• Bolus of 30 µg/kg IV followed by 4 µg/kg/min infusion for at least 2 hours or the duration of the procedure (whichever is longer) • In the transition from cangrelor to a thienopyridine, the thienopyridine should be administered immediately after discontinuation of cangrelor with an LD (clopidogrel 600 mg or prasugrel 60 mg); to avoid a potential DDI, prasugrel may also be administered 30 minutes before the cangrelor infusion is stopped. Ticagrelor (LD 180 mg) should be administered at the time of PCI to minimize the potential gap in platelet inhibition during the transition phase
GP IIb/IIIa receptor inhibitors (IV)	
Eptifibatide	• Double bolus of 180 µg/kg IV (given at a 10-minute interval) followed by an infusion of 2.0 µg/kg/min for up to 18 hours • *For CrCl 30–50 mL/min:* First LD, 180 µg/kg IV bolus (max. 22.6 mg); maintenance infusion, 1 µg/kg/min (max. 7.5 mg/h). Second LD (if PCI), 180 µg/kg IV bolus (max. 22.6 mg) should be administered 10 minutes after the first bolus, contraindicated in patients with end-stage renal disease and with prior ICH, ischemic stroke within 30 days, fibrinolysis, or platelet count <100,000/mm^3
Tirofiban	• Bolus of 25 µg/kg IV over 3 minutes, followed by an infusion of 0.15 µg/kg/min for up to 18 hours • For CrCl ≤60 mL/min; LD. 25 µg/kg IV over 5 mm followed by a maintenance infusion of 0.075 µg/kg/min continued for up to 18 hours • Contraindicated in patients with prior ICH, ischemic stroke within 30 days, fibrinolysis, or platelet count <100,000/mm^3

(LD: loading dose: MD: maintenance dose)

Box 1 Academic Research Consortium-high bleeding risk criteria.

High bleeding risk according to the Academic Research Consortium for high bleeding risk

Major criteria:
- Anticipated use of long-term oral anticoagulation
- Severe or end-stage CKD (<30 mL/min)
- Hemoglobin <11 g/dL
- Spontaneous bleeding requiring hospitalization or transfusion in the past 6 months or at any time, if recurrent
- Moderate or severe baseline thrombocytopenia (<100 × 10^9/L)
- Chronic bleeding diathesis
- Liver cirrhosis with portal hypertension
- Active malignancy in the past 12 months
- Previous spontaneous ICH/traumatic ICH within 12 months/brain AV-malformation/ischemic stroke within 6 months
- Nondeferrable major surgery on DAPT
- Recent major surgery or major trauma within 30 days before PCI

Minor criteria:
- Age >75 years
- Moderate CKD (30–59 mL/min)
- Hemoglobin 11–12.9 g/dL for men and 11–11.9 g/dL for women
- Spontaneous bleeding requiring hospitalization or transfusion within the past 12 months not meeting the major criterion
- Long-term use of oral nonsteroidal anti-inflammatory drugs or steroids
- Any ischemic stroke at any time not meeting the major criterion

High bleeding risk–At least one major criterion or more than 2 minor criterions.[10]

Prasugrel

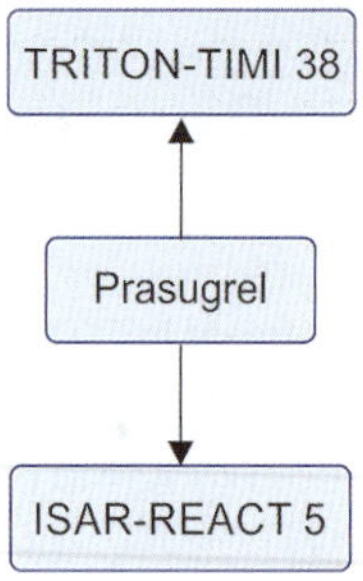

Cangrelor

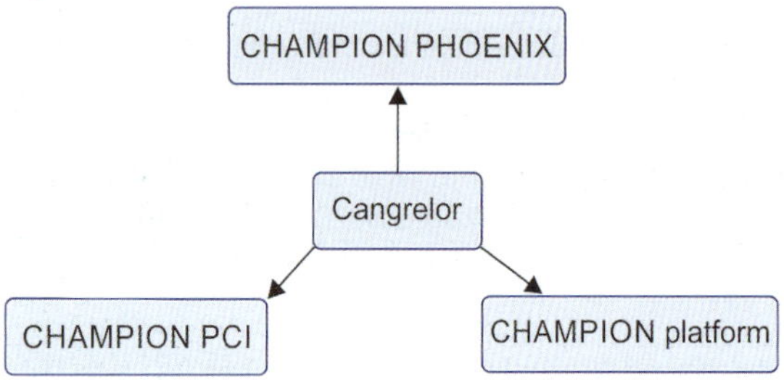

WHAT THE GUIDELINE SAYS?

Flowcharts 1 and 2 describe decision making for the selection of the $P2Y_{12}$ inhibitors in DAPT combination with aspirin for patients with NSTE-ACS and STEMI, respectively, according to the ACC/AHA and ESC guidelines.

2023 ESC guidelines for the management of acute coronary syndromes **(Table 3)**.

ABBREVIATED DUAL ANTIPLATELET THERAPY

Despite the recent advances in revascularization strategy and medical therapies, ACS including acute MI still has high mortalities, morbidities, and needs for rehospitalizations. Along with appropriate revascularization, if needed, medical therapy, including antiplatelet therapy, is the primary treatment strategy for patients with ACS. Novel treatment strategies of DAPT escalation and de-escalation have been evaluated recently in randomized trials showing potential advantages compared with standard DAPT regimens **(Fig. 3)**.[11-14] The escalation consists of switching from a

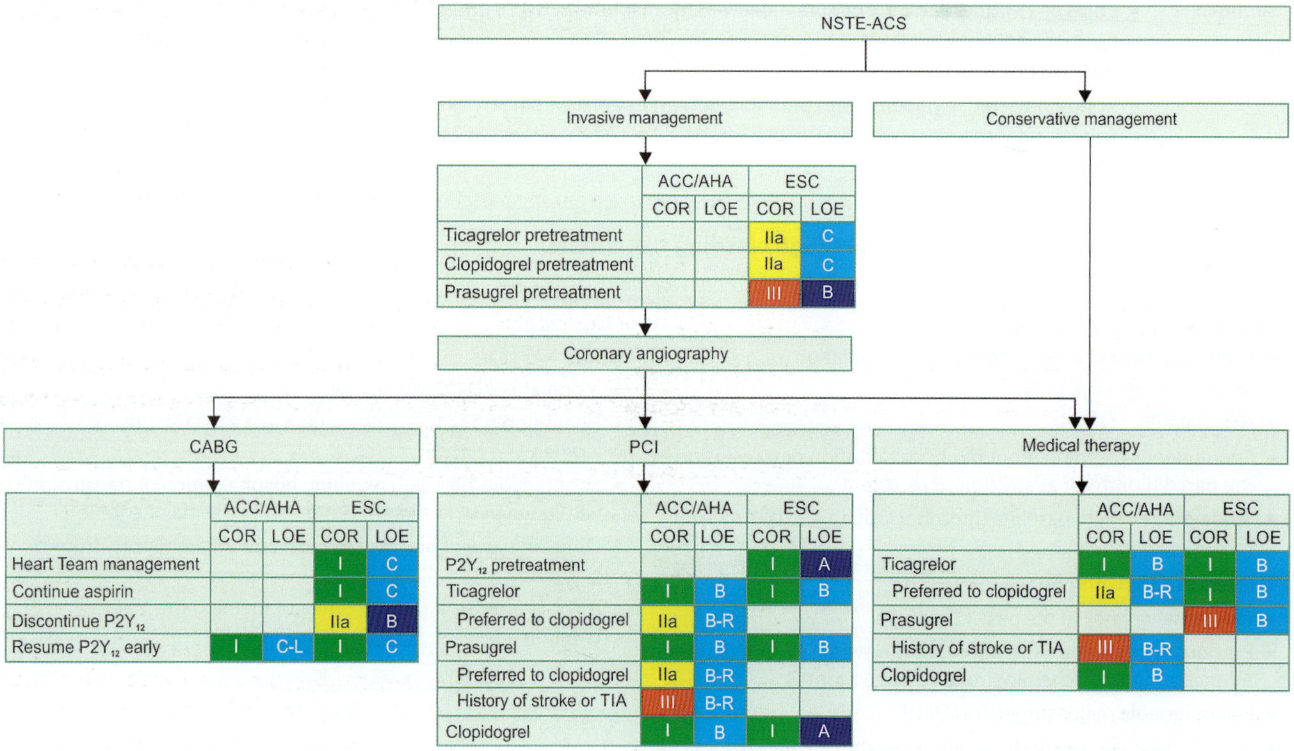

Invasive management:

	ACC/AHA		ESC	
	COR	LOE	COR	LOE
Ticagrelor pretreatment			IIa	C
Clopidogrel pretreatment			IIa	C
Prasugrel pretreatment			III	B

CABG:

	ACC/AHA		ESC	
	COR	LOE	COR	LOE
Heart Team management			I	C
Continue aspirin			I	C
Discontinue $P2Y_{12}$			IIa	B
Resume $P2Y_{12}$ early	I	C-L	I	C

PCI:

	ACC/AHA		ESC	
	COR	LOE	COR	LOE
$P2Y_{12}$ pretreatment			I	A
Ticagrelor	I	B	I	B
Preferred to clopidogrel	IIa	B-R		
Prasugrel	I	B	I	B
Preferred to clopidogrel	IIa	B-R		
History of stroke or TIA	III	B-R		
Clopidogrel	I	B	I	A

Medical therapy:

	ACC/AHA		ESC	
	COR	LOE	COR	LOE
Ticagrelor	I	B	I	B
Preferred to clopidogrel	IIa	B-R	I	B
Prasugrel			III	B
History of stroke or TIA	III	B-R		
Clopidogrel	I	B		

FLOWCHART 1: Decision making for the selection of the $P2Y_{12}$ inhibitors in DAPT combination with aspirin for patients with NSTE-ACS according to the ACC/AHA and ESC guidelines.

STEMI → Primary PCI; Fibrinolysis

Primary PCI:

	ACC/AHA		ESC	
	COR	LOE	COR	LOE
$P2Y_{12}$ pretreatment	I	B	I	A
Ticagrelor			I	B
Prasugrel			I	B

→ Coronary angiography → CABG; PCI; Medical therapy (Fibrinolysis → Medical therapy)

CABG:

	ACC/AHA		ESC	
	COR	LOE	COR	LOE
Heart Team management			I	C
Continue aspirin			I	C
Discontinue $P2Y_{12}$			IIa	B
Resume $P2Y_{12}$ early	I	C-L	I	C

PCI:

	ACC/AHA		ESC	
	COR	LOE	COR	LOE
Ticagrelor	I	B	I	B
Preferred to clopidogrel	IIa	B-R		
Prasugrel	I	B	I	B
Preferred to clopidogrel	IIa	B-R		
History of stroke or TIA	III	B-R		
Clopidogrel	I	B	I	A

Medical therapy:

	ACC/AHA		ESC	
	COR	LOE	COR	LOE
Ticagrelor	I	B	I	B
Preferred to clopidogrel	IIa	B-R	I	B
After thrombolysis	I	B-R		
Prasugrel			III	B
History of stroke or TIA	III	B-R		
Clopidogrel	I	R		
After thrombolysis	I	B-R	I	A

FLOWCHART 2: Decision making for the selection of the $P2Y_{12}$ inhibitors in DAPT combination with aspirin for patients with STEMI according to the ACC/AHA and ESC guidelines.

TABLE 3: Recommendations for antiplatelet therapy in acute coronary syndrome.

Recommendations	**Class**[a]	**Level**[b]
Antiplatelet therapy:		
Aspirin is recommended for all patients without contraindications at an initial oral LD of 150–300 mg (or 75–250 mg IV) and an MD of 75–100 mg OD for long-term treatment	*I*	*A*
In all ACS patients, a $P2Y_{12}$-receptor inhibitor is recommended in addition to aspirin, given as an initial oral LD followed by an MD for 12 months unless there is HBR[c]	*I*	*A*
A proton pump inhibitor in combination with DAPT is recommended in patients at high risk of gastrointestinal bleeding	*I*	*A*
Prasugrel is recommended in $P2Y_{12}$-receptor inhibitor-naïve patients proceeding to PCI (60 mg LD, 10 mg OD MD, 5 mg OD MD for patients aged ≥75 years or with a body weight <60 kg)	*I*	*B*
Ticagrelor is recommended irrespective of the treatment strategy (invasive or conservative) (180 mg LD, 90 mg BID MD)	*I*	*B*
Clopidogrel (300–600 mg LD, 75 mg OD MD) is recommended when prasugrel or ticagrelor are not available, cannot be tolerated, or are contraindicated	*I*	*C*
Prasugrel should be considered in preference to ticagrelor for ACS patients who proceed to PCI	*IIa*	*B*
GP IIb/IIIa receptor antagonists should be considered if there is evidence of no-reflow or a thrombotic complication during PCI	*IIa*	*C*
In $P2Y_{12}$-receptor inhibitor-naïve patients undergoing PCI, cangrelor may be considered	*IIb*	*A*
In older ACS patients,[d] especially if HBR,[c] clopidogrel as the $P2Y_{12}$-receptor inhibitor may be considered	*IIb*	*B*
Pretreatment with a $P2Y_{12}$-receptor inhibitor may be considered in patients undergoing a primary PCI strategy	*IIb*	*B*
Pretreatment with a $P2Y_{12}$-receptor inhibitor may be considered in NSTE-ACS patients who are not expected to undergo an early invasive strategy (<24 hours) and do not have HBR[c]	*IIb*	*C*
Pretreatment with a GP IIb/IIIa receptor antagonist is not recommended	*III*	*A*
Routine pretreatment with a $P2Y_{12}$-receptor inhibitor in NSTE-ACS patients in whom coronary anatomy is not known and early invasive management (<24 hours) is planned and not recommended	*III*	*A*

[a] Class of recommendation.

[b] Level of evidence.

[c] HBR should be assessed in a structured manner, e.g., presence of single major or two minor characteristics as defined by ARC-HBR.

[d] The definition of older patients varies across trials, ranging from 70–80 years of age. Frailty and comorbidities should also be taken in consideration.

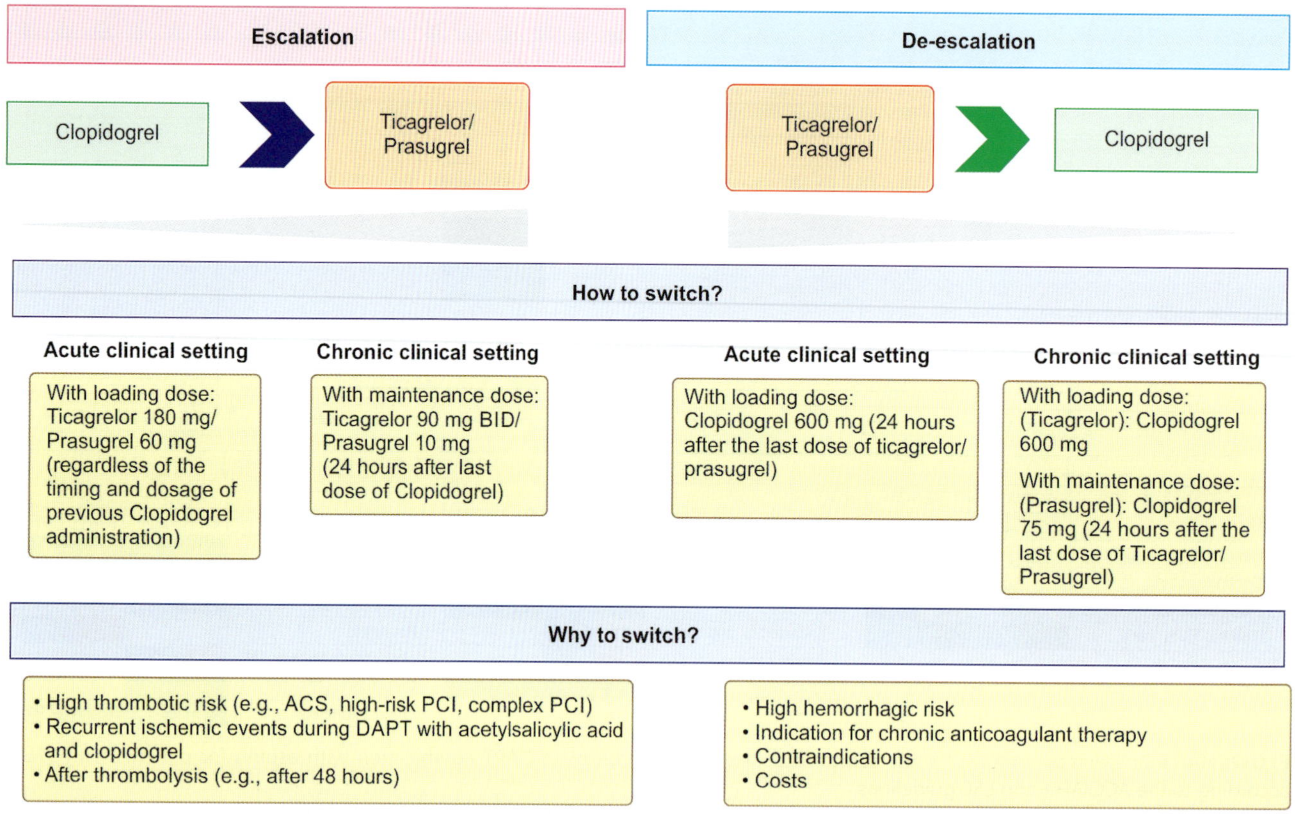

FIG. 3: DAPT score and precise DAPT score.

less potent (i.e., clopidogrel) to a more potent oral $P2Y_{12}$ inhibitor (i.e., ticagrelor or prasugrel) with the goal of reducing thrombotic risk after ACS and/or PCI. At variance, the de-escalation consists of switching from ticagrelor or prasugrel to a reduced dosing regimen or switching to clopidogrel in order to decrease bleeding risk.[11-15] Both escalation and de-escalation approaches can be guided or unguided **(Table 4)**. The guided approach involves the use of genetic or platelet function tests to identify carriers of LoF alleles of CYP2C19 or assess the HPR status, respectively. The unguided approach involves escalating or de-escalating DAPT based on clinical considerations only (i.e., not informed by genetic or platelet function tests). For the de-escalation strategies, (1) Discontinuation [stopping one of the two antiplatelet agents and transitioning to single antiplatelet therapy (SAPT) such as aspirin or a $P2Y_{12}$ inhibitor monotherapy] **(Table 5)**, (2) Switching (changes from potent $P2Y_{12}$ inhibitors to less potent $P2Y_{12}$ inhibitors), and (3) Dose reduction (reducing the dose of prasugrel or ticagrelor in DAPT). There are different scores that can be used for stratification of HBR and high thrombotic risk such as DAPT score, PARIS score, Precise DAPT score, and ARC bleeding score for the determination of short versus long duration DAPT. DAPT score and Precise DAPT score as described in **Figure 3**. Short DAPT trial as shown in **Table 4**. **Table 6** shows what the ACC and ESC guidelines say for the monotherapy **(Figs. 4 and 5)**.

ISCHEMIC RISK

The clinical presentation is a critical factor to consider in the assessment of the individual ischemic risk profile. In addition to the pattern of CAD and the complexity of PCI, ACS inherently has a higher ischemic risk compared to chronic coronary syndrome.

Over the past four decades, endovascular devices and interventional techniques have undergone an extraordinary evolution, enabling the treatment of increasingly complex patterns of CAD as well as challenging patient populations. Clinical and angiographic characteristics associated with a higher risk of thrombotic events need to be considered when evaluating the type and duration of antiplatelet therapy. These considerations refer not only to DAPT following PCI but also to chronic maintenance antiplatelet therapy in the long-term period. The thrombotic risk stratification aids in identifying patients who would benefit from intensified antithrombotic treatment following standard DAPT duration.

Higher Thrombotic Risk Condition

- *Clinical characteristics:* Elder age, diabetes mellitus, current smoking, moderate-to-severe chronic kidney disease (CKD), previous MI or stent thrombosis, multivascular atherosclerotic disease, etc.

TABLE 4: Randomized clinical trials that evaluated DAPT escalation or de-escalation strategies (guided or unguided).

Test	Strategy	Study	Year	Patients enrolled	Clinical presentation	Follow-up	Experimental arm versus control	Primary endpoint	Primary endpoint reached?
Platelet Function Test	*Escalation*	PATH-PCI	2019	2,285	ACS: 0% CCS: 100%	6 months	Ticagrelor in patients nonresponders to clopidogrel versus standard therapy.	Cardiovascular death, MI, stent thrombosis, urgent revascularization BARC 1–5	Yes
		TRIGGER-PCI	2012	421	ACS: 0% CCS: 100%	6 months	Prasugrel vs. clopidogrel in clopidogrel nonresponders	Cardiovascular death or MI	No
	De-escalation	*ANTARCTIC*	2016	877	ACS: 0% CCS: 100%	12 months	Therapy guided by platelet function testing versus standard DAPT	Cardiovascular death, MI, stent thrombosis, urgent revascularization stroke, bleeding BARC 2–5	No
		TROPICAL-ACS	2017	2,610	ACS: 0% CCS: 100%	12 months	Therapy guided by platelet function testing versus standard DAPT	Cardiovascular death, MI, stroke, bleeding BARC 2–5	Yes
Genetic Testing	*Escalation*	*ADAPT*	2020	54 M	ACS: 50% CCS: 50%	16 months	Prasugrel or ticagrelor in patients nonresponders to clopidogrel versus standard therapy	Cardiovascular death. MI, urgent revascularization, stent thrombosis	No
		PHARMCLO	2018	888	ACS: 97% CCS: 3%	12 months	Prasugrel or ticagrelor in patients nonresponders to clopidogrel versus standard therapy	Cardiovascular death, MI, stroke, bleeding BARC 3–5	Yes
		TAILOR-PCI	2020	5,302	ACS: 69% CCS: 31%	12 months	Prasugrel or ticagrelor in patients nonresponders to clopidogrel versus Standard therapy	Cardiovascular death, MI, stroke, stent thrombosis, recurrent severe ischemia	No
	De-escalation	*POPular Genetics*	2019	2,488	ACS: 100% CCS: 0%	12 months	Genotype-driven de-escalation versus standard DAPT	Death from all causes, MI, stent thrombosis, stroke, major bleeding according to PLATO criteria	Yes
Unguided Approach	*De-escalation*	*HOST- REDUCE POLYTECH- ACS*	2020	3,429	ACS: 100% CCS: 0%	12 months	DAPT with prasugrel 5 mg versus DAPT with prasugrel 10 mg	Death from all causes, MI, stent thrombosis, repeat revascularizations, stroke, bleeding BARC 2–5	Yes
		TALOS-MI	2021	2697	ACS: 100% CCS: 0%	12 months	DAPT with clopidogrel versus DAPT with ticagrelor	Cardiovascular death, MI, stroke, bleeding BARC 2–5	Yes
		TOPIC	2017	646	ACS: 100% CCS: 0%	12 months	DAPT with clopidogrel versus standard DAPT	Cardiovascular death, urgent revascularization, stroke, bleeding BARC 2–5	Yes

Source: Thomas A, Gitto M, Shah S, et al. Antiplatelet Strategies Following PCI: A Review of Trials Informing Current and Future Therapies. JSCAI. 2023;2(3):100607.

TABLE 5: Randomized clinical trials evaluating the efficacy and safety of $P2Y_{12}$ inhibitor monotherapy.

Trials	Number of patients	Main inclusion	ACS patients	Timing of randomization	Experimental group		Control group	Primary endpoint (hypothesis)
					Duration and $P2Y_{12}$ inhibitor for DAPT	$P2Y_{12}$ inhibitor for SAPT	$P2Y_{12}$ inhibitor for DAPT	
GLOBAL LEADERS	15,986	CCD or ACS	47%	After DAPT	1 month, ticagrelor	Ticagrelor	Ticagrelor for ACS, clopidogrel for CCD	All-cause mortality or new Q-wave MI at 24 months (superiority)
TWILIGHT	7,119	High-risk patients	65%	After DAPT	3 months, ticagrelor	Ticagrelor	Ticagrelor	BARC bleeding type 2, 3, or 5 at 15 months (superiority)
SMART-CHOICE	2,993	CCD or ACS	59%	After PCI	3 months, any types	Any types	Any types	Death, MI, or stroke at 12 months (noninferiority)
STOPDAPT-2	3,045	CCD or ACS	38%	After PCI	1 month, clopidogrel	Clopidogrel	Clopidogrel	Cardiovascular death, MI, stroke, ST, or major or minor bleeding at 12 months (noninferiority)
STOPDAPT-2 ACS	4,169	ACS	100%	After PCI	1–2 months, clopidogrel	Clopidogrel	Clopidogrel	Cardiovascular death, MI, stroke, or ST or major or minor bleeding at 12 months (noninferiority)
STOPDAPT-3	5,966	ACS or high bleeding risk	75%	After PCI	Aspirin was discontinued immediately after PCI	Prasugrel	Prasugrel	BARC 3 or 5 bleeding at 1 month (superiority)
TICO	3,056	ACS	100%	After PCI	3 months, ticagrelor	Ticagrelor	Ticagrelor	Death, MI, ST, stroke, TVR, or major bleeding at 12 months (superiority)
T-PASS	2,850	ACS	100%	After PCI	<1 month, ticagrelor	Ticagrelor	Ticagrelor	Death, MI, ST, stroke, or major bleeding at 1 year

(ACS: acute coronary syndrome; BARC: bleeding Academic Research Consortium; CCD: chronic coronary disease; DAPT: dual antiplatelet therapy; MI: myocardial infarction; PCI: percutaneous coronary intervention; SAPT: single antiplatelet therapy; ST: stent thrombosis; TVR: target-vessel revascularization).

TABLE 6: Current guidelines for the use of potent $P2Y_{12}$ inhibitor monotherapy.

Guidelines	Recommendations
2021 ACC/AHA/SCAI guideline for coronary artery revascularization	In selected patients undergoing PCI, shorter duration DAPT (1–3 months) is reasonable, with subsequent transition to $P2Y_{12}$ inhibitor monotherapy to reduce the risk of bleeding events (Class 2a, level of evidence A)
2023 ESC guidelines for the management of acute coronary syndromes	In patients who are event-free after 3–6 months of DAPT and who are not high ischemic risk, single antiplatelet therapy (preferably with a $P2Y_{12}$-receptor inhibitor) should be considered (Class IIa, level of evidence A)
	In HBR patients, aspirin or $P2Y_{12}$-receptor inhibitor monotherapy after 1 month of DAPT may be considered (Class IIb, Level of evidence B)

(ACS: acute coronary syndrome; DAPT: dual antiplatelet therapy; HBR: high bleeding risk)

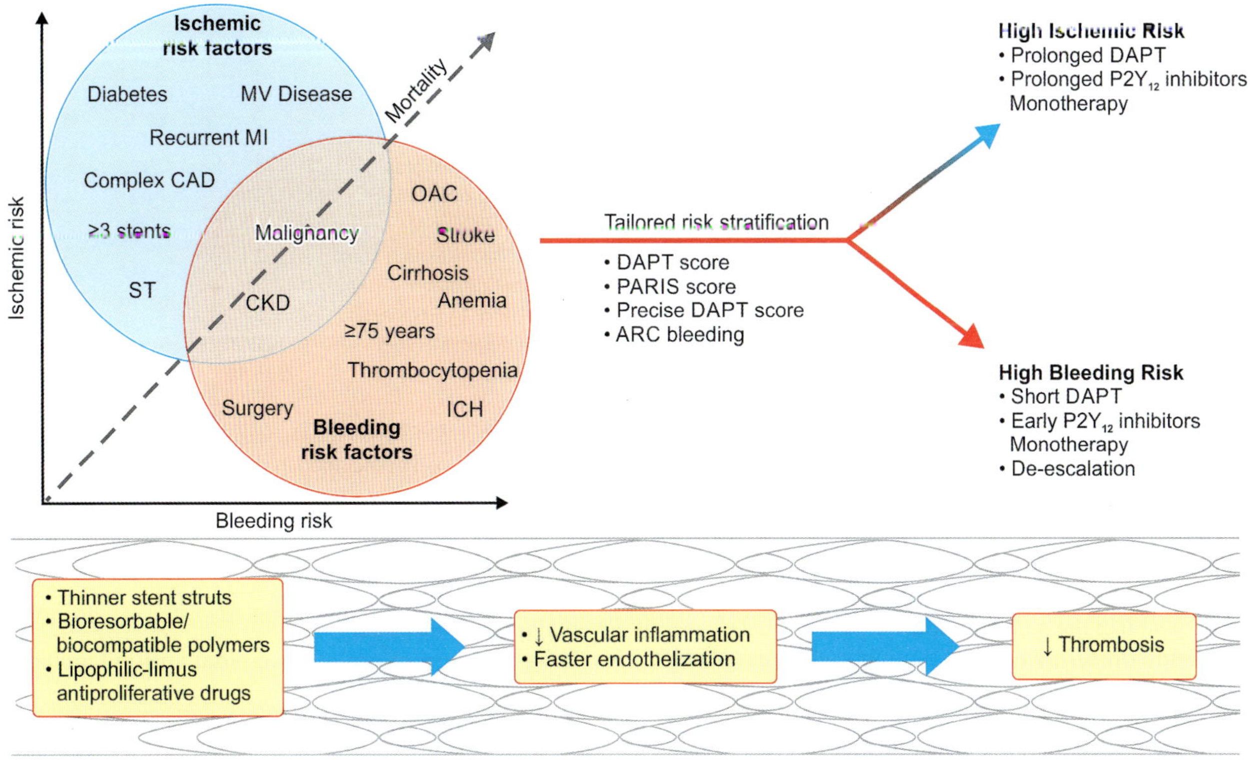

FIG. 4: Central illustration. Tailored antiplatelet strategies in the contemporary drug-eluting stents era.

(ARC: Academic Research Consortium; CAD: coronary artery disease; CKD: chronic kidney disease; DAPT: dual antiplatelet therapy; ICH: intracranial hemorrhage; MI: myocardial infarction; MV: multivessel; OAC: oral anticoagulation; PZY12: P2Y purinoceptor 12; PARIS: patterns of nonadherence to antiplatelet regimen in stented patients; ST: stent thrombosis)

Source: Adapted from Thomas A, Gitto M, Shah S, et al. Antiplatelet Strategies Following PCI: A Review of Trials Informing Current and Future Therapies. JSCAI. 2023;2(3):100607.

- *Procedural characteristics:* Implantation of three or more stents, treatment of three or more lesions, multivessel CAD, stenting of the last remaining patent coronary artery, treatment of the left main coronary artery, treatment of bifurcation disease with two stents, treatment of chronic total occlusion, stented length >60 mm, and mainly suboptimal results of PCI (stent malapposition, stent underexpansion, residual dissection, etc.).

Bleeding Risk

Major criterion for ARC-HBR include clinical diagnoses, which confer BARC 3 or 5 bleeding risk ≥4% at 1 year or a risk of intracranial hemorrhage (ICH) of ≥1% at 1 year:

- Long-term oral anticoagulation
- Severe or end-stage CKD [estimated glomerular filtration rate (eGFR) <30 mL/min]

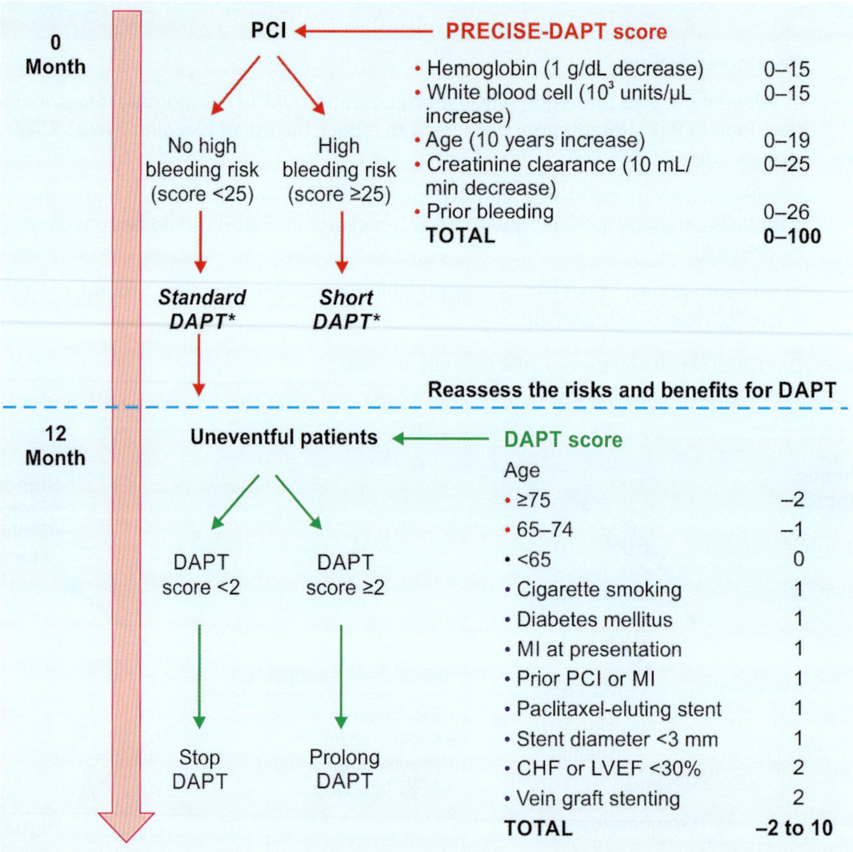

*In the validation study, short-term DAPT consisted of 3–6 months of therapy and standard DAPT consisted of at least 12 months of DAPT.

FIG. 5: Decision making on DAPT duration based on PRECISE-DAPT and DAPT scores. Variables included in the scores are associated with increased bleeding risk (red dot), increased ischemic risk (blue dot) or neutral effect (black dot).

- Hemoglobin <11 g/dL
- Spontaneous bleeding requiring hospitalization and transfusion in the past 6 months
- Moderate-to-severe baseline thrombocytopenia (platelet count <100 × 109/L)
- Chronic bleeding diathesis
- Liver cirrhosis with portal hypertension
- Active cancer in the past 12 months
- Previous spontaneous ICH (at any time)
- Previous traumatic ICH within the past 12 months
- Presence of known brain arteriovenous malformations
- Moderate-to-severe ischemic stroke within the past 6 months
- Nondeferrable major surgery on DAPT
- Recent major surgery or trauma within 30 days before PCI

Minor criterion for ARC-HBR is defined as any criterion that, in isolation, is considered to confer increased bleeding risk, with a BARC 3 or 5 bleeding rate of <4% at 1 year:

- Age >75 years
- Moderate CKD (eGFR 30–59 mL/min)
- Hemoglobin 11–12.9 g/dL for men and 11–11.9 g/dL for women.
- Spontaneous bleeding requiring hospitalization or transfusion within the past 12 months not meeting major criterion.
- Long-term use of oral nonsteroidal anti-inflammatory drugs or steroids.
- Any ischemic stroke at any time not meeting major criterion.

SWITCHING BETWEEN ORAL $P2Y_{12}$ INHIBITORS

The transition from clopidogrel to ticagrelor is the only switch between $P2Y_{12}$ inhibitors that has been investigated in a trial powered for the clinical endpoint, even if the study was not explicitly designed to assess the safety and efficacy of the transition from clopidogrel to ticagrelor. As the need to switch between $P2Y_{12}$ inhibitors may arise for clinical reasons (i.e., side effects or drug intolerance), and registry data indicate that switching is not infrequent in practice, switching algorithms based on pharmacodynamic studies are provided in both acute and chronic setting according to ESC guideline **(Figs. 6A and B)**.

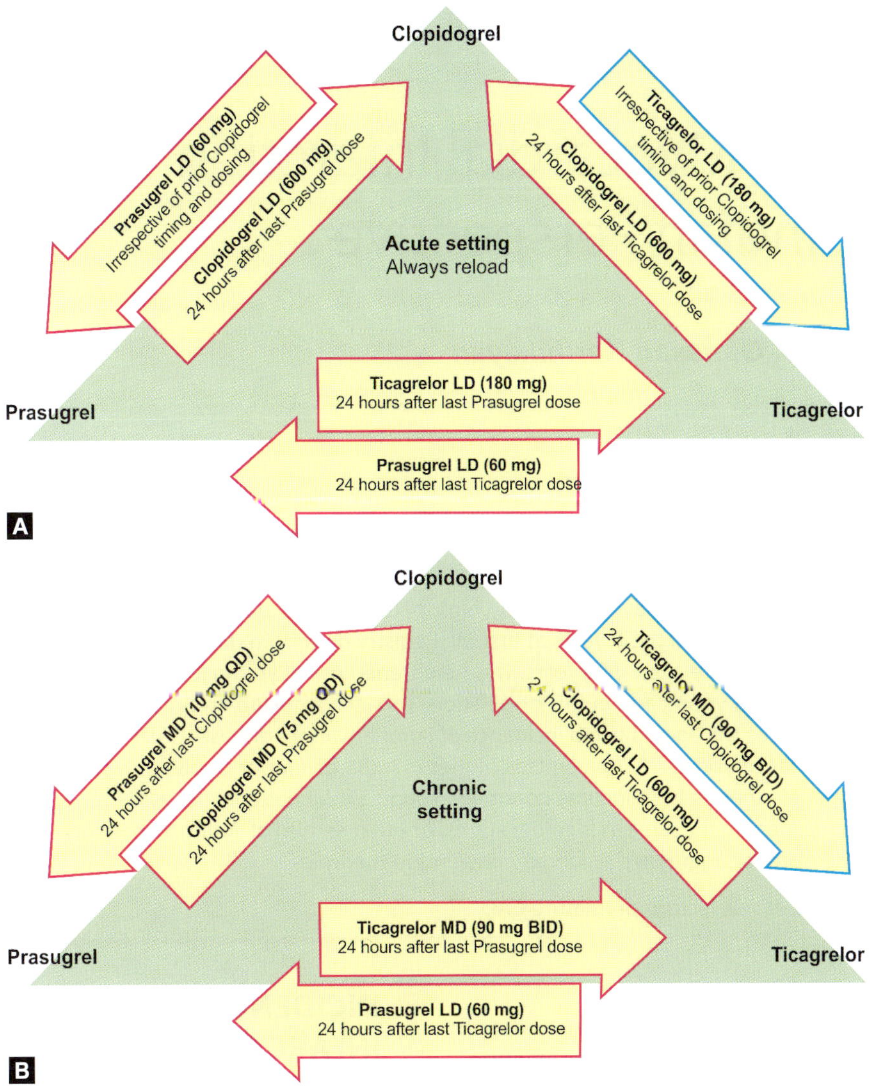

FIGS. 6A AND B: Switching algorithms based on pharmacodynamic studies are provided in both acute and chronic setting according to ESC guidelines.

CONCLUSION

- The net benefit of dual antiplatelet therapy depends on the balance between the individual risks of thrombosis and bleeding.
- Current European guidelines recommend for most patients undergoing PCI with DES implantation a period of DAPT of 6 months with aspirin and clopidogrel if the index clinical presentation is a chronic coronary syndrome and 12 months with aspirin and ticagrelor or prasugrel if an acute coronary syndrome (ACS).
- Advances in DES technology and PCI optimization have substantially reduced the risk of target lesion failure and several recent randomized trials have shown that 1–3 months of DAPT can be sufficient.
- In the setting of ACS, DAPT de-escalation is a viable alternative to short DAPT duration.
- There is still uncertainty about the preferred antithrombotic monotherapy after DAPT, with recent data indicating a possible advantage of using a $P2Y_{12}$ inhibitor over the traditional therapy with aspirin.
- Patients with high thrombotic risk may benefit from prolonged DAPT and potent $P2Y_{12}$ inhibitors.

ONLINE REFERENCES

Please scan the QR code provided at the end of the table of contents for References of this chapter.

CHAPTER

125

ST-elevation Myocardial Infarction in Young: Indian Perspective

Mohsin Raj Mantoo, Ganesan Karthikeyan

ABSTRACT

South Asian countries including India have a relatively high percentage of patients with "young" myocardial infarction (MI), defined as age less than or equal to 50 years at first MI. Registry data from different parts of India report that around 20–30% of ST-elevation MI cases are aged < 50 years. This heightened risk of young MI is largely explained by early accrual of conventional risk factors at a young age in this population. Tobacco smoking and dyslipidemia are the most common risk factors for young MI. While the age-adjusted incidence of coronary artery disease (CAD) in young patients is not higher in India, the overall number of young CAD patients is higher in India given our population structure, which has a larger proportion of young people than in high-income countries. Young STEMI patients generally have less extensive coronary disease. Treatment guidelines are the same as for older adults. About one third of young MI patients get a recurrent ischemic event, highlighting the need for aggressive secondary prevention therapies.

Keywords: Young MI, STEMI, risk factors, premature CAD

INTRODUCTION

There is no single age cut-point for defining "premature" or "young" myocardial infarction (MI). First MI at an age of ≤50 years is considered "young" and MI at ≤40 years is considered "very young" as per YOUNG-MI registry.[1] A more traditional teaching considers coronary artery disease (CAD) as premature if it occurs before 55 years of age in men or 65 years of age in women. South Asians are at a higher risk of premature CAD and are reported to experience their first MI at an average 5 years younger age than other populations.[2] South Asians living in developed countries have a higher age-adjusted incidence of MI as well as rates of hospitalizations and mortality as compared to other ethnic groups.[3,4] Premature CAD affects the most productive years of life and has enormous economic implications for the patient and nation as a whole. This chapter gives an overview of the available literature on young MI, with special emphasis on data from India.

INCIDENCE OF MYOCARDIAL INFARCTION IN YOUNG

Age is an important risk factor for CAD. The 10-year incidence rates of MI in the landmark Framingham heart study (n = 5,127) were 12.9, 38.2, and 71.2 per 1,000 for men in the age groups 30–34, 35–44, and 45–54 years, respectively, and 2.2, 5.2, and 13 per 1,000 for women in the corresponding age groups. In comparison, the incidence rates were much higher in the age groups 55–64 and 65–74 years as 108 and 141 per 1,000 for men, and 47 and 56 per 1,000, respectively.[5] The proportion of young patients in different MI registries varies from 5 to 20% depending on the age cutoffs used. In the relatively older Coronary Artery Surgery Study (CASS) registry enrolling 8,839 patients with MI, there were 294 men <35 years of age and 210 women <45 years of age, i.e., around 5% patients were young MI.[6] In the YOUNG-MI registry which enrolled 2,097 consecutive young patients in 2 large academic hospitals of the United States, 431 (20.5%) patients were 40 years old or younger at the time of first MI.[1] Further, this proportion of very young MI patients increased over the study period (2000–2016) at an average rate of 1.7% per year.

MYOCARDIAL INFARCTION IN THE YOUNG—INDIAN DATA

In a multinational case-control study, the mean age at first MI in South Asians (53 ± 11.4 years) was 5 years less than in their counterparts (58.8 ± 12.2 years).[2] In a large acute coronary syndrome (ACS) registry from the state of Kerala with data on 25,748 consecutive ACS admissions, around 22% cases were <50 years old.[7] Similarly, in another large prospective multicenter registry (CREATE) enrolling >20,000 ACS patients from India, 30% of all cases were <50 years old. ST-elevation myocardial infarction (STEMI) was the most common diagnosis (60.6% of ACS) and 34% of these patients were <50 years old.[8] **Table 1** depicts the proportion of young MI patients reported in different ACS registries from India.

The proportion of young people with MI in cross-sectional studies does not provide data regarding the incidence of young MI. There are no prospective studies that have reported on the risk of MI in young people in India. The Global Burden of Disease (GBD) Study reports data on the incidence of CAD (a large proportion of which could represent MI). Despite the obvious limitation in the interpretation of these data, they provide the only information on the occurrence of new MI by age groups. These data suggest that the incidence of CAD in India is 341 new cases per 100,000 which is same as that of high-income countries—344 new cases per 100,000. However, the overall burden of CAD in India is on a rising trend in contrast to that in high-income countries where it is declining **(Fig. 1A)**. The age-adjusted incidence rate of CAD in the age group 50–69 years is much higher in India than in high-income countries, 1,267 versus 453 new cases per 100,000 **(Fig. 1B)**. Same is true for population older than 70 years, with incidence of ischemic heart disease (IHD) 3,128 new cases per 100,000 versus 1,519 per 100,000 in high-income countries. The incidence of CAD in the age group 15–49 years is 60 new cases per 100,000 in India which is similar to that of high-income countries—57 per 100,000 **(Fig. 2)**. Therefore, the incidence of CAD is higher in India in people aged 50 years and older and not in young Indians, contrary to the popular belief. Also, the rate of CAD in young population is not rising in particular, in contrast to conventional thinking. The overall number of young patients with CAD will be higher in India given our population structure which has a larger proportion of young people than in high-income countries.

THE RISK FACTORS OF MYOCARDIAL INFARCTION IN YOUNG

The risk factors for MI in young adults are generally the same as in older individuals with a few key differences. Smoking, dyslipidemia, substance abuse, and a positive family history are more common risk factors in young MI patients, while hypertension and diabetes are relatively less common.[13] Tobacco smoking is the most common risk factor for premature CAD, present in 50–60% of subjects enrolled in registries.[14,15] Smokers are more likely to present with STEMI, and have high rates of substance abuse and a trend toward higher mortality. Smoking cessation produced an overwhelming 75% relative risk reduction in all-cause and cardiovascular mortality in patients enrolled in YOUNG-MI registry.[15]

A significant proportion of premature CAD patients have inherited dyslipidemias.[13] Familial hypercholesterolemia (FH), familial combined hyperlipidemia (FCH), and elevated lipoprotein(a) were present in 9.1%, 12.5%, and 19.4% of young (men < 50 years old and women < 55 years old) CAD patients, respectively, in a recent prospective study.[16] In another series of 382 young MI patients (age < 40 years), 21.2% had definite or probable heterozygous FH, characterized by high levels of low-density lipoprotein (LDL) cholesterol, ApoB, and lipoprotein(a). This subgroup of patients had more extensive CAD angiographically.[17] Several studies point to a significant association of elevated lipoprotein(a) level and premature MI. The blood level of Lp(a) is based on the genetic expression of its gene, and tends to remain stable in an individual's lifetime. Therefore, individuals with high Lp(a) level are predisposed to accumulating CAD risk from a very early age. In an analysis from YOUNG-MI registry, 20% of enrolled subjects had Lp(a)

TABLE 1: Proportion of "young" MI patients in Indian registries.

Study and year	Place	Sample size	Age cutoff (years)	Young MI (%)
Siwach et al.[9]	Rohtak	338	<40	19.2
Xavier et al. (CREATE)[8]	50 cities	20,937	<50	30
Mohanan et al. (Kerala ACS)[7]	Kerala	25,748	<50	22.2
Deora et al.[10]	Bengaluru	8,268	<40	10
Sharma et al.[11]	Jaipur	4,672	<55	25
Singh et al.[12]	Ludhiana	977	<45	12.8

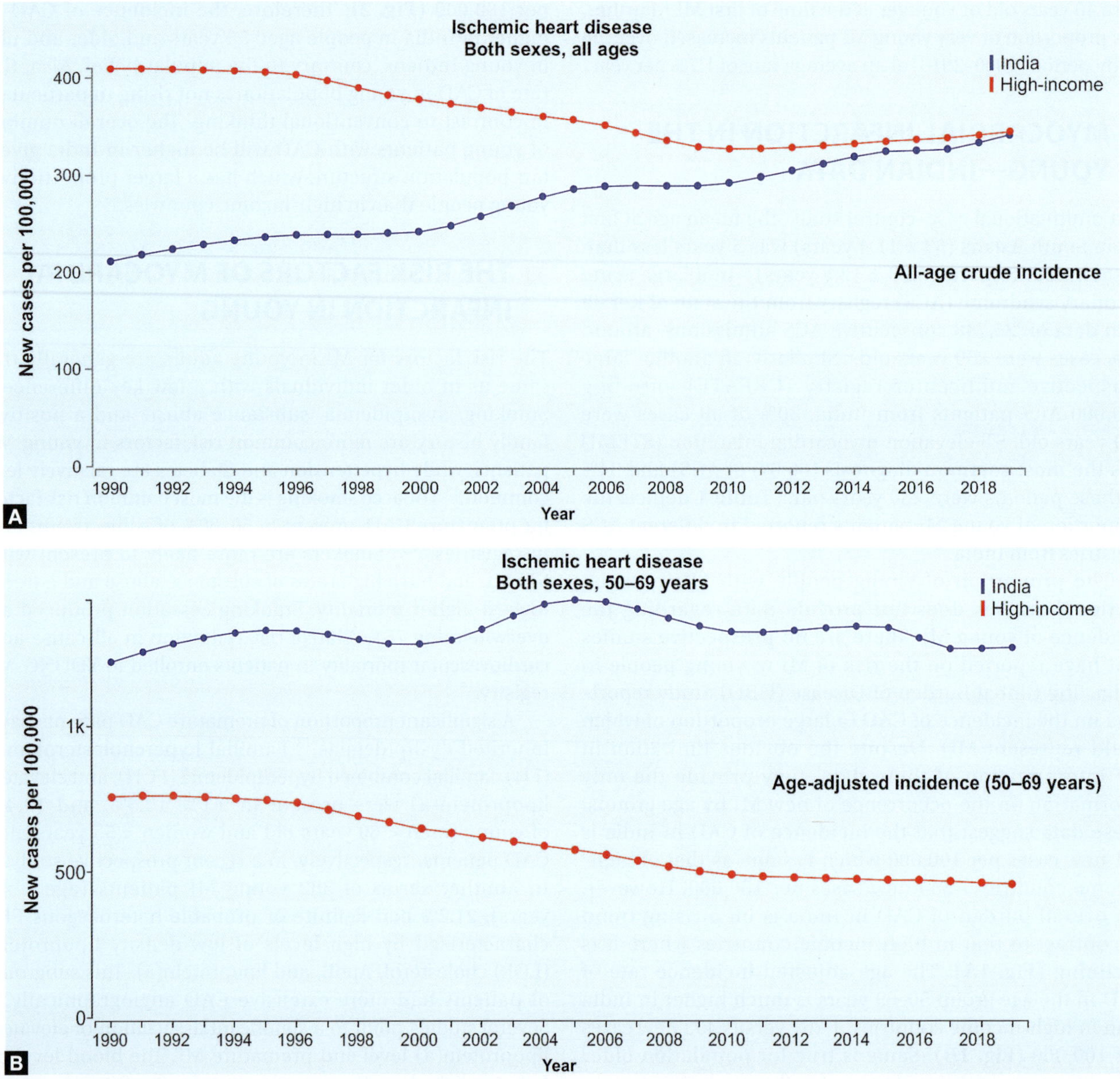

FIGS. 1A AND B: (A) Crude all-age incidence of ischemic heart disease (IHD) in India as compared to that in high-income nations; (B) Age-adjusted (age group 50–69 years) incidence of IHD in India compared to high-income nations. Note the higher incidence of IHD in India compared to high-income nations where the incidence is decreasing over the past couple of decades.

Source: IHME. GBD compare. [online] Available from https://vizhub.healthdata.org/gbd-compare/. [Last accessed September, 2024].

levels measured. Nearly one in three young MI patients had elevated Lp(a) (value greater than 80th percentile), yet two thirds of these individuals were classified as low or borderline risk by conventional atherosclerotic cardiovascular disease (ASCVD) risk estimator.[18] Elevated Lp(a) has been reported to increase the risk of premature CAD by threefold over and above other risk factors.[19] In a recent systematic review by Tian et al., including 51 studies and >100,000 individuals, higher Lp(a) values were significantly associated with premature CAD [odds ratio (OR) 2.44; 95% CI 2.06–2.90). Lp(a) increased CAD risk in patients with FH and diabetes mellitus as well. Further, South Asians had a higher odds of premature CAD due to raised Lp(a) than Caucasians.[20] The societal guidelines on managing dyslipidemia also label elevated Lp(a) (>50 mg/dL) as a risk modifier and advise a discussion about statin initiation in individuals who otherwise may have borderline risk of ASCVD by conventional risk estimator.[21] Further, guidelines also recommend Lp(a) estimation in individuals with personal or family history of premature CAD or at least once in lifetime in every adult patients to identify those with highly elevated Lp(a) levels who may have an equivalent lifetime ASCVD risk as heterozygous FH.[22]

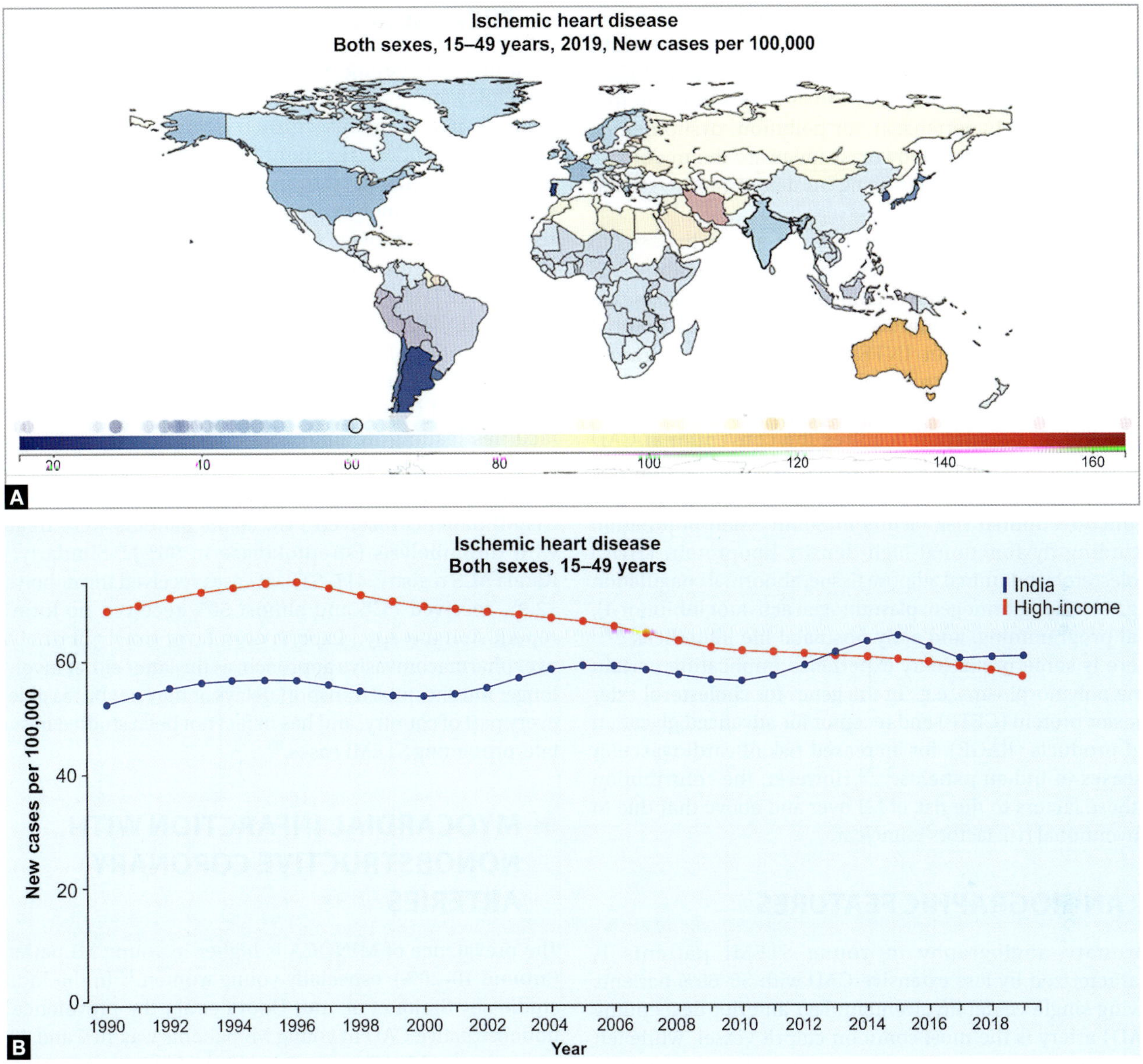

FIGS. 2A AND B: Age-adjusted (age group 15–49 years) incidence of premature ischemic heart disease (IHD) in India compared to high-income nations. Therefore, the incidence (number of new cases per 100,000 at-risk people) of young IHD in India is roughly the same as in high-income countries.

Source: IHME. GBD compare. [online] Available from https://vizhub.healthdata.org/gbd-compare/. [Last accessed September, 2024].

Substance abuse has been implicated as one of the risk factors for premature MI, besides other cardiovascular outcomes like stroke, arrhythmias, and cardiomyopathies. In a retrospective study of 2,097 patients who experienced first MI at <50 years of age, history of cocaine and/or marijuana abuse was present in 10.7%. This subgroup of young MI patients also had higher rates of tobacco use and worse cardiovascular and all-cause mortality.[23] There are also data that point to a significant association of lower socioeconomic status (SES) with higher rates of MI and deaths due to CAD. About half of this excess risk is attributed to higher prevalence of traditional CAD risk factors in the lower SES group.[24]

The age-adjusted incidence of CAD as well as cardiovascular death is higher in low- and middle-income nations including India. However, there is lack of large prospective registry data from such nations to understand specific risk factors. The INTERHEART study fills this gap in literature by enrolling patients from 52 different countries (covering all inhabited continents).[25] This study enrolled 15,152 cases of first AMI (irrespective of age) and 14,820 age- and gender-matched controls. The median age at first AMI was 53 years in South Asia as compared to 59 years in North America and 63 years in Europe. Raised ApoB/ApoA1 ratio, smoking, diabetes, psychosocial factors, hypertension, abdominal obesity, physical inactivity, and abnormal diet pattern collectively accounted for >90% MI risk in all patients, irrespective of age, gender, or country of origin.[25] Data from GBD Study from different Indian states indicate that unhealthy diet, hypertension, air pollution, dyslipidemia, dysglycemia, and high body mass index are the major risk factors responsible for increasing burden of cardiovascular diseases in India.[26]

Whether South Asian ethnicity per se predisposes to premature CAD is debatable. Studies done on South Asians living in Western countries highlighted their predisposition to get first MI at a younger age.[27,28] However, as pointed above, the data from INTERHEART study elegantly showed that >90% of this predisposition is explained by the cumulative effect of conventional CAD risk factors.[25] Asian Indian population acquires the conventional CAD risk factors at a young age, with a more exponential rise after the age of 30 years.[29] Recent reviews also highlight role of unconventional risk factors in South Asian population including dysfunctional high-density lipoprotein (HDL) cholesterol, abdominal adipose tissue, abnormal coagulation (e.g., elevated fibrinogen, plasminogen activator inhibitor-I), fetal programming, and early postnatal life influences.[30,31] There is some preliminary experience implicating certain gene polymorphisms, e.g., in the genes for cholesterol ester transfer protein (CETP) and receptor for advanced glycation end products (RAGE), for increased risk of cardiovascular diseases in Indian patients.[32,33] However, the contribution of these factors to the risk of MI over and above that due to conventional risk factors is unclear.

ANGIOGRAPHIC FEATURES

Coronary angiography in young STEMI patients is characterized by less extensive CAD with 50–60% patients having single vessel involvement. Left anterior descending (LAD) artery is the most common culprit vessel, while left main CAD is generally seen in <5% cases. There is a higher prevalence of myocardial infarction with nonobstructive (<50% diameter stenosis) CAD (MINOCA) in younger patients (approximately one in eight). Spontaneous coronary artery dissection (SCAD) accounts for about one third of women with young MI, especially in the peripartum period.[13,34] An intravascular imaging study in premature CAD patients reported that such patients have shorter target lesion length, less plaque burden, and more fibrotic, less necrotic, and less calcified coronary lesions.[35]

In an Indian study by Deora et al., including 611 young STEMI cases (age <40 years), single vessel disease was found in 56.6% of cases on angiography, while 29% had nonobstructive CAD. Double vessel and triple vessel disease were present in 10.8% and 3.6% of cases, respectively. LAD was the most common culprit vessel.[10] Similar findings are reported by other ACS registries enrolling young patients in India.[12,36]

TREATMENT

Treatment of young STEMI patients follows the same principles and guidelines as that of older adults.[37] Timely primary percutaneous coronary intervention (PPCI) is the recommended treatment for STEMI. In patients with anticipated delay of >120 minutes in PPCI, thrombolysis with a bolus fibrinolytic agent is advised. In the YOUNG-MI registry, STEMI patients aged <40 years had similar all-cause and cardiovascular mortality at 1 year and long-term follow-up (median 11.2 years) as patients who were aged 41–50 years at the time of first MI.[1]

Treatment of STEMI patients in India is suboptimal in general, characterized by long prehospital delays, interhospital transport, and lack of PPCI or thrombolysis facilities leading to almost 50% STEMI cases getting no revascularization at all. In the CREATE registry, median time to hospital presentation was 360 minutes and only 8% STEMI patients received PCI. 58.5% patients were treated with thrombolysis (streptokinase in 96%).[8] Similarly, in Kerala ACS registry, 41% STEMI cases received thrombolysis, 12.9% received PCI, and almost 50% received no form of reperfusion therapy.[7] Experts even favor timely fibrinolysis over pharmacoinvasive approach, as the latter either involves longer interhospital transport delays or may not be feasible in every part of country, and has in fact not been studied in such late-presenting STEMI cases.[38]

MYOCARDIAL INFARCTION WITH NONOBSTRUCTIVE CORONARY ARTERIES

The prevalence of MINOCA is higher in young MI patients (around 10–20%), especially young women.[13] In the Indian studies by Sinha et al. and Deora et al., the prevalence of nonobstructive CAD in young MI patients was 18% and 20%, respectively. MINOCA mostly arises due to acute plaque changes (rupture or erosion) with superimposed thrombosis in these otherwise nonobstructive coronary lesions. Such distinction of acute plaque changes is possible with the use of intravascular imaging modalities like optical coherence tomography (OCT).[39] The optimum treatment strategy of these nonobstructive culprit lesions is not clear. Aggressive lipid-lowering therapy is warranted in all cases. Dual antiplatelet therapy (DAPT) with aspirin and a P2Y12 inhibitor is reasonable in cases with plaque disruption. Initiation of other guideline-directed medical therapy (GDMT) agents like beta blockers and RAAS blockers may also be considered on an individual basis.[13] A randomized study evaluating beta blockers and RAAS blockers in MINOCA is ongoing (MINOCA-BAT trial). Whether to stent these culprit lesions or not is controversial. A small study (EROSION study) used OCT to identify ACS patients with plaque erosion of the culprit lesion and demonstrated safety of DAPT therapy while avoiding stenting of these lesions.[40] However, a recent consensus paper favors treatment of such nonobstructive ACS culprit lesions with a drug-eluting stent.[41]

PROGNOSIS

In the YOUNG-MI registry, in-hospital mortality rate of ACS patients in age groups <40 and 41–50 years was 1.4% and 2.2%, respectively. At a median follow-up of 11.2 years, all-cause mortality in these subgroups was 8.5% and 10.7%, respectively.[1] Collet and colleagues followed 888 premature CAD patients (aged ≤45 years) for 20 years and reported a recurrent event (mostly a second MI) in about one third cases. A small study from north India reported 1-year mortality and major adverse cardiovascular event (MACE) rates of 3.2% and 18.4%, respectively, in STEMI patients aged <45 years.[12]

CONCLUSION

The age-adjusted incidence of CAD as well as cardiovascular death is higher in India than in more developed countries. This higher burden of CAD at a relatively young age is explained by early accrual of conventional risk factors in the Indian population, rather than the ethnicity per se. Tobacco use and dyslipidemia are the most common risk factors of premature MI, besides unhealthy diet, ambient air pollution, central obesity, hypertension, and diabetes. Treatment protocols of young STEMI are the same as those for older adults. Only half of STEMI cases get any form of urgent revascularization therapy (mostly fibrinolysis) in India. About one third of young MI patients get a recurrent ischemic event in studies with available long-term follow-up. This emphasizes the need for aggressive secondary prevention therapies in young MI patients.

ONLINE REFERENCES

Please scan the QR code provided at the end of the table of contents for References of this chapter.

Invasive versus Conservative Management of Older Patients with Non-ST-elevation Acute Coronary Syndrome

CHAPTER 126

Dibya Kumar Baruah, P Chakradhar, D Anuradha

ABSTRACT

Diagnostic and therapeutic advances during the past decades have substantially improved health outcomes for patients with acute coronary syndrome (ACS). Older patients with non-ST-elevation acute coronary syndrome (NSTE-ACS) carry significant risk due to the complexities of coronary lesions, associated comorbidities, and bleeding risk. They are also less likely to receive guideline-directed treatment including invasive coronary angiography and revascularization. Though evidence-based recommendations for invasive treatment in this cohort are scarce, recent studies and meta-analyses support invasive strategy in older patients with NSTE-ACS with documented benefits of reduced reinfarction and repeat revascularization.

Keywords: Acute coronary syndrome, revascularization, percutaneous coronary angioplasty, older adults

INTRODUCTION

Coronary artery disease is the leading cause of death worldwide, with the greatest mortality burden observed in the older population.[1] It is predicted that the percentage of the global population aged 65 years and above is expected to rise from 10% in 2022 to 16% in 2050, with double the number to 1.5 billion by 2050.[2] With this global rising trend of older population, more patients are being treated for ACS including non-ST-elevation acute coronary syndrome (NSTE-ACS) worldwide. Adults ≥ 75 years of age constitute about 30–40% of all hospitalized patients with ACS, and the majority of ACS-related death is observed in this segment of the population.[3-5] However, guideline-directed treatment including coronary angiography and percutaneous coronary intervention (PCI) is less likely to be delivered to this group of patients due to the scarcity of data regarding the recommendation of different strategies in this cohort.

RATIONALE AND BACKGROUND FOR PCI IN PATIENTS WITH NSTE-ACS

Atherosclerosis is a chronic disease with the development of fibrofatty plaques in the coronary arterial wall, which usually remains silent for many years and may eventually result in the development of "vulnerable plaque" which is prone to rupture or erosion resulting in acute coronary syndrome.[6] ACS includes troponin-negative unstable angina (UA) and troponin-positive NSTE-ACS and ST-elevation acute coronary syndrome (STE-ACS). Long-term outcomes of NSTE-ACS are similar to STE-ACS and worse than UA likely due to the high prevalence of multivessel disease and a higher incidence of recurrent ischemia.[7] Evaluation of causes of ACS is essential when interventional treatment is considered, knowing the fact that PCI is not necessarily the only appropriate treatment option for all cases of ACS. Treatment of NSTE-ACS is based on two principles: (1) Immediate relief of ischemia, and (2) Prevention of progression to acute STEMI and cardiac death. This can be achieved with guideline-directed therapy that includes anti-ischemic, antiplatelet, and antithrombotic therapies with or without percutaneous coronary intervention **(Flowchart 1)**.

STRATEGY OF INVASIVE MANAGEMENT IN PATIENTS WITH NSTE-ACS

Various cardiological societies have extensively studied the pathophysiology of ACS and elucidated the strategy of an invasive approach in NSTE-ACS.[8-11] Recent updates have

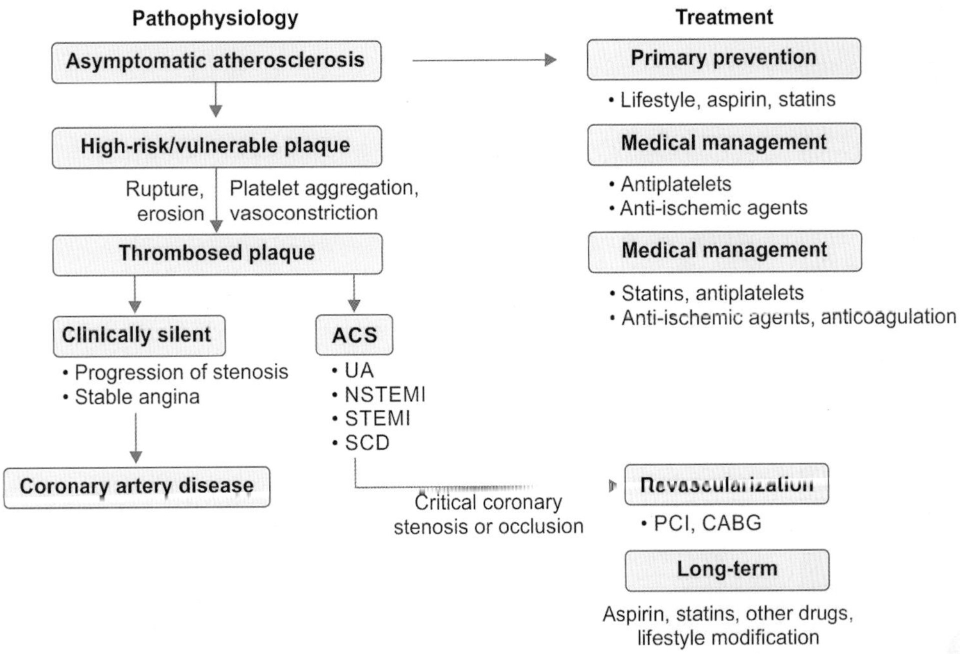

FLOWCHART 1: Pathophysiologic mechanisms of acute coronary syndrome (ACS) and treatment.
(CABG: coronary artery bypass surgery; PCI: percutaneous coronary intervention)

discussed and recommended the invasive strategy in a time-frame manner as well as in accordance with the risk status of the patient. However, no specific recommendation could be found concerning the older population who presented with NSTE-ACS, and most of the patients are being treated as per the general recommendations.

INVASIVE CORONARY ANGIOGRAPHY AND REVASCULARIZATION

Coronary angiography in ACS helps to diagnose the origin of chest pain due to myocardial ischemia, as a consequence of a culprit lesion or not. In the presence of a culprit lesion, revascularization with PCI or CABG can be performed in the same sitting based on the morphological features of coronary disease and risk factor profile of the patient. In the latter case, the exclusion of a culprit lesion paves the way to further diagnostic evaluations ultimately revealing the cause of chest pain and/or myocardial ischemia. However, invasive coronary angiography carries certain procedure-related risks and should be considered in the management decision.

ROUTINE INVASIVE VERSUS SELECTIVE INVASIVE APPROACH

In the strategy of a routine invasive approach, all patients undergo coronary angiography, whereas in the selective angiography strategy, coronary angiography will only be performed in patients with recurrent symptoms, objective evidence of inducible ischemia on noninvasive testing, or detection of obstructive CAD by coronary computed tomography angiography (CCTA).[12] Available evidence indicates that routine invasive strategy reduces the risk of composite ischemic endpoints, particularly in high-risk patients; does not reduce the all-cause mortality risk; and increases the risk of periprocedural complications such as periprocedural MI and bleeding.[13,14] In summary, risk stratification in the decision process and application of invasive strategy in high-risk patients are recommended which are supported by various randomized controlled trials (RCTs) and their meta-analyses.

Timing of the invasive strategy is based on the risk factor analysis, and immediate revascularization, within 2 hours of presentation, is recommended in very high-risk group of NSTE-ACS as per guidelines of various cardiological societies **(Fig. 1)**.

Internationally, an invasive strategy is being followed in the high-risk substrate of NSTE-ACS as per these guidelines; however, evidence-based recommendations for the care of older patients with NSTE-ACS are scarce and this is being highlighted as a significant gap in the evidence.[15] Older patients are at the highest risk of in-hospital deaths, bleeding complications, ischemic events, and renal complications and are underrepresented in various studies. In contemporary practice, older patients presenting with ACS are a heterogeneous group with clinical characteristics such as frailty, multimorbidity, and cognition that influence outcomes.[16] Coronary artery disease in older patients also has more complex and calcified lesions requiring complex

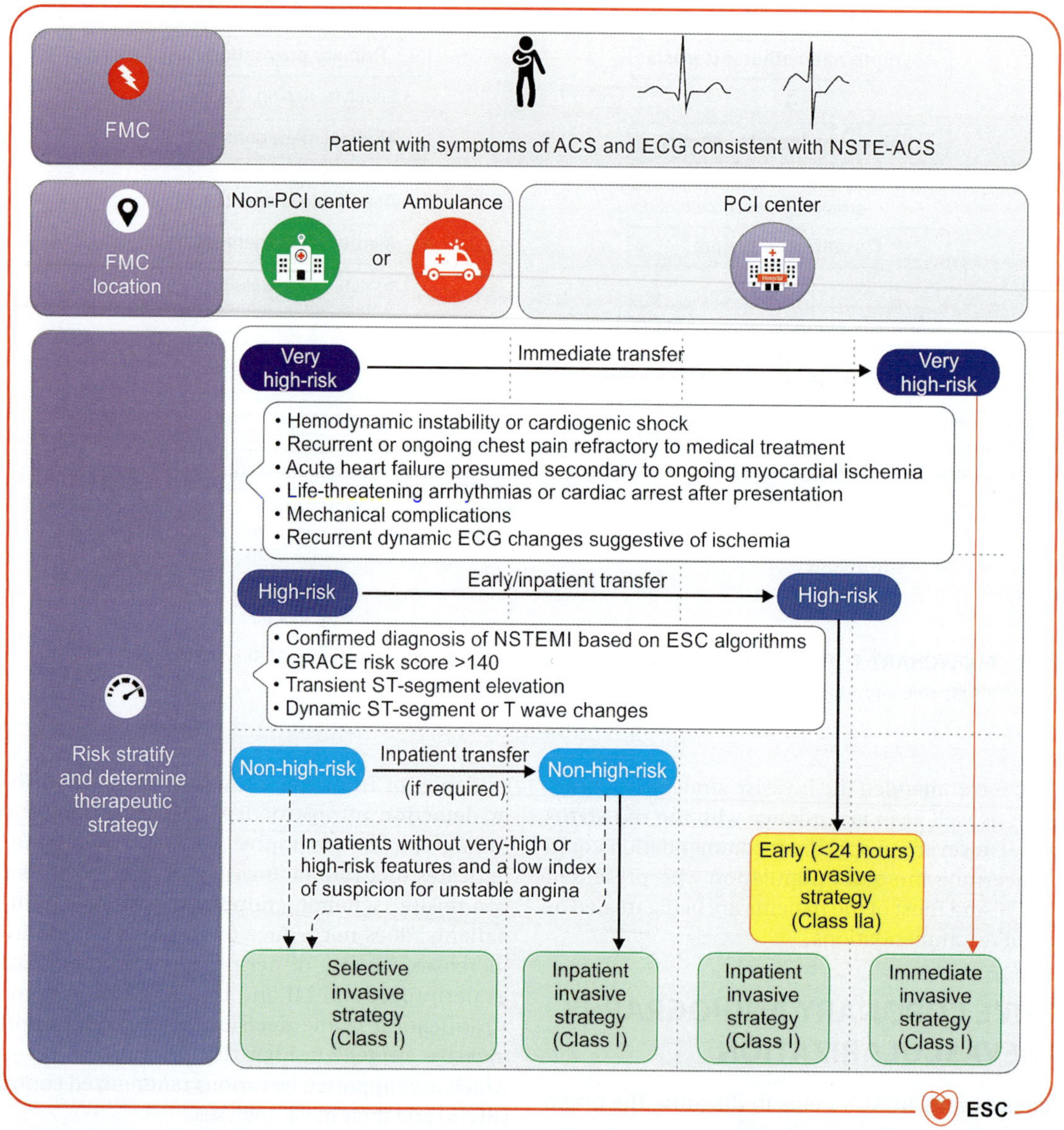

FIG. 1: Selection of invasive strategy and reperfusion therapy in patients presenting with NSTE- ACS.

(ACS: acute coronary syndrome; CS: cardiogenic shock; ECG: electrocardiogram; FMC: first medical contact; GRACE: Global Registry of Acute Coronary Events; NSTE-ACS: non-ST-elevation acute coronary syndrome; NSTEMI: non-ST-elevation myocardial infarction)

Source: Adapted from 2023 European Society of Cardiology (ESC) Guidelines for the Management of Acute Coronary Syndromes.

intervention in the presence of multiple comorbidities and high bleeding risk.[17] International guidelines recommend the same strategy of treatment in older patients as applied in the case of younger ones, and an invasive approach is indicated in patients with NSTE-ACS having a high risk of adverse outcomes based on risk factors.[18] However, older age itself is considered a negative predictor, and with frailty and the presence of comorbidities, they are less likely to receive evidence-based medication, coronary angiography, and interventions.[8,19]

There are limited studies comparing invasive treatment with a conservative approach in older patients presented with NSTE-ACS. Only six RCTs have been published comparing an interventional versus conservative approach in older patients with NSTE-ACS. Although limited by selection bias, registry data and subgroup analysis indicate that older patients with NSTE-ACS are likely to benefit from an invasive approach.[20] In the historical landmark FIR trial, a meta-analysis was performed of patient-pooled data from the FIR (FRISC-II, ICTUS, RITA-3) studies.[21] Results regarding a 5-year composite outcome of cardiovascular death or MI was associated with lower hazard in patients aged 65–74 years (HR 0.72; 95% CI 0.58–0.90) and those aged ≥75 years (HR 0.71; 95% CI 0.55–0.91), but not in patients aged

< 65 years (HR 1.11; 95% CI 0.90–1.38; p = 0.001) for interaction between strategy and age, and driven by an excess early myocardial infarction (MI) in patients < 65 years of age. In another largest randomized trial of 457 patients, invasive versus conservative treatment in elderly patients (≥80 years) who presented with NSTE-ACS was studied in the "After Eighty study" with a median follow-up of 1.5 years.[22] The primary outcome of death, MI, stroke, or urgent revascularization occurred in 41% of the invasive group versus 61% of the conservative group (p < 0.0001). Invasive therapy was beneficial for patients ≤ 90 years (HR 0.47), while it appeared harmful for patients > 90 years (HR 1.21, p for interaction = 0.033). Among elderly patients with NSTE-ACS, invasive therapy was beneficial in reducing adverse cardiovascular events compared with conservative therapy. This was due to a reduction in recurrent MI and urgent revascularization procedures. However, no mortality benefit was found in this study.

Given the paucity of adequate data, there have been significant discrepancies in the treatment of NSTE-ACS in elderly patients and deficiency has been always felt for proper scientific evidence regarding invasive versus conservative treatment in older individuals. A recent meta-analysis involved six randomized trials—Italian Elderly ACS, After Eighty study, MOSCA, 80 + study, RINCAL, and MOSCA-FRAIL, in which 1,479 patients of >70 years of age were studied for routine invasive strategy versus initial conservative strategy with 1 year follow-up.[23] This study is the first individual patient data (IPD) meta-analysis including all available trials that specifically enrolled older patients with NSTE-ACS. Compared to a previous meta-analysis (FIR study), consistent application of inclusion criteria in this study helps maintain the homogeneity of the included studies, ensuring that the pooled results accurately reflect the targeted research question, minimizing the risk of post hoc decisions that could introduce bias.

This study did not find significant treatment difference for the composite endpoint of all-cause mortality or MI during a 1-year follow-up period, with an incidence of 24.5% in the early invasive management group and 28.9% in the conservative management group and an unadjusted HR of 0.87 (95% CI 0.63–1.22; p = 0.43) using a random-effects model. A possible explanation could be related to the short follow-up restricted to 1 year or the heterogeneity of the population studied. However, MI was significantly lower in the invasive arm compared to the conservative arm (12.2% vs. 19.1%), indicating that early invasive treatment in older patients substantially reduces the hazard of a further MI within the first year (HR 0.62; 95% CI 0.44–0.87; p = 0.006). In addition, the need for repeat revascularization within a year of NSTE-ACS was substantially reduced in the early invasive management group compared to the initial medical treatment group [HR from random-effect model 0.41 (95% CI 0.18–0.95; p = 0.037)]. In conclusion, this study provides robust evidence that a routine invasive strategy is superior to a conservative approach in reducing the risk of MI and urgent revascularization at 1 year. It supports and strengthens the strategy of a routine invasive approach in the treatment of NSTE-ACS in older individuals.

CONCLUSION

Older individuals frequently have complex coronary artery lesions and present with competing risks of comorbidities, altered physiology, and vulnerability to both ischemic outcomes and bleeding events. Therefore, elderly patients presented with NSTE-ACS should undergo initial risk stratification, and a decision regarding treatment strategy should be reached based on the risk factors. Available scientific evidence supports a routine invasive strategy in older patients who presented with NSTE-ACS with the benefits of reduced risk of reinfarction and urgent revascularization, without significant mortality benefit.

ONLINE REFERENCES

Please scan the QR code provided at the end of the table of contents for References of this chapter.

CHAPTER

127

Latest Clinical Practice Guidelines for Non-ST-elevation Acute Coronary Syndrome: What is New

AN Patnaik, Soumya Patnaik

ABSTRACT

The American Heart Association/American College of Cardiology (AHA/ACC) has not published any full-scale "Clinical practice guidelines on management of NSTE-ACS" after its 2014 document. The European Society of Cardiology (ESC) published two guidelines in 2021 and 2023, which have recommended some modifications in the existing clinical practices in managing acute coronary syndrome (ACS). The main issues dealt with in this appraisal of these documents are role of cardiac troponins, early invasive versus noninvasive strategies, role of imaging, dual antiplatelet therapy (DAPT) issues, management of special subsets and comorbidities, and new approaches in secondary prevention. The endorsement for complete revascularization in index hospitalization is stronger than earlier recommendations for multivessel disease presenting as non-ST-elevation acute coronary syndrome (NSTE-ACS). Routine use of intravascular imaging and personalized antithrombotic therapies are possible recommendations in the near future in light of the exciting data emerging in recent years.

Keywords: Non-STE-acute coronary syndrome, clinical practice guidelines, antiplatelet therapy, intravascular imaging, multi-vessel disease, colchicine

INTRODUCTION

Acute coronary syndrome (ACS) is a spectrum of manifestations due to myocardial ischemia, ischemic injury, and the release of biomarkers to varying extents. It is traditionally been categorized into *unstable angina*, *non-ST-elevation (NSTE) myocardial infarction*, and *ST elevation (STE) myocardial infarction*. The 2018 joint task force of the American College of Cardiology (ACC), American Heart Association (AHA), European Society of Cardiology (ESC), and World Heart Federation (WHF) defined myocardial infarction (MI) as the presence of acute myocardial injury detected by abnormal cardiac biomarkers in the setting of acute myocardial ischemia. The fourth universal definition labels acute myocardial damage due to atherothrombosis (secondary to plaque rupture, ulceration, fissuring, or dissection as ACS). This encompasses two ECG descriptors—STE-ACS and NSTE-ACS, both clubbed as *type I MI* in universal definition. Unstable angina is a clinical syndrome like non-ST-elevation acute coronary syndrome (NSTE-ACS) but with no evidence for myocardial damage; however, it has the potential to progress to NSTE-MI or STE-MI and can be considered as a subtype of NSTE-ACS. In essence, any presentation of ACS not qualifying as STE-ACS can be considered as NSTE-ACS evaluated for myocardial injury and extent of the release of biomarkers of myocardial damage, risk-stratified, and follow an appropriate treatment.

The AHA/ACC has not published any clinical practice guidelines on the management of NSTE-ACS after its 2014 document. However, the guidelines by AHA on chest pain and revascularization in 2021 had a few newer messages for change in practices. The ESC published two guidelines—in 2021 (Collet et al.)[1] and 2023 (Byrne et al.)[2] which have significant practice updates **(Table 1)**. The recent guidelines preferred to consider STE-ACS and NSTE-ACS as a continuum of the same pathological process and condensed the management principles wherever relevant. In this chapter, we present an issue-based analysis of these clinical practice guidelines in the management of NSTE-ACS. The main issues dealt with in this chapter are early invasive versus noninvasive strategies, multivessel disease, role of imaging, dual antiplatelet therapy (DAPT) modulations, special subsets and comorbidities, and new approaches in secondary prevention.

TABLE 1: Major guidelines having a bearing on NSTE-ACS clinical practice.

AHA 2023	Chronic coronary disease
AHA 2021	• Coronary artery revascularization • Chest pain
AHA 2018	Blood cholesterol
AHA 2016	DAPT in patients with coronary artery disease (focused update)
AHA 2014	NSTE-ACS
ESC 2023	ACS
ESC 2021	• 2020 ESC guidelines for the management of ACS in patients presenting without persistent ST-segment elevation • CVD prevention
ESC 2019	• Dyslipidemias • Chronic coronary syndromes
ESC 2018	• ESC/EACTS myocardial revascularization • Fourth universal definition of myocardial infarction
ESC 2017	Focused update on DAPT

(ACS: acute coronary syndrome; AHA: American Heart Association; CVD: cardiovascular disease; DAPT: dual antiplatelet therapy; ESC: European Society of Cardiology; EACTS: European Association for Cardio-Thoracic Surgery; NSTE: non-ST-elevation acute coronary syndrome)

CARDIAC TROPONINS

As per recent ESC guidelines, one blood sample for troponins on admission is highly recommended (results expected in 60 minutes). A 1- or 2-hour sample is recommended to rule out NSTE-ACS. If earlier results are inconclusive, the additional sample is sent for analysis at 3 hours of admission.

Is Early-invasive Strategy Preferable?

The ESC 2023 advocates early (within 24 hours) invasive strategy for NSTE-ACS, if recurrent chest pain or dynamic ST changes are present, transient/intermittent ST elevation, in-hospital life-threatening arrhythmias, acute heart failure, or a GRACE (Global Registry of Acute Coronary Events) risk score > 140 [Class IIa; Level of Evidence (LOE) B].[2] This was a step down from Class I with LOE A, in earlier recommendations despite a large meta-analysis with more than 10,000 patients who underwent early invasive strategy showing reduced risk of recurrent ischemia and re-hospitalizations.[3] This approach is based on the lack of conclusive superiority of a routine early invasive strategy and the need to address the real-world logistics in patient—referrals to percutaneous coronary intervention (PCI)-enabled centers. Prior coronary artery bypass grafting (CABG) is generally considered a marker of higher risk when a patient presents with NSTE-ACS. There is a tendency for early invasive management even though there is no supportive evidence for such a practice. A recent meta-analysis of randomized controlled trials (RCTs) spanning 24 years found no significant clinical benefit of a routine invasive strategy in this group of patients.[4]

STAGING PERCUTANEOUS CORONARY INTERVENTION FOR MULTIVESSEL DISEASE

In STE-ACS, it is no longer a dispute to do preventive revascularization of all nonculprit lesions after successful primary PCI of the culprit lesion to reduce cardiovascular (CV) mortality and re-MI.[5] In patients presenting with NSTE-ACS and multivessel disease, staged PCI of all significant lesions should be considered preferably during the index procedure itself [Class IIa; LOE C] (ESC 2023). The strength of earlier ACC recommendation was weaker that suggested to consider multivessel PCI during index hospitalization [Class IIb; LOE B].

ROLE OF IMAGING AND OTHER TESTS

In stable suspected ACS patients, it was an accepted practice to do computed tomography coronary angiogram (CT-CAG) and exercise testing liberally. Their indication has been downgraded from Class I LOE B to IIa LOE A.[2] In MINOCA (myocardial infarction with nonobstructive coronary arteries), cardiac magnetic resonance (CMR) is recommended if the diagnosis is uncertain [Class I; LOE B].

To Guide PCI: Intracoronary imaging, especially optical coherence tomography (OCT) and intravascular ultrasound (IVUS) improved the precision in diagnosing the complexity of lesions and guiding the complex PCIs. Despite a number of trials favoring the use of OCT/IVUS, the older guidelines were not clear about their use for guiding the management of non-infarct-related artery (IRA) lesions. The 2023 ESC guidelines recommended the use of angiographic severity of non-IRA lesions to decide on PCI [Class I; LOE B]. In case of suspected spontaneous coronary artery dissection (SCAD), intracoronary imaging should be considered as per the prior guidelines [Class IIa; LOE A]. These guidelines also advised to consider coronary computed tomography angiography (CCTA) or noninvasive stress imaging as the initial workup, when a patient presents with ACS with equivocal ECG, high-sensitivity cardiac troponin (hs-cTn), and no recurrent anginal episodes.

Current guidelines, however, recommend OCT to clarify the atherosclerotic cause of ACS [Class IIb; LOE C] and to optimize PCI outcomes [Class IIa; LOE A]. The much-discussed four intracoronary trials—ILUMIEN IV, OPTIMAL PCI, OCTOBER, and OCTIVUS—have provided evidence for the incremental value of the use of intracoronary imaging techniques in complex PCI. These were also followed by a popular meta-analysis favoring the use of OCT/IVUS in complex PCI. Surprisingly, these robust findings did not influence the upgrading of the class of recommendation in the 2023 ESC guidelines. Some authorities felt that it was a missed opportunity in this document.[1]

DUAL ANTIPLATELET THERAPY AND ANTICOAGULATION ISSUES

There are no new recommendations on the initial loading doses of P2Y12 inhibitors or the established indications and contraindications in the recent guidelines. Ticagrelor or prasugrel is preferred over clopidogrel as per previous recommendations. Despite accumulating evidence of shorter DAPT, especially in patients with high bleeding risk (HBR), no recommendations were made on routine treatment personalization. The decade-old recommendation to give a P2Y12 receptor inhibitor in addition to aspirin [initial loading followed by maintenance for 12 months unless contraindicated or in the event of excess bleeding (Class I; LOE A)] remains unchanged in recent ESC guidelines.

For any patient with low ischemic risk, DAPT can be used for 3–6 months followed by aspirin or P2Y12 inhibitor [Class IIa; LOE A]. In the SMART-DATE trial (2018), 2,700 patients with ACS were assigned to 6-month DAPT followed by aspirin versus 12-month DAPT. The former arm was associated with an increase in nonfatal ischemic events with no significant difference in bleeding outcomes.[6] The authors recommended the 12-month DAPT be continued after drug-eluting stent (DES) implantation. In the STOP-DAPT 2 ACS trial (n = 4,169), clopidogrel monotherapy after 1–2-month DAPT was not proven equivalent to 12-month DAPT with respect to reduced CV events, even though bleeding episodes were lesser.[7] However, in a recent meta-analysis (2023) that included 11 trials (n = 9,006 patients) of HBR after PCI, a 1- or 3-month DAPT showed lower bleeding and CV mortality without increased ischemic events compared to a 6-month DAPT group.[8] In HBR patients, a 1-month DAPT followed by a single antiplatelet agent—aspirin or a P2Y12 inhibitor—is suggested as a possibility in the recent guidelines [Class IIb; LOE B].

The latest guidelines recommended that switching from potent P2Y12 to clopidogrel [de-escalation] may be considered after 1-month DAPT with ticagrelor or prasugrel [Class IIb; LOE A]. However, de-escalation before 1 month is contraindicated [Class III; LOE B]. The novel strategy of de-escalation was supported by two recent meta-analyses of similar patients.[9,10] In-patients who may require oral anticoagulant (OAC), antiplatelet therapy may be stopped after 6 months [Class IIb; LOE B]. Pretreatment (adding of oral P2Y12 receptor blocker to aspirin, even before coronary angiography is done) is often practiced, but there is no definitive evidence in its favor. The guidelines degraded this practice since 2020. The ACCOAST trial (2013) studied whether 30 mg of prasugrel before the coronary angiography could reduce the primary events of CV death, MI, stroke, urgent revascularization, or glycoprotein IIb/IIIa inhibitor rescue therapy. However, the results were not favorable to recommend such practice, and the bleeding complications were higher by pretreatment. When there may be a longer delay between pretreatment and coronary angiography, the potential for benefits is not ruled out. The pretreatment with Class IIb continues in the current guidelines.[11] The recent guidelines have not changed this recommendation. Similarly, pretreatment with GP-IIa/IIIb inhibitors is not recommended before knowing the coronary anatomy. In NSTE-ACS where early (<24 hours) invasive angiography is not anticipated, fondaparinux is recommended [Class I].[2] The new recommendations were included in the 2023 ESC guidelines for patients who had stopped DAPT before CABG. It recommends that DAPT should be restarted soon after surgery and continued for 12 months [Class I; LOE C].[2]

ATRIAL FIBRILLATION

If the $CHAD_2DS_2$-VASc score is >1 in men or >2 in women, an initial triple antithrombotic therapy (aspirin, clopidogrel, and NOAC), followed by NOAC and clopidogrel for 12 months is recommended following an ACS event. During PCI in such a patient, appropriate use of unfractionated heparin is recommended. Ticagrelor and prasugrel are not recommended as a part of triple therapy.[2]

ISSUES IN ELDERLY AND FRAIL PATIENTS

It is well established that patients more than 75 years are more likely to have more diffuse disease and severe coronary disease. Elevated cTn levels in the elderly are less specific and may cause error in assessment. Both ischemic and bleeding risks are high in the elderly. The elderly have higher adverse outcomes both in-hospital and within the first 6 weeks after discharge. A sizable proportion of ACS patients are elderly, but those above 75 years are under-represented in most trials. In the absence of robust data, the treatment approach is best individualized. As per the recent ESC guidelines, in the elderly who are potentially HBR patients, clopidogrel is the recommended choice over ticagrelor or prasugrel [Class IIb; LOE B].[2] The frail patients with NSTE-ACS have complex coronary disease, longer hospital stay, and higher mortality but less frequently receive full guideline-directed medical therapy (GDMT). Multi-comorbidities add to the challenges in the elderly and frail patients.

NON-ST-ELEVATION ACUTE CORONARY SYNDROME IN SHOCK

In those presenting with ACS and cardiac shock, an initial transthoracic echocardiography (TTE) is recommended [Class I]. Routine early CT-CAG is not recommended. However, in those with hemodynamic instability or shock, a conventional angiogram is recommended to provide early invasive therapy.[2] If multivessel disease is found, a staged PCI of non-IRA should be considered [Class IIa; LOE C] (ESC 2023) unlike earlier recommendations advising not to follow this strategy.[2]

SUDDEN CARDIAC DEATH SURVIVORS

Guidelines advise against routine immediate angiography in stable sudden cardiac death (SCD) survivors without persistent ST-segment elevation [Class III; LOE A]. This recommendation is mainly based on the results of the COACT trial.[12,13] Those who were comatose after surviving from cardiac arrest need a thorough neurological evaluation after 72 hours of admission [Class I; LOE C].[2]

NON-ST-ELEVATION ACUTE CORONARY SYNDROME IN PATIENTS WITH CHRONIC KIDNEY DISEASE

One in three patients of ACS has impaired renal function of significance. In the presence of CKD, there is lesser utilization of interventional and noninterventional therapies compared to those with normal renal function. An old analysis of 19,000 patients with NSTE-ACS with estimated glomerular filtration rate (eGFR) < 70 mL/min showed higher mortality at 30 days and at 6 months (10.5 vs. 3.4%).[14] There are data showing that early invasive therapy may be more beneficial than medical management in patients of CKD with NST-ACS.[15]

PREGNANCY

The diagnostic criteria and management algorithms are not to be much influenced by the presence of pregnancy. It is established that spontaneous coronary dissections occur more frequently in pregnant women. These situations need a multidisciplinary approach. Delivery may be postponed by 2 weeks if it can be achieved to reduce maternal mortality.[2]

CANCER PATIENTS

If cancer therapy is suspected to be contributing to ACS, such therapies may be temporarily interrupted [Class I; LOE C]. If the platelet count is <10,000/μL, aspirin is not recommended. If the count is < 30,000/μL, clopidogrel is not recommended; when the count is <50,000/μL, prasugrel and ticagrelor are not recommended.[2] Invasive strategy should not be denied if a high-risk ACS situation occurs in cancer patients who have expected survival > 6 months [Class I; LOE B]. If expected survival is <6 months or very HBR, a noninvasive strategy is preferred [Class IIa; LOE C].[2]

LOW-DOSE COLCHICINE

The role of inflammation in ACS has been rediscovered following the CANTOS trial. COLCOT and LoDoCO2 trials provided evidence for consistent benefits of colchicine in reducing CV events irrespective of the timing of prior ACS. Based on the recent evidence, a dose of 0.5 mg once a day may be considered if other risk factors are not satisfactorily controlled or if recurrent events occur despite optimal therapy [Class IIb; LOE A].[16]

POLYPILL

The recent guidelines considered poly pill as a good secondary preventive strategy to ensure medication adherence and better long-term outcomes [Class IIa]. This recommendation for secondary prevention following ACS gained strength from the results of the SECURE trial.[17] For long-term secondary prevention, evidence-supported medications like statins, beta-blockers, and antihypertensive and antidiabetic drugs have to be used as per standard guidelines and individualized to the clinical profile and tolerability of the patient. It goes without saying that lifestyle modification components are to be taken care of during secondary prevention.

CONCLUSION

Evidence-based new recommendations or modification of old strategies periodically is inherent to the practice of CV care; NSTE-ACS is no exception. An updated comprehensive guideline from the AHA/ACC is still awaited. The ESC is in favor of considering STE-ACS and non-STE-ACS as a continuum of the same pathological process and condensing the management of these two conditions into a single document. The endorsement for complete revascularization for NATE-ACS is stronger than before for multivessel disease. Routine use of intravascular imaging and personalized antithrombotic therapies are issues for the near future in light of new data.

ONLINE REFERENCES

Please scan the QR code provided at the end of the table of contents for References of this chapter.

CHAPTER

128

Hemodynamics of Cardiogenic Shock

Anil Dhall, Ayush Malhotra, Mahendra Chouhan

ABSTRACT

Monitoring in cardiogenic shock (CS) involves clinical, noninvasive, and invasive modalities, including clinical parameters, echocardiography, arterial catheterization, central venous pressure, and advanced hemodynamic monitoring for appropriate diagnosis, timely intervention, circulatory support, escalation, and de-escalation.

First-line monitoring is crucial for evaluating indicators of reduced blood flow and assessing symptoms. Echocardiography can identify etiologies such as left or right systolic dysfunction, severe valvular disease, or LV outflow tract obstruction. Advanced hemodynamic monitoring, such as pulmonary artery catheterization (PAC), is recommended for patients nonresponsive to initial therapies or those with RV dysfunction.

Broadly, we know that CS can complicate ST-elevation myocardial infarction (STEMI), can be seen in decompensation of known heart failure, or can occur as primary acute heart failure. The etiology is important as the therapy has to be directed toward the primary etiology. However, physiological variables help define prognosis and guide us on the path across various therapeutic options available. The advent of hemodynamics and etiology assessment by echocardiography was a landmark development but remains infrequent. Despite challenges in large trials, PAC and hemodynamic assessments offer the most accurate, continuous, and real-time evaluation. PAC is the mainstay of invasive hemodynamic monitoring, accurately determining filling pressures, diagnosing CS, and identifying normotensive CS in patients with clinical hypoperfusion and SBP >90 mm Hg.

Keywords: CS, noninvasive, clinical, invasive modalities, crucial, STEMI

INTRODUCTION

Hemodynamic monitoring in cardiogenic shock (CS) is cornerstone of its management. Though CS can have diverse etiologies, classically, there are two major subsets of CS, i.e., ST-elevation myocardial infarction (STEMI)/ACS shock and decompensated HF shock. The widespread use of mechanical circulatory support (MCS) is changing CS management and outcomes. Effective hemodynamic monitoring with pulmonary artery catheterization (PAC) can guide clinical decision-making for optimizing therapies for CS patients. Along with development of echocardiography, rampant use of PAC without standardized protocols with its inability to constructively use its hemodynamic data led to its failure to alter outcomes in clinical trials. The ESCAPE trial highlighted the same. The invasive and noninvasive data needed to be used in complementary fashion and it may be noted that ESCAPE trial did not recruit patients with CS. However, this had a demoralizing effect on routine PAC use in CS.

CARDIOGENIC SHOCK

Cardiogenic shock (CS) is defined by a cardiac index of <1.8 L/min/m^2 without support and <2.0–2.2 L/min/m^2 with support. Additionally, it is characterized by a systolic blood pressure below 90 mm Hg and indications of systemic hypoperfusion, such as elevated lactic acid levels, in the absence of hypovolemia. The European Society of Cardiology (ESC) defines CS as "the presence of clinical signs of hypoperfusion, such as cold sweated extremities, oliguria, mental confusion, dizziness, and narrow pulse pressure. In addition, biochemical manifestations of hypoperfusion, elevated serum creatinine, metabolic acidosis, and elevated serum lactate are present and reflect tissue hypoxia and alterations of cellular metabolism leading to organ dysfunction." CS may arise due to various dysfunctions, including myocardial, valvular, electrical, pulmonary arterial, or pericardial abnormalities, either individually or in combination.[1]

Despite more than two decades of advances in interventional techniques, the development of rapidly deployable temporary mechanical circulatory support (tMCS) devices, and systems-of-care strategies to treat AMI, patients with CS continue to fare poorly with 30–50% risk of 30-day mortality and associated multiorgan dysfunction.[2-7]

INDICATIONS OF HEMODYNAMIC ASSESSMENT

Heart Failure

Indications of hemodynamic assessment in heart failure are as follows:

- Differentiating between hemodynamic and permeability pulmonary edema or dyspnea when trial or diuretic or vasodilator has failed or is associated with high-risk
- Differentiating between cardiogenic and noncardiogenic shock when trial or intravascular volume expansion has failed or is associated with high-risk guidance of pharmacologic or mechanical therapy
- Guidance of therapy in patients with features of both forward and backward heart failure
- Determination of pericardial tamponade when clinical exam and echocardiography are conclusive
- Per operative management of patients with heart failure, undergoing intermediate or high-risk surgery
- Detection of pulmonary hypertension and guidance of therapy
- Indication of hemodynamic assessment

Myocardial Infarction

Indications of hemodynamic assessment in myocardial infarction are as follows:

- Differentiating between CS and hypovolemic shock when initial therapy with trial or intravascular volume and low-dose inotropes has failed
- Management of CS with pharmacologic and/or mechanical therapy
- Pharmacologic or mechanical management of acute mitral regurgitation
- Preoperative assessment of left-to-right severity in VSD
- Management of RV infarction associated with hypertension and or signs of low cardiac output, not responsive to intravascular volume low-dose, inotropes, and restoration of heart rate and AV synchrony
- Management of pulmonary edema, not responsive to diuretics, vasodilators, and low-dose inotropes

MONITORING IN CARDIOGENIC SHOCK

Clinical, noninvasive, and invasive modalities are used to determine the hemodynamic status of the patient. Clinical parameters are based on assessment of volume status, BP, congestion, and organ perfusion or organ system dysfunction. The clinical assessment alone can have several limitations (**Flowchart 1**).

Goals of monitoring:

- Characterization of the type of cardiac dysfunction and the degree of its severity

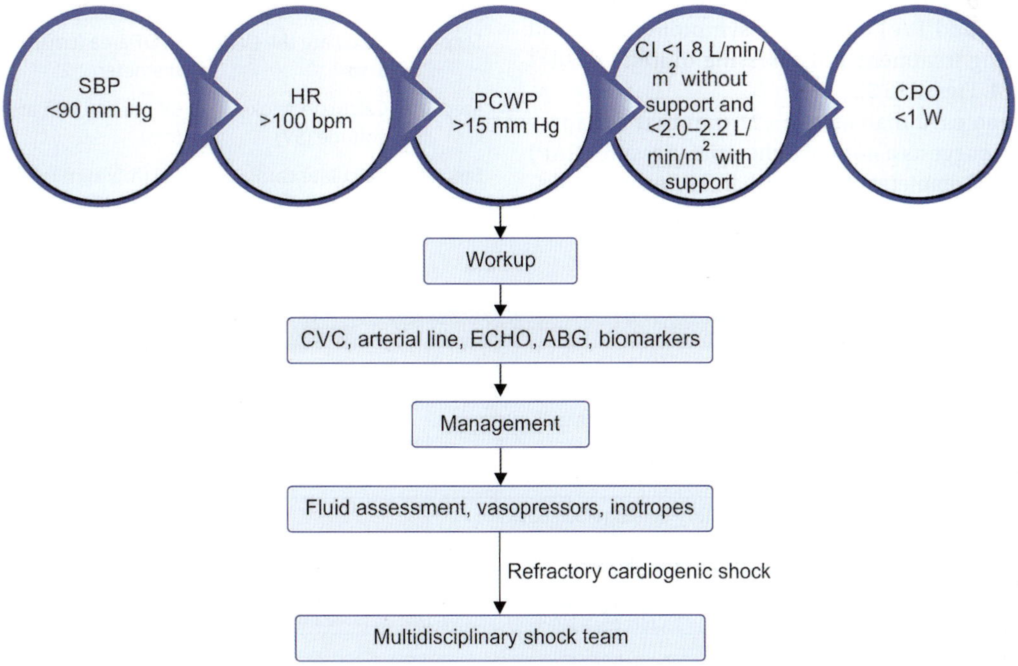

FLOWCHART 1: Diagnosis and management of cardiogenic shock.

- Very early detection of associated vasoplegia
- Detection and monitoring of organ dysfunction and tissue oxygenation
- Guidance for the introduction and optimization of inotropes and vasopressors as well as the timing of mechanical support

First-line Monitoring

In addition, it is essential to monitor urine output and conduct frequent electrocardiograms. Nevertheless, clinical examinations may be unable to estimate cardiac output, which is an essential parameter in the management of CS patients **(Fig. 1)**.[2]

Echocardiography

Echocardiography can identify the etiology, such as left or right systolic dysfunction (secondary to acute myocardial infarction, myocarditis, acute or chronic heart failure, or rhythm or conduction disturbances), severe valvular disease (endocarditis, aortic dissection, or chordae or papillary muscle rupture), or LV outflow tract obstruction.

Step-by-step Guide to Cardiac Output Measurement

A step-by-step guide to cardiac output measurement is given in **Tables 1 and 2**.

Echocardiography measures right and left filling pressures, fluid responsiveness, and pulmonary artery pressure. While most CS patients have increased LV end-diastolic pressure, hypovolemia may also be present in some situations. The assessment of right [inferior vena cava (IVC) diameter, respiratory changes, and hepatic vein] and left (mitral E/A and E/é) congestive symptoms is crucial for personalizing treatment and assessing diuretic need[3,4] **(Tables 3 and 4, Figs. 2 to 5)**.

Inferior vena cava diameter of <21 mm that collapses >50% with sniff suggests a normal right atrial pressure (RAP) (0–5 mm Hg). IVC diameter of greater than 21 mm with <50% collapsibility suggests elevated RAP (10–20 mm Hg). **Fig. 4A** shows IVC diameter is 17 mm and collapses >50%, suggesting normal RAP. In contrast, the **Fig. 4B** has a measured IVC of 30.4 mm and collapsibility is >50%, suggesting elevated RAP.

Echocardiographic evaluation of LV antegrade flow is given in **Figure 6**.

Per beat parameters:
- *Stroke distance (SD):* Represents LV contraction The most accurate in predicting mortality if ≤ 18 cm.
- *Stroke volume (SV)*: Represents volume ejected by LV in each beat.
- *Stroke volume index (SVI)*: Represent if the volume ejected is adequate for body surface area (BSA), has prognostic implication; normal: > 30 mL/m^2

Per-minute outflow parameters:
- *Minute distance (MD):* Independent from LVOT area, heart rate (HR) is taken into account; influenced by valve regurgitation
- *Cardiac output (CO):* Volume ejected by LV in 1 minute; depends on the LVOT area and is influenced by HR
- *Cardiac index (CI):* Represent if the volume ejected in 1 minute is adequate for BSA; normal > 2.0 L/min/m^2

Mitral Annular Plane Systolic Excursion

Mitral annular plane systolic excursion (MAPSE) is measured by M-mode echocardiography from four sites of the atrioventricular plane corresponding to the septal, lateral, anterior, and posterior walls using the apical four- and two-chamber views. The M-mode cursor should always

TABLE 1: Step-by-step guide to cardiac output measurement.

Step 1	Calculate the LVOT area	LVOT area (cm^2) = π × (LVOT diameter/2)2
Step 2	Calculate stroke volume (SV)	SV (mL) = LVOT area (cm^2) x VTI (cm)
Step 3	Calculate cardiac output	CO (mL/min) = SV (mL/cycle) × HR (bpm)

		Volume status	
		Wet	Dry
Peripheral circulation	Cold	Classic cardiogenic shock (↓CI; ↑SVRI; ↑PCWP)	Euvolemic cardiogenic shock (↓CI; ↑SVRI; ↔PCWP)
	Warm	Vasodilatory cardiogenic shock or Mixed shock (↓CI; ↑SVRI; ↑PCWP)	Vasodilatory shock (Not cardiogenic shock) (↓CI; ↑SVRI; ↑PCWP)

FIG. 1: The 2×2 Matrix for evaluation of cardiogenic shock.

TABLE 2: Various ECHO Doppler-based useful calculations.

Echocardiography parameters	How to calculate?	Normal values
Stroke volume (SV)	LVOT VTI × LVOT area	50–100 mL
Cardiac output (CO)	(LVOT VTI × LVOT area) × HR	5–6 L/min
CPO	(CO × MAP)/451	1 W
RAP	• Nondilated IVC with >50% inspiratory collapse = 3–5 mm Hg • Dilated IVC with >50% inspiratory collapse = 8–10 mm Hg • Nondilated IVC with <50% inspiratory collapse = 8–10 mm Hg • Dilated IVC wlth <50% inspiratory collapse = 13–15 mm Hg	3–5 mm Hg
Pulmonary artery systolic pressure (PAPS)	$(4 \times Vmax^2) + RAP$	<35
LV filling pressure [Medial early mitral valve inflow velocity to early diastolic annular velocity ratio (E/e' ratio)]	E/e'	<14

TABLE 3: Modalities to address perfusion parameters.

Perfusion parameters	Utility	Normal values
IVOT VTI and CI	A reliable quantitative parameter that truly reflects circulatory status and global end-organ perfusion	LVOT VTI2 = 18 cm CI> 2.5 L/min/m^2
LV GLS	A valuable and sensitive tool for follow-up examinations	LV GLS <-20%
RVOT VTI	Gives information about the right ventricle function and pulmonary vascular resistance	RVOT VTI = 12 cm
RV 2D FAC	Provides an estimate of global RV systolic function	RV FAC = 35%
TAPSE	Represents a measure of RV longitudinal function	TAPSE = 17 mm
TDIS'	Correlates well with other measures of global RV systolic function	S>9.5 cm/s
Global longitudinal RV-free wall strain	Useful for estimating RV global and regional systolic function	RV-free wall strain

TABLE 4: Modalities to approximate congestion parameters.

	IVC diameter	Used to estimate RA pressures	IVC <21 mm that collapses > 50%
Congestion parameters	TDIe'	Associated with increased mortality in the critically ill patients	Average e' ≥ 10 cm/s lateral e' <8 cm/s
	E/e'	A load-independent marker of LV filling pressure	E/e' < 15
	PASP	The most used noninvasive tool for estimating PAP	PASP > 35 mm Hg
	PAAT	Represents pulmonary flow acceleration, which increases as the vascular resistance is augmented	PAAT 136–153 ms
	PALS	An additional index of congestion to optimize therapeutic management	PALS ≥ 15%

be aligned parallel to the LV walls. The systolic excursion of mitral annulus should be measured from the lowest point at end-diastole to aortic valve closure (end of the T-wave on the electrocardiogram).[5,6] MAPSE represents the amount of displacement of the mitral annular plane toward the apex, and thus assesses the global change in size of the LV cavity (in the long-axis direction). The average normal value of MAPSE derived from previous studies for the four annular regions (septal, anterior, lateral, and posterior) ranged between 12 and 15 mm, and a value of 8 mm was associated with a depressed LVEF (<50%). A mean value for MAPSE of 7 mm could be used to detect an EF <30%. Note that the association between MAPSE and EF is only valid in case of normal or dilated left ventricle, but the correlation is rather poor in patients with LV hypertrophy **(Figs. 7A to D)**.[7,8]

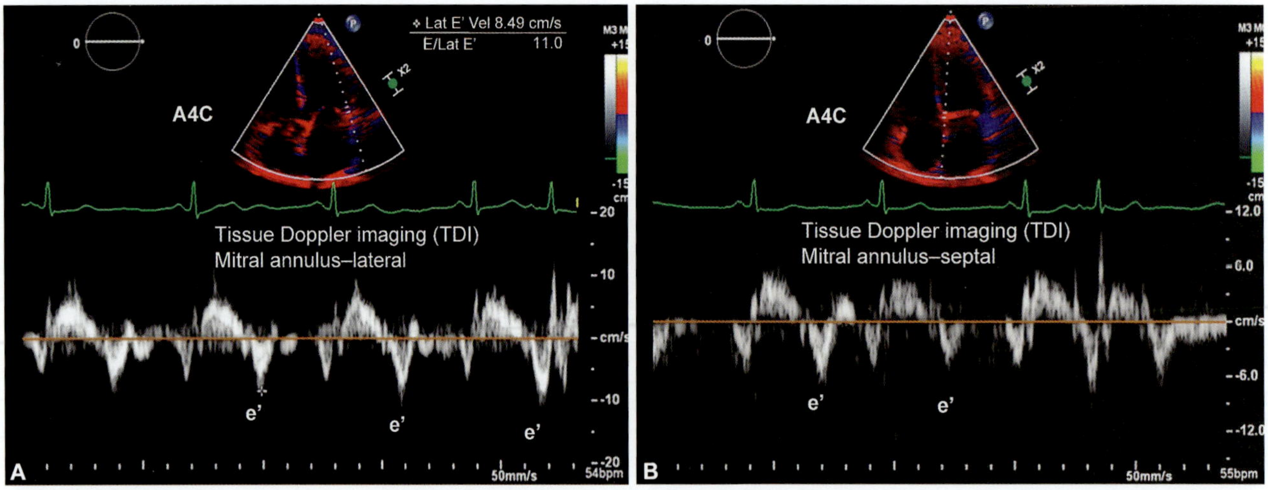

FIGS. 2A AND B: Lateral and septal mitral annular e' velocities using tissue Doppler imaging (TDI). The e' velocity corresponds to the velocity of tissue relaxation in early diastole. The average of lateral and septal velocities corresponds to the velocity of tissue relaxation in early diastole. The average of lateral and septal mitral e' velocities is used to calculate the E/e' ratio, which can be used to estimate LAP.

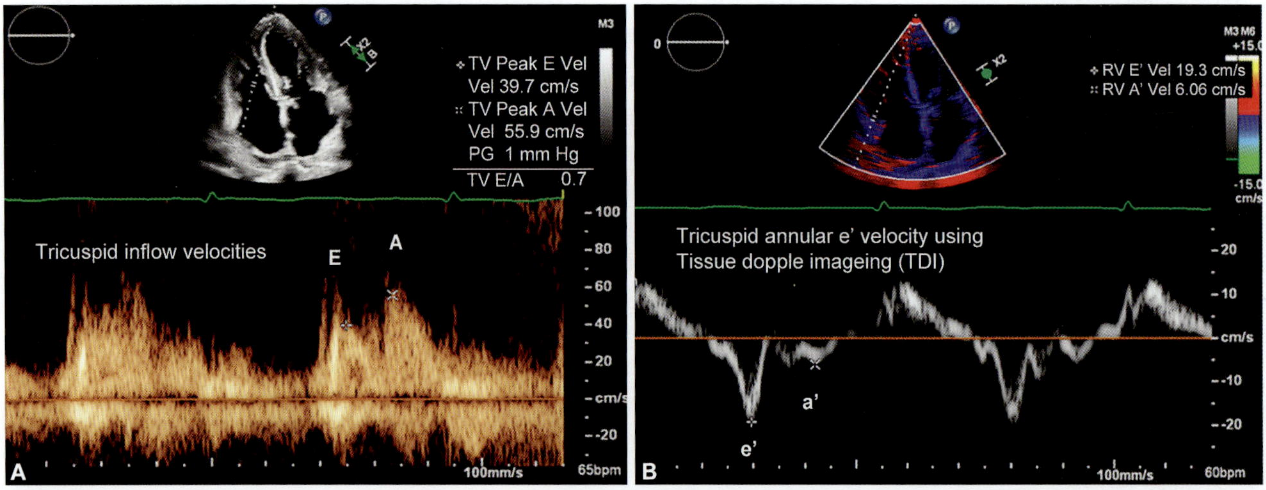

FIGS. 3A AND B: (A) Tricuspid inflow velocities. Apical four-chamber view. Pulse-wave Doppler sample volume is placed between the tricuspid valve leaflets at the level of the leaflet tips. Velocity tracing volume is placed between the tricuspid valve leaflets at the level of the leaflet tips. Velocity tracing below. E wave corresponds to rapid right ventricular filling. A wave corresponds to the right atrial systole. (B) Tricuspid annular velocity using tissue Doppler imaging. Tricuspid e' corresponds to velocity of right ventricular tissue relaxation. Tricuspid E/e' can be used to estimate RAP.

Arterial Catheterization

While the utilization of cuff arm pressure in a noninvasive manner is generally effective in evaluating mean arterial pressure (MAP), it is important to note that instances of severe hypotension and hypothermia can impact the consistency between noninvasive and invasive MAP measurements. A study conducted by Burstein et al. demonstrated that an MAP below 65 mm Hg, as measured using a combination of invasive and noninvasive methods, within the initial 24 hours of care for patients with CS, was correlated with an increased death risk.[8]

VExUS

Accurate measurement of central venous pressure (CVP) is critical for improving volume management in HF patients. In this context, measuring the IVC is the most popular noninvasive technique. CVP may be measured by measuring IVC diameter and inspiratory variability, which has been found to predict rises in RAP more frequently and accurately than physical inspection of the jugular venous pulse. In addition, there are various limitations in its analysis, such as mechanical ventilation, pulmonary hypertension, varied breathing patterns during spontaneous ventilation, and lung

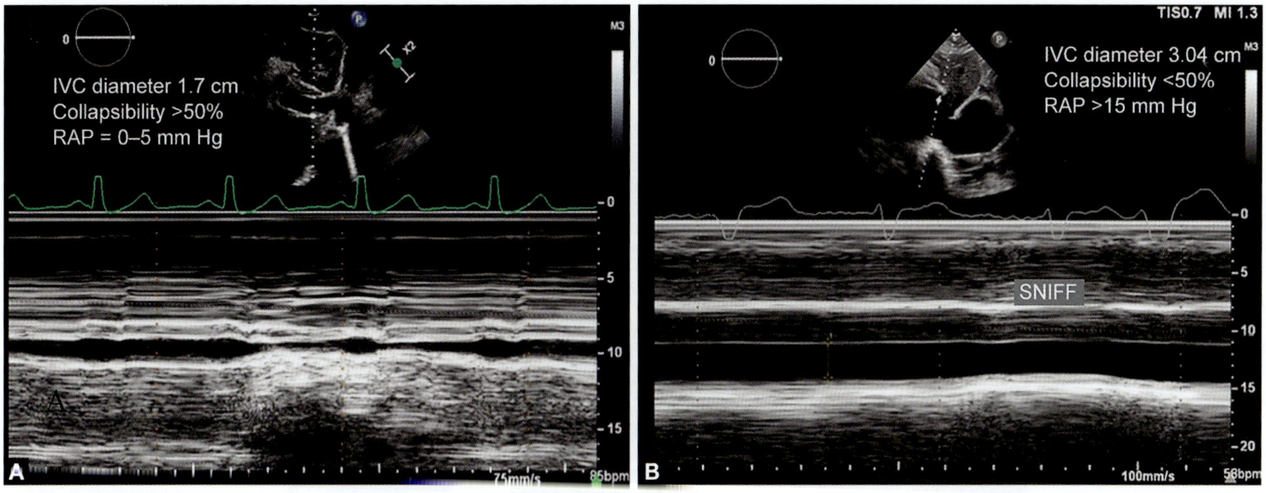

FIGS. 4A AND B: (A) Normal and (B)dilated IVC.

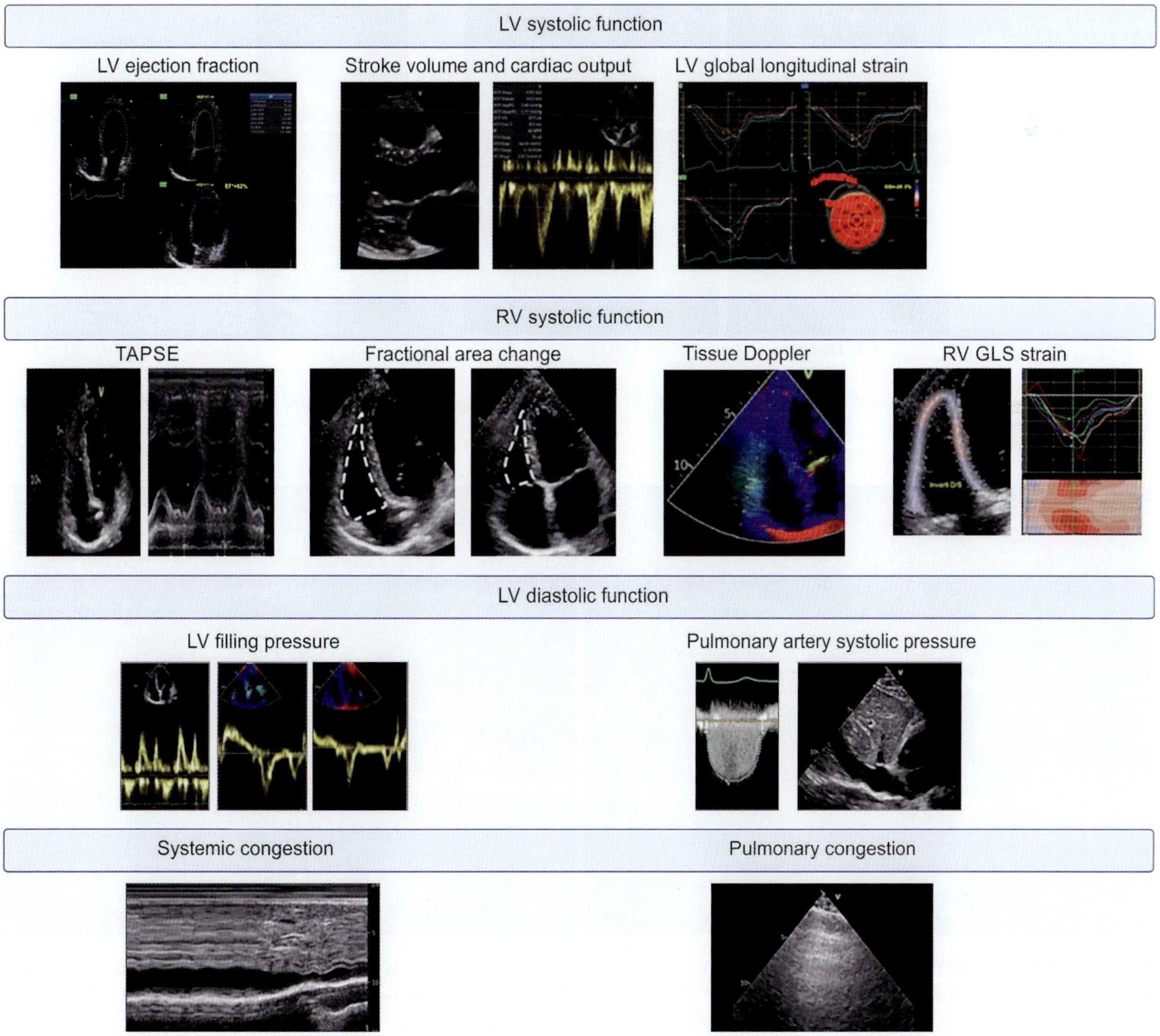

FIG. 5: Some measurements in echocardiography.

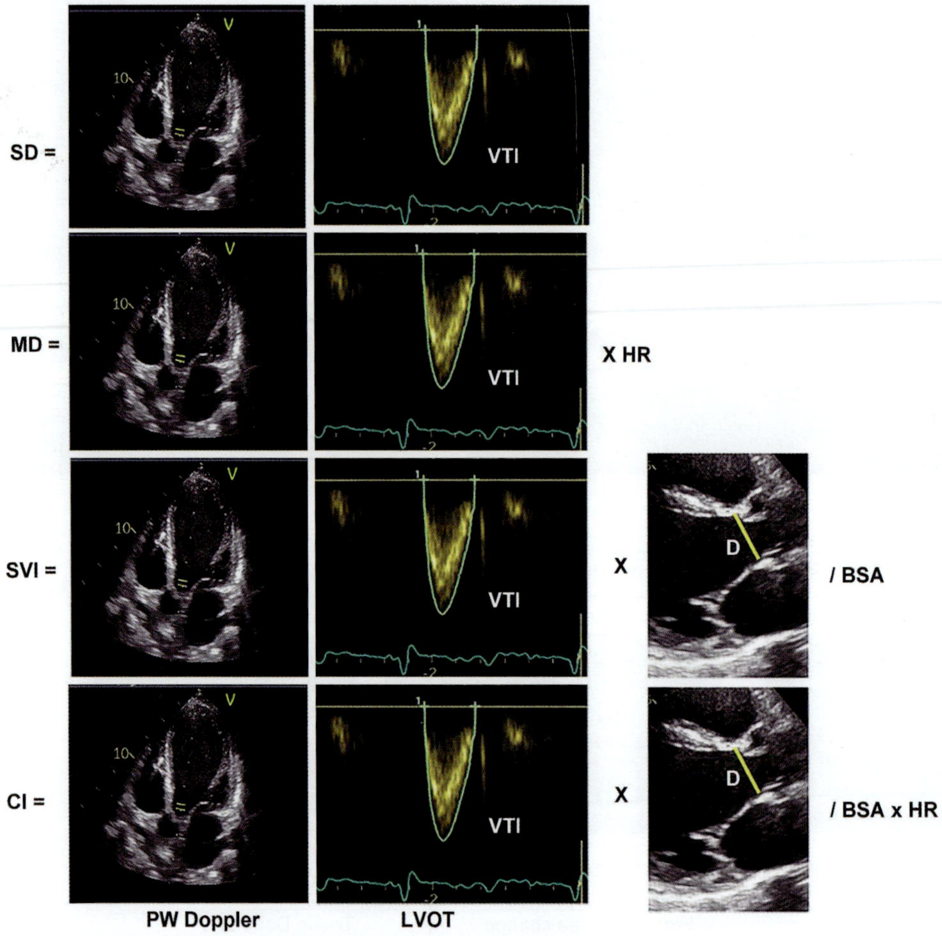

FIG. 6: Echocardiographic calculation of LV blood ejection in apical five-chamber view. Per beat and per minute outflow parameters.

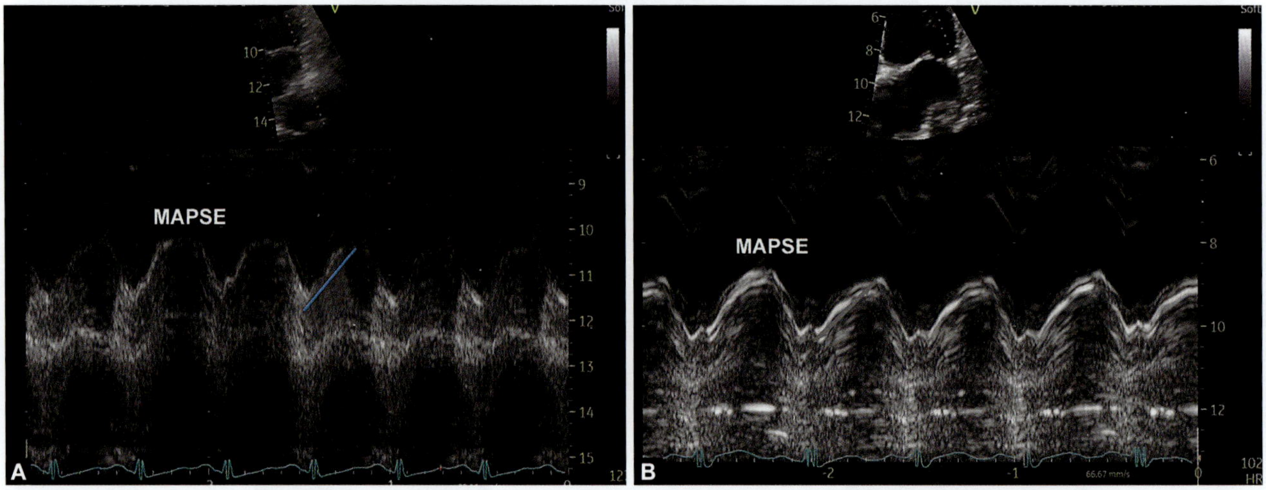

FIGS. 7A TO D: *Continued*

Continued

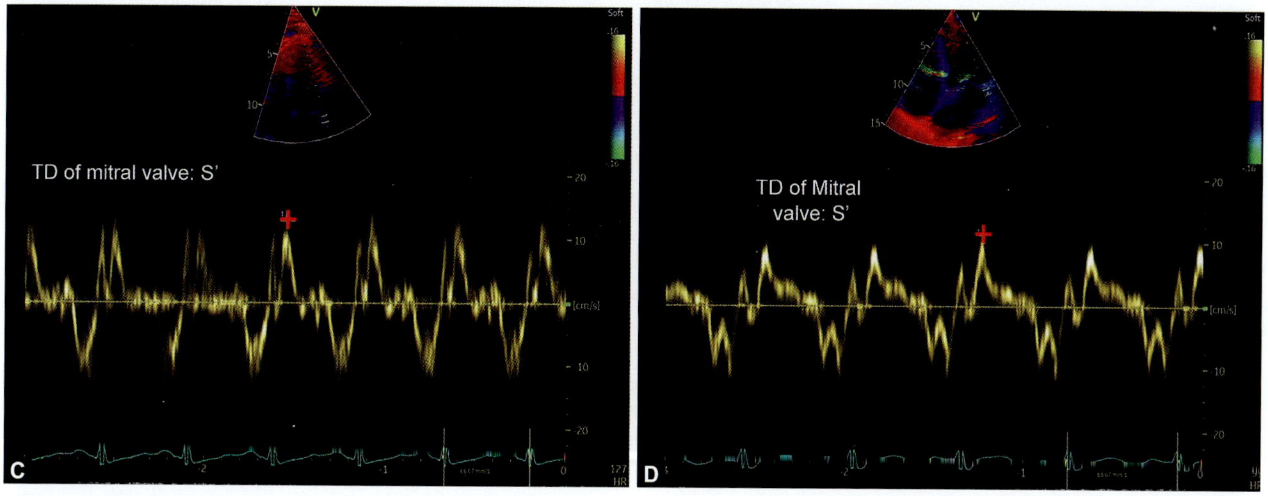

FIGS. 7A TO D: Left ventricular ejection fraction surrogates. (A and B) Mitral annulus plane systolic excursion (MAPSE) and (C and D) Tissue Doppler peak systolic wave at the mitral lateral annulus (S′).

hyperinflation in patients with obstructive lung disease.[9] Venous congestion leads not only to dilation of the IVC but also to pressure transmission to peripheral organs, altering the pattern of venous blood flow predictably In this regard, VExUS has emerged as a significant advancement in the assessment of systemic venous congestion **(Tables 5 and 6, Fig. 8)**.[10,11]

Left Atrial Strain

Left atrial (LA) strain is a more sensitive parameter than LA volume for early detection of LA structural and functional impairment. In early phase of LV diastolic dysfunction, LA volume can be normal, but the progressive and chronic increase of left ventricle filling pressures (LVFP) leads to LA structural abnormalities, which are detected by reduced LA strain as reduced compliance and LA dilatation that occurs in the last phase. Considering the thin wall of LA, cavity deformation mechanics—PALS (Global peak longitudinal strain) are impaired in patients with hypertension or diabetes despite normal LVEF even when LA indexed volume (LAVi) is normal. LA strain offers a quick analysis of cavity deformation and is correlated with invasively assessed LVFP.[3] It also provides additional value for diastolic function classification and HFpEF diagnosis. In the latest European Association of Cardiovascular Imaging (EACVI) consensus document for use of multimodality imaging in evaluating HFpEF, use of LA strain is suggested in case of missing with only two criteria available, one positive and another negative, with the cutoff value of LA reservoir strain (PALS) <18% to define elevated LVFP **(Flowchart 2)**.[12-14]

TABLE 5: Hepatic vein measurement parameters.

Clinical condition	Hepatic vein pressures (mm Hg)	Hepatic vein wedge pressures (mm Hg)	Hepatic venous pressure gradient (mm Hg)
Normal	6	8	2
Portal hypertension and no venous congestion	6	18	12
Venous congestion and no portal hypertension	18	22	4
Portal hypertension and venous congestion	18	28	10

TABLE 6: VExUS scoring.

VExUS score	Criteria
0 (No congestion)	<2 cm
1 (Mild congestion)	≥2 cm and absence of severe flow pattern in all three veins
2 (Moderate congestion)	≥2 cm and presence of one severe pattern in any of the three veins
3 (Severe congestion)	≥2 cm and presence of ≥2 severe patterns in the three veins

Advanced Hemodynamic Monitoring

Advanced hemodynamic monitoring is recommended for patients nonresponsive to initial therapies or those with RV dysfunction **(Figs. 9 and 10)**.[2]

Right heart catheterization, which is essential for patients with heart failure throughout the whole spectrum from ambulatory patients to those in cardiogenic shock, as well as those undergoing left ventricular device treatment and heart transplantation, can evaluate hemodynamic parameters.

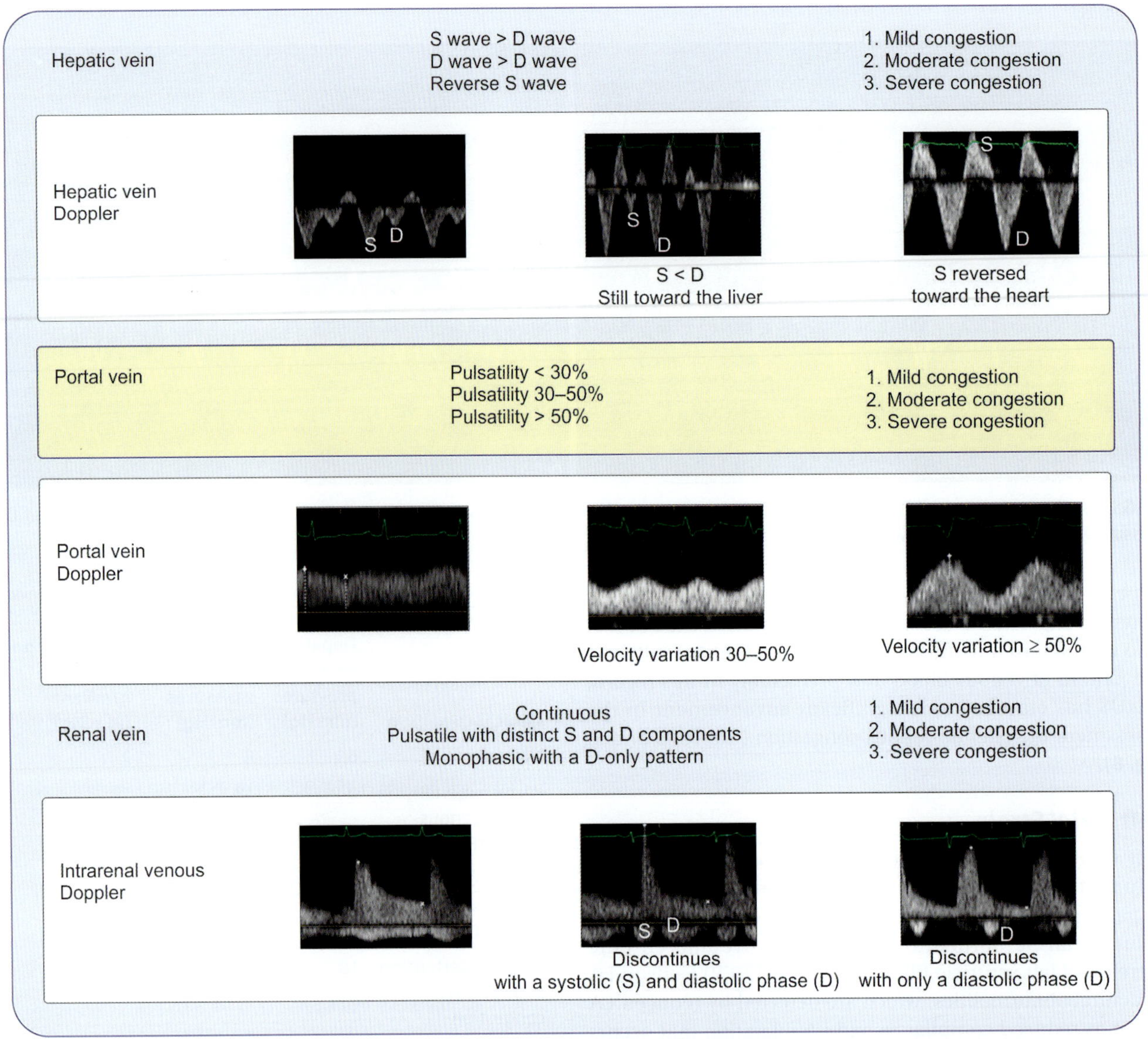

FIG. 8: Hepatic vein, portal vein, and intrarenal venous Doppler measuring modalities.

The use of PAC has not been studied in the context of CS, evaluated in patients receiving MCS, or used to drive an algorithm that improves outcomes in a prospective study.[15] Recent retrospective registry studies found that PACs improved CS outcomes in Impella pump patients.[16,17]

A second study using the National Inpatient Sample database found that PAC use improved survival in CS patients but worsened outcomes in ESCAPE (Evaluation Study of Congestive Heart Failure and Pulmonary Artery Catheterization Effectiveness)-acute decompensated congestive heart failure patients.[18,19] Based on such findings, PACs are being added to CS-treatment algorithms being evaluated at US centers.[20,21] Current society guidelines and scientific statements recommend limited PAC use in cardiovascular disease and CS (with or without MCS) patients due to limited evidence.

Factors influencing utility of PAC in CS (**Table 7**):
- Importance of accurate pressure signal acquisition and interpretation
- Characterizing different phenotypes of CS: LV-dominant, RV-dominant or biventricular shock
- Understanding hemodynamics for selection and management of MCS devices using
- PAC-derived data to drive a treatment algorithm

HEMODYNAMIC MONITORING USING PULMONARY ARTERY CATHETERIZATION

Hemodynamic monitoring using PAC is described in **Tables 8 and 9**.

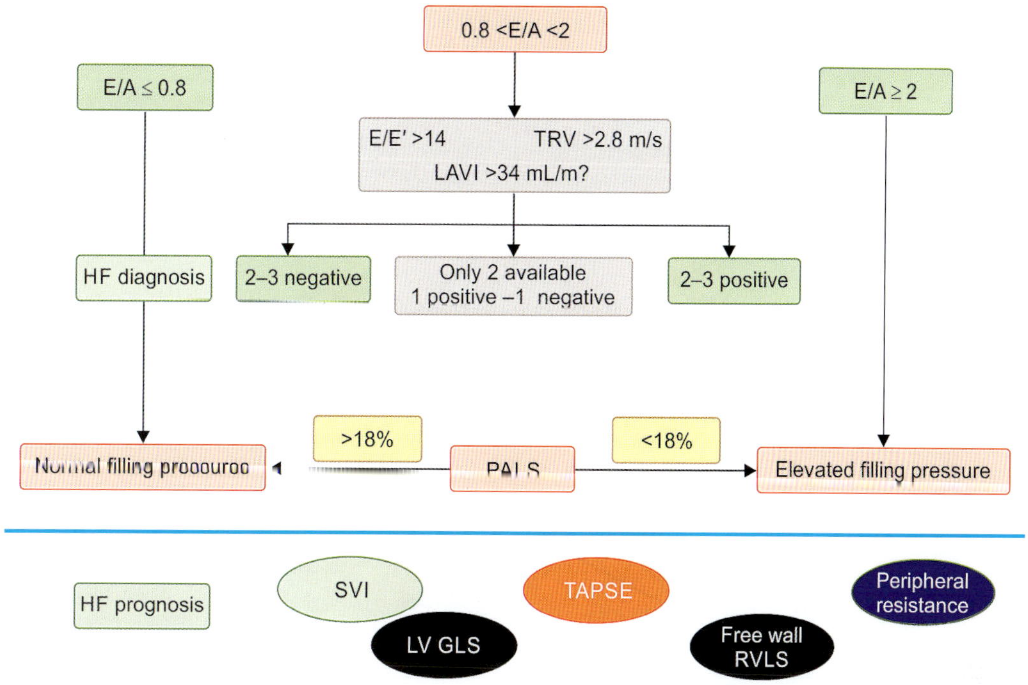

FLOWCHART 2: Role of LA strain.

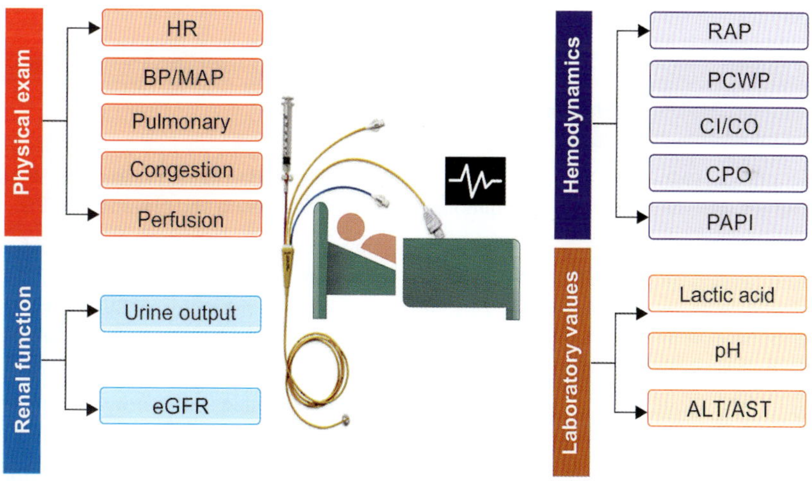

FIG. 9: Framework of clinical parameters to follow in patients with heart failure-related CS.

Direct Parameters with Pulmonary Artery Catheterization

Refer to **Table 8**.

Derived Parameters

Refer to **Table 9**.

CARDIAC POWER OUTPUT

Tan et al.[22] have shown that the resting cardiac power output (CPO) for a hemodynamically stable average-sized adult is approximately 1 W. However, during stress or exercise, cardiac power reserve can be recruited to increase the heart's pumping ability up to 6 W. Cardiac power is a novel hemodynamic measure. Cardiac power is the strongest hemodynamic correlate of outcome for patients in cardiogenic shock. Increasing age and female gender are independently associated with lower cardiac power.

$$\text{Cardiac power index (CPI)} = \text{MAP} \times \text{CI}/451$$
$$(\text{Cutoff.} = 0.32\ \text{W/m}^2)$$

Cardiac power output (CPO) and CPI are two significant derived parameters that have demonstrated a robust

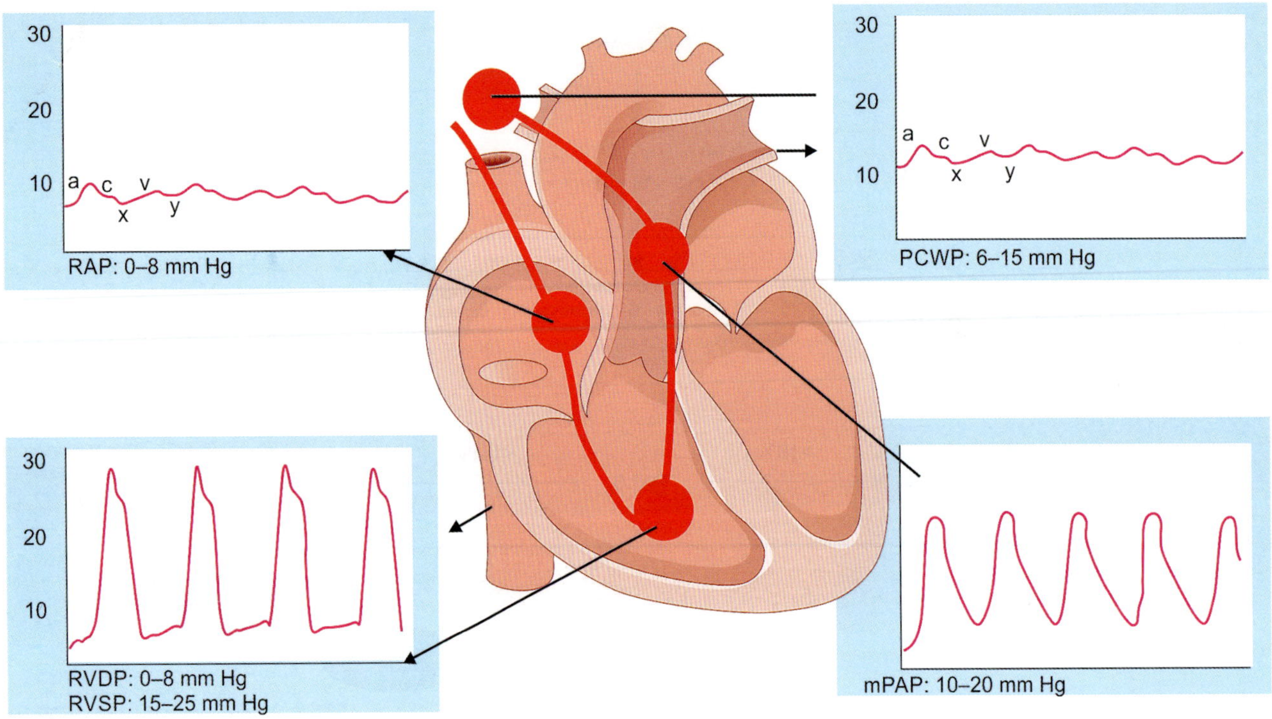

FIG. 10: Right heart catheterization pressure modalities.

TABLE 7: Calculations to be done during PAC.

	Formula	Normal range	Significance
Transpulmonary gradient (mm Hg)	Mean PAP – PCWP	<12	Chronic elevations in left-sided filling pressures in HF can lead to reactive pulmonary vascular remodeling and elevation in TPG
Pulmonary vascular resistance (WUs)	TPG/CO	<2	• PVR can be elevated with chronic HFrEF and HFpEF and is associated with increased CV mortality • Elevated PVR >3 WUs is a risk factor for RV failure after heart transplantation and acute pulmonary vasodilator testing is recommended to assess for reversibility
Systemic vascular resistance (dyne-s/cm)	MAP – RAP × 80 CO	900–1,200	Owes ence ay indir deconentag i am matory response or active infection
Pulmonary artery pulsatility index	PA systolic – PA diastolic	>2.0	• Estimates RV pulsatile load and contractile Strength, and by using RAP, also incorporates a measure of RV congestion • PAPI < 1.85 is a risk factor for RV failure after LVAD
	RAP		
Right ventricular stroke work index, g × m/m'/beat PAP–RAP) × (CI/HR × 1,000) × I		>8	• Estimates RV workload and contractility through measurement of RV pressure (mean PAP) and flow (cardiac index) • Low RVSWI is associated with RV failure after LVAD
Cardiac power output (Watts)		>1.0	Incorporates measures of both pressure and flow to estimate cardiac pumping capability
	(MAP – BAP) = CO		Used in cardiogenic shock as prognostic factor and in decision to escalate therapy

TABLE 8: PAC-derived parameter calculations.

Hemodynamic parameters	Normal range
Central venous pressure (CVP)	2–6 mm Hg
Right atrial pressure (RAP)	0–8 mm Hg
Right ventricular systolic pressure (RVSP)	15–25 mm Hg
Right ventricular diastolic pressure (RVDP)	0–8 mm Hg
Pulmonary artery systolic/diastolic pressure (PASP/PADP)	15–25 mm Hg; 8–15 mm Hg
Mean pulmonary artery pressure [mPAP: PADP + (PASP – PADP/3)]	10–20 mm Hg
Pulmonary capillary wedge pressure (PCWP)	6–15 mm Hg
Diastolic pulmonary gradient (DPG: PADP – PCWP)	<7 mm Hg
PAPi [(PASP – PADP)1/RAP]	>2
Transpulmonary gradient (TPG: mPAP – PCWP)	<12 mm Hg
Mean systemic arterial pressure [mSAP: DBP + 1/3(SBP – DBP)]	65–110 mm Hg
Cardiac output (CO)	4–8 L/min
Cardiac index (CI: CO/BSA)	2.5–4 L/min/m^2
Stroke volume (SV)	60–100 mL/beat
Stroke volume index (SVI: SV/BSA)	33–47mL/m^2/beat
Systemic vascular resistance [SVR: (mSAP – RAP)/CO × 80)	700–1600 dyn.s/cm^5
SVR index (SVRI: SVR/CI)	1,330–3,040 dyn.s/cm^5.m^2
Pulmonary vascular resistance (PVR: [mPAP – PCWP]/CO × 80)	20–120 dyn.s/cm^5
PVR index (PVR1: PVR/CI)	38–228 dyn.s/cm^5.m^2

correlation with the risk of inhospital mortality in CS. The concepts of CPO and CPI are utilized to measure and assess the amount of external mechanical work performed by the left ventricle. A CPO value below 0.6 W, calculated as the difference between MAP and right atrial pressure multiplied by cardiac output, is indicative of poorer prognoses in patients with acute myocardial infarction complicated by CS, even when receiving treatment in accordance with established guidelines.

Similar to how the indices function as substitutes for LV function, indices such as RV stroke work, RV stroke work index, and the ratio of CVP to PCWP serve to quantify RV function. An elevated CVP/PCWP ratio greater than 0.86 indicates impaired RV function, if the CVP is also above the normal range. In a similar vein, RV CPO and RV CPI can be quantified, albeit to a lesser extent, akin to LV parameters. The evaluation of systemic blood flow can be accomplished through the utilization of thermodilution or Fick methods, both of which assess cardiac output. Cardiac index, which is calculated by dividing cardiac output by BSA, is a valuable

TABLE 9: PAC-derived parameters.

Indirect measurements	Formula
Cardiac output (CO) (per Fick)	(125 × BSA)/[Hb × 1.36 × (SaO_2 – SvO_2)]
Cardiac power output	(MAP × CO)/451
Mean pulmonary artery pressure (mPAP)	[PASP+(2 × PADP)]/3
Transpulmonary pressure gradient (TPG)	MPAP–PCWP
Diastolic pulmonary gradient (DPG)	PADP–PCWP
Cardiac index (CI)	CO/BSA
Stroke volume (SV)	CO/HR × 1,000
Stroke volume index (SVI)	CI/HR × 1,000
Systemic vascular resistance (SVR)	80 × (MAP – RAP)/CO
Systemic vascular resistance index (SVRI)	80 × (MAP – RAP)/CI
Pulmonary vascular resistance (PVR)	(mPAP – PCWP)/CO
Pulmonary vascular resistance index (PVRI)	80 × (MPAP – PCWP)/CI
Pulmonary artery pulsatility index (PAPI)	(PASP – PADP)/RAP

metric for normalizing cardiac output. Additionally, mixed venous oxygen saturation (SvO_2) serves as an indicator of systemic blood flow.

The SHOCK Trial Registry data suggests that cardiac power is the strongest hemodynamic correlate of mortality in cardiogenic shock.

Transpulmonary Thermodilution

Transpulmonary thermodilution (TPTD) technique-based devices have emerged as an interesting monitoring approach that differs from the use of PACs. Indeed, this system allows for the assessment of cardiac output in two different ways. First is a thermodilution technique that measures cardiac output by using the Stewart-Hamilton principle. Here, a cold saline bolus is injected in the right central vein and the blood temperature is measured in the femoral artery. Second is the pulse contour analysis of the arterial curve sampled through the arterial catheter, which allows real-time monitoring of cardiac output and is calibrated by TPTD each time thermodilution is performed, which makes this technique very precise. TPTD devices also allow the assessment of other parameters, particularly two indices of cardiac systolic function, i.e., cardiac function index (CFI) and the global ejection fraction.

The combination of TPTD and pulse contour analysis makes it an alternative to using PACs, especially in complex situations like hemodynamic instability or acute respiratory distress syndrome **(Box 1)**.

Right Ventricular Function Assessment

The indices of right ventricular (RV) function encompass RV stroke work, RV stroke work index, and the ratio of CVP to PCWP. In typical circumstances, CVP is notably lower than PCWP. A CVP/PCWP ratio greater than 0.86 indicates potential impairment of RV function. However, this ratio is more accurate in identifying RV dysfunction when CVP is elevated beyond the normal range. In recent times, the utilization of the pulmonary artery pulsatility index [PAPi = (PAS - PAD)/CVP] has demonstrated its utility in providing a more precise assessment of RV dysfunction. A PAPi value of <0.9 is indicative of a notable decline in RV function. When combined with other observations, this finding may imply the necessity for additional RV support.[11,3]

Hemodynamic Classifications of Cardiogenic Shock

Cardiogenic shock is typically defined by systolic blood pressure <90 mm Hg or the need for inotropic, vasopressor, or mechanical support to maintain it above 90 mm Hg, along with end-organ hypoperfusion.[23,24] It requires an abnormally low cardiac index and normal or elevated intracardiac filling pressures (CVP and PCWP). Medically refractory CS does not resolve within 30–60 minutes of volume optimization and recommended inotrope or pressor doses. CS can be LV-dominant, RV-dominant, or biventricular shock, each with its own treatment strategy **(Table 10)**.

- *LV-dominant CS* has high PCWP and normal or reduced CVP in reduced LV function.
- *RV-dominant CS* has elevated CVP, normal-to-low pulmonary artery pressure, PCWP, and preserved LV function. RV-dominant CS is a variant affecting patient with pulmonary artery hypertension, high pulmonary arterial pressure, CVP, and PCWPs, but low cardiac index and blood pressure.
- *Biventricular CS* involves hypotension, elevated CVP, PCWP, and reduced LV function. Recent literature suggests *that biventricular shock is present in as many as 40% of patients who, based on clinical assessments alone, were suspected of having LV-dominant CS.*[25,26]

BOX 1 TPTD measurements and PAC measurements.

- Transpulmonary thermodilution:
  - Intermittent cardiac output
  - Continuous cardiac output
  - Cardiac function (CFI and GEF)
- Pulmonary artery catheterization:
  - Intermittent cardiac output
  - Semicontinuous cardiac output
  - PCWP
  - MPAP
  - SvO_2 and PCO_2 gap from the pulmonary artery

SCAI CLASSIFICATION

The SCAI classification is given in **Table 11**.

TABLE 10: Hemodynamic profiles in cardiogenic shock.

	RV-dominant shock	Biventricular shock	LV-dominant shock
CVP (mm Hg)	>14	>14	>14
PCWP (mm Hg)	<18	Variable	>18
CVP/PCWP	>0.86	>0.86	<0.86
PAPi	<1.5	<1.5	>1.5

(CVP: central venous pressure; LV: left ventricle; PAPi: pulmonary artery pulsatility index; PCWP: pulmonary capillary wedge pressure; RV: right ventricle)

TABLE 11: 2019 SCAI classification of cardiogenic shock.

Stage of shock	Biochemical markers	Hemodynamics	Description
Stage A "At Risk"	Normal renal function and lactate	Normotensive CI ≥ L/min/m², CVP <10 mm Hg PAsat ≥65%	Patients currently not in CS, but are at risk of developing CS. These include those with STEMI, NSTEMI, and acute or acute-on-chronic CHF
Stage B "Beginning" cardiogenic shock	Normal renal function and lactate; elevated BNP	SBP <90 or MAP <60 or >30 mm Hg drop from baseline. Pulse ≥ 100 bpm CI ≥ 22.2 L/min/m² PA sat ≥ 65%	Clinical evidence of hypotension or tachycardia without hypoperfusion
Stage C "Classic" cardiogenic shock	*Lactate ≥ 2 mmol/L:* • Serum creatinine doubling or >50% drop in GFR • Elevated LFTs and BNP	SBP <90; MAP <60 or >30 mm Hg drop from these targets CI <2.2 L/min/m², PCWP > 15 mm Hg, RAP/PCWP ≥20.8, PAPi <1.85, and CPO ≤50.6 W/m²	Clinical evidence of hypoperfusion requiring baseline and medications/MCS beyond volume resuscitation to restore perfusion
Stage D "Deteriorating or Doom"	Stage C and deteriorating	Stage C + requires multiple pressors or MCS devices to maintain perfusion	Like stage C but getting worse and failing to respond to initial interventions
Stage E "Extreme"	pH ≤ 7.2 Lactate >5 mmol/L	Hypotensive despite maximal support	Cardiac arrest (PEA or refractory VT/F) with ongoing CPR or ECLS placement

MECHANICAL CIRCULATORY SUPPORT DEVICES

Mechanical circulatory support devices have evolved as novel treatments to restore systemic perfusion for cardiac recovery in the short term or as durable support devices for refractory heart failure. CS has a growing number and variety of MCS devices to improve efficacy or replace pharmacotherapy to avoid side effects.

In recent years, MCS, such as IABP, Impella, TandemHeart, and ECMO, are gradually more used in this setting to increase SV and/or to unload LV **(Flowchart 3 and Table 12)**.

HEMODYNAMIC-BASED MECHANICAL CIRCULATORY SUPPORT SELECTION

Hemodynamic-based MCS selection is given in **Flowchart 4** and **Figure 11**.

HEMODYNAMIC-BASED PATIENT MANAGEMENT DURING MECHANICAL CIRCULATORY SUPPORT

The use of MCS is dependent on the hemodynamics derived from PAC. SvO_2 offers supplementary assessment of flow

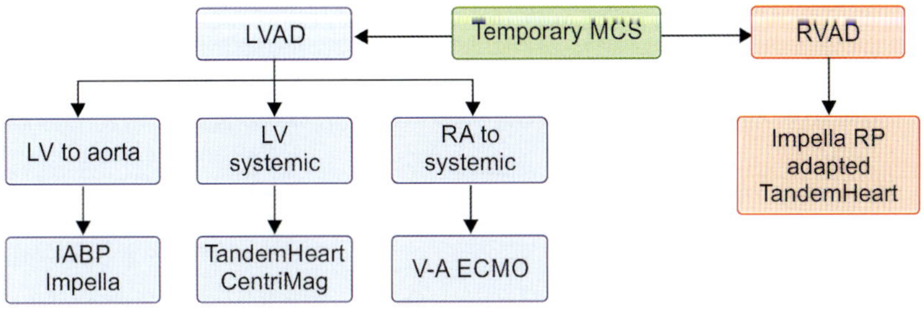

FLOWCHART 3: Use of temporary MCS in CS.

TABLE 12: Common clinical occurrences during right heart catheterization.

Clinical occurrences	Mechanism	Troubleshooting
Improper zeroing	If pressures are consistently higher or lower than expected, the level of the transducer may be incorrect	• Pressure transducer should be zeroed to atmospheric pressure at the left of the right atrium, which is located at midthorax level • Lines should he flushed to remove any air bubbles
Overdamping	• Can result in false reduction of systolic pressures and elevation of diastolic pressures • Clues are waveforms that appear "rounded" and loss of dicrotic notch in PA waveform • Causes include catheter kinking or thrombus, air in the system, or loose connections	Catheter and the tubing leading to pressure transducer should be inspected and flushed.
Catheter whip	Excessive movement of catheter in vessel can cause erratic reposition catheter waveforms	• Partial or complete deflation of balloon • Ensure tubing between catheter and transducer is not being moved or manipulated during waveform acquisition
Underwedged PCWP tracing	• Pressure waveform will interfere with PCWP waveform leading to false elevation of recorded PCWP • PCWP waveform may look similar to PA waveform	• If balloon catheter is inadequately wedged, the higher PA • Measure PCWP saturation in all cases, and saturation should be within 5% of systemic saturation • If unable to wedge, consider direct measurement of LVEDP

Continued

Continued

Clinical occurrences	Mechanism	Troubleshooting
Overwedged PCWP tracing	• Characterized by loss of waves and v waves and lack of • Avoid full inflation of balloon in distal PA • Respiratory variation • Inflating balloon fully in distal PA may result in overwedging and false elevation of PCWP • Can occur when end-hole of catheter is not parallel to the vessel but compressed against side wall • Overwedging can cause pulmonary artery rupture	Deflate balloon, withdraw catheter to the proximal PA, inflate balloon and advance
Significant respiratory variation	More commonly offered in patients with obesity or lung disease	• Report should note the presence of significant respiratory variation • Report average pressure over entire respiratory cycle as well as pressures at end-expiration_ • Avoid sedation
Mitral regurgitation leading to tall v-waves in PCWP	Higher than end-diastolic PCWP, which is typically what is recorded, because it corresponds to LVEDP	• With large v-waves. mean PCP may be significant • Large v-waves contribute to the increase in mean PAP, and therefore, mean PCW should be used to calculate PVR • Report should note presence of v-waves as well as mean PCWP and end-expiratory PCWP
Inaccurate CO (thermodilution)	• Direct Fick CO is considered gold standard but usually not • On average, take 3–5 measurements and ensure reproducibility available because of inability to directly measure oxygen consumption • Changes in preload caused by large changes in intrathoracic pressures (respiratory variation) • Operator error is possible, particularly among new operators/trainees, leading to variation in volume of saline solution injected • Thermistor abutting vessel wall	• Injection of saline solution at same point in respiratory cycle • Good PA tracing indicates thermistor is not against a vessel wall • Inaccurate in intracardiac shunts and should not be reported directly measured to calculate Fick CO
Inaccurate CO (Fick)	• Oxygen consumption should be directly measured • Assumed oxygen consumption values available in most laboratories are not reliable in patients with obesity or systemic disease such as HF	Avoid reporting Fick CO if oxygen consumption is not directly measured

adequacy in relation to the physiological condition. The measurement of serum lactate offers additional information; however, the time it takes for lactate to be cleared from the body and the delay in obtaining laboratory results make the measurement of SvO_2 more advantageous in terms of guiding therapeutic interventions **(Fig. 12)**.

ESCALATION OF MECHANICAL CIRCULATORY SUPPORT

Escalation refers to the process of transitioning from one MCS to another that has a greater flow capacity. This transition may also involve the addition or removal of a secondary device, which is necessitated by insufficient support provided by the initial MCS. When contemplating the escalation of therapy, it is imperative to acknowledge that as the duration of critical illness extends, there is an increased probability of advancing toward multiorgan failure **(Fig. 13)**.

It can be questioned whether such rapid and decisive clinical decision-making can be made without a PAC in place?

This phenomenon is exemplified in the PCWP tracings, which depict a case study of a patient who exhibited CS accompanied by increased PCWP and subsequently received ECMO therapy.

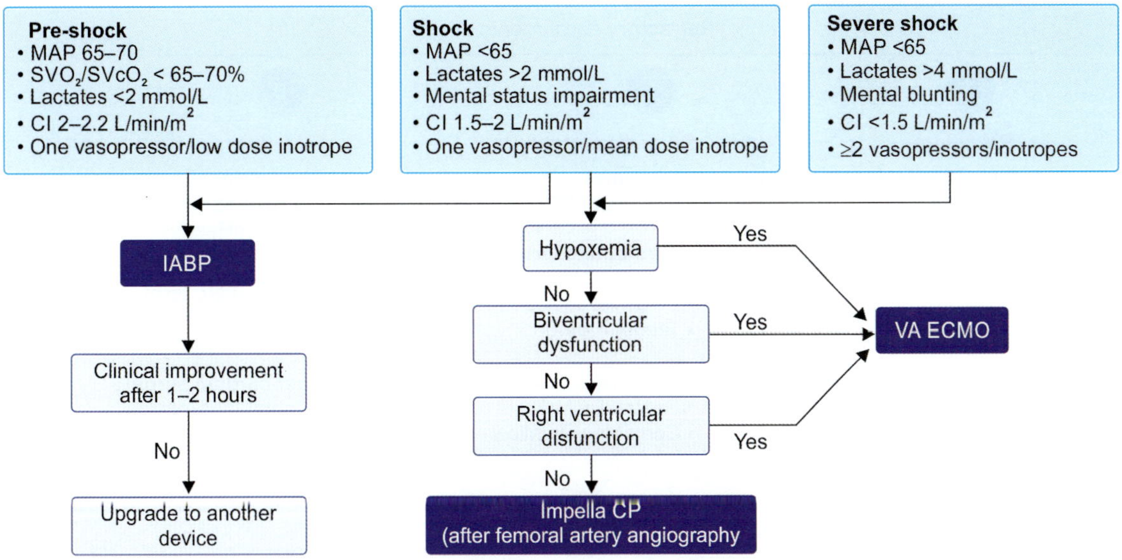

FLOWCHART 4: MCS selection based on hemodynamics.

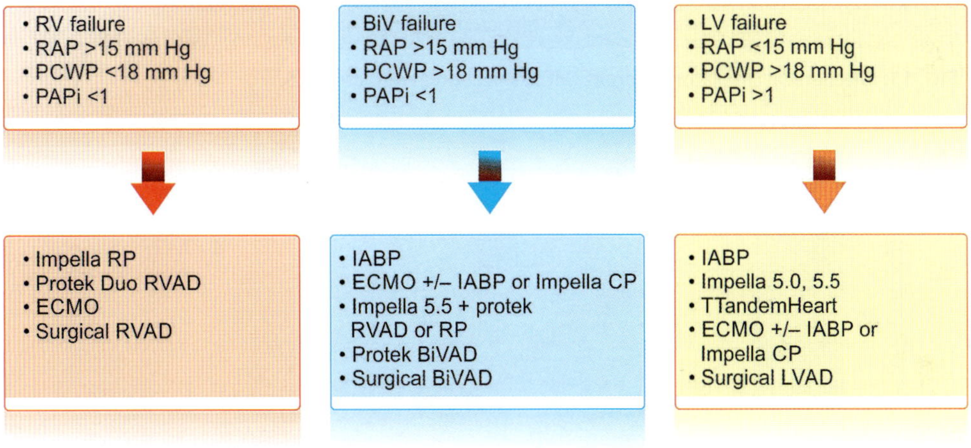

FIG. 11: Device configuration according to hemodynamics.

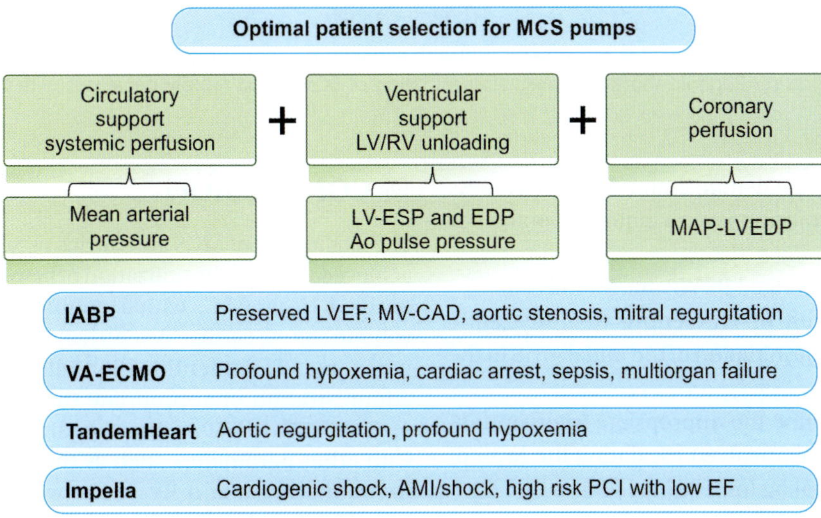

FIG. 12: Considerations for invasive hemodynamic assessment in HF-CS.

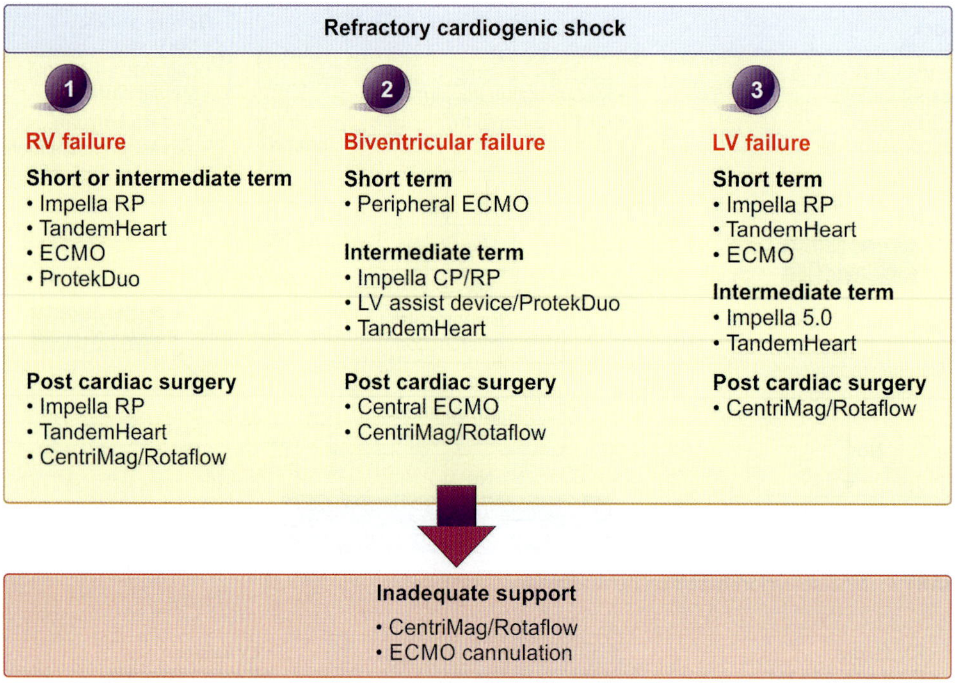

FIG. 13: Mechanical circulatory support (MCS) selection in refractory CS.

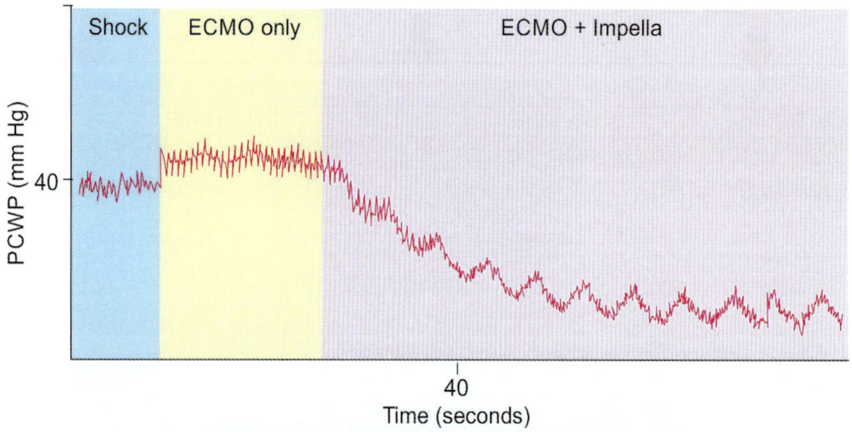

FIG. 14: Changes in pulmonary capillary wedge pressure (PCWP) with extracorporeal membrane oxygenation (ECMO) and Impella. PCWP at the time of presentation in cardiogenic shock increases after initiation of ECMO and rapidly decreases with the initiation of Impella support.

In a broader sense, this case demonstrates the effectiveness of utilizing the PAC in achieving several important outcomes **(Fig. 14)**:

- Prompt detection of elevated PCWP upon admission
- Prompt identification of worsening hemodynamic condition following the initiation of the initial MCS in the form of ECMO
- The ability to determine the appropriate intervention, which in this instance, involved escalating the level of support and incorporating Impella
- Confirmation of the swift resolution of the issue

CONCLUSION

The facilitation of MCS and device escalation optimization is achieved through the utilization of hemodynamic parameters derived from PAC, which enables the identification of volume status, cardiac biventricular function, cardiac power index, etc. This identification allows for the appropriate administration of appropriate therapy. The measurement of CVP and PCWP, either separately or in conjunction with other parameters such as the CVP/PCWP ratio, PAPi, RV stroke work, and RV stroke work index, offers crucial insights into volume status and the extent of RV dysfunction.

This information can help determine the necessity for fluid administration, diuretic therapy, renal replacement therapy, or the initiation of RV mechanical support.

The elucidation of the hemodynamic profile, encompassing parameters such as cardiac index, systemic vascular resistance (SVR), and volume status, in individuals of this nature can provide valuable guidance for medical interventions aimed at expediting the enhancement of end-organ perfusion. Moreover, this approach has the potential to mitigate the progression of the condition into overt CS.

ONLINE REFERENCES

Please scan the QR code provided at the end of the table of contents for References of this chapter.

Percutaneous Coronary Intervention in Acute Myocardial Infarction with Shock: Current Strategies of Management

CHAPTER 129

Ajay S Chaurasia, Shreyak P Kadu, Arjun Mali, Pankaj Kashyap, Nikhil Borikar, Sandeep Kamat

ABSTRACT

Acute myocardial infarction (AMI) complicated by cardiogenic shock (CS) is a critical challenge in cardiovascular medicine with high mortality rates despite advancements in management strategies. This chapter looks over the latest evidence, methods, and clinical guidelines for managing AMI patients with CS. AMI complicated by CS is characterized by reduced systolic blood pressure, elevated intracardiac pressures, and target organ damage due to cardiac dysfunction. The incidence of AMI complicated by CS is nearly 7–10%, and in-hospital mortality rates are around 50%, despite advances in percutaneous coronary intervention (PCI) strategies and techniques. CS is defined by systolic blood pressure <90 mm Hg, reduced cardiac index, and the need for inotropic or vasopressor support. The classification of shock provides a basis for risk stratification, triage, and planning the management strategies. Management includes immediate triage to PCI-capable facilities, early stabilization, and if needed, the use of mechanical circulatory support (MCS). PCI has been shown to improve outcomes, though the use of devices like intra-aortic balloon pumps and venoarterial ECMO remains debated. Early revascularization and individualized mechanical support are the keys to improving survival in acute myocardial infarction with cardiogenic shock.

Keywords: Acute myocardial infarction with shock, PCI in cardiogenic shock, mechanical circulatory support, culprit artery revascularization, Impella, ECMO

INTRODUCTION

Acute myocardial infarction (AMI) and associated cardiogenic shock (CS) are critical situations in the field of health where death is very high despite modern approaches in management. On this note, percutaneous coronary intervention (PCI) has shown remarkable progress in this setting as a means of restoring circulation. This chapter is focused on managing PCI in AMI patients with shock, and reviews the latest evidence, methods, and clinical guidelines concerning the issue. Acute myocardial infarction is the most common cause of CS.[1] Although ST-segment elevation myocardial infarction (STEMI) incidence is decreasing, the incidence of CS-complicating AMI (AMICS) remains relatively stable (7–10%).[2] Cardiogenic shock is a combination of a systolic blood pressure of <90 mm Hg, elevated intracardiac filling pressures, and target organ damage secondary to cardiac dysfunction. Early case series of CS has shown in-hospital mortality of nearly 80% and even with the advances in treatment modality and strategies; CS continues to have an in-hospital mortality of around 50%. The integration of PCI into the management of AMI with CS has significantly improved outcomes, yet numerous challenges persist.

CARDIOGENIC SHOCK

The shock state has been difficult to define. The National Cardiovascular Data Registry's Cath PCI registry defines shock as >30 minutes of systolic blood pressure < 90 mm Hg, cardiac index < 2.2 L/min/m^2 determined to be secondary to cardiac dysfunction, or the requirement for inotropic or vasopressor agents or MCS.[3] Pathophysiologically, CS is a state of end-organ hypoperfusion due to cardiac failure. Presenting manifestations of CS include cold extremities, decreased urine output (<30 mL/h), alteration in mental status, and low systemic arterial blood pressure. LV pump failure is the primary mechanism in AMI leading to CS.

Systolic dysfunction leads to decreased stroke volume and decreased CO. In an attempt to maintain the blood pressure, the body increases the heart rate and there is peripheral vasoconstriction leading to temporary stabilization but at the cost of increased myocardial work and as a result decreased coronary perfusion. The diastolic filling period decreases as the heart rate increases and further decreases the coronary perfusion leading to myocardial ischemia. The lower blood pressure also triggers the renin-angiotensin-aldosterone system (RAAS) and results in fluid retention and peripheral vasoconstriction. Diastolic dysfunction leads to an increased LV end-diastolic pressure (LVEDP), which leads to pulmonary congestion and hypoxia. Right ventricular (RV) dysfunction can contribute to CS as RV failure can decrease LV filling via a reduced cardiac output (CO) or ventricular interdependence, or both.[2] Shock secondary to isolated RV dysfunction carries a mortality risk as high as shock due to LV failure. In AMI mechanical complications such as ventricular septal rupture and papillary muscle rupture can cause CS without severe reduction in LV function **(Flowchart 1)**.

The Society for Cardiovascular Angiography and Intervention (SCAI) has introduced a classification scheme for a patient's hemodynamic state. Multiple series have shown a stepwise increase in the risk of hospital mortality with increments of SCAI shock stages A to E **(Fig. 1)**.[4] An important aspect of the SCAI classification is a cardiac arrest modifier. At every stage of SCAI shock, the presence of cardiac arrest significantly increases mortality, and this makes it useful to stratify risk in hospitalized patients. Studies are required to prospectively test the clinical utility of this classification scheme.

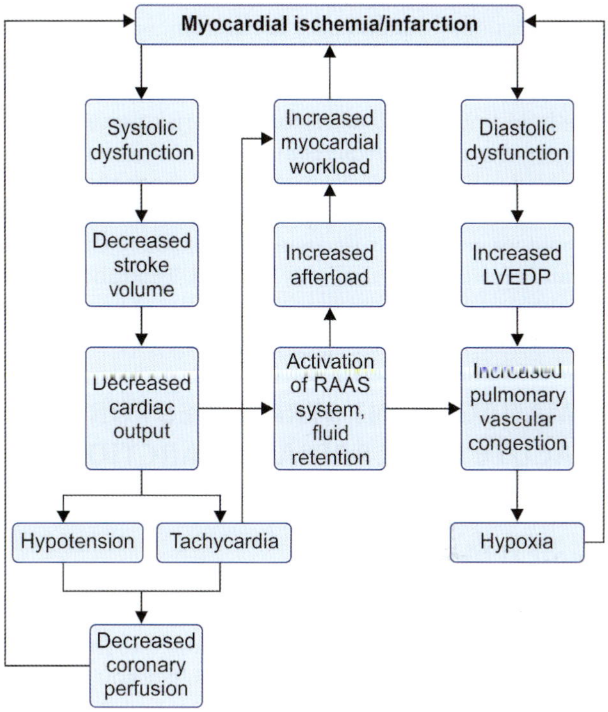

FLOWCHART 1: Pathophysiology of cardiogenic shock in acute myocardial infarction.

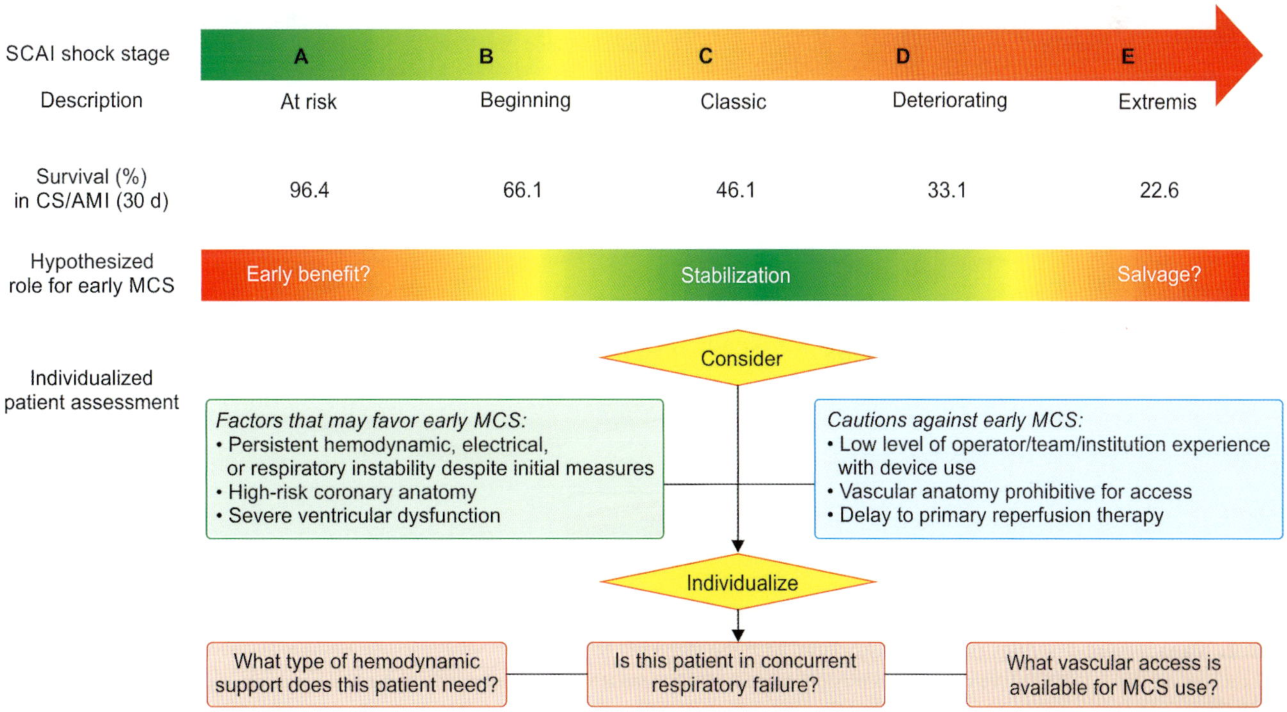

FIG. 1: Classification of shock.

CLINICAL PRESENTATION AND DIAGNOSIS

The majority of patients with CS and AMI have (1) peripheral hypoperfusion, (2) pulmonary congestion, and (3) arterial hypotension. Nearly 25% of patients with hypotension and hypoperfusion do not have pulmonary congestion and should not be mistaken for a low-risk presentation.[2] Although a very small percentage of AMI have CS as a presentation but majority who developed shock after AMI do so within the initial 24 hours of presentation. In the SHOCK (SHould we emergently revascularize Occluded Coronaries for cardiogenic shocK) trial, only 9% had CS and about 46.6% who developed shock did so within 6 hours of presentation and 25.9% had a late-onset shock (>24 hours).[5]

MANAGEMENT STRATEGIES FOR ACUTE MYOCARDIAL INFARCTION WITH SHOCK

Medical Management

Triage and Classification

Patients with AMI with CS should be shifted to the cardiac catheterization laboratory of a PCI-capable hospital as early as possible.[1,2] Initial bedside examination and recognizing red flag signs help in risk stratification as well as further triage. Early echocardiography and laboratory examination (arterial blood gas, lactate) are important. Stable patients with risk factors for shock (stage A) or early shock (stage B) may be shifted directly to the catheterization laboratory for coronary angiography and culprit lesion revascularization. Patients presenting in shock (stages C–E) will first require hemodynamic stabilization with attention to blood pressure, end-organ perfusion status, oxygenation, and acid–base status. In cases of STEMI, all the necessary efforts must be expedited to stabilize and minimize delay to reperfusion therapy.[6] Patients with late or extreme stages of shock (stage E) in whom invasive management has not shown any benefit and should instead be evaluated for palliative care. It is important to note that early engagement of palliative care services and aggressive early invasive management are not mutually exclusive **(Fig. 2)**.[7]

Initial Stabilization

Blood Pressure

The minimum dose of vasopressor that needs to maintain mean arterial blood pressure >65 mm Hg must be initiated; norepinephrine is preferred as first-line therapy.[9,10] Alternative agents may be preferred in specific circumstances such as unstable bradycardia for which the effect of dopamine or epinephrine may be desired; in case

	A: At Risk	B: Beginning CS	C: Classic CS	D: Deteriorating	E: Extremis
Clinical	• Normotensive • With risk factors of CS	Hypotension*	• Hypotension* • Inotropes or vasopressors to maintain blood pressure	Deterioration from stage C despite appropriate intervention	Circulatory collapse
Biomarker	Lactate <2.0 mmol/L		Lactate ≥2.0 mmol/L		
Hemodynamics	• LVEDP ≤18 mm Hg • Cardiac index ≥2.2 L/min/m²		• LVEDP >18 mm Hg • Cardiac index <2.2 L/min/m²		

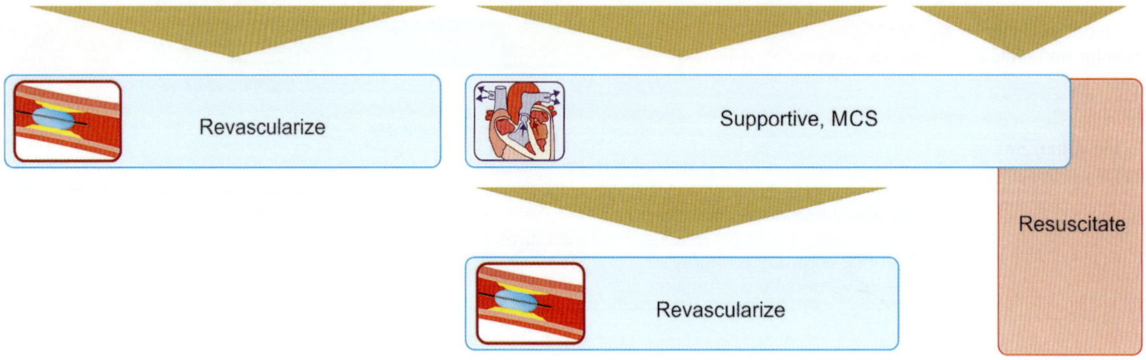

*Level of consensue: 100% agree; 0% neutral; 0% disagree. "SBP <90 mm Hg OR MAP <60 mm Hg >30 mm Hg drop from baseline.

FIG. 2: Management strategies as per risk associated with the stage of CS.[8]

(CS: cardiogenic shock; LVEDP: left ventricular end-diastolic pressure; MAP: mean arterial pressure; MCS: mechanical circulatory support; SBP: systolic blood pressure)

Source: Contains images from Servier Medical Art by Servier, licensed under a Creative Commons Attribution 3.0 Unported License of dynamic left ventricular (LV) outflow tract obstruction a pure vasopressor such as phenylephrine or vasopressin may be preferred. Even if the mean arterial blood pressure target of 65 mm Hg is established the clinical perfusion status must be evaluated. While escalating the vasopressor and inotrope therapy it must be kept in mind that higher levels of pharmacological support are associated with higher mortality in observational studies, and this also reflects the severity of the illness.[11] Studies for evaluating the adjunctive role of milrinone, levosimendan, and dobutamine in different shock settings are ongoing. However, these inotropic agents are of limited value for initial stabilization in AMI and CS as they may worsen myocardial ischemia.

Respiratory Function

AMICS leads to hypoxemia (resulting from cardiogenic pulmonary edema) and metabolic acidosis (caused by lactic acidosis and acute kidney injury), and patients are at risk for acute respiratory failure.[1] Continuous hypoxemia and acidosis increase the risk of ventricular fibrillation and death during attempted coronary revascularization.[12] Hence, it is recommended to start early mechanical ventilation as it may support revascularization by improving oxygenation and enhancing metabolic profile. Caution is advised in patients with predominant right ventricular failure initiation of positive pressure ventilation can abruptly lower systemic arterial pressure.

Diagnostic Evaluation

Physical Examination

Focused physical examination will provide immediate insight into a patient's hemodynamics.[1,2]

- Rales and difficulty in lying supine suggest pulmonary venous congestion.
- Jugular venous distention suggests systemic venous congestion.
- Cool and clammy extremities, rapid thready pulses, and altered level of consciousness may represent hypoperfusion.
- A systolic murmur may hint toward mechanical complications.

Echocardiography

Echocardiography should be performed as soon as possible, either before or simultaneously with invasive evaluation. Special attention must be on the evaluation of left and right ventricular systolic function, significant valvular stenosis or regurgitation, pericardial effusion/tamponade, and evidence of mechanical complications, including septal, papillary muscle, or free wall rupture.

Right-sided Heart Catheterization

Right-sided heart catheterization can provide quantitative data on individual patient hemodynamics over time. ESCAPE trial examined the role of routine right heart catheterization in acute decompensated heart failure patients and did not reveal a mortality difference between patients treated with invasive monitoring compared with those treated without invasive monitoring.[13] This study also confirmed the lack of sensitivity of physical examination findings in predicting the hemodynamic state of the CS patient.

Key parameters to assess and monitor include central venous pressure, pulmonary capillary wedge pressure, cardiac output, cardiac power output, pulmonary artery pulsatility index, and mixed venous oxygen saturation. Invasive measures, including central venous pressure >10 mm Hg, central venous pressure/pulmonary capillary wedge pressure >0.63 mm Hg, pulmonary artery pulsatility index <2.0, and right ventricular stroke work index <450 g/m^2, may help identify right ventricular dysfunction complicating AMICS.[14] Right-sided heart catheterization is not required to diagnose shock. Performance of right-sided heart catheterization can cause an undue delay in timely reperfusion therapy and should be done after completing the revascularization.

MECHANICAL CIRCULATORY SUPPORT IN ACUTE MYOCARDIAL INFARCTION WITH CARDIOGENIC SHOCK

Patients with AMICS and persistent hemodynamic compromise even after initial stabilization can benefit from immediate MCS. Early initiation of MCS in AMICS aims to alleviate ventricular workload (by unloading), boost systemic and myocardial perfusion, and offer hemodynamic support during PCI procedures.

Persistent clinical hypoperfusion, hypotension, vasopressor requirement, or cardiac power output <0.6 W with adequate filling pressures provides a rationale for MCS as an additional support for stabilization before coronary revascularization.[1]

Mechanical circulatory support options available for patients with predominant LV failure **(Fig. 3)**:

- Intra-aortic balloon counterpulsation (IABP)[15]
- Transvalvular axial flow pump (Impella LP/CP/5.0/5.5)[16]
- TandemHeart percutaneous LV assist device

Mechanical circulatory support options for patients with predominant right ventricular failure:

- Transvalvular axial flow Impella RP pump
- TandemHeart ProtekDuo percutaneous right ventricular assist device

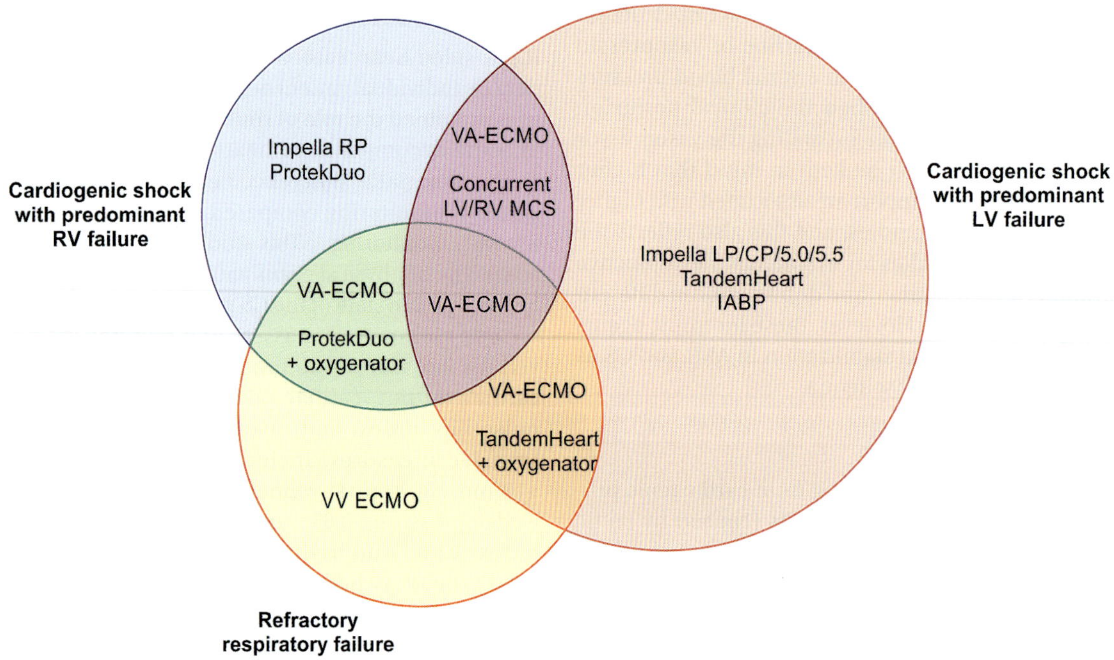

FIG. 3: Matching of mechanical circulatory support (MCS) platforms with clinical presentations.

Mechanical circulatory support options for patients with biventricular failure **(Fig. 3)**:

- Bilateral Impella pumps
- VA-ECMO with a concomitant LV venting mechanism

In patients with concurrent refractory respiratory failure, VA-ECMO should be considered. Observational studies of AMICS systems of care incorporating early MCS have reported improved survival compared with historical controls, but no randomized controlled trial has provided evidence in support of routine use for any short-term MCS platform.

DanGer SHOCK TRIAL[17]

The DanGer Shock trial showed that routine implantation of Impella CP along with standard care is superior to standard care alone in decreasing 6-month mortality in patients presenting with STEMI and cardiogenic shock. The complications included bleeding, limb ischemia, need for RRT, and sepsis, and the risk of these complications was high with Impella CP. Impella CP was placed prior to revascularization in >50% of patients. This is an important trial as the population it addresses has been challenging to study. Many observational studies suggested that it was harmful to use Impella CP in this patient population.

Multiple randomized studies of VA-ECMO in AMICS are also ongoing:

- EURO SHOCK (Testing the Value of Novel Strategy and Its Cost Efficacy in Order to Improve the Poor Outcomes of Cardiogenic Shock)
- ECLS-SHOCK (Extracorporeal Life Support in Cardiogenic Shock)
- ECMO-CS (Extracorporeal Membrane Oxygenation in the Therapy of Cardiogenic Shock)
- ANCHOR (Assessment of ECMO in Acute Myocardial Infarction Cardiogenic Shock)

These trials and others will provide additional insights into managing patients with AMICS.

The STEMI-DTU pivotal (Primary Unloading and Delayed Reperfusion in ST-Elevation Myocardial Infarction) trial will investigate whether initiating MCS before reperfusion can limit myocardial damage in patients with anterior STEMI who do not have cardiogenic shock (CS).[18] It remains unclear whether findings from STEMI without shock can be generalized to AMICS. Emerging observational data among AMICS patients suggest that early MCS might enhance outcomes in specific patient groups rather than worsening them.

REPERFUSION THERAPY AND STRATEGIES FOR ACUTE CORONARY SYNDROME COMPLICATED BY SHOCK

As per ESC 2023 guideline for acute coronary syndrome (ACS) early revascularization (either PCI or CABG) is recommended for patients with AMI complicated by CS **(Table 1)**. SHOCK trail[5,19,20] corresponds to a number needed to treat (NNT) of fewer than eight patients to save one life.

TABLE 1: ECS 2023 guidelines for revascularization in acute myocardial infarction with cardiogenic shock.

Recommendations	Class	Level of evidence
Immediate coronary angiography and PCI of infarct-related artery (IRA) (if indicated) is recommended in patients with CS-complicating ACS	I	B
Emergency CABG is recommended for ASC-related CS if the PCI of the IRA is not feasible/unsuccessful	I	B
In cases of hemodynamic instability, emergency surgical/catheter-based repair of mechanical complications of ACS is recommended, based on the Heart Team discussion	I	C
Fibrinolysis should be considered in STEMI patients presenting with CS if a PPCI strategy is not available within 120 minutes from the time of STEMI diagnosis and mechanical complications have been ruled off	IIa	C

TABLE 2: ECS 2023 guidelines for mechanical circulatory support in AMI with CS.

Recommendations	Class	Level of evidence
In patients with ACS and severe/refractory CS, short-term mechanical circulatory support may be considered	IIb	C
The routine use of an IABP in ACS patients with CS and without mechanical complications is not recommended	III	B

As per IABP-SHOCK II, if CS is not associated with mechanical complications, the routine use of an IABP is not recommended for AMI with CS.[15] Currently the role of the mechanical circulatory devices [venoarterial extracorporeal membrane oxygenation (VA-ECMO), micro-axial pump] in the AMI setting is not established and large-scale randomized trials are warranted.

Mechanical circulatory support may be considered in selected patients with ACS and severe/refractory CS,[20] caution should be exercised in this regard until further randomized data are available **(Table 2)**.

Several studies have proven the advantages of emergency PCI over fibrinolytics in obtaining stable TIMI grade 3 flow in STEMI, thus significantly reducing mortality rates and maintaining the functionality of LV function.[5,19] In the SHOCK trial, the most common mode of revascularization was PCI, 84 of 132 patients were randomized to immediate revascularization with PCI.[5] The definition of successful PCI was, the combination of a residual stenosis <50%, a >20% reduction in stenosis, and TIMI grade 2- or 3-flow and it was achieved in 76% of patients.[2,5] The survival in the PCI group was 54% at 30 days and 50% at 1 year. 30-day survival was 65% after successful PCI. The patency and TIMI grade 3 flow in the IRA was associated with survival and No patient with an occluded IRA (TIMI flow grade 0 or 1) after PCI survived. Patients who presented in the first 6 hours after symptom onset were associated with lower mortality rates among CS patients undergoing primary PCI in the Arbeitsgemeinschaft Leitende Kardiologische Krankenhausarzte (ALKK) registry and it had a door-to-angiography time less than 90 minutes in approximately 75% of patients.[21] SHOCK trial also showed an increase in long-term mortality rates with increase in the time to revascularization (from 0 to 8 hours) but a survival benefit was noticed if the revascularization was performed within 48 hours after MI and 18 hours after shock onset.[2,5,19] The age of the patient is an important factor that may influence the outcome in patients with AMI and CS however, The American College of Cardiology (ACC)/ American Heart Association (AHA) guidelines recommend early revascularization in CS for those younger than 75 years of age (class I) and for suitable candidates over 75 years of age (class IIa).[22]

MANAGEMENT OF MULTIVESSEL DISEASE IN ACUTE CORONARY SYNDROME COMPLICATED BY CARDIOGENIC SHOCK

Complete coronary occlusion can cause CS in patients with ACS, which occurs in 4–11% of the patients with ACS.[1,23] Ischemia-related HF, acute severe mitral regurgitation, and mechanical complications are the important precipitating causes of CS in ACS. No matter what the presentation is, with or without ST-segment elevation or equivalent ECG patterns, patients must be moved quickly to a tertiary care center where they can undergo Invasive Coronary angiography and interventions can be done **(Flowchart 2)**.[24]

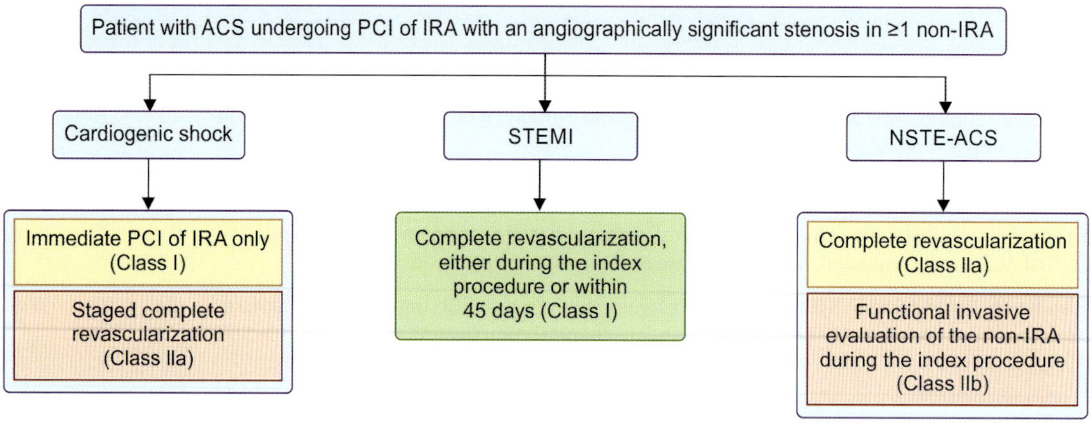

FLOWCHART 2: Algorithm for treatment of infarct-related artery in case of AMI.

TABLE 3: ESC 2023 recommendation for treatment of infarct-related artery in case of AMI.

Recommendations	Class	Level
It is recommended to base the revascularization strategy (IRA PCI, multivessel PCI/CABG) on the patient's clinical status and comorbidities, as well as their disease complexity, according to the principles of management of myocardial revascularization	I	B
Multivessel disease in ACS patients presenting in cardiogenic shock		
IRA-only PCI during the index procedure is recommended	I	B
Staged PCI of non-IRA should be considered	IIa	C

In the SHOCK trial which compared the usage of emergency revascularization with initial medical stabilization in 302 patients who had acute MI complicated by CS, 85% had MVD. Among those patients who were assigned to emergency revascularization, 64% of them were treated with PCI, and the others 36% underwent CABG.[2,5] The 30-day mortality in both groups (medical stabilization vs. early revascularization) did not differ but at 6 months mortality was lower in the early revascularization group than in the medical therapy one. Hence, this evidence points out the necessity for immediate coronary angiography followed by PCI and for patients with coronary artery anatomy not suitable for PCI, or emergency CABG **(Table 3)**.

The CULPRIT-SHOCK trial included patients with both ACS with and without ST-segment elevation or equivalent, and it suggested PCI during index procedure should be restricted to infarct-related artery (IRA) only.[25] In the CULPRIT-SHOCK trial, PCI of the infarct-related artery was associated with significantly less all-cause death or renal replacement therapy at 30-day follow-up (RR 0.83; 95% CI 0.71–0.96). The mortality rate was similar in both groups at the 1-year follow-up.[25] In recent data from the Korea Acute Myocardial Infarction National Health Registry, the multivessel PCI was associated with a lower risk of all-cause death than culprit artery-only PCI at 3 years.[26] This suggested the possible benefit of complete revascularization during the index hospitalization on long-term clinical outcomes.

ASIAN PACIFIC SOCIETY OF CARDIOLOGY CONSENSUS STATEMENTS ON THE DIAGNOSIS AND MANAGEMENT OF ACUTE MYOCARDIAL INFARCTION-CARDIOGENIC SHOCK

The APSC convened an expert consensus panel to review the literature on the diagnosis and management of AMI-CS, discuss gaps in current management, determine areas where further guidance is needed, and develop consensus recommendations on the diagnosis, assessment, and management of AMI-CS.[8] The 21 experts on the panel are members of the APSC who were nominated by national societies and endorsed by the APSC consensus board or invited international experts **(Table 4)**.

TABLE 4: Asian Pacific Society of cardiology consensus statements.

Consensus recommendation	Level of consensus	Level of evidence (%)		
		Agree	Neutral	Disagree
Immediate point-of-care echocardiography should be considered to assess ventricular and valvular functions, and loading conditions and to detect mechanical complications. However, this should not delay reperfusion	Moderate	90.5	0	0.5
Hemodynamic assessment of left ventricular end-diastolic pressure (LVEDP) may be considered for guiding therapy. It should not delay reperfusion	Low	82.6	8.7	8.7
Hemodynamic assessment with pulmonary artery catheterization (PAC) may be considered for guiding therapy. It should not delay reperfusion	Low	87	8.7	4.3
AMI patients with hypotension but with blood lactate < 2.0 mmol/L, LVEDP ≤ 18 mm Hg and cardiac index ≥2.2 L/min/m^2 should be classified as being in Stage B CS	Moderate	100	0	0
AMI patients who require the use of inotropes/vasopressors to prevent hypotension should be classified as being in Stage C CS	Very low	91.4	4.3	4.3
AMI patients with hypotension and with blood lactate ≥2.0 mmol/L, LVEDP >18 mm Hg or cardiac index <2.2 L/min/m^2 should be classified as being in Stage C CS	Very low	100	0	0
Immediate revascularization is recommended for AMI patients with Stage B CS	Moderate	100	0	0
The majority of patients only require revascularization of the culprit lesion	Low	78.3	17.4	4.3
Patient stabilization is recommended before revascularization in AMI patients with Stage C CS or worse	Very low	74	21.7	4.3
For patients in Stage C CS, ensuring adequate oxygenation should be considered before transfer to the cardiac catheterization laboratory	Very low	78.3	21.7	0
Hemodynamic assessment with PAC should be considered for guiding therapy in patients with Stage C and D CS	Moderate	95.7	0	4.3
Temporary MCS [e.g., intra-aortic balloon pump (IABP), Impella, or venoarterial extracorporeal membrane oxygenation (VAECMO)] may be considered in AMI patients in Stage C and D CS	Low	95.7	4.3	0
The use of MCS for patients in Stage E CS is considered futile. VA-ECMO may be considered in highly selected patients based on clinical imperatives	Low	78.3	13	8.7
For patients in Stage C or D, PCI (over emergency coronary artery bypass grafting) may be considered as the mode of revascularization	Low	91.3	8.7	0
A multidisciplinary team approach is recommended in the management of patients with CS due to AMI	Moderate	100	0	0
A protocolized treatment is recommended in the management of patients with CS due to AMI	Moderate	100	0	

CONCLUSION

The management of PCI in AMI complicated by cardiogenic shock is an evolving field and management is always challenging. Timely reperfusion with PCI, supported by correct hemodynamic management and adjunctive therapies, is critical for improving outcomes. The incorporation of advanced MCS devices, personalized medicine approaches, and ongoing research into novel therapies offers hope for further advancements in the care of these critically ill patients. Continued efforts to refine and optimize these strategies will be essential in reducing the high mortality associated with AMI and cardiogenic shock.

ONLINE REFERENCES

Please scan the QR code provided at the end of the table of contents for References of this chapter.

CHAPTER

130

STEMI! Strategic Difference in the Treatment and Management in Men and Women

Subroto Mandal, B Shukti, Rajeev Gupta

ABSTRACT

Cardiovascular disease is a leading cause of death worldwide, but its impact on health of women and men may affect significantly. Multiple factors are responsible for these disparities. Significant proportion of women presenting with acute coronary syndromes (ACS). Women often experience different symptoms, risk factors, and outcomes compared to men.

In general population, communities and healthcare providers cardiovascular disease to be considered as preferably men's disease and that women are at low risk. Women are different from men by their physical, anatomical, mental, and psychological aspect. Unlike men they have menarche, menstrual cycle, and menopause. They have the extraordinary responsibility to give birth to offsprings.

Deficiency of awareness is not only at the gender or social level but also at family physician level. Which makes the outcome even worse in cases with female genders. Cardiovascular risk and symptoms, often atypical with women, and therefore females receive delayed medical attention.

Specially in case of ST-elevation MI (STEMI), even with medical emergency where it is a part of training and teaching that "time is muscle", women with ACS receive delays in diagnosis and management strategies.

Incorrectly judgement by the physicians often estimates wrongly leading to a slowdown in diagnosis, which leads to further risk of ACS in women. Incorrect diagnosis affects appropriate treatment in proper time, including coronary angiography, revascularization, and primary percutaneous coronary intervention (PCI), with intervention get hampered. In comparison to men, women receive less guideline-directed medical therapy along with increased mortality rates, higher cardiovascular events and bleeding rates in women.

It is the need of the hour to review the sex disparities in presentation, risk factors, pathophysiology, diagnosis, management, and end results cardiovascular disease in both sexes in their context.

Because of the knowledge gap, the treatment remains same for men and women both, results into the inferior outcomes in women. Yet these differences have historically been under-researched and under-recognized. This is the need of time to bridge this knowledge gap.

Keywords: Cardiovascular disease, risk factors, death worldwide, diagnosis, and STEMI

INTRODUCTION

Cardiovascular disease (CVD) remains the leading cause of mortality across the globe in both sexes.[1] Coronary artery disease (CAD) in a patient may present with acute coronary syndromes (ACSs), and unstable angina (UA), with variable ST changes (NSTEMI) and (STEMI). Immediate diagnosis and revascularization strategies are critical to minimize ischemia-related complications.[2]

Significant increment witnessed in the cases of CAD in women.[3] Interestingly in all income groups, CVD is the prime cause of mortality across nations.[4] Although mortality after ACS has been dramatically reduced in the recent years due to improvement in medical sciences over the past decade.[5]

But recent data revealed important issues related to CVD in women that in comparison to men women have poor outcomes after MI in all ethnicities and age groups.[6-8]

Lack of awareness is one of the important factor for this disparity. Problem with awareness is not only at the gender or social level but also at family physician level. Which makes the outcome even worse in cases with female genders. Cardiovascular risk and symptoms, often atypical with women, and therefore females receive delayed medical attention.

Another principal reason is that CAD in women is underdiagnosed and undertreated, with unacceptable use of medical therapy and revascularization strategy. In general, CVD to be considered as "men's disease" and that women are at low risk. Women are different from men by their physical, anatomical, mental, and psychological aspect. Unlike men they have menarche, menstrual cycle, and menopause. They have the extraordinary responsibility to give birth to offsprings.

It is the need of the hour to review the sex disparities in presentation, risk factors, pathophysiology, diagnosis, management, and end results CVD in both sexes in their context.

Because of the knowledge gap the treatment remains same for men and women both, results into the inferior outcomes in women. Yet these differences have historically been under-researched and under-recognized. This is the need of time to bridge this knowledge gap of biological or pathophysiological issues with sex or difference in healthcare in physician level.

CARDIOVASCULAR DISEASE IN WOMEN—PATHOPHYSIOLOGY

The pathophysiology of CVD in women is very complex and affected by many unique factors such as biological and hormonal factors which differentiate from men. These differences are crucial for proper diagnosis, treatment, and prevention for the disease profiling.

In many studies, the pathogenesis of MI in women have revealed a number of biological and hormonal factors are responsible in comparison with opposite gender.[9,10] One of the important factor is estrogen hormonal influences. This hormone during menstruation period women has a lower risk of CVD than men, partly due to the protective effects of estrogen, by maintaining a favorable lipid profile, promotes vasodilation, and reduces inflammation. But postmenopause, reduction in estrogen levels is linked with an increased risk of CVD.

Endothelial dysfunction in women is more prone to CAD, which contributes to the development of atherosclerosis. Estrogen's protective effects on endothelial function are diminished after menopause. Compared to men, the microvascular disease and dysfunction may responsible along with diminish coronary flow reserve are strongly associated with cardiovascular events in women.[11]

In MINOCA (myocardial infarction with non-obstructive coronary arteries) approximately 6–15% of all MIs in women these two factors are primarily responsible.[12-14] Patients with MINOCA have significantly higher rates of mortality and morbidity compared to age-matched controls with a hazard ratio (HR) of 4.6 (95% CI 3.54–6.10) for cardiovascular events of 2 years duration.[15] Pathology behind the MINOCA includes mainly plaque erosion, microvascular dysfunction, coronary spasm, coronary embolism, coronary dissection, etc. MINOCA is considered a phenomenon in women because the presentation of MINOCA in women is five times compared to men.[14,16] In general population, MINOCA includes of nearly 50% women, although only 25% in MI due to obstruction in coronary artery.

There is challenge in MINOCA patients in women due to is the least numbers of randomized controlled trials and studies. In a registry from the Swedish Web System for Enhancement of Evidence-based Care in Heart Disease Evaluated According to Recommended Therapies (SWEDEHEART) concluded a beneficial results of lipid lowering therapy and angiotensin-converting enzyme (ACE) inhibitors or angiotensin receptor blockers (ARBs).[17]

The culprit mechanism for an MI is more often plaque erosion in young females, and another pathophysiological factor plaque rupture is common in elderly women.[18,19] Spontaneous coronary artery dissection (SCAD) is another crucial pathophysiological factor for cardiovascular event in women comparing to men. And responsible for about 1% cases with ACS.[20] Interestingly its increased up to 25% in women of >60 years of age.[21,22]

CARDIOVASCULAR DISEASE IN WOMEN—RISK FACTORS

Common risk factors for both men and women are same for CVD such as diabetes, smoking, and hypertension but it affects more and are associated with increased relative risk in women. High blood pressure in women compared to men in women extend to 1.8 times more the risk for MI, similarly with smoking, the risk in women is doubled, and in diabetes mellitus, its three times that of opposite sex.[23]

Interestingly women have nontraditional risk factors which are very peculiar to the female genders. Other gender-specific risk factors conditions such as polycystic ovary syndrome (PCOS), preeclampsia, gestational diabetes, and autoimmune diseases (e.g., lupus and rheumatoid arthritis) are associated with an increased risk of CVD in women.

Hormonal and pregnancy-related risk factors are small-for-gestational age births, menopause and pregnancy-related complications, preterm delivery, gestational diabetes, pregnancy-induced hypertension, preeclampsia, and eclampsia **(Fig. 1)**.

Hypertensive disorders during gestational period led to a markedly increased risk for cardiovascular mortality with younger age that risk carries in later life up to the age of 70 years and more.[24]

Higher levels of blood sugar in fasting during gestational period has significant effect on cardiovascular health in women during pregnancy and later life also.[25] Young women with CAD have higher risk of 16% compared to men, in spite of the fact the healthcare providers discuss lesser with them about their cardiovascular health and strategy to lower and modify the risk of acute events.[26]

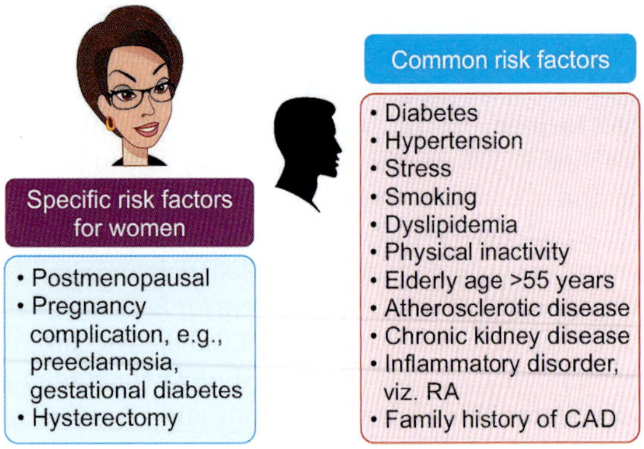

FIG. 1: Cardiovascular risk factors in men and women.
(CAD: coronary artery disease; RA: rheumatoid arthritis)

CARDIOVASCULAR DISEASE IN WOMEN—CLINICAL PRESENTATION

The clinical presentation of CVD in women can differ significantly from that in men. Heart attack is the men's disease is the false impression that only men suffer with heart disease is strong in our society, which results into miscalculate risk of heart attack in women.[27] Women often experience more subtle or atypical symptoms, which can sometimes lead to underdiagnosis or delayed treatment.

Atypical symptoms are experienced by mostly women compared to men. Presentation-associated symptoms are mainly palpitations, pain irradiating into the arm, neck, between shoulder blades and the jaw, and shortness of breath, nausea, or vomiting.[28] Because of these atypical symptoms and interpretation by healthcare provider results into the delay in the treatment.[28,29]

In fact, 85% of men and women experience typical symptoms of heart attack, yet receive different attentions and interpretation. Young patients with MI and chest pain.[28] Although the prevalence of prodromal symptoms is lesser in men than women. Prodromal symptoms can be more prominent in women, such as sleep disturbances, arm weakness, coughing, neck pain, headache and unusual fatigue, etc.[30]

Women with typical symptoms also receive longer delay in medical care in both the women, and their treating physicians and healthcare providers.[28] In a study in Australia and globally showed remarkable delays in presentation and PCI of women with ACS and MI.[31,32] Delay in time is very critical for the strategy for the management, may be in two situations. Primarily delay for the patient seeks first medical contact (FMC) from the onset of clinical symptoms. Secondarily delay or "SYSTEM-DELAY" in the final management is performed (i.e., PCI) or revascularization of target vessel. Multiple factors are responsible for this delay from onset of symptoms to final strategy or revascularization.[28,29,33]

Socioeconomic status is another important issue that affect the awareness. Study showed that women with lower

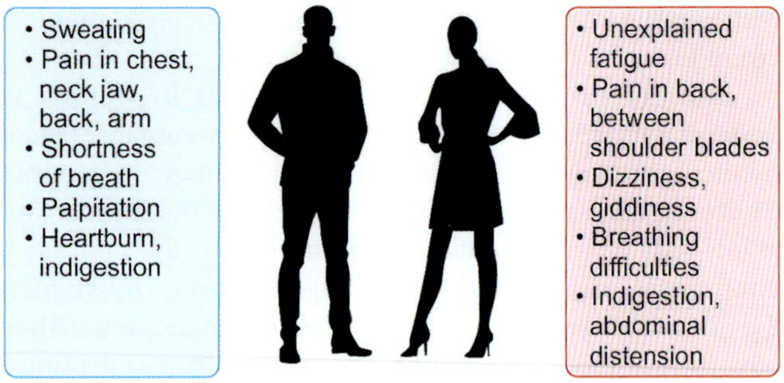

FIG. 2: Heart attack signs in men versus women.

socioeconomic status is associated with low socioeconomic status have less MI awareness and emergency presentation. Gender role in the family also have a significant role to receive medical care specially in developing country.[34] Significant delay in the treatment receives by female patients regardless of transportation facility healthcare center and support system with prehospital ECG transmission that delays the FMC **(Fig. 2)**.[35]

Prehospital delays are the main reason to seek the invasive treatment from FMC. Prehospital delay can be multifactorial components. Which starts from availability of basic facility to revascularization facility which affects door-to-balloon (DTB) time.[36]

To diagnose MI in women, there are a basic electrocardiograph (ECG)-based diagnosis is also difficult during emergency presentation. Women tend to have less J-point elevation compared to men, hence STEMI can be more easily be misdiagnosed. Interestingly right coronary artery as disease appears more with women, leading to less significant ECG changes then left anterior coronary artery occlusion, usually presents in MI with men.[31]

A randomized trial in Italy revealed that female patient treated with early revascularization receives less benefit compared medical management to women with in-hospital and 1-year mortality.[37] Comparing to men about 12.5% less women receive revascularization in time, which is crucial to the prognosis and long-term events.[38]

CARDIOVASCULAR DISEASE IN WOMEN—DIAGNOSIS

Anatomical and physiological factors play an important role in women, which produces significant impact on pathological and biochemistry tests. These biochemical parameters are crucial for the diagnosis and management strategies for any cardiovascular events. Unfortunately, the cut-off value for the cardiac-specific tests are some for both sexes.

In compared to men, women with MI receive fewer invasive testing, less timely revascularization procedures. This observation confirmed by many large registries as, Myocardial Ischaemic National Audit Project (MINAP, conducted in England and Wales).[38,39] The Swedish Web System for Enhancement of Evidence-based Care in Heart

Disease Evaluated According to Recommended Therapies (SWEDEHEART).[40] Another study, Australian Cooperative National Registry of Acute Coronary Care, Guideline Adherence and Clinical Events (CONCORDANCE) also confirmed the same results.[32]

Retrospective analyses revealed that women diagnosed with an MI has been doubled when it used of gender linked troponin cut-offs values, and diagnosis further confirmed higher risk of reinfarction or death.[41] Differences observed in both type of MI (Type-1 MI, i.e., atherosclerotic plaque disruption and subsequent thrombosis) (type-2 MI preexisting plaque of the coronary artery with recent onset discrepancy in oxygen supply).[42]

After using a high-sensitivity troponin assay for the diagnosis a notable sex inconsistency in troponin cut-offs has been observed. It has been recommended to take lower cut-offs for sensitivity troponin assays in females with suspected MI or ACS from the publication of Fourth Universal Definition of Myocardial Infarction, without providing any cut-off values.[43] Irony is even after the diagnosis with recommendation for the women with new troponin cut-off with higher number of registrations. Still the invasive testing was haft compared to men.[42] Regrettably the survey data from across the globe indicated that the in real world follow of gender-dependent cut-off values has not been practiced generously. It has been observed five times more additional women than men with MI when it used sex-linked thresholds to diagnose the disease.

Many factors paly role for the lower adherence to guideline-directed diagnosis and treatment in women, but the responsibility of healthcare professionals to estimate of risk of MI is misjudged.

Females are receiving 15% less invasive therapy compared to male, even after a large awareness campaign and the inadequate use of an invasive therapy in female with MI has not been improved.[44] Few factors have the impact in a smaller number of PCI is higher risk of bleeding in women has observed during undergoing invasive testing and treatment compared to opposite sex.

MANAGEMENT AND POST-MI CARE

Outcome depends on the management planning, support system, and optimal care by healthcare providers. The European Society of Cardiology (ESC) developed a model for optimal care with quality indicators to correlate with short-term and long-term morbidity and mortality rates. In the optimal model care, women achieved 13 out of 16 recommend quality parameters.[45] Adherence to antiplatelet therapy was observed less with women.[46] Adverse effects of drug such as bleeding and dyspnea are the important factors leading to lack of adherence early drop of antiplatelet therapy.[46,47] Interestingly, the bleeding rates with P2Y12 inhibitors were found to be equal in men and women in a large meta-analysis post-MI between both sexes.[48]

This is established the benefits of ticagrelor to mortality reduction, unfortunately registry data does not manifest that, it showed that prescription of potent P2Y12 inhibitors was less often women with MI.[49-51] Another important observation made in GLOBAL LEADERS subanalysis data that women with stable CAD showed increased bleeding events comparing with women with MI after prescribing P2Y12 inhibitors.[52] P2Y12 inhibitors were reportedly safe and effective even in older women with MI **(Fig. 3)**.

In invasive parameters, indicators of diagnostic angiogram and PCI where women were seen insufficient in numbers, for STEMI and NSTEMI.[39,53,54] Benefits of PCI are equal to both sexes, in spite of that invasive therapy received by women was than men.[55] Reason for the less invasive therapy described by late presentation in women is another factor to miss the window of for revascularization therapy and the higher rates of SCAD, MINOCA, and takotsubo cardiomyopathy in women and lower diagnostic yield in women.[44]

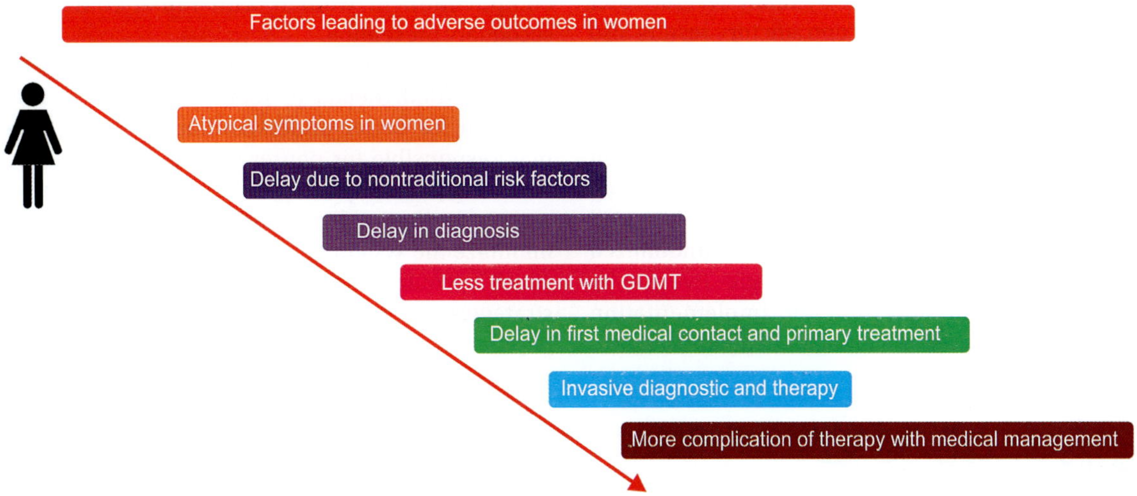

FIG. 3: Factors responsible for the worse outcome in heart attack in women.
(GDMT: guideline-directed medical therapy)

European and American guidelines for both sexes recommend radial access for the interventional procedures in primary or elective procedures.[56,57] However, Australian data demonstrate persistently lower radial access use in women compared to men.[58] Recently, radial arterial access for the intervention has become popular, due to reduction in major bleeding. Interestingly, it has been noted in various study that less procedure has been performed via radial route in women compared to men. In fact, benefits radial access has been found to better in women than men.[59-61]

It is established that optimal guideline-directed medical therapy (GDMT) has the benefits in secondary prevention and still, women are receiving less GDMT than men.[38,62] Despite the fact specially women with MINOCA receiving less medical therapy in secondary prevention. Nonadherence of therapy and socioeconomic factors in women may be the causes the for lesser use of GDMT in women.[63,64] It is proven that cardiac rehabilitation program carries a significant role in secondary prevention, yet women are less often referred by physicians for the rehabilitation program and less likely participate by women.[65,66]

CARDIOVASCULAR DISEASE IN WOMEN—COMPLICATIONS AND CONSEQUENCES

In all age groups, female gender has an independent predictor including octogenarians of mortality. Women lose 8% less expected life years after a STEMI than men do.[67-70]

Recent data suggest the matter of concern with rise in higher mortality rates in younger group of females,[71] which can be minimize by delivering equal cardiovascular care by healthcare providers based on protocols and ESC quality indicators.[38,40,72]

Women has lower risk of (MACE) major adverse cardiovascular events and mortality after adjustment for comorbidities observed in large meta-analysis of TIMI-trials data and similar conclusion made by many several other studies.[37,53,54,73] In many studies contradictory results also observed that despite coordinate with propensity, female has the faced inferior outcomes even after treating with an invasive therapy earlier.[74]

Lower rate of radial access used in women is important factors for major bleeding and worse outcomes in women presenting with both STEMI and NSTEMI, during and postprocedures.[46,75] In MATRIX study a large, randomized trial (Minimizing Adverse Hemorrhagic Events by TRansradial Access Site and Systemic Implementation of angioX) clearly showed advantage of radial access in women.[61] Sadly, procedure with radial access is less often used in women than men.[58] Thrombolytic agents and medication are another reason for major bleeding in women results into higher rates of blood loss.[76] In the first 12 months after interventions, women suffer with higher bleeding events, namely, hemorrhagic stroke with P2Y12 inhibitor.[52,67]

New-onset heart failure after STEMI in women is more prevalent than men which affects the outcome with increased mortality regardless of adjustment with treatment and comorbid differences,[50] which leads to a greater number of hospitalizations in women with 26–29% more admission compared to men.[77] Post-MI complications with women shown to higher with reduction in quality of life, more pain sensation, depression, and anxiety.[66]

Another important factors to note that the fact is women have less representation in clinical trials, in fact that participation to prevalence ratio of only 0.6, which limits our analysis and insights in gender-based studies.[78]

CONCLUSION

In conclusions, all factors to be considered with cardiovascular care in women, biological and pathophysiological variations need to be reviewed. The prime challenges that required to address to increase the awareness amongst women patients, and healthcare providers including nurses', and doctors. Recently check-list based approaches by artificial intelligence and machine learning could help healthcare providers.[79,80]

To improve women's awareness of their risk factors and warning signs for a CVD and heart attack and to provide knowledge and demonstration to seek help as and when required need a public campaign on heart disease.

Healthcare professionals need to be educated with public awareness programmed with gender-related cardiovascular risk and the differences in management and outcomes. Education related with understanding of gender-specific troponin level and their values, early invasive diagnostic testing, and interventional procedures. Also access related complication in women with radial route along with secondary prevention.

The CVD in women is under-researched and understudied, needs to focus on more cardiovascular research for better understanding of all the factors that may responsible for poorer outcomes compared to men. Including pathophysiology of MI and under lying causes in women for the implementation for the better healthcare to minimize the system delay. This is high time for a guideline which is required to clarify the all the steps and management strategies and recommendations appropriate for female, required to implement into clinical practice successfully.

ONLINE REFERENCES

Please scan the QR code provided at the end of the table of contents for References of this chapter.

CHAPTER

131

Diagnostic and Management Dilemmas in Women Presenting with Acute Coronary Syndrome

Sarita Rao, Roshan Rao, Vaibhav Shukla, Achukatla Kumar

ABSTRACT

Acute coronary syndrome (ACS) remains a leading cause of mortality globally, with significant diagnostic and management challenges, especially in women. This chapter explores the unique presentation and treatment dilemmas faced by women with ACS, highlighting disparities in outcomes compared to men. Women often present with atypical symptoms, leading to delays in diagnosis and treatment initiation. Traditional risk factors like diabetes, hypertension, and smoking have a more pronounced impact on women, complicating their clinical management.

Gender disparities extend to treatment, with women being less likely to receive revascularization procedures and guideline-recommended medications, resulting in poorer outcomes. The chapter also discusses the higher prevalence of myocardial infarction with nonobstructive coronary arteries (MINOCA) in women, a condition requiring tailored diagnostic and therapeutic approaches.

Addressing these disparities requires increased awareness among healthcare providers, refined diagnostic criteria, and patient education to ensure timely and effective care. The chapter underscores the need for continued research into sex-specific differences in ACS pathophysiology and treatment responses. By understanding and addressing these issues, the goal is to improve health outcomes for women with ACS and enhance overall cardiovascular care.

Keywords: Acute coronary syndrome, gender, women, outcomes

INTRODUCTION

Acute coronary syndrome (ACS) is a critical condition associated with significant mortality rates. Despite advancements in the diagnosis and treatment of ACS, cardiovascular disease (CVD) remains the leading cause of death globally.[1] In India, CVD accounts for a quarter of all deaths, with an age-standardized CVD death rate higher than the global average (272 vs. 235 per 100,000 population).[2] The incidence of ACS globally is estimated to be around 100–200 cases per 100,000 people per year.[3] Developed countries often report higher incidence rates due to better surveillance systems. The incidence of ACS in India is estimated to be between 50 and 100 cases per 100,000 people per year.[4] This is likely an underestimation due to limited healthcare access and reporting in rural areas. Men typically have a higher prevalence of ACS compared to women, especially in younger age groups. However, the gap narrows with increasing age, and postmenopausal women show a prevalence closer to that of men.[5]

RISK FACTORS AND PRESENTATION IN WOMEN

Young people with ACS often exhibit cardiovascular risk factors such as smoking, hyperlipidemia, obesity, and a family history of coronary artery disease (CAD). In urban India, the prevalence of these risk factors has surged over the past 25 years. Women presenting with ACS are older and more likely to be diagnosed with diabetes, hypertension, and congestive cardiac failure than men.[5]

Women presenting with ACS often exhibit traditional risk factors, but the impact of individual components such as smoking, diabetes, and obesity is more pronounced in women than in men.[5] For instance, a woman diagnosed with diabetes has a fourfold increased risk of myocardial infarction (MI), while in men, the risk is only increased by 2.5 times. Similarly, the relative risk of MI in female smokers is 3.3, compared to 1.9 in male smokers.[6] Hypertension and obesity also have greater impacts on women. Furthermore, a maternal family history of MI before age 65 years is linked to a fourfold higher risk of ACS in female offspring compared to women of the same age or older.[7]

Chest pain remains the predominant symptom for ACS in both sexes, with "cardiac" symptoms showing greater predictive value in women compared to men. Studies have produced mixed results on whether women experience different symptoms compared to men with ACS. Some studies emphasize that the symptom overlap between men and women. Women with ACS often exhibit a broader range of symptoms, including epigastric discomfort, palpitations, and shortness of breath, more frequently than similarly aged men.[6] They are also more likely to present later after symptom onset and receive initial reassurance that their symptoms are not cardiac in nature, leading to further delays. Commonly used high-sensitivity troponin (hsTn) thresholds for diagnosing non-ST-segment elevation myocardial infarction (NSTEMI) may be less sensitive in women than in men.[8]

TREATMENT DISPARITIES AND OUTCOMES

Gender disparities in the treatment of ACS are well-documented. Women are less likely to undergo revascularization procedures such as PCI or coronary artery bypass grafting (CABG) compared to men. For example, a study in the United States found that women were 34% less likely to receive PCI and 25% less likely to undergo CABG compared to men.[9] When PCI is performed, radial access is less common in women, with only 22% of women receiving radial access compared to 34% of men.[10] Older women experience higher rates of significant postprocedural bleeding compared to men, with bleeding rates of 8.6% for women versus 5.1% for men.[11] Additionally, women are less likely to receive guideline-recommended secondary prevention medications at discharge, with 58% of women receiving statins compared to 75% of men, and 42% of women receiving ACE inhibitors or angiotensin receptor blockers (ARBs) compared to 56% of men.[12] These disparities may contribute to the smaller reductions in recurrent MI rates over time in women.

Delays in ST-segment elevation myocardial infarction (STEMI) treatment for women are often greater than for men, partly due to longer times from symptom onset to first medical contact. A study from Vienna involving 4,593 patients found notable delays in the time from pain onset to first medical contact for female STEMI patients.[13] Similarly, Stehli et al. identified significant delays between symptom onset and hospital presentation in women with STEMI, even after accounting for age and comorbidities.[14] Women also have a lower priority for ambulance transport, experience greater delays upon hospital arrival, and less frequently receive reperfusion therapy, leading to poorer outcomes. A recent review of 43 studies reported that over 90% of them found longer symptom-to-balloon or door-to-balloon (DTB) times for female STEMI patients compared to men.[15] Despite these challenges, rapid reperfusion therapy benefits both sexes equally, prompting international societies to launch campaigns to educate women on recognizing and responding to common STEMI symptoms to reduce patient delays. In terms of treatment disparities, women are less likely to receive evidence-based ACS treatment, including early dual antiplatelet therapy, heparins, reperfusion therapy, and secondary prevention treatment. For instance, a study from China found that women with ACS were 21% less likely to receive reperfusion therapy compared to men.[16] In Germany, women were reported to be 25% less likely to undergo PCI and 17% less likely to receive CABG.[17] Similarly, research from Switzerland indicated that women were 19% less likely to be admitted to intensive care units for ACS.[18] Recent data on mechanical circulatory support (MCS) in women with ACS shows significant gender disparities. Women are 20% less likely to receive intra-aortic balloon pump (IABP) and 30% less likely to receive extracorporeal membrane oxygenation (ECMO) compared to men. When MCS is used, women have higher inhospital mortality rates (35% vs. 25%) and greater complications, such as major bleeding (12% vs. 7%) and vascular issues (14% vs. 9%).[19,20]

Sex-specific differences in outcomes following ACS have yielded conflicting results. Women are at higher risk of bleeding due to factors like smaller body volume, older age, and smaller blood vessels. Data from Australia indicates higher adjusted 30-day mortality rates for women following PCI in STEMI cases, with women experiencing a 30-day mortality rate of 6.1% compared to 4.2% for men.[21] Other studies have identified female sex as an independent predictor for inhospital mortality in STEMI but not NSTEMI patients, with women having a 20% higher risk of inhospital mortality for STEMI.[22] Research from the USA and other regions highlights a higher risk-adjusted inhospital mortality for women treated with PCI or CABG for STEMI, showing a 25% higher inhospital mortality rate for women undergoing PCI and a 30% higher rate for those undergoing CABG.[23] However, no sex differences were found in NSTEMI patients treated with PCI.[24] Higher mortality risks for women treated with CABG have been attributed to factors like smaller coronary vessels and treatment delays.

Long-term mortality outcomes for ACS have also been inconsistent. While several large studies report no sex-specific differences after adjusting for clinical risk factors, some recent studies suggest a higher long-term mortality risk for women. For instance, a single-center study from Portugal found a significantly higher 5-year mortality risk for female STEMI patients, even after propensity score matching, with women experiencing a 5-year mortality rate of 18.3% compared to 12.7% for men.[25] ACS includes unstable angina (UA), (NSTEMI, and STEMI), forming substantial parts of ischemic heart disease (IHD).

ST-SEGMENT ELEVATION MYOCARDIAL INFARCTION

Women exhibit a higher incidence of atherosclerotic plaque erosion, whereas men more commonly experience plaque rupture leading to acute myocardial infarction (AMI). Studies show higher mortality rates in women suffering from AMI. A meta-analysis of 18,555 women with STEMI found that women had double the risk of inhospital mortality and 1.5 times the risk of 1-year mortality compared to men.[26] Despite improvements in ACS care, advancements specifically for women have plateaued. Data from the ACS Israeli Surveys (2000–2013) indicated that women had longer delays in seeking medical care and had worse risk profiles (e.g., higher GRACE and Killip scores) than men, despite a lower proportion of STEMI cases.[27] Age acts as an effect modifier; young women with ACS are a particularly high-risk group. One study noted that younger women with STEMI had higher inhospital mortality compared to men, but this difference was not observed in non-ST-elevation acute coronary syndrome (NSTE-ACS) patients.[28] The YOUNG-MI registry, which followed 2,097 patients with a first MI before age 50 years for a median of 11.2 years, found women had similar cardiovascular mortality but worse all-cause mortality compared to men after adjusting for risk factors.[29]

Timely STEMI treatment requires early symptom recognition, quick access to healthcare, and rapid reperfusion (measured by DTB time). An analysis of the International Survey of Acute Coronary Syndromes in Transitional Countries found that women experienced longer prehospital delays than men (mean time from symptom onset to inhospital diagnosis was 270 minutes for women vs. 240 minutes for men).[30] No significant difference in DTB times was observed. The Victorian Cardiac Outcomes Registry also reported longer symptom-to-door times for women, and a smaller proportion of women achieved a DTB time of <90 minutes compared to men (64.5% vs. 69.8%, $p = 0.005$).[31] The VIRGO study indicated that women were more likely to attribute symptoms to stress or anxiety (20.9% vs. 11.8% in men). Additionally, 53% of women who sought medical care prior to their AMI reported that their physician did not recognize their symptoms as cardiac-related, compared to 37% of men.[32]

Thrombolytic therapies are recommended for patients at non-PCI-capable hospitals when PCI delay exceeds 120 minutes. In the GUSTO-I trial, women who received thrombolytic therapy had higher risks of nonfatal complications (e.g., shock, congestive heart failure, serious bleeding, and reinfarction) and a higher mortality rate. Despite the higher complication rates, thrombolytics were equally effective in both sexes with similar post-thrombolysis ejection fractions and ventricular function.[33] Revascularization of the obstructed artery is crucial for STEMI treatment. The GUSTO-II-B PTCA sub-study showed that women benefitted similarly to men from direct angioplasty.[34] Although some studies indicate higher mortality rates in women treated with primary PCI, these findings are confounded by the higher baseline cardiovascular risk factors in women. Lower revascularization rates in women might be due to less severe obstructive CAD and other MI etiologies. Women presenting with STEMI have been found to receive fewer PCIs, resulting in higher mortality rates compared to men.[35]

NON-ST-SEGMENT ELEVATION MYOCARDIAL INFARCTION

Women with NSTE-ACS also experience higher inhospital mortality rates compared to men. Despite guidelines recommending an invasive strategy for high-risk NSTE-ACS patients, studies have shown mixed results for women. The ISAR-REACT trial reported an increased risk for women undergoing CABG, and the FRISC II trial showed an increased risk of invasive strategies in women at 12 months.[36,37] However, some trials, like TACTICS-TIMI 18, found a significant benefit for women with elevated troponin undergoing invasive strategies.[38] Women are often undertreated, receiving fewer revascularization procedures and pharmacological treatments like heparin and ACE inhibitors.[39]

Sex-specific differences in long-term outcomes have been inconsistently reported. Women in the FRISC II trial showed a higher mortality risk with an invasive strategy, while other trials indicated similar outcomes between sexes.[37] Women have lower medication adherence, contributing to worse long-term outcomes.[40] Studies have highlighted the need for further research into sex-specific barriers to medication adherence and treatment.[41]

The 2014 ACC/AHA NSTE-ACS guidelines recommend that women receive the same pharmacological treatments as men, with attention to weight and renal dosing to reduce bleeding risks.[42] The 2020 ESC NSTE-ACS guidelines similarly emphasize dose adjustments based on body weight and renal function, especially in women.[43] The CRUSADE National Quality Improvement Initiative revealed lower acute treatment rates with heparin and ACE inhibitors for women with NSTE-ACS.[44] Persistent disparities at discharge included lower rates of aspirin, ACE inhibitors, and statin prescriptions for women.[45] Women also have lower adherence rates to prescribed medications, highlighting the need for further investigation into structural barriers to medication adherence.[37]

MYOCARDIAL INFARCTION WITH NONOBSTRUCTIVE CORONARY ARTERIES

Myocardial infarction with nonobstructive coronary arteries involves MI signs or symptoms with angiographic evidence of normal or <50% stenosed coronary arteries. Individuals with ischemia but no obstructive CAD face higher risks of adverse outcomes compared to those without ischemia.[46] Diagnosing and treating MINOCA is more challenging than obstructive CAD. Subcategories of MINOCA, such as spontaneous coronary artery dissection (SCAD), have better-defined investigation and management pathways. SCAD should be suspected, especially in young women, to prompt intravascular imaging, guide tailored management, and adjust the approach for subsequent chest pain episodes.[47]

Treatments vary based on the underlying etiology. Calcium channel blockers may treat epicardial coronary vasospasm, while beta-blockers, statins, ACE inhibitors, and ARBs are preferred for coronary microvascular dysfunction.[48] Statins can reduce exercise-induced ischemia by inhibiting oxidative stress, reducing inflammation, and stabilizing atherosclerotic plaque.[49] Anti-ischemic agents, including nitrates, show variable efficacy for angina caused by microvascular dysfunction due to etiologic heterogeneity.[50] Additional therapies like ranolazine, ivabradine, phosphodiesterase inhibitors, metformin, and L-arginine show variable efficacy and require further large, randomized trials to determine their effectiveness for MINOCA.[51]

STABLE ISCHEMIC HEART DISEASE IN WOMEN

In women, stable IHD is often due to nonobstructive atherosclerosis rather than flow-limiting epicardial stenosis. Other causes include coronary spasm, inflammation, and endothelial and microvascular dysfunction.[52] Traditional risk factors for IHD are similar between men and women, but factors like hypertension, diabetes, and physical inactivity are more predictive of MI risk in women.[53] Sex-specific risk factors for IHD in women include pregnancy-related hypertension, gestational diabetes, preterm delivery, small-for-gestational age birth, recurrent miscarriages, premature ovarian failure, early menopause or menarche, and polycystic ovarian syndrome.[54] Autoimmune disorders like rheumatoid arthritis and systemic lupus erythematosus (SLE) are more prevalent in women and lead to accelerated atherosclerosis, with IHD being the leading cause of mortality in SLE patients.[55] Breast cancer, more common in women, is also linked to higher CVD risk due to overlapping risk factors and cancer treatments.[56]

Diagnostic criteria for IHD in women are similar to those for men and include stress testing, echocardiography, and coronary computed tomography angiography (CCTA). The 2021 ACC/AHA Chest Pain Guidelines recommend estimating the pretest probability of obstructive CAD to guide diagnostic testing. Intermediate-to-high risk patients should undergo CCTA or stress testing, with CCTA preferred for those under 65 years of age and not on optimal preventive therapies, and stress testing for those 65 years or older in age.[57]

Women with IHD have worse outcomes than men, including lower quality of life, higher hospitalization rates, increased repeat coronary angiography, and higher mortality.[58] Studies have shown women are less likely to receive aspirin, ACE inhibitors/ARBs, and statin therapy for stable IHD.[59] While the role of statin therapy in primary prevention for women has been debated, two large meta-analyses confirmed its benefits for both sexes in secondary prevention.[60,61]

CONCLUSION

The diagnosis and management of ACS in women present unique challenges that contribute to significant disparities in outcomes compared to men. Women often present with atypical symptoms, which can delay accurate diagnosis and treatment initiation. Traditional diagnostic criteria and risk assessment tools may be less effective in women, leading to under-recognition of ACS and delayed treatment.

Management dilemmas arise from several factors, including gender-specific differences in risk profiles, symptom presentation, and treatment responses. Women are more likely to experience comorbid conditions such as diabetes and hypertension, which complicate the management of ACS and may contribute to worse outcomes. Additionally, women often face delays in receiving timely and evidence-based treatments like revascularization and guideline-recommended medications. Disparities in the application of these treatments reflect broader issues of gender bias and differences in healthcare access.

Addressing these challenges requires a multifaceted approach. Enhancing awareness among healthcare providers about the diverse presentations of ACS in women is crucial for improving diagnostic accuracy. Tailoring diagnostic criteria and treatment guidelines to account for sex-specific differences can help ensure that women receive appropriate and timely care. Furthermore, targeted educational initiatives for both patients and healthcare professionals can help bridge gaps in recognition and response to ACS symptoms.

Ultimately, improving outcomes for women with ACS involves a concerted effort to overcome diagnostic and management dilemmas, ensuring that all patients receive equitable and effective care. Continued research into sex-specific differences in ACS pathophysiology, treatment responses, and outcomes will be essential for refining guidelines and reducing disparities in ACS management. By addressing these issues, we can work toward achieving better health outcomes for women with ACS and enhancing overall cardiovascular care.

ONLINE REFERENCES

Please scan the QR code provided at the end of the table of contents for References of this chapter.

CHAPTER

132

Ventricular Tachycardia after Myocardial Infarction

Nishad Chitnis, B Hygriv Rao

ABSTRACT

Ventricular tachycardia (VT) following myocardial infarction (MI) is the leading cause of sudden cardiac death (SCD). The electrophysiological basis of VT is the substrate resulting from the myocardial scar caused by the infarct. The risk of VT and SCD is determined by the size and characterization of this scar. Cardiac magnetic resonance imaging (CMRI) has evolved as a very dependable tool to assess the myocardial scar. The extent of late gadolinium enhancement (LGE) predicts the occurrence of ventricular arrhythmias and SCD. Recent advancements in the software have enabled the characterization of scar and profiling of the arrhythmogenic border zones (BZs) of the scar which contain the pathological electrograms like the late and fragmented potentials. The characterization of scar heterogeneity has refined and demonstrated incremental benefits over LVEF in the risk stratification of post-MI SCD. The combination of LVEF and myocardial scar are useful parameters to recommend ICD for primary prevention of SCD in post-MI patients. Radiofrequency ablation has proven to be effective in treating recurrent VT and rescuing patients from the electrical storm of VT. Ablation involves targeting abnormal electrograms in the scar and BZs. Neuromodulation by modifying sympathetic innervation of the heart by various techniques is another tool to treat recurrent VT episodes.

Myocardial scar is the essential electrophysiological substrate leading to ventricular arrhythmias and sudden death following myocardial infarction. CMRI is an established modality to identify, quantify, and characterize the scar. Assessment of myocardial scar in addition to estimation of LVEF helps in risk assessment of SCD following MI. ICD implantation, radiofrequency ablation, and neuromodulation are major treatment modalities for post-MI VT apart from guideline-directed medical management (GDMT).

Keywords: Ventricular tachycardia, myocardial infarction, scar, CMRI, ICD, catheter ablation

INTRODUCTION

Ventricular tachycardia (VT) following myocardial infarction is the most important cause of sudden cardiac death (SCD). In the prehospital phase and early period following acute coronary syndromes, SCD results more often due to polymorphic ventricular arrhythmias while it is caused by monomorphic VT anchoring around the substrate of healed scars in the later phases of myocardial infarction. This chapter outlines the pathology of the myocardial substrate, its assessment, risk prediction and management of VT, and prevention of SCD.

TEMPORAL CLASSIFICATION OF MYOCARDIAL INFARCTION-RELATED VENTRICULAR ARRHYTHMIAS

Myocardial infarction (MI)-related VA may occur at different times during the course of an MI. The temporal relation of VA to MI is of critical importance, as the early and late prognosis, as well as management protocol, differs as per the time of occurrence.

- *Prehospital VA*: A small but significant minority of ACS patients present with out-of-hospital cardiac arrest

(OHCA), but ACS is the most common cause of OHCA. These patients have a high immediate and early mortality, which can only be reduced by increased awareness in the general population, increased basic CPR education, improved EMS systems, and strengthened ACLS training among EMS services. However, those who survive rarely have recurrent events if the ischemia is corrected. These patients need immediate CPR and ACLS as per standard guidelines. This should be followed by emergency revascularization strategies, with early coronary intervention providing the best results.[1]

- *VA occurring within 48 hours of acute MI*: VA occurring within 48 hours of ACS is due to ischemic substrate. These patients have high 30-day mortality and need aggressive drug therapy till their rhythm stabilizes. However, the long-term arrhythmic risk remains low, and no specific long-term therapy is needed (barring beta-blockade).[2]
- *VA occurring after 48 hours of acute MI*: Sustained VT/VF occurring beyond 48 hours of acute MI is a marker of long-term arrhythmic risk.[3] These patients need evaluation for ICD placement or a wearable defibrillator along with antiarrhythmics, especially if VA occurs even after complete revascularization. This is in contradistinction to primary prevention recommendations where ICD is not recommended in the first 40 days.[2]
- *VA occurring late after MI*: Patients who have sustained monomorphic VT beyond 40 days after MI have scar VT and should undergo ICD implantation along with antiarrhythmic drug therapy.[2]

PATHOLOGY OF MYOCARDIAL SCAR FORMATION

Adult mammals are unfortunate in losing the ability to regenerate the myocardium, unlike neonatal rodents, teleostean fish, and newts which can completely regenerate myocardial damage. As a result, MI in adult mammalian hearts can only heal by scar formation. After an MI, mechanical stress, as well as stimulation by hormones, growth factors, and cytokines, stimulates fibroblast proliferation, migration, and transdifferentiation into myofibroblasts. The extracellular matrix (ECM) stimulates the proliferation of, and collagen synthesis by, fibroblasts via biochemical signaling. Matrix metalloproteinases, fibronectin, thrombospondins, tenascins, and connective tissue growth factors all play a role in the formation of myocardial scar.[4]

The healing process after MI has three phases: (1) Inflammatory phase, where an influx of cytokines, chemokines, and immune cells results in phagocytosis and proteolysis of necrotic tissue; (2) Reparative or proliferative phase, which is characterized by the proliferation of fibroblasts and synthesis of collagen to form a scar; and (3) Maturation phase, when cross-linking of collagen results in the formation of a stable scar. These phases are seen at the site of infarct **(Fig. 1)**. Optimum control of inflammation is necessary to form a healthy scar, and both reduced and increased inflammation can result in adverse cardiac remodeling with resultant arrhythmogenic substrate and worsening heart failure, if not outright rupture.[4,5]

The second type of fibrosis occurs in remote myocardium, a phenomenon called reactive fibrosis. Compensatory cardiomyocyte hypertrophy and increased collagen deposition result in stiffening of uninfarcted myocardial territory and diastolic dysfunction which eventually worsens cardiac function and causes progressive heart failure more often than scarring at the MI site itself **(Fig. 2)**.[4]

Sustained monomorphic VT is the most common arrythmia leading to SCD post MI. It results from a reentry around a scar with a central slow-conducting isthmus **(Fig. 3)**. The isthmus most often is the border zone (BZ).

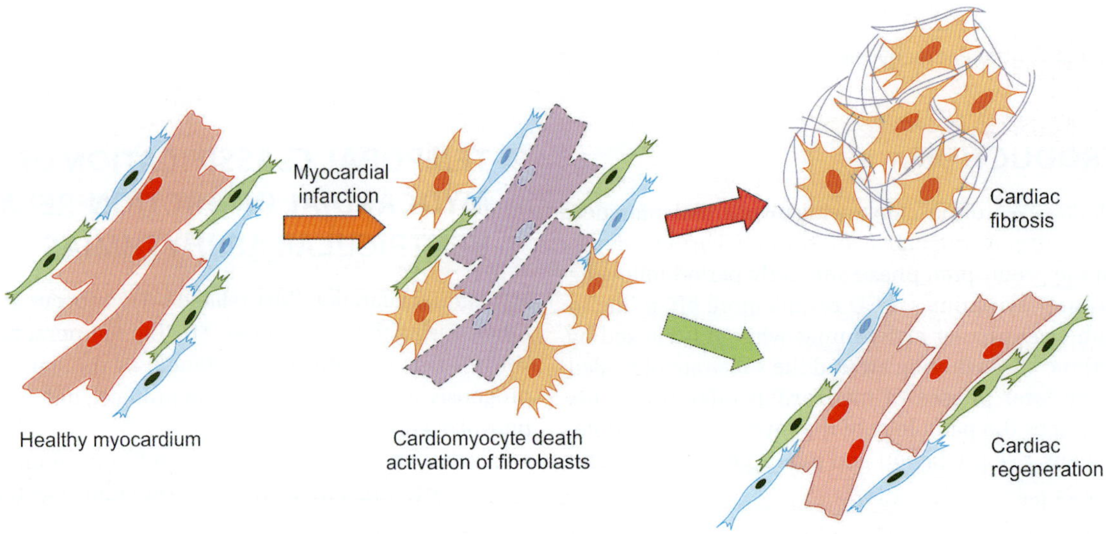

FIG. 1: Myocardial reparative response. The figure shows the response of myocardium to injury. Cardiomyocyte death is followed by infiltration of tissue by fibroblasts. In mammals, this is followed by fibrosis, while some animals like newts have complete regeneration of cardiomyocytes.

Source: With permission from Talman and Ruskoaho (2016).[4]

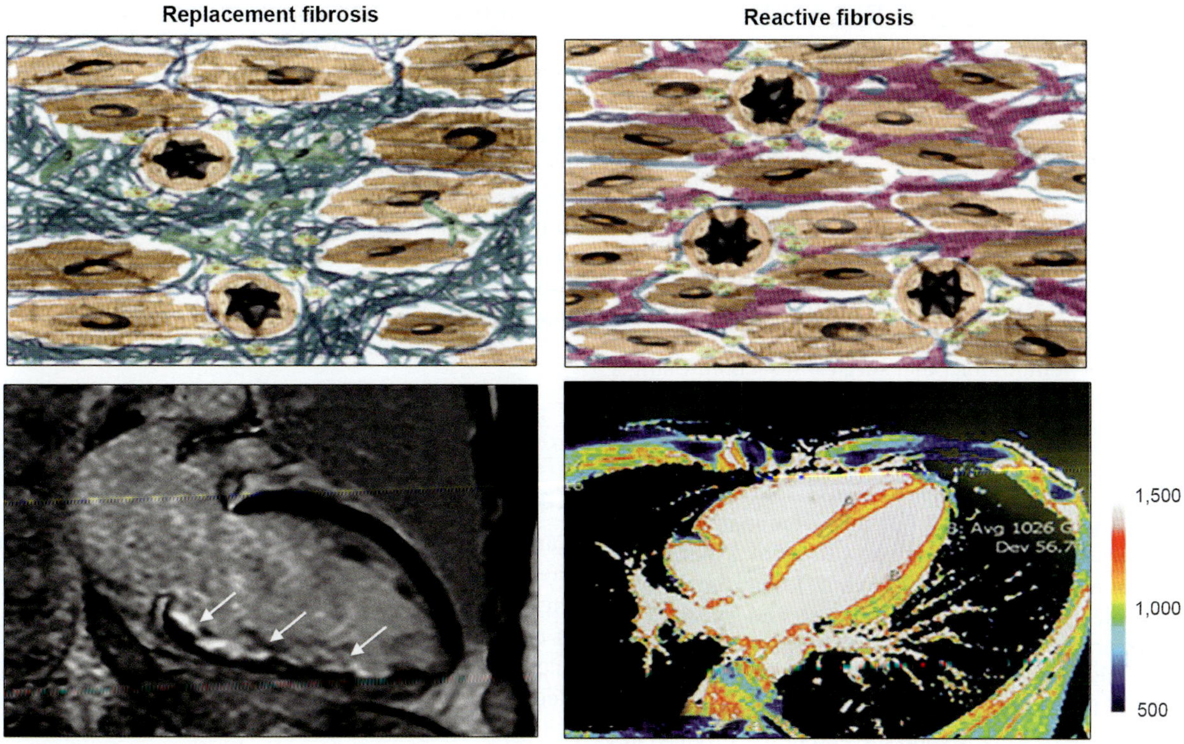

FIG. 2: Replacement fibrosis versus reactive fibrosis. The figure shows the difference between replacement fibrosis and reactive fibrosis. Replacement fibrosis is seen in infarcted territory and collagen replaces dead myocytes to form a scar. Reactive fibrosis occurs in remote territory and cardiomyocyte hypertrophy and thickening of collagen tissue occur resulting in stiffening of the myocardium.

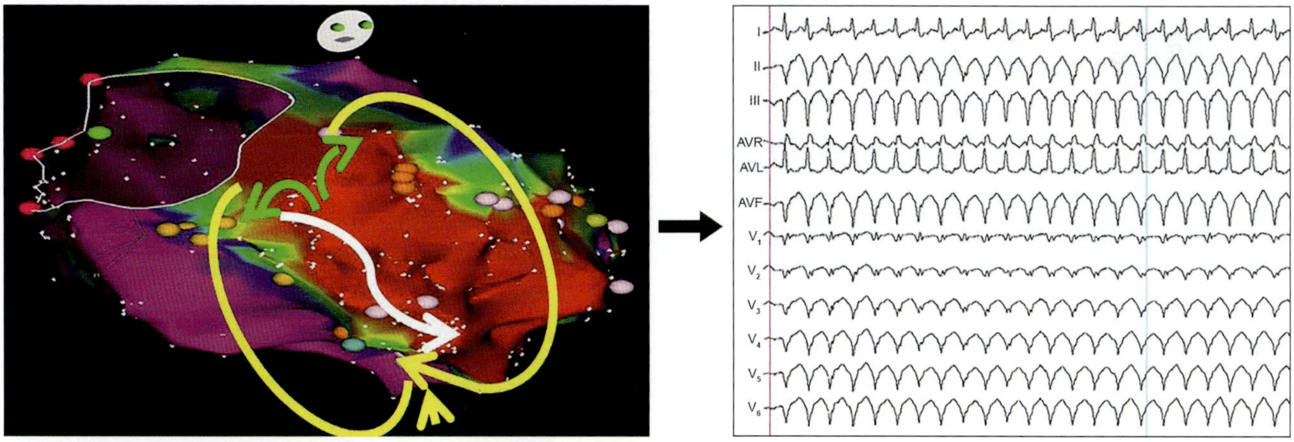

FIG. 3: Mechanism of scar VT in a post-MI patient. The figure represents an electroanatomical map of the left ventricle of a patient with remote myocardial infarction and recurrent VT. The large scar caused by infarct is shown in red. The central white line denotes slow conducting isthmus. The re-entry circuit of VT is seen going around the scar.

While infarct zone fibrosis is electrically inactive, providing an anchor for the re-entry VT, BZ contains electrically active myocytes which are separated by nonconducting fibrous septa, providing foci for ectopic activity as well as reentrant circuits.[5]

In ACS patients in India, STEMI is more common, and the mean time to presentation is longer. It follows that myocardial scars are larger which are expected to result in more events of SCD and heart failure.[6]

MYOCARDIAL SCAR-RELATED ELECTROGRAMS AS PREDICTORS OF VENTRICULAR TACHYCARDIA

Electrophysiological hallmark of the infarcted substrate of the myocardium is the presence of abnormal electrograms which are responsible for the generation and perpetuation of sustained ventricular arrythmias **(Fig. 4)**. The earliest demonstration of the correlation of VT with abnormal electrograms is attributed to the work of Miller who studied 18 patients with anteroseptal MI with VT. All these patients underwent endocardial surgical resection. Using a stainless-steel endocardial mesh, he elegantly demonstrated abnormal ventricular electrograms which were abolished following resection of segments of the left ventricle. This study not only confirmed the causative role of abnormal electrograms in post-MI VT but also demonstrated that removal of electrically abnormal subendocardial areas could potentially cure VT.[7] Subsequently, Josephson showed that these electrograms could be mapped endocardially by electrophysiology catheters without the need for surgical resection. The abnormal electrograms identified by these groups were fractionated (prolonged, multicomponent, low amplitude), late (lasting beyond the end of the surface QRS complex), and split (having two or more discrete electrogram components). In particular, fractionated and fragmented electrograms appear to be important in the BZs which result from the separation of myocytes by fibrous tissue.[7,8] This led to the era of endocardial mapping and ablation of VT. Refinements in mapping of substrates of VT uncovered the importance of channels which are tiny corridors of high-voltage areas within low-voltage myocardial scars. These channels sometimes show isolated late potentials which are responsible for the perpetuation of sustained VT. Hence, these are important targets of ablation.[9]

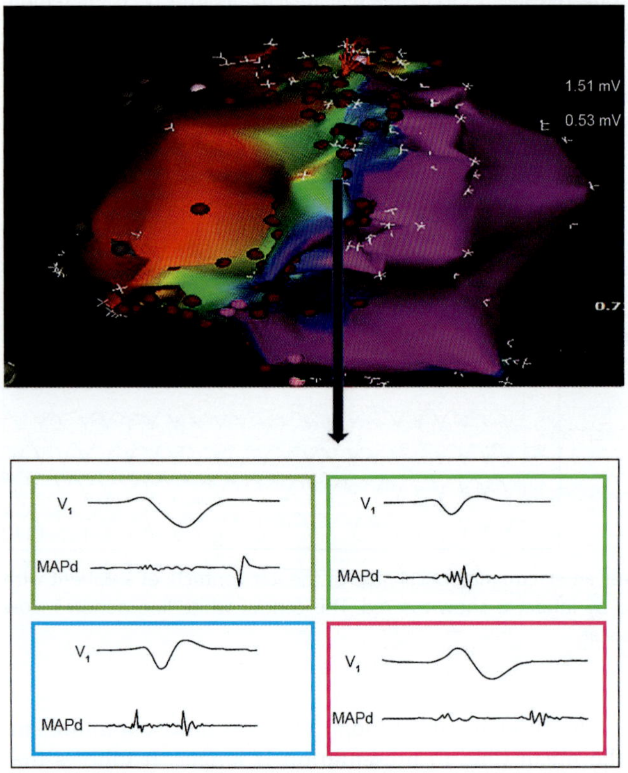

FIG. 4: Illustration of abnormal electrograms. Late potentials and fractionated potentials in the border zone of a scar in a post-MI patient with VT. These electrograms are important in perpetuating VT.

IMAGING OF VENTRICULAR TACHYCARDIA SUBSTRATE

Cardiac Magnetic Resonance Imaging

Cardiac magnetic resonance imaging has evolved to be the most effective imaging tool to identify and quantify the myocardial scar. Late gadolinium enhancement (LGE) is used to visualize scar tissue with a very high level of accuracy, permitting quantification of the scar **(Fig. 5)**. Recent studies have shown the correlation of scar burden with the occurrence of sudden cardiac death (SCD). This is particularly important as using the guideline-dictated LVEF ≤30% as a criterion for ICD implantation has a lot of limitations.[10] Several studies have shown the incremental benefit of CMRI-detected myocardial scar over LVEF for risk assessment of patients with prior MI.

Klem et al. enrolled 137 patients who were under evaluation for ICD placement for CMRI assessment of LVEF and scar quantification. The study demonstrated scar size > 5% as an independent predictor of all studied adverse events. Patients with scar size > 5% had a higher incidence of inducible VT, a higher incidence of appropriate ICD discharges, and an increased risk of sudden death, compared

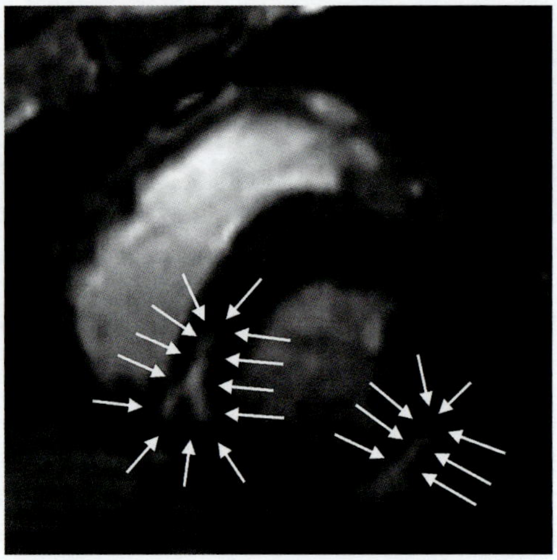

FIG. 5: Cardiac magnetic resonance imaging of a patient with ischemic cardiomyopathy. The arrows depict the scar.

to patients with scar size < 5%. When scar size was compared to LVEF as a risk marker, the study showed that patients with LVEF > 30% (otherwise considered low risk), in the presence of scar size > 5%, had a similar high risk for VT as did patients with LVEF ≤ 30%. Conversely, patients with LVEF ≤ 30%, but with scar size < 5%, had a similar low risk to patients with LVEF > 30%. This suggests that scar size may be superior to LVEF as a risk marker to recommend prophylactic ICD placement.[10] Our data of 133 heart failure patients with a mean LVEF of 34% showed that the presence of LGE (myocardial scar) of 5% or more correlated with HF events, appropriate shocks, and total mortality.[11] As it was known that the scar BZ and channels within the scar contained arrhythmogenic areas, identifying these areas on CMRI gained increasing interest. Hence, characterization of the myocardial scar by imaging its heterogeneity with advanced software was the next advancement in CMRI. Demirel et al. in 99 post-MI patients with low LVEF attempted to correlate scar heterogeneity with risk prediction of SCD in a small series of 99 patients with prior infarction and LV dysfunction. They showed that a high ratio of peri-infarction to core infarction zone was found to have a strong association with arrythmia incidence, ICD discharge, and sudden death.[12] A larger study, the GAUDI-CRT study, established these concepts emphatically in a clinical setting. The investigators evaluated scar mass, core and BZ quantity and distribution, and the presence, mass, and characteristics of BZ channels. These channels are conductive areas in the BZ that connect territories of viable myocardium which are otherwise separated by scar. Scar mass > 10 g and the presence of BZ channels were found to be very specific and sensitive for the prediction of future arrhythmic events. Two algorithms were developed. The first algorithm is of two steps based on scar mass > 10 g and the presence of BZ channels and predicted at-risk patients with 100% sensitivity and 81.3% specificity. The second algorithm, also of two steps, based on scar mass > 10 g and BZ mass > 5.3 g showed 100% sensitivity and 79.3% specificity. These CMRI algorithms show great promise in refining ICD recommendations.[13] These results are promising as current LVEF-based prophylactic ICD placement not only subjects many people to the device who never experience an appropriate shock, but also leaves many high-risk patients unprotected.

THERAPY OF POST MYOCARDIAL INFARCTION VENTRICULAR TACHYCARDIA

Device Therapy

Though guideline-directed medical therapy (GDMT) has been shown to decrease SCD and improve survival, it is not adequate to protect the high-risk post-MI population from SCD. These patients merit implantation of an implantable cardioverter-defibrillator (ICD). Beta blockers and antiarrhythmic agents are useful in reducing the incidence of appropriate shocks and in VT storm. The AHA/ACC/HRS guidelines for ICD implantation post-MI are detailed in **Table 1**.[14]

Catheter Ablation

Radiofrequency catheter ablation provides a significant reduction in recurrent VT, reduces ICD shocks, and may be lifesaving in VT storm.[15] The primary goal is the interruption of critical areas of slow conduction (isthmus) responsible for the development and maintenance of the re-entrant

TABLE 1: Indications for ICD implantation.

Type of prevention	Recommendation class	Level or evidence	Indication
Secondary	I	B-R, B-NR	In patients with ischemic heart disease, who either survive SCA due to VT/VF or experience hemodynamically unstable VT (LOE: B-R) or stable sustained VT (LOE: B-NR) not due to reversible causes, an ICD is recommended if meaningful survival greater than 1 year is expected
	I	B-R	A transvenous ICD provides intermediate value in the secondary prevention of SCD, particularly when the patient's risk of death due to a VA is deemed high and the risk of nonarrhythmic death (either cardiac or noncardiac) is deemed low based on the patient's burden of comorbidities and functional status
	I	B-NR	In patients with ischemic heart disease and unexplained syncope who have inducible sustained monomorphic VT on electrophysiological study, an ICD is recommended if meaningful survival of greater than 1 year is expected
Primary	I	A	In patients with LVEF of 35% or less that is due to ischemic heart disease who are at least 40 days post-MI and at least 90 days postrevascularization, and with NYHA class II or III HF despite GDMT, an ICD is recommended if meaningful survival of greater than 1 year is expected
	I	A	In patients with LVEF of 30% or less that is due to ischemic heart disease who are at least 40 days post-MI and at least 90 days postrevascularization, and with NYHA class I HF despite GDMT, an ICD is recommended if meaningful survival of greater than 1 year is expected

Continued

Continued

Type of prevention	Recommendation class	Level or evidence	Indication
	I	B-R	A transvenous ICD provides high value in the primary prevention of SCD, particularly when the patient's risk of death due to a VA is deemed high and the risk of nonarrhythmic death (either cardiac or noncardiac) is deemed low based on the patient's burden of comorbidities and functional status
	I	B-R	In patients with NSVT due to prior MI, LVEF of 40% or less, and inducible sustained VT or VF at electrophysiological study, an ICD is recommended if meaningful survival of greater than 1 year is expected
	IIa	B-NR	In nonhospitalized patients with NYHA class IV symptoms who are candidates for cardiac transplantation or an LVAD, an ICD is reasonable if meaningful survival of greater than 1 year is expected
	III	C-EO	An ICD is not indicated for NYHA class IV patients with medication-refractory HF who are not also candidates for cardiac transplantation, an LVAD, or a CRT defibrillator that incorporates both pacing and defibrillation capabilities

Source: With permission from Al-Khatib et al. (2018).[14]

circuit. Identification of the VT isthmus is best achieved by VT activation and entrainment mapping. Various methods of substrate modification have been demonstrated which majorly include targeting abnormal electrograms.[8,16] One of the very successful techniques is ablation of local abnormal ventricular activities (LAVA) which are sharp, high-frequency ventricular potentials. Complete elimination of LAVA has been shown to eliminate VT.[17] Elimination of all channels is a similar technique where abnormal "channels" in the scar are ablated selectively.[18] Elimination of all abnormal potentials leads to scar homogenization which has been shown to reduce VT recurrence to 19% in comparison to 47% by standard ablation.[19] Linear ablation lesions, which replicate the effect of surgical subendocardial resection, were described by Marchlinski et al. for patients with multiple unmappable VTs.[20] Patients with LV aneurysm which is the focus of VT circuits can be treated by ablation of neck of aneurysm resulting in electrical isolation of an arrhythmogenic substrate.[21] A multicenter study by Komatsu et al. has demonstrated an 84% success rate in eliminating in-hospital VT storm by catheter ablation, thus confirming a consistent benefit in mortality and morbidity reduction.[22]

SPECIAL SITUATIONS: ELECTRICAL STORM AND INCESSANT VENTRICULAR TACHYCARDIA

Electrical storm (ES) is defined as "the occurrence of three or more distinct episodes of ventricular tachycardia (VT) or ventricular fibrillation (VF) in 24 hours, requiring the intervention of the defibrillator (antitachycardia pacing or shock)." While the electrical storm is defined by recurrent ventricular arrhythmia episodes or recurrent ICD therapies, incessant VT is defined as hemodynamically stable VT lasting longer than 1 hour.[23] ES has high mortality and needs urgent management.

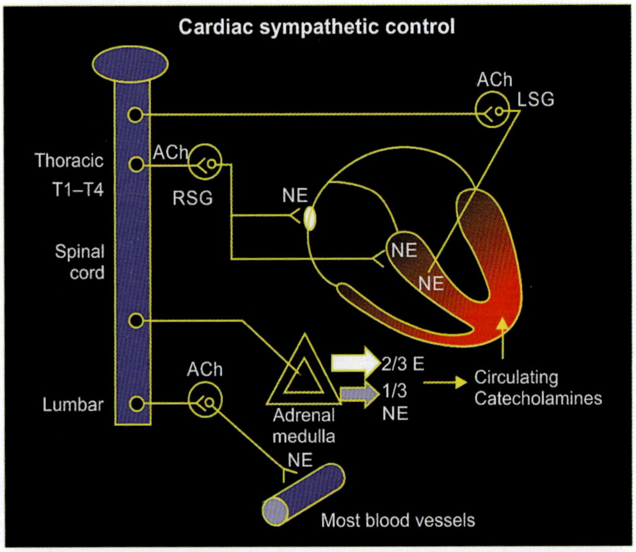

FIG. 6: Illustration summarizing the sympathetic innervation of the heart which is the basis of neuromodulation in recurrent VT.

Electrical storm patients need intensive care admission, deep sedation, and mechanical ventilation (to control the hyperadrenergic state). ICD, if present, should be switched off to avoid battery depletion and an external defibrillator should be attached. Antiarrhythmic agents are the first-line therapy for ES. In the case of refractory ES, catheter ablation is used.[23]

It is evident that sympathetic innervation of the myocardium has an important role in the perpetuation of ventricular arrhythmias. Neuromodulation by modifying sympathetic input has been used in refractory ES along with or instead of catheter ablation **(Fig. 6)**. Various techniques of neuromodulation are thoracic epidural anesthesia (TEA), sympathetic denervation, and stellate ganglionectomy via thoracoscopy. Rao et al. have demonstrated an alternative method of radiofrequency ablation of the stellate ganglion using fluoroscopy-guided conventional RFA delivered via a needle electrode. This is a percutaneous procedure and avoids risks associated with the surgical approach.[24]

The STAR study was a multicenter trial that demonstrated impressive results of a percutaneous stellate ganglionic block for the therapy of ES. Around half of the patients enrolled had ischemic heart disease.[25]

CONCLUSION

Ventricular arrhythmias are a major cause of mortality and morbidity in patients after myocardial infarction. The risk of VA post MI has been estimated by LVEF alone till recently. However, LVEF is not an adequate risk marker. CMRI has shown promise in detecting heterogenous scars and abnormal electrical channels in scars which have been shown to be much better predictors of VA risk than LVEF and may be superior to decide about ICD implantation for primary prevention. Secondary prevention of VA involves antiarrhythmic drugs (especially beta-blockers and amiodarone), ICD (for all sustained and recurrent VA occurring after 48 hours of MI), and catheter ablation. Electrical storm is a high mortality condition that needs aggressive urgent therapy.

ONLINE REFERENCES

Please scan the QR code provided at the end of the table of contents for References of this chapter.

CHAPTER

133

Open Artery Ischemia: Comprehensive Management

Mainak Mukhopadhyay, Sandipta Ray, Kajal Ganguly, Subhasis Roy Chowdhury, Arijit Ghosh

ABSTRACT

The MINOCA (myocardial infarction with nonobstructive coronary arteries) and INOCA (ischemia and nonobstructive coronary artery disease) are both terms used in cardiology to describe conditions where patients present symptoms suggestive of myocardial ischemia (reduced blood flow to the heart) but do not have significant blockages (<50% stenosis) in their epicardial coronary arteries.[1] These conditions are of clinical importance as they may require different management strategies compared to typical myocardial infarctions with obstructive coronary artery disease. Managing these conditions can be challenging and typically involves comprehensive approaches.

Keywords: MINOCA, INOCA, myocardial ischemia, epicardial, management

INTRODUCTION

Conventional diagnostic coronary angiography is like "missing the forest for the trees", i.e., we can see only the larger epicardial coronary trees but cannot see the forest of coronary microvasculature. Around 10–15% patients with ACS can have nonobstructive lesion in invasive or CT coronary angiography.[1,2] There lies the concept of open artery ischemia. INOCA and MINOCA are the two ends of the spectrum of the disease, chronic or acute presentation, respectively. Although female patients are more prone to suffer from the microvessel disease, male smokers are affected more with epicardial coronary vasospasm.

MYOCARDIAL INFARCTION WITH NONOBSTRUCTIVE CORONARY ARTERIES

Definition

Myocardial infarction with nonobstructive coronary arteries refers to cases where there is evidence of myocardial infarction (heart attack) based on clinical symptoms, electrocardiogram (ECG) changes, and biomarkers (such as troponin elevation), but without significant epicardial coronary artery obstruction (typically defined as <50% stenosis of any coronary artery).[1]

Causes

Myocardial infarction with nonobstructive coronary arteries can be caused by coronary microvascular dysfunction (CMD), coronary vasospasm, or a combination of both. CMD can be due to a variety of conditions including atherosclerosis, spasm, dissection, capillary rarefication, microvascular inflammation, embolism, etc. It is important to identify the underlying cause because treatment may vary. Causes such as myocarditis or takotsubo cardiomyopathy must be excluded before the diagnosis of MINOCA.[1,2]

ISCHEMIA AND NONOBSTRUCTIVE CORONARY ARTERY DISEASE

Definition

INOCA is a broader term that encompasses cases where patients have symptoms of myocardial ischemia (such as chest pain or discomfort) and evidence of ischemia on diagnostic tests (such as stress tests or imaging), but with epicardial nonobstructive coronary artery disease (NOCAD).[1]

Causes

Like MINOCA, causes of INOCA include CMD, coronary artery spasm, endothelial dysfunction, and other less common causes such as myocardial bridging.[1,2]

SYMPTOMS

Patients with microvascular angina often experience chest pain or discomfort that may be similar to typical angina, but it can also present differently. Symptoms may include chest tightness, pressure, burning sensation, or even shortness of breath (angina equivalent). Patients with symptoms suggestive of angina should seek evaluation by a healthcare provider for proper diagnosis and management, as there are various conditions that can cause similar symptoms, including other forms of coronary artery disease (CAD).

COMPREHENSIVE EVALUATION AND DIAGNOSIS

Diagnosis can be challenging because standard tests such as angiography may not show significant blockages in the large coronary arteries. Tests used to diagnose microvascular angina may include stress testing, echocardiography, cardiac MRI, or coronary reactivity testing.

Detailed History and Physical Examination

This helps in understanding the patient's risk factors, symptoms, and bedside clinical cardiac findings. ECG often reveals ischemic changes but many times can be normal also, but stress ECG (TMT) can show objective changes due to ischemia.

Cardiac Imaging

Apart from echocardiography techniques such as cardiac MRI or stress testing may help in assessing myocardial function and detecting ischemia.

- *Echocardiography*: In a better window mid LAD flow can be assessed at rest and after hyperemia to evaluate for the resting and maximum diastolic coronary blood flow (CBF), thus coronary flow velocity ratio (CFVR) can be calculated. CFVR, in the absence of epicardial stenosis, gives us an idea of microvascular status. If it is <2–2.5 then there is microvascular dysfunction. Myocardial contrast echo is also effective in diagnosing microvascular perfusion.
- *CT angiography*: CT CAG not only gives a detailed description of the epicardial fixed lesions but also CT perfusion imaging if done will detect microvascular function.[3-5]
- *Cardiac MRI*: CMRI with gadolinium contrast is extremely helpful in detecting microvascular function. Delayed signal increase and persistently hypointense regions are suggestive of impaired microvascular perfusion.[3-6]
- *Cardiac PET*: Nuclear tracer molecules are taken up by the myocardial cells in proportion to the perfusion that can be taken up by the PET scanner. Myocardial flow reserve (MFR) and myocardial perfusion reserve (MPR) can be derived from a cardiac PET scan.[3-5]
- *Coronary angiography*: To confirm the absence of significant CAD and to evaluate for potential causes such as coronary microvascular dysfunction or spontaneous coronary artery dissection invasive CAG is the gold standard. In MINOCA/INOCA, there will be <50% stenosis in epicardial arteries, but sometimes slow flow can be detected. Intracoronary imaging (IVUS/OCT) can detect layered plaque/thrombus in some cases even with a good luminogram. Intracoronary acetylcholine challenge test can detect epicardial coronary spasm.[3-5] FFR value should be high in MINOCA/INOCA cases. With the thermodilution technique, CFR and IMR (index of microvascular resistance) can be calculated. CFR < 2 and IMR > 25 are suggestive of microvessel resistance. HMR (hyperemic microvascular resistance) is Doppler-based index and a value > 1.9 indicates microvessel dysfunction.

MANAGEMENT

Both MINOCA and INOCA require careful evaluation to determine the underlying cause and appropriate management strategies. They represent challenges in cardiology because they involve conditions with significant symptoms of ischemia but without the typical atherosclerotic CAD seen in traditional myocardial infarction. Comprehensive management of open artery ischemia involves a combination of medical therapies, interventions, and lifestyle modifications aimed at improving blood flow to the affected area and preventing further complications.[2,7] Here is a structured approach.

Lifestyle Modifications

- *Smoking cessation*: Crucial to reduce cardiovascular risk factors.
- *Healthy diet*: Low-fat, low-sodium, and high-fiber—promotes heart health and manages cholesterol levels.
- *Cardiac rehabilitation programs*: Exercise training, education, and counseling—facilitate recovery and improve long-term outcomes.
- *Weight management*: Maintain a healthy BMI—reduces strain on the heart and lowers risk of developing atherosclerosis.
- *Stress management*: Relaxation techniques, counseling—help reduce emotional stress which can impact cardiovascular health.

Complication Prevention

- *Education and awareness*: Patient education—symptoms of ischemia, importance of medication adherence, and when to seek medical help.

- *Complication management*: Monitoring for arrhythmias and heart failure—prompt identification to prevent further deterioration.

Monitoring and Follow-up

Regular medical check-ups: Blood pressure monitoring, lipid profile, and glycemic status checks—ensure treatment effectiveness and adjust medications as needed.

Medical Management

- *Antiplatelet therapy*: Antiplatelets are recommended as per standard protocol in IHD. Ticagrelor increases adenosine level in plasma which is effective in microcirculatory dilatation.
- *Calcium channel blocker*: They have got a potent role in reducing vasospasm. Diltiazem and verapamil also reduce heart rate that decreases the myocardial oxygen demand.
- *Vasodilators*: Although nitrates improve blood flow by dilating coronary arteries and reduce angina symptoms, their role is more in epicardial CAD s than in microvessel disease. Nicorandil has got role in arteriolar dilatation and hence has some effective niche.
- *Statins*: Reduce cholesterol levels, stabilize plaques, and have anti-inflammatory effects, thereby preventing further atherosclerotic progression. Statin also reduces capillary inflammation.
- *Beta-blockers*: Reduce heart rate and myocardial oxygen demand, especially beneficial in angina management.
- *ACE inhibitors/ARBs*: They are recommended in MINOCA/INOCA for their significant role over plaque remodeling as well as anti-remodeling agents.
- *Others*: Super saturated oxygen therapy has got some role in microvascular obstruction associated with ACS. Role of ECP might be evolving but yet to be recommended in routine practice. Ranolazine and trimetazidine are often prescribed agent in these subgroup patients but without much significant favorable data. Role of low-dose anticoagulant has not been established yet in INOCA/MINOCA.

By integrating these strategies, healthcare providers can effectively manage open artery ischemia, reduce symptoms, prevent complications, and improve long-term outcomes for patients.

PROGNOSIS

The prognosis for microvascular angina varies. It is generally considered to be a chronic condition that requires ongoing management. While it is not typically associated with the same risk of ACS as obstructive CAD, it can significantly impact quality of life due to ongoing symptoms. Few patients will culminate into HFpEF, AF, chronic persisting symptoms, or develop ACS (MINOCA from INOCA) in spite of all possible therapies.

CONCLUSION

Managing MINOCA and INOCA requires a multidisciplinary approach, involving cardiologists, imaging specialists, and sometimes other specialists depending on the underlying cause identified. Individualized care is key due to the diverse spectrum of conditions encompassed by these terms. Therapy of open artery ischemia is an evolving science, till then good control of risk factors are of paramount importance.

ONLINE REFERENCES

Please scan the QR code provided at the end of the table of contents for References of this chapter.

CHAPTER

134

Dilemma of Asymptomatic Three-vessel Coronary Artery Disease after Myocardial Infarction

Kamal K Sethi, Kabir Sethi

ABSTRACT

Coronary artery bypass grafting (CABG) is the preferred modality of treatment over medical therapy in patients with established three-vessel coronary artery disease with the aim of providing a survival benefit. However, the survival benefit with CABG largely depends on the quantum of myocardium at risk [i.e., the extent of coronary artery disease (CAD)], the coronary flow reserve, and the myocardial reserve. Symptomatic patients with three-vessel disease are easier to deal with as there is substantial evidence in favor of revascularization in such patients. It is the asymptomatic patient in whom there is a dilemma in choosing the right modality of treatment. Evidence that prophylactic revascularization is beneficial in such patients is lacking.

This chapter aims to synthesize the approach to treatment in asymptomatic patients according to latest guidelines and recent trials and also attempts to understand the role of prophylactic revascularization in such patients.

Keywords: Asymptomatic three-vessel coronary artery disease, coronary artery bypass grafting, triple territory major vessel disease

INTRODUCTION

Coronary artery disease is the dominant cardiovascular disease worldwide and continues to be among the first few causes of mortality. For over four decades, coronary artery bypass grafting has been the default strategy in patients with established three-vessel disease (TVD) with the idea to derive survival benefits.[1] Despite the large number of studies that define the natural history of symptomatic patients with angiographically-proven coronary artery disease, there is little known about the prognosis in asymptomatic individuals. Thought to fare better than their symptomatic counterparts, there have been studies that have demonstrated annual mortality rates as high as 4–5% in asymptomatic patients with TVD, especially if they have had prior myocardial infarction (MI). This has reiterated the views of those who emphasize more aggressive medical or surgical therapies in patients with established TVD, especially if they have suffered MI in the past. This chapter will help us to understand the prognosis in asymptomatic individuals with established coronary artery disease and lay emphasis on the role of prophylactic revascularization in such patients.[2-7]

DEFINITION OF THREE-VESSEL DISEASE

Three large early RCTs defined TVD as "a reduction of at least 50% luminal diameter in the three major arteries" [Veterans Administration Cooperative Study (VA study)],[8] "a 50% or more obstruction in three major arteries" [European Coronary Surgery Study (ECSS)],[9] and "a 70% or greater reduction in the internal diameter of the right, left anterior descending, and left circumflex coronary artery" [Coronary Artery Surgery Study (CASS)].[10] However, among the three, the VA study was the only RCT that demonstrated a survival benefit with CABG over medical therapy in patients with left main involvement. This was in part due to the difference in the characteristics of the study population as the CASS trial excluded patients with left main stenosis of more than 70% and the enrolment of such patients was much lower in the ECSS.

Although the CASS did not demonstrate a survival benefit with CABG in patients with good left ventricular (LV) function (reflecting the protective effect of better coronary flow reserve), this benefit was clearly apparent in patients

TABLE 1: Trials of patients with triple-vessel disease and good LV function.

Randomization (N)	VA trial (686)	ECSS (768)	CASS (780)	CASS registry (24,179)	ISCHEMIA (5,179)
MT (*n*)	47	188	90	127	316
CABG (*n*)		219	70	507	112
Survival % MT/CABG	93/92	82.4/94	95/95	74/92	93.2/–
p value	NS	0.0003	0.91	<0.0001	NS

Note: ECSS EF >50%, VA trial and CASS EF normal. ISCHEMIA LV function not stated.

(CABG: coronary artery bypass grafting; CASS: Coronary Artery Surgery Study; ECSS: European Coronary Surgery Study; ISCHEMIA: International Study of Comparative Health Effectiveness with Medical and Invasive Approaches trial; MT: medical therapy; NS: not statistically significant; VA: veterans' administration)

with moderately impaired LV function (35–49%).[11] This was contrary to the results shown in the ECSS trial, which did demonstrate a survival benefit with CABG in patients with preserved LV function **(Table 1)**.[9]

Subsequently, 20% of the patients in the CASS trial switched from the medical therapy arm to the CABG arm within 14 months of randomization; this number rose to 40% by 5 years.[10] This clearly reiterates the fact that patients with TVD, preserved LV function, low level of symptoms, and minimal demonstrable ischemia should initially be subjected to optimized medical therapy with a low threshold for offering revascularization if there is a change in the symptoms, functional class, LV function, or observable ischemia.

DEFINING SURVIVAL BENEFIT FROM CORONARY ARTERY BYPASS GRAFTING

Among the patients living with CAD, those with triple territory major vessel disease and/or left main involvement demonstrate a higher risk of sudden cardiac death in comparison to those living with less severe forms of CAD.[12] This is primarily due to the large volume of myocardium at risk in these patients, in addition to the impaired coronary flow reserve.[13]

When MI occurs in one territory, the workload on the other territories of the heart is enhanced by default. This is of utmost relevance in patients with extensive TVD since the limited coronary reserve in these patients is unable to adequately meet the demands of the increased workload, which in turn leads to symptoms of ischemia. A poor LV function backed by a poor coronary flow reserve further worsens the outcome.[13] Revascularization with CABG for survival benefit should be the goal in these patients as demonstrated in the early RCTs.[8,10,11] The importance of LV function and the survival benefit is further backed by the study of Hammermeister et al.[6] which noted a 2% annual mortality in patients with TVD and a well-preserved ejection fraction greater than 50% in contrast to the 5% annual mortality in patients with ejection fraction between 31 and 50%. Most patients in this study had a prior MI but only a few suffered from congestive heart failure.

PROGNOSIS IN ASYMPTOMATIC CORONARY ARTERY DISEASE

Even though the early angiographic studies noted the difference in prognosis in patients with one-vessel, two-vessel, or three-vessel disease, with more ominous prognosis with three-vessel coronary artery disease,[14] none of these studies defined the effect of lack of symptoms in these patients. In the mid-1970s, a number of surveys were conducted in the United States for understanding the prognosis in patients with asymptomatic coronary artery disease. The annual mortality rates in these surveys ranged from 1 to 3%. However, the major adverse cardiac events (MACE) occurred at similar rates irrespective of whether the patient suffered from one-vessel, two-vessel, or three-vessel disease[2] reiterating the fact that it is the volume of jeopardized myocardium and not merely the number of vessels involved that decides the outcome. **Table 2** summarizes the prognosis in asymptomatic patients with angiographically-confirmed coronary artery disease.

ASYMPTOMATIC VERSUS SYMPTOMATIC PATIENTS

The earlier angiographic studies demonstrated the annual mortality rates in asymptomatic patients to be half of that of symptomatic patients.[8,15,16] Amongst them was the Duke Harvard Data Bank Study that was unique in its attempt to evaluate the prognosis in a comparable group of 44 symptomatic patients who were matched with the 127 asymptomatic patients for their coronary anatomy, left ventricular function, and the number of prior MIs. The annual mortality rate for the symptomatic patients was found to be 5.7%, which was twice of the asymptomatic patients, much in accordance with the early angiographic studies. From these limited studies, it appeared that asymptomatic patients fare better than their symptomatic counterparts. However, these conclusions were drawn from a specific kind of patient population, and do not necessarily reflect the prognosis in all asymptomatic patients as a number of these patients experience either a nonfatal MI or a sudden cardiac death as their first overt clinical event. This was clearly evident in a study by Sharma et al.,[17] which included 19 patients who

TABLE 2: Prognosis in asymptomatic patients with established coronary artery disease.

Reporting institution	Number of patients	Mean follow-up (months)	Total cardiac events*	Mortality
US Air Force, School of Aerospace Medicine	78	36	22 (29%)	3 (1% per year)
Yale University	12	57	4 (33%)	0
National Institutes of Health (NIH)	147	25	27 (17%)	8 (3% per year)
Duke-Harvard†	44	42	13 (30%)	4 (2.7% per year)
University of Washington†	217	66	NA	NA for entire group
Green Lane†	50	54	24 (49%)	5 (~2% per year)

*Angina, myocardial infarction, death.

†Includes patients with prior myocardial infarction (NIH and University of Washington studies also included mildly asymptomatic patients).

(NA: not available)

were successfully revived from out-of-hospital ventricular fibrillation (VF). Eleven of these 19 patients had no symptoms prior to the episode and nearly all exhibited painless electrocardiographic and wall motion changes on bicycle ergometry. On angiography all patients showed multivessel disease, further rendering the belief of asymptomatic patients doing better than symptomatic patients, rather tentative.

ASYMPTOMATIC POSTINFARCTION PATIENTS

Among the asymptomatic patients, there is a subgroup of asymptomatic post-infarction patients who often times go undetected as they have no symptoms prior to or after the episode of MI. These patients are usually picked up on exercise testing. Short-term survival statistics based on these post infarction exercise tests indicate that among these patients, those who exhibit exercise-induced ST depression have higher 1–2 year mortality rates in comparison to those who do not.[18-20] Theroux et al.[18] showed that 1-year mortality rate in those without ST depression on exercise stress test was much lower than those with ST changes on exercise (2.1% vs. 27%). The presence or absence of angina during the stress test did not contribute to the prognostic importance of ST depression. Because this study was not specifically designed to prognosticate symptomatic patients, more data is needed in this subgroup of patients.

So, how should we treat these patients? What do the guidelines recommend?

The 2019 ESC guidelines,[21] keeping in mind the relevant clinical scenarios, clearly point out the need for revascularization irrespective of the symptom status, in the following scenarios **(Flowchart 1)**:

- Documented ischemia (ischemia should be >10% in asymptomatic patients)
- Diameter stenosis > 90%
- FFR <0.80 or instantaneous wave-free ratio (iFR) <0.89 in major vessels
- Left ventricular ejection fraction (LVEF) <35% due to coronary artery disease[21]

The 2021[22] American guidelines emphasize the indication of revascularization in stable ischemic heart disease (SIHD) as follows:

- For symptom relief (class of recommendation 1) or to improve prognosis in multivessel disease, left ventricular dysfunction LVEF <35% (class of recommendation 1) and 36–50% (class of recommendation 2a) or in case of significant left main stenosis
- If the anatomy is suitable, PCI is recommended for left main stenosis (class of recommendation 2a)
- In case of SIHD and a normal left ejection fraction, the impact of revascularization on survival is uncertain except in multivessel disease and proximal left anterior descending stenosis (class of recommendation 2b).

CONCLUSION

Even though asymptomatic patients living with coronary artery disease show a low annual mortality rate, there is a high chance of developing angina or myocardial infarction in such patients. This suggests that the asymptomatic state might just only be a forerunner of the clinical state in these patients. Despite low annual mortality, these patients are always at risk of developing MACE, which even though nonfatal, can be severely incapacitating. As a result, a more aggressive approach may be needed in some of these patients with a low threshold for offering revascularization, especially if there is demonstrable myocardial ischemia.

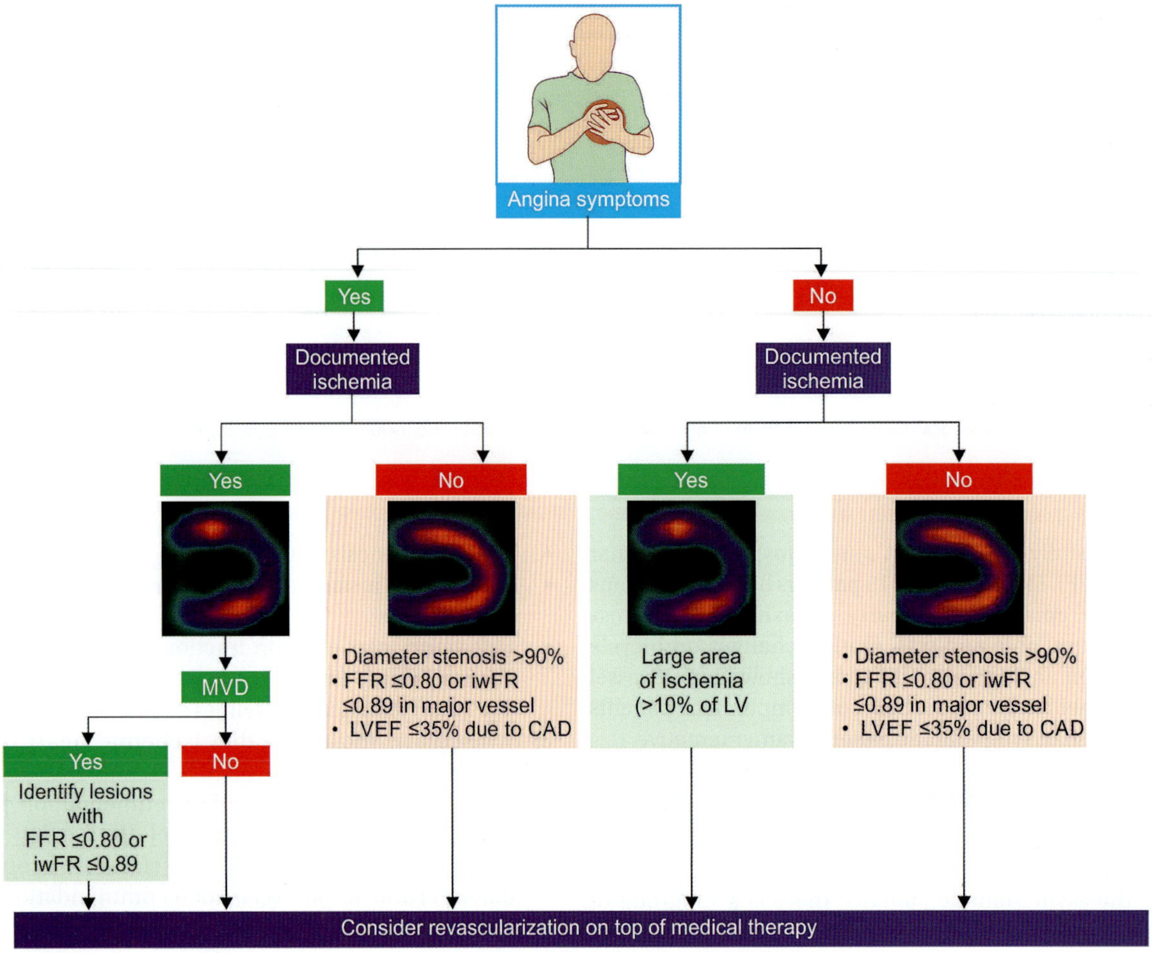

FLOWCHART 1: Decisions for revascularization based on clinical presentations.

Source: European Society of Cardiology, 2019.

ONLINE REFERENCES

Please scan the QR code provided at the end of the table of contents for References of this chapter.

CHAPTER

135

Current Status of Biomarkers in Reinfarction

Rajeev Gupta, Manu Gupta, Anuj Gupta, Pooja Sharma Gupta

ABSTRACT

For early detection of patients for reinfarction, assessment of various biomarker levels may enhance early diagnosis. The review provides an overview of the role of cardiac biomarkers in early diagnosis of myocardial reinfarction. Novel biomarkers are incorporated into multibiomarker strategies, linked to pathophysiological processes such as inflammation, neurohormonal activation, myocardial stress, myocardial necrosis, cardiac remodeling, and vasoactive mechanisms. Provide additional value for AMI prognosis.

Keywords: Biomarkers, acute myocardial infarction, reinfarction

INTRODUCTION

Temporal changes in biomarkers have relationships to reinfarction and to its clinical outcomes among patients with ST-segment elevation myocardial infarction (STEMI).

Biomarkers are indices of pathophysiological assessments[1] and rise/fall of cardiac troponin (cTn) (at least one value above the 99th percentile of the upper reference limit) helps in diagnosis of acute myocardial infarction (AMI)[2] with one of the following—(1) symptoms of ischemia, (2) electrocardiogram (ECG) changes of new ischemia, (3) new pathological Q waves, or (4) imaging evidence of new loss of viable myocardium.

Biomarkers play a crucial role in the diagnosis and management of reinfarction, particularly in the context of myocardial infarction (MI). Here are some key biomarkers and their current status in relation to reinfarction:

- *Cardiac troponins (cTn)*: Troponins are proteins released when there is damage to cardiac muscle cells. They are the cornerstone biomarkers for diagnosing MI, including reinfarction. High-sensitivity troponin assays allow for earlier detection and better prognostic assessment. Persistent elevation or a new rise in troponin levels can indicate reinfarction.
- *Creatine Kinase-MB (CK-MB)*: Although less commonly used now, CK-MB is another biomarker that can indicate myocardial damage. Its role in reinfarction diagnosis has been largely replaced by troponin assays.
- *Myoglobin*: This biomarker is less specific than troponins but can be elevated early after myocardial injury. It is more useful in ruling out MI when levels are normal.
- *Brain natriuretic peptide (BNP) and N-terminal prohormone BPN (NT-proBNP)*: BNP and its NT-proBNP are released in response to ventricular wall stress, often due to heart failure secondary to MI. They are not specific to reinfarction but provide valuable information on cardiac function and prognosis.
- *Inflammatory biomarkers*: High-sensitivity C-reactive protein (hs-CRP) and interleukins (such as IL-6) can indicate ongoing inflammation and are associated with increased cardiovascular risk. They may have a role in assessing the inflammatory response in reinfarction.
- *Lipid profile*: Elevated lipid levels, especially LDL cholesterol, are risk factors for cardiovascular events, including reinfarction. Monitoring lipid profiles is crucial in managing risk factors post-MI.
- *Genetic biomarkers*: Genetic variants (e.g., certain polymorphisms related to clotting factors) may predispose individuals to reinfarction. Genetic testing is not routine but may be considered in select cases for risk assessment.

DISCUSSION

What Makes a Good Biomarker Amongst Diagnostic Biomarkers?

Biomarker are surrogate marker for disease and its severity.[3] A good biomarker should have high specificity and sensitivity, newer biomarkers and their relationship to various pathophysiological processes. Glycated hemoglobin (HbA1c) monitors blood sugar control while blood sugar is used to diagnose diabetes.[4]

Cardiac Troponin

With a history of ischemic pain or ECG changes reflecting ischemia cTn is useful in diagnosis of MI and reinfarction. cTn a protein released from myocytes when irreversible myocardial damage occurs. It is highly specific to cardiac tissue and accurately diagnoses MI. cTn replaced CK-MB as the biomarker of choice for diagnosing a MI.[5]

Cardiac troponin level is dependent on infarct size.[6] Troponin levels peak at 10 hours or more, and stay elevated for 10 days or more. Newer, more sensitive troponin assays[7] have been introduced to rectify this limitation. MI is associated with the loss of myocardiocytes, fibrosis, and cardiac remodeling.

Cardiospecific troponins are preferred biomarkers for diagnosing an ACS due to their high sensitivity and virtually absolute specificity for myocardial injury.[8] High-sensitivity methods[9] have observed a dose-dependent relationship between the values of cardiospecific troponins and the subsequent risk of death and HF.

NATRIURETIC PEPTIDES

The natriuretic peptides, and particularly BNP, NT-proBNP, and mid-regional atrial natriuretic peptide (MR-proANP), the evidence in support of assessment for prognostication of patients after a MI is now well established.[10,11]

Interleukin-33

Interleukin-33 as the functional ligand of ST2, and the discovery of the pivotal role of the IL-33/ST2L complex for preventing the development of HF after myocardial injury, series of clinical studies that investigated the concentration of sST2 in patients with MI. An increased concentration of sST2 subtracted IL-33 from its physiological binding to ST2L and thereby increased the risk of progression toward adverse cardiac remodeling.[12]

Galectin-3

Galectin-3 is a soluble, beta-galactoside-binding lectin that plays an important role across several profibrotic pathways.

A number of biological studies have clearly shown that galectin-3 is upregulated in hypertrophied hearts and exerts stimulatory effect on macrophage migration and fibroblast proliferation, and thereby promotes the subsequent development of fibrosis.[13] Nevertheless, despite a large number of studies designed to assess the prognostic role of galectin-3 in patients with established HF, there is limited information on its role in predicting HF in patients with reinfarction.

CYTOKINES AND GROWTH FACTORS

Growth differentiation factor-15 (GDF-15), also known as macrophage inhibitory cytokine-1, belongs to the family of transforming growth factor beta. This cytokine is mainly synthesized and upregulated in myocardium in response to ischemia and proinflammatory cytokines, thus reflecting its putative role as a biomarker of multiple stress pathways in the heart, where it also exerts an antihypertrophic activity. The concentration of GDF-15 increases rapidly after an episode of MI, peaks at 90 minutes, and persists at an elevated level up to 52 hours after the onset of myocardial ischemia[14] serial values are useful in reinfarction.

OSTEOPROTEGERIN

Osteoprotegerin is a 401 amino acid protein that belongs to the tumor necrosis factor superfamily. This cytokine is highly expressed in a large number of tissues, is a powerful inhibitor of cancer cell apoptosis, and also exerts a crucial function in bone metabolism. Emerging evidence has also been provided that this protein may participate in the pathogenesis of cardiovascular disease and reinfarction through some putative mechanisms such as positive modulation of the inflammatory response and amplification of atherosclerotic plaque calcification.[15]

Osteopontin

Osteopontin is a glycoprotein (gp) that has recently been implicated in the pathogenesis of cardiovascular diseases, reinfarction, and other acute and chronic inflammatory disorders. The cardiac synthesis of this protein is enhanced after myocardial ischemia, and reinfarction with evidence suggesting that a significant relationship may exist between osteopontin production and LF dysfunction or cardiomyocyte hypertrophy, especially in patients with dilated cardiomyopathy.[16]

Neopterin

Neopterin, a member of the pteridines family, is synthesized by macrophages upon stimulation by the cytokine interferon-gamma. It is, therefore, a marker of macrophage/monocyte activation, exerting a physiological role in enhancing macrophage cytotoxicity. Since HF has an inflammatory component, the concentration of this biomarker has also been primarily investigated in patients with diagnosed HF;[17] however, only one study has assessed its prognostic role in patients with previous ischemic heart disease and reinfarction.

Matrix Metalloproteinase-8

Matrix metalloproteinase-8 (MMP-8), also known as neutrophil collagenase, is released by leukocytes in the atherosclerotic plaque, where it promotes fibrous cap thinning and plaque rupture, ultimately supporting the transformation of atherosclerotic lesions from stable to unstable[18] and reinfarction.

Matrix Metalloproteinase-9

There is growing evidence that MMP-9 may be a crucial actor in the complex pathway of cardiac remodeling via mechanisms that are probably independent from its collagenase properties. In fact, enhanced expression of this protein promotes neutrophil infiltration and degranulation in the atherosclerotic plaque, thus amplifying the adverse consequences of myocardial ischemia by favoring ventricular dilatation and increasing infarct wall thinning.[19]

Interleukin-6

Some studies have previously shown that IL-6 may participate in the pathogenesis of MI and LVR, although it has also been reported that knockdown of the *IL-6* gene does not influence infarct size, LVR, LV function, or mortality during long-term follow-up after permanent coronary occlusion in animal models, thus suggesting that the role of this cytokine is probably not substantial for long-term adaptation of LV postinfarction.[20]

Cardiotrophin-1

Cardiotrophin-1 is a 201 amino acid protein that belongs to the IL-6 cytokine family. This protein displays hypertrophic and cardioprotective properties and acts through leukemia inhibitory factor receptor b/gp130-coupled signaling pathways. The mechanical stretch in reinfarction is an important trigger of cardiotrophin-1 production by cardiac fibroblasts, and it has also been shown that the expression of this protein often anticipates the onset of contractile dysfunction that accompanies pathological hypertrophy and HF.[21]

Glycoprotein 130

Glycoprotein 130 (gp130) is the signal-transducing receptor subunit of the IL-6 family. The activation of gp130 is associated with generation of hypertrophic and cytoprotective signals in cardiomyocytes and promotion of cardiac extracellular matrix deposition, two separate pathways characterized by a convergence toward HF.[22]

C-reactive Protein

Although the clinical significance of CRP as a useful biomarker of CVD and, even more importantly, as an active player in the pathogenesis of atherosclerosis, is now well established,[23] there is emerging evidence that its role may extend beyond acute myocardial ischemia, with an effective contribution to reinfarction and development or progression of post-MI complications.

BIOMARKERS OF NEUROHORMONAL ACTIVATION

Copeptin

Copeptin is a 39 amino acid protein that originates from the precursor preprovasopressin along with the arginine vasopressin peptide (AVP). This neurohormone is actively secreted by the neurohypophysis in response to a drop in blood pressure or a change in osmotic pressure. As such, copeptin has received major focus in clinical practice as a marker of cardiovascular (i.e., HF and MI) and extracardiac (i.e., sepsis and infection) conditions.[24]

Cystatin C

Myocardial ischemia and reinfarction typically triggers an increase in the production and release of cystatin C. Interestingly, in ischemic myocardial tissue, the increase of this protein effectively inhibits cathepsin B and also promotes accumulation of fibronectin and collagen, thus representing a potential causal factor of cardiac dysfunction.[25]

Red Blood Cell Distribution Width

Anisocytosis, which is typically expressed as red blood cell distribution width (RDW) (i.e., the ratio between standard deviation of erythrocyte volume and mean corpuscular volume), has been increasingly found to be associated with a number of acute and chronic disorders including myocardial ischemia and relative complications. Although it has not been clearly established whether RDW may be a simple biomarker of disease and reinfarction or an active player in the pathogenesis of myocardial ischemia, a number of studies have assessed its prognostic role in patients with MI.[26]

Inflammatory Biomarkers

Inflammatory processes in patients with AMI not only influence the extent of atherothrombosis and vulnerability of a single lesion and predisposes to reinfarction but also affect cardiac repair mechanisms and the severity of myocardial tissue damage.[27-29] IL-6, a soluble proinflammatory cytokine and central hub in cardiometabolic signaling,[30] has been suggested to play a relevant part in these processes.[27,31] On average, patients with acute STEMI and reinfarction have higher levels of circulating IL-6. However, the clinical relevance of circulating IL-6 in patients with STEMI remains incompletely understood. IL-6 has been linked to microvascular dysfunction,[32] myocardial damage,[33] and adverse outcome,[34] but no differences in the extent of infarct severity and outcome between patients with low- or high-IL-6 levels have been described as well.[34,35]

CONCLUSION

Biomarkers estimation helps in diagnosis of myocardial infarction and reinfarction.

Cardiac troponins (especially high-sensitivity assays) remain the primary biomarkers for diagnosing reinfarction due to their high specificity and sensitivity. Other biomarkers and tests, such as BNP/NT-proBNP and inflammatory markers, provide additional information on cardiac function and prognosis after infarction. Integrating these biomarkers with clinical assessment and imaging (e.g., ECG and echocardiography) is crucial for managing patients at risk of or experiencing reinfarction.

ONLINE REFERENCES

Please scan the QR code provided at the end of the table of contents for References of this chapter.

CHAPTER

136

Post-PCI Physiology: Current Concepts

Rajiv C, Abraham Paul

ABSTRACT

Physiological assessment of coronary lesions prior to PCI has been well validated. Post-PCI functional assessment, though much less widely used, carries a similar prognostic implication. Both hyperemic and nonhyperemic indices can be used post-PCI. Although there are no guideline recommendations, a general consensus between different studies is that a higher value often translates to better clinical outcomes. It can be an additional tool for quantification of functional results, identifying potential causes of poor physiology, and acts as a guide to imaging and appropriate post-PCI steps for final good physiological results.

Keywords: Post-PCI, FFR, iFR, and functional PCI

INTRODUCTION

Physiological guidance has shown better outcomes when compared to luminographical assessments in terms of long-term outcomes when planning for PCI in intermediate coronary stenotic lesions. Invasive functional assessment of intermediate stenosis currently has class Ia recommendation by European guidelines and class IIa according to American guidelines. The commonly used modalities are fractional flow reserve (FFR) and iFR for epicardial vessel assessment. However, these modalities are less validated in complex anatomies, including tandem disease, microvascular disease, and long lesions.[1] FFR works on the assumption of minimal pharmacologically induced microvascular resistance. Thus, microvascular dysfunction can produce false FFR values, including in other situation such as in the presence of proximal stenosis, LV dysfunction, reduced myocardial viability, or modest distal territory, STEMI, or in the case of elevated diastolic pressure,[2] situations where iFR trumps over FFR. Modalities to assess microvascular resistance include CFR and IMR.

Physiological assessment, in addition to preprocedural planning, is also useful in post-PCI setting. There is growing evidence that post-PCI physiological assessment can be used for prediction of long-term outcomes, adequacy of PCI, and even provide real-time data for post-PCI optimization.

THE CONCEPT OF POST-PCI FUNCTIONAL ASSESSMENT

The FFR and nonhyperemic pressure ratios (NHPR) are useful in post-PCI target vessel analysis for optimizing functional result after a successful angiographic result,[3] as relying on lumiography alone is often associated with suboptimal functional results. Angiographically, pleasing results may have suboptimal epicardial physiology in up to 25% of patients, referred to as residual ischemia.[4,5] The reason for this could be either stent related or vessel related:

- Stent under expansion
- Stent malapposition
- Plaque protrusion
- Thrombus within stent
- Inadequate lesion coverage
- Incorrect stent sizing
- Edge dissection
- Bystander diffuse disease
- Untreated focal lesion

These functionally suboptimal PCIs are associated with adverse clinical outcomes,[6] which may or may not be amenable to further correction. Thus, unsatisfactory post-PCI physiology warrants further evaluation with intravascular imaging to identify correctable causes. Conversely, imaging-guided PCI shows good correlation to ideal post-PCI physiology.[7] Thus, post-PCI vessel interrogation by imaging or physiology is complimentary. The techniques and benefits are briefly mentioned in **Table 1**.

Longitudinal Physiological Vessel Analysis

Conventional physiology assessment with FFR calculates the cumulative effect of lesions in the distal vessel as a single value. Longitudinal assessment of FFR, iFR, or resting full cycle ratio (RFR), using pressure wire pullback, done either manually or using dedicated software, allows for accurate length measurement of lesion of interest. Such a measurement also allows for differentiation of discrete or diffuse disease. Analysis can be done either by visual inspection of the pullback curve, or objectively with the pressure pullback gradient index (PPG index) or dFFR(t)/dt index, an automated algorithm that analyzes the instantaneous FFR gradient per time unit. Pre-PCI proven diffuse disease has poorer prognosis than discrete lesions. Post-PCI, a discrete pattern of pressure drop identifies functionally significant areas amenable to post dilation, while a diffuse pattern identifies a vessel where further manipulation may be futile. The patterns of variation in physiological indices in different settings are mentioned in **Table 2**.

Physiological Endpoints

The therapeutic cut-offs for physiological indices have been well defined during lesion assessment. However, a definitive value to predict post-PCI outcomes has yet to be fully defined. Rimac et al. has proposed a post-PCI FFR of ≥0.90 to predict lower incidence of MACE.[8] A more recent study with drug eluting stents by Hwang et al. proposes a value of 0.86 for target lesion failure and 0.8 for myocardial infarction or death.[9] For iFR, a value of ≥0.95 has been proposed, based on the DEFINE PCI study[5] below which rates of MACE were significantly higher. Cut off values in various studies are given in **Table 3**[10] for FFR derived, and **Table 4** for NPHR.

TABLE 1: Post-PCI physiology assessment.[3]

Objective	Technique	Benefit
Ensuring an optimal functional result of PCI	Physiological measurements in PCI target vessel after satisfactory angiographic result, and jailed side-branch interrogation	Early identification of residual flow-limiting disease in the PCI target vessel after the intervention
Identifying potential targets of functional optimization of PCI	Post-PCI longitudinal vessel analysis	• Establishing the cause of suboptimal functional PCI results • Establishing the feasibility and mode of PCI optimization
Assessing the impact of PCI optimization	Repeat physiological measurements after physiology-based optimization	Residual disease not amenable to PCI may identify need for directed medical therapy or surgical revascularization

TABLE 2: Post-PCI physiology assessments.[3]

Pattern	FFR	NHPR	FCA
Focal	FFR with abrupt pressure loss at the stented site or elsewhere within the treated vessel	Abrupt drop of iFR/RFR/DFR values at the stented site or elsewhere within the treated vessel	Abrupt drop of QFR/vFFR values at the stented site or elsewhere within the treated vessel
Tandem	Abrupt drop of FFR values at the level of an untreated tandem stenosis	Abrupt drop of iFR/RFR/DFR values at the level of an untreated tandem stenosis	Abrupt drop of QFR/vFFR values at the level of an untreated tandem stenosis
Diffuse	Progressive and linear loss in FFR values over length of stented vessel during pullback	Progressive and linear loss in iFR/RFR/DFR values over length of stented vessel during pullback	Progressive and linear loss in QFR/vFFR values over length of stented vessel

(FFR: fractional flow reserve; NHPR: nonhyperemic pressure ratio)

TABLE 3: Clinical studies evaluating cut-off value of post-PCI FFR and clinical outcome.[10]

First author	Year	Device	Endpoint	Follow-up (months)	Event rate		*P* value	FFR cut-off value
					<Cut-off value	≥Cut-off value		
Leesar et al.	2011	DES/BMS	MACE	24	28%	6%	0.02	0.96
Dupouy et al.	2005	BMS	Angina	–	52%	19%	0.05	0.95
Klauss et al.	2005	BMS	MACE	6	26.4%	6.0%	0.04	0.95
Piroth et al.	2017	DES	VOCE	24	8.7%	4.2%	0.011	0.92
Kasula et al.	2016	DES	MACE	28.8/31.2	30%	19%	0.03	0.91

Continued

Continued

First author	Year	Device	Endpoint	Follow-up (months)	Event rate		*P* value	FFR cut-off value
					<Cut-off value	≥Cut-off value		
Reith et al.	2015	DES	MACE	20	35.9%	5.3%	0.01	0.905
Bech et al.	1999	BA	MACE	24	41%	12%	0.012	0.90
Pijls et al.	2002	BMS	MACE	6	20.2%	5.5%	<0.05	0.90
Nam et al.	2011	DES	MACE	12	12.5%	2.5%	<0.01	0.90
Ito et al.	2014	DES	MACE	17.8	17%	2%	0.02	0.90
Azzalini et al.	2019	DES/BMS/BVS	MACE	12	31.6%	9.1%	0.047	0.90
Van Bommel et al.	2019	DES	MACE	1	2.0%	1.5%	0.636	0.90
Doh et al.	2015	DES	TVF	36	39%	11%	0.03	0.89
Li et al.	2017	DES	TVF	36	12.3%	6.1%	0.002	0.88
Agarwal et al.	2016	DES/BMS	MACE	31	23%	17%	0.02	0.86
Hoshino et al.	2019	DES	VOCE	24	–	–	0.002	0.86
Hakeem et al.	2019	DES	MACE	30	23%	17%	0.02	0.86
Lee et al.	2018	DES	TVF	24	9.1%	2.6%	0.006	0.84
Hwang et al.	2019	DES	TVF	24	8.3%	3.1%	< 0.001	0.84
Shin et al.	2020	DES	TVF	24	10.3%	2.5%	< 0.001	0.80

(BA: balloon angioplasty; BVS: bioresorbable vascular scaffolds; BMS: bare-metal stent; DES: drug-eluting stent; FFR: fractional flow reserve; MACE: major adverse cardiovascular events; PCI: percutaneous coronary intervention; TVF: target vessel failure; VOCE: vessel oriented composite events)

TABLE 4: Clinical studies evaluating cut-off value of post-PCI NHPR and clinical outcome.[10]

First author	Year	Device	Endpoint	Follow-up (months)	Event rate		*P* value	Post-PCI NHPR cut-off value
					<Cut-off	≥Cut-off value		
Hakeem et al.	2019	DES	MACE	30	24%	15%	0.0005	Resting Pd/Pa 0.96
Shin et al.	2020	DES	TVF	24	6.2%	2.5%	0.029	Resting Pd/Pa 0.92
Patel et al.	2022	DES	MACE	12	5.7%	1.8%	0.04	iFR 0.95

(DES: drug-eluting stent; iFR: instantaneous wave-free ratio; MACE: major adverse cardiovascular events; NHPR: nonhyperemic pressure ratio; PCI: percutaneous coronary intervention; Pd/Pa: distal coronary pressure to aortic pressure ratio; TVF: target vessel failure)

In addition to final post-PCI FFR, FFR gains (post-PCI FFR – pre-PCI FFR = ΔFFR) is also independently associated with MACE **(Table 5)**.

Emori et al.[11] proposed an intrastent FFR gradient of 0.04 as ideal, above which results are deemed to be suboptimal.

These indices can be complimentary. A trans-stent FFR gradient of <0.04 can still have a suboptimal FFR, in the presence of additional lesions outside the stented segment.

VESSEL-RELATED DIFFERENCES

One confounding factor that needs consideration is the normal anatomical factors that may contribute to lower functional indices. Post-PCI FFR is lower in LAD than other vessels. This variation is possibly due to higher prevalence of intramuscular coronary tracts in LAD, hydrostatic effect due to the relative position of the concerned coronary artery in relation to the aorta,[12] or the high-flow rate in LAD due to a larger myocardial area of supply,[13] with a resultant significant pressure drop across otherwise minor plaques when it is a long segment lesion. Taking these into consideration, a normal post-PCI FFR for LAD has been proposed to be a lower value of 0.92, as opposed to non-LAD vessels with value of 0.96.[3]

PREDICTION OF POST-PCI PHYSIOLOGY

The concept of in silico PCI refers to prediction of post-PCI anatomical and physiological results during the pre-procedural planning phase. This aids in proper strategizing to prevent suboptimal results. These can be simulated from baseline longitudinal vessel analysis. CT angiography derived FFR values can be used for prediction of post PCI FFR with dedicated softwares.[14,15] Such predictions can also be modeled from iFR and QFR.

TABLE 5: Clinical studies evaluating FFR gains and clinical outcome.[10]

First author	Year	Device	Endpoint	Follow-up (months)	Event rate		*P* value	Post-PCI index
Nishi et al.	2018	DES	QoL	12	ΔFFR	EQ-5D at 1 month	0.013	Tertiles of ΔFFR
					≤0.18	0.037		
					0.19–0.32	0.069		
					≥0.33	0.086		
					ΔFFR	EQ-5D at 1 year	0.022	
					≤ 0.18	0.033		
					0.19–0.32	0.063		
					≥0.33	0.085		
Fournier et al.	2019	DES	Angina severity	24	ΔFFR	Odds ratio, 1.33	0.02	Increase of ΔFFR
			VOCE	24	ΔFFR	VOCE	0.01	ΔFFR ≤ 0.24
					≤0.18	9.0%		
					0.19–0.30	7.1%		
					>0.31	4.7%		
Lee et al.	2018	DES	TVF	24	ΔFFR ≤ 15%	ΔFFR > 15%	0.003	ΔFFR > 15%
					9.2%	3.0%		
Yang et al.	2020	DES	MACE	72	ΔFFR ≥ 0.04	ΔFFR < 0.04	0.031	Trans-stent FFR gradient ≥ 0.04
					30.4%	6.6%		

(DES: drug-eluting stent; FFR: fractional flow reserve; MACE: major adverse cardiovascular events; PCI: percutaneous coronary intervention; QoL: quality of life; TVF: target vessel failure; VOCE: vessel oriented composite events)

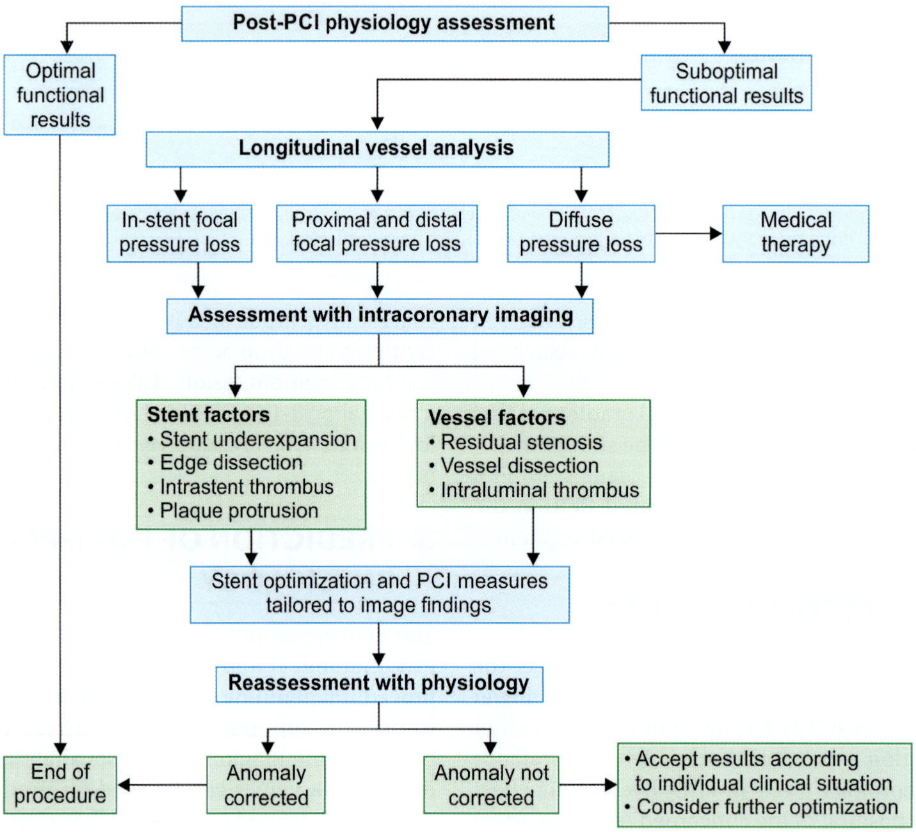

FLOWCHART 1: Proposed algorithm for postprocedural assessment and optimization of functional PCI results based on physiological interrogation.[3]

CONCLUSION

Although it may not be superior to imaging in terms of long-term outcomes,[16] post-PCI physiology can be an added assessment modality to angiography and imaging, termed as triregistration, where a longitudinal pullback identifies physiologically significant residual lesion while the imaging identifies the cause of pressure drop.[17] The final aim of PCI should be to attain a physiologically good result, which conventional luminography-only strategies may fail to achieve **(Flowchart 1)**.

ONLINE REFERENCES

Please scan the QR code provided at the end of the table of contents for References of this chapter.

CHAPTER 137

Non-ST-elevation Acute Coronary Syndrome in Previous Coronary Artery Bypass Graft: Management

Avinash Mani, Vishal Rastogi, Vijay Kumar, Ashok Seth

ABSTRACT

Non-ST-elevation acute coronary syndrome (NSTEACS) in post-coronary artery bypass graft (CABG) patients presents a unique challenge in our routine clinical practice. Management of these patients involves shared decision making while considering their clinical status and associated comorbidities. Invasive testing with coronary angiography followed by revascularization is usually recommended, unless patients have several comorbidities and poor life expectancy. CT coronary angiography also plays an important role in evaluation of these patients. Revascularization strategies include redo CABG, PCI of saphenous venous grafts or PCI of native coronary vessels.

Keywords: NSTEMI, CABG, saphenous venous graft, percutaneous coronary intervention

INTRODUCTION

Non-ST-elevation acute coronary syndrome (NSTEACS) in postcoronary artery bypass grafting (CABG) patients represents a challenging clinical situation. These patients constitute around 10% of the total cohort of patients presenting as NSTEACS.[1] They are usually older and have more comorbidities as compared to their counterparts. The management strategy in such patients is dependent on a number of factors including clinical profile, anatomic, and hemodynamic factors. These patients are usually managed with either a conservative medical strategy or invasive strategy with revascularization. Individualized decision making is required during management of these cases.

CLINICAL PRESENTATION

Post CABG patients with NSTEMI usually present with chest pain and shortness of breath. Many of these post CABG patients have previous myocardial infarction (MI) with left ventricular dysfunction. They can also present with features of acute decompensated heart failure (ADHF) including orthopnea, PND, and leg swelling. Presentation with cardiogenic shock is uncommon in this subset of patients. Around one-third of these patients usually have renal impairment in the form of chronic kidney disease or acute kidney injury.[2] ADHF in these CKD patients can lead to further worsening of renal function causing oliguria or anuria.

INVESTIGATIONS

The 12-lead electrocardiogram (ECG) usually shows ST segment depression with/without T-wave inversion. T-wave inversion can also be present in isolation. New onset q waves with T wave changes can also be seen in some cases, indicative of recent ACS. The localization of ECG changes provides a clue regarding the location of the culprit lesion and possible graft failure. New onset ventricular arrhythmias can be seen in these patients. These are usually the result of ventricular scar and dysfunction along with ongoing myocardial ischemia. These patients are also predisposed to development of atrial fibrillation due to their old age and associated comorbidities. In a registry of post CABG patients presenting with ACS, cardiac arrhythmias were noted in 36% of the cohort.[2]

The 2D echocardiogram in these patients usually shows presence of left ventricular dysfunction with a reduced LV ejection fraction (LVEF). New onset regional wall motion abnormalities (RWMA) can help localize the lesion and plan management strategies. Quantification of mitral regurgitation (MR) is important in such cases as these patients can have significant MR secondary to papillary muscle dysfunction or ventricular dilatation. Estimation of pulmonary artery pressures and right ventricular function becomes important to determine hemodynamic status of the patient.

Elevated cardiac enzymes (CK-MB and troponin I/T) denote myocardial injury and aid in diagnosis of NSTEMI. Rising titer of cardiac enzymes gives a more accurate estimation of myocardial injury as compared to a single raised value. Interpretation of elevated cardiac enzymes should be done cautiously in patients with baseline renal dysfunction and those with associated sepsis as these can cause falsely high troponin levels.

Anemia is commonly noted in these patients owing to old age, chronic kidney disease, and use of antiplatelet drugs. Severe anemia can lead to type II MI due to demand-supply mismatch. Very high or extremely low total leukocyte counts indicate sepsis, which affects the overall prognosis of the patient. Elevated serum creatinine levels can be a result of acute kidney injury or secondary to chronic kidney disease.

MANAGEMENT

Management of post CABG patients presenting with NSTEMI involves initial medical stabilization followed by evaluation for subsequent invasive testing. As these patients are elderly and have several comorbidities, shared decision making becomes important in choosing between conservative and invasive strategy.

Antiplatelet Therapy

The ESC guidelines recommend use of dual antiplatelet therapy including aspirin and a newer generation P2Y12 inhibitor, i.e., ticagrelor or prasugrel (if invasive strategy) in patients presenting with NSTEMI. In post CABG patients, who are usually elderly, the increased bleeding risk needs to be balanced with high thrombotic risk owing to high platelet reactivity on antiplatelet drugs. In such situations, the antiplatelet strategy needs to be tailored to individual patients depending on their individual bleeding risk. Prasugrel is not recommended in patients >75 years of age as it is associated with higher bleeding events. There was no difference noted in ischemic and bleeding endpoints between prasugrel 5 mg versus clopidogrel 75 mg in TRILOGY ACS substudy and elderly ACS-2 substudy which included elderly patients presenting with ACS.[3,4]

After an ACS event, the risk of ischemic events is high in the acute and subacute period—usually 1–3 months. Hence, most potent platelet inhibition is usually required in this period. This concept has led to the development of tailored DAPT strategy which includes more potent antiplatelet therapies in the initial period post ACS followed by de-escalation to a less potent drug subsequently. This helps to balance the ischemic and bleeding risks in these patients. In the first 3 months, DAPT with aspirin and ticagrelor followed by de-escalation to clopidogrel is a good strategy in these patients, especially those who undergo revascularization post ACS. The TOPIC study evaluated this strategy of aspirin with ticagrelor for 1 month followed by aspirin with clopidogrel in comparison to no de-escalation strategy. No difference in ischemic endpoints were noted at 12 months whereas significant bleeding rates were significantly lower in the de-escalation group.[5] Aspirin-free strategy can also be considered in patients who have undergone revascularization post ACS. This approach is hypothesized to reduce bleeding risk in elderly patients while preventing ischemic events.[6] In summary, the antiplatelet therapy in these patients needs to be tailored according to the situation, balancing the thrombotic and bleeding risk.

Antithrombotic Therapy

Unfractionated heparin (UFH) should be initiated in all patients after diagnosis of NSTEMI has been made. Low molecular weight heparin (LMWH) can also be used as an alternative to UFH as it does not require regular monitoring of clotting times. In a meta-analysis comparing UFH with LMWH, no difference was noted in mortality and major bleeding events between the two groups.[7] Parenteral anticoagulation should be continued till the period of index hospitalization or until the patient undergoes invasive coronary angiography (ICA). Postrevascularization, parenteral anticoagulation is not routinely recommended and should be continued only in presence of left ventricular thrombus or atrial fibrillation.

Management of Heart Failure and Arrhythmias

The ADHF management involves intravenous diuretics, oxygen therapy, noninvasive positive pressure ventilation, and inotropes. Guideline directed medical therapy (GDMT) needs to be initiated at the time of discharge. Intravenous antiarrhythmic therapy may be needed in case of new onset ventricular and atrial arrhythmias. In case of arrhythmias with hemodynamic instability, DC cardioversion is recommended to restore sinus rhythm.

Conservative versus Invasive Strategy

After initial stabilization, a routine invasive strategy has been shown to be beneficial in patient presenting with NSTEMI as it reduces death and MI.[8] In elderly patients presenting with NSTEMI, a systematic review and meta-analysis of available studies showed that a routine invasive strategy showed significant reduction in MI and unplanned revascularization at the expense of increased major bleeding events and no mortality difference.[9] As discussed earlier, post CABG patients with NSTEMI are usually elderly and have a number of comorbidities. Invasive management is less frequently performed in these patients due to higher bleeding risk, technical challenges during multiple graft cannulation and presence of renal dysfunction. There are no clear guidelines regarding management strategies in post CABG patients presenting with ACS. Similarly, there is paucity of data in the literature regarding the superiority of routine invasive strategy as compared to selective invasive strategy.

The CABG-ACS study was a randomized control trial (RCT) which included 60 post CABG patients who had unplanned hospitalization due to NSTEMI.[2] In this study, early invasive strategy was compared with conservative management. At the end of follow-up period of 2 years, the composite efficacy outcome of all-cause mortality, MI, rehospitalization for MI, or heart failure was similar in both the groups (HR 0.85, 0.39–1.83). The composite safety outcomes of bleeding, major stroke, and renal derangement was also same in both groups. Only 32% patients in the invasive group received PCI. This shows the inherent complexities associated with post CABG patients as identification of culprit vessel/lesion may be difficult in some cases.

The TACTICS-TIMI 18 was a randomized study evaluating early invasive strategy in all comers NSTEMI patients. In the CABG subgroup of this study, 484 patients demonstrated reduction in composite outcome of death, MI, or rehospitalization in the early invasive strategy group. Early invasive approach also led to significant reduction in MI rates at the end of 6 months (OR 0.44; 95% CI 0.21–0.93; $p = 0.032$). This study favored the use of early invasive approach in these high-risk patients.

In a retrospective analysis of post CABG patients from Canada, 1,487 patients who presented with NSTEMI were evaluated.[10] At the end of 1 year, the primary composite outcome of death or recurrent MI was highest in patients who were conservatively managed without invasive testing as compared to those who underwent coronary angiography followed by PCI (27.3% vs. 14.8%; $p < 0.001$). Among patients who underwent revascularization, native vessel PCI was most commonly performed (71%) followed by graft PCI (21%).

In a recently performed meta-analysis of post CABG patients with NSTEMI, 897 patients from 11 RCTs were included and evaluated for a superiority of a routine invasive strategy in all patients.[11] All-cause and cardiac mortality was similar in both routine invasive and conservative group. There was no difference in MI and cardiac hospitalization rates on follow-up. This meta-analysis showed that there is no definite benefit of a routine invasive strategy in post CABG patients who present with NSTEMI. The main limitation of this meta-analysis was that it included <1,000 patients over 11 RCTs. This shows the fact that this population is significantly under-represented in clinical studies. Considering the small patient population represented in the existing trials, there is no concrete data at present in the literature with different studies showing conflicting results. More RCTs involving larger population is required to determine the best management strategy in these patients.

Role of Computed Tomography Coronary Angiography

ICA is technically challenging in post CABG patients due to the variable graft anatomy, lack of expertise at all centers for graft cannulation, and presence of renal dysfunction. This is one of the main reasons for low rates of angiography and subsequent revascularization in post CABG patients. In many circumstances where prior information about graft anatomy is unavailable, searching for grafts during invasive angiography becomes time consuming with increased levels of contrast and radiation exposure.

Computed tomography coronary angiography (CTCA) is a useful noninvasive clinical tool for evaluation of graft anatomy in stable patients. CTCA has shown to be highly sensitive and specific for detection of graft stenosis (98%).[12] BYPASS-CTCA trial was a single center RCT which compared the strategy of CTCA before ICA versus ICA alone for post CABG patients. 688 patients were randomized in this trial among whom 37% had NSTEMI on presentation. There was significant reduction in procedure time and radiation dosage in the CTCA + ICA group. Overall contrast usage was lower in the CTCA + ICA group, even when the contrast used during CTCA was included (148.9 ± 50.6 vs. 173.0 ± 68.0 mL; $p < 0.001$). Procedural complications including periprocedural MI and vascular access complications were lower in the combined CTCA + ICA group. The primary outcome of MACE at 1 year was lower in the CTCA followed by ICA group as compared to direct ICA group (16% vs. 29.4%, $p < 0.001$). The difference in outcomes was mainly driven by lower rates of nonfatal MI. There was no difference in major adverse kidney events including new onset renal dysfunction at 1 year follow-up. This study showed that upfront use of CTCA followed by ICA helps in reducing procedural time and complications with favorable MACE events on follow-up.

Use of CTCA before ICA helps in determining the number and location of bypass grafts along with their status (patent or occluded). This helps to reduce contrast volume and time during ICA as it avoids seeking of grafts which are already occluded. It also helps to focus attention on the particular graft stenosis noted on CTCA, if any, and plan for the revascularization procedure. However, this strategy may not be feasible in patients who are unstable and have baseline severe chronic kidney disease. CTCA need to be performed and interpreted with significant expertise in order to replicate the potential benefits shown by the combined approach. Thus, in unstable patients and those with severe renal dysfunction, direct ICA remains the gold standard investigation of choice.

REVASCULARIZATION IN POSTCORONARY ARTERY BYPASS GRAFT PATIENTS

Redo Coronary Artery Bypass Graft

Redo CABG is usually indicated in patients with multiple diseased grafts, left ventricular dysfunction, and ischemic symptoms.[13] The incidence of redo CABG ranges around 2–3% in the current practice.[14] Some recent studies suggest similar outcomes after redo CABG as compared to first CABG during periprocedural period and continuing up to 5 years. However, 5 year mortality was noted to be higher in the redo CABG cohort.[15] Immediate periprocedural outcomes after redo CABG have improved with time as experience among surgeons have increased—operative mortality was reduced from 6.0 to 4.9% between 2000 and 2009.[16] However, redo CABG is associated with its own set of challenges. Redo sternotomy is one of the most challenging steps which can cause injury to adjacent cardiac structures which may be adherent to the sternum.[17] Injury to previous internal mammary graft during redo sternotomy is also a potential complication with serious consequences. Hence, the decision for redo CABG in such patients needs to be taken by a heart team after considering need for revascularization, patient's comorbidities and previous graft status. Considering these challenges, PCI is the most common revascularization strategy seen in clinical practice in this subset of patients. Either PCI of the graft vessels or native arteries can be done depending on the culprit lesion and complexity of the procedure.

Percutaneous Coronary Intervention of Graft Vessels

PCI of saphenous venous grafts (SVG) have been performed traditionally to treat post CABG patients presenting with acute coronary syndrome. However, initial reports with SVG stenting were not very encouraging. In the SOS study, graft occlusion were more commonly seen with bare metal stents as compared to 1st generation paclitaxel eluting stents (51% vs. 9%, $p < 0.0001$).[18] Long-term outcomes after SVG stenting are not very encouraging. In an analysis from the VA health system, SVG stenting was associated with higher rates of mortality and MI as compared to native vessel PCI [hazard ratio (HR) 1.3 and 1.6, respectively]. Repeat revascularization rates were also significantly higher in the SVG group (HR 1.6; 95% CI 1.5–1.71).[19] However, there is paucity of data on the outcomes of SVG stenting with latest generation drug eluting stents (DES).

Stenting of saphenous grafts is associated with high rates of periprocedural events including slow flow, no flow, and periprocedural MI.[20] This is attributed to the unique pathophysiology of SVG lesions. After CABG, intimal hyperplasia occurs within the SVG as an adaptive response to high arterial pressures. Atherosclerosis progresses faster in the venous grafts when compared to the native vessels. The atherosclerotic lesions in SVG are more concentric and diffuse as compared to native vessels and usually lack a fibrous cap. This makes these lesions prone to rupture and distal embolization.[21] Hence, SVG stenting requires expertise and a meticulous approach **(Figs. 1A and B)**.

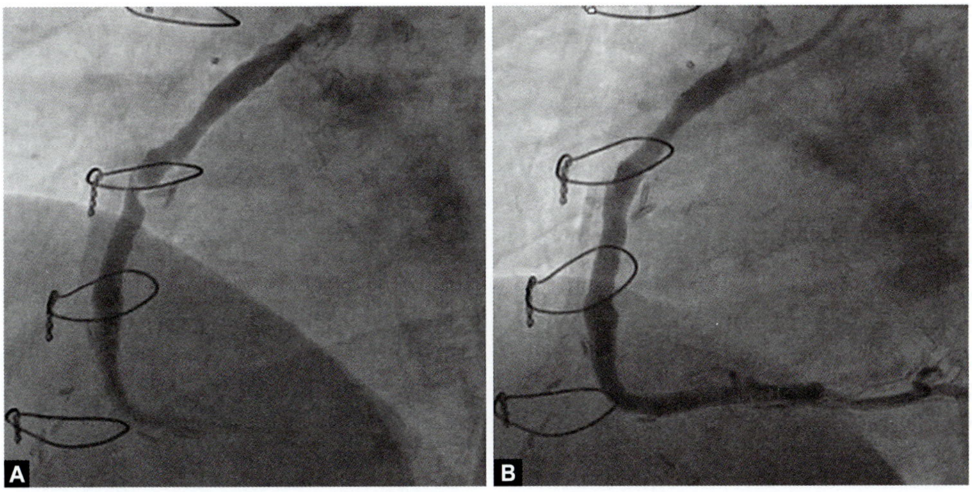

FIGS. 1A AND B: (A) SVG to RCA shows an eccentric hazy 90% lesion in the mid segment. These lesions have very high propensity for distal embolization. (B) A distal protection filter, spider (5 mm) was deployed distally followed by direct stenting of the SVG lesion using a 3.5 × 15 mm DES. Final result showed good result with TIMI III flow distally.

Few tips and tricks that should be used during SVG PCI are as follows:

- *Guide selection:* Proper guide selection is important for adequate support. Amplatz (AL) and multipurpose guides work well for both left and right-sided grafts. They can be used for both transradial and transfemoral approach. Guide extension catheters may be needed when coaxial cannulation of graft ostium is not feasible for delivery of hardware. In very distal graft lesions, short length guide catheters are required to ensure adequate length of balloon shaft for delivery to target.[22]
- *Embolic protection devices (EPD):* EPD have been provided a class IB recommendation during PCI of SVG lesions.[23] They help in reducing distal embolization during procedure and are associated with significant reduction of periprocedural MI and early mortality. Contemporary use of EPD has reduced with time and are currently used in only one-third of SVG PCI cases. Different types of EPD are available and should always be used whenever technically feasible.
- *Use of microvascular vasodilators*: Adequate preparation of coronary bed is important before starting PCI in venous grafts. Nitroglycerin, diltiazem, nicorandil, adenosine, or sodium nitroprusside can be used to prevent slow flow during procedure. Distal infusion of drugs into the vessel using a microcatheter, infusion catheter, or slit balloon is always more effective.
- *Pre- and postdilation:* Direct stenting is preferred in SVG lesions as it reduces risk of distal emboli. Predilation should only be done if the lesion is very stenotic causing impediment to stent and EPD delivery. Similarly, postdilation should be avoided when possible. If postdilation is required, it should be done using a 1:1 sized balloon with gradual inflation to nominal pressures followed by slow deflation. High pressure postdilation is not recommended.
- *Stent choice*: Latest generation DES are recommended for SVG PCI. It is prudent to use a longer stent to ensure complete coverage. Use of an undersized stent during SVG PCI was associated with lesser tissue protrusion in a study by Hong et al.[24] However, no difference in clinical outcomes were noted in comparison with 1:1 sizing at 1-year follow-up.
- *Managing high thrombus burden*: SVG lesion often present with high thrombus burden owing to the underlying friable lipid rich plaque. Presence of significant thrombus on angiography increases the risk of slow flow/no flow during the procedure. Mechanical thrombectomy can be considered in such situations to reduce the thrombus burden. Angiojet and CAT RX systems are commercially available for effective thrombus aspiration.

In the current clinical practice, SVG stenting is usually recommended in acute coronary syndrome in patients with critical graft stenosis, where native vessel PCI is technically complex. It is also recommended in cases where SVG graft can be used as conduit for native vessel PCI in the future.

Percutaneous of Native Vessels

Despite the advances in techniques of graft PCI along with use of embolic protection devices, high ischemic events are noted after graft PCI as compared to native vessel PCI. In an analysis of patients who underwent PCI in the ADAPT DES study, outcomes of SVG PCI were compared with native vessel PCI. At 2 years follow-up, SVG PCI was associated with higher risk of cardiac death (6.9% vs. 1.9%; $p < 0.0001$), stent thrombosis (2.6% vs. 0.8%; $p = 0.0006$) and target vessel revascularization (21.3% vs. 9.2%; $p < 0.0001$).[20] Bleeding rates were similar in both groups. Another study of SVG PCI in elderly patients showed that MACE rates were high at 2 years (18.6%) with repeat revascularization rates of 7.1%.[25] Hence, it is always advisable to undertake PCI of native vessels wherever feasible. Majority of patients have high calcified lesions or chronic total occlusion in their native vessels. With significant advancement of device therapy for managing severely calcified lesions (intravascular lithotripsy, rotational atherectomy, and orbital atherectomy), good short-term and long-term outcomes can be obtained in post CABG patients. CTO PCI success rates are more than 90% when performed at high volume centers by experienced operators.[26] Use of intravascular imaging in complex lesions helps to reduce MACE events including cardiac death and target vessel revascularization on follow-up.[27] Hence, PCI of native vessels should be favored, wherever technically feasible, during decision making for revascularization in post CABG patients **(Figs. 2A to C)**.

SELECTING THE OPTIMAL STRATEGY

An algorithm for deciding optimal management strategy in post CABG patients presenting with NSTEMI has been described in **Flowchart 1**. Patients presenting with NSTEMI should be medically managed initially. Once stabilized, treatment strategy should depend on clinical and anatomical variables. In very elderly patients with other associated comorbidities (renal dysfunction, sepsis, etc.), it may be reasonable to adopt a conservative approach during the index hospitalization. In patients who do not have associated comorbidities or continue to have ischemia-induced symptoms, invasive strategy is recommended with coronary angiography. CTCA before an invasive angiography is a good strategy. After invasive CAG, revascularization of native vessels should be preferred wherever technically feasible. SVG PCI should be considered if a critical stenosis is noted in the graft and native vessel PCI is not feasible in the acute setting. SVG PCI can also be done to use the graft as an epicardial conduit for PCI of the native vessel (retrograde approach) in the future.

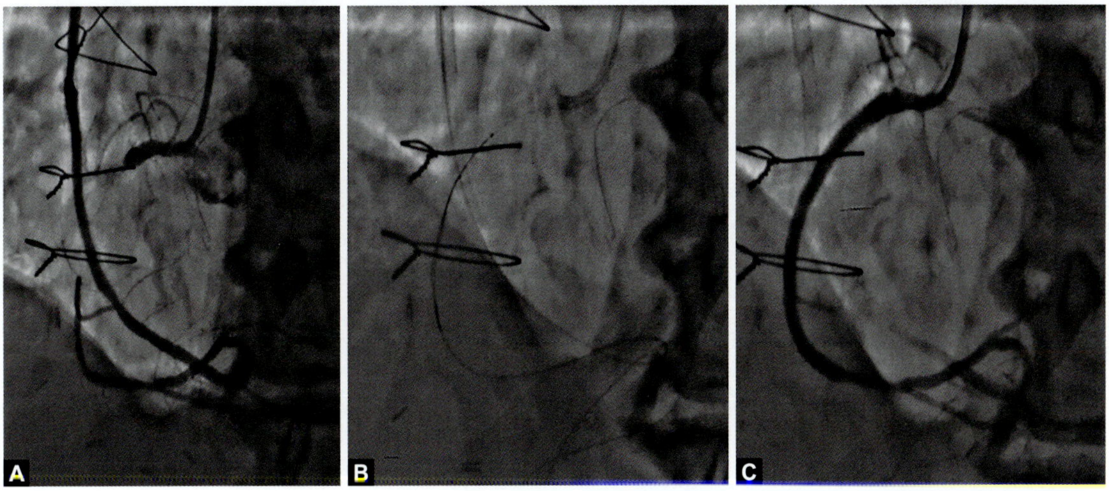

FIGS. 2A TO C: A 65-year-old gentleman, post CABG, presented with complaints of angina on exertion. He had a lesion in his SVG to RCA graft which was stented with a view to perform native vessel PCI in future. (A) Native RCA CTO was planned for a retrograde approach via the saphenous venous graft of RCA. (B) Retrograde wire via SVG kept in distal true lumen as marker for antegrade wire. (C) Successful RCA CTO PCI done using SVG as a conduit.

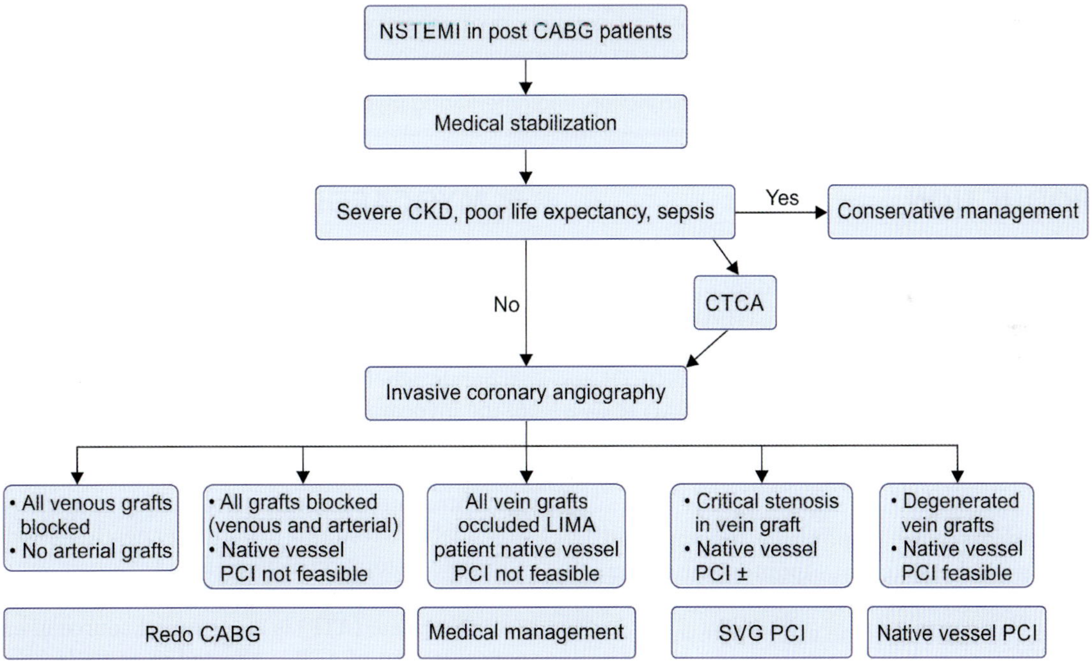

FLOWCHART 1: Decision making algorithm in post CABG patients presenting with NSTEMI.

CONCLUSION

NSTEMI in post CABG patients is a common situation seen in our clinical practice. The optimal treatment strategy should be selected through informed decision-making while taking the clinical profile of the patient into account. CTCA is a good adjunct tool to help decide revascularization strategy. PCI of native vessels is favored to SVG PCI during revascularization in these patients.

ONLINE REFERENCES

Please scan the QR code provided at the end of the table of contents for References of this chapter.

CHAPTER 138

Myocardial Hibernation: Clinician Perspective

Puneet Rastogii

ABSTRACT

Coronary artery disease (CAD) is the leading cause of morbidity and mortality, affecting around 126 million people worldwide. Coronary artery disease is the primary cause, accounting for two-thirds of left ventricular dysfunction cases. Early recognition of impaired LV function (chronic hibernating myocardium) can be reversible with appropriate therapy, and restoring blood flow can improve LV ejection fraction, depending on the duration of hibernating myocardium.

Keywords: Morbidity and mortality, CAD, LV dysfunction, and hibernating myocardium

INTRODUCTION

Coronary artery disease (CAD) is one of the common causes of morbidity and mortality. The incidence of ischemic cardiomyopathy (ICM) and heart failure (HF) is increasing across the globe. Currently, approximately 126 million people in the world are suffering from ischemic HF. Of the total cases of left ventricular (LV) dysfunction, CAD is seen in two-third cases. Major contributors to HF after myocardial infarction are LV remodeling and hemodynamic changes.

Multiple processes are responsible for impaired LV function after an ischemic event. Apoptosis and necrosis are irreversible causes of cell death; however, other processes may be reversible to some extent with appropriate therapy. Restoration of adequate blood flow in hibernating (viable myocardium) can restore myocardial contractility leading to improved LV function. A series of transitions, from stunned to hibernating myocardium to necrosis with scar formation, is seen in patients having ischemic cardiomyopathy.

Various types of viable myocardium after an ischemic insult are:

- Stunned myocardium
- Short-term hibernation
- Chronic hibernation

MYOCARDIAL HIBERNATION

The hibernation term was coined by Diamond et al.[1] in 1978 and the pathophysiologic concept was first given by Rahimtoola[2] in early 1980s. He described hibernating myocardium as "a subacute or chronic stage of myocardial ischemia where contractility, metabolism, and function of the myocardium is reduced to match the reduced blood supply". In other words, hibernating myocardium is a stage seen in myocardial ischemia, where myocardial necrosis is prevented and the contractility and function of myocardium are capable of restoring to normal or nearly normal state after adequate restoration of blood flow.[3]

For proper contractile function of myocytes, adenosine 5-triphosphate (ATP) is an essential source of energy. The concentration of ATP is affected in acute ischemia, which is responsible for acute ischemic contractile dysfunction **(Box 1)**.[3]

BOX 1 Mechanism of contractile dysfunction after acute myocardial ischemia.

- Reduction of ATP concentration in myocardium
- Cardiac potassium channel activation
- Acidosis
- Changes in calcium handling of sarcoplasmic reticulum
- Desensitization of myofibrils for calcium
- Collapse of coronary arteries

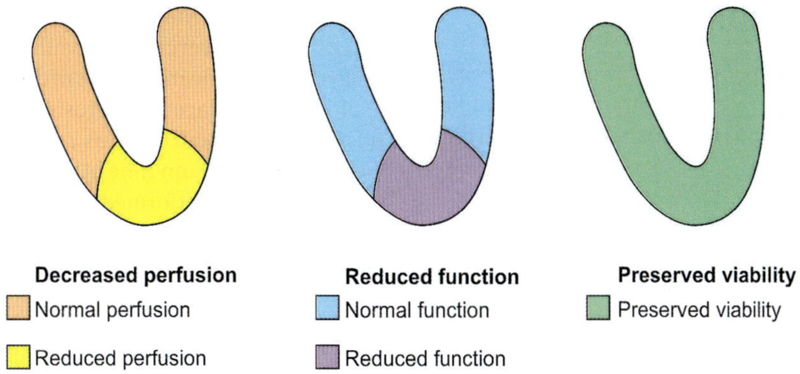

FIG. 1: Schematic representation of hibernating myocardium. The conical structure is heart with apex at bottom, base at top, and ventricular cavity in the middle. At apex, there is decreased perfusion, which results in reduced function after months to years. The viability is demonstrated by PET in both myocardium with normal function and reduced function

Clinical evidence of hibernating myocardium can be demonstrated by the following:

- Demonstration of viability in areas of reduced perfusion using nuclear imaging techniques like positron emission tomography (PET) and magnetic resonance imaging
- Recovery of left ventricular (LV) ejection fraction and motion abnormality after restoration of blood flow
- Biopsy showing dedifferentiated cardiac myocytes in areas of reduced perfusion and motion abnormality

There is a contraction of dyskinetic or akinetic myocardium after giving inotrope and nitroglycerin, thus suggesting a potential to contract and viability.[4]

Figure 1 shows image finding of hibernating myocardium.[4]

BOX 2 Features of short-term hibernating myocardium.

- Regional myocardium with reduced blood flow becomes dysfunctional (contraction–perfusion matching)
- Improvement of metabolic status after reperfusion, that is reduction of lactate and return of creatine phosphate to normal values
- Increased contractile function on giving inotrope, at the expense of worsening metabolic status
- Return of contractile function after reperfusion
- Absence of irreversible myocardial damage, i.e., necrosis

MECHANISMS OF HIBERNATION

A series of dynamic processes that follow prolonged ischemia and myocardial infarction determine the fate of myocardium, whether it will recover or undergo necrosis. The metabolic adaptations seen in stunned and hibernating myocardium are believed to play a vital role in the recovery of salvageable myocardium. The "smart heart" theory postulated that decreased myocardial blood flow (MBF) at rest is responsible for cardiac myocytes switching to a state of hibernation; however, other theories suggest decreased myocardial flow reserve (MFR) might be the cause.[5]

The pathophysiologic triad seen in hibernating myocardium is the presence of reduced MBF and MFR, significant coronary artery stenosis limiting the flow to myocardium causing myocardium dysfunction, and presence of viable myocardium, which is irreversibly damaged myocardium. It is also important that following revascularization, patient is restudied for several months, since recovery of hibernating myocardium may take several months after revascularization and early assessment might miss it.

SHORT-TERM HIBERNATION

When the limitation of blood flow to myocytes is not severe enough to cause infarction, the myocardium becomes reversibly dysfunctional as adaptive mechanism as seen in myocardial ischemia. Restoration of blood flow can result in the reduction of infarct size leading to recovery of myocardial function, and thus improved survival **(Box 2)**.

CHRONIC HIBERNATION

In chronic hibernation, there is chronic contractile dysfunction for months or years, which occur after flow-limiting CAD. The myocardial dysfunction is reversible after reperfusion, as evidenced by clinical studies. Chronic hibernation can occur after repeated small ischemia, that is stable and unstable angina or can occur after acute myocardial infarction. Thus, clinical conditions associated with chronic hibernation are shown in **Box 3**.[3]

Morphological features of chronic hibernation are given in **Box 4**.

VIABLE MYOCARDIUM

Viability of myocardium depends not only on the severity of occlusion of blood flow but also on duration of blood flow limitation. If revascularization is done when the myocardium is in a state of hibernation, recovery of myocardial contraction can be seen. However, if revascularization and treatment are delayed for significant periods of time, the viable myocardium is ultimately replaced by fibrosis and irreversible myocardial dysfunction occurs. Thus, outcome after myocardial ischemia depends on time at which adequate treatment and intervention are performed.

BOX 3 Clinical conditions associated with chronic hibernation.

- Unstable and stable angina
- Acute myocardial infarction
- Congestive heart failure and/or left ventricular (LV) dysfunction
- Anomalous left coronary artery from pulmonary artery (ALCAPA)

BOX 4 Morphological features of chronic hibernation.[2,3]

- Cardiomyocyte alternations
    - Loss of myofilaments (thin filament complex, myosin, and titin)
    - Numerous small doughnut-like mitochondria
    - Loss of sarcoplasmic reticulum
    - Sequestration of cellular particles into extracellular space
    - Disorganization of cytoskeleton (desmin, vinculin, and tubulin)
    - Atrophy and apoptosis
    - Increased number of glycogen deposits
- Interstitial alterations
    - Increased number of macrophages and fibroblasts
    - Increased amount of matrix and structural proteins (fibronectin and all collagen)
    - Fibrosis

After patients suffer from CAD, myocardial viability is assessed by noninvasive stress imaging (dobutamine stress echocardiography, cardiac magnetic resonance imaging, PET, and single photon emission computed tomography) as recommended by ESC guidelines (class IIb, level of evidence B) for guiding revascularization.

The ACC/AHA also recommend checking for myocardial viability for making decisions regarding revascularization in patients with high surgical risk or with complex medical problems **(Flowchart 1)**.

IDENTIFICATION OF HIBERNATING MYOCARDIUM

In all patients with CAD and chronic LV dysfunction, presence of hibernating myocardium should be suspected. The severity and extent of CAD does not directly correlate with severity and extent of LV dysfunction. Patients with CAD may have normal LV function due to presence of newly developed vessels and collateral vessels in coronary vasculature.

Hibernating myocardium is identified using various imaging techniques. These imaging techniques are based on the concept that hibernating myocardium is capable of increasing contractility when appropriately stimulated and also shows presence of metabolic activity in the imaging used. Hibernating myocardium has the potential to improve its function following revascularization, which is, however, not seen if the myocardium is irreversibly damaged. Thus,

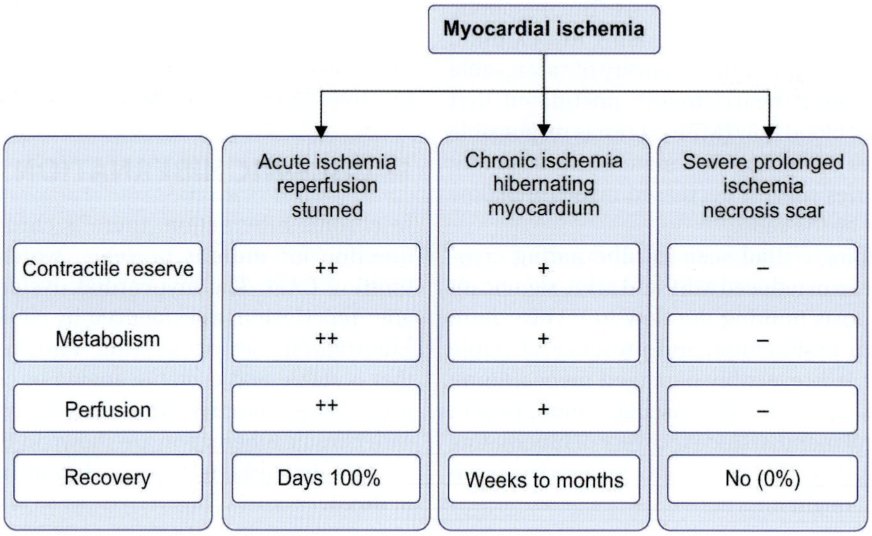

FLOWCHART 1: Myocardial ischemia.

by identification of hibernating myocardium, decision can be made on whether patient will benefit from revascularization or not. Various groups have published data predicting of improvement of myocardial function following revascularization.[6]

For identification of viability in hibernating myocardium following approaches can be used:

- *For assessing the integrity of membrane, metabolism, and perfusion:*[7]
  - 99mTc-sestamibi (MIBI), 201TI scintigraphy, and 99mTc-tetrafosmin
  - *PET:* 13NH3, 18FDG, 14C-acetate, and 82Rb
  - MRI for assessment of wall function and regional perfusion
- *For assessing regional function*:
  - Postextrasystolic potentiation (PESP)
  - Dobutamine stress echocardiography
  - Low-dose catecholamine administration
  - Exercise testing
  - Nitroglycerine administration

REASONS FOR NONRECOVERY OF VIABLE MYOCARDIUM AFTER REVASCULARIZATION

Recovery of viable myocardium is affected by a number of factors; therefore, failure of a dysfunctional but viable myocardial segment to recover function after revascularization may not necessarily mean there is an error in the test.

Possible reasons are as follows:

- *Preprocedure factors*:
  - Increased duration of hibernation
  - Presence of severe LV dysfunction
  - Presence of subendocardial scar
- *Periprocedure*:
  - Procedure-related necrosis
  - Incomplete revascularization
- *Postprocedural*:
  - Time at which repeat LV assessment is done
  - Development of graft occlusion or in-stent restenosis

PREVENTION AND MANAGEMENT OF HIBERNATION

Animal models have shown that in chronic hibernation occurring after 3 months of progressive coronary stenosis, when intracoronary injection of allogenic mesenchymal stem cells or cardiospheres are given, it leads to increase in cardiomyocyte nuclear size and reduced cardiomyocyte size (indicative of proliferation), increase in capillary density. and also improvement of regional contractile function even when blood flow was not improved.

Studies showed that 4 weeks after cell therapy, the size of anterior LV wall thickness remained depressed in 34% of the vehicle group, whereas in both the allogenic mesenchymal stem cell group and cardiosphere-derived cell group it recovered to 51%.

In the pig model, when the chronic hibernation was treated with pravastatin over 2 weeks, it lead to mobilization of bone-marrow derived progenitor cells into the circulation, and thus promoted the cardiomyocyte regeneration, thus resulting in improvement in regional contractile function even in the absence of improved blood flow.[4,8]

CLINICAL APPROACH TO MANAGEMENT OF ISCHEMIC HEART FAILURE PATIENTS

Flowchart 2 shows algorithm for management of ischemic heart failure.

*After revascularization, response can be assessed as given in **Flowchart 3**.*[10]

EVIDENCE FROM CLINICAL TRIALS

STITCH trial is the only prospective, randomized controlled trial that has given some positive results on revascularization benefits in ICM among many observational studies on chronic myocardial hibernation in patients with coronary artery disease.[9]

A total of 1,212 patients having ejection fraction of ≤35% and CAD were included in the STITCH trial. Patients were randomly assigned to undergo CABG plus medical therapy (CABG group) and medical therapy alone (medical therapy group). A total of 610 patients were included in CABG group and 602 patients in medical therapy group. Death from any cause was the primary outcome. Patients were followed up for a period of 9.8 years. The study demonstrated that the primary outcome event occurred in 398 patients (66.1%) in the medical therapy group and in 359 patients (58.9%) in the CABG group (hazard ratio with medical therapy vs. CABG 0.84 and $p = 0.02$ by log-rank test)

Cardiovascular cause of death was seen in 297 patients (49.3%) in the medical therapy group and in 247 patients (40.5%) in the CABG group ($p = 0.006$ by log-rank test; hazard ratio 0.79). In the study, hospitalization for cardiovascular causes or death from any cause was seen in a total of 467 patients (76.6%) in the CABG group and 524 patients (87.0%) in the medical therapy group ($p < 0.001$ by log-rank test; hazard ratio 0.72)

The results from the trial showed that in a cohort of patients with CAD and ejection fraction of ≤35%, patients who underwent CABG plus medical therapy had significantly lower rates of death from any cause, hospitalization for cardiovascular causes, and death from cardiovascular causes in a follow-up period of 10 years, when compared to patients who received medical therapy alone.[9]

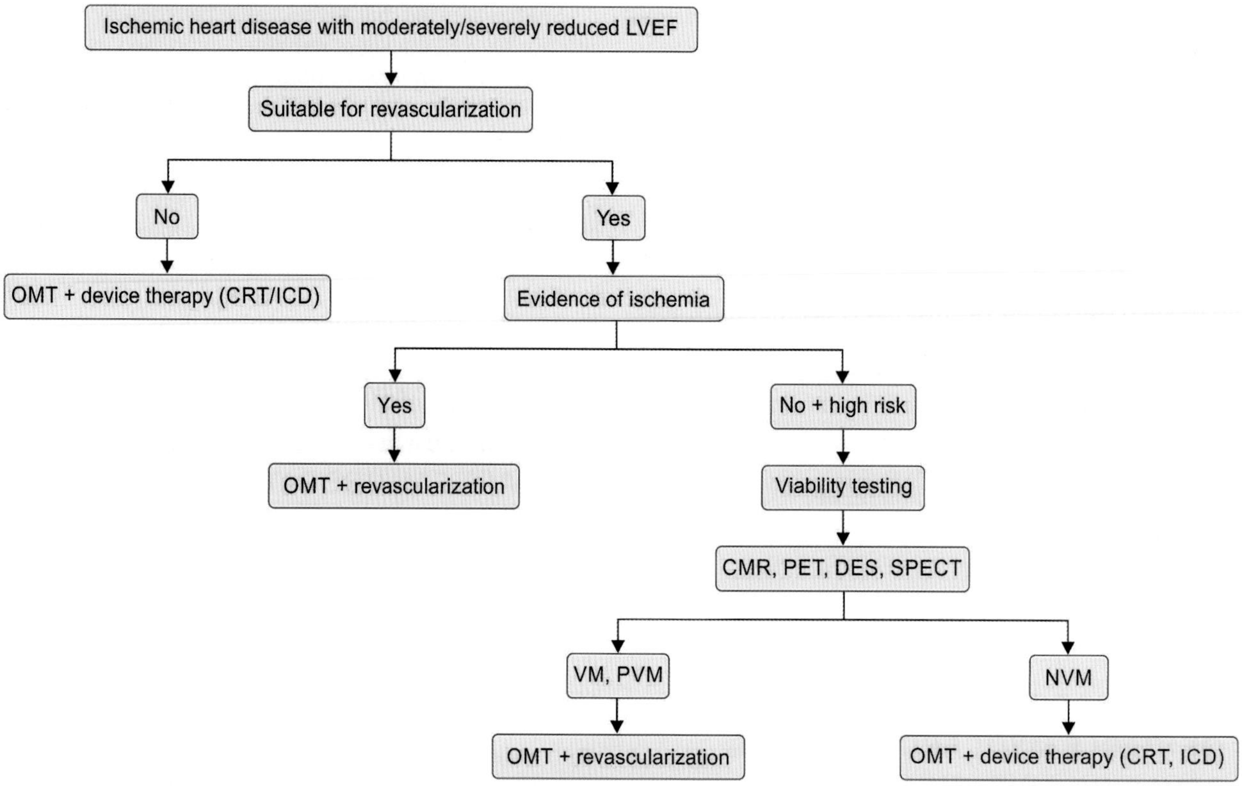

FLOWCHART 2: Treatment algorithm for management of patients with ischemic heart failure with moderately/severely reduced ejection fraction.

(CMR: cardiac magnetic resonance; CRT: cardiac resynchronization therapy; PET: positron emission tomography; DES: dobutamine stress echocardiography; ICD: implantable cardioverter defibrillator; NVM: nonviable myocardium; PVM: partially viable myocardium; OMT: optimal medical therapy; SPECT: single-photon emission tomography; VM: viable myocardium)

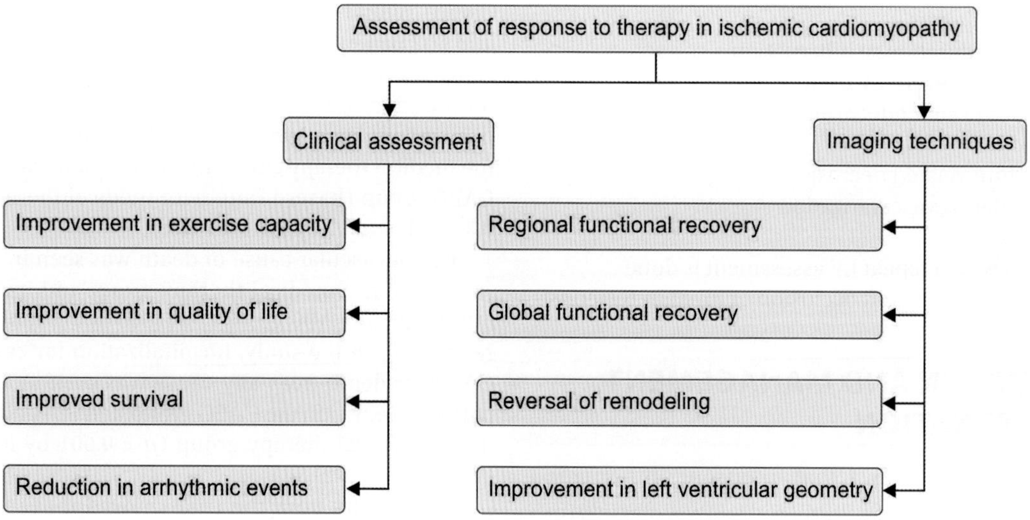

FLOWCHART 3: Assessment of response to therapy in ischemic cardiomyopathy.

ALTERNATIVES TO REVASCULARIZATION IN ISCHEMIC CARDIOMYOPATHY

Revascularization for ICM carries great risk despite pharmacological, technological, and surgical advances, and must be balanced against the putative benefits. Pharmacological therapy for HF as per current recommendations must also be given in all ICM patients. Despite medical therapy, high mortality rate persists in patients having ICM.

In comparison to optimal medical therapy (OMT), cardiac resynchronization therapy (CRT) is better in improving LVEF, reducing mechanical dyssynchrony, decreasing severity of mitral regurgitation, decreasing ventricular volume, improving QoL, and thus reducing mortality in patients with HF. This benefit is seen more in non-ICM patients and to a lesser extent in ICM patients. Clinical and echocardiographic benefits seen after CRT are directly correlated with degree of hibernating myocardium and less benefit is seen in the presence of scar in posterolateral wall (LV lead of CRT is positioned) in patients of ICM.[11]

CONCLUSION

Despite decades of research, patient management with hibernating myocardium remains a challenge. From a clinical point of view, the outcome in patients with ICM depends on duration, magnitude, and presence of hibernating myocardium, LV remodeling, subendocardial scar, procedure-related necrosis, incomplete revascularization, timing of repeat LV function assessment, graft occlusion or in-stent restenosis, optical medical therapy, and other concomitant comorbidities.

None of the imaging modalities accurately predict viable myocardium in ischemic LV dysfunction and regional or global functional recovery.

As none of the methods has been shown to be different in predicting hibernating myocardium, cost, local expertise, availability, and risk associated with the technique should determine which technique is to be utilized. However, experimental studies suggest that a novel therapy for hibernating myocardium involves stem cell therapy. Till the time definite guidelines come, the cardiologists are likely to continue on the existing evidence base to guide management.

ONLINE REFERENCES

Please scan the QR code provided at the end of the table of contents for References of this chapter.

CHAPTER

139

Takotsubo Syndrome

Madhu Sreedharan

ABSTRACT

Takotsubo syndrome (TTS) was first described in 1990 by Japanese cardiologists. It is an acute reversible heart failure syndrome characterized by presentation with chest pain or breathlessness, ECG changes, troponin elevation, and unobstructed coronary arteries. It has typical wall motion abnormalities involving the apical and mid-ventricular myocardium and is precipitated by physical or emotional stressors. The incidence has been rising due to increased awareness. It represents a form of neurocardiogenic myocardial stunning though the pathophysiological mechanism remains unclear. Long-term prognosis is similar to that of acute coronary syndrome but has no effective therapy to improve survival.

Keywords: Takotsubo syndrome, etiopathogenesis, management and prognosis

INTRODUCTION

The term Takotsubo syndrome (TTS) was first coined in 1990 by Saito et al. who published a series of five cases in Japan.[1] It derives its name from the Japanese word for octopus trap, from the shape of LV at the end of systole. There are various terms used to describe this entity including stress cardiomyopathy, broken heart syndrome, or apical ballooning syndrome. TTS shares many common features with acute coronary syndrome (ACS) such as presentation with chest pain, ECG changes, and elevated cardiac markers. The triggers include a wide spectrum of emotional or physical stressors, and hence it is best described as a syndrome.[2] Though initially considered to be benign due to the absence of obstructive coronary artery disease, it is associated with increased mortality, not dissimilar to ACS.[3]

A TYPICAL CASE

A 61-year-old lady presented with acute onset of chest discomfort and breathlessness to the emergency department at 1 AM. She was on treatment for type 2 diabetes mellitus, hypertension and dyslipidemia. She had features of LVF with bibasal crackles and so was shifted to the coronary care unit. Her pulse rate was 76 beats/minute and blood pressure was 150/80 mm Hg. Her ECG at admission showed J-point elevation in V_{1-4}, which evolved to a deep T inversion across the precordial leads **(Figs. 1 and 2)**. She was treated with IV diuretics and noninvasive ventilatory support for the LVF along with beta-blockers, ACEi, diuretics, MRA, dual antiplatelets, statins, and OHA.

Her serial high sensitivity troponins were elevated 51.7 → 10,930 → 5,819 pg/mL, suggestive of myocardial injury. But, the levels were not very high and the rapid decline of cardiac markers was not consistent with that seen in ACS. Her echocardiogram (echo) showed apical ballooning with strain imaging, confirming wall motion abnormality of the apical segments **(Figs. 3 to 5)**.

She was taken up for a coronary angiogram, which showed normal epicardial coronaries **(Figs. 6 and 7)**.

On further questioning, she admitted to having emotional stress secondary to conflict in family related to alcoholism of her husband. With her presentation with chest pain and LVF, ECG changes, elevated cardiac markers, apical ballooning on echo, normal epicardial coronaries, and being precipitated by emotional stress in a postmenopausal stage, a diagnosis of TTS was made. As is typically seen in TTS, a repeat echo after a week showed almost complete recovery of LV function **(Fig. 8)**.

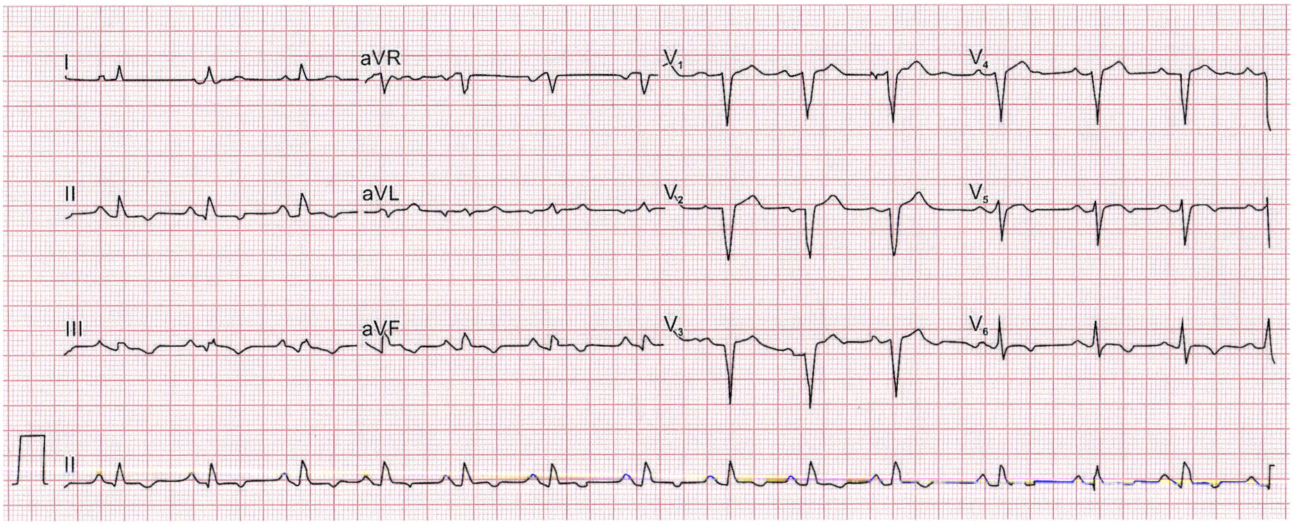

FIG. 1: ST elevation in V_{1-4}.

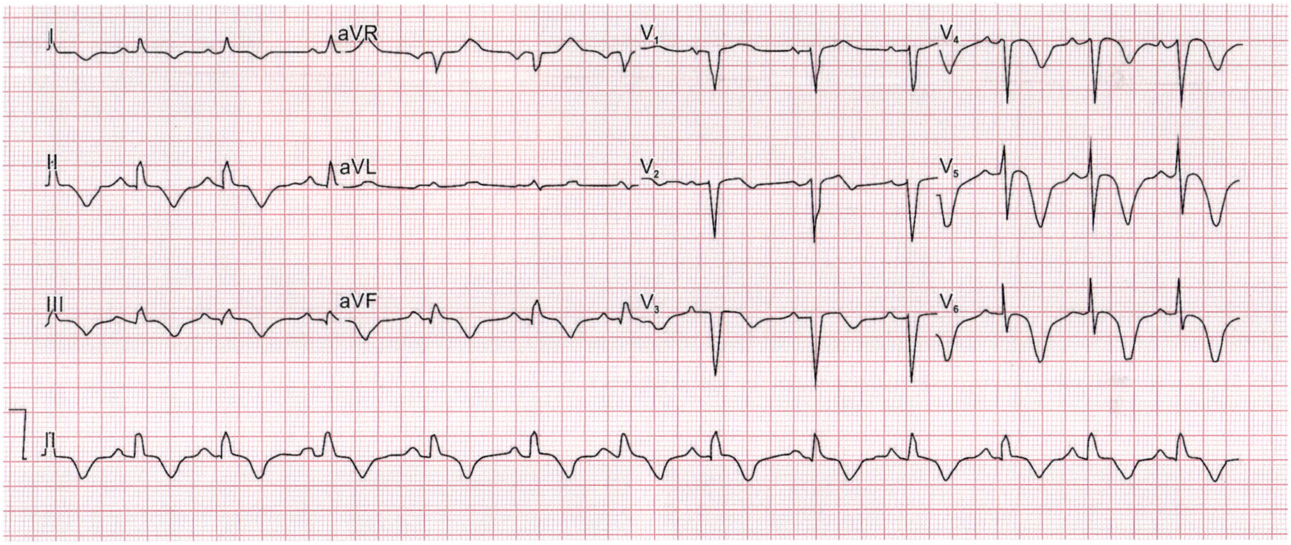

FIG. 2: Deep T inversion at V_{2-6}, II, III, and aVF.

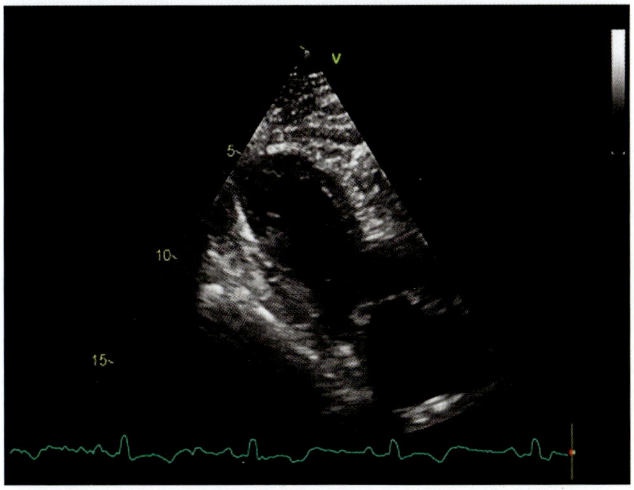

FIG. 3: pLAX showing apical ballooning.

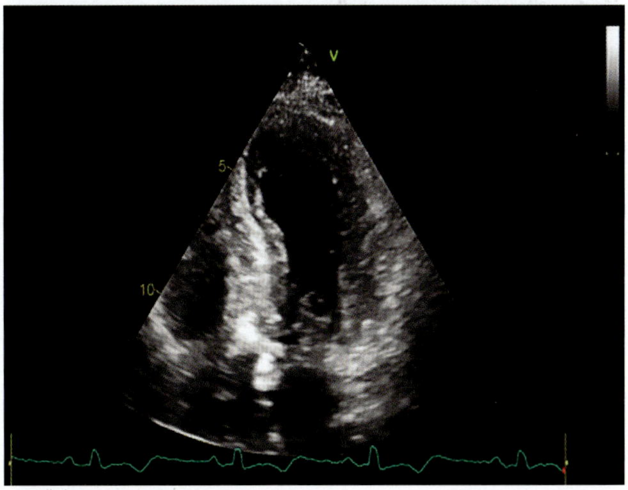

FIG. 4: Apical four-chamber view.

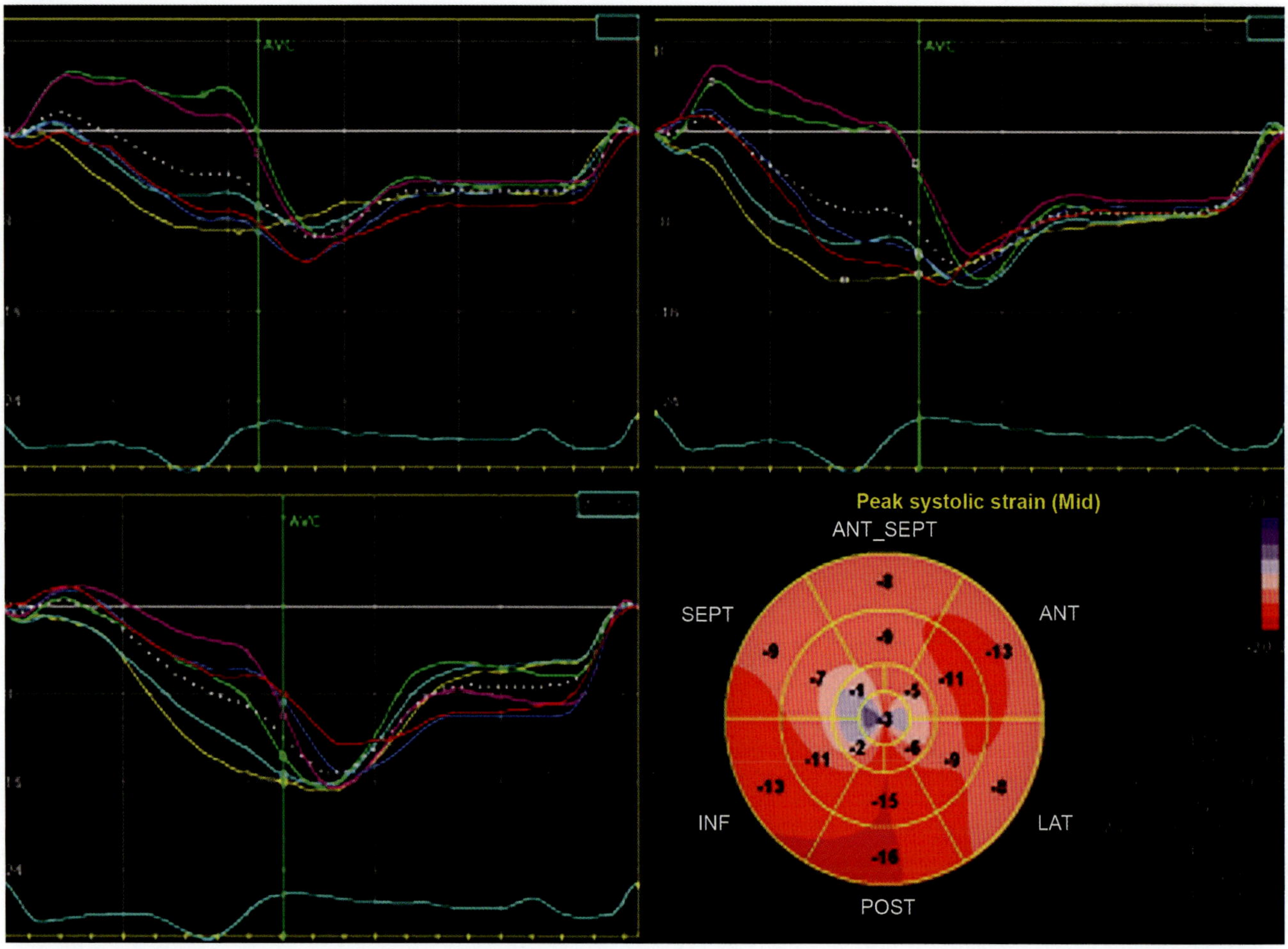

FIG. 5: Strain imaging showing hypokinesia/akinesia of the apical segment.

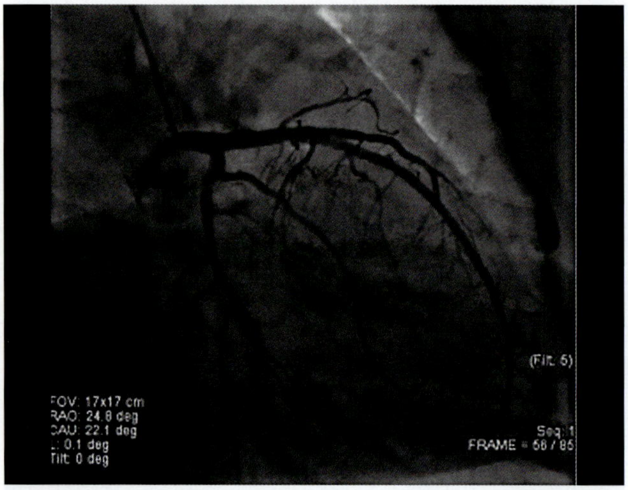

FIG. 6: Normal LAD and LCx.

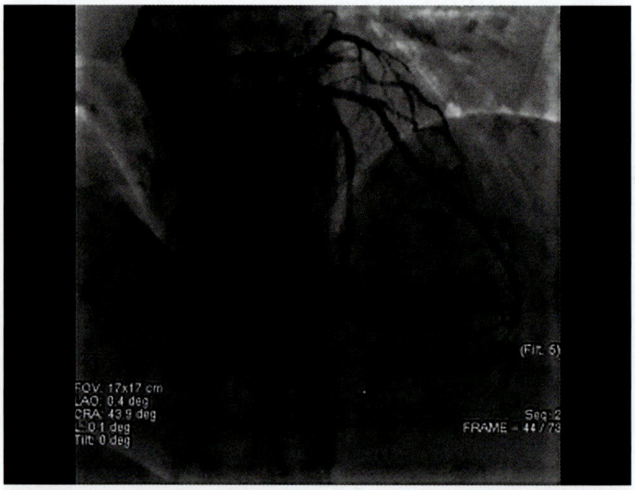

FIG. 7: Normal LAD and D1.

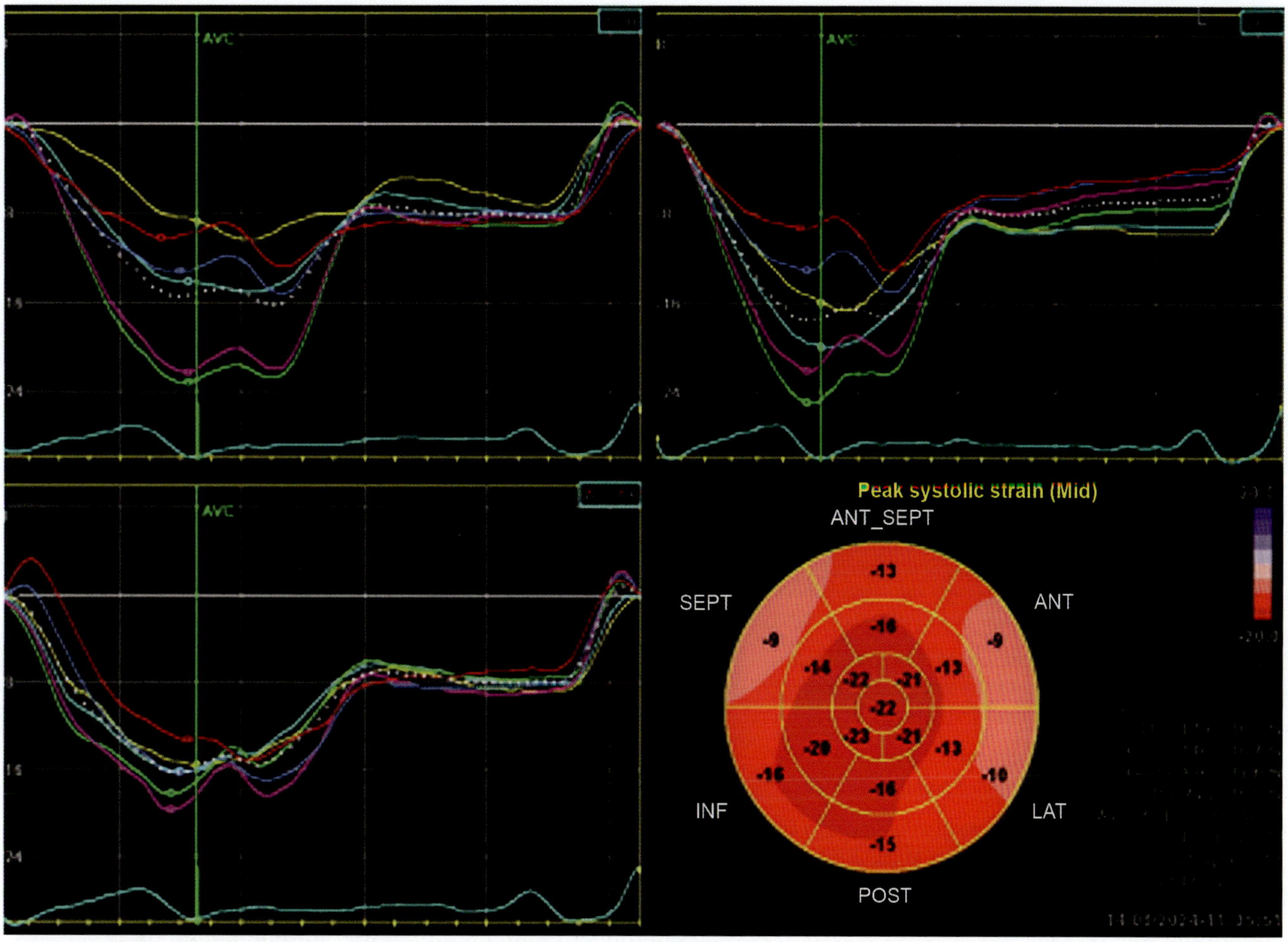

FIG. 8: Repeat echocardiogram showing almost complete recovery of LV function.

EPIDEMIOLOGY

Takotsubo syndrome accounts for up to 5–6% of female patients presenting with ACS. It typically affects women in the sixth decade of life. Younger patients are likely to be males, have atypical TTS, fewer comorbidities with neurological or psychiatric disorders, and develop inhospital complications.[4]

PATHOPHYSIOLOGY

The pathophysiology of TTS is not well established. Predisposing factors of TTS include older age, female sex, stressors, and mental health. Emotional or physical stressors precipitate the episode. Activation of hypothalamic–pituitary–adrenal axis results in epinephrine and norepinephrine release from the adrenal medulla. It results in increased ventricular afterload, coronary vasospasm, and microvascular dysfunction. Increased responsiveness of the left ventricular (LV) apex to catecholamines could explain the apical ballooning. Direct myocardial injury resulting in catecholamine stunning and contraction band necrosis via altered beta-adrenergic receptor signaling is another postulate.[5]

DIAGNOSTIC CRITERIA

Diagnosis of TTS is challenging because the presentation and phenotypes resemble that of ACS. Apical TTS was seen in 81.7%, mid-ventricular type was seen in 14.6%, and basal and focal forms were seen in 2.2% and 1.5% patients in a study of 1,750 patients.[6] Though troponins were elevated in both ACS and TTS, it was significantly more in patients with ACS ($p < 0.001$). A diagnostic criterion for the diagnosis of TTS, International takotsubo diagnostic criteria (InterTAK diagnostic criteria), has been developed **(Box 1)**.[2]

CLINICAL FEATURES

Patients typically present with acute onset chest pain, dyspnea, and changes in the ECG after a stressful event. It is often treated as an ACS. Rarely, it may present as STEMI, heart failure, or cardiogenic shock. Stressors are usually emotional though physical stressors may also precipitate TTS. Neurological conditions like subarachnoid hemorrhage, pheochromocytoma, epilepsy, or severe critical illness can also trigger it. Mental illnesses like depression and anxiety are present in 30% of TTS patients. Psychiatric or neurologic

BOX 1 International Takotsubo diagnostic criteria (Inter TAK diagnostic criteria).

- Patients show transient left ventricular dysfunction (hypokinesia, akinesia, or dyskinesia) presenting as apical ballooning, mid-ventricular, basal, or focal wall motion abnormalities
- Right ventricular involvement can also be present
- RWMA extends beyond a single vascular territory though rarely it may be present in the myocardial territory of a single coronary artery (focal TTS)
- Emotional, physical, or combined triggers can precede the event, though not obligatory
- Neurological disorders (SAH, stroke, TIA, or seizures) as well as pheochromocytoma may serve as triggers for TTS
- New ECG abnormalities are present (ST elevation or depression, T inversion, or QTc prolongation). Rarely ECG may be normal
- Cardiac biomarkers (troponin and creatinine kinase) are moderately elevated in most cases. Elevation of BNP is also common
- Significant coronary artery disease is not a contraindication in TTS
- Patients have no evidence of infectious myocarditis
- Cardiac MRI is recommended to exclude myocarditis
- Postmenopausal women are predominantly affected

TABLE 1: Mimics of Takotsubo syndrome (TTS).

	Takotsubo	Myocarditis	Acute MI (STEMI/Non STEMI)
Clinical features	Acute chest pain or dyspnea with preceding stressors and preexisting psychiatric illness	Acute chest pain, dyspnea, and heart failure preceded by respiratory infection or gastroenteritis	Acute chest pain or dyspnea and risk factors for atherosclerosis
ECG	• ST–T changes • QT prolongation	Nonspecific ST–T. ST elevation in all leads to myopericarditis	Ischemic changes—corresponding to the vascular territory
Cardiac markers	Moderate elevation of troponin and marked elevation of BNP/CRP	Elevated troponin	Marked elevation of troponin and moderate elevation of BNP/CRP
Echo	Transient LV dysfunction	Global systolic dysfunction (rarely regionals/segmental)	Normal/persistent RWMA
CAG	Normal/nonobstructive CAD and apical ballooning on LV angio	Normal/nonobstructive CAD	Obstructive CAD
Cardiac MRI	No persistent late gadolinium enhancement	Late gadolinium enhancement with focal or patchy subepicardial or noncoronary distribution	Late gadolinium enhancement—infarct pattern and regional wall motion abnormality

(CAG: coronary angiogram; echo: echocardiogram; MI: myocardial infarction)

illnesses in TTS patients are 7-fold higher than in patients with ACS.

Patients with emotional stressors are more likely to be females, present with chest pain, and have better outcomes. Those with physical stressors are more likely to be men, have associated comorbidities, present with syncope or dyspnea, have basal pattern of LV dysfunction, and have acute complications.[7] The various differential diagnoses of TTS are given in **Table 1**.

There are various anatomical variants of TTS.[8] The typical pattern with narrow neck and globular lower portion in the apical ballooning form is present in 75–80% of patients. The other variants include mid-ventricular, basal or inverted TTS, biventricular, isolated RV, and localized focal forms **(Table 2)**.

INHOSPITAL MANAGEMENT

There is no clinical trial or evidence-based management for the treatment of TTS. Extrapolation of treatment is known to be effective after acute myocardial infarction, e.g., beta-blockers and ACE inhibitors have been used. In the acute setting, the focus is on supportive care and to prevent complications. It may broadly be divided into treatment of complications, predischarge, and long-term management **(Table 3)**.

In patients presenting with shock, treatment is challenging. Inotropic agents can worsen LV dysfunction due to the excess catecholamines involved in the pathogenesis of the condition. Mechanical approaches to provide hemodynamic support like intra-aortic balloon pump,

TABLE 2: Anatomical variants of Takotsubo syndrome.

Type	Prevalence	Features
Apical ballooning (typical)	75–80%	It may be associated with left ventricular (LV) tract outflow obstruction and apical thrombus. It has variable prognosis
Mid-ventricular	10–20%	Severe LV dysfunction and acute heart failure
Basal or inverted	5%	Less severe hemodynamic compromise
Biventricular	<0.5%	Severe hemodynamic compromise and shock
Focal	Rare	Benign course, associated with chest pain

TABLE 3: Management of Takotsubo syndrome.

	Consider	Avoid
Acute complications		
Heart failure/pulmonary edema	• Diuretics • IV nitroglycerine	
Left ventricular outflow tract obstruction	• IV fluids • Beta-blockers (BB) (if no heart failure)	Inotropes
Ventricular arrhythmias	BB and magnesium	QT-prolonging drugs
High-grade AV block	Temporary pacing	• BB • Permanent pacemakers
Thromboembolism LV thrombus	Anticoagulation for 3 months, prophylactic anticoagulation for apical ballooning and LVEF <30%	
Predischarge		
Bystander CAD	Secondary prevention—antiplatelet and statin	
LV dysfunction	BB, ACEi/ARB, diuretics, MRA, and SGLT-2i	
Tachycardia	BB and ivabradine (if sinus rhythm and can not tolerate BB)	
Assessment for LV thrombus	Cardiac imaging and assessment for anticoagulation	
Long-term management		
Prevent recurrence	Treatment of cardiovascular risk factors	
Address risk factors	Underlying mental health issues	

(CAD: coronary artery disease; LV: left ventricular)

extracorporeal membrane oxygenation, or ventricular assist devices are recommended. Identification of left ventricular outflow tract obstruction (LVOT) obstruction is important as it may be worsened with IABP. If mechanical support is not available, levosimendan may be used as a catecholamine-sparing inotrope.

Long-term management of TTS, if associated with coronary artery disease, should include antiplatelet, statin, and ACE inhibitors. Those with LV dysfunction should be managed as per guidelines. However, in those whose LV function has normalized, there is no clear evidence of the benefit of using beta-blockers or ACE inhibitors to improve survival or to prevent the recurrence of TTS.[6]

NATURAL HISTORY AND PROGNOSIS

Patients with TTS have transient LV dysfunction with nonobstructed coronaries, which spontaneously recover without fibrosis or scarring. Despite this, the long-term prognosis of patients with TTS is comparable to that of patients with acute myocardial infarction in many registries.[9] In a case-control study of 620 patients with TTS compared with matched post-myocardial infarction (n = 620) and general population (n = 2,480) followed up for a median of 5.5 years from Scotland, 25% patients died. This was lower than the mortality for those with myocardial infarction (31% $p = 0.012$) but was higher than that of the general population (15% $p < 0.0001$). The reduced survival was due to excess mortality due to cardiovascular as well as noncardiovascular causes. Cardiovascular mortality was mostly due to heart failure—a significant proportion of patients evolve toward heart failure with preserved ejection fraction after recovery from the acute phase. Mortality from noncardiovascular causes was predominantly due to pulmonary conditions. Despite comparable medications, treatment was associated with better survival in patients with myocardial infarction but not in those with TTS. Patients on diuretics and anti-inflammatory and psychotropic therapies had worse outcomes.[10]

Depending on the triggering factors, TTS may have differing prognoses. TTS patients with emotional stress had a favorable short- and long-term prognosis. Those secondary to neurological disease had the worst short-term prognosis. TTS secondary to neurologic diseases, physical activities, medical conditions, or procedures had significantly higher mortality compared with ACS during long-term follow-up.[9] Recurrences are common at 2–4% per year and up to 20% at 10 years.

CONCLUSION

Takotsubo syndrome is an acute cardiac disorder with transient LV dysfunction. It must be differentiated from ACS for appropriate management. Multimodality imaging helps in this regard. Emotional stress with catecholamine excess is implicated in its pathogenesis. Despite recovery of LV function and absence of myocardial fibrosis, it is not benign and has a mortality significantly higher than that of the general population. It remains a poorly understood condition with no proven or effective treatment.

ONLINE REFERENCES

Please scan the QR code provided at the end of the table of contents for References of this chapter.

CHAPTER 140

Spontaneous Coronary Artery Dissection

K Sivaprasad, Manju Bhargav BR

ABSTRACT

Spontaneous coronary artery dissection (SCAD) is becoming an increasingly important cause of acute coronary syndrome and sudden cardiac death, particularly among young women and often with sparse conventional atherosclerotic risk factors. Invasive coronary angiography with imaging and conservative therapy are generally recommended, with percutaneous or surgical revascularization reserved for clinical instability, high-risk anatomy, or as a last resort. Robust evidence on optimal medical therapy is scarce, posing unique challenges. The follow-up plan is crucial because recurrent SCAD is not uncommon, long-term planning for pharmacological therapy and lifestyle modifications is necessary, and SCAD-related conditions need to be treated. This chapter aims at a practical management approach to SCAD patients.

Keywords: SCAD, ACS, women, fibromuscular dysplasia, pregnancy

INTRODUCTION

Spontaneous coronary artery dissection (SCAD) is an emerging cause of acute coronary syndrome (ACS) in young women. First case was reported by Harold C pretty 1931, in the British Medical Journal in 1931 in a 42-year-old woman with severe chest pain and died unexpectedly, and autopsy showing ruptured dissecting right coronary artery.[1] SCAD primarily affects young and middle-aged women. Even though SCAD accounts for <5% of all ACS cases, it accounts for one-third of cases in women under the age of 50.[2-4] This chapter will discuss the understanding of pathophysiology, clinical presentation, diagnosis, and management of SCAD.

DEFINITION AND CLASSIFICATION OF SCAD

The SCAD refers to the nontraumatic, noniatrogenic development of a false lumen within the coronary artery wall unrelated to atherosclerotic disease or primary aortic dissection. The dissection may originate from an intimal tear leading to dissection into the arterial wall or from spontaneous bleeding from ruptured vasa vasorum without an intimal tear.[5] SCAD is typically characterized by the sudden formation of an intramural hematoma (IMH) between the coronary artery wall's three layers (intima, media, and adventitia). An intimal tear may form a communication between the IMH and the true lumen of the artery. SCAD may cause abrupt mechanical obstruction to coronary blood flow, resulting in ACS and, less commonly, acute arrhythmia and sudden cardiac death.

Saw et al.[6,7] proposed three distinct types of SCAD based on angiographic appearance. Type 1 SCAD has visible contrast in both true and false lumens, giving the pathognomonic appearance of multiple lumens on angiography. In type 2 and type 3 SCAD, contrast is seen in the true lumen only with the appearance of a diffuse (type 2) or short (type 3), often tubular stenosis. Using coronary angiography (CAG) alone can make it challenging to distinguish between type 3 SCAD and an atherosclerotic lesion. Confirmation of the diagnosis may require intravascular ultrasound (IVUS) or intracoronary optical coherence tomography (OCT). Type 2 SCAD is classified into two types—(1) type 2a, in which the hematoma is located between normal artery segments proximal and distal to the affected segment, and (2) type 2b, in which the SCAD/hematoma extends to the vessel's very distal aspect. Type 4 SCAD refers to complete occlusion of the coronary artery. It is difficult to distinguish from other causes of coronary occlusion, but it can be diagnosed with intracoronary imaging following vessel opening or subsequent angiography demonstrating complete vessel healing **(Table 1 and Figs. 1A to E)**.

TABLE 1: Coronary angiography classification of SCAD.

Type of SCAD	Description
Type 1 (29–48%)	A multilumen appearance with visible contrast in both true and false lumens
Type 2 (52–67%): • 2a • 2b	• A diffuse stenosis (>2 cm) with contrast visible in the true lumen • SCAD does not extend to the tip of the vessel • SCAD extends to the tip of the vessel
Type 3 (0–3.9%)	Appearance of short stenosis (<20 mm). Contrast visible in the true lumen only may mimic atherosclerotic lesion
Type 4	Total occlusion of the coronary artery. Need to exclude thrombus as the cause, and subsequent angiography should demonstrate healing of the vessel

EPIDEMIOLOGY AND RISK FACTORS FOR SCAD

The SCAD was once thought to be a rare condition, but its incidence has risen due to increased clinician awareness and better access to intracoronary imaging. SCAD occurs in 1–5% of cases of ACS, with women accounting for 80–95% of SCAD cases.[8] In women under 50 years of age with MI, the prevalence of SCAD is up to 35%.[2] SCAD is the leading cause of MI in pregnant women, with the majority of cases occurring during the third-trimester or the first month after delivery. SCAD results from a combination of a precipitating factor and an underlying arteriopathy that weakens the arterial wall **(Table 2)**.

PATHOPHYSIOLOGY OF SCAD

Two primary theories elucidate the mechanism of SCAD—the "inside-out" and "outside-in" theories. The inside-out theory states that the initial insult is a tear in the coronary intimal layer, which causes blood to dissect into the subintimal space and form a hematoma. The outside-in theory, on the other hand, holds that the initial insult is the rupture

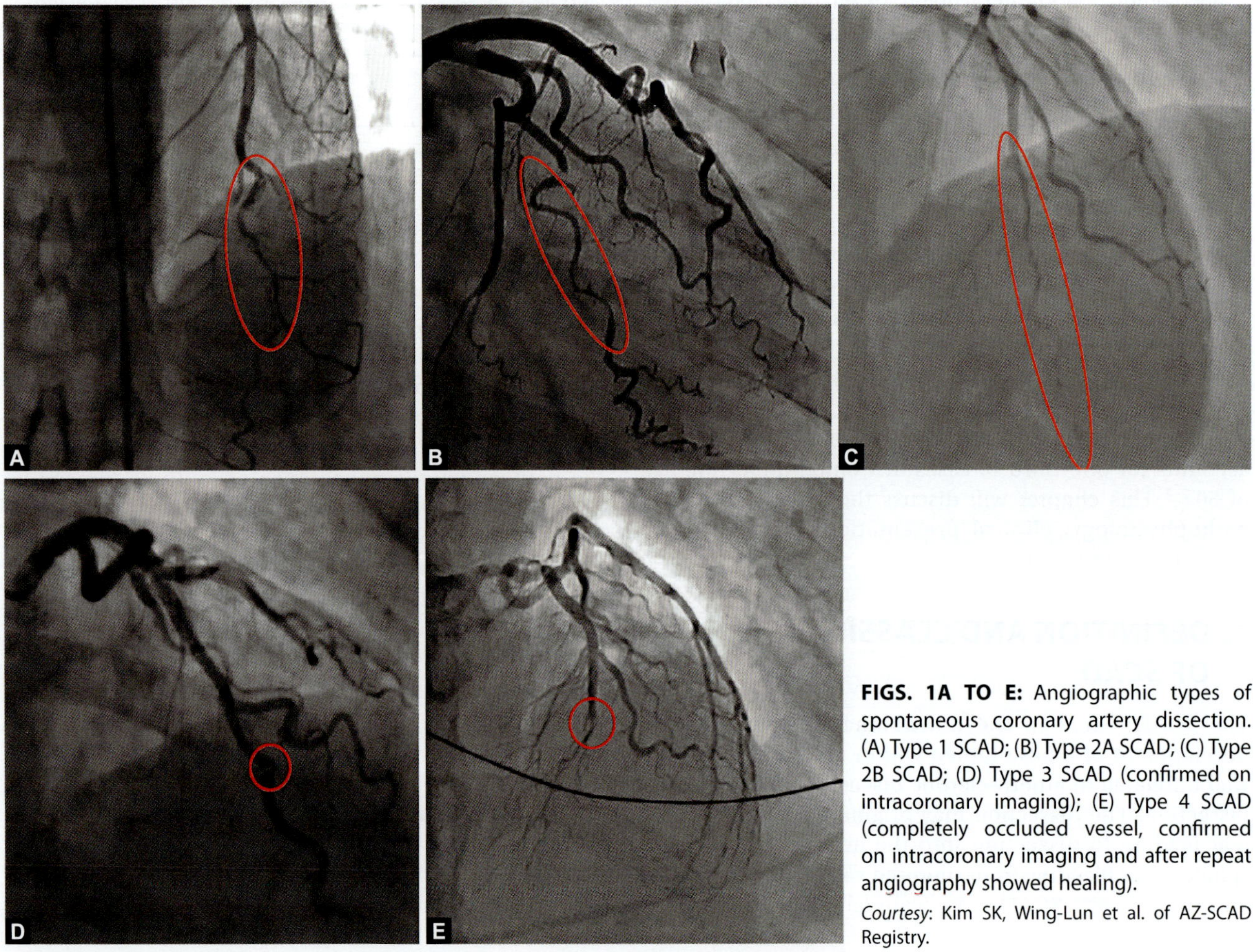

FIGS. 1A TO E: Angiographic types of spontaneous coronary artery dissection. (A) Type 1 SCAD; (B) Type 2A SCAD; (C) Type 2B SCAD; (D) Type 3 SCAD (confirmed on intracoronary imaging); (E) Type 4 SCAD (completely occluded vessel, confirmed on intracoronary imaging and after repeat angiography showed healing).

Courtesy: Kim SK, Wing-Lun et al. of AZ-SCAD Registry.

of the vasa vasorum, resulting in a hematoma within the arterial wall that may later rupture into the true lumen. This is supported by OCT imaging, which has shown a lack of communication between the true and false lumen.[9-11] The outside-in theory is more common, implying that bleeding is the primary mechanism rather than dissection or tearing.

Regarding the link between women and SCAD, it is known that the estrogen hormone influences angiogenesis, vasodilation, and autonomic regulation.[12] These effects may explain its association with SCAD, though the mechanism is unknown. Structural weakness in the arterial wall predisposes to SCAD. Multiple arteriopathies have been identified in SCAD cases, with fibromuscular dysplasia (FMD) being the most common.[13] SCAD is linked to several common variants, implying complex polygenic interactions.[14] SCAD is linked to an allele in the PHACTR1 (phosphatase and actin regulator 1) common genetic locus on chromosome 6p24, according to a genome-wide analysis of more common genetic variants.[15] Interestingly, this allele is also linked to FMD, which may help to explain the link between the two conditions. A recent genome-wide association meta-analysis has identified 16 risk loci for SCAD, which are enriched in vascular smooth muscle cells and fibroblasts **(Flowchart 1)**.[16]

TABLE 2: Predisposing conditions and precipitating triggers for SCAD.

Predisposing conditions	Precipitating factors
Fibromuscular dysplasia	Extreme emotional stress
Connective tissue disorders (Marfan, Ehlers-Danlos, Loeys–Dietz syndrome, and polycystic kidney disease)	Intense physical stress (strenuous exercise, labor, and delivery)
Systemic inflammatory disease (SLE, IBD, celiac disease, sarcoidosis, and rheumatoid arthritis)	Recreational drugs (cocaine and amphetamines)
Pregnancy-related	
Hormonal therapy (oral contraceptive pill)	

(IBD: inflammatory bowel disease; SLE: systemic lupus erythematosus)

CLINICAL PRESENTATION AND NATURAL PROGRESSION OF SCAD

According to the Canadian SCAD registry, ACS is the most common presentation, accounting for 28% of STEMI, 70% of NSTEMI, and 0.5% of unstable angina. Chest discomfort is the most common symptom (92%), while arrhythmia is uncommon (1%).[13] Sudden cardiac death is a rare

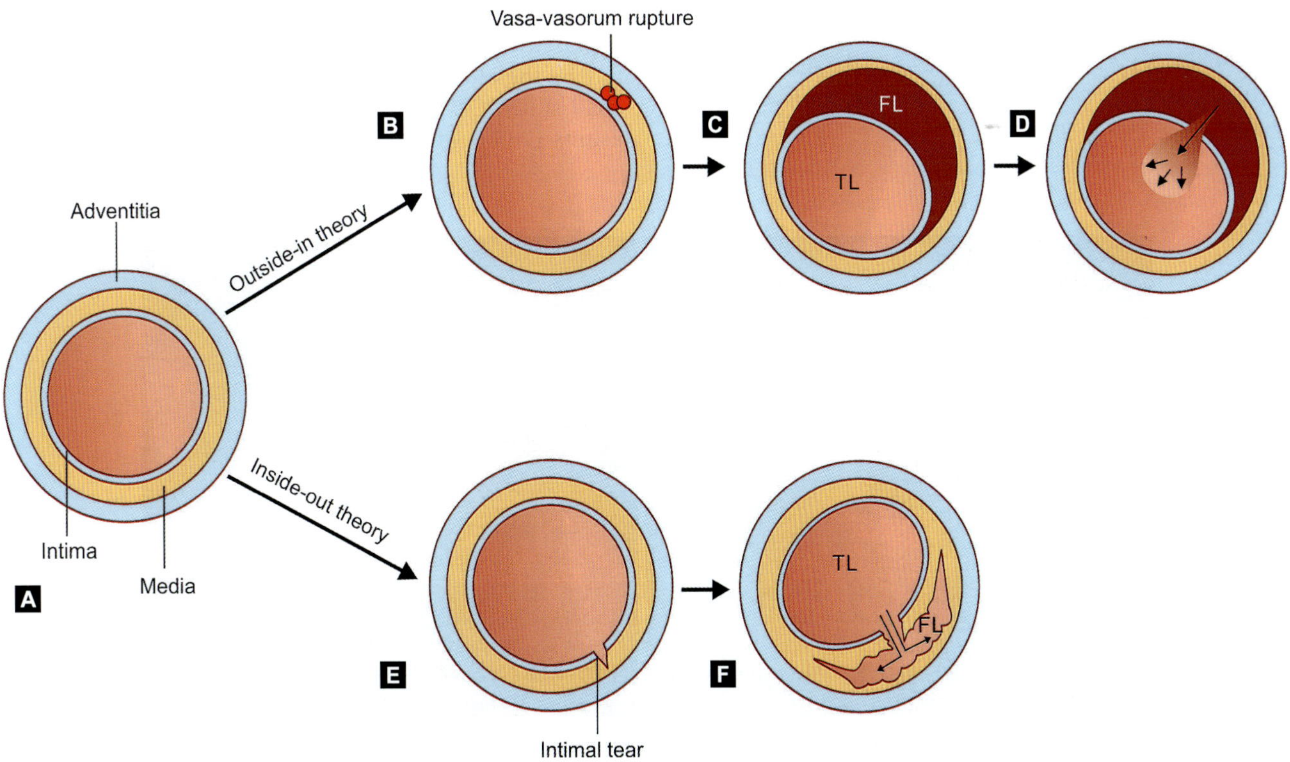

FLOWCHART 1: Pathophysiology of SCAD. Schematic representation of the cross-section of a normal coronary artery with three layers. (A) In the outside-in theory, a vasa-vasorum ruptures in the media, causing a small intramural hematoma. (B) This hematoma may increase in size and compress the true lumen, (C) and /or result in rupture of the intima, leading to a hematoma emptying into the true lumen. (D) In the inside-out theory, a tear first appears in the intima, (E) followed by subintimal dissections caused by blood entering the lumen, creating a false lumen. The false lumen may expand as the dissection spreads further between layers of the arterial wall.[17]

occurrence; in a recent autopsy study of people who died unexpectedly, only 0.3% had SCAD.[18] The majority of SCAD cases heals spontaneously over time, with a median duration of 5–39 months.[19]

DIAGNOSIS AND ROLE OF MULTIMODALITY IMAGING INVASIVE CORONARY ANGIOGRAPHY

Invasive CAG is the current gold standard test for diagnosing SCAD. **Table 3** shows the characteristics that distinguish SCAD from atherosclerosis plaques. In cases of diagnostic uncertainty, intracoronary GTN, intravascular imaging, CT coronary angiogram, and cardiac MRI can be used.

TABLE 3: SCAD and atherosclerosis on invasive coronary angiography.

Characteristics	SCAD	Atherosclerosis plaque
Appearance of the lesion	Linear, tubular, and contrast staining of double lumen	Irregular
Typical location	Mid to distal	Proximal
Nonculprit coronary arteries	Normal arteries, free of significant stenoses	Multiple stenoses in coronary arteries
Lesion length	Usually >10 mm	<10 mm
Calcification	Uncommon	Possible
Coronary artery tortuosity	Common	Less common

INTRACORONARY IMAGING IN SCAD

Although not always used, intracoronary imaging modalities such as IVUS and OCT can help resolve diagnostic uncertainty and provide guidance for treatment. Both imaging modalities, OCT and IVUS, have advantages and disadvantages in SCAD. OCT has a higher spatial resolution and greater ability to visualize an intimal tear. IVUS has better depth penetration and is, therefore, more useful in larger vessels. The benefit of IVUS is that it does not require contrast injection to obtain images, as this could lead to the hematoma spreading. The size of these devices (approximately 1 mm) is another drawback of intravascular imaging, which makes it difficult to use in small, tortuous, and distal vessels—areas that are frequently involved in SCAD cases. Either modality can aid in diagnosis confirmation when there is diagnostic uncertainty, especially in larger, more proximal vessels or type 3 SCAD. When percutaneous intervention is required in cases of SCAD, intracoronary imaging can confirm wire position (luminal or subintimal), guide stent size and length, and reduce the risk of stent malapposition following intramural hematoma reabsorption **(Figs. 2A and B)**.

CT CORONARY ANGIOGRAM IN SCAD

One benefit of CTCA is that it is a noninvasive diagnostic technique that can show whether coronary calcification or plaque is present, which suggests that atherosclerosis may be the alternative cause of coronary narrowing. In a small study, CTCA correctly identified SCAD in 14 of 18 lesions (78%), with the majority of misses occurring in

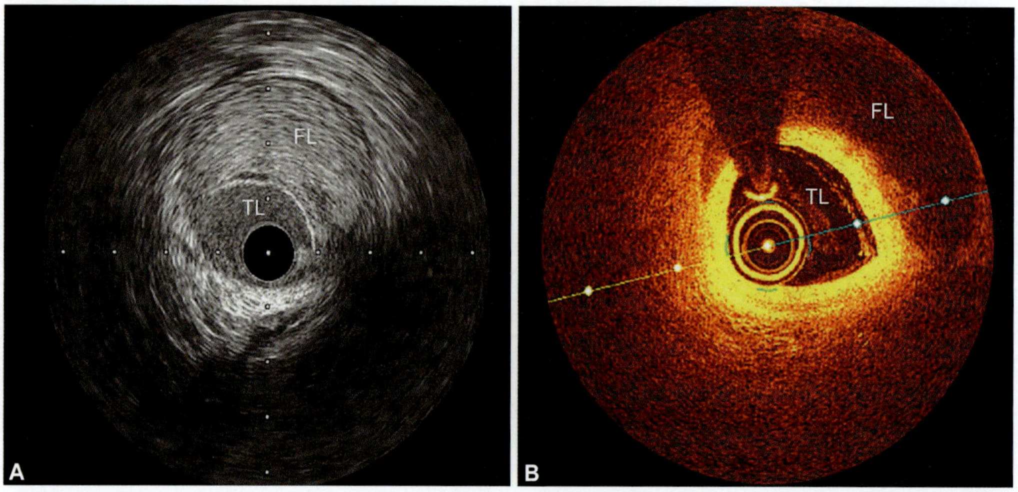

FIGS. 2A AND B: Intracoronary imaging of SCAD. (A) Intravascular ultrasound image of SCAD; (B) Optical coherence tomography of SCAD. (FL: false lumen; TL: true lumen)

Courtesy: Kim SK, Wing-Lun et al. of AZ-SCAD Registry.

small vessels.[20] This demonstrates CTCA's main limitation in SCAD—the lower spatial resolution, which limits SCAD detection in smaller vessels, prevents CTCA from excluding the diagnosis. As a result, CTCA's primary diagnostic strategy is limited and serves as an adjunctive test for ICA in people with suspected SCAD. Furthermore, there is no consensus on using CTCA as a follow-up modality.

ACUTE MANAGEMENT OF SCAD

Most cases of SCAD heal on their own, so it is best to adopt a conservative approach whenever possible. Percutaneous intervention in SCAD has a high risk of causing catheter-induced coronary dissection, and procedures such as wiring, ballooning, and stenting can all worsen the dissection or intramural hematoma. Guidewires and/or stents may be accidentally inserted into a false lumen, and stent sizing may be difficult due to a large intramural hematoma. This can result in late stent malapposition once the SCAD heals, restenosis, and stent thrombosis. The American College of Cardiology/American Heart Association and European Society of Cardiology guidelines for ACS management recommend an early invasive strategy for revascularization of culprit lesions over conservative therapy in high-risk situations such as left main disease or proximal two vessel disease, hemodynamic instability, active ongoing ischemia and in recurrent symptoms after conservative management.[21-23] This stent-based lesion pacification technique lowers the risk of recurrent lesion occlusion and associated adverse events in atherosclerotic MI. There have been no randomized studies or subgroup analyses of treatment outcomes, nor have there been any comparisons of acute revascularization strategies for SCAD-induced ACS **(Flowchart 2)**.

Conservative Management

Because the natural history of conservatively treated SCAD is typically benign, with progressive and complete healing of the involved vessel, taking a conservative approach with medical therapy and in-hospital monitoring appears to be safer than intervention in the majority of SCAD presentations. Hence, noninvasive treatment is preferred for stable and even symptomatic patients at presentation. Following the diagnosis, it is critical to avoid aggressive antithrombotic strategies that may aggravate the condition. This means that glycoprotein (GP) IIb/IIIa inhibitors should be avoided, and anticoagulants should be discontinued following CAG. To counteract the prothrombotic activity caused by intimal fenestrations or flaps and prevent thrombosis of the true lumen due to the expanding IMH and/or false lumen, the majority of experts advises taking both aspirin and clopidogrel. Other P2Y12 inhibitors have not been widely used, and their strong antiplatelet effects may be unneeded or even hazardous. The majority of guideline-directed pharmacological therapies for atherosclerotic ACS is unclear in SCAD-associated ACS, with the exception of antithrombotic agents. The cornerstone of treatment is beta-blockers, which lower cardiac shear stress and contractility. Other antianginal medications such as ranolazine, nitrates, and calcium channel blockers are also helpful in managing symptoms. When left ventricular dysfunction develops, angiotensin-converting enzyme inhibitors (ACEIs), angiotensin receptor blockers (ARBs), mineralocorticoid receptor antagonists (MRAs), and sodium-glucose cotransporter-2 inhibitors (SGLT-2i) should be taken into consideration. Statins should be prescribed based on the estimated cardiovascular risk for patients undergoing primary prevention.[22]

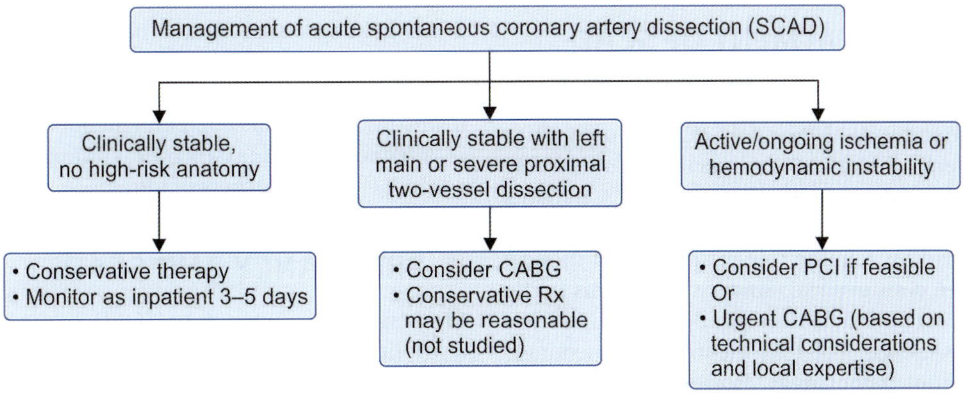

FLOWCHART 2: Algorithm for management of acute SCAD.

(CABG: coronary artery bypass graft; PCI: percutaneous intervention; SCAD: spontaneous coronary artery dissection)

Source: Adapted with permission from: Hayes SN, et al. (2018);[22] and Hayes S, et al. (2020).[23]

Optimizing the Technique for Percutaneous Coronary Intervention

In SCAD, it is crucial to employ precise angiographic and instrumentation techniques in order to maximize the results of percutaneous coronary intervention (PCI). This entails avoiding deep catheter engagement, making sure the catheter tip is positioned coaxially, avoiding catheter dampening, and using contrast agents with caution. It might be preferable to use femoral access in possible SCAD cases, or to use extreme caution when using radial catheterization. A retrospective study found that SCAD patients who underwent CAG via radial access had a threefold higher risk of catheter-induced iatrogenic dissection than those who used femoral access. The following approaches have proven effective in treating IMH—(1) use of smaller sized balloons for dilatation and implanting long drug-eluting stents covering >5–10 mm on both the proximal and distal edges of the IMH to allow the hematoma to spread when compressed by the stent. (2) Direct stenting without balloon predilation to lower the risk of IMH extension. (3) Restoring coronary flow with balloon angioplasty alone, without stenting. (4) Cutting balloon fenestration of the IMH is performed to allow decompression of the false lumen blood pool into the true lumen, with or without additional stenting. It is critical to recognize the theoretical risk of coronary rupture, so cutting balloon inflation should be done with caution and an undersized balloon. (5) Using a multistent approach, first sealing the distal and proximal ends with stents before inserting a stent in the middle to reduce IMH propagation.

Coronary Artery Bypass Grafting

Venous grafts are the recommended option if CABG is done. The affected vessel will likely heal within a few months, after which the graft will occlude. This presents an opportunity to preserve arterial conduits for future use.

LONG-TERM TREATMENT OF SCAD AND PREVENTION OF RECURRENCE

According to one study, the 3-year risks of SCAD recurrence and extension were 2.4% and 3.5%, respectively.[24] According to the most recent ESC ACS guidelines from 2023, patients with SCAD should receive the same pharmaceutical treatments as those with ACS.[25] The role of antiplatelet therapy in SCAD has been controversial. Since SCAD results in the formation of an intramural hemorrhage, using antiplatelets or anticoagulants used in ACS may theoretically encourage further dissection or hemorrhage. However, SCAD is also prothrombotic due to the potential exposure of blood to the subintimal tissue and reduced coronary flow from true lumen obstruction. Thrombus formation in the hematoma and the true lumen has been observed.[26] Antiplatelet use may, therefore, be beneficial in reducing this thrombus burden. In their scientific statements, the AHA and ESC suggested that at least a single antiplatelet agent (aspirin) be used acutely. According to a European observational study, among patients receiving conservative treatment, MACE occurred in 18.9% of cases with dual antiplatelet use and 6% with single antiplatelet use at 1 year.[27] Observational registries indicate that the most widely used treatment for SCAD worldwide is 3 months of dual antiplatelet therapy (aspirin and clopidogrel), which is followed by lifetime single antiplatelet therapy.[28] A systematic review involving 4,206 SCAD patients found that beta-blockers were significantly associated with a reduced risk of SCAD recurrence after adjusting for other factors. As a result, beta-blockers are recommended for all SCAD patients.[29] This significant and unmet knowledge gap will be addressed by the beta-blockers and antiplatelet agents in patients with SCAD (BA-SCAD) trial, which is currently enrolling participants. A small retrospective study found that using statins was linked to a 50% versus an 8% increased risk of SCAD recurrence.[30] This, however, was not replicated in other research, and a different systematic review (n = 295) failed to discover a correlation between statins and recurrent SCAD.[29] Therefore, even though statins are not usually advised for individuals with a confirmed diagnosis of SCAD, they may be used in cases where the patient has atherosclerosis or hypercholesterolemia, or if the diagnosis is unclear. Patients with SCAD-related ACS and left ventricular ejection fraction (LVEF) impairment should be treated with ACEIs or ARBs, MRAs and SGLT-2i in keeping with current guidelines. The use in patients without LVEF impairment has not been well established. As untreated hypertension is a risk factor for SCAD recurrence, ACEI or ARB could be considered as an option to treat hypertension.

Greater than half of survivors of SCAD encounter persistent chest pain after the event. This pain could be due to ongoing ischemia (lack of blood flow) caused by the nonhealing of SCAD, microvascular dysfunction, or unknown reasons. >70% of survivors with persistent chest pain despite SCAD healing were found to have microvascular dysfunction, as demonstrated by abnormal coronary flow reserve or index of microcirculatory resistance, in a recent study involving 17 survivors.[29] Treatment options for chronic post-SCAD chest pain may include antianginal drugs such as calcium channel blockers or nitrates.

PREGNANCY AND SCAD

Pregnancy or postpartum SCAD has a 4% in-hospital mortality rate. Pregnant-related SCAD (P-SCAD) usually has higher ST-elevation myocardial infarction incidences, reduced LVEF, and involvement of the left main artery or multivessel SCAD.[31] Aspirin is safe and can be continued by women who are breastfeeding, planning a pregnancy, or who are already pregnant. Except for atenolol, the majority of beta-blockers is safe to use during pregnancy. Most medications have not been thoroughly tested in pregnancy.

As a result, other commonly used SCAD medications should be used cautiously during pregnancy or are not recommended at all during pregnancy or breastfeeding. These include P2Y12 inhibitors such as clopidogrel (category B) or ticagrelor (category C), statins (category X), and ACEI/ARBs (category C or D). Special consideration is required when using these medications in pregnant women.

CARDIAC REHABILITATION AND PHYSICAL ACTIVITY WITH SCAD

The SCAD can be caused by strenuous physical activity because it increases shear stress in the coronary arteries. This has raised concerns about physical activity in people with SCAD, particularly during cardiac rehabilitation. It is recommended that people with SCAD engage in low-intensity activities, moderate aerobic exercise, interval training, and weight training with low resistance and high repetition. It is critical to monitor symptoms and gradually increase activity levels while engaging in moderate-intensity activities. High-intensity activities that involve sudden movements and extreme head positions should be avoided.

CONCLUSION

The SCAD is an emerging cause of ACS in young, otherwise healthy patients especially females, but the etiopathogenesis is not completely elucidated. Although conservative therapy produces positive short-term results, there is a high recurrence rate and long-term morbidity, necessitating close monitoring for cardiac events. Prospective studies are needed to investigate the underlying pathways and the efficacy of disease-specific interventions in improving the prognosis for SCAD.

ONLINE REFERENCES

Please scan the QR code provided at the end of the table of contents for References of this chapter.

CHAPTER

141

Myocarditis as an Acute Coronary Syndrome Mimicker: Diagnosis and Management

Gopal Chandra Ghosh, Suvro Banerjee

ABSTRACT

Myocarditis, an inflammatory condition of the heart muscle, often presents a significant diagnostic challenge due to its ability to mimic acute coronary syndrome (ACS). This comprehensive chapter explores the intricate relationship between myocarditis and ACS, focusing on key aspects of differentiation and management. We delve into the pathogenesis, clinical presentation, and diagnostic approaches that aid in distinguishing myocarditis from ACS. The chapter emphasizes the crucial role of advanced imaging techniques, particularly cardiac magnetic resonance imaging, in achieving accurate diagnosis. Furthermore, we discuss current management strategies, highlighting the importance of etiology-specific treatments and supportive care. By enhancing understanding of myocarditis as an ACS mimicker, this chapter review aims to improve diagnostic accuracy and patient outcomes in clinical practice.

Keywords: Myocarditis, acute coronary syndrome, differential diagnosis, cardiac magnetic resonance imaging, troponin, electrocardiography, management

INTRODUCTION

Myocarditis, an inflammatory condition of the heart muscle, often presents a significant diagnostic challenge due to its ability to mimic acute coronary syndrome (ACS). Both conditions can manifest with similar symptoms, including chest pain, dyspnea, and fatigue, making initial differentiation difficult.[1] However, distinguishing between myocarditis and ACS is crucial, as their management strategies and prognostic implications differ substantially.

The importance of accurate diagnosis cannot be overstated. Misdiagnosis can lead to inappropriate treatments, potentially exposing patients to unnecessary risks or delaying vital interventions. For instance, administering thrombolytic therapy to a patient with myocarditis mistaken for an acute myocardial infarction could have severe consequences.[2]

This chapter aims to provide a comprehensive overview of the clinical presentations, the diagnostic challenges in differentiating acute myocarditis from ACS, the role of various diagnostic tools, and the implications for management.

CLINICAL PRESENTATION

The clinical presentation of myocarditis can be remarkably similar to that of ACS, contributing to the diagnostic challenge. Both conditions often present with chest pain, which may be described as sharp, pressure-like, or squeezing. However, certain characteristics can help differentiate between the two **(Tables 1 and 2)**.

- *Age and risk factors*: Myocarditis tends to affect younger individuals, often without traditional cardiovascular risk factors.[1] On the contrary, ACS is more common in older adults and those with established cardiovascular risk factors such as hypertension, diabetes, and hyperlipidemia.[3]
- *Prodromal symptoms*: Patients with myocarditis frequently report a recent history of upper respiratory or gastrointestinal infection,[4] whereas these prodromal symptoms are typically lacking in ACS.[5]
- *Nature of chest pain*: In myocarditis, chest pain may be positional or pleuritic, often worsening with inspiration

TABLE 1: Comprehensive comparison of acute myocarditis and acute coronary syndrome.

Parameter	Acute myocarditis	Acute coronary syndrome (ACS)
Clinical presentation	*Age*: Younger individuals	*Age*: Older adults
	Cardiovascular risk factors: Often absent	*Cardiovascular risk factors*: Usually present (e.g., hypertension, diabetes, hyperlipidemia)
	Prodromal symptoms: Recent history of upper respiratory or gastrointestinal infection	*Prodromal symptoms*: Typically, absent
Nature of chest pain	May be positional or pleuritic; worsens with inspiration or lying flat	More constant; may radiate to left arm or jaw
Associated symptoms	Fever, fatigue, myalgias	Diaphoresis, nausea
Electrocardiography (ECG)	*ST-segment changes*: Diffuse ST-segment elevations, often concave upward	ST-segment elevations or depressions in a coronary distribution
	Other ECG findings: PR segment depression in multiple leads; T wave inversions; occasional conduction abnormalities	*Other ECG findings*: Q waves may develop in evolving myocardial infarction; T wave inversions in ischemic territories
Cardiac biomarkers	*Troponin pattern*: Elevation may be out of proportion to ECG changes; levels may remain elevated for a prolonged period	*Troponin pattern*: Rise and fall in a characteristic pattern; magnitude often correlates with extent of myocardial damage
	Other biomarkers: C-reactive protein (CRP) and erythrocyte sedimentation rate (ESR) may be prominently elevated	*Other biomarkers*: Less prominent elevation of inflammatory markers
Imaging techniques	*Echocardiography*: Global hypokinesis or regional wall motion abnormalities not corresponding to coronary territories; pericardial effusion may be present	*Echocardiography*: Regional wall motion abnormalities corresponding to specific coronary artery territories
	Coronary angiography: Normal coronary arteries or nonobstructive coronary artery disease	*Coronary angiography*: Significant coronary artery stenosis or occlusion

TABLE 2: Key differentiating factors between acute myocarditis and acute coronary syndrome.

Factor	Acute myocarditis	Acute coronary syndrome
Age	Typically, younger patients	Often older patients
Cardiovascular risk factors	Usually absent	Often present
Recent history	Viral illness common	No specific prodrome
Chest pain	Often pleuritic or positional	Typically constant, may radiate
Associated symptoms	Fever, fatigue, myalgias	Diaphoresis, nausea
ECG changes	Diffuse ST elevations, PR depression	ST changes in coronary distribution
Troponin elevation	May be disproportionate to ECG changes	Correlates with extent of infarct
Echocardiography	Global or noncoronary regional wall motion abnormalities	Regional wall motion abnormalities in coronary distribution
Coronary angiography	Normal coronaries or nonobstructive disease	Significant stenosis or occlusion
CMR findings	Edema on T2, patchy late gadolinium enhancement	Subendocardial or transmural late gadolinium enhancement
Response to nitrates	Limited effect	Often provides relief

or when lying flat.[6] ACS-related chest pain is typically more constant and may radiate to the left arm or jaw.[7]

- *Associated symptoms*: Myocarditis patients may experience fever, fatigue, and myalgias.[8]

ACS is more commonly associated with diaphoresis and nausea.[7]

Despite these differences, the overlap in symptoms can be significant, necessitating further diagnostic evaluation.

DIAGNOSTIC APPROACHES

Electrocardiography

Electrocardiography (ECG) plays a crucial role in the initial evaluation of patients with suspected myocarditis or ACS. However, interpretation can be challenging due to overlapping features:

- *Myocarditis*:[9]
  - May show diffuse ST-segment elevations, often concave upward
  - PR segment depression in multiple leads
  - T-wave inversions
  - Occasional conduction abnormalities
- *ACS*:[10]
  - Typically presents with ST-segment elevations or depressions in a coronary distribution
  - Q waves may develop in evolving myocardial infarction
  - T-wave inversions in ischemic territories

It is important to note that ECG changes in myocarditis can mimic those of ACS, particularly in the early stages. Therefore, while ECG is a valuable tool, it should not be used in isolation for definitive diagnosis.

Cardiac Biomarkers

Cardiac troponins (cTn) are elevated in both myocarditis and ACS, reflecting myocardial injury. However, the pattern of elevation can provide diagnostic clues:

- *Myocarditis*:
  - Troponin elevation may be out of proportion to ECG changes.
  - Levels may remain elevated for a prolonged period.[11]
- *ACS*:
  - Troponin levels typically rise and fall in a characteristic pattern.
  - The magnitude of elevation often correlates with the extent of myocardial damage.[12]

Other biomarkers, such as C-reactive protein (CRP) and erythrocyte sedimentation rate (ESR), may be more prominently elevated in myocarditis due to the inflammatory process.

Imaging Techniques

Echocardiography

Transthoracic echocardiography is often the first imaging modality used in the evaluation of suspected myocarditis or ACS:

- *Myocarditis*:
  - May show global hypokinesis or regional wall motion abnormalities not corresponding to coronary territories
  - Pericardial effusion may be present.[13]
- *ACS*: Typically shows regional wall motion abnormalities corresponding to specific coronary artery territories[14]

Coronary Angiography

Coronary angiography plays a crucial role in differentiating myocarditis from ACS:

- *Myocarditis*: Generally shows normal coronary arteries or nonobstructive coronary artery disease
- *ACS*: Reveals significant coronary artery stenosis or occlusion

However, it is important to note that the presence of normal coronary arteries does not definitively rule out ACS, as conditions such as coronary vasospasm or spontaneous coronary artery dissection can cause ACS with angiographically normal coronaries.[15]

Cardiac Magnetic Resonance Imaging

Cardiac magnetic resonance (CMR) imaging has emerged as the gold standard noninvasive diagnostic tool for myocarditis:

- *T2-weighted imaging*: Demonstrates myocardial edema in acute myocarditis
- *T1-weighted imaging with early gadolinium enhancement*: Myocardial hyperemia and capillary leak
- *Late gadolinium enhancement (LGE)*:
  - Reveals patterns of myocardial necrosis or fibrosis
  - In myocarditis, LGE typically shows a patchy, mid-wall or subepicardial distribution
  - In ACS, LGE follows a subendocardial or transmural distribution in a coronary territory

Cardiac magnetic resonance has a sensitivity of 81% and a specificity of 71% for diagnosing myocarditis when using the Lake Louise Criteria, which combines these three tissue characterization techniques.[16]

Endomyocardial Biopsy

While considered the gold standard for diagnosing myocarditis, endomyocardial biopsy is not routinely performed due to its invasive nature and risk of complications. It may be considered in cases of unexplained new-onset heart failure, particularly if associated with hemodynamic compromise.[16]

Differential Diagnosis Strategies

A systematic approach to differentiating myocarditis from ACS involves:

- Thorough history and physical examination
- ECG analysis
- Cardiac biomarker assessment
- Echocardiography
- Coronary angiography in cases with high suspicion of ACS
- CMR for suspected myocarditis or inconclusive cases

Clinical decision-making algorithms, such as the SAMY (SAlzburg MYocarditis) score, have been developed to aid in this differentiation. The SAMY score incorporates age, CRP levels, and absence of ST-segment elevation in lead

V2, achieving a sensitivity of 90% and specificity of 95% for diagnosing myocarditis.[17]

MANAGEMENT IMPLICATIONS

The management of myocarditis and ACS differs significantly, underscoring the importance of accurate diagnosis.

Acute Management of Myocarditis[6]

- Supportive care is the mainstay of treatment
- Heart failure management with diuretics, ACE inhibitors/ARBs, and beta-blockers as tolerated
- Arrhythmia management
- Mechanical circulatory support in severe cases
- Immunosuppression in specific cases (e.g., giant cell myocarditis)

Acute Management of ACS[7]

- Immediate reperfusion therapy (primary percutaneous coronary intervention or thrombolysis)
- Antiplatelet and anticoagulant therapy
- Pain management
- Secondary prevention measures

Prognosis and Follow-up

Prognosis varies significantly between myocarditis and ACS:

- *Myocarditis*:
  - Generally good prognosis in uncomplicated cases
  - Risk of progression to dilated cardiomyopathy in a subset of patients
  - Fulminant myocarditis, paradoxically, often has a better long-term prognosis if patients survive the acute phase[18]
- *ACS*:
  - Prognosis depends on the extent of myocardial damage and timeliness of reperfusion
  - Long-term risk of recurrent events and heart failure[18]

CONCLUSION

Differentiating acute myocarditis from ACS remains a significant challenge in clinical practice. While these conditions share many similarities in their presentation, key differences in clinical features, biomarker patterns, and imaging findings can guide accurate diagnosis. The advent of advanced cardiac imaging techniques, particularly CMR, has greatly enhanced our ability to distinguish between these entities.

Accurate diagnosis is crucial, as the management strategies for myocarditis and ACS differ substantially. Misdiagnosis can lead to inappropriate treatments and potentially adverse outcomes. A systematic approach to evaluation, incorporating clinical assessment, ECG, biomarkers, and appropriate imaging studies, is essential for optimal patient care.

As our understanding of these conditions continues to evolve, future research should focus on developing more specific diagnostic biomarkers and refining imaging techniques. Additionally, exploring novel therapeutic approaches for myocarditis and improving risk stratification strategies for both conditions will be crucial in advancing patient care.

By enhancing our ability to differentiate between myocarditis and ACS, we can ensure that patients receive timely and appropriate treatment, ultimately improving outcomes in these challenging cardiac conditions.

ONLINE REFERENCES

Please scan the QR code provided at the end of the table of contents for References of this chapter.

CHAPTER

142

Ischemic Mitral Regurgitation: Mechanisms and Management

S Shanmugasundaram, Ilayaraja U, Samuel Jebavaram, BG Vinodkumar

ABSTRACT

Ischemic mitral regurgitation is a form of ventricular functional mitral regurgitation, in which regional or global remodeling of left ventricle due to ischemia/infarction will result in tethering of leaflets and failure of coaptation. Tethering may be asymmetric or symmetric depending on whether the ventricular remodeling is regional as in inferolateral infarction or global as in large anterior wall infarction. The presence of MR, even of mild severity, worsens the prognosis by increasing mortality and heart failure hospitalizations. Clinically, it may present with dyspnea or heart failure of acute or chronic onset and the murmur may be misleadingly faint or absent. Echocardiogram confirms the diagnosis, quantifies the regurgitation, and identifies poor responders to surgical annuloplasty or transcatheter edge-to-edge repair. Management includes guideline-directed therapy for heart failure, biventricular pacing when indicated, surgical repair or replacement or transcatheter edge to edge repair. Reduction of MR and improvement of exercise tolerance occur with both surgery and intervention, provided the anatomy is suitable but mortality benefit is seen with transcatheter therapy not surgery. Repair in the form of mitral annuloplasty has the disadvantage of recurrence in one third. Additional procedures such as chordal cutting and papillary muscle approximation are evolving.

Keywords: Tethering, functional mitral regurgitation, papillary muscle rupture, papillary muscle dysfunction, edge-to-edge repair, asymmetric tethering, symmetric tethering, annuloplasty, proportionate MR, disproportionate MR

INTRODUCTION

Mitral regurgitation (MR) is classified into primary (organic) and secondary (functional). Primary MR is due to intrinsic disease of the leaflets and or the core components of the subvalvular apparatus, namely chordae and papillary muscles (PMs). Secondary MR is due to dilatation and dysfunction of the left ventricle [ventricular functional MR (vFMR)] or that of left atrium [atrial functional MR (aFMR)]. vFMR is mostly induced by tethering of leaflets due to remodeled LV as in idiopathic dilated cardiomyopathy (ventricular nonischemic functional MR) or regional or global LV remodeling after myocardial infarction (MI) (ventricular ischemic functional MR) **(Flowchart 1)**. In primary MR, it is the diseased valve that makes the ventricle sick and in secondary MR, it is the sick ventricle that makes the valve leaky.

Secondary MR constitutes 65% of all cases of MR, affecting 16,250 individuals per million. Moderate-to-severe MR seems to occur in 15–20% of heart failure patients. MR of any severity is detected in 25–50% of patients with acute myocardial infarction (AMI) and 12% of AMI patients have moderate to severe MR. In chronic ischemic heart disease with left ventricular dysfunction, ischemic MR (IMR) occurs in about 50%. Presence of MR of even mild degree adversely affects the prognosis. The risk of dying or getting hospitalized for heart failure is almost doubled in the presence of moderate to severe MR, both in ischemic and in idiopathic dilated cardiomyopathy.[1-4] Fortunately, the incidence of IMR and the mortality related to it are coming down, owing to early reperfusion. In a prospective registry, the rates of moderate-to-severe IMR was 17.2% in the year 2001–2010 and 9.3% in the year 2011–2020. After 3 months, 48.5% had persistent MR in the first decade versus 9.5% in the second decade. Death rates at 2 years was 17.8% and 9.6% respectively.[5] Pathophysiology and management of IMR are complex and evolving and this chapter reviews the contemporary issues regarding this common problem.

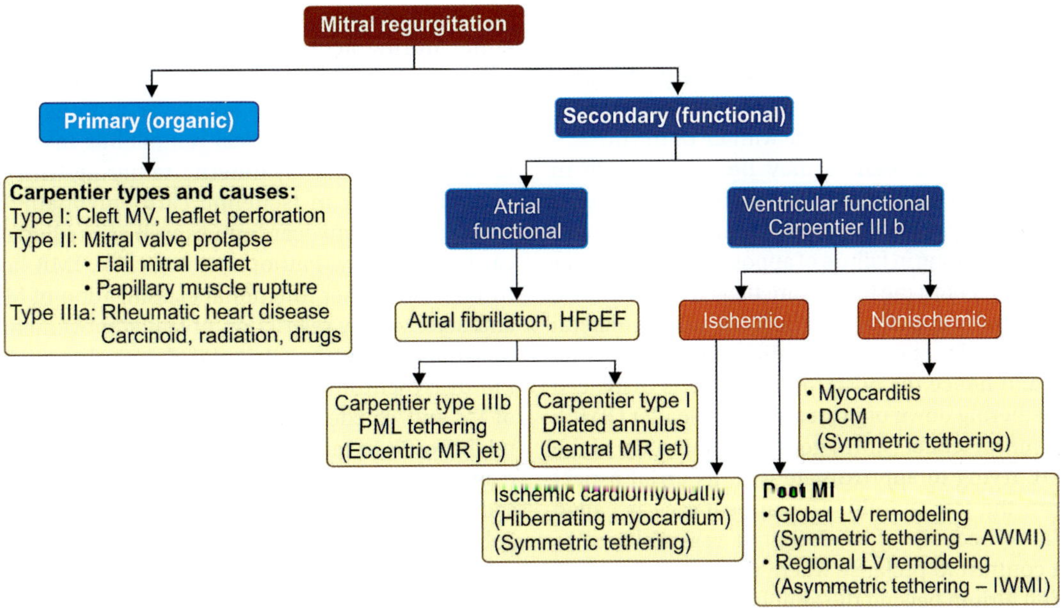

FLOWCHART 1: Morphofunctional classification of mitral regurgitation.

PATHOPHYSIOLOGY

For many years, it was believed that papillary muscle dysfunction (PMD), i.e., failure of contraction or elongation of ischemic/infarcted PM was the cause of IMR. But the contemporary evidence is in favor of adverse LV remodeling of LV with the resultant tethering of mitral leaflets as the major determinant of IMR. Neither experimentally induced isolated PM ischemia nor the presence of LV dysfunction without remodeling resulted in MR in experimental models. If PMD were the cause, the mitral leaflets would be expected to move beyond the annulus, prolapsing into LA (Carpentier type II), but the leaflets of IMR are pulled down toward the apex. If at all PMD causes MR, it may account for the transient MR and flash pulmonary edema that occur during reversible ischemic episodes. Actually when the mitral leaflet is tethered down, superadded episodic ischemia resulting in PMD should minimize or abolish MR because of decreased tethering forces. At the best, only 5% of MR occurring in CAD could be caused by PMD.

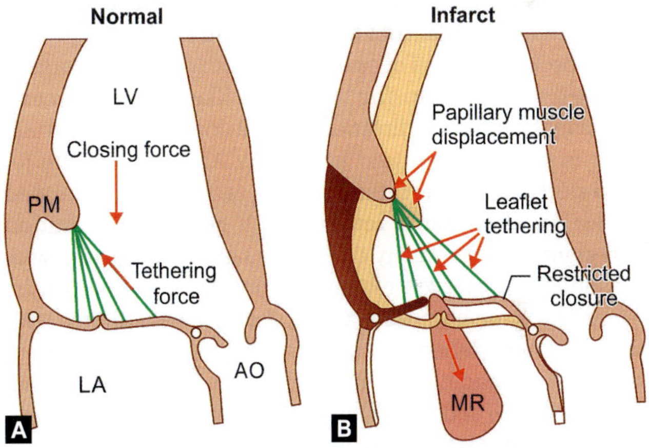

FIGS. 1A AND B: Regional remodeling of inferobasal myocardium in inferolateral infarct augmenting tethering forces, restricting systolic movement of posterior leaflet; reduced closing forces are due to LV dysfunction.

Mitral regurgitation that is due to post-MI remodeling of LV is typically called as IMR, or more appropriately functional IMR. In this condition, there is imbalance between the mitral valve closing forces and tethering forces **(Figs. 1A and B)**. Atrial contraction creates vortices around the ventricular aspect of mitral leaflets and float up the leaflets thereby initiating mitral valve closure. As the left ventricle starts contracting, the rising ventricular pressure (closing force) completes the approximation of leaflets while the PM contraction pulling the taut inextensible chordae prevent the leaflets from prolapsing into left atrium (tethering force). The net result is effective sealing of mitral orifice. These opposing forces that are timed appropriately and exerting balanced forces of equal magnitude prevent prolapse of the leaflets and at the same time preclude excessive pulling down of the leaflets. The leaflets approximate not at the free margin but a few mm proximal to it, thereby offering some reserve mechanism in case the annulus dilates or the free margin of leaflets is damaged by disease process. In IMR, the leaflets are tethered down (increased tethering forces) by regional or global distortion of LV cavity which displaces the PM(s) apically and laterally. Simultaneously, decreased contractile forces of LV due to post-MI LV dysfunction results in decreased closing forces thereby contributing to defective approximation of leaflets. In an experimental study done in dogs, acute LCX ligation (acute model) results in trivial MR despite a low EF (23 ± 8%) if LV expansion was limited by pericardial restraint. MR became severe once the LV expansion was permitted to occur by removing the pericardial restraint. In the chronic model, LCX branches were ligated. MR which was trivial to start with, became severe with progressive LV remodeling that developed over the next 8 weeks. MR did not correlate with EF or dP/dt.[6]

Tethering of mitral leaflets may be asymmetric in which the posterior leaflet is selectively pulled down posterolaterally (with respect to midline of LV long axis) and toward the apex resulting in failure of apposition with AML or symmetric in which both the leaflets are tugged toward apex, restraining the leaflet apposition. In IMR due to inferolateral MI, the ischemic (akinetic or dyskinetic) inferolateral wall is deformed and hence the posteromedial PM is displaced resulting in tethering down of posterior mitral leaflet (PML). The anterior mitral leaflet (AML) goes behind the tip of the tethered PML trying to approximate with its atrial aspect far away from the free margin. This appearance is called pseudoprolapse because of its deceptive resemblance to prolapse. In contrast to prolapse where the leaflets bulge or buckle into left atrium beyond the annulus plane, in IMR the AML would still be on the ventricular side of annulus. When tethering is asymmetrical (closure point is more posterior) the MR jet in color Doppler echo is eccentric, directed toward the posterolateral wall of LA **(Figs. 2A and B)**.

In prolapse or flail of posterior leaflet, MR jet is anteriorly directed as the prolapsing leaflet acts like a hood directing the jet in the opposite direction. In IMR due to PML tethering, PML is pulled down and hence the AML directs the jet posteriorly, i.e., in the same direction as that of the deformed leaflet. In asymmetric tethering, LV geometry alteration is regional and LV cavity dimensions are near normal with reasonably preserved global function. In contrast, in the event of a large anterior wall MI, the LV cavity dilates with spherical remodeling. This leads to apicolateral displacement of both PMs, leading to symmetrical tethering of both leaflets **(Figs. 3A to C)** causing a central jet of MR. LV dilatation and LV dysfunction are likely to be more severe in this type.

While MR due to asymmetric tethering of PML occurs either during acute phase or at least in the first 1 or 2 weeks of inferolateral MI, symmetric tethering of both leaflets manifests later—weeks or months after anterior wall MI, as global spherical remodeling takes longer time to develop. Similar symmetric tethering with central MR may also occur in ischemic cardiomyopathy caused by hibernating LV myocardium as well as in idiopathic dilated cardiomyopathy. Pathophysiologically, IMR belongs type III b of Carpentier functional classification of MR, which is characterized by restriction of leaflet movement in systolic phase alone. Intraventricular dyssynchrony, particularly PM dyssynchrony due to differential ischemia or scarring of LV and/or coexisting left bundle branch block (LBBB) might result in temporally uneven tethering forces thereby contributing to MR. Annular dilatation with flattening (loss of saddle shape) caused by LV dilatation along with ineffective sphincteric contraction of posterior annulus plays a minor role in causation of IMR (Carpentier type I). Atrial dilatation due to increased ventricular filling pressures, MR and/or atrial fibrillation may add to the preexisting MR (combined ventricular and atrial functional MR).

Even in the absence of significant remodeling of ventricle, acute IMR could be severe, particularly the one that occurs with inferolateral MI. A 3D echocardiography study[7] looked at the dynamics of mitral valve apparatus in 87 patients with acute IMR, 87 acute MI patients without MR and 44 patients in chronic post-MI state. Though annulus dimensions and tethering appeared to be more in acute IMR when compared to controls, they are not different from what occurred in chronic post-MI state. Annulus dynamicity was also not very much affected in acute IMR. Increased PM angulation (38.4 ± 6.2° for moderate vs. 33.5 ± 7.3° for mild vs. 31.4 ± 6.3° for no IMR) and increased interpapillary distance (21.7 ± 4.9 mm acute MR vs. 20.0 ± 3.4 mm no MR) were found to correlate with the severity of MR and these values were significantly more than that occurred in chronic MI group. Failure of contraction of

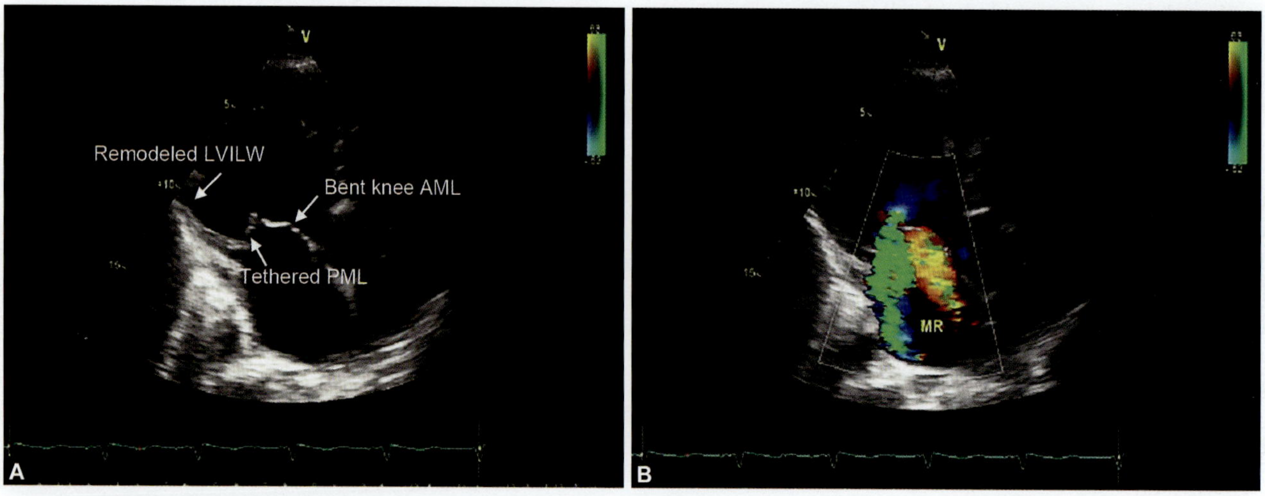

FIGS. 2A AND B: Regional (inferobasal) remodeling of LV with asymmetrical tethering of PML and eccentric MR.

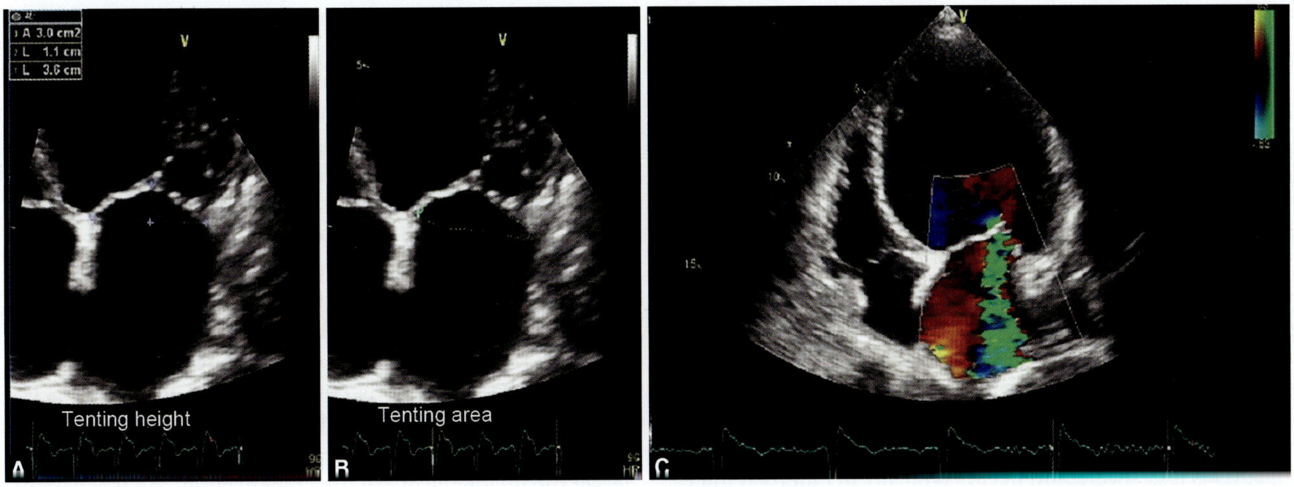

FIGS. 3A TO C: Remote anterior wall infraction with remodeled, spherical LV with symmetrical tethering and central MR.

the myocardium in relation to the posteromedial PM could thus result in MR even before deformation occurs.

Ischemic mitral regurgitation is likely to be more frequent and more severe in inferior MI (IWMI) than in anterior MI, despite mild or no global LV dysfunction. Regional LV remodeling of inferolateral wall readily occurs when compared to the anterolateral segment, probably because of solitary blood supply (posterolateral branch of either RCA or LCX) to the inferolateral wall adjoining the posteromedial PM in contrast to the dual blood supply (diagonal and marginal branches) to the anterolateral wall adjoining the anterolateral PM. Since regional LV distortion can occur within the first few hours, IMR of ILMI may begin quite early, often within first few hours to days. When IMR occurs in anterior wall MI (AWMI), the infarct is usually large leading to spherical remodeling of LV causing nearly equal displacement of both PMs (apically and laterally). Hence symmetrical tethering of both leaflets occurs which leads to a central jet of MR. Global systolic function is near normal in IWMI with IMR while it is significantly reduced in AWMI with IMR. Since global LV remodeling requires long time to occur, IMR of AWMI presents weeks or months after MI. In an outcome study of STEMI with MR[8] who had undergone primary PCI, 17.8% of AWMI and 21.8% of IWMI manifested MR. Among those with MR, severity was more (Grade 4) in IWMI group (4.6%) than in AWMI group (1.3%). LV volumes were similar but EF was lower in AWMI group (36.3 ± 14% vs. 44.6 ± 12.3%). Direction of MR jet was posterior in 70.9% and central in 26.9% in IWMI and central in 88.8% and posterior in 3.4% in AWMI. 30 days and 3 years mortality was 14.9% and 39.7% in AWMI and 6.8% and 24.8% in IWMI.

Though symmetric tethering of both leaflets is typical of AWMI and asymmetric tethering of PML is typical of IWMI, PML (asymmetric) tethering may also occur with antero-apical MI, which is attributed to extension of anterior wall MI to the inferior apex. It results in bulging of the dilated apex which exerts traction force on the posteromedial PM

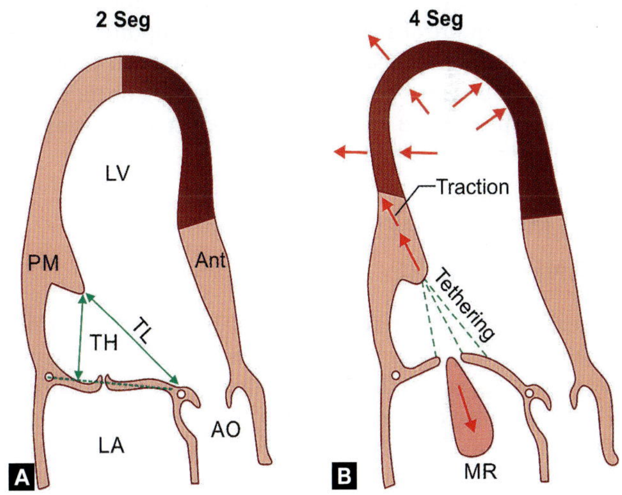

FIGS. 4A AND B: Anteroapical MI with apicoinferior extension stretches posterior papillary muscle thereby tethering posterior leaflet.

(TH: tethering height; TL: tethering length)

(Figs. 4A and B). In this condition, there may not be contractile abnormality of the underlying inferobasal myocardium. This concept has been suggested by Yosefy et al.[9] who did a retrospective and human mechanistic study along with animal experimental model of LAD ligation. In those with anterior wall MI with apical inferior extension, the tethering length (distance between PM tip to annulus opposite to the tethered PM) was more in those with moderate-to-severe MR and there was diminished systolic shortening.

Leaflet adaptation in the form of increasing size of leaflets in response to stretch caused by tethering appears to protect against functional MR. Animal experiments and 3D echo studies in patients with fMR suggest that absence of leaflet adaptation or growth contributes to worsening of MR in the chronic phase. On the other hand, progressive thickening and stiffening of leaflets (maladaptation) in the chronic phase may worsen MR.[10] Chaput demonstrated a 35% increase in leaflet area in patients with LV dysfunction compared to normal suggesting that leaflet growth occurred in these patients.[11] If the leaflet growth does not match with increase in annulus size, MR would result. Leaflet to annulus ratio of <1.7 seemed to predict secondary MR.

Another important but uncommon cause of acute MR in MI is rupture of papillary muscle (PMR) or one of its heads. In the strict sense, PMR has to be considered as a mechanical complication of acute MI (Carpentier type II) and it should be viewed as one form of primary MR. PMR is encountered in 0.05% of MI. Posteromedial PM is commonly affected, because of solitary blood supply (either right coronary or left circumflex) and occurs with posterolateral MI. The infarct is often small, overall LV function is good, the extent of CAD is less severe and occurs typically in elderly females. It usually occurs in the first week of MI, often in the first 24 hours. Pathological spectrum includes (1) PM thinning and lengthening (like a taffy candy) with or without partial rupture, (2) rupture of a head of PM, and (3) rupture of entire PM. Echocardiographically, type 1 presents with prolapse of the leaflet because of inadequate anchoring or tethering force and types 2 and 3 manifest as flail leaflet that carries the PM head or the entire body along with it.

CLINICAL PRESENTATION AND COURSE

Clinically, IMR may have an acute or subacute/chronic presentation, the latter being the commoner variety. Acute IMR typically occurs with acute inferolateral MI, often caused by occlusion of left circumflex artery or right coronary artery. Patients with acute IMR present with dyspnea that occurs within the first week onset of MI, often in the first 24–48 hours, called as "whistling angina". Patients with mild IMR may be asymptomatic while those with moderate-to-severe acute IMR manifest rapidly worsening dyspnea and may even progress to cardiogenic shock (CS). Because of acute onset of MR, preload compensation (dilatation of LV with increased end diastolic volume) is inadequate, leading to marked reduction of forward stroke volume and hence CS. At the same time, larger amount of regurgitation into a nondilated noncompliant LA may result in marked rise of LA pressure leading to pulmonary edema. In patients with moderate-to-severe IMR, physical examination may reveal an orthopneic individual with tachycardia, tachypnea, low blood pressure with narrow pulse pressure, and rales in the lung fields. Murmur due to acute MR may be deceptively faint or may be absent because of rapid equalization of LV and LA pressures in mid-late systole, LV dysfunction, low stroke volume, and masking by lung signs. Clinical presentation of post-MI MR (PMR or acute IMR), may be classified into four types. Type 1, often caused by of rupture of entire PM, presents in the form of CS and pulmonary edema or even cardiac arrest. Lactate levels are high. Type 2 may manifest as severe heart failure with pulmonary edema, reduced cardiac index but with maintained blood pressure. Lactate levels are usually normal. Type 3 is a less severe form, manifesting as episodes of pulmonary congestion and flash pulmonary edema. In type 4, heart failure is mild-to-moderate. Echocardiography performed within 30 days of AMI in a cohort of 1,331 patients, identified MR in 50% of cases (38% mild, 12% moderate-to-severe). Nearly half of those with mild IMR and one-third of those with moderate-to-severe MR did not have a clinically detectable murmur. Moderate-to-severe MR increased the risk of heart failure by 3.44-fold and death by 1.55-fold.[2]

Early restoration of blood flow either by thrombolysis or primary percutaneous coronary intervention (PCI) has resulted in decrease of incidence of IMR. PCI fares better than thrombolysis and shorter the door to balloon time, lesser the incidence of MR. In a recent study of 4,005 patients with STEMI undergoing PCI within 12 hours of symptom onset, Grade 1, 2, 3, and 4 MR was present in 10.7%, 6.5%, 2.3%, and 0.7%. More severe MR was associated with older age, female sex, lower body mass index, inferior location of MI, and longer door to balloon time. The 30-day mortality rates were 7.3%, 8.8%, 19.8%, and 26.1%, respectively while mortality of those with no MR was 6.8%. In those with grade 4 MR, culprit artery was RCA or LCX in 94% and the infarct location was inferior in 85%.[12]

Long-term outlook was also poor in those with IMR, particularly in those with moderate-to-severe MR. In a prospective registry of 1,036 patients with STEMI, moderate-to-severe MR was seen in 11.5%. It was associated with older age, female sex, and lower EF. After a median follow-up of 2.8 (1.7–4.3) years, hazard ratio for death and heart failure was 3.1 and 3.3, respectively.[13] In a study which looked at the temporal trends of IMR after MI, moderate-to-severe MR was seen at the time of admission in 17.2% and 9.3% in the study period of 2001–2010 and 2011–2020, respectively. The decline in the occurrence of post-MI-MR in the second phase is attributed to timely reperfusion. By the end of 3 months, MR improved or nearly disappeared in half of them, particularly in those who presented with mild MR. 2-year mortality was 17.8% in those with MR while it was 9.3% in those without MR.[5] MR may complicate non ST-elevation MI (NSTEMI) as well. In a study of 237 patients with NSTEMI, MR was seen in 40%. Roughly one-third of them had moderate-to-severe MR. LV dysfunction rather than leaflet tethering seemed to the determinant of IMR in this group. Cardiovascular death and heart failure were nearly two-fold in those with moderate-to-severe MR during a follow-up of 3 years.[14] MR was present in 29% of Sharma's series of 1,000 patients with AMI treated by PCI. 76% of them had mild MR, 21% moderate MR, and 3% severe MR. Prevalence did not differ between NSTEMI and STEMI—29% versus 30%. Patients with MR were older, had worse LV function, higher rates of hypertension, heart failure, and remote MI. LCX or RCA occlusion was more frequently encountered among them. Delayed revascularization (>72 hours) in NSTEMI group was associated with higher incidence of IMR. At a median follow-up of 3.2 years, mortality among patients without MR was 6% and in those with MR of any severity it was 19%. Mortality in those with mild MR was 17% and was worse in those with moderate-to-severe MR.[15]

MR tends to be more dynamic in IMR than in primary MR as the severity is influenced by many factors such as medical treatment, volume status, dynamic ischemia, and perturbations in afterload. Exercise increased the mitral regurgitant orifice (MRO) by >20 mm^2 in 30% of patients studied by Lancellotti.[16] Neither the resting MR severity nor the degree of LV dysfunction was the determinant of exercise induced increase in IMR. On the contrary, the exercise induced increase in MRO correlated with the extent of mitral valve deformation and the degree of LV remodeling—regional or global. There was reduction in IMR after exercise in some but occurred only in those with inferior MI with IMR. In the preoperative period, reduction of afterload by anesthetic agents/vasodilators may reduce the severity of MR as assessed by intraoperative transesophageal echo (TEE), making decision regarding mitral valve repair difficult. Moreover, IMR exhibits dynamic behavior even within the same cardiac cycle, with the regurgitant orifice being larger in early and late systole and smaller in midsystole. The later has implications in severity assessment by proximal isovelocity surface area (PISA) method. Apart from being dynamic, MR, particularly of ischemic cause is likely to be progressive. The volume overload induced by MR results in progressive LV remodeling and increased sphericity which in turn accentuate leaflet tethering and the resultant MR. Annular dilatation and flattening will also increase with progressive LV enlargement leading to worsening of MR. When the basic ischemic cause is not corrected because of poor target vessels for revascularization, LV dysfunction tends to worsen which in turn mat accentuate MR.

DIAGNOSIS

Mechanical complications such as PMR, ventricular septal rupture (VSR), or contained free wall rupture (pseudoaneurysm) as well as IMR should be considered in those with ACS (acute or recent) presenting with heart failure and or CS. Transthoracic echo (TTE) should be done in such individuals before shifting to angiographic suite. TTE with 3D features is usually needed to confirm the diagnosis and assess the mechanism and severity of IMR. Not uncommonly one may need TEE, particularly 3D TEE with mitral valve quantification software (4D auto MVQ of GE, mitral valve navigation of Philips to mention a few) for a precise analysis. Before focusing on mitral valve, a comprehensive evaluation has to be done which includes assessment of LV volumes/dimensions, regional and global LV function, LVEF and GLS, left atrial volume and strain, mitral annulus size, shape and function, pulmonary artery pressure, and RV function. Then the next step is to differentiate secondary MR from primary MR. In patients with acute MR differentiation between PMR and IMR due to leaflet tethering is important because therapeutic options and prognosis are different. PMR may be diagnosed when a flail leaflet with the attached chordae and PM head is seen making swift flipping to and fro movements (a sort of "yo yo" motion) between LA and LV along with torrential MR. The structures flip into LA in systole and back to LV in diastole. Rarely, when a small head of the PMRs, the diagnosis may be difficult and in such circumstance TEE may be worthwhile to consider. Sensitivity for diagnosis of PMR by TTE is 65–85% while it is 95–100% with TEE. In contrast to PMR in which there is excessive motion of the leaflets (type II), in IMR there would be leaflet tethering with restricted motion in systole (III b) caused by displacement of PM(s). Regional or global remodeling of LV can be identified.

Once it is confirmed as secondary MR, differentiating vFMR from aFMR is the next task. aFMR typically occurs in those presenting clinically with AF or HFPEF. Significant LA enlargement with preserved LV function raises the suspicion of aFMR. It may manifest as one of the two phenotypes—(1) dilated annulus with a central MR jet or (2) tethering of PML from left atrial side with posteriorly directed MR jet. In the latter type, basal posterior leaflet is pulled up and would appear as if it is flushed with the crest of LV posterior wall. In contrast to aFMR, leaflet tethering toward ventricular apex is the primary mechanism in vFMR which exhibits Carpentier type III b physiology. The morphological features of the two phenotypes of IMR are depicted in **Table 1**.

In order to define the phenotype of IMR, the following measurements of mitral valve apparatus should be routinely done **(Fig. 5)**. In 2DE, length of AML and PML in diastole, tenting depth (annulus to coaptation point in midsystole) and area (area delimited by annulus plane, the atrial surface of mitral leaflets, and the coaptation point), coaptation length (apposed portion of leaflets-distance between the leaflet tips and coaptation point), angle of AML and PML in relation to the annulus plane in A4C view, tethering distance between posteromedial PM to anterior annulus (LAX or A3C) and distance between anterolateral PM to the medial annulus (A4C), interpapillary distance (SAX view), anteroposterior (PS LAX or A3C), and medial to lateral dimensions (A2C) of mitral annulus and AML/annulus ratio should be measured. In 3DE, annulus area in diastole and systole, mitral leaflet area, diameter of the annulus (A4C and A2C in end systole), AML annulus ratio, vena contracta (VC) area, angle between PMs, and tenting volume should be measured. Mitral apparatus dimensions in normal subjects and those with CAD with no MR versus asymmetric and symmetric tethering phenotypes are tabulated in **Table 2**.[17,18] Mitral annulus dilatation is diagnosed when the ratio of AP diameter of the annulus to AML length exceeds 1.3 or the annulus diameter exceeds 35 mm. In a 3DE study with a special software, maximum tenting depth in IMR versus control was 9.8 ± 2.0 mm versus 3.1 ± 1.2 mm and tenting volume was 4.09 ± 1.22 mL versus 0.45 ± 0.29 mL.[19]

TABLE 1: Morphological changes in tethering phenotypes.

Feature	Asymmetrical tethering	Symmetrical tethering
LV remodeling	Regional (inferolateral wall)	Global (increased sphericity index)
Global LV function	LVEF normal or slightly reduced	LVEF is significantly reduced ~30%
Causative infarction	Inferobasal/inferolateral	Anterior
Culprit artery	Right coronary/left circumflex	Left anterior descending
Time course of development	Often acute may be subacute or chronic	Often subacute—chronic
Papillary muscles	Asymmetric, posteromedial PM is displaced laterally (and apically), interpapillary distance increased slightly and PM angle is widened	Symmetric, both PMs are displaced apically (and laterally). Interpapillary muscle distance increased very much and PM angle is near normal
Annulus	Slightly dilated	Dilated and flat; dysfunctional
Coaptation	Displaced posteriorly, AML apposes with the atrial aspect of PML—pseudoprolapse	Displaced apically, coaptation length decreased
Anterior leaflet	Bent knee (sea gull) appearance due to traction by strut chordae	Shape preserved
Posterior leaflet	Curved with concavity toward LV inferior wall, tip faces inferior wall	Shape preserved
Leaflet angle	Posterior angle > anterior angle	Both leaflet angles are equal
Tethering distance, Area and volume	Slightly increased	Very much increased
MR jet	Eccentric—posterolateral	Central—ellipsoid in short axis
MR relative severity	More severe	Less severe

The term "asymmetric tethering" is classically used for selective tethering of PML often involving P2 segment, leaving AML unaffected. In this situation, the asymmetric tethering is posteroanterior, diagnosed by a larger ratio of posterior leaflet angle/anterior leaflet angle of >1.5 (normal being 1.0–1.2) in PS LAX or apical LAX views of TTE or in Midesophageal (ME) long axis or three-chamber view (120°) in TEE. The other type of asymmetric tethering involves selectively S3 segment, called as "mediolateral asymmetric tethering" which is caused by apical displacement of posterior PM. It is diagnosed in TEE by measuring the tenting area of S3 segment (advancement/retroflexion at ME 0°) and that of S1 segment (withdrawal/flexion at ME 0°). A ratio of medial (S3) tenting area/lateral (S1) tenting area > 1.52 is considered abnormal. In a study of 178 functional MR patients,[20] 37.9% had posteroanterior tethering and 27.5% had mediolateral tethering. MR reduction was less effective after device therapy with posteroanterior tethering and increased all-cause mortality was seen in both types (HR 2.77).

The following are the imaging predictors of failure of surgical repair in the form of restrictive annuloplasty—thickened deformed leaflets, tenting depth of >10 mm, tenting area of >2.5–3.0 cm^2, interpapillary distance > 20 mm, posterior papillary-fibrosa distance of >40 mm, global LV remodeling with LV EDD > 65 mm, LV ESD > 51 mm, ESV > 140 mL and systolic sphericity index of >0.7, posterolateral angle > 45° and complex MR jets originating centrally and posteromedially.[21]

Quantification of MR is somewhat similar to that of primary MR. The caveats are that VC dimension may underestimate MR severity because of the ellipsoidal shape of regurgitant orifice, the jet may be eccentric in asymmetrical tethering which may deceptively underestimate the disease severity and EROA by PISA method may again underestimate the severity, as the orifice size is larger in early and late systole and smaller in midsystole. PISA measurements are mostly done in midsystole at which phase the orifice size is the smallest. Moreover the size of LV and LA cannot be used to diagnose severe MR because the degree of ventricular remodeling may be the primary determinant of LV size rather than severity of MR. E wave amplitude may not be useful as elevated LV filling pressures in vFMR, by itself may increase E amplitude.

Measuring the MR jet area or the ratio of MR jet to that of LA is a qualitative measure of severity of MR. This method is used to make out the mere presence of MR and may at the most be useful to differentiate mild MR from severe MR. VC of >7 mm is considered to indicate severe MR and a value of 4–7 mm moderate MR. Usually, VC is best measured from PS LAX view. Because of the ellipsoidal shape of regurgitant orifice in IMR, an average of VC dimension obtained from A2C and A4C views seems to be more reliable. An average value of VC > 8 mm indicates severe MR, 5–7 moderate MR

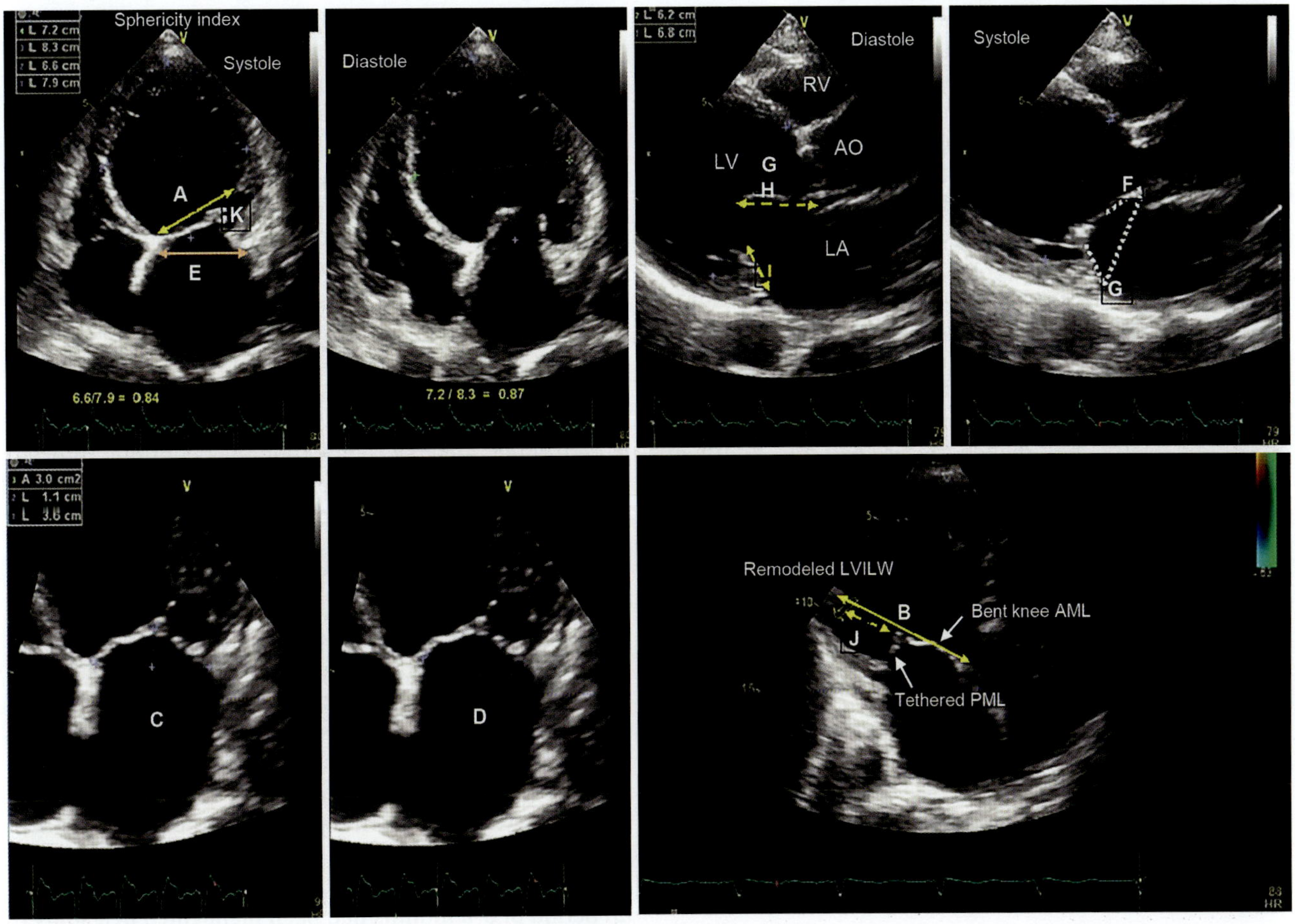

FIG. 5: Measurements of mitral apparatus: A—anterolateral PM to annulus distance; B—posteromedial PM to annulus distance. C—Tenting distance. D—tenting area. E—annulus diameter. F—anterior leaflet angle. G—posterior leaflet angle. H—length of anterior leaflet. I—length of posterior leaflet. J—tethering distance. K—coaptation length.

TABLE 2: Measurements of mitral valve apparatus in normal and tethering phenotypes.

Parameter	Normal/No MR	Symmetric tethering	Asymmetric tethering
Anterior leaflet angle	25°	25–45°	25–45°
Posterior leaflet angle	36°	30–45°	40–60°
Tenting height mm	4–6	9.3	7.7
Tenting area cm^2	<2.5	3.0–3.2	4.0–4.1
Tenting volume (mL)	<2.3	4.4–5.5	2.5–4.3
Coaptation length (mm)	6–10	<5	<5
Interpapillary distance (cm)	2.1–2.5	3.5–3.8	3.0
Mitral annulus diameter (A4C) (cm)	2.5–3.8 (Male) 2.3–3.3 (Female)		
Mitral annulus diameter (A2C) (cm)	2.5–3.5 (Male) 2.2–3.4 (Female)		
Annulus height (mm)	6–8	8.5	10.3
Annulus area (cm^2)	6.4	11.1–12.3	9.0–10.8
Systolic annulus area change	56%	13.9%	30.7%
LV sphericity index (minor axis/major axis) A4C	<0.7	>0.7	≥0.7

and 3–4 mild MR. Because of poor outcomes associated with EROA of >20 mm^2 and RV > 30 mL, these values were initially recommended for defining severe lesion in vFMR. However, the present consensus is to diagnose severe MR irrespective of the etiology when EROA is >40 mm^2, regurgitant volume (RV) is >60 mL and regurgitant fraction (RF) is >50%. A subcategory of moderate MR with an EROA 30–40 mm^2, RV of 45–60 mL and RF of 40–50% qualify for grade III MR or moderate-to-severe MR and may be considered for mitral valve procedures because of the poor prognosis of secondary MR. Multiparametric assessment is often necessary and limitations of each method should be kept in mind during assessment of severity of the lesion.[22] If intraoperative TEE is used for assessment, it should be remembered that anesthetic agents may reduce the preload and afterload leading to underestimation of MR. In such circumstances, increasing preload by fluid boluses or increasing afterload by IV phenylephrine may be done to overcome the effect of anesthesia on MR severity assessment.

Cardiac MR Imaging

Cardiac MR (CMR) is emerging as a more precise imaging method in assessment of IMR. Apart from proving reliable measurements of LV volumes, EF, RV and tenting volumes, the extent of viable myocardium, and scar burden can be assessed.

MANAGEMENT

Management decisions are as complex as the pathophysiology and diagnosis. Revascularization alone is enough for patients with mild IMR, but a close follow-up with imaging surveillance is required as some of these patients may progress to moderate-to-severe MR later. For those with moderate and severe MR, surgery or intervention is offered with the hope of improving symptoms and exercise tolerance and reducing heart failure hospitalizations and death. Though either of the procedures lead to prompt reduction of MR in majority, reverse remodeling of LV in sizeable number, reduction of all-cause or cardiovascular mortality remains to be confirmed.

Those who present with acute MR often accompanied by heart failure or CS, should be stabilized medically using vasodilators (if in heart failure with adequate arterial pressure) or vasopressors/inotropes (if in CS) and mechanical circulatory support. Mechanical ventilation with positive end-expiratory pressure may improve the oxygenation and reduce the impact of acute severe MR by reducing the preload and afterload.

For PMR, emergency surgery is the treatment of choice but the in-hospital mortality may be as high as 25%. MVR with preservation of the chordae is the surgery of choice but repair is possible in selected instances. If hemodynamics is precarious, transcatheter edge-to-edge repair (TEER) may be considered as a bridge to surgery or destination therapy. The results of recently published case reports and small series of TEER in PMR are encouraging.[23] In IREMMI, 23 patients with acute MR (nine with complete rupture, nine with partial rupture, and five with chordal rupture), procedural success rate was 87%, MR reduction was achieved in 20, 70% were discharged from hospital and five required reintervention in the form of surgical MVR.[24]

If acute MR due to leaflet tethering is encountered within the time window of primary PCI, prompt restoration of blood flow in the culprit artery (most often LCX or RCA) should be done. While MR improves in some, it may remain as such or may worsen in others. Time delay in reperfusion determines the natural history of acute IMR. If considerable myocardial damage and remodeling of LV have occurred by the time PCI is performed, adverse remodeling may continue to occur thereby worsening MR. Generally, moderate-to-severe MR at baseline tends to persist or worsen during follow-up. In a study of 174 patients who had undergone primary PCI within 12 hours of onset of chest pain, mild MR was seen in 34% and moderate-to-severe MR in 11%. IMR seen in the immediate post-PCI period was predicted by an ischemic time of >540 minutes (OR 2.92) and female gender. At a median follow-up of 366 days, 44% were found to have IMR with moderate-to-severe MR in 15%. MR regressed by at least 1 grade in 18% but progressed in 22%. Actually 7% of patients with mild or no MR progressed to moderate-to-severe grade. Moderate-to-severe MR was an independent predictor of MACE (HR 2.58).[25]

The long-term course of IMR after AMI during a follow-up period of 6–8 months had been highlighted in a study of 546 patients managed successfully with PCI. IMR was found in 36% of patients on arrival—mild in 24%, moderate in 10%, and severe in 2%. Before discharge, mild MR was present in 28%, moderate MR in 9%, and severe MR in 1%. In the chronic phase (6–8 months), mild MR was seen in 23%, moderate MR was seen in 4%, and severe MR was seen in 1%. In those with baseline moderate-to-severe MR, the severity did not change in roughly half and showed improvement in the other half after PCI. In the chronic phase, half of those with left with moderate-to-severe MR at discharge showed improvement. However, it is important to note that 17% of patients with mild MR at baseline developed moderate-to-severe MR post-PCI. Moreover, 4% of those with mild MR at discharge developed moderate-to-severe MR in chronic phase.[26]

In those with chronic IMR and LV dysfunction, who continue to be symptomatic despite maximal medical therapy for at least 3 months, device therapy/surgery may be considered. Rhythm control for those with AF, preferably by ablative therapies is useful in those with IMR and heart failure. Cardiac resynchronization therapy (CRT) or left bundle branch area pacing (LBBA pacing) should be considered for those with LBBB (QRS duration of > 120 ms) or IVCD (QRS duration of >150 ms). Improvement of MR may be biphasic with immediate postprocedure reduction of MR (by about 35%), possibly due to correction of dyssynchrony and improvement of dP/dt resulting in augmented closing forces.

Late progressive improvement is attributed to reduction of LV size resulting in diminished tethering forces. Moderate to severe MR (EROA of >20 mm^2) and marked LV enlargement appear to be predictors of lack of improvement of MR after CRT. In a study of 277 patients with secondary MR (ischemic in 40%), the presence of mechanical dyssynchrony in the form of septal flash and apical rocking seemed to predict improvement of MR after CRT. 30% of the entire cohort had grade 3–4 MR. MR improved by at least one grade in 62% of them. Reverse remodeling of LV was more frequent in those with MR reduction. Among the many variables studied, baseline severity of MR, apical rocking, and septal flash were significantly associated with MR improvement, with an odds ratio of 1.4, 3.8, and 3.6, respectively.[27]

CABG alone does not correct IMR in the majority. On the other hand, additional mitral valve procedures increase the surgical risk of CABG. Generally, mitral valve surgery is recommended for those undergoing CABG when there is moderate-to-severe MR (EROA > 30 mm^2) with EF > 30%. It may also be considered in those with severe MR when EF is <30%. Rarely, isolated mitral valve surgery may be considered in those who are not candidates for CABG, when EF is >30% and symptoms are attributable to severe MR. Mitral valve surgery may be considered for those with moderate MR (EROA 20–30 mm^2) undergoing CABG, only when repair is feasible. Those with mild IMR may require only revascularization procedure (PCI or CABG) unless there is evidence that there is exercise induced increase in MR with EROA increasing by >3 mm^2 with exercise.

The standard repair technique that is offered for chronic IMR is reducing the annulus size with an undersized rigid or semirigid ring, preferably with a saddle shape **(Figs. 6A to C)**.

If there are predictors for failure of repair such as coaptation distance of >10 mm, tenting area > 2.5–3.0 cm^2, posterolateral angle of >45° which indicate that tethering is the dominant cause for MR, valve replacement may be considered. Presence of complex multiple jets of MR and annulus diameter of >37 mm also predict failure of repair.[28]

Obviously, mitral annuloplasty would help patients with Carpentier type I (isolated annulus dilatation) or a mixed pathology with type I and III b. Type II pathology with PMD causing mitral valve prolapse or PMR would require replacement rather than repair. When there is marked LV remodeling (LVEDD > 65 mm, LVESD > 51 mm) or when there are multiple nonviable segments, any form of mitral valve surgery is futile and cardiac transplant should be seriously considered. Observational and randomized studies of combined CABG and mitral annuloplasty were heterogenous in nature but mortality benefit could not be demonstrated in most of these studies despite reduction of MR, reverse LV remodeling and improvement of functional status.[29] Similarly, there has been no difference between mitral valve replacement and repair in terms of survival benefit but recurrence of MR occurs in a large proportion of patients who underwent repair. Nearly 30–40% of patients with IMR may have persistence or recurrence of MR in the repair group which predict poor outcome. Subvalvular repair in the form of PM approximation along with annuloplasty seems to offer better results and some survival benefit.[30] Chordal cutting[31] has also been proposed as an additional procedure for those with AML tethering by strut chordae particularly in those with the bending angle < 145° **(Figs. 7A to C)**.

Role of Transcatheter Edge-to-edge Repair

Transcatheter repair of MR using devices like Mitraclip (Abbott Vascular, Santa Clara, California) has been found to be useful in reducing the severity of MR in both primary and secondary MR. The ideal imaging findings for a successful TEER include regurgitation occurring at A2-P2 segments, coaptation depth of <11 mm, coaptation distance of >2 mm, flail width of <15 mm, flail gap of <10 mm, absence of mitral annulus calcification or marked annulus dilatation, MVA in diastole > 4.0 cm^2, absence of marked LV enlargement (LV dimension in diastole < 70 mm) or severe LV dysfunction (LVEF 20–50%), absence of severe PH (PA systolic pressure

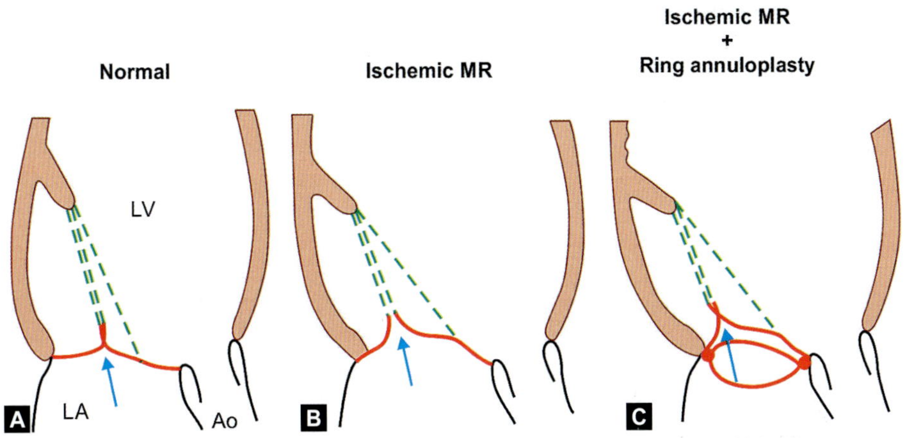

FIGS. 6A TO C: Ring annuloplasty restores loss of coaptation length and reduces MR.

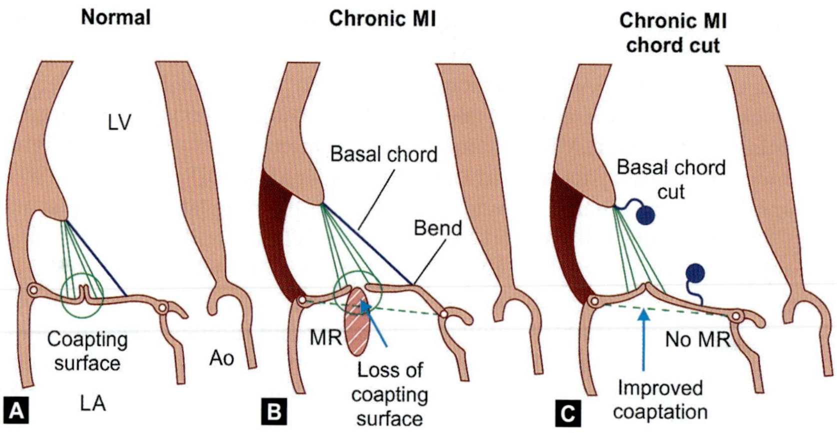

FIGS. 7A TO C: Cutting the strut chordae to anterior leaflet allows it to fall down toward tethered posterior leaflet thereby restoring proper coaptation.

< 70 mm Hg), or RV dysfunction. Bicommissural MR, shorter PML length, larger anteroposterior annulus diameter (>3.5 cm) and intercommissural diameter (>3.7 cm), and smaller MVA area/LVEDV ratio (3.60 ± 1.93 vs. 5.04 ± 2.69 mm^2/mL) were found to be the echo predictors of suboptimal results with TEER.[32] Asymmetric tethering of PML is a feature that is associated with persistence or recurrence of MR after Mitraclip. Those patients with proportionate MR (RV/EDV of ~0.10; EROA/EDV < 0.15) mostly have symmetric tethering and respond to medical therapy and those with disproportionate MR (RV/EDV ~0.20; EROA/EDV > 0.20) mostly have asymmetric tethering and respond better to Mitraclip. Generally, those with severe LV remodeling with EDV > 250 mL respond poorly and those with less severe LV remodeling with EDV < 200 mL respond better to Mitraclip. These facts need to be incorporated in decision making regarding management.

CONCLUSION

Ischemic MR is common and correctable. Any degree of MR imposes higher risk to patients with acute and remote MI. Recognition of the phenotype and mechanism of MR is important to choose the appropriate management. Lower thresholds may be considered for diagnosing severe MR because of poor prognosis of functional MR. The limitations of conventional echo parameters for severity assessment in MR of ischemic etiology should be recognized. Multimodal imaging and multiparametric assessment are often needed for flawless decision making. A checklist of predictors of improvement of MR or lack of response to surgical or percutaneous treatment will be of help in deciding appropriate management. Heart team approach and shared decision making are important while planning for management strategies.

ONLINE REFERENCES

Please scan the QR code provided at the end of the table of contents for References of this chapter.

CHAPTER

143

Cardiac Rehabilitation after Acute Myocardial Infarction

Madhuvanthi Rajendran, Thomas Alexander

ABSTRACT

Cardiac rehabilitation (CR) plays an important part in the management of patients after an acute myocardial infarction. A comprehensive CR care comprises exercise training for cardiac patients; dietary counseling; pharmacological modification of their cardiovascular risk factors such as hypertension, diabetes, and dyslipidemia; and therapeutic lifestyle modification. Participation in a center-based CR program improves the quality of life and reduces the risk of future cardiac events.

Keywords: Cardiac rehabilitation, therapeutic lifestyle modification, exercise training, secondary CVD prevention, Yoga-based cardiac rehabilitation

INTRODUCTION

Cardiac rehabilitation (CR), also referred to as cardiovascular (CV) rehabilitation, has an imperative role in the comprehensive management of patients recovering from an acute coronary syndrome (ACS) or acute worsening of heart failure (HF). It is a multidisciplinary, systematic, yet personalized approach to providing evidence-based secondary prevention therapies for patients with CV disease.

Exercise training forms the core component of CR. Other components include assessment of CV risk profile, control of modifiable risk factors, implementing therapeutic lifestyle and dietary changes, behavioral modification, and providing psychosocial support to patients.

Participation in CR programs reduces mortality, morbidity, and unplanned hospitalizations, and improves exercise capacity, psychosocial well-being, and quality of life.[1-3]

DEFINITION OF CARDIAC REHABILITATION

The British Association for Cardiovascular Prevention and Rehabilitation (BACPR) defines CR as "the coordinated sum of activities required to influence favorably the underlying cause of CVD, as well as to provide the best possible physical, mental and social conditions, so that the patients may, by their own efforts, preserve or resume optimal functioning in their community and through improved health behavior, slow or reverse progression of disease."

Cardiac rehabilitation by commonly accepted terminology is defined as "a physician-supervised program that furnishes physician-prescribed exercise, cardiac risk factor modification, psychosocial assessment, and outcomes assessment."

The multidisciplinary CR team generally consists of physicians, nurses, exercise physiologists, dietitians, social workers, and psychologists.

EVOLUTION OF CARDIAC REHABILITATION

The first documented anecdote of exercise as treatment for angina dates back to 1772, when Heberden, a British physician, reported that a patient with angina who sawed wood 30 minutes daily for 6 months "was nearly cured."

The roots of modern CR can be traced to the 1950s with the development of hospital-based exercise regimens. Observations by Levine et al.[4] showed that armchair exercise was both safe and beneficial for hospitalized patients recovering from myocardial infarction. Later, Kennedy et al.[5] in their small but important study showed that an outpatient exercise training program for patients with stable angina improved oxygen consumption for a repetitive workload, which mirrored Heberden's observation. A meta-analysis by Oldridge et al.[6] of 10 randomized control trials that included 4,347 patients showed a 25% reduction in CV mortality among patients randomly assigned to CR.

With emerging evidence, the practice of CR has evolved into a dedicated service that not only focuses on exercise training but also includes nutrition counseling and educational and psychological support sessions according to patients' individualized treatment plan under the guidance of the CR team.

GOALS OF CARDIAC REHABILITATION

The broad goals of CR are to improve physical fitness, functional capacity, and psychosocial well-being of patients with cardiac disease and to reduce the risk of future cardiac events. The specific goals are given in **Box 1**.

INDICATIONS FOR CARDIAC REHABILITATION

Cardiac rehabilitation as a structured, center-based exercise training program is approved for the indications given next. Eligible patients enter the CR pathway when referred after a qualifying event or diagnosis, ideally beginning within 1–2 weeks after the event. HF patients on optimal medical therapy and stable New York Heart Association (NYHA) class II or III symptoms should be considered for supervised exercise training **(Box 2)**.

BOX 1 Various goals of cardiac rehabilitation.

Medical goals:
- Improve cardiac function
- Lower the risk of SCD and future cardiac events
- Relieve angina and improve symptoms
- Increase exercise capacity
- Prevent progression of ASCVD

Psychological goals:
- Restore self-confidence
- Relieve anxiety and depression
- Relieve or manage stress
- Restore good sexual health

Behavioral goals:
- Cessation of smoking
- Inculcate heart-healthy eating behavior
- Adopt a physically active health style
- Adhere to prescribed medications

Social goals:
- Facilitate return to work
- Promote independence in activities of daily living

Health service goals:
- Reduce medical cost
- Promote early mobilization and early discharge from hospital
- Minimize hospital readmissions

CARDIAC REHABILITATION PATHWAY

The three parts of the CR pathway include steps to help patients initiate CR, components of an effective CR program, and steps to help patients maintain progress over time **(Flowchart 1)**.

BOX 2 Current indications for cardiac rehabilitation.[7]

- ACC-AHA: Coronary artery revascularization
- ACC-AHA: Chest pain
- ACC-AHA: Heart failure
- ISHLT: Heart transplantation
- Heart valve repair/replacement

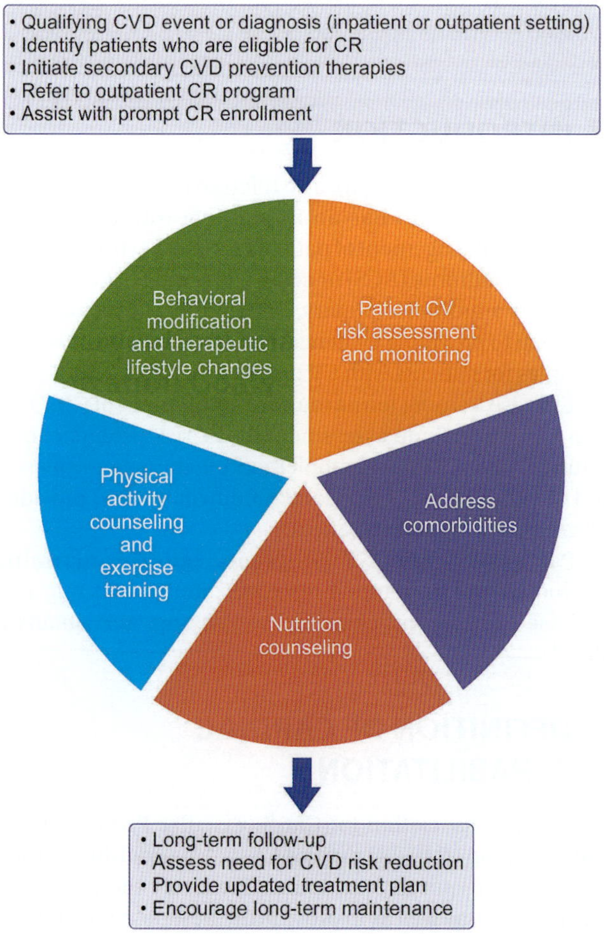

FLOWCHART 1: The three parts of cardiac rehabilitation pathway.

CARDIAC REHABILITATION: CONTINUUM OF CARE

Initiation of secondary prevention begins shortly after resolution of the acute event. Early mobilization and assessment for activities of daily living (ADL) such as walking, using toilet, bathing, and stair climbing constitute early inpatient rehabilitation. An important handover occurs at the time of hospital discharge when issues regarding driving, return to work, exercise, sexual activity, and recreational activities are discussed. The continuum of care follows through the phases mentioned in **Flowchart 2**.

INITIAL ASSESSMENT AND CARDIAC RISK STRATIFICATION

All individuals prior to undertaking exercise should be thoroughly assessed as a first step, which enables cardiac risk stratification and prior goal setting **(Table 1)**.

PHYSICAL ACTIVITY COUNSELING

All cardiac patients should be assessed for ADL and encouraged to gradually increase the volume of physical activity with relevance to age and gender, and to adopt practices such

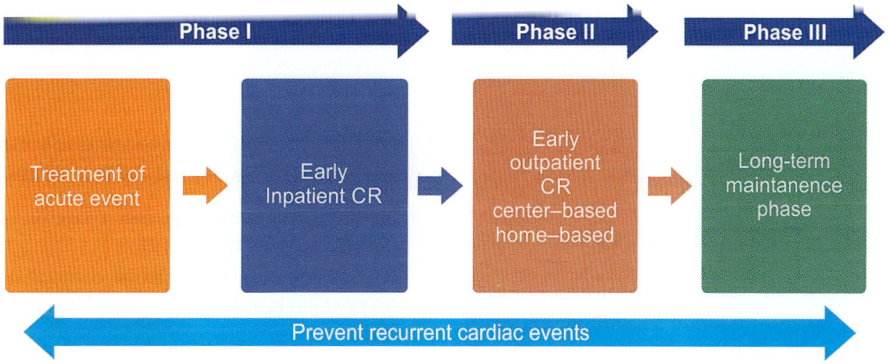

FLOWCHART 2: The three phases of cardiac rehabilitation.

TABLE 1: The components of initial cardiac assessment.

History	• Complete medical history • Past cardiac conditions and procedures • Cardiovascular risk profile • Immunization status (flu and pneumococcal vaccine) • Dietary pattern • Current functional status • List of medications • Educational background • Socioeconomic status • Behavioral pattern—tobacco use, alcohol indulgence	• Look for presence of relevant symptoms: angina, dyspnea, orthopnea, cough and PND, palpitations, claudication • Any unhealthy dietary pattern • Identify psychosocial barriers
Physical examination	• Heart rate and BP • Oxygen saturation level • Weight, height, BMI • Waist circumference • JVP, peripheral edema • Cardiovascular system examination • Respiratory system examination • Muscle power and tone • Signs of peripheral vascular disease	• Look for: ○ Signs of decompensated heart failure ○ Signs of peripheral vascular disease ○ Signs of neuromuscular weakness ○ Physical disability and orthopedic conditions ○ Relative contraindications to exercise testing

Continued

Continued

Baseline investigations	• Resting 12-lead ECG • Complete hemogram • Glycemic profile • Baseline RFT, LFT • Lipid and thyroid profile	• Initiate GDMT • Set LDL targets • Glycemic control
Functional capacity testing	• Submaximal testing or • Maximal testing as appropriate	• *Establish endpoints*: Submaximal/symptom-limited • *Training heart rate*: Low/moderate/high intensity
Cardiac risk stratification	Low, moderate, and high risk based on baseline cardiac functions and exercise testing	• Assess risk of future cardiac events • Need for supervised exercise training • Need for ECG monitoring during exercise
Setting goals	*S*pecific, *m*easurable, *a*chievable, *r*elevant, *t*imely goals that can be *e*valuated and *r*evised	• Physical activity and exercise goals • Vocation and return to work, sports • Heart-healthy diet and lifestyle • Behavior modification

as lunchtime walks, parking further away to get more steps, and taking up simple gardening tasks **(Box 3)**.

CARDIAC RISK STRATIFICATION

The information on baseline cardiac status, abnormal hemodynamic, procedural complications, and functional capacity is useful for stratifying patients in two ways:

1. Risk for adverse cardiac events during exercise
2. To determine the degree of clinical supervision/ECG monitoring required during the initial training period when the risk of adverse events is the highest

The AACVPR model of cardiac risk stratification is given in **Table 2**.

BOX 3 The EACPR[8] recommendations for physical activity in post-ACS patients.

- Following an uncomplicated procedure, patients can begin physical activity the next day
- Following a large myocardial damage, patients should start PA post-clinical stabilization, and increase gradually as per the symptoms
- Patients with preserved exercise capacity can resume routine PA, like brisk walking for a period of 30–60 minutes, along with increase in daily activities
- For other patients, it is recommended that PA be resumed at 50% of maximal exercise capacity, and slowly increased
- PA counseling should be provided based on wound healing and exercise capacity

TABLE 2: The AACVPR[9] model of cardiac risk stratification.

High risk (presence of one or more characteristics)	Low risk (presence of all the following characteristics)	Moderate risk (presence of neither high-risk nor low-risk criteria)
• LVEF < 40% • Survivor of cardiac arrest • Complex VT at rest or with exercise • MI complicated by cardiogenic shock, CHF, postprocedural ischemia • Abnormal BP response to exercise/chronotropic incompetence • Silent ischemia (≥2-mm ST-segment depression with exercise or in recovery) • Maximum functional capacity <5 METS	• LVEF > 50% • No resting or exercise-induced arrhythmias • Uncomplicated MI/PCI/CABG • Normal hemodynamics with exercise and in recovery • Asymptomatic with exercise and in recovery • Maximal functional capacity ≥7 METS	• LVEF: 40–50% • Signs/symptoms of angina during moderate levels of exercise (60–70% of maximum functional capacity) • Mild to moderate silent ischemia (ST-segment depression <2 mm) with exercise or in recovery
• At least 18–36 exercise sessions • 90 days postevent/procedure • Begin with continuous ECG monitoring and decrease to intermittent monitoring as appropriate	• At least 6–18 sessions • 30 days postevent/procedure • Begin with continuous ECG monitoring and decrease as appropriate	• At least 12–24 exercise sessions • 60 days postevent/procedure • Begin with continuous ECG monitoring and decrease as appropriate

EXERCISE TRAINING

A structured exercise includes all aspects of physical fitness: aerobic training, resistance training (RT), body composition, and flexibility. Specific training plans are prescribed according to the acronym FITT (Frequency, intensity, time, and type) **(Table 3)**.

Aerobic or endurance training helps in reversal of left ventricular remodeling and improves functional capacity and peak oxygen uptake (VO_2). It can trigger multiple physiological adaptations and improve various facets of CV health **(Fig. 1)**. Continuous moderate-intensity training (MCT) is safe and well tolerated as compared to high-intensity interval training (HIIT). HIIT produces larger improvement in cardiorespiratory fitness,[11] but requires careful patient selection and extra staff effort. In the HF-ACTION trial,[12] heart rate reserve [resting heart rate + 0.6 (peak heart rate – resting heart rate)] was used to guide exercise intensity.

TABLE 3: Summary of recommendations for exercise training.

	Frequency (days per week; how often?)	Intensity (how much to exert?)	Time (minutes per day)	Type (what activity?)
CV fitness	3 times per week	• Moderate • 40–70% HRR • BORG RPE 11–14	20–60 minutes (plus 15-minute warm up and 10-minute cool down)	• Treadmill • Cycle ergometer • Swimming
Resistance training	2–3 times per week	• *Upper body*: 30–40% 1RM • *Lower body*: 50–64% 1RM	Minimum 1–3 sets 8–10 repetitions	• Activities using resistance • Bands, dumbbells, pulleys
Flexibility and balance	2–3 times per week	To mild discomfort	Each stretch for 30 seconds	Main joint/muscle groups
Deconditioned individuals unable to attain 3 METS	Incorporate into daily routine	• Moderate • 40% HRR • BORG RPE 11	5- to 10-minute bouts (gradually increase to 30 min/day)	Walking low step-ups; sit-to-stand seated activities

[HRR: heart rate reserve (HRR = HRmax – HRrest); 1RM: one-repetition maximum; RPE: rate of perceived exertion; METS: metabolic equivalents]

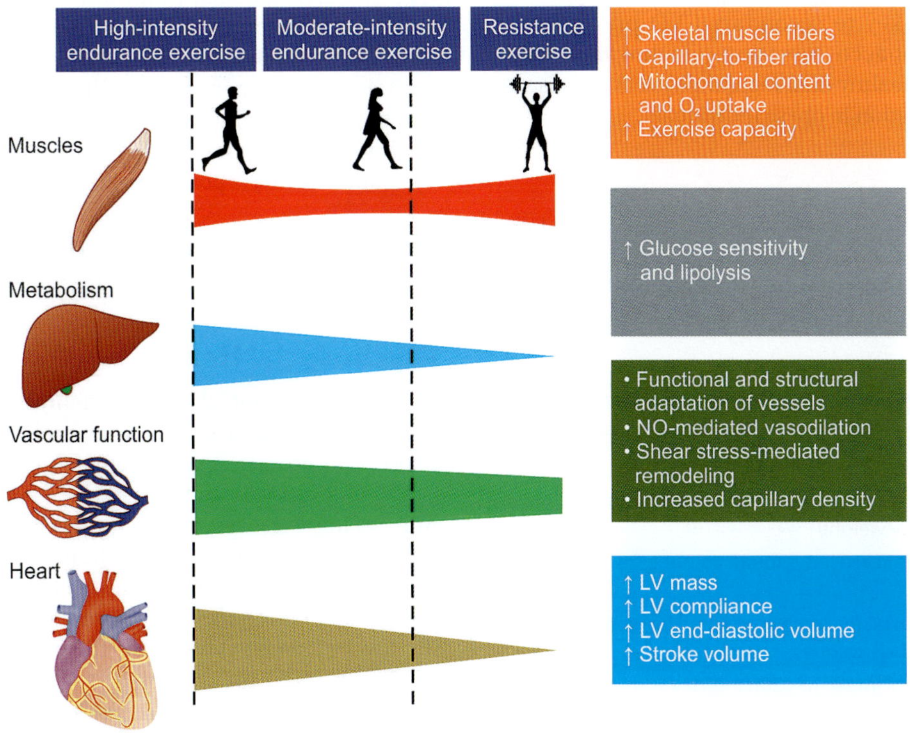

FIG. 1: Exercise-triggered physiological adaptations and cardiovascular benefits.[10]

Dynamic RT improves muscle strength and thereby cardiorespiratory endurance. It is a suitable strategy for patients with sarcopenia, as it increases muscle mass[13] and bone strength which increase physical independence in ADL. RT is commonly done in a gym-based setting utilizing weight training, pulley systems, resistance bands, kettle balls, free weights, etc.

NUTRITIONAL COUNSELING

Dietary recommendations to reduce CV risk generally involve calorie restriction and reduction of saturated fat consumption. A prudent diet[14] characterized by a higher intake of whole grains, vegetables, fruits, legumes, fish, and poultry is heart healthy compared to Western diet which includes red and processed meat, refined grains, sweets, and desserts. A low-carbohydrate diet (<40% of total energy) might be an effective weight loss strategy in insulin-resistant individuals as against a low-fat diet. An elevated triglyceride/HDL-C ratio (>3.5) is suggestive of insulin resistance.[15] Marine omega-3 fatty acids[16] decrease triglycerides and are effective in reducing mortality and coronary events **(Box 4)**.

BEHAVIORAL MODIFICATION AND THERAPEUTIC LIFESTYLE MODIFICATIONS

Apart from pharmacological modification of major coronary risk factors (i.e., systemic hypertension, diabetes, dyslipidemia, and obesity), lifestyle and behavioral modifications are the key to secondary CVD prevention.[17,18] These include tobacco cessation, alcohol moderation, adopting a heart-healthy diet, regular physical exercise, and active weight reduction in obese individuals.

Tobacco Use

In individuals with coronary artery disease, cessation of smoking reduces all-cause mortality by 36%.[19] Nicotine is the most important by-product of smoking. It increases oxygenation of LDL and promotes atherogenesis. The risk of an acute coronary event decreases by 50% within 2 years of cessation.[20]

The combination of counseling and medication is more effective for smoking cessation than either one alone. Intensive personalized interventions (IPANR)[21] such as the "5Rs + 5As" may be adopted.

Pharmacologic interventions such as nicotine receptor partial agonist (e.g., varenicline), nicotine replacement therapy (nicotine patch, gum, nasal spray, lozenge, inhaler), or bupropion should be considered when appropriate. Nicotine replacement products can precipitate serious arrhythmias in patients within 2 weeks of an MI.

BOX 4 Key features of the therapeutic lifestyle changes diet recommended by the US National Institutes of Health.

- An individual must consume only enough calories to achieve or maintain a healthy weight
- Calories from saturated fat should account for <7% of total calories
- Calories from total fat (including saturated fat) should comprise 25–35% of total daily calories
- Restrict cholesterol intake to <200 mg/day
- Options for lowering LDL-cholesterol include plant sterols or sterols (2 g/day) and increased viscous fiber (10–25 g/day)

Alcohol and Illicit Drug Use

Increase in alcohol intake >3 U/day is related to increase in blood pressure levels as well as risk of cardiac arrhythmias, cardiomyopathy, sudden death, and hemorrhagic stroke.[22] In patients who consume alcohol, it is recommended[23] to limit alcohol consumption to two glasses per day (20 g/day) for men and one glass per day (10 g/day) for women, with a minimum of 2 alcohol-free days per week.

Illicit drug use—especially heroin, cocaine, and methamphetamine—contributes to the development of various CV complications.[24] Recognition of such drug use and prompt referral to a psychiatrist/deaddiction program is important.

Weight Management

Central obesity is independently associated with CAD risk. CVD risk is heightened with waist circumference ≥90 cm in males and ≥80 cm in females.[25] Setting reasonable short-term targets such as dietary caloric restriction (1,000 kcal/day), increased energy expenditure and physical activity, and daily 60–90 minutes of walking can be practical. Long-term goal of achieving weight reduction >10% at the rate of 1–2 pounds/week is possible with persistent motivation.

Management of Comorbid Conditions

Table 4 explains the recommendations.

Psychosocial Health

Various psychosocial factors including social isolation, marital distress, stress at work and/or home, hostility, depression, anxiety, sexual dysfunction, and substance abuse can hinder recovery and lead to a worse prognosis of CVD.[30] Addressing these psychosocial risk factors, in particular treatment of depression after MI, has been associated with improved CVD outcomes. Creating a supportive rehabilitative environment and providing community resources improves the level of social support for the patient and family. Use of standardized measurement tools to identify clinically significant psychosocial distress helps in early referral to appropriate mental health specialists.

TABLE 4: Recommendations for management of comorbid conditions.

Dyslipidemia	Very high-risk group LDL-C goal <50 mg/dL (LAI recommendation for secondary CVD prevention)[26]	• Recommended ratio of LDL-C to HDL-C ≤ 1.5[27] • Addition of ezetimibe/PCSK9 inhibitors to maximum tolerated dose of statins to achieve LDL-C targets[26] • If triglycerides are 200–499 mg/dL after LDL-C target is reached, add a fibrate
Hypertension	The risk of mortality due to CAD or stroke increases linearly with increasing BP levels from 115/75 mm Hg[21]	• *In hypertensive patients*: Systolic BP < 140 mm Hg and diastolic BP < 90 mm Hg • In hypertensive patients with CKD, HF, or diabetes: Systolic BP < 130 mm Hg and diastolic BP 90 mm Hg[28] • To adopt a DASH eating plan • Regular aerobic physical activity • Moderation of alcohol consumption—limit consumption to no more than two drinks per day • Management of obstructive sleep apnea
Diabetes	In patients with chronic coronary syndrome, T2DM is associated with an increased risk of CV death, MI, and stroke	• Achieve fasting blood glucose levels of 90–130 mg/dL and HbA1c < 7 g% • Decrease episodes of hypoglycemia or hyperglycemia at rest or with exercise • SGLT-2 inhibitors and/or GLP-1 receptor agonists are recommended in patients with T2DM and CAD to reduce CV events[29]

Resumption of Sexual Activity

Sexual activity may increase the risk of CVD events; however, the absolute rate of events is negligible and accounts for a very minor proportion of the total time at risk for MI/ischemia. Patients may resume sexual activity 6–8 weeks after standard CABG if the sternum is well healed and 1–2 weeks after an uncomplicated PCI, provided there are no symptoms during mild/moderate physical activity (Class IIa).[31] Use of PDE5 inhibitors is effective in the management of erectile dysfunction among patients with stable CVD, but should not be administered to patients on nitrate treatment.

Yoga-based Cardiac Rehabilitation

Yoga is an Indian-origin, traditional mind-body practice which involves breathing practices (*pranayama*), postures (*asanas*), and meditation. Yoga-based CR (Yoga-CaRe)[32] program for post-MI patients typically comprises four phases and involves a total of 13 sessions conducted over 3 months, while encouraging patients to self-practice. Yoga-CaRe aligned to CR phases has been shown to improve self-rated quality of life and assist in resumption of daily activities after acute myocardial infarction.[33]

CONCLUSION

Advances in options for home-based CR or noncenter-based CR will likely play a prominent role in CR practice in the future. Technological developments including wearable devices, smart phone applications, artificial intelligence-guided clinical tools, HF devices, etc., have enhanced the scope of CR. It will continue to evolve and remain relevant and important in the spectrum of CV medicine.

In the Indian scenario, capacity building, community awareness programs, and government commitment toward CR services can bridge the gap in CR participation. Yoga is a feasible option and can have far-reaching benefits in terms of CR.

ONLINE REFERENCES

Please scan the QR code provided at the end of the table of contents for References of this chapter.

SECTION 14

Coronary Intervention

Section Outline

CHAPTER

144

Clinical Use of Intracoronary Imaging: Guidance and Optimization of Coronary Interventions

Sajan Narayanan

ABSTRACT

Historically, percutaneous coronary interventions (PCI) had been performed under angiographic guidance. In last two decades, there had been compelling evidence of limitations of angiographically guided coronary procedures, and imaging (intravascular ultrasound and optical coherence tomography)-guided PCI have been shown to have a superiority with regard to reduction in short- and long-term outcomes. Benefits of imaging-guided interventions are not only limited to high-risk complex lesion subsets, but also observed in patients with less complex lesions (low SYNTAX scores). Imaging-optimized PCI has been consistently associated with lowest event rates in all published clinical studies.

Keywords: Imaging, IVUS, under expansion, tissue prolapse, thrombus, OCT

INTRODUCTION

Over last two decades, there has been a deluge of data that convincingly proves that coronary percutaneous interventions (PCI) guided by imaging improve major adverse cardiac events (MACE). The European society of cardiology (ESC) has given class IIa recommendation for imaging guidance during complex PCI procedures, especially left main (LM) interventions.[1] Since over last 5 years, multiple randomized controlled trials have conclusively proven the superiority of imaging-guided PCI, irrespective of complexity of lesions treated.[2,3]

IMAGING TIMELINES DURING CORONARY INTERVENTION

An imaging-optimized PCI procedure involves specific timeperiods, during which imaging is employed during coronary intervention. Broadly, these timelines can be divided into prestent and poststent imaging. Parameters to be assessed during these imaging runs are illustrated in **Boxes 1 to 3**. Achieving optimal standardization criteria at the end of the procedure is critical to achieve lowest MACE rates.

BOX 1 **Prestent assessment with imaging. Imaging pullback should start from 5 to 10 mm distal to the lesion, where there are no major side branches and should be performed upto aortic ostium.**

- Distal reference segment:
    - Minimum lumen area (MLA)
    - Average minimum lumen diameter (MLD)
    - Plaque burden
    - Plaque characteristics
- Lesion:
    - Plaque characteristics, e.g., attenuation, fibrotic, calcification
    - Whether Lesion needs plaque preparation? e.g., calcium score
    - Any chance of stent underexpansion? e.g., fibrotic plaque especially at branch ostia
    - Risk of slow flow, e.g., plaque attenuation, thrombus score
- Proximal reference segment:
    - Minimum lumen area
    - Average MLD
    - Plaque burden
    - Plaque characteristics

BOX 2 **Imaging assessment of successful atherectomy procedure. Following atheroablative procedures (e.g., Rota ablation or orbital atherectomy) or predilatation with modified balloons (e.g., scoring/cutting balloons), imaging must demonstrate signs of adequate lesion preparation before stent placement.**

Assessment of adequate lesion preparation:
- Lumen gain
- Calcium fractures
- Reverberation artefacts

BOX 3 **Poststent optimization goals on imaging: In small vessels, where achievement of absolute MSA is impossible, operator can rely of relative expansion criteria.**

Minimum stent area (MSA):
- >5.5 mm^2 (IVUS), >4.5 mm^2 (OCT)
- >80–90% of average RLA
- No edge dissection: >60° (>2/3rd of 1 quadrant) and length > 2 mm, Thickness > 200 µm
- No major malapposition (>300–400 µm)
- No residual edge disease (<50% PB)
- No significant plaque protrusion which compromises final MLA

(MLA: minimum lumen area; PB: plaque burden; RLA: reference lumen area)

How can we Identify a Reference Segment?

Reference segment is that part of vessel which is relatively disease free and where the operator intends to land the proximal and distal stent edges. A reference segment should have adequate minimum lumen area (MLA) (>5–5.5 mm^2) and plaque burden (PB) at that site must be <40–50%. Angiographic assessment of reference segments is inaccurate. In a study of 884 angiographically normal segments, only 60 (6.8%) had normal or three-layered appearance on imaging. When assessed with intravascular ultrasound (IVUS), mean cross-sectional narrowing at angiographically normal segments was 50.7 ± 12.7%;[4] of 785 angiographically normal-looking proximal reference segments with poststenting diameter of stenosis of <20%, 290 (37%) had maximal plaque burden (PB) of >50%, while 21% of angiographically normal distal reference segments had PB of >50%.[5] These two studies highlight the limitation of angiographic assessment in selection of reference segments.

Reference segment MLA and PB, which predicted stent edge restenosis was 5.5 mm^2 and 50%, respectively on IVUS,[5] and 4.5 mm^2 on optical coherence tomography (OCT) imaging.[6] Plaque tissue characteristics determine edge restenosis, with worst outcomes when stent edge is placed in a lipid-rich area. Risk of stent failure was directly proportional to degree of lipid arc at edges with higher frequency of restenosis when lipid arc occupied more than three quadrants[7] **(Figs. 1A to C)**.

How can we Assess Successful Plaque Preparation?

Significant calcification is the most important indication for lesion preparation. Angiogram is a relatively less sensitive tool to detect coronary calcification. In a study of 1,155 target lesions with calcification, 73% contained gray scale IVUS calcium. Angiography defined moderate calcium (radiopacities noted only during the cardiac cycle before contrast injection) in 26% and severe calcium (radiopacities seen without cardiac motion, usually affecting both sides of arterial lumen) only in 12%. Overall sensitivity of angiography was only 48% and lowest in lesions with one quadrant calcium on IVUS. Angiography is not sensitive to detect isolated deep calcium. Overall specificity of angiogram to predict lesion calcification was 89% and correlated with severe calcification on imaging.[8] Calcium scores on IVUS and OCT have been proposed, which help in decision of upfront lesion preparation **(Figs. 2 and 3)**. After atherectomy procedure, imaging assessment must be performed to verify success of lesion preparation **(Figs. 4A to C)**. Imaging-based strategy would help operator to select the proper atherectomy device. If imaging catheter fails to cross the lesion, we need to employ an ablative strategy (e.g., rotational atherectomy). In PREPARE CALC study,[9] strategy success (successful stent delivery and expansion with attainment of <20% in stent residual stenosis of the target lesion in the presence of TIMI 3 flow without cross-over or stent failure) was better with rotational atherectomy (98% vs. 81%) while 9-month mean instent late lumen loss was 0.16 ± 0.39 mm in modified balloon-based strategy versus 0.22 ± 0.4 mm in rotational atherectomy ($p = 0.21$, $p = 0.02$ for noninferiority). This result conveys the message that an ablative strategy would be useful if we have an uncrossable lesion, while if we are able to successfully deliver the device (ablative or modified balloon) into the lesion, then long-term event rates are comparable between the devices.

Imaging would help to identify morphology of calcium which would help to choose the lesion preparation strategy. In a group of patients who underwent OCT-guided PCI of heavily calcified lesions, lower calcium thickness (0.35 ± 0.14 vs. 0.79 ± 0.13 mm), higher degree of calcification angle (256.3 ± 84.5° vs. 232.7 ± 74°) and convex-shaped calcium predicted successful lesion preparation with a balloon-based strategy.[10]

Superficial calcium, i.e., when calcified plaque is predominantly toward luminal aspect, most of ablative and balloon-based strategies would be successful while presence of calcified plaque toward adventitial aspect of the vessel wall, i.e., toward lateral one third of the vessel wall may need intravascular lithotripsy (IVL) **(Figs. 5A and B)**.

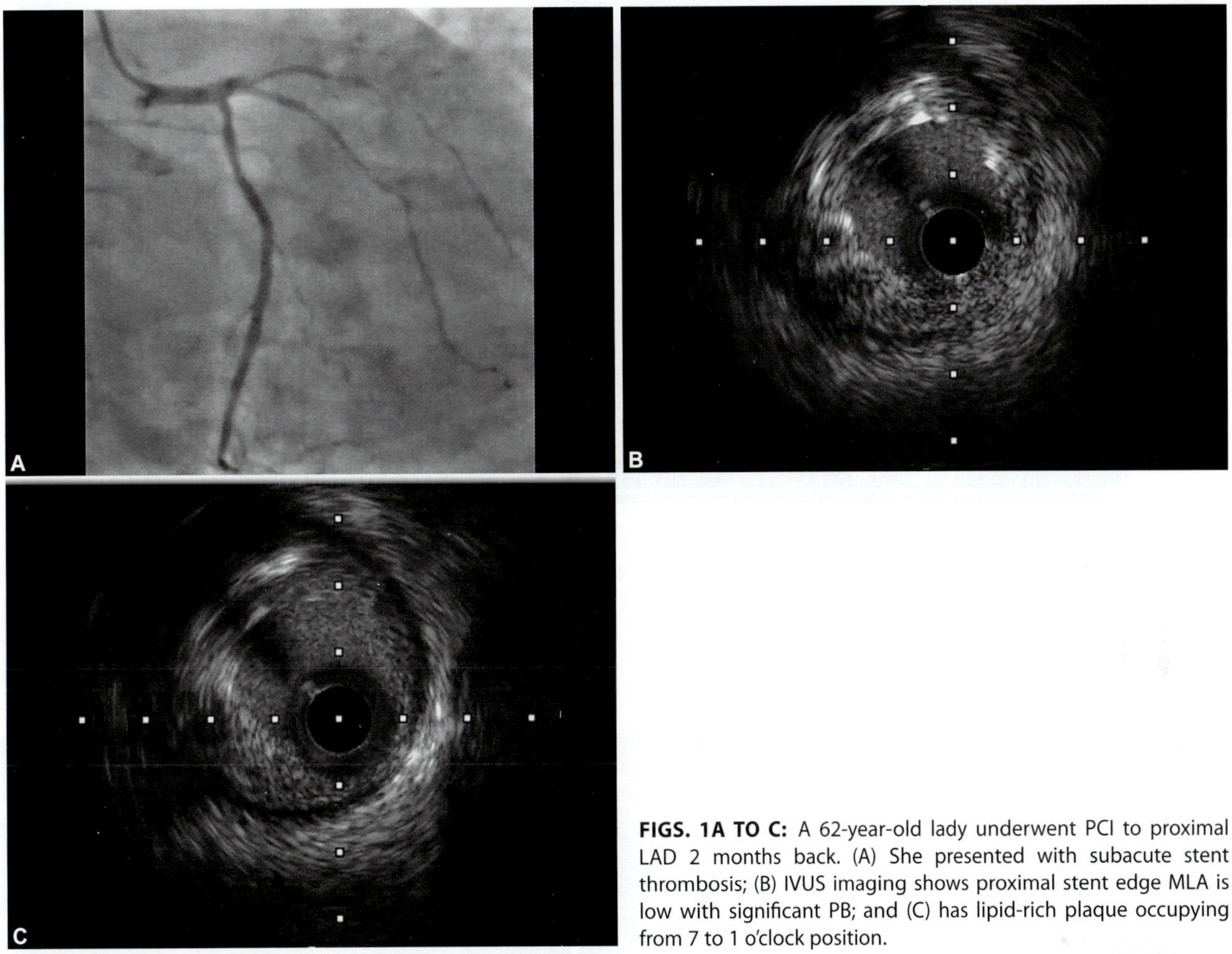

FIGS. 1A TO C: A 62-year-old lady underwent PCI to proximal LAD 2 months back. (A) She presented with subacute stent thrombosis; (B) IVUS imaging shows proximal stent edge MLA is low with significant PB; and (C) has lipid-rich plaque occupying from 7 to 1 o'clock position.

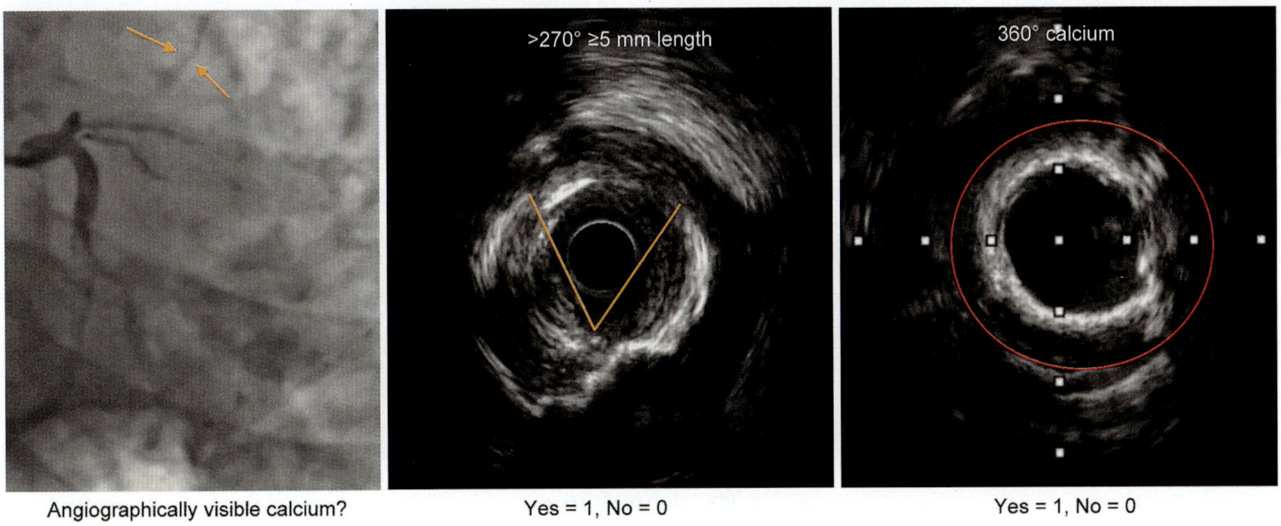

FIG. 2: *Continued*

Continued

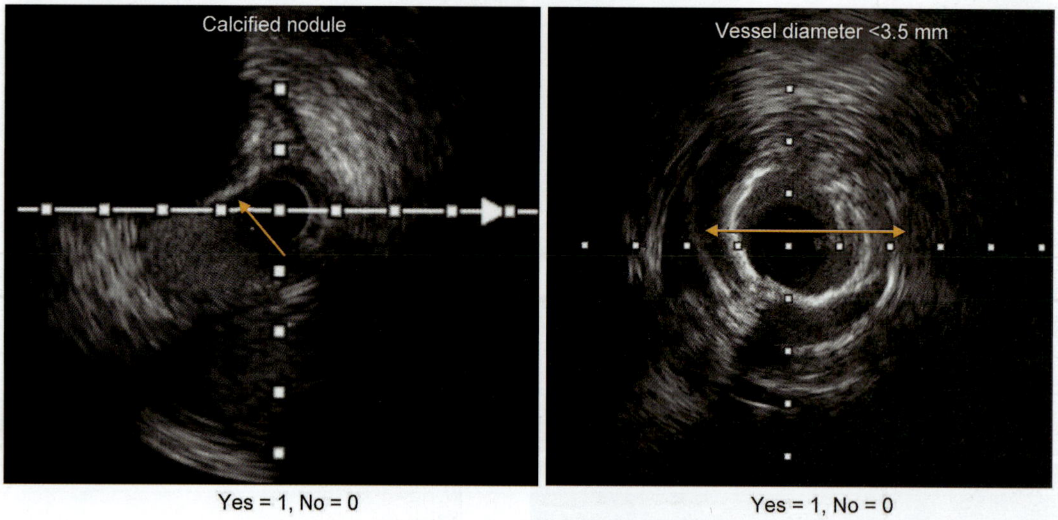

FIG. 2: Assessment of calcium burden on IVUS: If derived score is >2, predicts stent underexpansion without atherectomy with a sensitivity of 89% and specificity of 63%. Hence, if IVUS derived calcium score is >2, atherectomy may be considered before stent placement for optimal expansion.

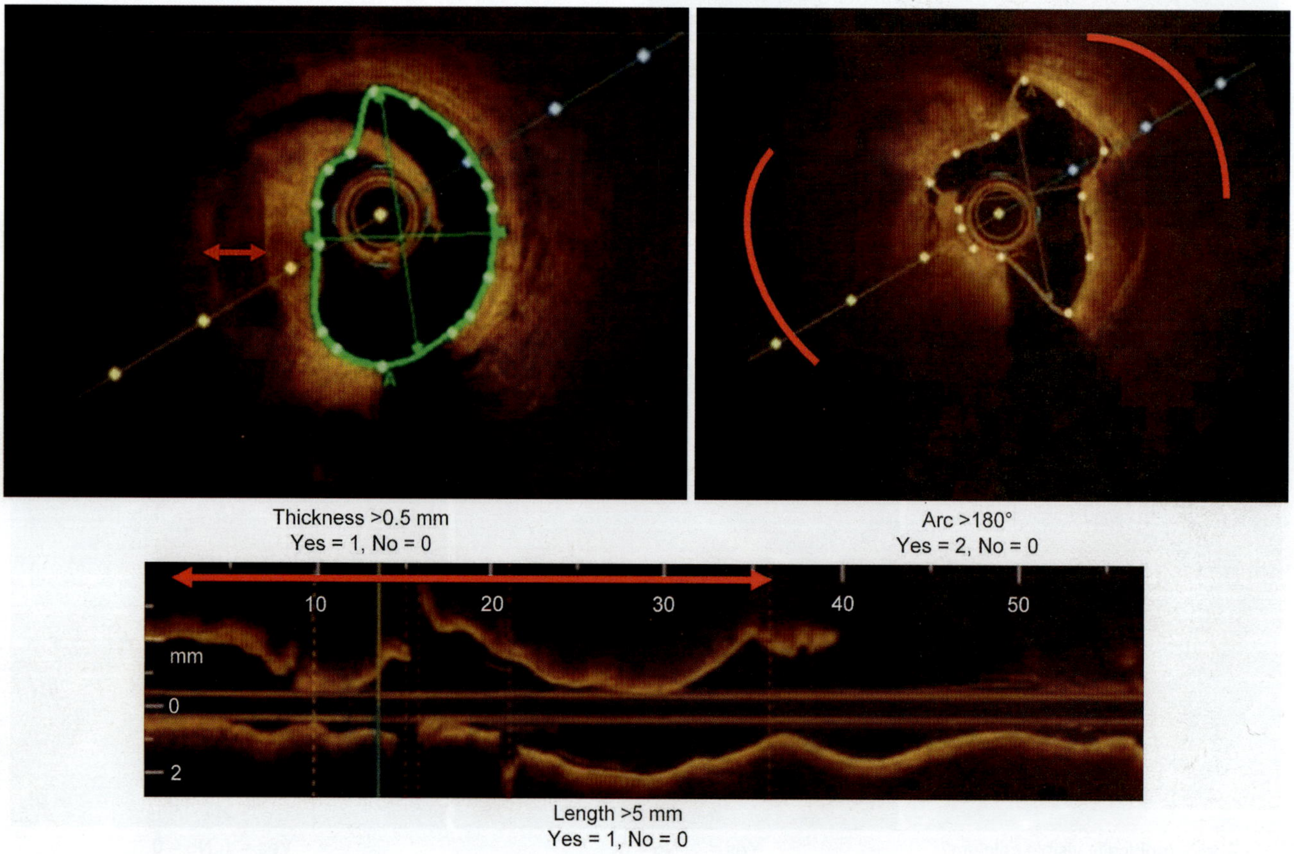

FIG. 3: Assessment of calcium burden on OCT: A calcium score > 4 predicts stent underexpansion and needs lesion preparation before stent placement.

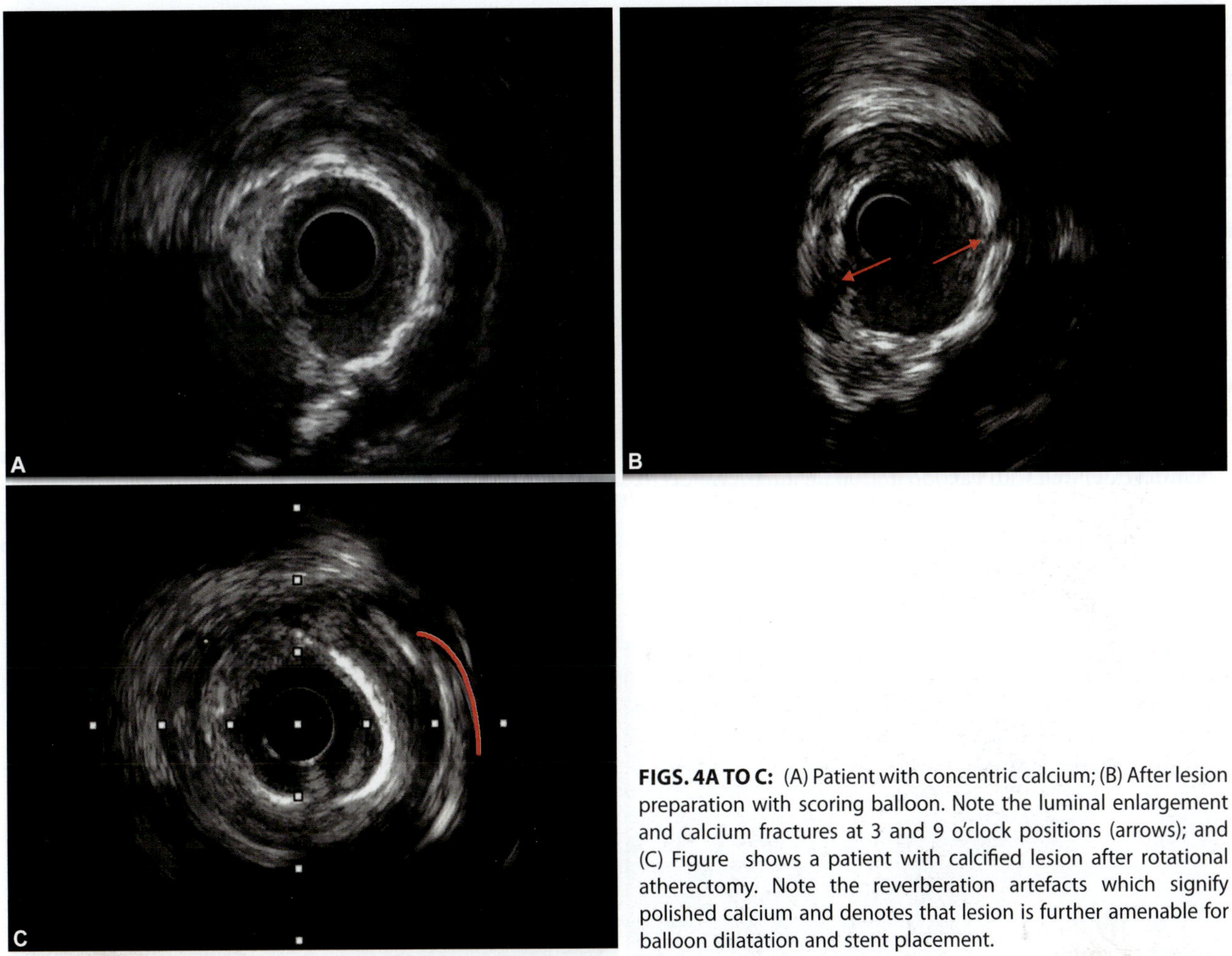

FIGS. 4A TO C: (A) Patient with concentric calcium; (B) After lesion preparation with scoring balloon. Note the luminal enlargement and calcium fractures at 3 and 9 o'clock positions (arrows); and (C) Figure shows a patient with calcified lesion after rotational atherectomy. Note the reverberation artefacts which signify polished calcium and denotes that lesion is further amenable for balloon dilatation and stent placement.

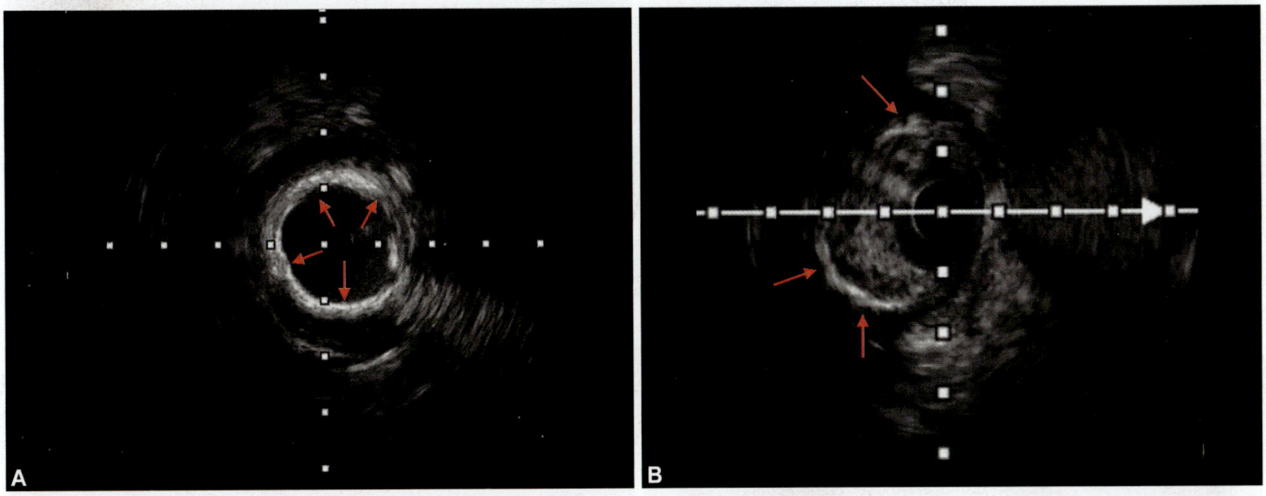

FIGS. 5A AND B: (A) Superficial calcium and (B) deep calcium. Note the location of calcium in relation to lumen. Calcification of leading edge of intima identifies superficial calcium.

Calcified nodules (CN) have important implications in deciding management strategies during PCI. Intracoronary imaging helps to identify two types of calcified protrusions, which have different pathobiological bases. Nodular calcified protrusion predicts poor stent expansion while eruptive calcified nodule is an important cause of acute coronary syndromes. Nodular calcified protrusion appears as projection with a smooth surface casting significant acoustic shadow. Eruptive nodules consist of small calcium fragments with an irregular surface **(Figs. 6A to D)**. Nodular protrusions need atherectomy procedures (rotablation if there is a favorable wire bias) or orbital atherectomy, while eruptive nodules, which happen due to rupture of fibrous cap through the calcified plates are eminently deformable with balloon dilatation. Even though eruptive nodules can be pushed back into vessel wall with balloon and stent, long-term event rates are higher in patients who harbor this pathology. In a post-hoc analysis of CLIMA registry, death and target lesion myocardial infarction occurred in 20% of patients with eruptive CNs versus 2.7% of those with noneruptive CNs and 3.3% of those without CNs ($p < 0.001$).[11] **Figures 7A to C** show significant ablation of nodular protrusion after rotablation.

Imaging-based algorithm helps to choose specific lesion-modifying strategies, which facilitate stent expansion and improve long-term outcomes **(Fig. 8)**.

Poststent Optimization with Imaging

Selection of stent size should be according to distal reference vessel diameter. Stent should be approximated proximally with appropriately sized balloon (proximal optimization or POT) according to proximal vessel diameter. Different definitions for optimal stent expansion have been proposed **(Table 1)**.

In DES era, an absolute minimum stent area (MSA) of > 5–5.5 mm^2 (IVUS) and ≥4.5 mm^2 (OCT) defines optimal stent expansion. In vessels where reference dimensions are smaller, relative criteria as defined by MSA > 80–90% of average reference lumen area (RLA) must be achieved.

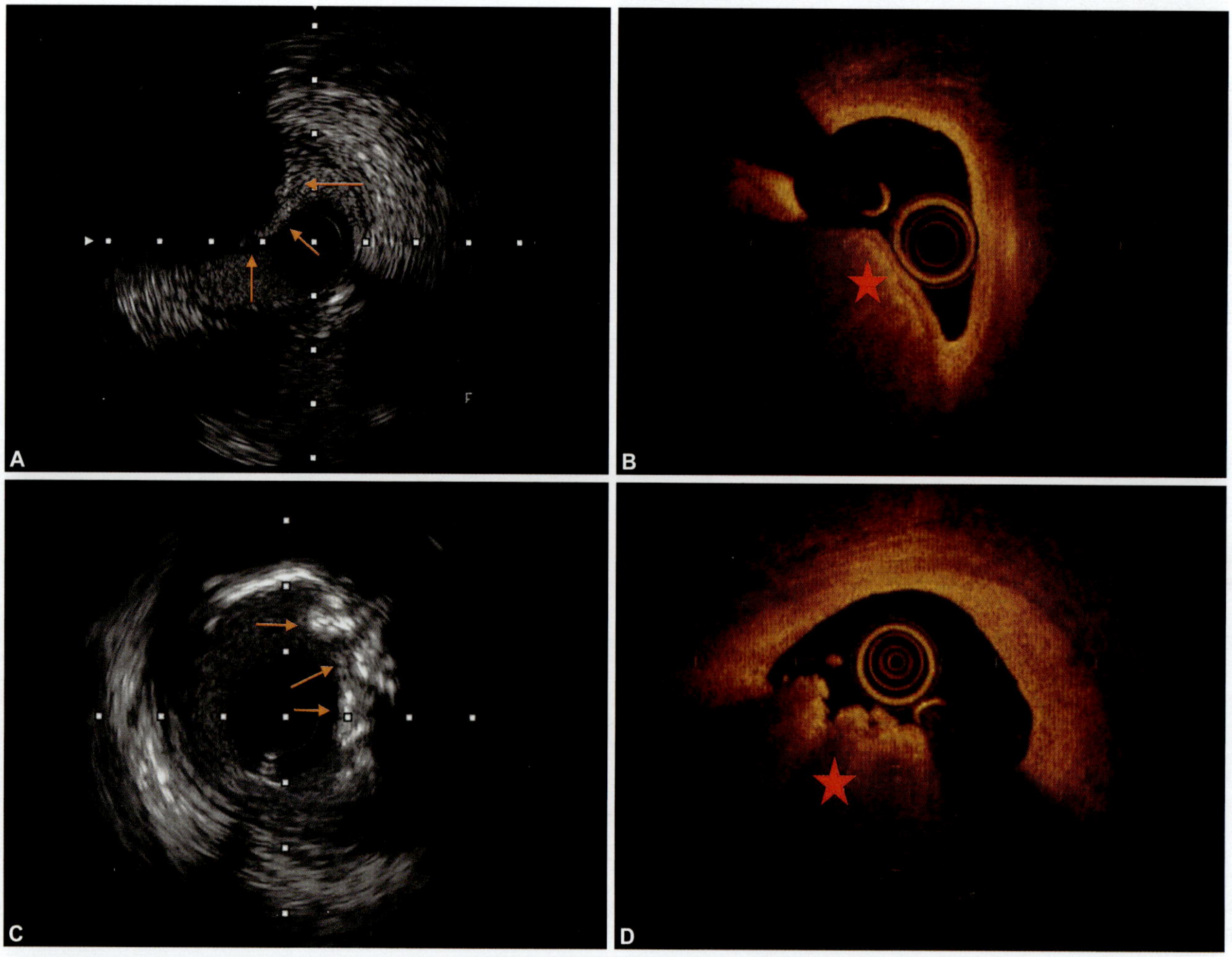

FIGS. 6A TO D: (A and B) Nodular protrusion—note smooth surface and significant shadowing on IVUS (A) and (B) signal attenuation on OCT; (C and D) Eruptive calcified nodules—(C) note irregular surface due to calcium fragments on IVUS; (D) Disrupted cap with fragments seen on OCT.

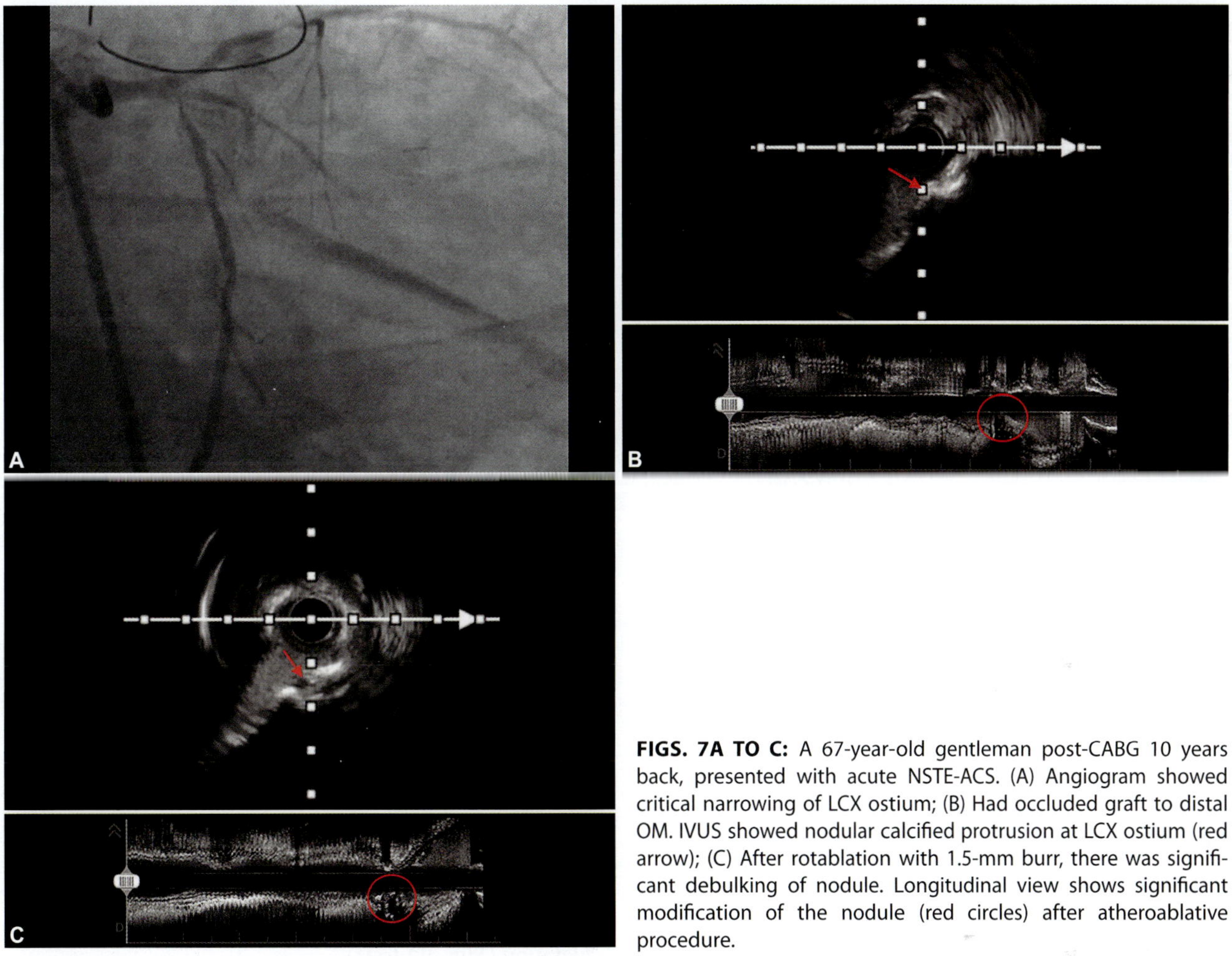

FIGS. 7A TO C: A 67-year-old gentleman post-CABG 10 years back, presented with acute NSTE-ACS. (A) Angiogram showed critical narrowing of LCX ostium; (B) Had occluded graft to distal OM. IVUS showed nodular calcified protrusion at LCX ostium (red arrow); (C) After rotablation with 1.5-mm burr, there was significant debulking of nodule. Longitudinal view shows significant modification of the nodule (red circles) after atheroablative procedure.

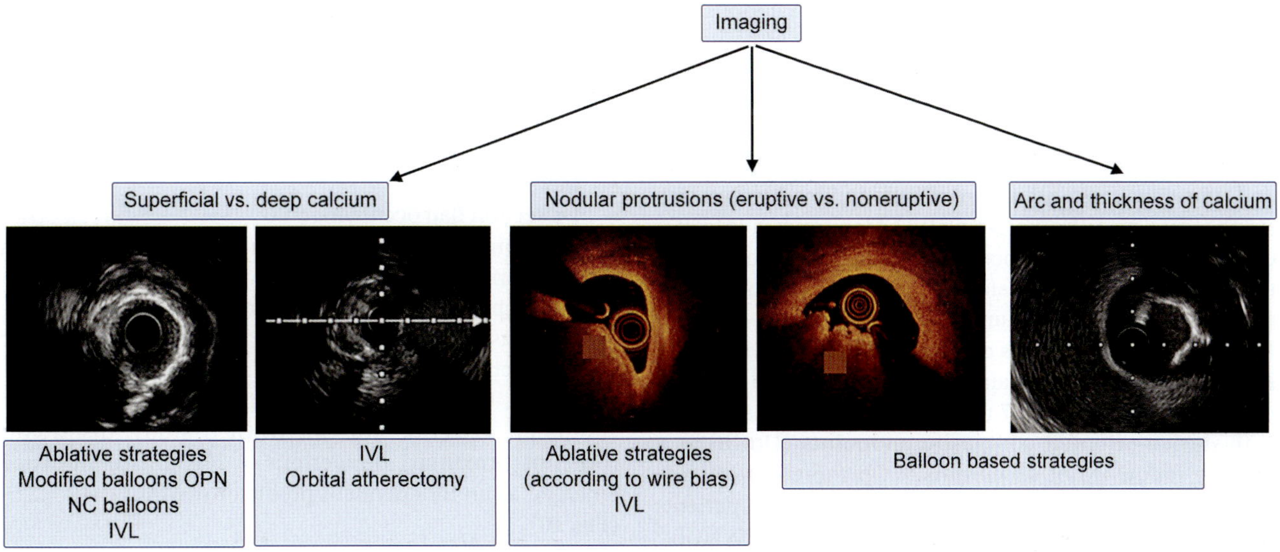

FIG. 8: Imaging helps to define specific morphology of calcified plaque and select plaque-modifying strategies. Concentric calcium, especially superficial are eminently modifiable with ablative or balloon-based strategies. Deep calcium, if occupying more than two quadrants need either IVL or orbital atherectomy. Nodular calcified protrusions need an ablative strategy (rotablation if there is a favorable wire bias and orbital atherectomy if wire bias is unfavorable). Eruptive nodules are amenable for balloon-based strategies. Arc of calcium defines need for further specific plaque modification with increasing need as calcium starts occupying more than two quadrants. Thick calcium (>0.5 mm) would need specific modification, especially with IVL.

TABLE 1: Studies which tested angiographic guidance versus imaging-guided PCI.

Criteria	Studies	Achieved mean MSA in group which showed clinical benefit
MSA > distal RLA	• IVUS XPL	5.9 mm^2 (MLA)
	• CTO IVUS	5.2 mm^2 (MSA)
	• OPTIVUS (stent > 28 mm)	5.7 ± 2.1 mm^2
MSA > 80% average RLA	• RESIST	7.49 ± 1.61 mm^2
	• TULIP	6 ± 3.3 mm^2
	• AIR-CTO	5.92 ± 2.16 mm^2
	• RENOVATE COMPLEX PCI	5.8 ± 2.1 mm^2
	• OPTIVUS (stent < 28 mm)	5.7 ± 2.1 mm^2
	• DOCTORS	6.41 ± 1.99 mm^2
MSA > 90% average RLA	• SIPS	7.95 ± 2.37 mm^2
	• OPTICUS	8.1 ± 2.3 mm^2
	• AVID	7.55 ± 2.82 mm^2
	• ILUMIEN III	5.89 mm^2
	• OPINION	5.28 ± 1.65 mm^2 (OCT) 6.12 ± 2.34 mm^2 (IVUS)
	• OCTACS	6 ± 1.6 mm^2
	• ILUMIEN IV	5.72 ± 2.04 mm^2
	• ULTIMATE	6.09 mm^2

(MSA: minimum stent area, RLA : reference lumen area)

Malapposition (Incomplete Stent Apposition)

Malapposition refers to lack of contact between stent strut and the vessel wall. Malapposition coexisting with underexpansion must be corrected. Broadly, studies have not been able to prove that isolated acute malapposition identified immediately after stent deployment is associated with stent failure. OCT identifies even minor degrees of malapposition due to superior image resolution.[12] Serial OCT analysis has revealed that incomplete stent apposition (ISA) distance reduces on follow-up by growth of endothelial cells and subsequent neointimal proliferation filling gap between stent struts and the vessel wall.[13] Maximum acute ISA distance which predicted persistent malapposition on follow-up for everolimus-eluting stents (EES) and sirolimus-eluting stents (SES) were >355 μm and >285 μm, respectively.[13] OCT evaluation of patients enrolled in a prospective registry identified that severe malapposition as defined by total malapposition volume ≥ 7 mm^3 was more often associated with device-oriented composite endpoints (DoCE) at a median follow-up of 43 months.[14] On the contrary, late incomplete malapposition is a frequent finding in patients whom present with stent failure. In two studies (PRESTIGE[15] and PESTO[16]), malapposition emerged as frequent finding in acute, subacute, and late stent thrombosis. Bern registry noted that persistent or late stent malapposition was an important finding in very late stent thrombosis.[17] So, a minor degree of malapposition (<300–400 μm) could be of no serious consequence, while extensive malapposition as defined by ISA distance of >400 μm extending axially for >1 mm may be corrected with appropriately sized balloon dilatation **(Figs. 9A to D)**.

Stent Edge Dissection

After stent deployment, edges should be free of significant dissection. Characteristics of a stent edge dissection (on IVUS),[18] which are associated with early stent thrombosis include:

- Medial extension
- Dissection flap occupying > 60°
- Flap compromising final lumen cross-section area (CSA) < 5.5 mm^2
- Axial length of dissection > 2–3 mm

OCT has more resolution and identifies more number of edge dissections compared to IVUS.

Hence, OCT identified dissections are twofold higher compared to IVUS.[12] In CLI-OPCI II study, distal edge (but not proximal) dissections > 200 μm in thickness emerged as an independent predictor of MACE (HR = 2.5)[6] **(Fig. 10)**.

Tissue Protrusion

Tissue or plaque protrusion (TP) appears as luminal filling defects after stent deployment. TP appears as prolapse of

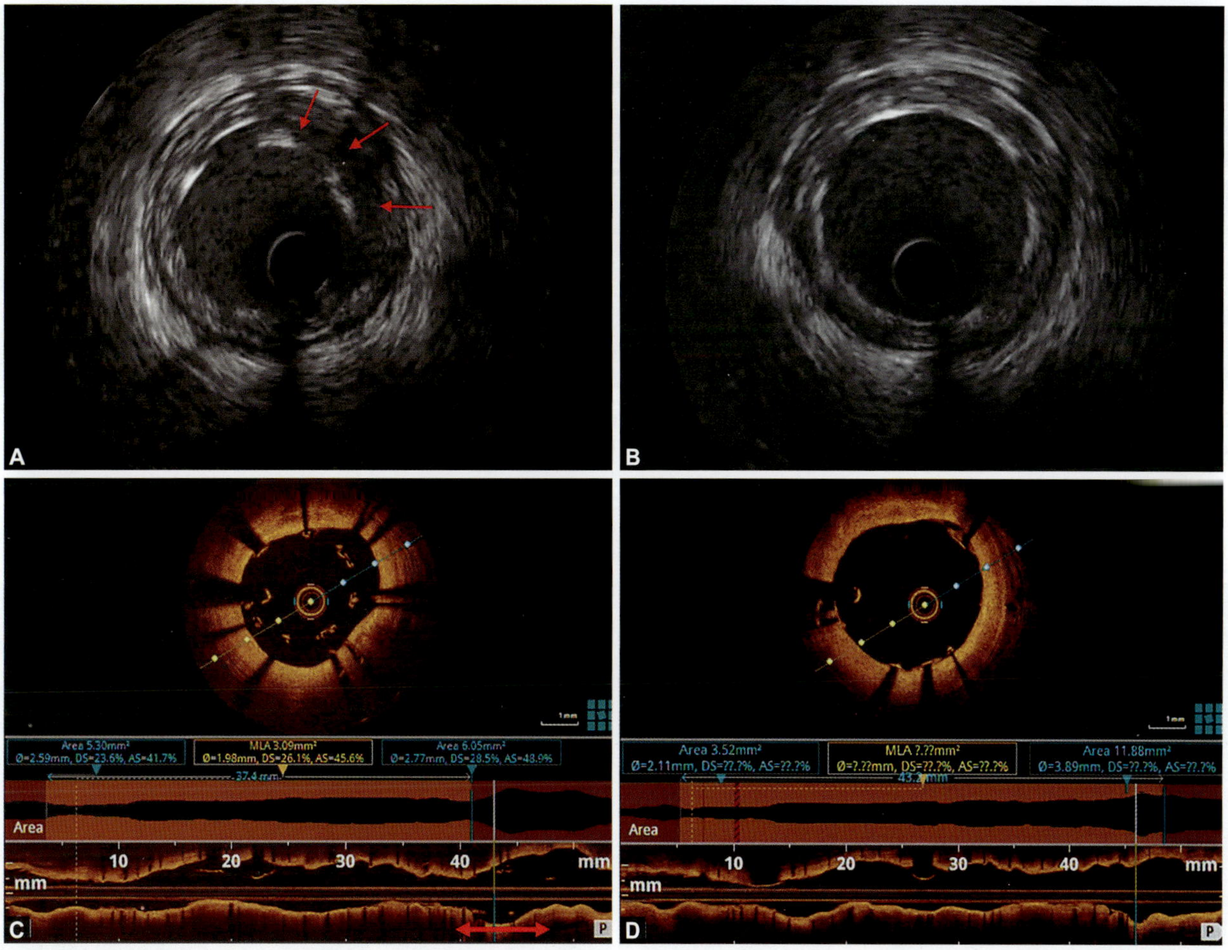

FIGS. 9A TO D: Significant malapposition on IVUS and OCT imaging. (A) Figure shows malapposition from 12 to 3 o'clock position (red arrows) at proximal stent; (B) Corrected with appropriately sized semicompliant balloon at nominal pressures; (C) Figure shows significant malapposition on OCT. Axial distance of incomplete malapposition is indicated in longitudinal view (double-headed red arrow—C); and (D) Malapposition was corrected with balloon dilatation.

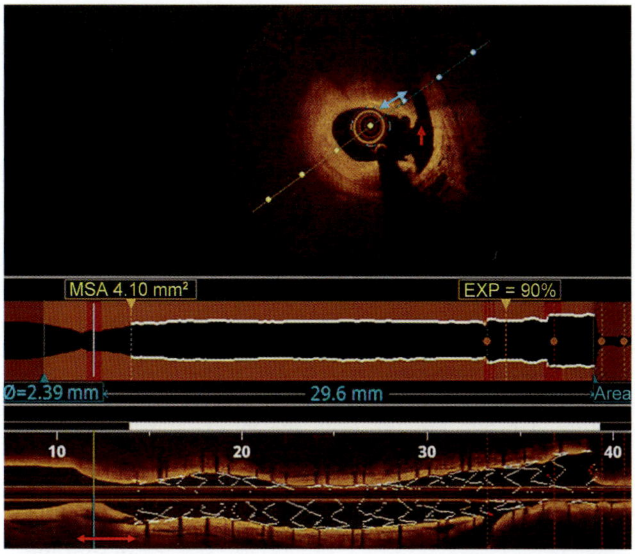

FIG. 10: Stent edge dissection on OCT. Note the dissection extending to media (red arrow) with thickness > 200 µm (double-headed arrow—blue) and axial length > 2 mm (double-headed arrow—red).

plaque material between the stent struts. Often, stent struts appear buried **(Figs. 11A to C)**. OCT can identify more details about TP. Three types of TP have been identified on OCT. Smooth protrusions (often observed after stent placement in stable angina) appear as prolapse with intact intimal surface. Disrupted fibrous tissue protrusion appear as disruption of underlying fibrous tissue protruding in between stent struts. Irregular TP appear as protrusion of material with an irregular surface. Latter two types of TPs are often observed in context of ACS **(Figs. 12A to C)**.

TP causing luminal compromise was an important predictor of early stent thrombosis in HORIZONS AMI study.[18] A 13-month imaging follow-up of same study confirmed that TP which were observed in 2/3rd of all cases following both paclitaxel-eluting stents (PES) and bare metal stent (BMS) implantation, all had resolved during follow-up; proving that most TP disappear over time[19] **(Figs. 13A to C)**. In a registry which analyzed poststent OCT images, presence of irregular TP and small MSA were predictors of DoCE at 1 year.[20]

Stent optimization targets are summarized in **Box 4**.

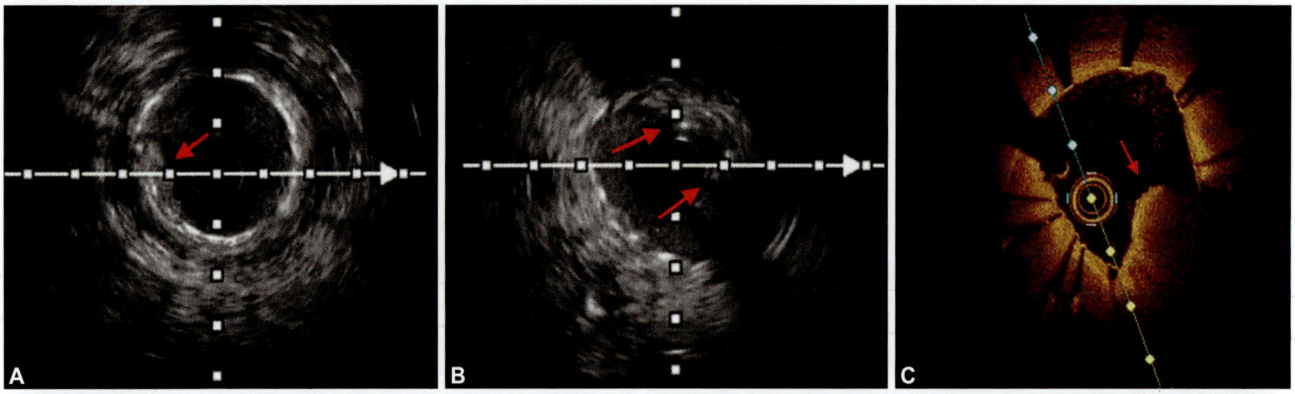

FIGS. 11A TO C: Tissue protrusion. (A) Figure shows small TP at 8 o'clock position; (B) Shows large TP between 11 and 2 o'clock positions (red arrows). Note the stent struts are not visible due to prolapse. (C) OCT image of tissue prolapse (red arrow).

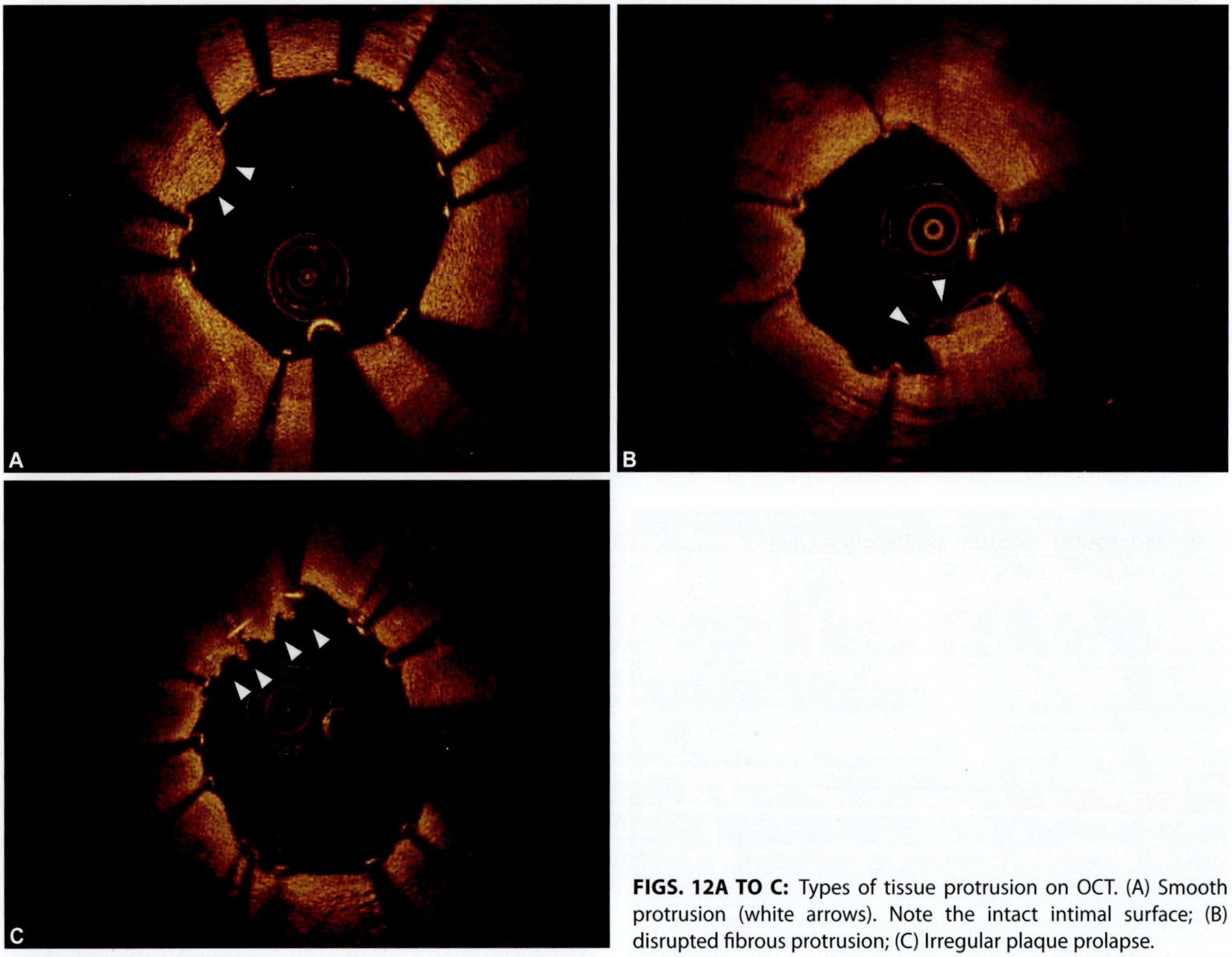

FIGS. 12A TO C: Types of tissue protrusion on OCT. (A) Smooth protrusion (white arrows). Note the intact intimal surface; (B) disrupted fibrous protrusion; (C) Irregular plaque prolapse.

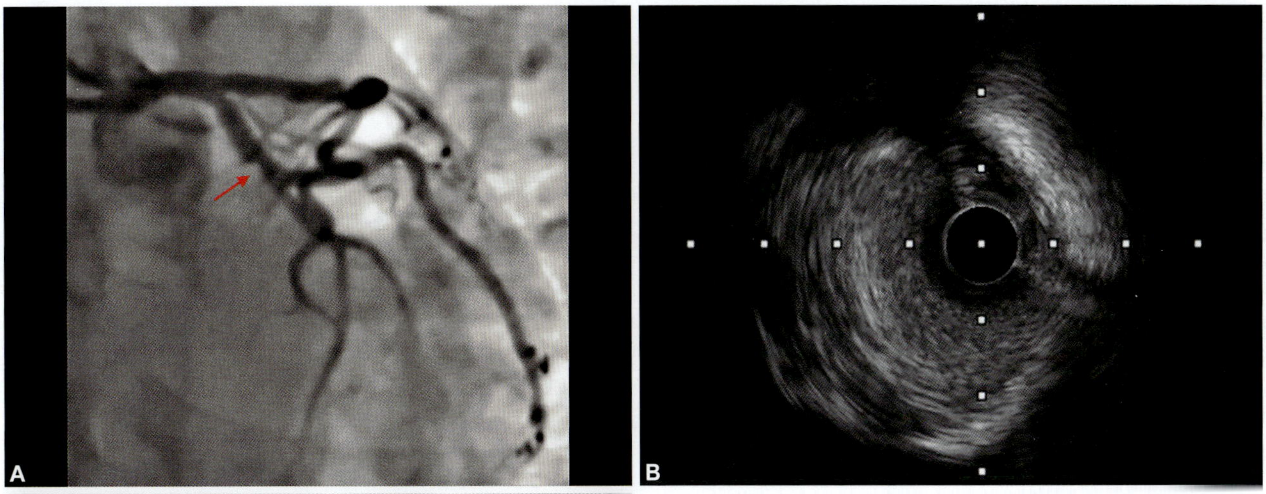

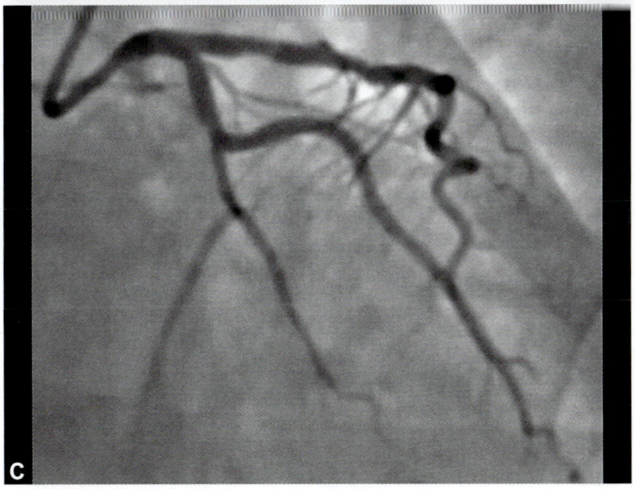

FIGS. 13A TO C: A 65-year-old gentleman presented with acute inferior wall STEMI. (A) After stent deployment from proximal LCX into OM1, there was filling defect seen (A—red arrow); (B) IVUS showed circumferential TP with stent struts fully buried; (C) Patient underwent repeat angiogram on day 10, which showed complete clearance of the filling defect.

BOX 4 Stent optimization targets after PCI.

- Minimum stent area > 5.5 mm^2 (IVUS) > 4.5 mm^2 (OCT)
  - >80–90% of average RLA
  - Malapposition < 400 µm, axial length < 1 mm
- Stent edges: PB < 40%
  - Attenuated plaque/lipid arc < 180°
  - Calcium arc < 180°
  - No thrombus
- Dissection—limited to intima
  - <60°, thickness <200 µm, axial length <2–3 mm
- Tissue protrusion: Not compromising target lumen area

(RLA: reference lumen area)

USE OF INTRACORONARY IMAGING IN INTERVENTIONS FOR ACUTE CORONARY SYNDROMES

Intracoronary imaging guidance improves outcomes after PCI in patients with acute coronary syndromes (ACS). In an all-comer population, there were significant reductions in 1-year rates of definite/probable stent thrombosis (0.6% vs. 1% HR 0.4, 95% CI 0.21–0.73, $p = 0.003$), MI (2.5% vs. 3.7%; HR 0.66, 95% CI 0.49–0.88, $p = 0.004$), and composite MACE (3.1% vs. 4.7%, HR 0.70, 95% CI 0.55–0.88, $p = 0.002$) with IVUS compared to angiographic guidance in patients with ACS undergoing PCI.[21] Imaging helps to distinguish between plaque erosion and plaque rupture. Among 55 patients who had imaging detected plaque erosion as mechanism of ACS, treatment with aspirin and ticagrelor without stent placement remained stable at both 30 days[22] and 1 year free of MACE[23] **(Fig. 14)**.

No reflow is an important complication in patients undergoing primary PCI. Presence of attenuated plaque at lesion site was significant predictor of slow flow and patients who developed this complication[24] have higher mean attenuation score derived from IVUS[25] **(Figs. 15A to C)**. In a study which studied 200 patients with ACS, those with IVUS detected plaque attenuation length of ≥5 mm randomized to distal protection with a filter device had significant reduction in slow flow versus conventional PCI and lower corrected TIMI frame counts (confirming lower microvascular obstruction).[26]

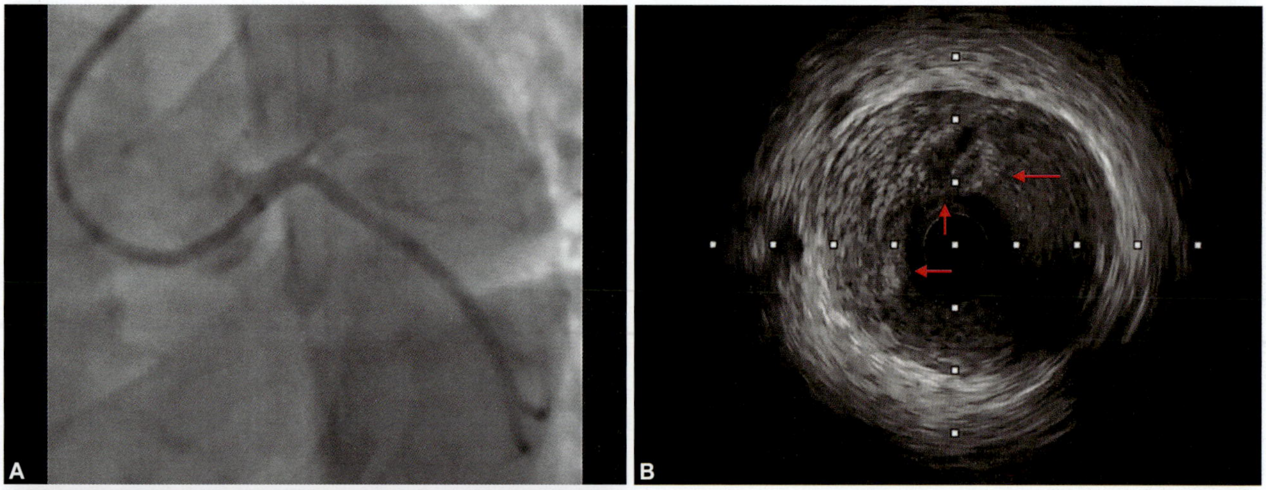

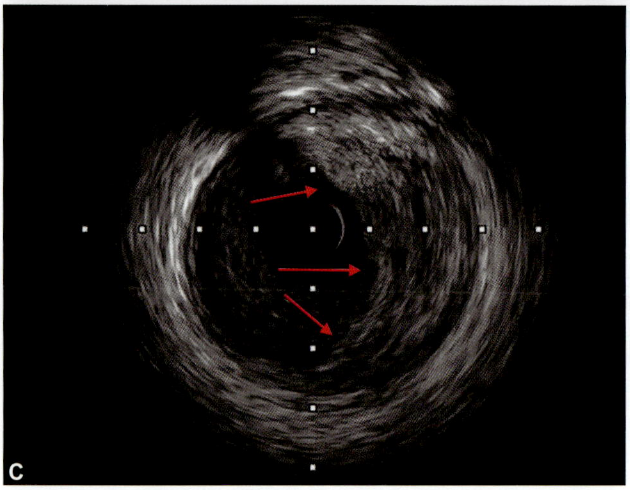

FIGS. 14A TO C: (A) A 33-year-old gentleman presented with acute anterior wall STEMI; (B) IVUS showed luminal thrombus. He was treated with DAPT, GP IIb/IIIa inhibitors and LMWH. Repeat IVUS on day 4; and (C) The figure shows complete clearance of thrombus with plaque from 12 to 6 o'clock position. IVUS shows no evidence of intimal disruption extending into media.

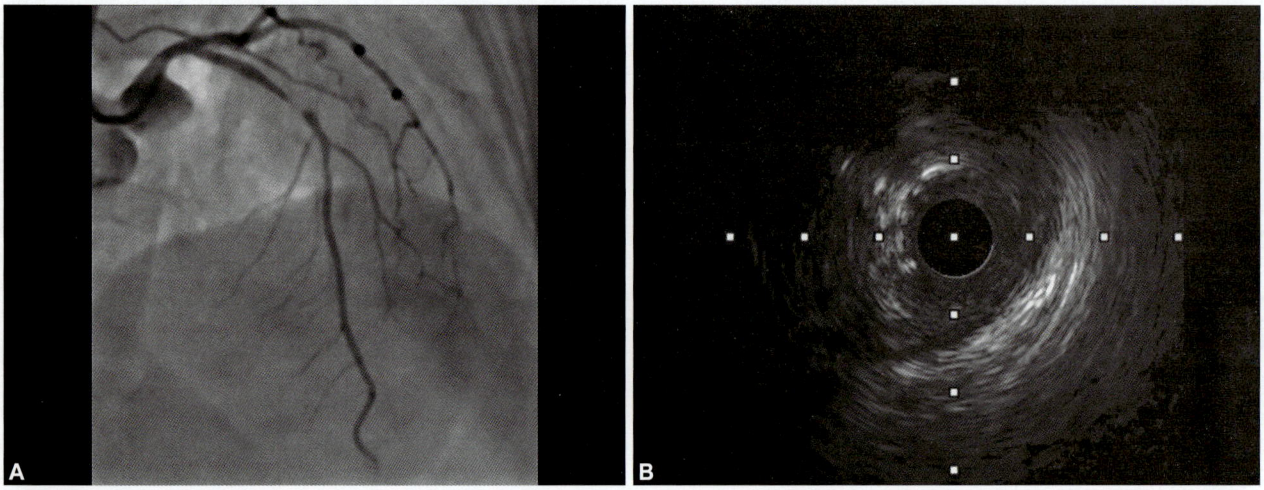

FIGS. 15A TO C: *Continued*

Continued

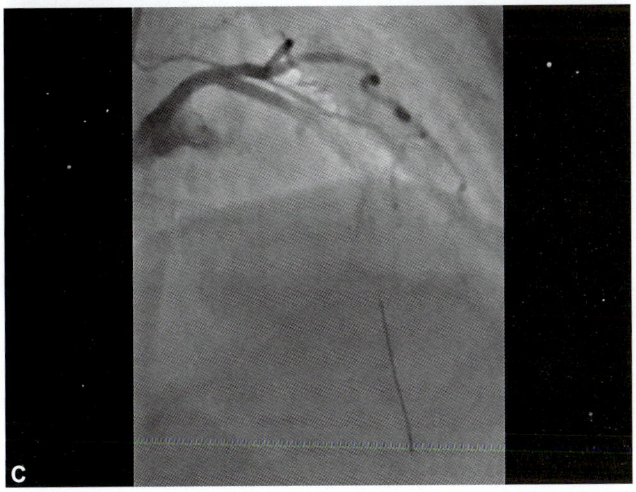

FIGS. 15A TO C: A 46-year-old lady presented with acute NSTE-ACS. (A) Angiogram showed proximal LAD tubular critical lesion; (B) IVUS showed significant ultrasound attenuation from 6 to 2 o'clock position; and (C) Patient developed severe slow flow after placement of stent.

Presence of thrombus is an important predictor of slow flow. High-definition IVUS (HD IVUS) helps to characterize age of thrombus[27] **(Figs. 16A to C)**. In a prospective single-center observational cohort study investigating impact of HD IVUS-guided primary PCI, presence of high thrombus burden (defined by thrombus score > 2 points) were associated with higher rates of impaired final TIMI flow after PCI.[28] Importantly, the study confirmed limitation of angiographic thrombus grading. Around 57.4% of patients who were classified as TIMI thrombus score 4–5 (high angiographic thrombus score) had low IVUS-derived thrombus score highlighting specificity of imaging assessment of thrombotic lesion.[29]

In a prospective multicenter randomized controlled trial assessing impact of IVUS-guided versus angiography-guided PCI for patients with ACS, imaging-guided optimized PCI was associated with significant reduction in primary endpoint of target vessel failure (composite of cardiac death, target vessel MI and clinically driven target vessel revascularization) at 1 year.[30]

Guidance and Optimization in Left Main Interventions

Left main (LM) disease is observed in 5–7% of patients undergoing coronary angiography, is a condition known for its higher mortality and morbidity.[31] PCI of LM disease is already recommended by the clinical guidelines, especially in those cases with low and intermediate SYNTAX scores.[1] IVUS use for procedural optimization of unprotected LM-PCI has been given Class IIa recommendation with level of evidence B.[1] An analysis from the National Society Database, intravascular imaging-guided unprotected LM-PCI was associated with significant reduction in 30-day and 1-year mortality.[32] In a subanalysis of a large RCT which tested benefit of imaging guidance for PCI to complex coronary lesions, LM subset showed statistically significant reduction in hard endpoint of cardiac death in imaging arm when compared to angiographic guidance[33] after a median follow-up of 2.1 years; confirming the importance of imaging during PCI to LM.

Procedural Guidance for LM-PCI

LM stenosis can occur in the ostial (23%), mid shaft (15%) and distal (61%) segments. Depending on the location and severity of the disease, treatment strategies differ.[34] When evaluating ostial LM lesions, its important to disengage the guiding catheter to avoid confusing with ostial stenosis and maintain a coaxial relationship between the IVUS catheter and the LM ostium **(Figs. 17A and B)**. OCT is generally not recommended to evaluate LM ostium (although there are recently described techniques[35]), while can be used for assessment of lesions involving shaft and distal parts. Always perform imaging pullbacks from both LAD and LCX to evaluate individual lesions and its not recommended to infer status of other vessel tangentially during pullback as ostial lumen dimensions and plaque burden can be misleading **(Figs. 18A to C)**. Proximal 5 mm of both daughter branches are segments of interest during the procedure. LM dimensions can be overestimated when performing pullback from angulated branch (usually LCX) due to oblique transducer position. Hence LM dimensions should be assessed from straighter branch **(Fig. 19)**. If no straight branches are available, smaller dimension is more accurate since dimensions can only be artificially large. When assessing lesions at distal LM (dLM) and proximal daughter branches, its important to consider the diffuse nature of atherosclerosis. In a systematic IVUS assessment of dLM, LAD and LCX, plaque was continuous from dLM into ostia of LAD and LCX in 62% of cases, irrespective of angiographic

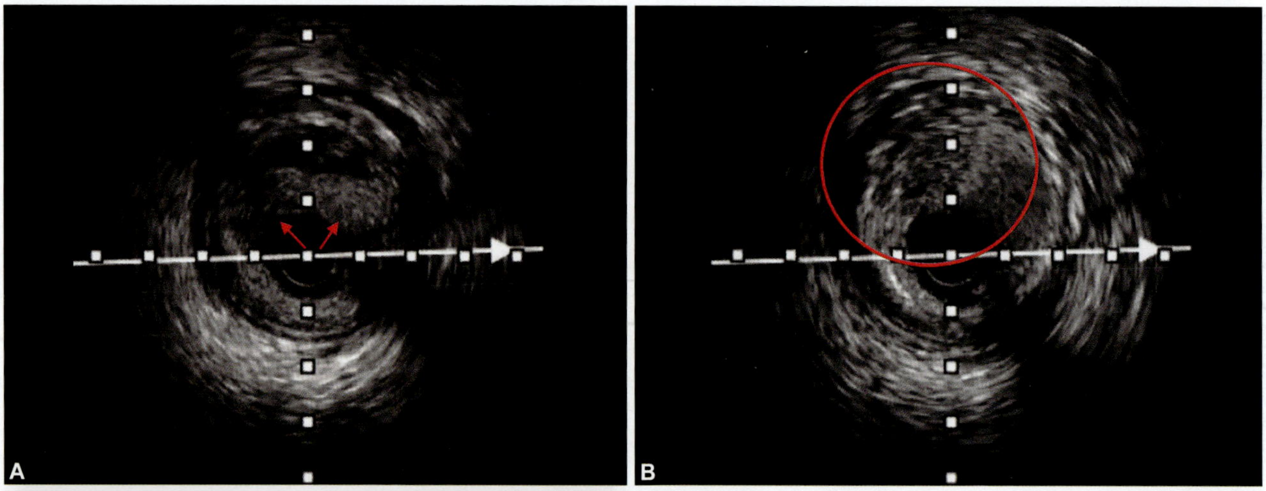

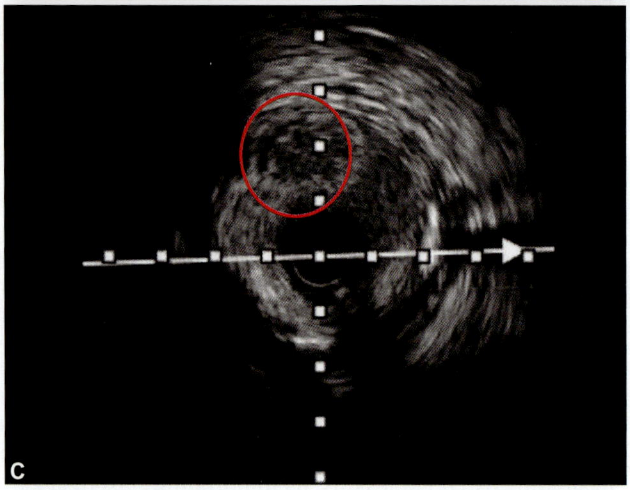

FIGS. 16A TO C: Imaging helps to detect the age of thrombus. (A) Acute thrombus reflect ultrasound with little signal attenuation, appear white with clear delineation; (B) Subacute thrombus contain a mixture of fibrin, RBCs and platelets will appear luminal shadow with mixed echo density; and (C) Organized thrombus contains predominantly RBCs and fibrin and will absorb ultrasound signals and appear dark.

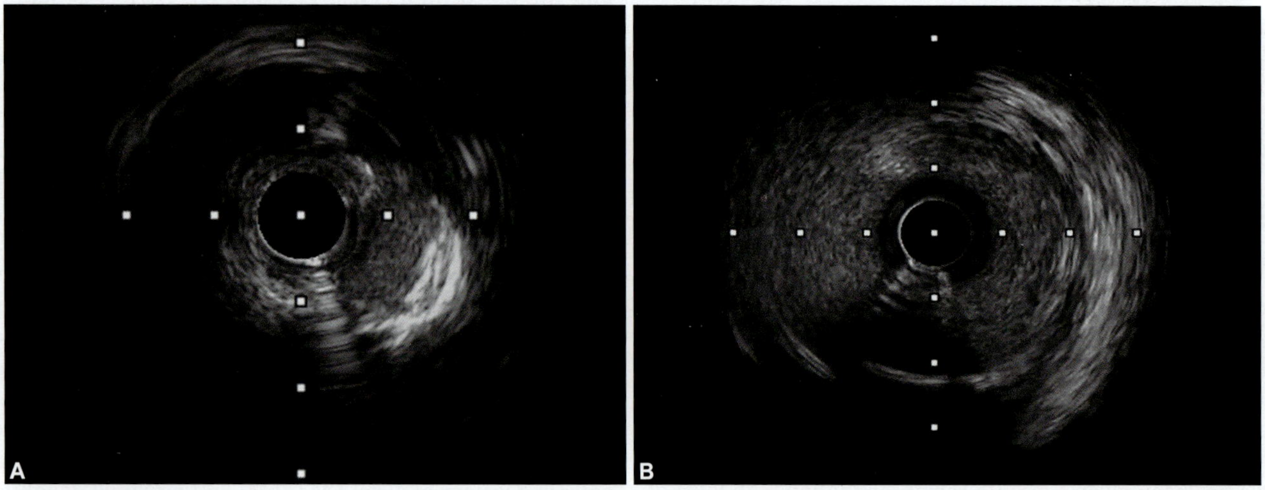

FIGS. 17A AND B: Importance of disengaging guide catheter from LM ostium. (A) On left with catheter engaging ostium shows artificial stenosis of the segment which (B) becomes clear after pullback is performed after disengaging the catheter

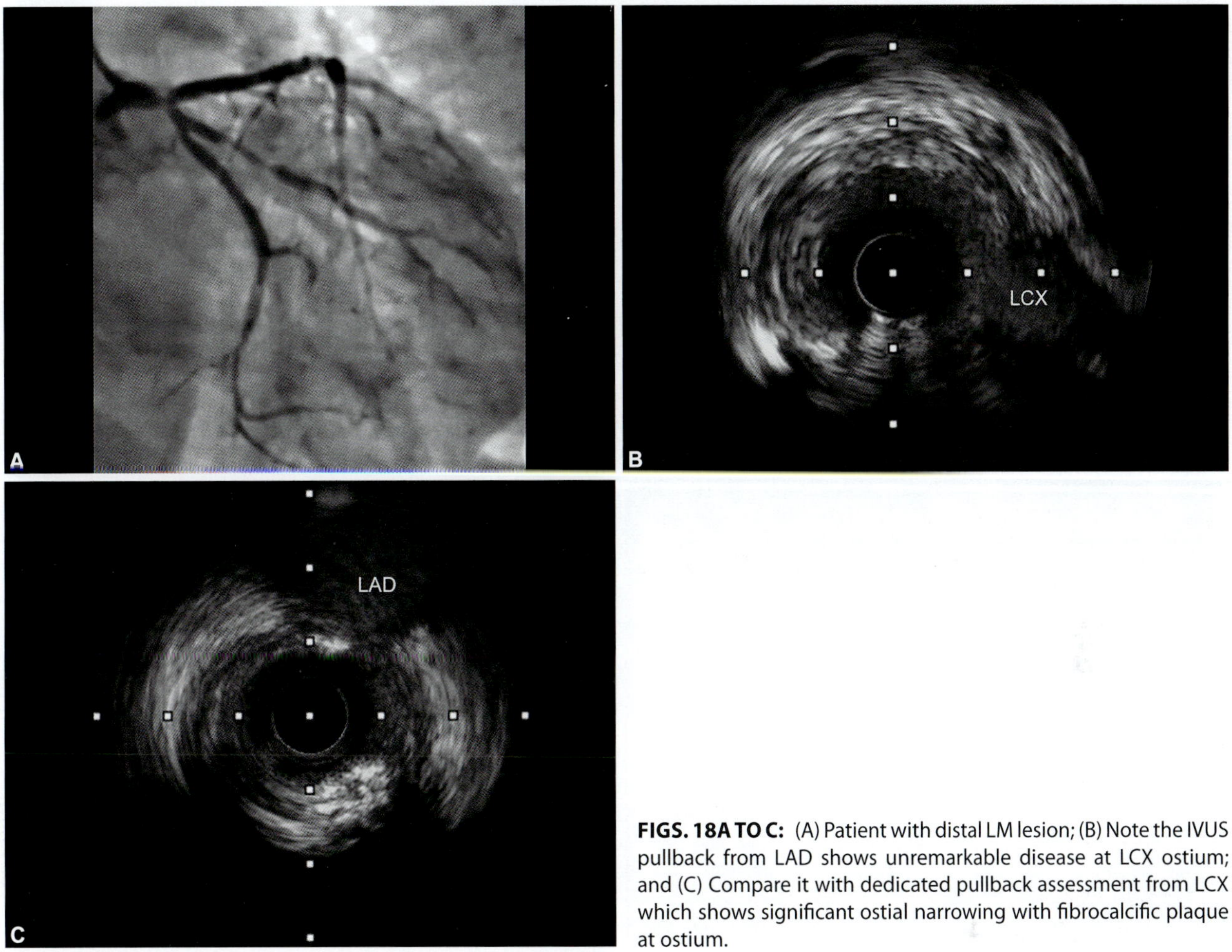

FIGS. 18A TO C: (A) Patient with distal LM lesion; (B) Note the IVUS pullback from LAD shows unremarkable disease at LCX ostium; and (C) Compare it with dedicated pullback assessment from LCX which shows significant ostial narrowing with fibrocalcific plaque at ostium.

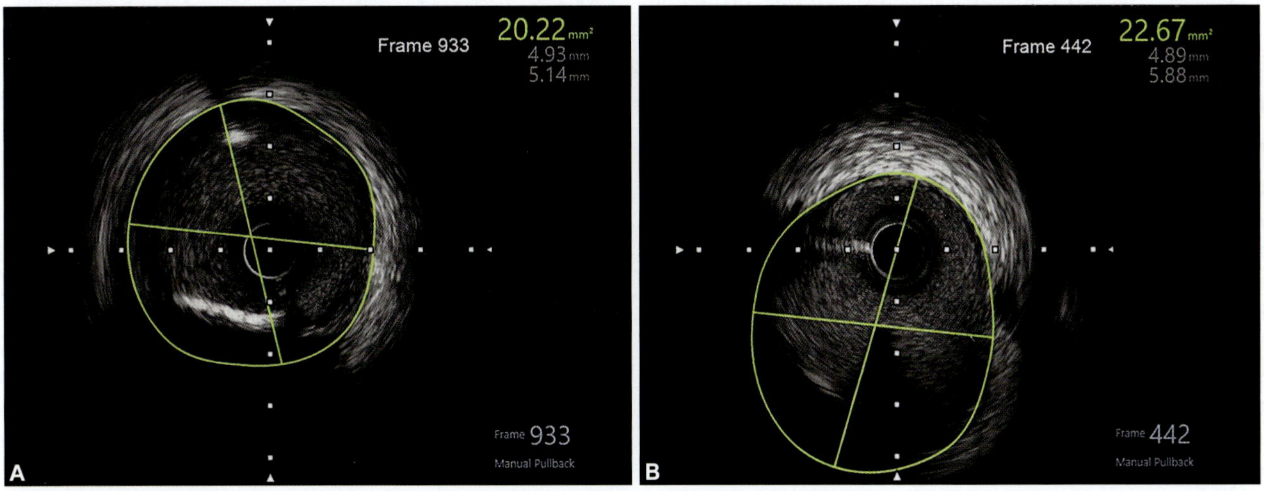

FIGS. 19A AND B: Difference in LM dimensions assessed from straighter branch (left—LAD) versus from an angulated side branch (right—LCX). Note the difference in LM diameter assessed from LAD (average 5 mm) versus from LCX (average 5.4 mm).

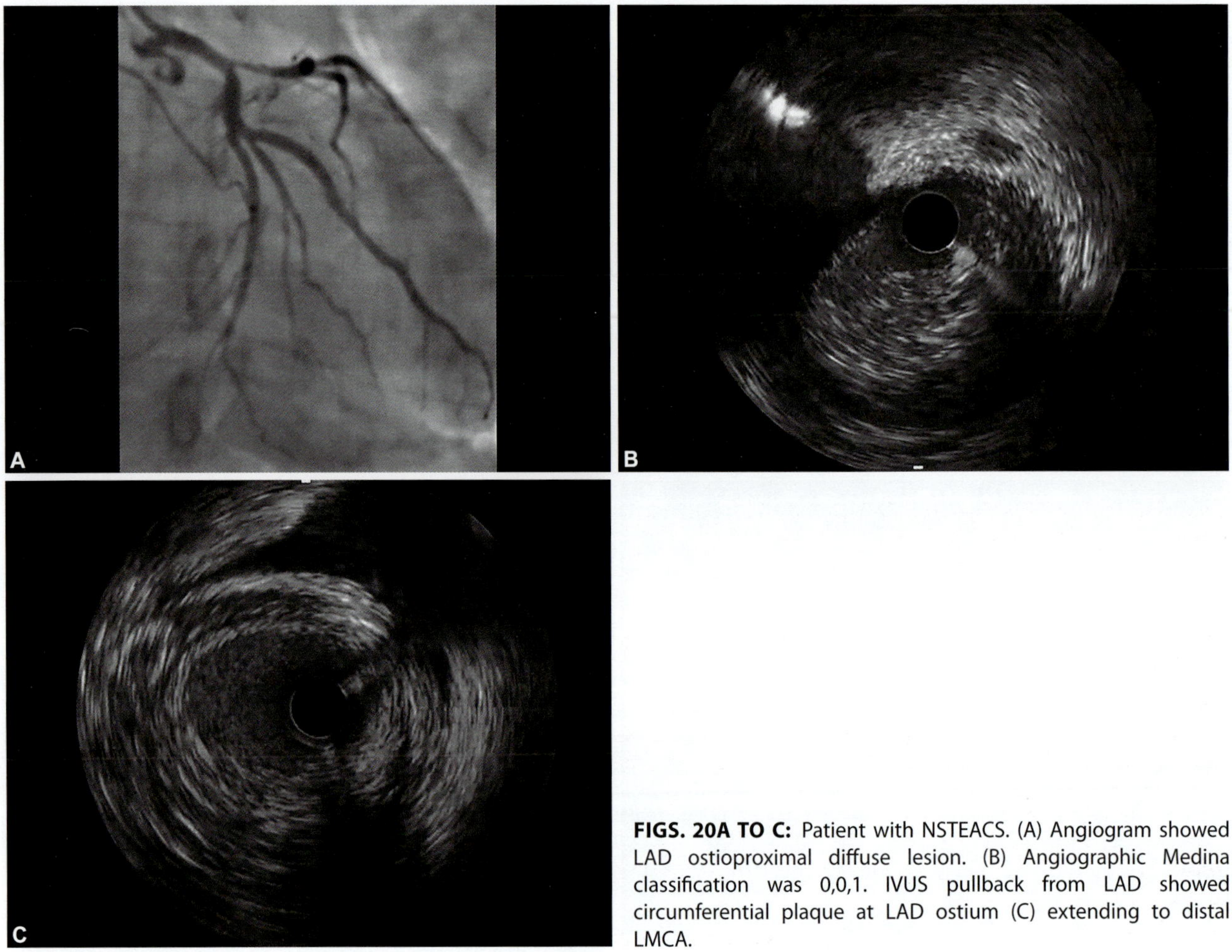

FIGS. 20A TO C: Patient with NSTEACS. (A) Angiogram showed LAD ostioproximal diffuse lesion. (B) Angiographic Medina classification was 0,0,1. IVUS pullback from LAD showed circumferential plaque at LAD ostium (C) extending to distal LMCA.

Medina classification,[36] confirming the point that isolated branch ostial disease is rare **(Figs. 20A and B)**.

Imaging Assessment of LMCA Disease: Indications for Treatment

Unlike other segments of coronary tree, LM has relatively constant area of myocardial supply. In majority of individuals, LM supplies 80% of myocardial territory. Hence, correlation between LM and MLA and physiological significance is predictable and subject to less variability. The three studies reported correlation between IVUS-derived MLA and fractional flow reserve **(Table 2)** and three other studies reported correlation between IVUS MLA cutoffs and long term clinical events **(Table 3)**. The strategy for selection of patients with angiographic intermediate LM lesions for revascularization based on IVUS is illustrated in **Flowchart 1**.

LM Intervention: Imaging-guided Optimization Goals

Imaging would help to provide following important information during PCI to LM:

- Vessel dimensions of proximal LAD and LCX
- Plaque burden and calcifications at ostia of SB
- Length of disease in LM and daughter branches
- Any tapering or reverse tapering morphology of LM trunk **(Figs. 21A to D)**

The EBC consensus recommends stepwise provisional side branch stenting strategy for most of distal LM bifurcation lesions.[43] Yet, when disease at SB ostia are extensive (>10 mm) or when operator feels that rescue of SB is difficult after MB stent placement, an upfront two-stent strategy may be considered.[44]

Imaging has identified predictors of SB compromise after MB stent placement in a crossover technique.

TABLE 2: Studies that reported correlation between IVUS parameters and FFR.

Study	FFR cutoff	IVUS parameters	Sensitivity/Specificity
Jasti et al.[37] *N* = 55	<0.75	• MLD < 2.8 mm • MLA < 5.9 mm^2 • AS > 50% • CSN > 67%	93%/98% 93%/94% 86%/80% 90%/88%
Kang et al.[38] *N* = 55	<0.8	• MLA < 4.8 mm^2 • PB > 72%	89%/83% 73%/79%
	<0.75	• MLA < 4.1 mm^2 • PB > 76% • Presence of plaque rupture	95%/83% 79%/81%
Park et al.[39] *N* = 112	<0.8	• MLA < 4.1–4.5 mm^2 • PB > 77% • Presence of plaque rupture	77%/82% 70%/82% 76%/88.9%

[AS: area of stenosis (reference lumen CSA – lesion CSA × 100/reference lumen CSA), CSN: cross-sectional narrowing (plaque + media CSA/external elastic membrane (EEM) CSA; MLA: minimum lumen area; PB: plaque burden]

TABLE 3: Clinical that reported correlation between IVUS-derived parameters and clinical endpoints.

Study/Duration	IVUS parameters	Clinical endpoints
Abizaid et al.[40] *N* = 122 Time : 12 months	• Lumen CSA: 6.8 ± 4.4 mm^2 • MLD: 2.3 ± 0.69 mm • Max lumen diameter: 3.07 ± 0.77 mm • CSN: 70 ± 14% • AS: 52 ± 21%	• Cardiac death: 3% • PTCA: 20% • CABG: 9%
LITRO[41] *N* = 354 Time: 2 years	• MLA: 4.8 ± 0.8 mm^2 • MLD: 2.2 ± 0.3 mm • Max LD : 3.1 ± 0.7 mm • EEM area: 16.1 ± 5 mm^2 • PB > 50%	• MLA < 6 mm^2 + revascularization: Cardiac death-free survival = 94.5% • MLA ≥ 6 mm^2 + deferral: Cardiac death-free survival = 97.7%
Fassa et al.[42] *N* = 121 Time: 3.5 ± 2.1 years	MLA < 7.5 mm^2	No difference in event rates between MLA < 7.5 mm^2 + revascularization vs. MLA ≥ 7.5 mm^2 + deferral

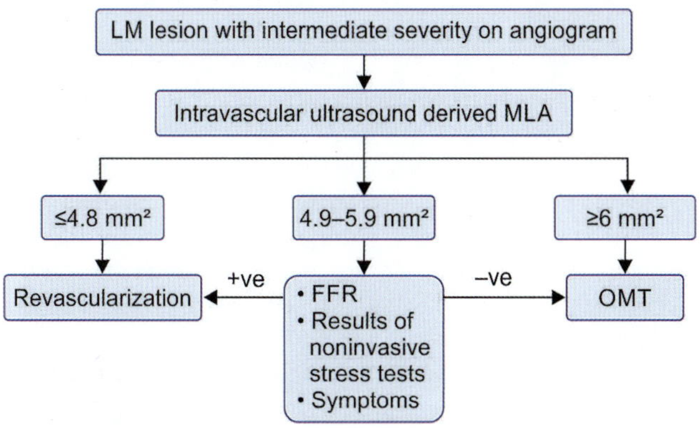

FLOWCHART 1: Management algorithm for patients with LM lesions and angiographic intermediate severity based on IVUS cutoffs.

- Preprocedural MLA of <3.7 mm^2 at SB ostium and PB of >56% predicted compromised SB post-PCI FFR of <0.8 in a series of patients undergoing LM stenting with crossover technique[45] **(Figs. 22A to D)**.
- A calcium arc of >60° at the MLA site in either distal LM or LAD ostium was an independent predictor of poststent narrowing at LCX ostium.[46]
- Patients with spiky/vulnerable carina—"eyebrow sign"—are at particular risk of adverse carinal shift toward SB ostium[47] **(Figs. 23A to C)**.

Poststent MSA optimization targets for LM PCI are indicated in **Table 4**. A good MSA at outflow regions, i.e., LAD and LCX ostioproximal regions are as important as target in LM. The current optimal stent expansion criteria, which define lowest MACE rates are at least 6 mm^2 at LCX ostium, 8 mm^2 at LAD ostium, and 12 mm^2 at LM.

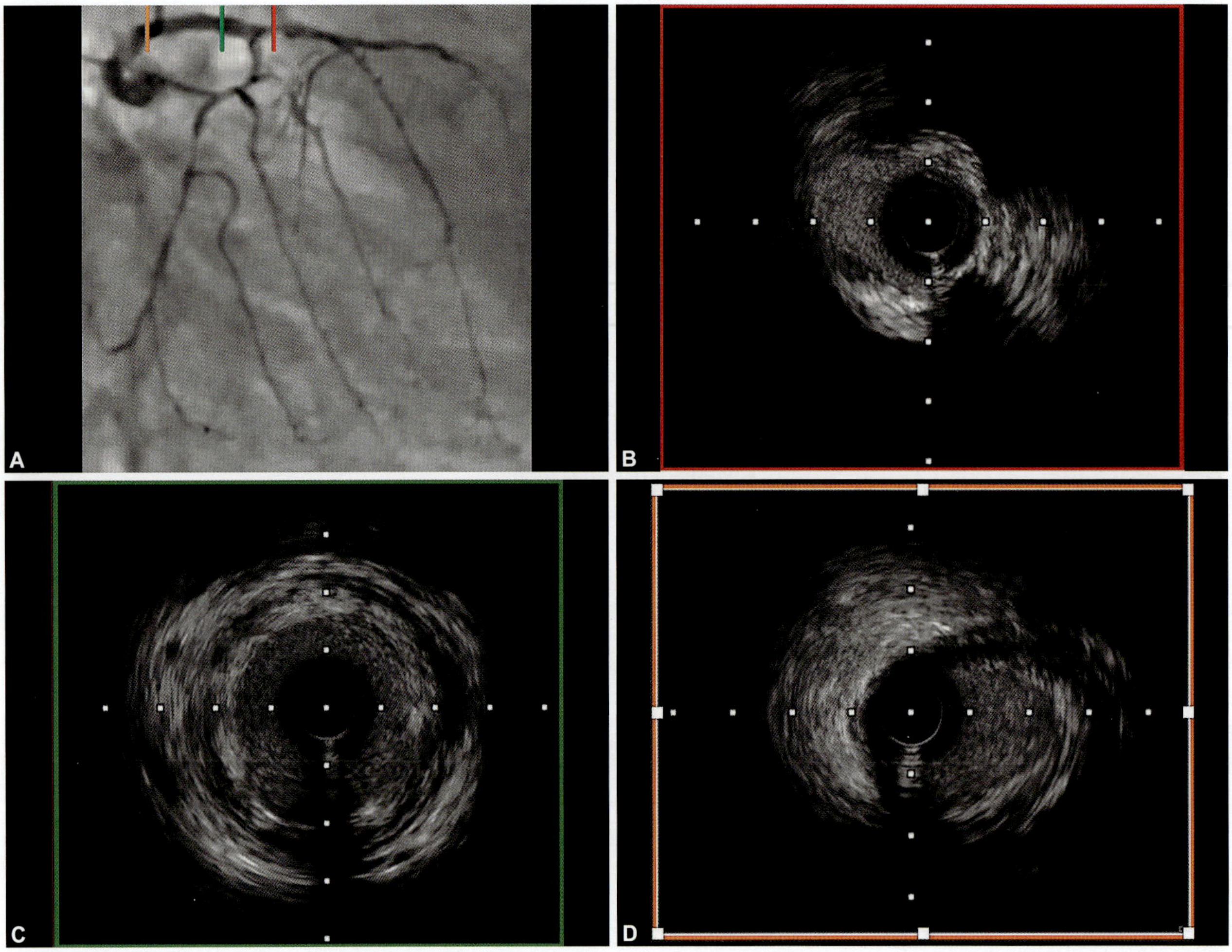

FIGS. 21A TO D: A 67-year-old lady presented with NSTE-ACS. (A) Angiogram showed ostial LAD tubular 90% lesion. IVUS sections from different segments indicated by color codes; (B) Ostial LAD has circumferential lipid-rich plaque; (C) Distal LM shows vessel size of 4 mm; (D) Ostial LM shows significant negative remodeling with vessel diameter of 3 mm. This particular anatomy of LM has funnel shape. Stent diameter has to be selected according to smaller segment dimensions and approximated at larger segments with appropriately sized balloon.

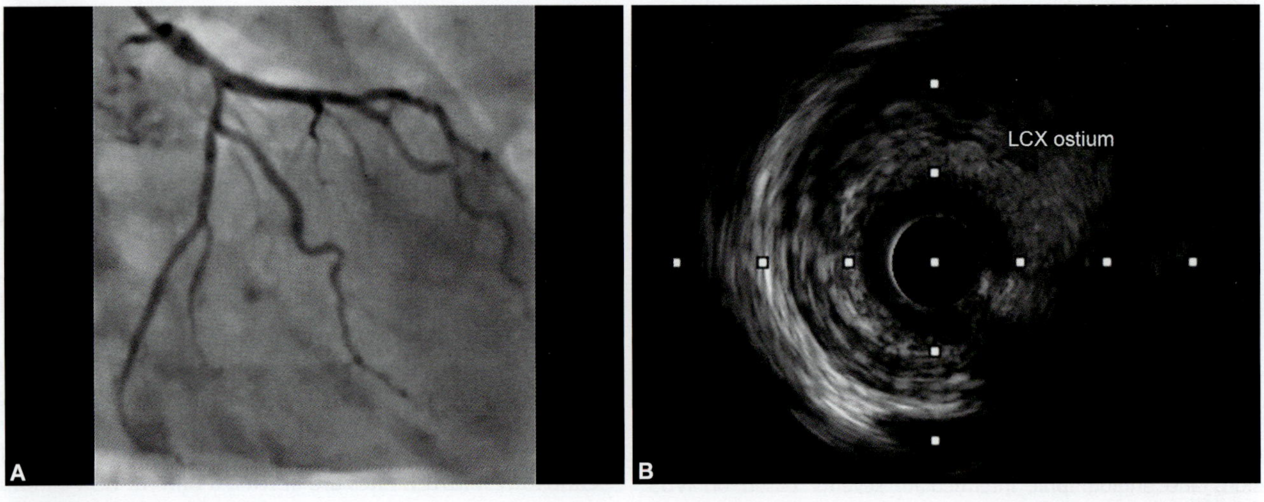

FIGS. 22A TO D: *Continued*

Continued

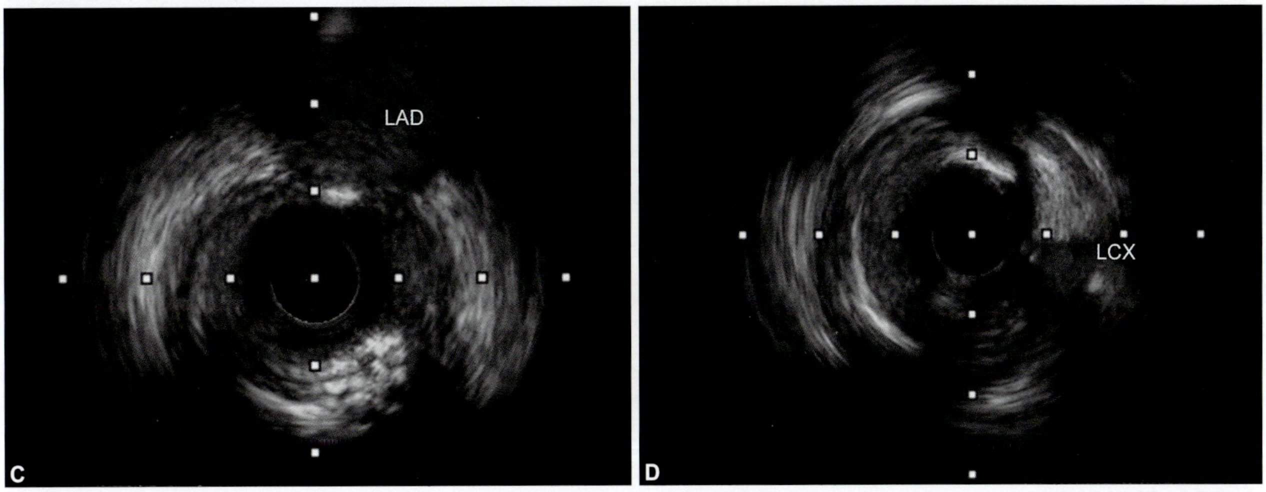

FIGS. 22A TO D: A 65-year-old gentleman presented with NSTE-ACS. (A) Angiogram showed hazy eccentric lesion at distal LM; (B) IVUS evaluation of LM showed hypoechoic plaque with lumen compromise at distal portion; (C) LCX ostium had MLA of 2.17 mm^2 with plaque burden of 74%. High plaque burden and MLA < 3.7 mm^2 at LCX ostium predict SB closure when a cross over stent is performed from LM in to LAD; (D) LAD ostium is shown in figure.

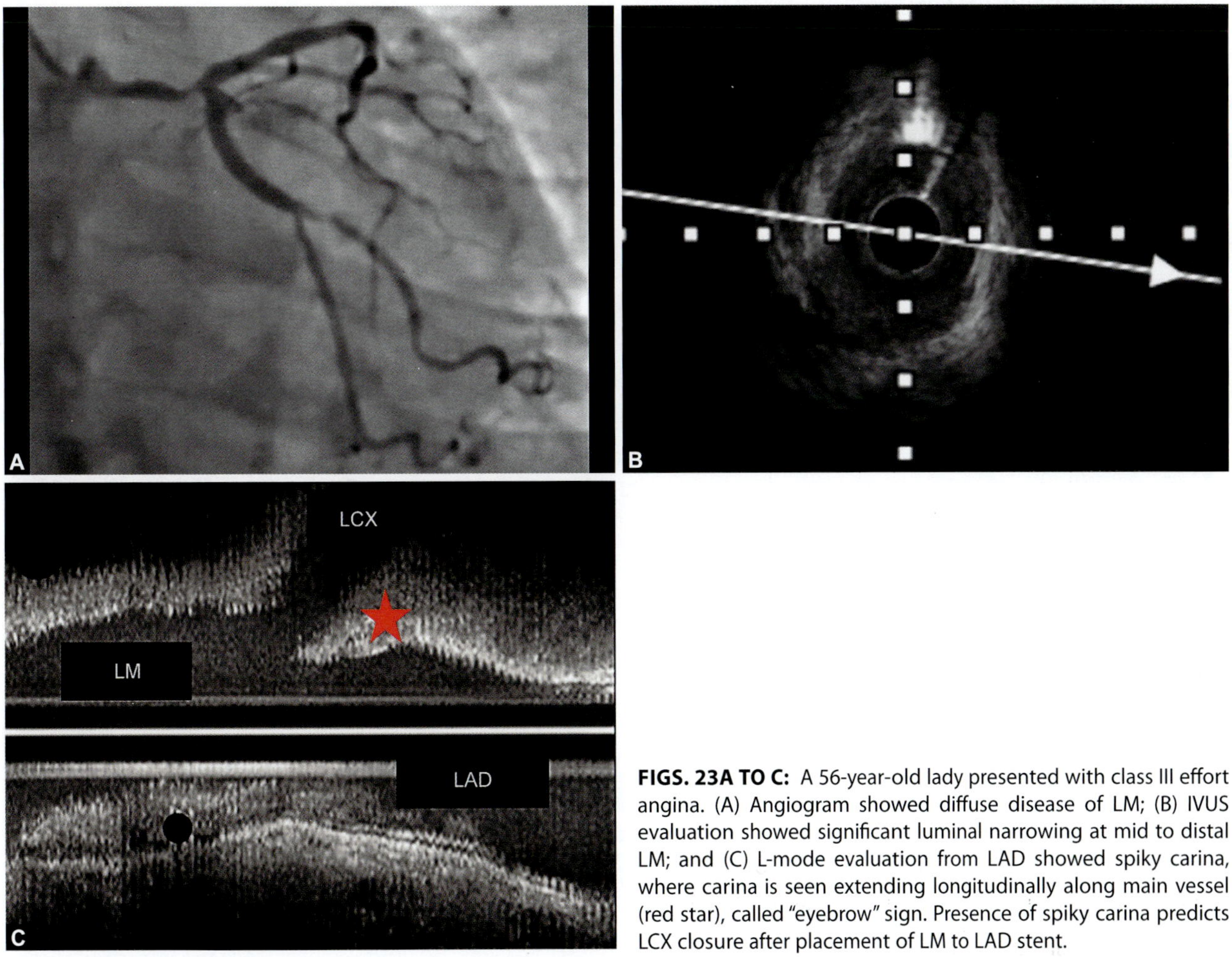

FIGS. 23A TO C: A 56-year-old lady presented with class III effort angina. (A) Angiogram showed diffuse disease of LM; (B) IVUS evaluation showed significant luminal narrowing at mid to distal LM; and (C) L-mode evaluation from LAD showed spiky carina, where carina is seen extending longitudinally along main vessel (red star), called "eyebrow" sign. Presence of spiky carina predicts LCX closure after placement of LM to LAD stent.

TABLE 4: Minimum stent areas and outcomes after LM-PCI.

Study	LAD	LCX	POC	LM	Endpoints	Time
Kang et al.[48]	6.3 mm^2	5.0 mm^2	7.2 mm^2	8.2 mm^2	Angiographic	9 months
Excel study[*49]	NA	NA	NA	9.8 mm^2	Death, MI, ST	3 years
NOBLE[*50]	10.1 ± 2.9 mm^2	9.6 ± 3.4 mm^2	16.9 + 4.2 mm^2	12.5 ± 3.0 mm^2	MACE	5 years
Hernadez et al.[¶28]	8.5 mm^2 (7.4–9.2)	7 mm^2 (6.3–7.6)	NA	11.8 mm^2 (10.2–12.6)	MACE	1 year
Kim et al[†51]	8.3 mm^2	5.7 mm^2	NA	11.8 mm^2	MACE	5 years

*EXCEL & NOBLE tested CABG versus PCI for LM lesions. IVUS substudy analyzed patients enrolled in PCI arm of the respective studies. Patients in lowest tertile of MSA (<9 mm^2 for EXCEL and <10.8 mm^2 in NOBLE) had higher event rates compared with patients who were in highest tertile (>11 mm^2 in EXCEL and >13.4 mm^2 in NOBLE).

¶Hernandez et al. prospectively assessed optimal relative expansion criteria (defined as > 90% of reference lumen area) and compared with subset from LM database who underwent PCI without optimization protocol. Absolute MSA achieved at individual segments is illustrated in the Table.

†Kim et al. assessed MSA outcomes which predicted MACE rates in patients who underwent upfront two-stent strategy.

CONCLUSION

Imaging-optimized PCI, which is defined as achievement of standard optimization criteria after intervention, has been associated with least MACE rates. Systematic use of imaging at different timelines—before, after lesion preparation, and post stent—helps to achieve optimal results.

ONLINE REFERENCES

Please scan the QR code provided at the end of the table of contents for References of this chapter.

CHAPTER 145

Step-by-Step Physiological Assessment to Accomplish Physiology Guide Percutaneous Coronary Intervention

S Selvamani, JS Thomas Xavier Paulsingh

ABSTRACT

The study of coronary physiology has progressed from a research focus to a crucial component of coronary artery disease management, encompassing both epicardial and microvascular segments. Implementing these methodologies requires using pressure wires alongside additional systems, which demands significant time and practice. This complexity contributes to the relatively low adoption rate. To maximize patient outcomes, it is essential to understand the latest evidence, available techniques, and their proper application. This chapter provides a practical overview of coronary physiology with the goal of ultimately improving the standard of patient care.

Keywords: Coronary artery disease, coronary physiology, pressure wire

INTRODUCTION

Coronary physiology has firmly established its role in percutaneous coronary intervention (PCI), notably through fractional flow reserve (FFR). Initially described by Pijls et al. in 1993, FFR determines the ratio of mean coronary pressure distal to a stenosis to mean aortic pressure, measured during pharmacological vasodilation to nullify resistance.[1] For example, an FFR of 0.70 indicates a 30% reduction in coronary flow from normal, whereas an FFR of 0.90 indicates only a 10% reduction, due to the presence of stenoses. FFR is ideally recommended for stenoses with 50–90% luminal narrowing when noninvasive evidence of ischemia is lacking.[2] The clinical significance of FFR-guided decisions for revascularization is highlighted by evidence from randomized clinical trials.[3] Recently, the instantaneous wave-free ratio (iFR) measured during wave-free period emerged as a nonhyperemic alternative to FFR.[4] During the diastolic phase of the cardiac cycle, a specific wave-free interval has been identified—from 25% after diastole begins to 5 ms before it ends—where coronary blood flow peaks and myocardial contraction ceases. This period mirrors conditions of maximal resting coronary flow and serves as an alternative to hyperemia, eliminating the need for pharmacological vasodilation. Instantaneous wave-free ratio (iFR) quantifies this by comparing the mean pressure distal to a coronary stenosis with the mean pressure at the aortic root during these intervals **(Fig. 1)**.

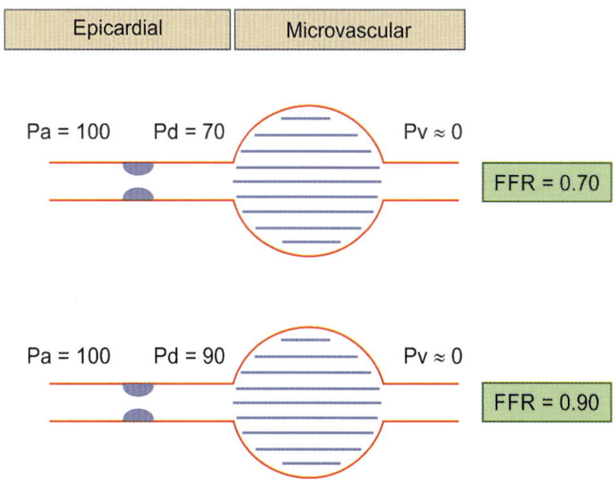

$$FFR = \frac{Pd - Pv}{Pa - Pv} \approx \frac{Pd}{Pa} \text{ (at maximal hyperemia)}$$

FIG. 1: Example of fractional flow reserve (FFR).

PERFORMING FRACTIONAL FLOW RESERVE MEASUREMENTS

Step 1: Patient Preparation

Patients should be informed about possible discomfort (like shortness of breath, angina, palpitations, heat sensation, and sweating) and potential risks, such as coronary injury from catheter or wire insertion, and side effects from hyperemia-inducing medications.

For intravenous hyperemia induction, patients should have adequate venous access (e.g., femoral sheath or cannula up to the cubital vein), or a peripheral location if using regadenoson, with concurrent saline infusion to ensure rapid medication onset. Anticoagulation therapy similar to PCI guidelines is recommended due to foreign body insertion into coronary arteries during measurements.

Patients generally continue their regular medications for FFR.[5] Caffeine's impact is minimal, especially if consumed in small quantities more than an hour before FFR. Theophylline should be stopped at least 12 hours before FFR.[6,7]

Step 2: Catheter Selection and Positioning

Guide catheters without side holes are preferred to avoid issues with adenosine administration and pressure calibration due to turbulence. It is crucial to select a proper catheter that aligns coaxially at the coronary ostium and does not obstruct ostial or proximal lesions, which could lead to inaccurate FFR measurements. When unsure, disengage the catheter from the ostium for proper pressure calibration and recording of pressures **(Fig. 2)**.[8]

Step 3: Calibration

First, ensure aortic pressure is zeroed by placing the pressure transducer at the heart level (one-third to two-thirds of the chest diameter), opening it to atmosphere, and zeroing the pressure. Prepare the FFR wire and connect it to the measurement system via cable or wireless connection.

Specific instructions vary:

- *For St. Jude Aeris® wire*: Lay the wire flat, flush the coil with saline, press "connect wirelessly" on the receiver, and activate the wire's transmitter for automatic pressure sensor zeroing.
- *For Volcano Verrata® wire*: Flush the wire, and then connect. Pressure sensor zeroing occurs automatically when the catheter remains flat and stationary.

If calibration is not done properly, it will delay the procedure as it will require removal of the guide wire and recalibration **(Fig. 3)**.

Step 4: Insert the Guidewire and Do Equalization

The tip of the wire should be carefully shaped to an appropriate curve before introducing it (generally not >45°). Advance the guidewire into the coronary artery until the pressure sensor present at the proximal end of radiopaque portion reaches the tip of the guide catheter. Flush the guide catheter with saline to replace the contrast agent; if needed, disengage it from the coronary artery ostium. Administer 200 µg of nitroglycerin to prevent spasm. Remove the introducer and close the Y connector valve completely. Then equalize the pressures. Avoid using a second wire to prevent artifacts. Ensure pressure curves are stable for several heartbeats before zeroing, as the mean pressure is averaged over three to five beats **(Fig. 4)**.

Step 5: Positioning of the Fractional Flow Reserve Wire

The introducer can be reinserted if necessary, and the guidewire is advanced through the target lesion(s); ideally, the sensor should be kept at least three vessel diameter lengths distal to the stenosis to allow for the phenomenon of pressure recovery. Turbulence in blood flow immediately downstream of the stenosis may lead to a relative drop in blood pressure, which can result in an overestimation of

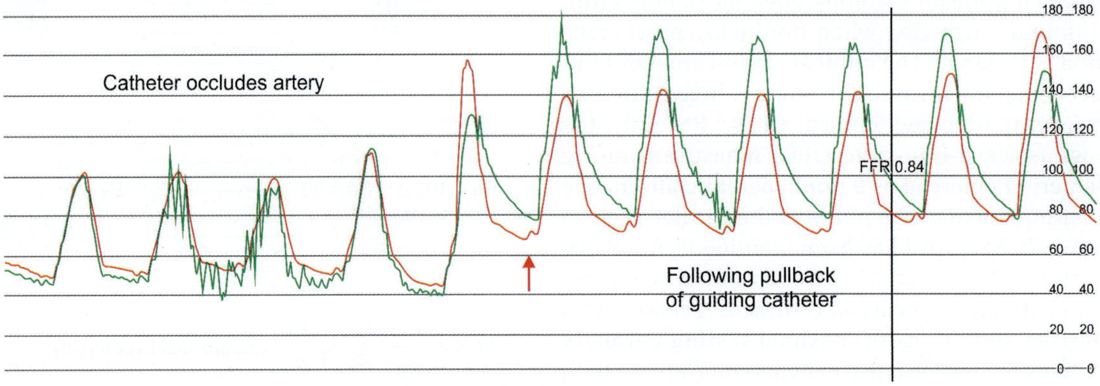

FIG. 2: Error due to catheter wedging. Initially, guide catheter rests on stenosis causing wedge pressure. It leads to underestimation of stenosis severity. Following withdrawal of the guide catheter into the ascending aorta (arrow), the correct pressure values are measured (FFR = 0.84).

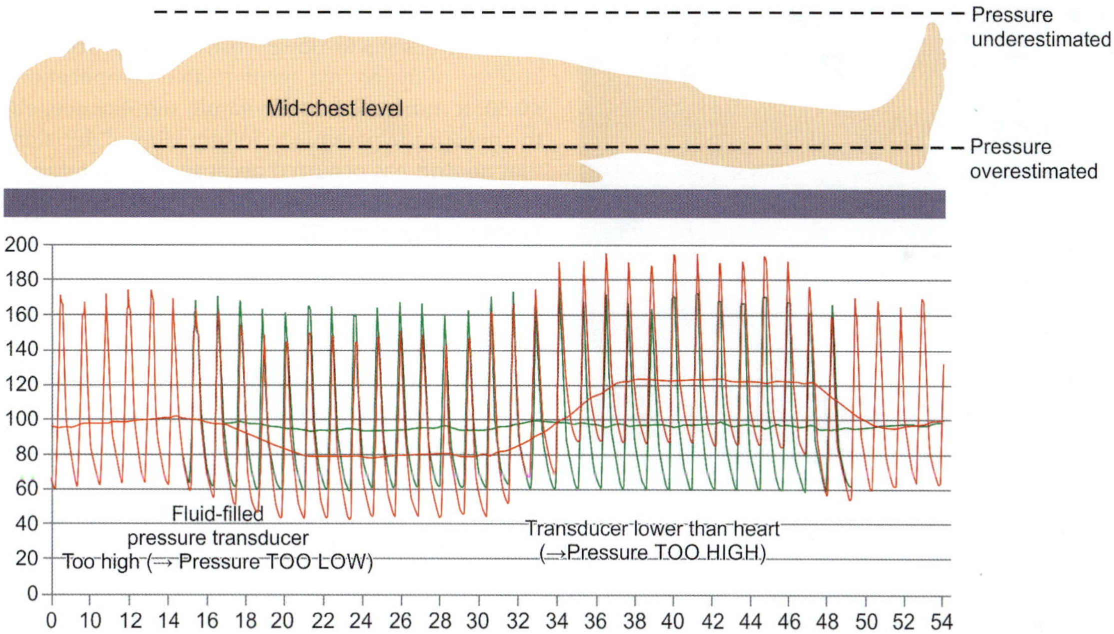

FIG. 3: The influence of an incorrect zero level on pressure recordings. If pressure transducer is kept too high, it will lead to underestimation of pressure. If it is kept too low, it will lead to overestimation of pressure.

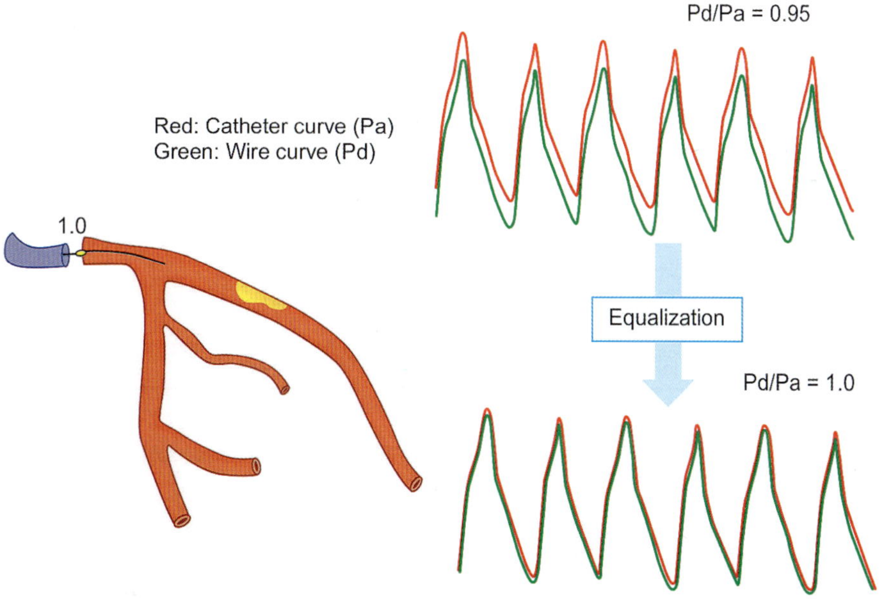

FIG. 4: Equalizing two pressures.

the stenosis's severity when using pressure measurements.[9] During measurement, be cautious of artifacts caused by the FFR wire's pressure sensor interacting with the vessel wall, particularly in small vessels or severely tortuous coronary segments.[10] To avoid these artifacts, avoid placing the sensor in areas with significant tortuosity **(Fig. 5)**.

Step 6: Measure a Resting Physiological Index (Pd/Pa)

Flush the catheter with normal saline because the presence of a viscous contrast can influence the resting indices. Then measure resting Pd/Pa and RFR. Resting Pd/Pa is calculated as mean Pd/Pa over the whole cardiac cycle. RFR is measured

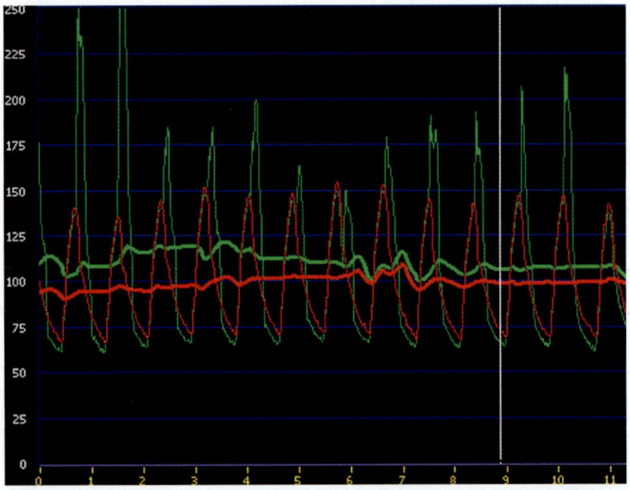

FIG. 5: Whipping artifact due to pressure wire sensor hitting the vessel wall.

as an instantaneous lowest Pd/Pa irrespective of cardiac cycle. Advantages are lower cost, shorter procedure time, and absence of hyperemia agent-related complications.[11] If it is ≤0.80, it indicates hemodynamic significance, eliminating the need for hyperemia to inform clinical decisions. Ensure that no drift has occurred because resting indices are much more influenced by pressure drift than hyperemic indices[12] **(Table 1; Figs. 6 and 7)**.

Step 7: Measure Hyperemic Fractional Flow Reserve

Contrast can induce submaximal hyperemia. Measure cFFR by injecting 8 mL contrast.[13] Then administer vasodilators to induce hyperemia and calculate Pd/Pa. FFR should be measured at stable maximum hyperemia. Maximum hyperemia is identified in the pressure wire tracings by the disappearance of dicrotic notch. Position the cursor to the

TABLE 1: Comparisons of wire-based coronary physiological indices: RCTs are available for FFR and iFR only.

Index	Vendor specific	Definition	Hyperemia required	Cutoff	RCT available
FFR	Generic	Mean Pd/Pa during the whole cardiac cycle	Yes	≤0.80	Yes
cFFR	Generic	Lowest mean Pd/Pa after injection of contrast medium	Yes*	≤0.83	No
Resting Pd/Pa	Generic	Mean Pd/Pa over the whole cardiac cycle	No	≤0.91	No
iFR	Philips	Mean Pd/Pa during the wave-free period	No	≤0.89	Yes
DFR	Boston Scientific	Mean Pd/Pa when Pa <mean Pa and downsloping Pa	No	≤0.89	No
dPR	ACIST	Pd/Pa at the peak-to-peak midpoint	No	≤0.89	No
	OpSens	Mean Pd/Pa during the entire diastole	No	≤0.89	No
RFR	Abbott	Lowest filtered Pd/Pa during the whole cardiac cycle	No	≤0.89	No

* Contrast medium produces submaximal hyperemia compared with adenosine.

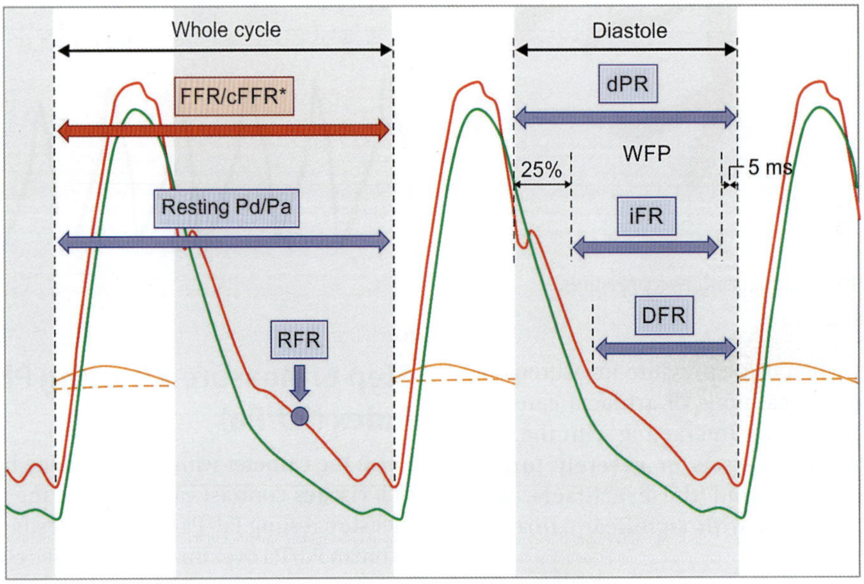

FIG. 6: Nonhyperemic pressure ratios based on the cardiac cycle.

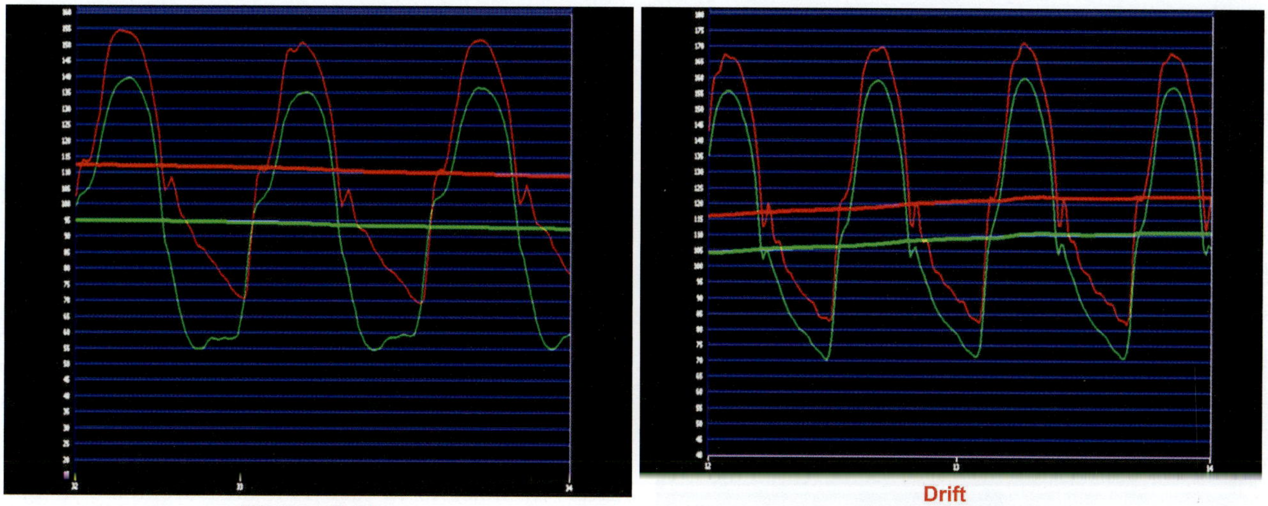

FIG. 7: Images of true gradient and inaccurate gradient due to drifting of resting index.

lowest value in pressure wire tracing during stable hyperemia to document FFR.

Adenosine is the most commonly used vasodilator agent. It can be given through intravenous or intracoronary route. If it given intravenously, Pd/Pa should be monitored for 1-3 minutes. Lowest FFR rarely occurs before the stabilization of hyperemia in some patients. If it is measured during this period, it will lead to overestimation of lesion severity. Wait for stable hyperemia and document FFR. SBP may drop up to 10 mm Hg and heart rate may increase by 5–10 beats/min during adenosine infusion. If intracoronary adenosine is administered, flush the catheter to ensure all the adenosine reaches the target coronary artery. Then measure the Pd and Pa pressures simultaneously until it returns to the baseline value and the lowest value is considered as FFR. If AV block occurs during intracoronary administration (especially in RCA), the measurement should be repeated with intravenous administration.

Other agents are regadenoson and papaverine. Regadenoson has fewer side effects than adenosine and is considered safer in COPD patients, though it has not been studied extensively.[14] Papaverine should not be used as the standard for inducing hyperemia due to limited research and a potentially higher risk of side effects, such as accumulation and ventricular arrhythmias.[15] If coronary spasm due to the FFR wire is suspected before injecting hyperemic agent, repeated injection of nitrates may be required **(Table 2; Figs. 8 and 9)**.[16-19]

TABLE 2: Doses of hyperemic agents.[16-19]

Drug	Dose
Adenosine intravenous	140–180 μg/kg/min
Adenosine intracoronary	*Left*: 200 μg *Right*: 100 μg
Regadenoson intravenous	400 μg irrespective of weight
Papaverine intracoronary	*Left*: 12 mg *Right*: 8 mg

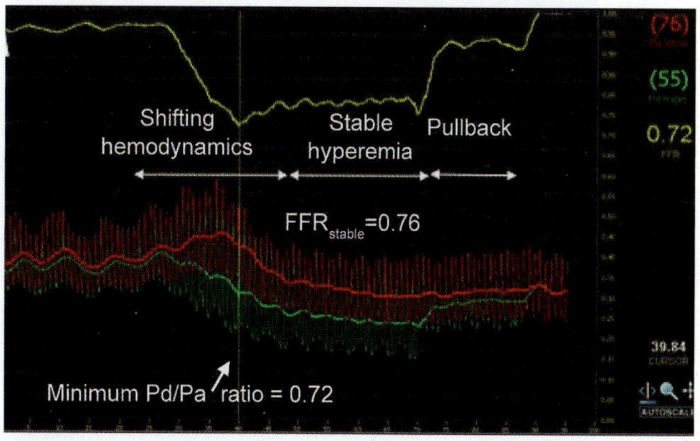

FIG. 8: Fractional flow reserve (FFR) tracing after giving intravenous adenosine: Initial FFR value may be low compared to FFR during stable hyperemia.

Step 8: Perform Pressure Wire Pullback While Recording Pressure

Determine the location of pressure drop(s) that suggest hemodynamically significant lesion(s). This is particularly important in patients with multiple lesions or diffuse disease.

Step 9: Confirm that No Pressure Drift has Occurred

Verify the calibration by checking the Pd/Pa when pressure sensor reaches the tip of the guide catheter. Ideally, the value should be 1. Pd/Pa >1.02, or <0.98, suggests significant pressure drift which often leads to inaccurate results.

Pressure drift is the loss of pressure equalization over time, unrelated to the effects of coronary stenosis.[9] Pressure drift is not an uncommon problem, affecting nearly 20% of FFR measurements.[20] If pressure drift is present, guide catheter and pressure wire pressures should be re-equalized and FFR should be repeated again. Most commonly, drift is related to changes in the piezoelectric sensor during the measurement and can be minimized by flushing the wire with saline before use **(Figs. 10A and B)**.

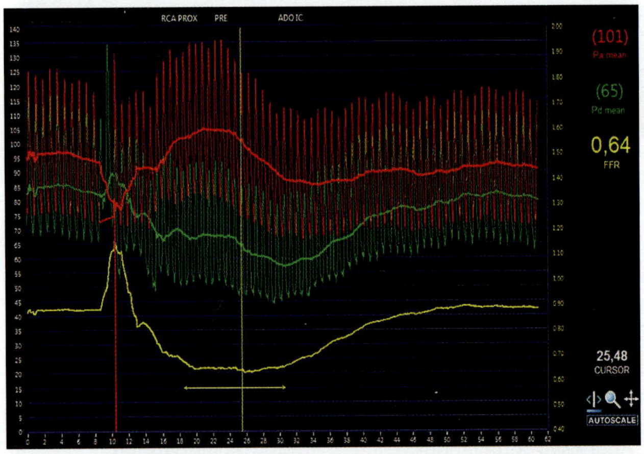

FIG. 9: Fractional flow reserve tracing after giving intracoronary adenosine—yellow arrow indicates stable hyperemia.

FRACTIONAL FLOW RESERVE IN SPECIAL SITUATIONS

Aorto-ostial Lesions

Prefer intravenous adenosine. Withdraw the guide catheter from the ostium for pressure equalization and FFR measurement **(Fig. 11)**.[21]

Left Main Coronary Artery Disease

Left main coronary artery diseases are rarely isolated. Mostly they will be having associated downstream disease. The flow and degree of hyperemia across the left main are determined by the outflow to both the LAD and the LCX.

The optimal method for assessing left main coronary artery stenosis is to take FFR measurements in both downstream vessels, unless one is very small.

In cases of isolated LMCA disease, measuring LMCA FFR in either branch theoretically yields similar results. However, it is advisable to perform an FFR pullback from both the distal LAD and the LCX, as the significance of downstream disease cannot be determined by visual estimation alone.[22]

If one downstream vessel has stenosis, LMCA FFR should be assessed in the proximal nondiseased downstream vessel only. First, check the severity of disease in the downstream vessel. If LAD has mild to moderate disease [stenosis <90% or FFR_{epi} (LMCA + LAD) >0.6], FFR of LMCA measured

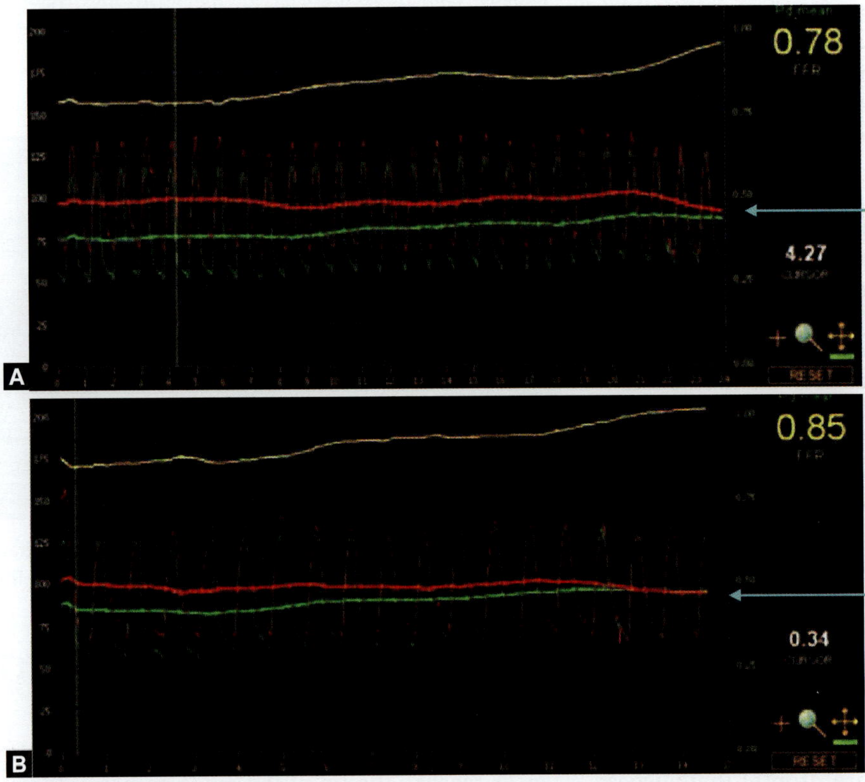

FIGS. 10A AND B: Impact of pressure drift on fractional flow reserve (FFR) measurements. Stenosis becomes insignificant after correcting pressure drift.

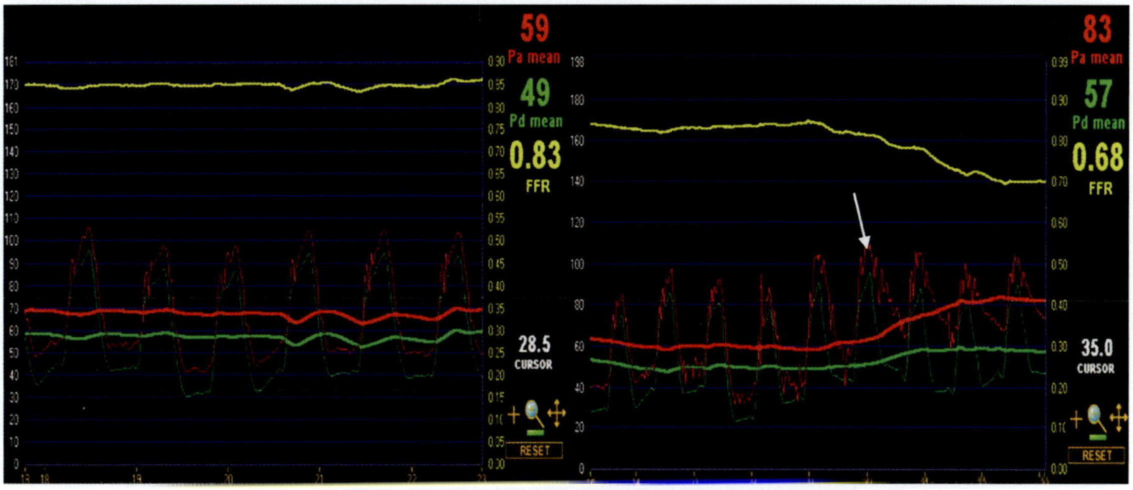

FIG. 11: Disengaging catheter in a patient with ostial lesion reveals positive FFR.

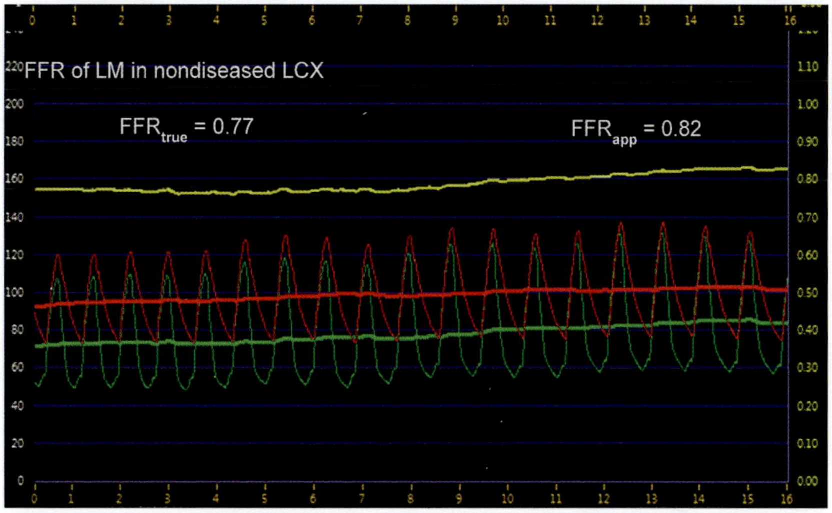

FIG. 12: FFR of LMCA is recorded from nondiseased LCX pressure wire before and after inflation of balloon in LAD ultimately leading to complete occlusion (simulating normal and stenotic LAD, respectively).

(FFR_{true}: Mimics FFR of LMCA in the absence of LAD lesion; FFR_{app}: apparent FFR: Mimics FFR value in the presence of diseased LAD; FFR_{app} will be falsely high compared to the FFR_{true} in the presence of severe stenosis in LAD)

in the LCX [apparent FFR (FFR_{app})] will be reliable.[23] In some studies, a total epicardial FFR of 0.45 was used as the cutoff value to diagnose severe disease in the downstream vessel. In the absence of severe disease in LAD, the FFR_{app} will reflect the true FFR. If LAD has severe disease [stenosis >90% or FFR_{epi} (LMCA + LAD) <0.6], it may impair maximal flow across the left main and falsely elevate the apparent LM FFR in the LCX. Here the FFR_{app} cutoff value is 0.85. It will correlate with true FFR of 0.80 in the absence of disease in LAD.[24] Another method for assessing FFR of the left main is to stent the LAD vessel first and then reassess FFR.

If both downstream vessels have stenosis, it is not possible to measure FFR for the left main coronary artery, as positioning the pressure sensor before these stenoses will not provide an accurate evaluation.[25] If they are considered for LMCA PCI, treat the distal vessel, and then reassess LMCA **(Fig. 12 and Flowchart 1)**.

Diffuse Lesions

Careful pullback of the FFR wire should be done to identify any localized pressure step-up. If such a pressure step-up is present, stenting should be considered, potentially in combination with intracoronary imaging. Consider medical management or surgical revascularization if no pressure step-up is found **(Fig. 13)**.

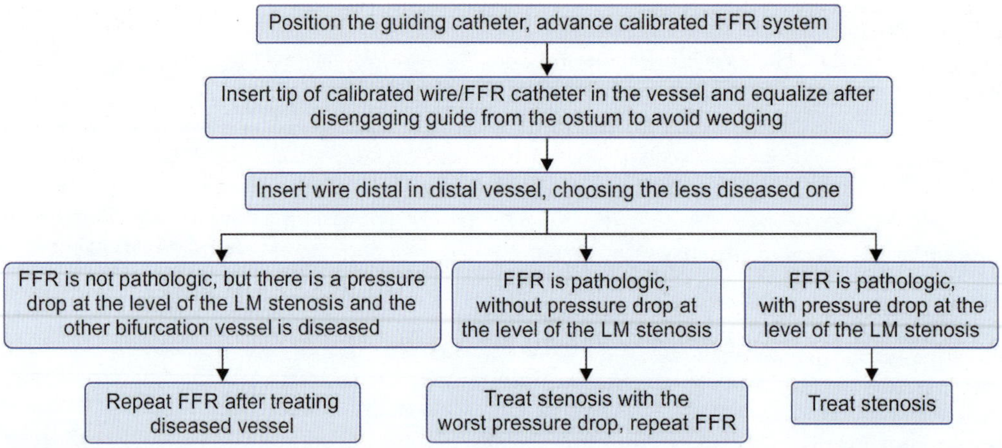

FLOWCHART 1: Assessment of LMCA lesion.

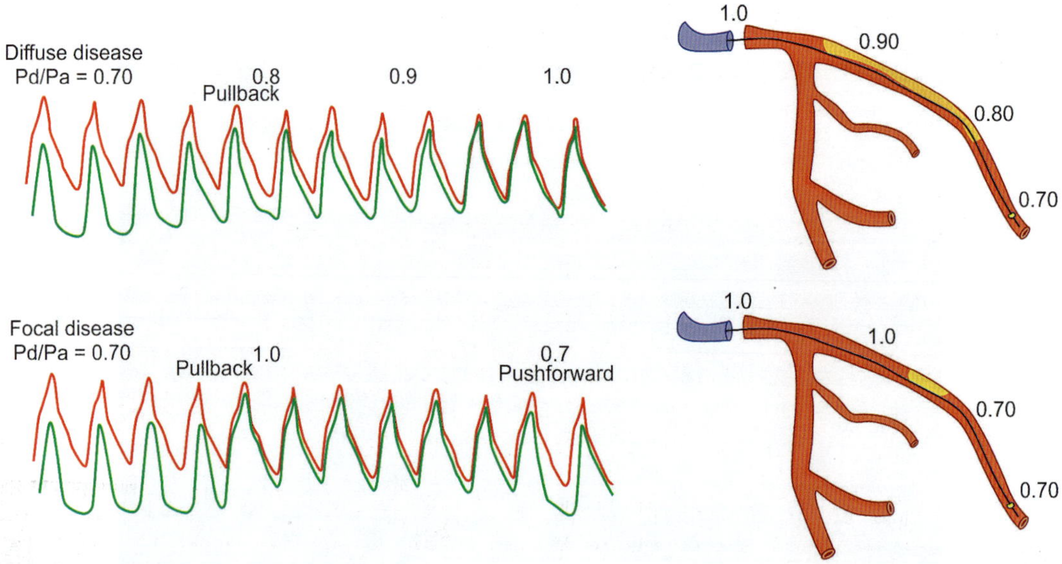

FIG. 13: Fractional flow reserve pullback in diffuse lesion: upper tracing does not have step-up. Lower tracing has significant step-up.

Tandem Lesions

Evaluating serial stenoses individually is not straightforward. For two successive stenoses, the distal measurement reflects the combined effect of both lesions. It is recommended to first revascularize the lesion with the higher pressure step-up during pullback. If it is unclear which lesion causes the greater pressure step-up, treat the distal lesion, and then reassess the remaining lesion **(Flowchart 2)**.[26]

Acute Coronary Syndrome (Based on ESC 2023 ACS Guidelines)

In STEMI, complete revascularization should be done based on angiogram only.[27] In NSTEMI, FFR may be considered to assess non-IRA severity during the index procedure.[28]

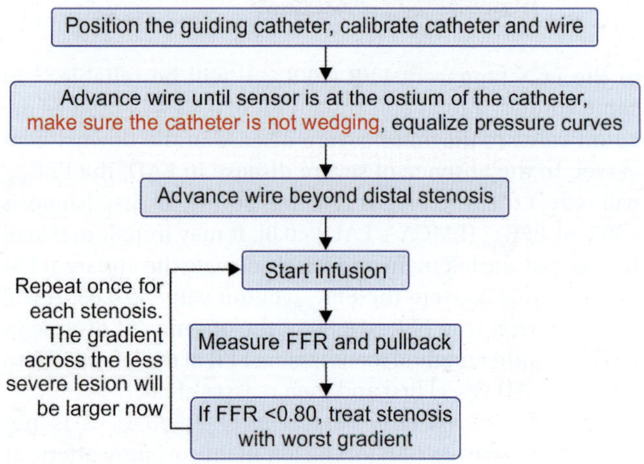

FLOWCHART 2: Algorithm in tandem lesion evaluation.

Multivessel Disease

Compared to the classic SYNTAX score, the functional SYNTAX score, which considers only ischemia-causing lesions, offers better reproducibility and prognostic value, and increases the number of multivessel CAD patients classified as low risk for adverse events after PCI.

Coronary Artery Bypass Grafts

When evaluating graft lesions, it is important to consider that the blood flow to the distal myocardial bed, where the pressure distal (Pd) is measured, comes from three sources: The native epicardial artery, the bypass conduit, and any developed collateral circulation. The measured FFR reflects the combined flow from these three sources during maximum hyperemia. Hence, graft FFR may be >0.80 even with significant graft stenoses if there is competitive flow via the native coronary artery **(Fig. 14)**.

Post-PTCA to Assess the Success of Revascularization

Post-PCI FFR >0.90 is linked to a lower risk of repeat PCI and major adverse cardiovascular events.[29] However, post-PCI FFR is rarely assessed in clinical practice.

Post-PTCA—Jailed Side Branch Assessment in Bifurcation Stenting

The hemodynamic significance of a jailed side branch stenosis during provisional stenting can be assessed using FFR. If FFR is ≤0.80 in the side branch, it should be stented.

Congestive Heart Failure

In patients with congestive heart failure who have high right atrial pressure and left ventricular end-diastolic pressure, adenosine FFR measurements will be affected.[30] FFR value may be falsely elevated. Although you can adjust the FFR calculation by including right atrial pressure [FFR = (Pd – Pv)/(Pa – Pv)], it is best to avoid functional assessment of coronary lesions in these patients **(Fig. 15)**.

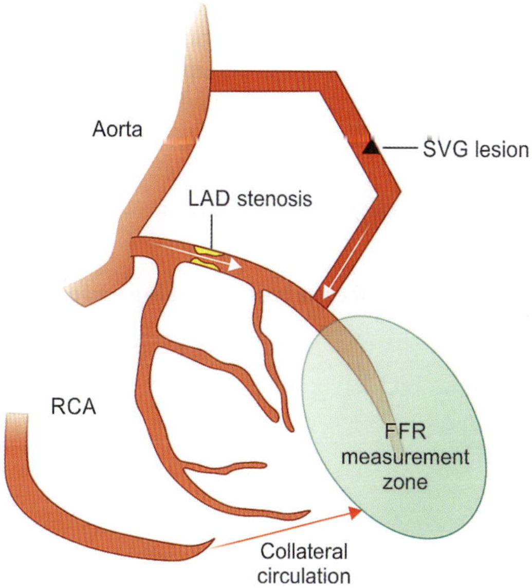

FIG. 14: Multiple sources of flow in the assessment grafts. Distal bed is perfused from three sources.

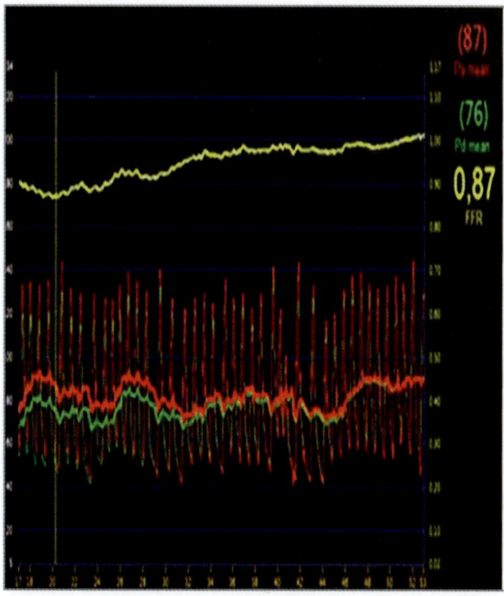

The FFR was 0.87. Pd at maximal hyperemia was 70 mm Hg, Pa 80 mm Hg. Based on the standard equation,

$$FFR = \frac{Pd}{Pa} = \frac{70}{80} = 0.875$$

Based on the concept of FFR, however, the true formula is:

$$FFR = \frac{Pd - Pv}{Pa - Pv}$$

Since Pd is by definition smaller than Pa, the results of the two formulas diverge for higher Pv values and for lower Pd and Pa values.

If Pv is 5 mm Hg, the result is:

$$FFR = \frac{70 - 5}{80 - 5} = 0.866$$

If Pv is 10 mm Hg, the result is:

$$FFR = \frac{70 - 10}{80 - 10} = 0.857$$

In a patient with an elevated Pv, 30 mm Hg, the result is:

$$FFR = \frac{70 - 30}{80 - 30} = 0.80$$

FIG. 15: Influence of CVP on FFR: An increase of CVP is related to a progressive reduction of FFR.

Chronic Total Occlusion

The hemodynamic significance of a lesion in a donor vessel supplying collateral to a CTO vessel may change after successful CTO recanalization. In a study by Sachdeva et al., 6 out of 9 donor vessels with baseline ischemia (FFR ≤0.80) showed nonischemic FFR values (>0.80) after successful CTO recanalization.[31]

Aortic Stenosis

The increased oxygen demand of hypertrophied ventricles in severe AS leads to partial microcirculatory vasodilation and increased resting coronary blood flow. This, along with a submaximal drug-induced hyperemic response may cause FFR significance to be underestimated.[32,33]

Discrepancy between Resting and Hyperemic Indices

Discordance between resting and hyperemic indices occurs in about 14% of cases, especially in large coronary arteries like the left main and proximal LAD, and in diabetic patients. Clinical presentation should guide decision making when discrepancies arise.

CONCLUSION

Clinical trials have shown that FFR improves outcomes in selected group of patients. This benefit is maximized with rigorous and standardized measurement and analysis of FFR.

ONLINE REFERENCES

Please scan the QR code provided at the end of the table of contents for References of this chapter.

Intravascular Imaging in Coronary Stent Restenosis: Prevention, Characterization, and Management

CHAPTER 146

Parayaru Kottayil Asokan

ABSTRACT

In-stent restenosis (ISR) remains the most common cause of stent failure after percutaneous coronary intervention (PCI). Intravascular imaging aids in managing ISR by optimizing stenting procedures, identifying underlying mechanisms, and evaluating treatment results through multiple stages.

Keywords: In-stent restenosis, target lesion revascularization, drug-eluting stent(s), intracoronary imaging, drug-eluting balloon, optic coherence tomography, intravascular ultrasound

INTRODUCTION

In-stent restenosis (ISR) is a common cause of stent failure after percutaneous coronary intervention (PCI), accounting for 5–10% of all PCI procedures. Although incidence has decreased with drug-eluting stents (DES) technologies, it remains the Achilles heel of modern PCI. Interventional cardiologists face significant challenges in managing ISR, a condition with high recurrent events, but developing strategies can improve patient outcomes, and reduce morbidity, and mortality. Intravascular imaging (IVI) offers valuable insights into stent-related mechanical issues, optimizing stenting procedures, guiding restenosis management, and evaluating reintervention results through multiple stages.

In-stent Restenosis

In-stent restenosis is a significant reduction in luminal diameter within the stented segment after a successful PCI, which remains the most common cause of stent failure. ISR is defined as a reduction of ≥50% of the luminal diameter within the previously stented segment or vessel segments 5 mm proximal and distal to the stent. Newer DES technologies have reduced ISR incidence compared to BMS, but ISR treatment still accounts for 5–10% of PCI procedures in clinical practice. Clinical restenosis occurs when luminal renarrowing exceeds 50% of the minimal luminal diameter, associated with ischemia symptoms or abnormal diagnostic testing results or IVI (<6 mm^2 for left main or <4 mm^2 for non-left main or luminal renarrowing of over 70% even without ischemia symptoms).[1-5]

ROLE OF INTRAVASCULAR IMAGING IN DETECTION OF MECHANISM OF IN-STENT RESTENOSIS

In-stent restenosis cases often lead to MI, with a 30-day mortality rate ranging from 10 to 25%. The incidence varies based on patient characteristics, angiography, and procedure as stated in **Table 1**, with a 5-year ISR rate ranging from 9 to 12%.

Second-generation DES has an ISR rate of 5.7% in nondiabetic individuals and 8.7% in diabetes patients. ISR is caused by neointimal tissue proliferation or hyperplasia, resulting from arterial wall damage during stent implantation. Factors include inflammation and hypersensitivity reactions to metals and early-generation DES polymers.[6-9]

BIOLOGICAL FACTORS OF IN-STENT RESTENOSIS

Biological factors of ISR include neointimal hyperplasia and neoatherosclerosis. Neointimal hyperplasia is defined as the accumulation of smooth muscle cells and extracellular matrix in the intima, while neoatherosclerosis is characterized by an accumulation of lipid-laden foamy macrophages, with or without necrotic core formation, and/or calcification within the neointima. Calcified neoatherosclerosis is challenging to manage, impacting percutaneous intervention decisions **(Figs. 1 and 2)**.

Optical coherence tomography (OCT) findings suggest neoatherosclerosis in DES-ISR within the 1st year post-PCI, compared to DES-ISR developing after 1 year post-PCI. Neoatherosclerosis advances faster than de novo atherosclerotic CAD, but the time of ISR formation affects OCT results.[6,9-17] Based on OCT appearances,[18] ISR can be classified into four groups **(Figs. 3A to F)**.

Neoatherosclerosis, a major cause of stent failure, is often diagnosed using optical coherence tomography (OCT). It is characterized by lipidic or calcified plaque in ≥3 consecutive frames or ruptured lipidic neoatherosclerosis. Calcified neoatherosclerosis could be primarily located within the stent (in-stent calcium) or surrounding the stent struts (peri-stent calcium) in ISR. A large amount of calcium levels exceeding 0.5 mm thick and 180° arc, including calcified neoatherosclerosis, were linked to poor stent expansion and worse outcomes.

TABLE 1: In-stent restenosis risk factors.

Patient factors	Angiographic factors	Procedural factors
• Diabetes mellitus • Renal insufficiency • ACS presentation • Female gender • Recurrent ISR	• Lesion length >20 mm • Diameter <3 mm • Chronic total occlusion • Ostial location • Bifurcation • Saphenous vein graft • Severe calcification • Multivessel CAD	• Underexpansion • Stent fracture • Bare metal stent • Stenoses proximal and distal to stent • Major arterial dissection involving media or >3 mm length • Multiple stent layers

Source: With permission form Klein et al. (2023).[6]

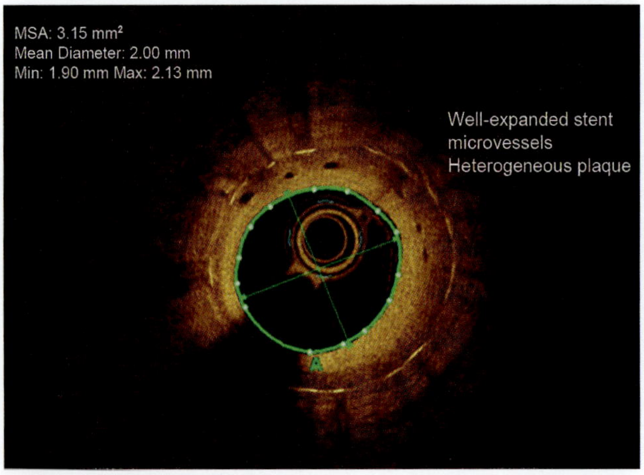

FIG. 1: Neoatherosclerosis.

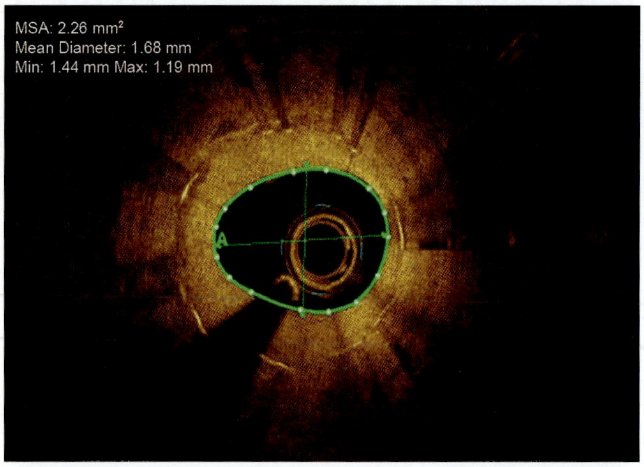

FIG. 2: Homogeneous plaque—NIH.

Intravascular imaging improves revascularization outcomes and reduces stent failure in complex lesions, allowing optimal stent sizing, detailed assessment, and identification of potential causes of ISR. Routine IVI is considered the most effective method for preventing ISR by identifying stent failure causes and optimizing PCI results. The 2018 ESC/EACTS Guidelines recommend intravascular ultrasound (IVUS) for unprotected left main lesions, while 2021 American College of Cardiology (ACC)/ American Heart Association (AHA)/SCAI guidelines classify IVUS for procedural optimization of left main or complex coronary stenting as Class IIA with OCT as a reasonable substitute. *ESC 2024* Guidelines recommend intracoronary imaging for complex lesions, in particular left main stem, true bifurcations, and long lesions as Class 1A.[11,19-28]

MECHANICAL FACTORS

Mechanical factors, such as stent undersizing, stent under-expansion, vessel calcification, stent fracture, and geographic miss, are also significant causes of ISR. Effective treatment requires precise diagnosis and cause understanding, with intracoronary imaging playing a crucial role. Adequate vessel preparation and imaging-guided stent implantation reduce ISR. Determining the underlying mechanisms is a key step in any ISR treatment **(Fig. 4)**.[13,17,29]

ROLE OF INTRAVASCULAR IMAGING IN PERCUTANEOUS CORONARY INTERVENTION PROCEDURE OPTIMIZATION

The ultimate trial found a lower 1-year risk for target vessel failure (TVF) in IVUS-guided patients undergoing second-generation DES implantation compared to angiography-guided patients. IVUS guidance significantly reduced TVF

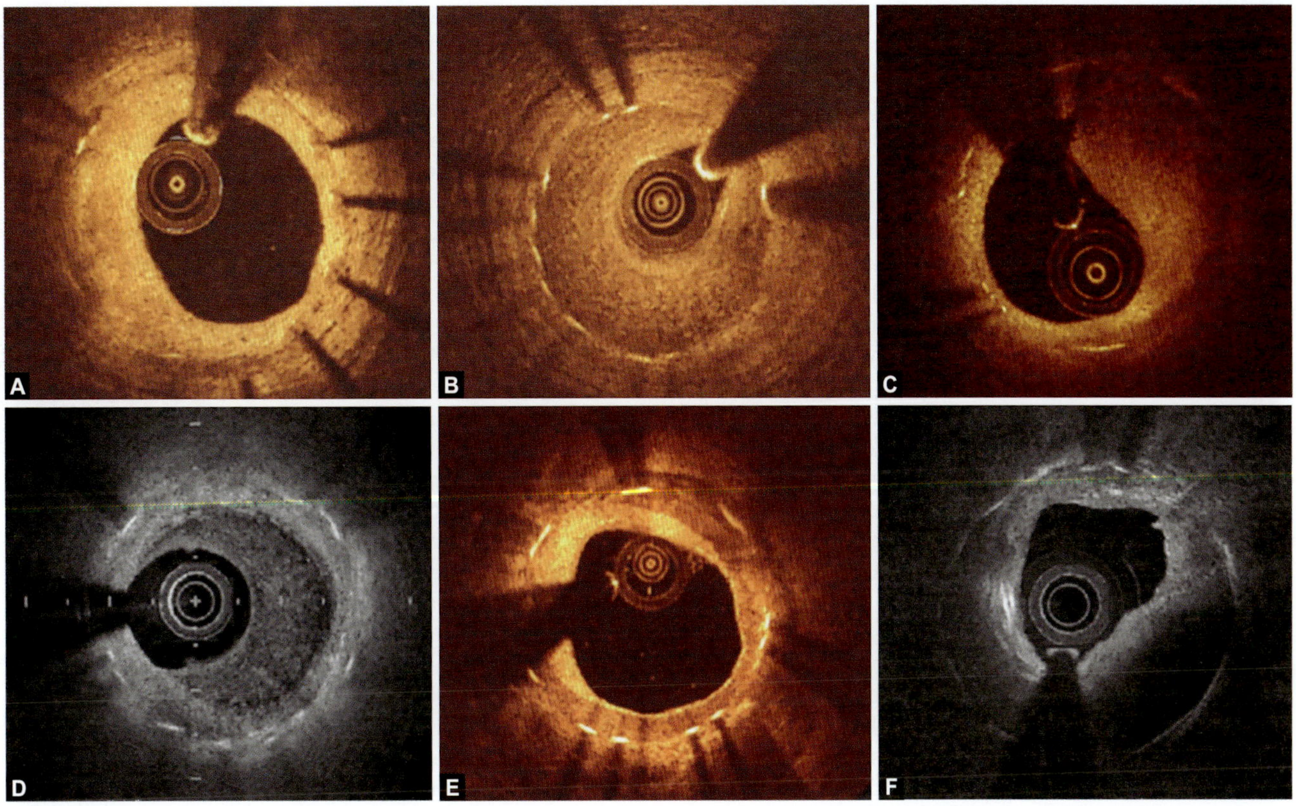

FIGS. 3A TO F: Neointima patterns. (A) Homogeneous intima; (B) Heterogeneous intima; (C) Layered pattern; (D) Neointima with Heterogeneous and Layered Pattern; (E) Calcific-rich neoatherosclerotic plaque; and (F) Lipid-rich neoatherosclerotic plaque.
Source: With Permission from Erdogan et al. (2022).[18]

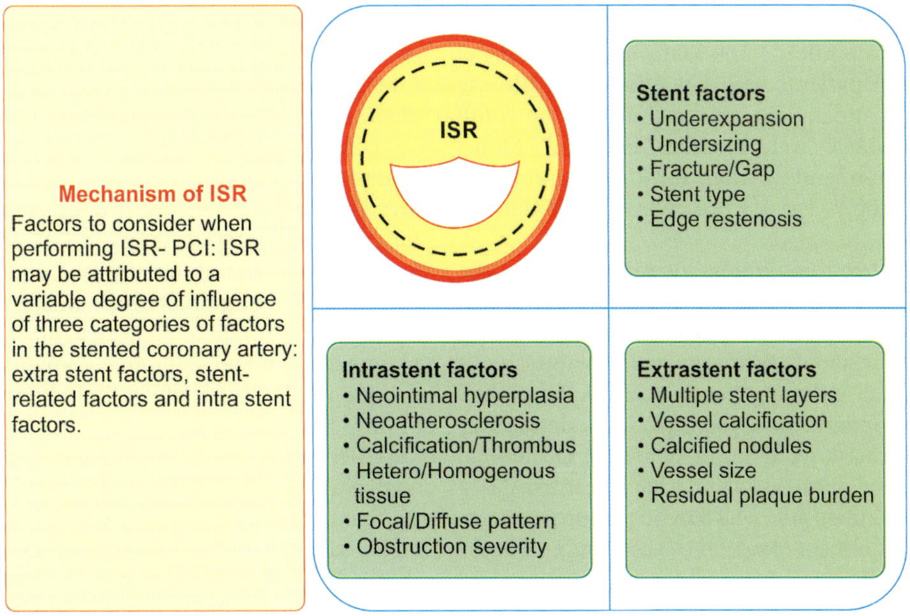

FIG. 4: Mechanism of ISR.
(ISR: in-stent restenosis; PCI: percutaneous coronary intervention)
Source: With permission from Alfonso et al. (2021).[17]

in patients, with optimal PCI resulting in better clinical outcomes. At 3 years, TVF occurred in 6.6% of IVUS-guided patients and 10.7% in angiography-guided patients, primarily due to decreased clinically driven target vessel revascularization.

The IVUS defined optimal criteria for DES implantation in this trial included: (1) Minimum luminal area in the stented segment >5.0 mm^2 or 90% of the minimal luminal area at the distal reference segments, (2) plaque burden 5 mm proximal or distal to the stent edge <50%, and (3) no edge dissection involving the media with length >3 mm. IVUS-defined optimal procedures were identified only if all three criteria were simultaneously met.[29]

A meta-analysis of nine randomized trials found that IVUS-guided DES implantation reduces cardiac death, coronary revascularization, and stent thrombosis compared to angiographic guidance. The IVUS-XPL study showed lower 5-year major adverse cardiac event (MACE) rates due to reduced ischemia-driven TLR. The ADAPT-DES registry found that IVUS guidance improved patient outcomes, particularly in reducing TVMI and revascularization, over a period of 1–2 years. Among patients with complex coronary-artery lesions, IVI-guided PCI led to a lower risk of a composite of death from cardiac causes, target vessel-related myocardial infarction, or clinically driven target-vessel revascularization than angiography-guided PCI (RENOVATE-COMPLEX-PCI).[19-21,30]

A study by Kang et al. found that intravascular ultrasound guidance improves outcomes in patients undergoing unprotected left main coronary artery stenting, especially in lesions with underexpansion of at least one segment. The optimal stent expansion is determined by the 5-6-7-8 rule of criteria, based on IVUS-measured minimal stent area, ostial left circumflex, LAD, POC, and LM. Kim et al. studied MSA in patients with LM bifurcation disease who underwent upstream two-stent technique. The cutoff values for 5-year MACEs were 11.8 mm^2 for distal LM, 8.3 mm^2 for LAD ostium, and 5.7 mm^2 for LCX ostium. OCT guidance reduces the 1-year risk of a composite containing TLR.[31,32]

Optical coherence tomography guidance reduces the 1-year risk of composite containing TLR, but suboptimal stent deployment increases the risk of MACEs, including TLR. Stent expansion should be maximized, malappositions should be minimized, and major stent edge dissection should be corrected. Suboptimal stent deployment is defined by quantitative OCT criteria, including in-stent minimal luminal area (MLA) <4.5 mm^2, distal dissection >200 μm, and distal or proximal reference lumen area <4.5 mm^2 in plaque presence, and accurate measurement of reference vessel/lumen size is crucial **(Fig. 5)**.[12,33,34]

The European Association of PCI's expert consensus defines optimal stent expansion as stent expansion (i.e., a minimum stent area versus average reference lumen area ratio) >80% of average reference lumen, MSA >5.5 mm^2 by IVUS and >4.5 mm^2 by OCT **(Fig. 6)**.[35]

In clinical practice, a relative expansion of >70% is achievable, with 80% or 90% being optimal criteria. Regions with a lipid arc >180° and lumen narrowing <4.5 mm^2 should be excluded for reference segments. IVI is crucial for therapy. Intraluminal diagnostic imaging is recommended to detect any inflow or outflow obstructions within 5 mm of the stent edge.[12,33-35]

A study by Yin et al. found that stent expansion increases myocardial infarction and TLR risk at 2-year follow-up. Optimizing stent expansion is crucial to reduce these risks. Suboptimal stent deployment is common in 31–58% of patients. The ILUMIEN study found similar stent expansion rates in both OCT and IVUS-guided stenting. Stent under expansion is the most common preventable mechanism of ISR in the DES era. Stent underexpansion can occur due to low deployment pressures, undersizing, or calcified lesions, requiring recognition of target lesion calcium and consideration of prestenting techniques.[13,18]

Severe target lesion calcium fracture is crucial for stent expansion and is achieved through calcium modification devices. IVUS calcium scores with length of superficial calcium more than >270 and longer than 5 mm, 360° of superficial calcium, presence of calcified nodule, and small vessel diameter less than 3.5 mm. Rotational or orbital atherectomy is recommended for lesions with high intravascular ultrasound calcium score 2. An OCT-based calcium scoring system predicts stent underexpansion with a maximum angle of 180°, maximal thickness >0.5 mm, and length >5 mm, slightly better than angiographic detection of severe calcium.[36,37]

The EAPCI consensus recommends distal lumen reference-based sizing for intracoronary imaging, optimizing for mid and proximal stent segments. IVUS is the gold standard due to superior EEL differentiation. Artificial intelligence-based methods, such as the ILUMIEN III and IV algorithm, can streamline stent sizing processes.[38,39]

Longitudinal geographic miss (GM) refers to an injured or diseased vessel segment not covered by the stent. IVUS and OCT help determine the appropriate landing zone for stent implantation to avoid GM and ensure adequate lesion coverage. A study of over 1,500 patients found that GM increased edge restenosis incidence and TVR rate at 1 year. IVUS predicts edge restenosis using poststenting plaque burden and reference segment MLA, with a 54.5% overall predictive cutoff. OCT studies found lipidic plaque in the stent edge segment and MLA (optimal cutoff was an arc ≥185 and 4.1 mm^2) as independent predictors of binary angiographic stent edge restenosis at 9–12 months.[42]

Stent edge dissection is a predictor of target lesion failure, and OCT helps determine its presence when angiography shows obscure findings. Postprocedural imaging may be more efficient than routine poststenting dilation with high-pressure balloons in preventing edge dissections. Previous studies have shown that media or adventitia involvement, a dissection angle of >60°, and a dissection length of >2 mm predict target lesion failure. In-stent tissue

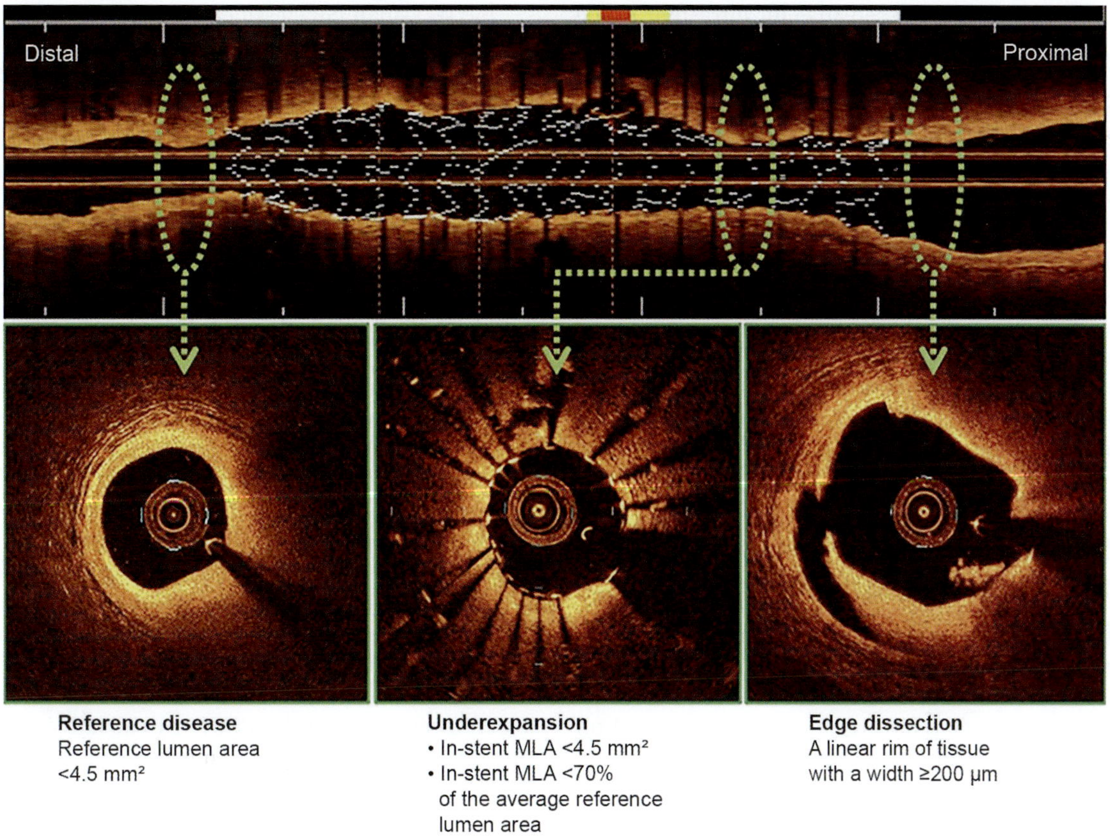

FIG. 5: Quantitative OCT metrics of suboptimal stent implantation. Stent underexpansion, reference disease, and stent edge dissection are associated with worse long-term PCI outcomes.

(MLA: minimum lumen area; OCT: optical coherence tomography; PCI: percutaneous coronary intervention)

Source: With permission from Kubo et al. (2022).[34]

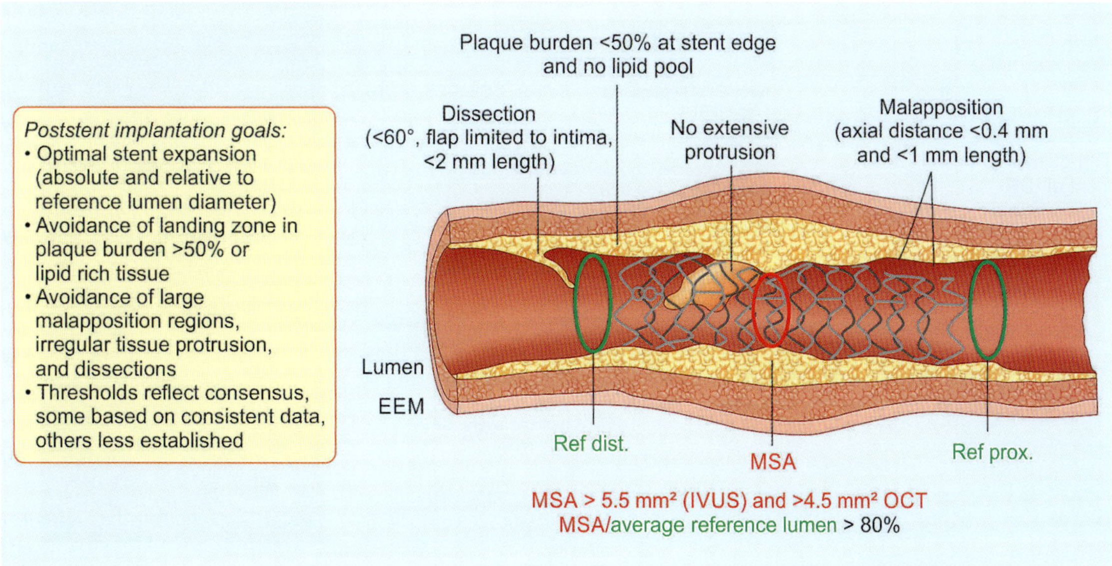

FIG. 6: Summary of post-PCI optimization in non-LM lesions.

Source: With permission from Räber et al. (2018).[35]

protrusion/prolapse is more sensitive for intrastent tissue protrusion detection than IVUS. Studies show no association between minor plaque prolapse and restenosis in coronary lesions.[15,33,34]

Stent fractures can cause damage to the scaffolding and local drug delivery in DES, leading to mechanical irritation of the vessel. IVUS can reveal recoil of strut edges near the fracture site, increasing the risk of ISR and TLR. An OCT-based classification was proposed, showing more complex stent fracture patterns are more common in device failure cases than incidentally discovered ones.[36,43]

Optical coherence tomography is more sensitive for intrastent tissue protrusion detection than IVUS, but studies show no association between minor plaque prolapse and restenosis in coronary lesions. IVUS-detected TP is associated with less clinically driven TLR.[12,13,18]

IN-STENT RESTENOSIS CLASSIFICATION: MORPHOLOGIC PATTERNS BASED ON INTRAVASCULAR IMAGING

The Mehran System classifies resenotic lesions based on morphology and extent of disease, with four subclasses based on location within the stented segment.[40]

The Waksman ISR classification is based on mechanistic considerations informed by intracoronary imaging **(Fig. 7)**.[41]

Intravascular ultrasound-OCT-based classifications have been proposed, with the SCAI recommending early, late, and very late timing categories for future diagnostic and therapeutic studies. This classification will be useful to determine best treatment options for DES ISR.

Kang et al. have proposed an IVUS-based classification that incorporates length of the restenosis as well as minimal luminal area. Gonzalo et al. and Ali et al. have proposed *OCT* classifications that rely on both quantitative and qualitative parameters.

The SCAI recommends that early (<30 days), late (30 days to 1 year), and very late (>1 year) timing categories be adopted for all future diagnostic and therapeutic studies. **Table 2** displays the proposed new SCAI classification incorporating the cause of ISR based on time from implantation.[6]

By integrating mechanistic etiology with timing, this classification will be useful to determine best treatment options. Regular IVI evaluation is crucial for managing restenosis, determining the cause, guiding therapeutic strategy, and confirming effective treatment after PCI. Identifying stent failure mechanisms is crucial for treatment selection and device durability as causative factors will influence the selection of treatment and devices to manage the ISR, ultimately impacting the durability of the repeat

Imaging-guided treatment of ISR

Type	Definition		Therapeutic guidance
I	Mechanical	Stent underexpansion (Type I A)	• High pressure balloon, ELCA, or IVL • Underexpansion must be treated prior to further stent implantation
		Stent fracture (Type I B)	DES
II	Biologic	Neointimal hyperplasia (Type II A)	Balloon, DCB, DES, or VBT
		Neoatherosclerosis, noncalcified (Type II B)	DCB, or DES
		Neoatherosclerosis, calcified (Type II C)	Scoring balloon, ELCA, CA or RA prior to DES
III	Mixed pattern: Combined mechanical and biologic etiology		High-pressure NC balloon with DCB, DES, or VBT
IV	Chronic total occlusion		DCB or DES: VBT for multiple layers, CABG as needed
V	>2 layers of stent		Balloon, DCB, VBT, or CABG

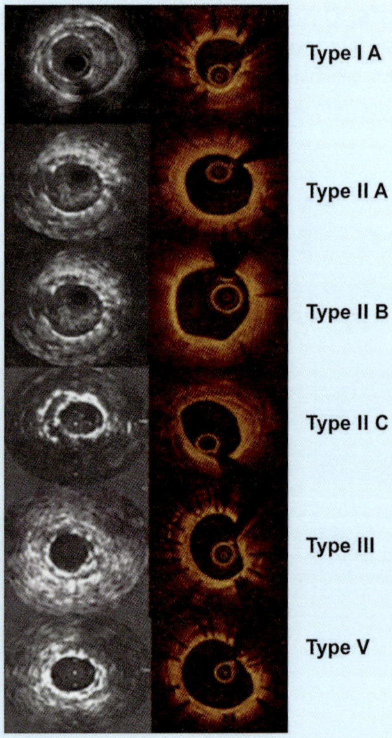

FIG. 7: Waksman in-stent restenosis (ISR) classification—image-guided treatment of ISR.

(CABG: coronary artery bypass graft; DCB: drug coated balloon; DES: drug-eluting stent; ELCA: excimer laser coronary atherectomy; IVL: intravascular lithotripsy; IVUS: intravascular ultrasound; NC: noncompliant; OA: orbital atherectomy; OCT: optical coherence tomography; RA: rotational atherectomy; VBT: vascular brachytherapy)

Source: With permission from Shlofmitz et al. (2019).[41]

revascularization. Angiography alone is often insufficient for assessing ISR in clinical practice. ISR treatment follows similar principles to native coronary stenoses, but with existing scaffolds, persistent issues leading to stent failure may need to be addressed to prevent recurrence.[6,19,41]

USE OF INTRAVASCULAR IMAGING IN MANAGEMENT OF IN-STENT RESTENOSIS: GENERAL STRATEGIC APPROACH

Restenosis management is crucial for determining the cause, guiding therapeutic strategy, and confirming effective treatment after PCI. Identifying stent failure mechanisms is essential for treatment selection and device durability, as causative factors influence the selection of treatment and devices to manage ISR, ultimately impacting the durability of the repeat revascularization. Angiography alone is often insufficient for assessing ISR in clinical practice.

TABLE 2: SCAI classification of in-stent restenosis—a system based on time interval and causative factor.

Early	<30 days	• Undersizing • Underexpansion
Late	30 days to 1 year	• Stent fracture • Delayed healing (including drug-induced) • Uncovered stent struts • Intimal hyperplasia (especially in BMS ISR)
Very late	>1 year	• Neoatherosclerosis • Stent fracture

Source: With permission from Klein et al. (2023).[6]

Current European guidelines recommend either DES or DCBs to treat ISR with a Class I indication. In the most recent ACC/AHA coronary revascularization guidelines, repeated DES has a Class 1A indication for the treatment of ISR with the use of PCI. Both the European and US guidelines recommend intracoronary imaging with IVUS or OCT to elucidate the mechanisms of ISR.[21,22]

The general strategic approach is to obtain the largest acute lumen gain as possible by maximizing the immediate postprocedural MLA. Quantitative coronary angiography measures and evaluates the antirestenotic efficacy of stent and balloon-based treatment modalities, including MLD, acute gain, and LLL. Drug-coated balloon therapy reduces acute gain and late loss compared to DES PCI, which increases acute gain but also late loss. Net gain is the most important parameter when comparing the two modalities.[17]

The temporal pattern of acute gain and LLL after PCI is shown in **Figure 8**.

Treatment modalities and mechanical factors influence acute gain and LLL in ISR settings. Stent underexpansion, often due to vessel calcification, is a significant factor in ISR lesions. Calcified neoatherosclerotic ISR can hinder maximal acute gain, and primary stent under expansion increases secondary stent underexpansion risk, which in turn increases the risk of MACE and ISR recurrence. Suboptimal treatment can cause multiple stent layers or the "onion skin phenomenon". Aggressively addressing mechanical factors before dedicated ISR treatment can prevent this

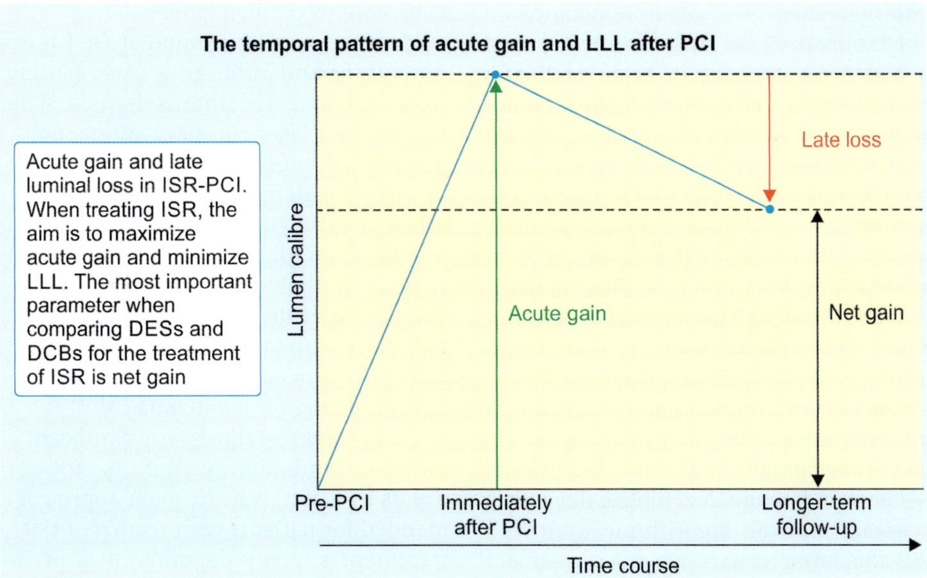

FIG. 8: Acute gain and late luminal loss in ISR-PCI.

(DES: drug-eluting stent; DCB: drug-coated balloon; ISR: in-stent restenosis; LLL: late lumen loss; PCI: percutaneous coronary intervention)

Source: With permission from Alfonso et al. (2022).[17]

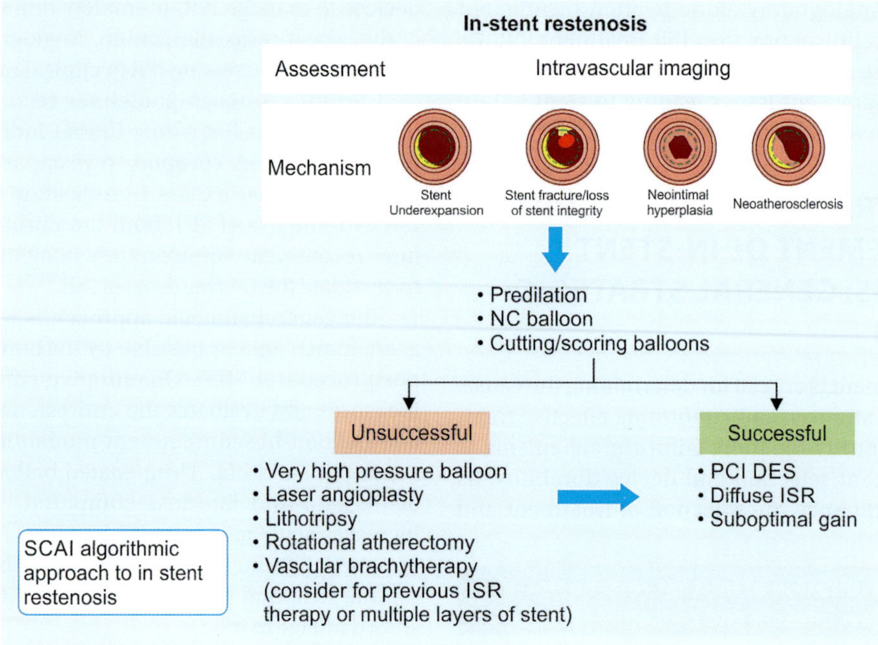

FIG. 9: SCAI algorithmic approach to in-stent restenosis.

(DES: drug-eluting stents; ISR: in-stent restenosis; PCI: percutaneous coronary intervention)

Source: With permission from Klein et al. (2023).[6]

issue.[17] The algorithmic approach suggests routine PCI after intracoronary imaging assessment to determine the cause of ISR, correct underlying mechanical factors, and image-guide a second stent for optimal stent expansion **(Fig. 9)**.[6]

High-pressure balloon angioplasty (BA) is crucial for treating DES-ISR due to underexpansion, often using short noncompliant balloons. Plain BA is inferior but important for treating DES-ISR. Twin-layer OPN™ highly noncompliant balloon (NCB) at high pressure (>30 atm) can correct stent underexpansion and increase luminal gain, leading to better clinical outcomes. High-pressure balloons also increase lumen gain by compressing neointimal tissue, which is often excessive in ISR lesions.[44,45]

Neointimal modification with CB before DEB reduces TLR rates at 5 years, consistent with bare-metal and DES, increasing lumen diameters and reducing elastic recoil in native lesions. The ISAR-DESIRE 4 trial found that patients receiving scoring BA plus DCB had lower rates of in-segment diameter stenosis and binary angiographic restenosis, and paclitaxel-coated scoring balloons performed better.[46-48]

Drug-eluting stents are the most effective treatment for DES-ISR, improving long-term patency in resenotic lesions with aggressive angiographic patterns at high risk of recurrent restenosis or stent fracture. A complete diagnostic evaluation is necessary, and an algorithmic approach suggests routine PCI after intracoronary imaging assessment to determine the cause of ISR, correcting underlying mechanical factors, and image-guiding a second stent for optimal expansion. The DAEDALUS study, involving 1,976 patients, found that DESs reduced the need for subsequent TLR compared to paclitaxel DCB. However, DES implantation may cause therapeutic challenges in ISR recurrence.[5,6,49,50]

Drug-coated balloons (CBs) are superior to plain BA in DES ISR and should be used in less complex restenotic lesions, multilayer ISR, BMS-ISR, and high-risk bleeding patients who cannot tolerate prolonged periods of DAPT.[21,44] Clinical safety and efficacy have been thoroughly studied, with current Japanese and Western guidelines providing consistent recommendations.

Intravascular ultrasound or OCT is essential for characterization, and rotational atherectomy (RA) is used to treat calcified neoatherosclerosis, which is resistant to BA. Excimer laser coronary atherectomy (ELCA) improves procedural success for difficult lesions like diffuse ISR or highly calcified, undilatable lesions. Intravascular lithotripsy (IVL) is a safe and effective treatment for calcium-mediated undilatable stents underexpansion or calcified NIH, potentially reducing vessel perforation or rupture. The CRUNCH-Registry confirms IVL's safety and efficacy in ISR. ELCA with in-stent NIH ablation in ISR has been linked to higher procedural success, lower complications, and improved long-term outcomes.[5,17,51-57]

Recurrent restenosis is a significant challenge in interventional cardiology, with up to 20% of patients reporting events in 1 year. A heart-team approach is strongly recommended for patients with recurrent ISR, and the preferred treatment strategy depends on a precise diagnosis and understanding of the cause.[17]

In-stent restenosis treatment strategies according to the underlying mechanism and neointima characteristics assessed by IVI are depicted in **Flowchart 1**.

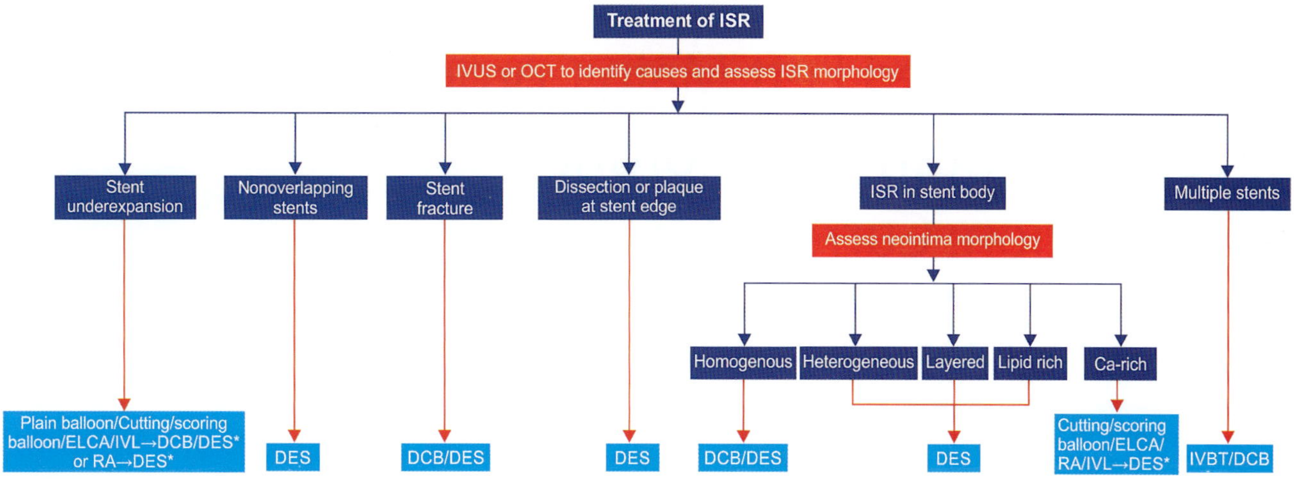

*Indicates use of DES only if there is optimal lesion preparation and expected optimal stent expansion.

FLOWCHART 1: In-stent restenosis (ISR) treatment according to the underlying mechanism and neointima characteristics assessed by intravascular imaging.

(Ca: calcific; DCB: drug-coated balloon; DES: drug-eluting stent; ELCA: excimer laser coronary atherectomy; IVBT: intravascular brachytherapy; IVL: intravascular lithotripsy; IVUS: intravascular ultrasound; OCT: optical coherence tomography; RA: rotational atherectomy)

Source: With permission form Erdogan et al. (2022).[18]

CONCLUSION

The mechanisms of ISR are heterogeneous and its management remains challenging. Characterization and identification of the underlying mechanisms and substrate of ISR are important. Intracoronary imaging should be performed to guide clinical management. Standardized use and optimal vessel preparation are needed for stent technology. Repeated DES implantation is the most effective treatment for single-layer ISR in reducing the need for repeated TLR, particularly in subsets of more severe patterns of ISR. DCBs are an attractive treatment option for multilayer ISR and restenosis within small vessel. The new ISR classification enables treatment tailored to specific lesion characteristics. In severely calcified lesions, intracoronary imaging along with adjuvant calcium debulking therapy should be considered. This approach aims to address the unique challenges posed by calcified lesions and optimize treatment outcomes. A heart-team approach is strongly recommended for patients with recurrent ISR. The preferred treatment strategy depends on a precise diagnosis and understanding of the cause. Consequently, identifying the mechanism in each case using intracoronary imaging and optimizing the interventional result are critical steps.

ONLINE REFERENCES

Please scan the QR code provided at the end of the table of contents for References of this chapter.

CHAPTER 147

Imaging-guided Left Main Coronary Artery Percutaneous Coronary Intervention: Current Concepts

Vijay Bang, Ashish Deshpande

ABSTRACT

Left main coronary artery (LMCA) disease has the highest mortality associated with it because it is responsible for supplying up to 80% of total blood flow to the left ventricle in a right-dominant coronary circulation. Due to the significant progress in technology, the modern drug-eluting stents have remarkably improved the prognosis of patients with LMCA disease treated invasively. Due to its bidimensional nature, angiography does not enable an accurate evaluation of the extension, distribution, and morphology of LMCA disease. Intravascular ultrasound (IVUS) is the invasive imaging modality of choice for the evaluation of LMCA disease, due to its ability to accurately characterize atherosclerotic disease in all the segments of LMCA bifurcation (including LMCA ostium). IVUS is therefore useful in each step of LMCA procedures, i.e., prestenting, during stenting, and poststenting. Several meta-analyses suggest the superiority of IVUS-guided LMCA percutaneous coronary interventions (PCI) as compared with LMCA PCI guided by angiography alone in terms of mortality, nonfatal myocardial infarction, stent thrombosis, restenosis, and target lesion revascularization.

Keywords: Left main coronary artery (LMCA), invasive coronary angiography, intravascular ultrasound (IVUS), optical coherence tomography (OCT), PCI

INTRODUCTION

Cardiovascular disease (CVD) remains the leading cause of death globally. Coronary artery disease (CAD), presented either as an acute coronary syndrome (ACS) or chronic coronary syndrome (CCS), is the main manifestation of CVD, affecting the majority of cardiac patients.[1-4]

Left main coronary artery (LMCA) disease is accompanied by highest mortality. When left untreated, the 3-year mortality is estimated at 63%, which is considerably higher than in coronary lesions located in other segments of the coronary artery tree.[5] Taking into consideration the anatomy and physiology of the coronary circulation, increased mortality is expected because LMCA is responsible for supplying up to 80% of total blood flow to the left ventricle (LV) in a right-dominant coronary system.[6] Thus, occlusion of the LMCA puts a significant portion of the myocardium in jeopardy. LMCA disease is a frequent finding in invasive coronary angiography (ICA). It is estimated that about 4% of ICA examinations reveal LMCA disease.[7] In addition, ICA reveals LMCA stenosis in about 5% and 7% of patients with stable angina and acute coronary syndrome, respectively.[8] About 5–10% of these patients present with isolated LMCA disease.[9]

The invasive treatment of LMCA disease has contributed to reduction in morbidity and mortality. Nowadays, both surgical and interventional revascularization have achieved comparable results in long-term follow-up; thus, a personalized approach is required for selecting the optimal therapeutic strategy.[10-12] The aim of this chapter is to review the main pathophysiological characteristics of LMCA disease, to present the imaging techniques during LMCA interventions and their impact on mortality, and, last, to shed light on the future directions in the management of this disease.

LEFT MAIN CORONARY ARTERY DISEASE: ANATOMIC AND PHYSIOLOGIC CHARACTERISTICS

The LMCA arises from the aorta, from the left sinus of Valsalva below the sinotubular junction. It runs between the pulmonary trunk and the left atrial appendage and ends up bifurcating into two major branches: The left anterior descending (LAD) and the left circumflex (LCx) artery.[13] A third branch, known as the ramus intermedius, arises from the LMCA in 30% of the general population.[13] The LMCA can be divided into three areas: The ostium, the trunk or shaft, and the distal vessel. The shaft and distal vessel present similar morphology; similar to epicardial vessels, they are composed of three layers (adventitia, media, and intima). However, the ostium lacks an adventitia and is more elastic, compared to other coronary vessels.[14] The total length of the LMCA is estimated at about 10.5 ± 5.3 mm, while the mean diameter is estimated at 3.9 ± 0.4 mm and 4.5 ± 0.5 mm in women and men, respectively.[15] Cases have been described in which the LMCA does not exist and the LAD and LCx have separate orifices; the prevalence of this anatomical variation is estimated between 0.2 and 1.6%.[16,17]

The composition of the atherosclerotic plaque of the LMCA differs significantly from lesions in other parts of the coronaries. LMCA plaques are characterized by minimal necrotic core content and thicker cap fibroatheroma.[18] The atherosclerotic plaques develop more frequently in segments with lower shear stress; thus, the most common locations of these lesions are the lateral walls of the bifurcation to the LAD and LCx.[19] Atherosclerotic lesions rarely appear on the carina of the bifurcation, probably due to the high shear stress at this location.[20] The vast majority of plaques are located in the distal part of the LMCA and are frequently extended to the proximal LAD and LCx, while the ostium is implicated in few cases,[21] especially in the short LMCA (<10 mm), probably due to the high shear stress and rheological laws.[22] The site of plaques has significant prognostic role because percutaneous coronary interventions (PCI) in lesions of the distal LMCA is technically more demanding and has poorer outcomes.[23] Due to all these factors, intravascular ultrasound (IVUS) or optical coherence tomography (OCT) is useful for choosing the optimal bifurcation strategy—an upfront two-stent or provisional stenting strategy in LMCA PCI, especially distal LMCA bifurcation stenting.[24]

IMAGING MODALITIES FOR LEFT MAIN CORONARY ARTERY PERCUTANEOUS CORONARY INTERVENTION

Current guidelines support PCI as an alternative and equivalent treatment to surgical revascularization in patients with LMCA disease and low or intermediate SYNTAX scores.[25] Patients with high (>32) SYNTAX score should be treated surgically. Intravascular imaging is considered mandatory before LMCA stenting, for the achievement of optimal results.[25] Imaging of LMCA stenosis is considered critical for its optimal evaluation and ideal management. As a result of progress in interventional cardiology, there exist both invasive and noninvasive methods to this end. Invasive assessment includes OCT and IVUS, whereas noninvasive includes mostly coronary computed tomography angiography (CCTA).[26] Each imaging modality has both advantages and disadvantages.

Invasive coronary angiography remains the gold standard and the first-line diagnostic tool used in LMCA disease. Historically, an angiographic diameter stenosis of >50% of the LMCA lumen has been established as a cutoff limit for distinguishing significant disease. However, the interpretation of angiographic views of the LMCA is frequently a challenge for invasive cardiologists. Several issues, such as overlap of branches, eccentric plaques, two-dimensional imaging, foreshortening of arteries, catheter displacement, and angle view of the LMCA, could lead to misinterpretation of disease severity. Moreover, angiographic evaluation remains subjective and may differ among operators. Taking the above into consideration, ICA remains the first step in the invasive assessment of LMCA disease, but is inadequate alone; thus, other techniques should accompany it for more accurate evaluation of the lesions, especially in patients with moderate stenosis (40–70%). IVUS or OCT also should be used for PCI guidance.

INTRACORONARY IMAGING GUIDANCE BEFORE, DURING, AND AFTER PERCUTANEOUS CORONARY INTERVENTIONS

Currently, intracoronary imaging has a class IIa recommendation in guiding LM treatment.[22] Moreover, in recent large randomized trials (although not specific for the LM setting),[27] intracoronary imaging was shown to improve long-term clinical outcomes, besides just the immediate procedural result. It is likely that the recommendation for its usage to guide complex PCI (including LM) will become even stronger in future consensus documents. IVUS is usually preferred to OCT, thanks to its ability to spare dye and to be independent from blood clearance, a well-known limitation of OCT in the evaluation of ostial lesions. The superior resolution of OCT can provide relevant advantages, especially when evaluating post-procedural results, and allows for an easier detection of stent malapposition. Still, at the moment, IVUS has an explicit recommendation in guidelines[28] based on available literature.

Intravascular Ultrasound

With over two decades of conventional use in LMCA disease evaluation, grayscale IVUS represents the mainstay of the LMCA intermediate lesions assessment. A small transducer is mounted at the tip of a flexible catheter, emitting ultrasound in the 10–60 MHz range, utilizing ultrasonography and acoustic properties for tissue characterization. Newer generation devices provide higher frequency and, as a result, improve the resolution.

Intravascular Ultrasound Measurements

Different measurements can be obtained by the IVUS, but the clinically relevant measurement of IVUS is the minimum luminal area (MLA). MLA has been studied extensively and can accurately predict whether revascularization is required or can be avoided.[29] Initial reports demonstrated that MLA >9 mm^2 or lumen stenosis greater than 50% constitute a hemodynamically significant stenosis. Fassa et al. decreased the lower limit of MLA to 7.5 mm^2 and major adverse cardiovascular events (MACE) rates in patients treated invasively and pharmaceutically did not show any differences in 3 years of follow-up, using this threshold.[30] Numerous trials have studied different MLA thresholds with comparable results, presented in **Table 1**.[30-34] Currents guidelines have set the cut-off at 6.0 mm^2, which could be applied globally.[31]

In the recent EXCEL trial, which compared PCI with CABG for LMCA disease, this value was used as the cutoff for MLA.[35] Smaller MLA thresholds have been studied in specific populations, and larger trials are required for validation of their results. According to the recent European position paper on intravascular imaging, LMCA IVUS-derived MLA >6 mm^2 could be safely deemed nonischemic, <4.5 mm^2 should be regarded as ischemia-generating, and the intermediate values are considered as "gray-zone", thus further assessment of ischemia should be performed.[36]

Calcium Assessment

Another feature of LMCA lesions is the existence of calcification, which is systematically underestimated in ICA. The identification and quantification of calcium is crucial because its presence is associated with poorer prognosis and suboptimal stent placement. Significant calcification could drive the carina to shift toward the LCx; thus, the kissing-balloon technique should be performed.[37] Indeed, calcium allocation affects the therapeutic algorithm; when the calcific arch surpasses 180°, a dedicated plaque modification strategy of calcified lesions is suggested. Rotational atherectomy remains a reliable approach for pretreatment of heavily calcified lesions, with acceptable inhospital results.[38] Intravascular lithotripsy could be also considered for lesion preparation in calcific distal LMCA disease.[38-42] When extensive calcification or high plaque load is located in bifurcations, the optimal technique is kissing-balloons. In the remaining cases, predilation with noncompliant balloons could be considered a sufficient treatment choice.[43]

TABLE 1: Studies comparing the optimal minimum lumen area (MLA) threshold.

Study	Year of publication	Number of patients	MLA threshold
Jasti et al.	2004	55	≤ 5.9 mm^2
Fassa et al.	2005	214	<7.5 mm^2
de la Torre Hernandez et al.	2011	354	<6 mm^2
Kang et al.	2011	403	<4.8 mm^2
Park et al.	2014	112	<4.5 mm^2

Percutaneous Coronary Interventions Guidance (Pre- and Post-stent)

In addition to the assessment of LMCA disease, IVUS is used for PCI guidance, before and after stent implantation. Prior to PCI, the operators should use IVUS, in order to:

- Characterize the plaque composition and distribution
- Select the suitable stent length and size
- Consider whether alternative interventions (lithotripsy or atherectomy) should be applied

After the stent's placement, IVUS should be performed to optimize the end result by assessing the plaque coverage and sufficient stent expansion.[44] Stent underexpansion has been demonstrated as the main risk factor for stent thrombosis and target lesion failure.[45] Moreover, suboptimal stent expansion has been correlated with hard endpoints, as it has been established as a serious prognostic factor for MACEs in 403 patients [Hazard ratio 5.56; 95% confidence intervals (CI) 1.99–15.49; $p = 0.001$].[32] The authors presented the minimum stent area (MSA) required in each segment of the LMCA to prevent significantly in-stent stenosis and MACEs. More specifically, the proposed MSA thresholds were 5.0 mm^2 for the LCx ostium, 6.3 mm^2 for the LAD ostium, 7.2 mm^2 for the polygon of confluence, and 8.2 mm^2 for the LMCA. These cutoffs, also known as the "5-6-7-8 rule", concern Korean patients, whereas in Caucasians, larger stent areas are needed, due to the greater body surface area. The prognostic role of MSA was validated by the recent EXCEL trial, which showed that the greater values of MSA are associated with less adverse events **(Fig. 1)**.

Real-world practice has shown that performing IVUS in LMCA disease management is highly beneficial. To the best of our knowledge, Saleem et al.[46] have conducted the

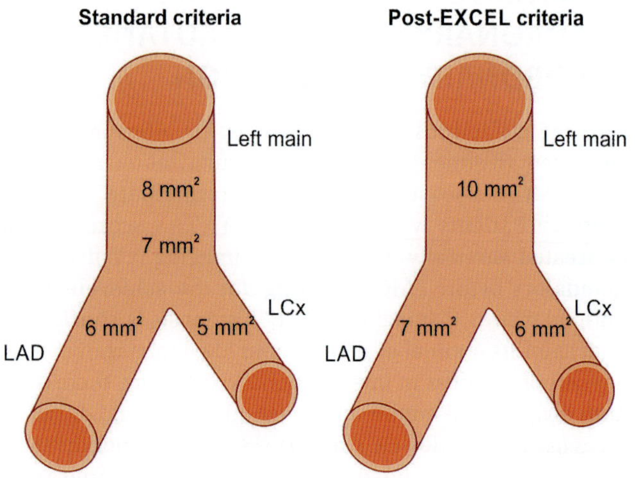

FIG. 1: Intravascular ultrasound criteria for stent optimization in the treatment of distal LM bifurcation.

largest meta-analysis about the prognostic role of IVUS on LMCA disease management. A total of 12 studies [2 randomized-controlled trials (RCTs) and 10 observational studies] were analyzed, resulting in considerable results; all-cause mortality (OR 0.57; 95% CI 0.46–0.70; $p < 0.00001$), cardiovascular mortality (OR 0.37; 95% CI 0.26–0.54; $p < 0.00001$), left-main revascularization (OR 0.63; 95% CI 0.45–0.89; $p = 0.009$), and myocardial infarction (MI) (OR 0.80; 95% CI 0.66–0.97; $p = 0.02$) were significantly lower in the IVUS-guided arm.[47] Moreover, Ye et al.[47] included ten studies totaling >6,400 patients, concluding that significant benefit from IVUS-guided PCI exists.

More specifically, IVUS-guided PCI was linked to a significantly lower risk of all-cause death [risk ratio (RR) 0.60; 95% CI 0.47–0.75; $p < 0.001$), cardiac death (RR 0.47; 95% CI 0.33–0.66; $p < 0.001$), target lesion revascularization (TLR) (RR 0.43; 95% CI 0.25–0.73; $p = 0.002$), and stent thrombosis (RR 0.28; 95% CI 0.12–0.67; $p = 0.004$).[48] These findings were confirmed by other smaller meta-analyses.[49,50] These metanalyses retrieved data from numerous observational studies and RCTs, which are reviewed in **Table 2**.[51-60]

One landmark meta-analysis is the "Meta-Analysis of Intravascular Ultrasound-Guided Drug-Eluting Stent Implantation for Left Main Coronary Disease" where a total of 11 studies (2 RCTs and 9 propensity-matched or adjusted observational studies) with 15,083 patients (7,668 in the IVUS group and 7,415 in the angiography group) were included. Follow-up in the included studies ranged from 1 to 10 years. Compared with angiography alone, IVUS-guidance was associated with a lower incidence of cardiovascular mortality (HR 0.39; 95% CI 0.27–0.58; $I^2 = 72\%$), all-cause mortality (HR 0.59; 95% CI 0.53–0.66; $I^2 = 0\%$), MI (HR 0.66; 95% CI

TABLE 2: Main studies comparing IVUS-guided and ICA-guided PCI in LMCA disease.

Study	Year of publication	Country	Design	Centers	Number of patients	Follow-up	Highlights
Park et al.	2009	Korea	Observational registry	Multicenter	756/219	3	↓ mortality rate in IVUS-guided arm ~ MI and TVF
de la Torre Hernandez et al.	2014	Spain	Pooled analysis of observational registries	Multicenter	505/1,165	3	↓ composite endpoint (cardiac death, MI, or TLR) in IVUS-guided arm ↓ all-cause mortality in IVUS-guided arm ↓ stent thrombosis in IVUS-guided arm
Gao et al.	2014	China	Observational	Single center	337/679	1	↓ composite endpoint (cardiac death, MI, or TLR) in IVUS-guided arm
Tan et al.	2015	Saudi Arabia	Randomized	Single center	61/62	2	~ MI and death ↓ TVF
Kim et al.	2017	Korea	Observational	Single center	122/74	3	~ all-cause, cardiovascular mortality, and MI
Andell et al.	2017	Sweden	Observational registry	Multicenter	621/1,847	10	↓ composite endpoint (all-cause death, restenosis, or definite stent thrombosis) in IVUS-guided amt ↓ all-cause death in IVUS-guided arm
Tian et al.	2017	China	Observational	Single center	713/1,186	3	↓ all-cause mortality in IVUS-guided arm ↓ MI in IVUS-guided arm
Liu et al.	2019	China	Randomized	Single center	167/169	1	↓ composite endpoint (cardiac death, MI, or TVF) in IVUS-guided arm ~ stent thrombosis
Choi et al.	2019	Korea	Observational	Single center	453/251	5	↓ cardiac death and adverse events in IVUS-guided arm
Kinnaird et al.	2020	United Kingdom	Observational Registry	Multicenter	5,056/6,208	1	↓ composite endpoint (death, stroke, or MI) in IVUS-guided arm ↑ 1 and 12 months survival in IVUS-guided arm
de la Torre Hernandez et al.	2020	Spain	Observational Registry	Multicenter	124/124	1	↓ composite endpoint (cardiac death, LMCA-related MI, and LMCA revascularization)

(ICA: invasive coronary angiography; IVUS: intravascular ultrasound imaging; LMCA: left main coronary artery; MI: myocardial infraction; PCI: percutaneous coronary interventions; TLR: target lesion revascularization; TVF: target vessel failure)

0.48–0.90, $I^2 = 0\%$), TLR (HR 0.51; 95% CI 0.39–0.68; $I^2 = 38\%$), and stent thrombosis (HR 0.38; 95% CI 0.26–0.56; $I^2 = 0\%$)[49] **(Table 2 and Fig. 2)**.

Another landmark study is the "Intravascular Imaging and 12-Month Mortality After Unprotected Left Main Stem PCI: An Analysis From the British Cardiovascular Intervention

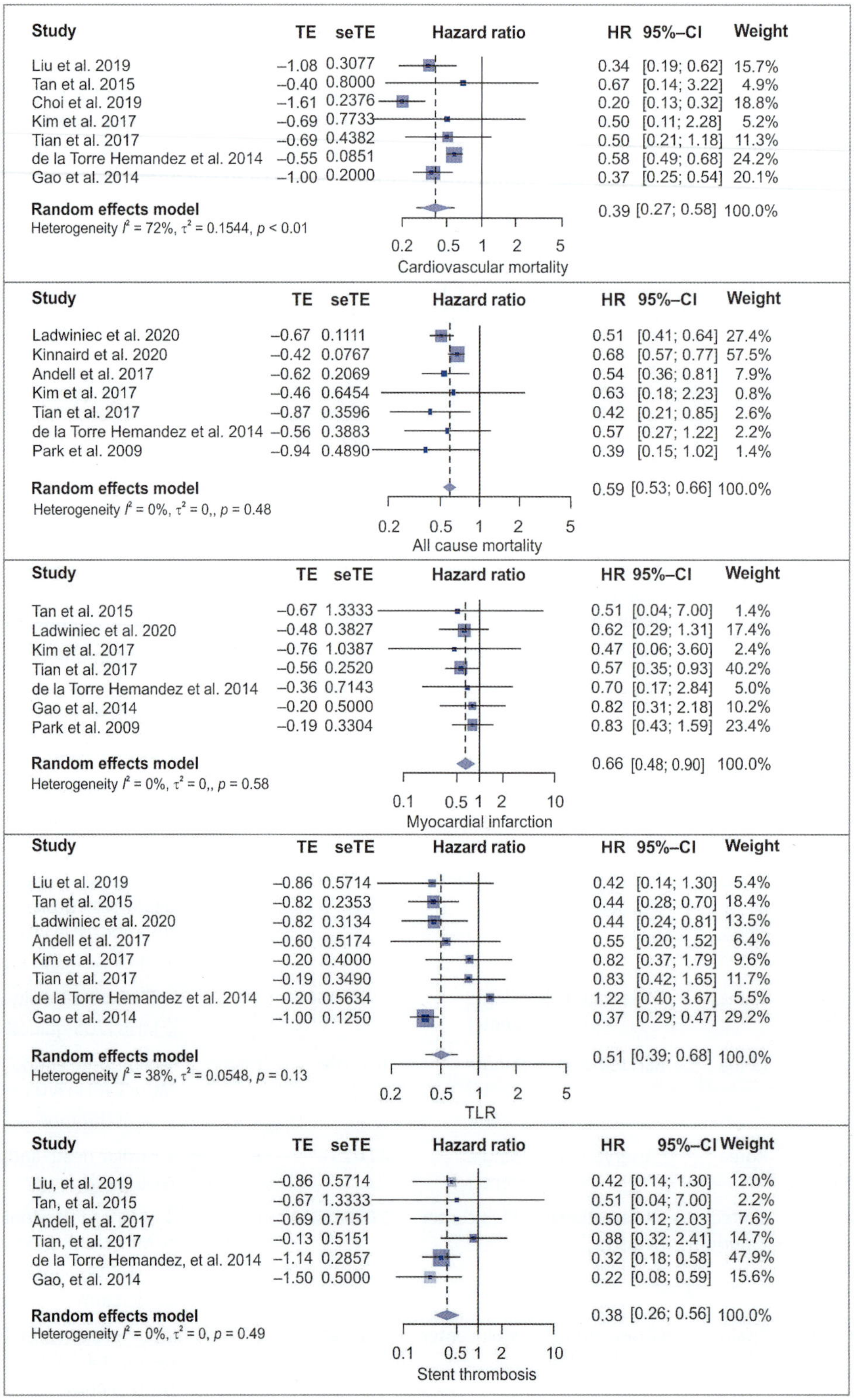

FIG. 2: Summary plot for outcomes: Meta-analysis of intravascular ultrasound-guided drug-eluting stent implantation for left main coronary disease.[49]

Society Database" where 11,264 patients undergoing LMCA PCI were studied out of which 5,056 patients underwent imaging (98% had IVUS), with imaging use increasing from 30% in 2007 to 50% in 2014 **(Fig. 3)**.[59]

A lower rate of coronary complications, lower inhospital MACE (OR 0.470; 95% CI 0.37–0.590; $p < 0.001$), and improved

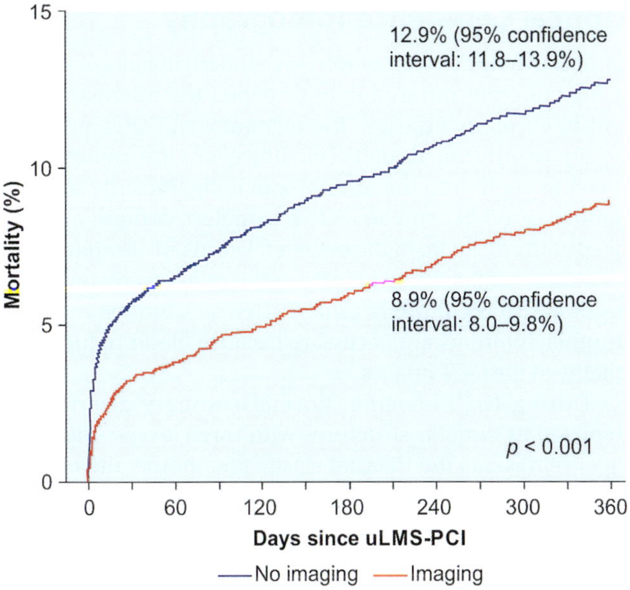

FIG. 3: Survival by intravascular imaging use after uLMS PCI in England and Wales from 2007 to 2014.[59]

30-day (OR 0.540; 95% CI 0.430–0.680; $p < 0.001$) and 12-month (OR 0.660; 95% CI 0.570–0.770; $p < 0.001$) mortality were observed with imaging use compared with no imaging use. Greater mortality reductions were observed with higher operator LMS PCI volume.[59]

Case example: Pre and postprocedural assessment of distal LMCA bifurcation PCI.[61]Following is a case example of the use of IVUS for preprocedure, intraprocedure, and postprocedure for LMCA PCI, which allows for lesion assessment, stent placements, and single versus two-stent strategy decision-making. **(Figs. 4 and 5).**

Center panel: Coronary angiography, showing severe disease of the distal LM, which involves the origin of both the LAD and the LCx. IVUS assessment allows accurate measurement of the reference vessel diameter of the LAD (**Fig. 4A**, of the LCx **(Fig. 4B)**, and of the LM **(Fig. 4F)**, minimum lumen diameter of the LAD **(Fig. 4C)**, of the LCx **(Fig. 4D)** and of the distal LM **(Fig. 5G)**, and longitudinal length of the lesion in both vessels **(Figs. 4E and H)** for LAD and LCx, respectively). Assessment of plaque morphology shows severe calcifications of both vessels, with an almost complete circumferential calcification at the level of the bifurcation.

The patient was treated with lithotripsy and implantation of two stents, with a T-and protrusion (TAP) technique. *Center panel:* Final angiographic view. Intravascular ultrasound shows good expansion and apposition of the stents and no residual dissection at the level of the distal landing of the LAD

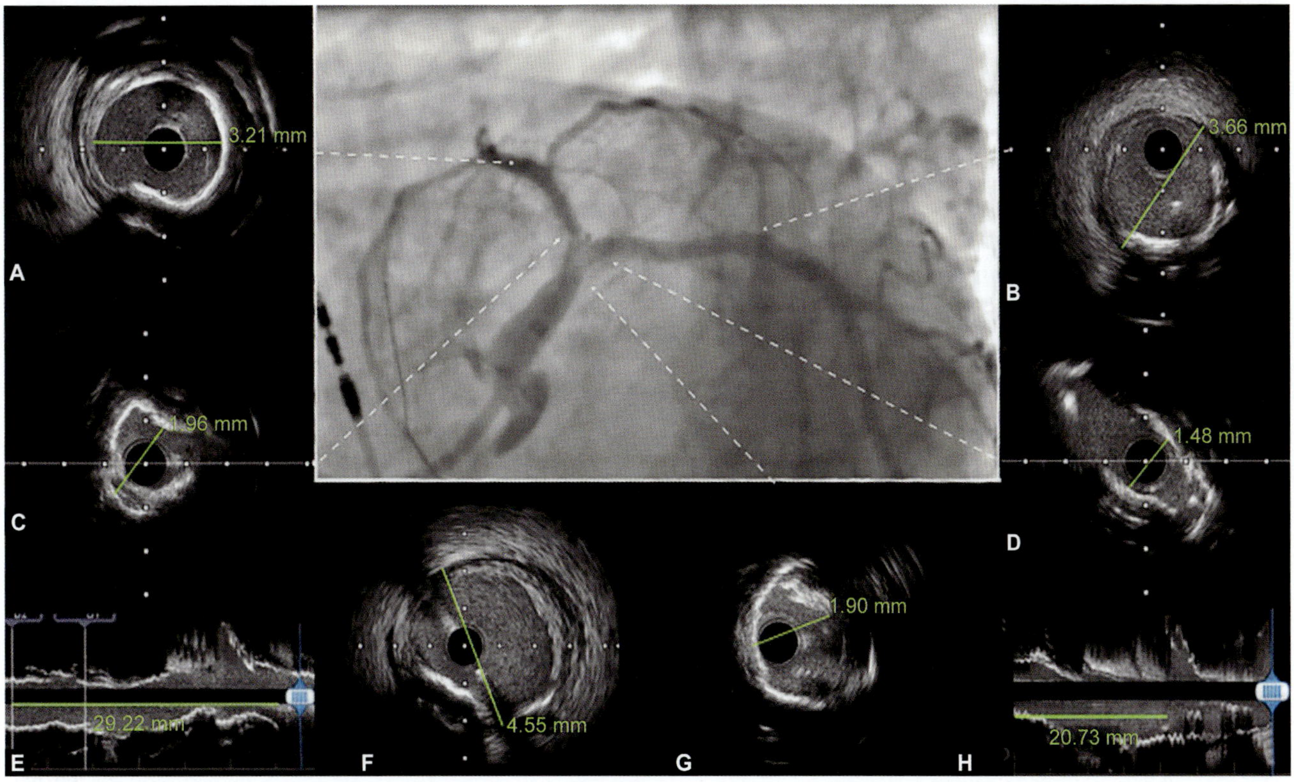

FIGS. 4A TO H: Preprocedural assessment of left main (LM) disease.[61]

and LCx arteries **(Figs. 5A and B**, respectively) at the level of the ostia **(Figs. 5C and D)** and at the level of the proximal and distal left main **(Figs 5 F and G)**. Neutral position of the neocarina is shown in panel **(Fig. 5G)** (red dotted line). Longitudinal view of the stents in the LAD and LCx are shown in panels **(Figs. 5E and H)**.

A recent study by Kim et al.[62] aimed to revise the IVUS-derived segmental MSA criteria for optimal stent expansion in patients undergoing an up-front two-stent strategy using the crush technique for LM bifurcation lesions to predict the 5-year clinical outcomes.

This study evaluated the IVUS-derived MSA criteria for optimal stent expansion based on the 5-year clinical events, including all-cause death, MI, and TLR in patients undergoing an up-front two-stent strategy using the crush technique for LM bifurcation lesions. This study found that the final MSA values within the LAD ostium (<8.3 mm^2) and LCx ostium (<5.7 mm^2) were significantly associated with the risk of 5-year MACE; however, MSA within the distal LM (<11.8 mm^2) was not predictive of long-term clinical events. In addition, patients with stent underexpansion in both the LAD and LCx ostium showed the highest rates of 5-year MACE (23.1%) and all-cause death (10.6%), whereas those with no or 1 underexpanded stent showed favorable 5-year clinical outcomes.

This study comprehensively analyzed the IVUS images from both LAD and LCx pullbacks, and stent underexpansion in the LAD and LCx ostium was significantly associated with long-term clinical outcomes after LM 2-stenting. These findings suggested the need to achieve a sufficiently large MSA, and the optimal MSA cutoff values proposed in this study could serve as a reference for stent optimization during LM PCI in the future **(Fig. 6)**.

Optical Coherence Tomography

Optical coherence tomography is a modern imaging modality using coherent infrared light to depict the microstructure within coronary arteries. The technology of OCT provides better resolution than IVUS; however, the penetrating imaging depth into the arterial wall is significantly smaller. Similar to IVUS catheters, OCT catheters contain an OCT head at the distal tip of the catheter. During the examination, automatic pullback and rotation of the catheter creates cross-sectional views of the coronary arteries. Contrast medium or other solutions are necessary because blood reduces the quality of the OCT images.[63]

During OCT imaging, normal coronary arteries are depicted as circular structures with three layers: The inner layer represents the internal elastic membrane; the middle, dark layer corresponds to the median layer; and the outer layer is the external elastic lamina.[64,65]

Optical coherence tomography is less studied than IVUS in LMCA disease. The ROCK I trial compared OCT-guided LMCA PCI with standard (angiographic ± IVUS) PCI,

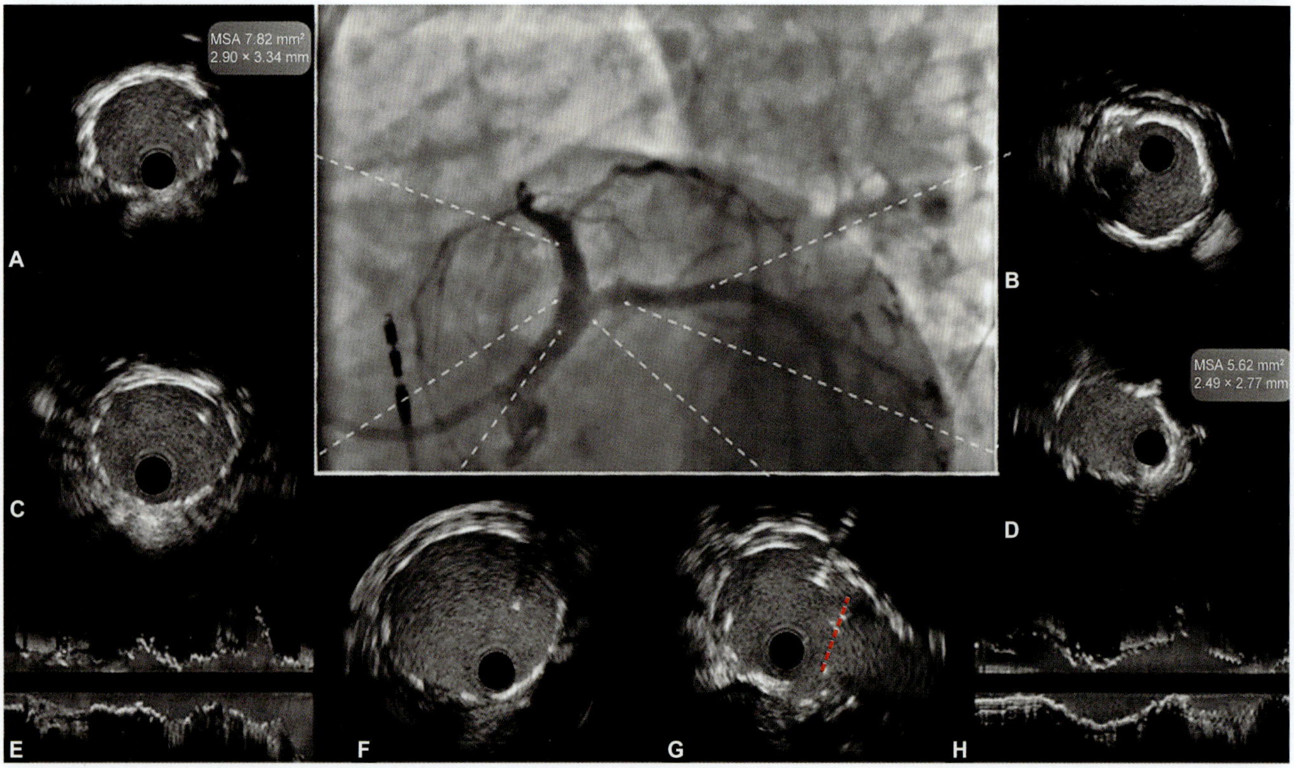

FIGS. 5A TO H: Final procedural assessment of the above case.[61]

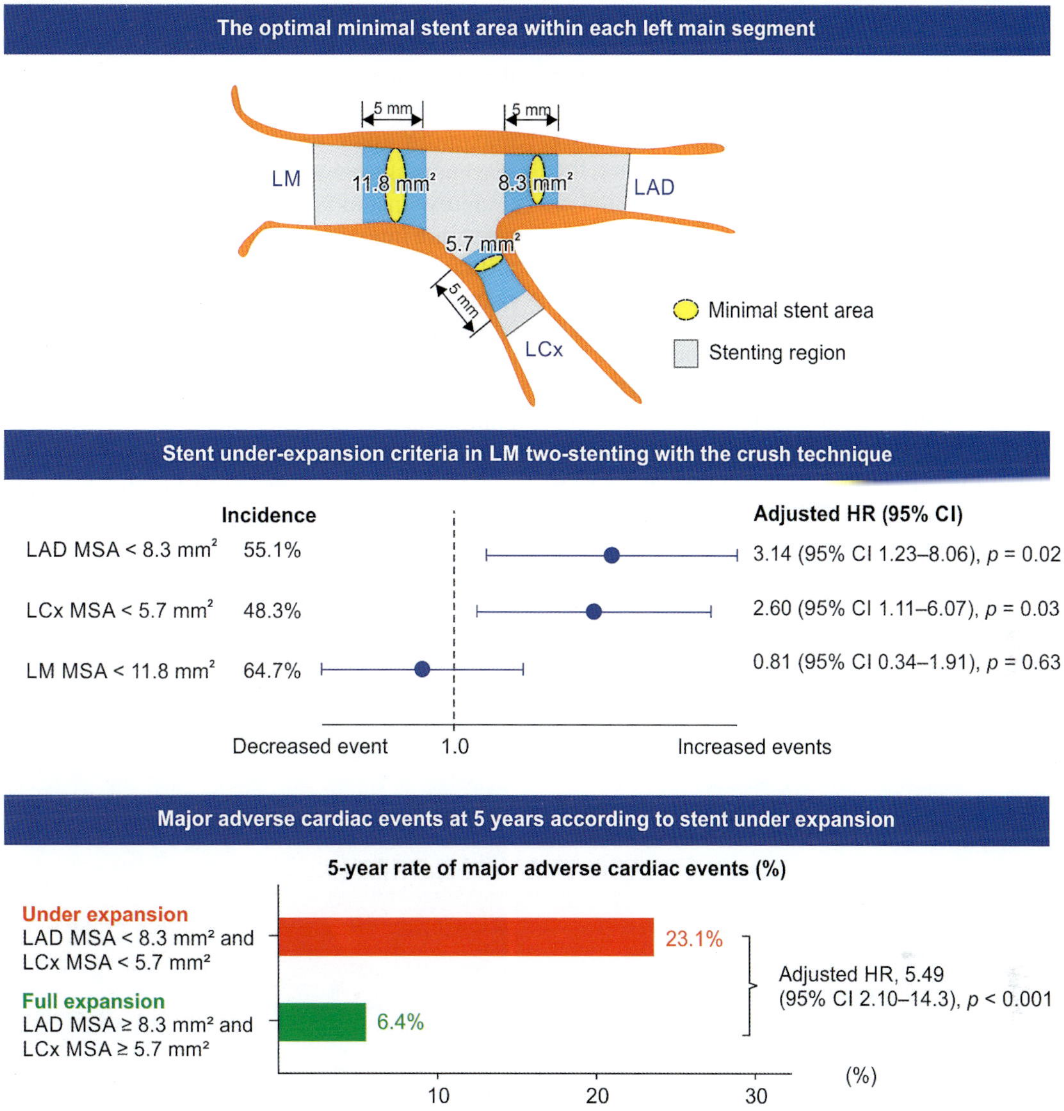

FIG. 6: Salient features from the study by Kim et al.[62]

retrospectively. Although no clinical difference was observed between the two groups, late lumen loss tended to be lower in the OCT arm and was significantly reduced in the distal part of the main vessel. Moreover, OCT guidance contributed to the detection of cases with underexpansion and malposition of stents.[66]

Roule et al.[67] supported that >90% of the quadrants of the LMCA were adequately assessable by newer-generation OCT, while most artifacts were located at the proximal part of the LM. A study by Burzotta et al.[68] confirmed that the OCT evaluation of the distal LM is more accurate and efficient, compared to the more proximal segments of the LMCA, where the diagnostic ability of OCT is poor.

Bouki et al.[69] confirmed the inability of OCT to evaluate proximal lesions, as only half of the plaques located in the proximal LMCA could be analyzed. Moreover, they claimed that the OCT-derived MLA of ≤5.38 mm^2 accurately predicts the functional severity of LMCA disease. Nevertheless, further studies with OCT should be conducted for defining OCT-derived MLA criteria and not extrapolating data by IVUS, due to the existing discrepancy between the two methods.

Optical coherence tomography is more effective in detecting thrombus, dissection, extent of calcification, and incomplete apposition of stent struts. The LEMON study[70] is the first to assess the role of OCT in LM PCI according to a standardized protocol. This study included 70 patients with nonostial LM stenosis from 10 centers in France. The prespecified protocol consisted of three OCT runs. The first one was performed prior to stent implantation to evaluate plaque features, landing zones, lesion length, dimensions of the reference segment and stent, and balloon diameter for proximal optimization technique (POT). After stent placement, POT, and side branch (SB) rewiring, the second run was carried out with the goal of assessing the recross wire in the jailed SB. After PCI optimization, a third run was conducted to analyze stent expansion and identify significant strut malapposition and edge dissection. Further PCI optimization was carried out in 26% instances following the second and third runs, indicating that OCT guidance altered the PCI approach in a quarter of patients.

To overcome the inherent difficulties in stent expansion assessment within bifurcated lesions, a novel OCT criterion called the "LEMON criteria" was established. The stent was divided into two sections, using the carina as the cutoff point. The MSA was then measured in the proximal (upstream carina) and distal (downstream carina) sections. The ratio between MSA and reference MLA was calculated for both sections. The expansion was considered successful if the MSA/reference MLA was ≥80% in both proximal and distal stent sections. The primary endpoint of procedural success was a combination of residual stenosis of <50% by quantitative coronary angiography and TIMI III flow in all arteries. Adequate stent expansion was achieved in 86% of the cases. The MACE rate at 1 year was 1.4%.[70]

Although IVUS can provide decent information about calcified lesions, OCT is more precise in estimating calcium thickness and whether it can affect stent expansion. It has been reported that patients with calcium deposit with a maximum angle greater than 180°, length >5 mm, and maximum thickness higher than 0.5 mm were at risk of stent underexpansion and subsequent stent stenosis.[71] In such cases, the interventional cardiologists could perform special techniques, such as rotational atherectomy, balloon dilation, or lithotripsy, in order to appropriately modify the plaques.

Optical coherence tomography is useful for evaluating stent failure. Specifically, OCT could provide critical information regarding the underlying mechanism of failure, such as neoatherosclerosis, neointimal hyperplasia, stent thrombosis, underexpansion, or fracture. Thus, the appropriate treatment could be chosen and preventive measures for repetitive stent failure could be applied.[72]

Case example: OCT in LM bifurcation PCI[61]

It depicts the use of OCT in LMCA PCI, especially bifurcation lesions, with excellent demonstration of stent apposition and the final result poststenting **(Figs. 7A to D).**

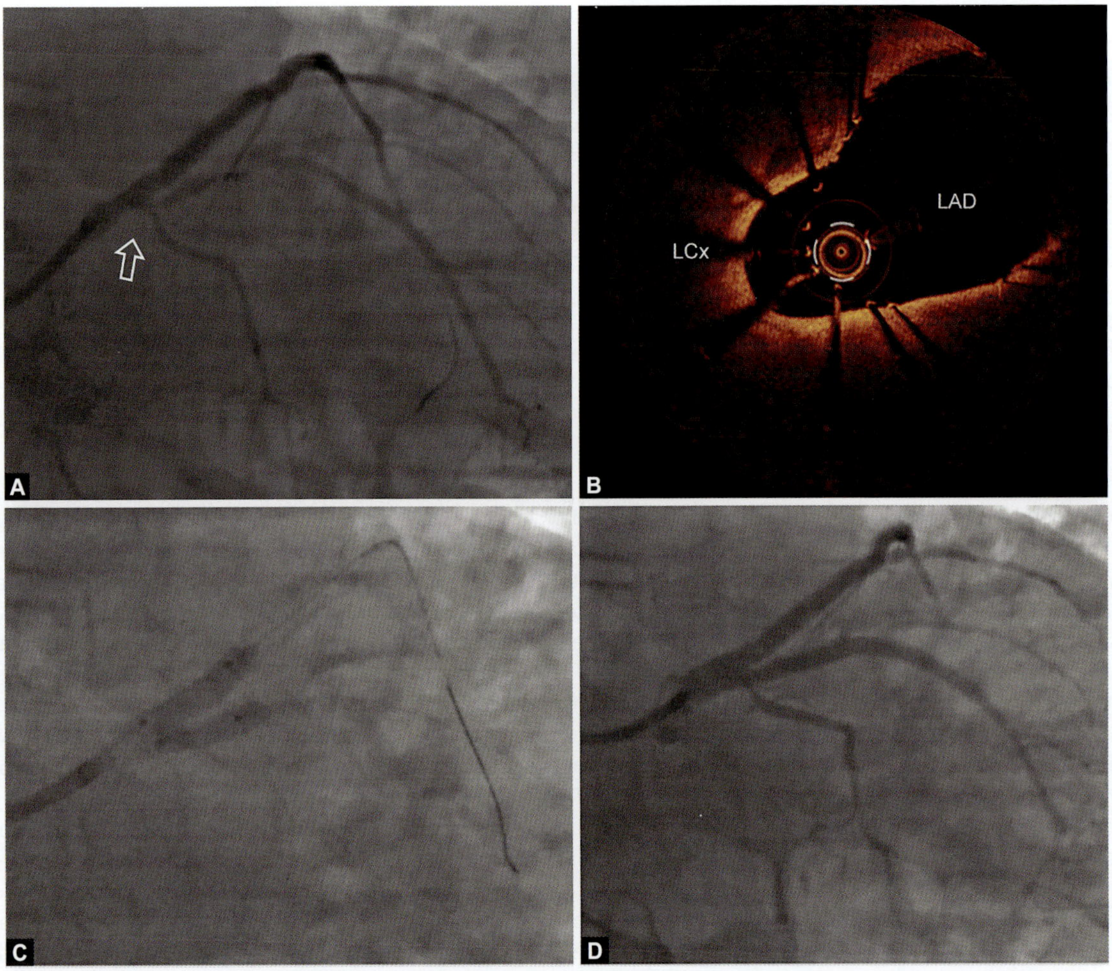

FIGS. 7A TO D: Intravascular detection of unintentional stent protrusion in the left main.

The patient had a previous intervention in the LAD, with stents trying to nail the ostium of the vessel. A staged procedure of the LCx was planned due to severe stenosis up to the ostium **(Fig. 7A**, arrow**)**. Due to difficult delivery of devices in the LCx, OCT was performed **(Fig. 7B)**, showing unintentional protrusion of the "ostial" stent from the LAD in the LM, with good expansion but extensive malapposition and intraluminal passage of the LCx wire. The lesion was then treated with kissing-balloon inflation **(Fig. 7C)** and implantation of a new stent from the LCx to the LM to complete a culotte technique. After final kissing-balloon inflation, a good result was achieved in both vessels **(Fig. 7D)**.

EUROPEAN BIFURCATION CLUB CONSENSUS STATEMENT: SALIENT POINTS[73]

Intravascular Ultrasound Assessment of Left Main Coronary Artery

Three considerations are important from a technical standpoint when evaluating LMCA lesion severity.

First, when studying an ostial LMCA stenosis, it is important to disengage the guiding catheter to avoid confusing the guiding catheter with an ostial stenosis, and it is important to maintain a coaxial relationship between the IVUS catheter and the LMCA ostium.

Secondly, it is not reliable to use IVUS imaging of either the LCx or the LAD to infer the status of the other vessel tangentially during pullback, as either ostial lumen dimension or plaque burden assessment can be misleading.

Third, a discrepancy in the MLA in the LMCA when imaging from the LAD or LCx can be generated by the oblique plane of the IVUS beam when the transducer turns from the daughter vessel with the greatest angle into the LMCA. This oblique transducer position can create an artificially large MLA, but not one that is artificially small; therefore, the smallest MLA is the most accurate.

As part of procedure planning, IVUS can be used before stent implantation to assess the following:

- *Risk of SB compromise:* Lesions proximal or distal to the SB or ostial SB stenoses affect the risk of SB compromise after main vessel stenting. Patients who have a "vulnerable" carina—the eyebrow sign or significant calcium identified by IVUS longitudinal reconstruction—are at particular risk of adverse carina shift toward the LCx.
- *Stent length:* When using automated pullback, proposed stent length can be measured to limit residual stenosis in adjoining segments (i.e., geographic miss).
- *Stent diameters:* Segmental stent diameters can be based on proximal and distal reference size measurements.
- Reference size and length measurements can be used to plan the size and length of the "POT balloon" to ensure that it fits within the stent from carina to the proximal stent edge.

Summary statements/recommendations:

- A "provisional" approach is the default treatment strategy for the LMCA.
- Sizing of the stent should be based on the diameter of the branch vessel. The selected stent type should allow POT as the final dilation of all LMCA procedures (POT or re-POT). IVUS can be used before stenting to inform the operator about the likelihood of needing a two-stent technique
- POT and kissing-balloon postdilation are mandatory in two-stent bifurcation procedures.

Conclusions of the EBC consensus: The EBC believes that IVUS guidance is useful at each step of an LMCA interventional procedure—

- To decide whether or not revascularization is necessary
- To decide whether a one-stent crossover technique (the default strategy) is sufficient or whether a two-stent technique may be more appropriate
- To size the stent (diameter and length) and select the optimum landing zones
- To optimize the final result (expansion, apposition, and geographic miss). While randomized trials are limited, data suggest that IVUS guidance is superior to angiographic guidance in terms of death, MI, TLR, ISR, and ST.

SUGGESTED ALGORITHM FOR LMCA BIFURCATION LESION TREATMENT

After reviewing all the available data on LM bifurcation PCI randomized controlled trials and considering the provisional stenting technique and escalation to two-stent strategies in LMCA bifurcation lesions, with technical characteristics of optimal provisional LMCA stenting technique and angiographic and intravascular determinants of escalation, the following is a suggested algorithm for LMCA bifurcation PCI with imaging guidance upfront and also after crossover stenting **(Fig. 8)**.[74]

FUTURE PERSPECTIVES

During the two last decades, intravascular imaging modalities have developed remarkably, but further steps are required for the better depiction, evaluation, and management of LMCA lesions. The progress in technology and biophysics will significantly contribute to the evolution of IVUS. The first devices combining IVUS with near-infrared spectroscopy (NIRS) have been recently released. Although the existing literature is limited, integrated IVUS–NIRS systems are thought to provide more detailed information regarding atherosclerotic plaque morphology and erosion risk.[75]

The combination of IVUS with OCT may attract attention in the near future. Simultaneous performance of OCT and IVUS examination as coregistration has been applied in some

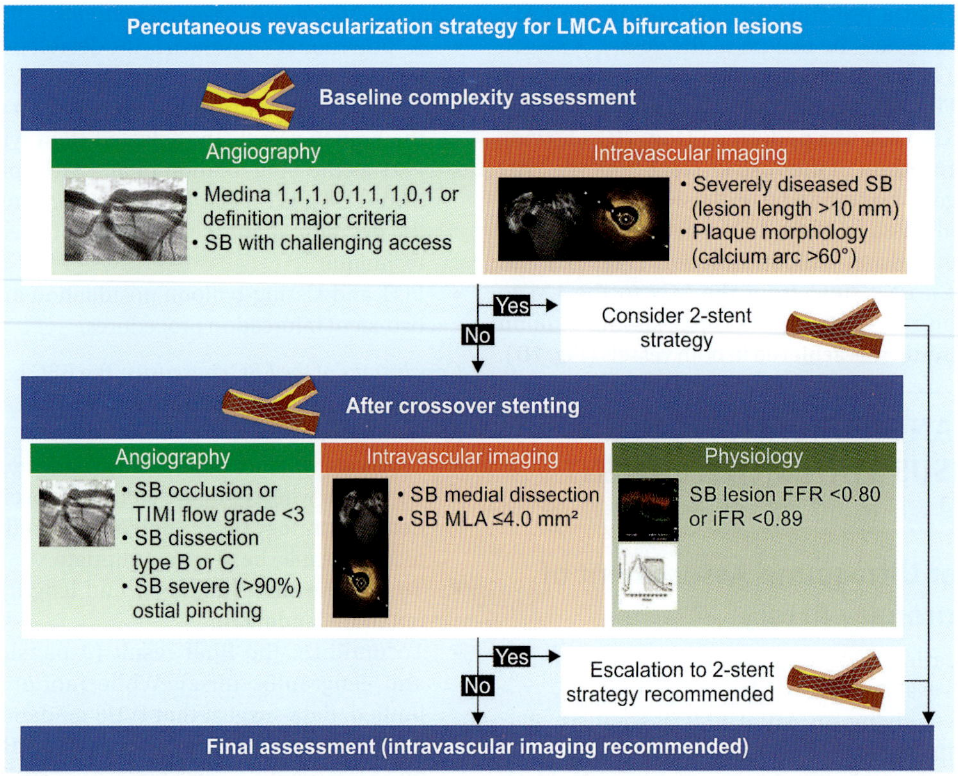

FIG. 8: Percutaneous revascularization strategy for LMCA bifurcation lesions.

catheterization laboratories.[75,76] Moreover, IVUS and OCT were integrated into a hybrid, single-catheter system. The novel, hybrid OCT-IVUS catheter aims to achieve optimal depiction of lesions in the coronary arteries.

For "gray-zone" lesions, in which the optimal management remains unclear, the IVUS "virtual histology" option could be helpful. This is an IVUS-based postprocessing modality for spectral interpretation of the primary raw backscattered radiofrequency. After the processing of black and white images, the tissues are color-coded as four major components; dense calcium (white), necrotic core (red), fibro-fatty (light green), and fibrous tissue (dark green).[77,78] Newer technologies will allow artificial intelligence (AI) enabled three-dimensional (3D)-reconstruction to achieve a more realistic depiction of the anatomy and morphology of the lesions.[79,80] Moreover, AI and deep learning systems will expand intravascular imaging capabilities.[81,82]

CONCLUSION

Imaging plays a vital role in LMCA PCI, enhancing procedural success and patient outcomes. Coronary angiography, IVUS, OCT, fractional flow reserve, and 3D imaging and reconstruction each offer unique insights and benefits. By integrating these modalities, interventional cardiologists can optimize stent placement, expansion, and apposition, reducing complications and improving long-term results. As technology continues to evolve, we can expect even more advanced imaging tools to emerge, further revolutionizing the field of interventional cardiology.

ONLINE REFERENCES

Please scan the QR code provided at the end of the table of contents for References of this chapter.

CHAPTER 148

Physiological Assessment of Intermediate Left Main Coronary Artery Lesion

Arun Mohanty, Ashish Kumar Jain, Sonal Jain

ABSTRACT

The left main coronary artery (LMCA) is responsible for supplying the majority of left ventricular myocardium. Visual estimation of stenosis has major limitations. Assessment of intermediate lesions, particularly those with 50–70% involvement, is crucial for diagnostic and therapeutic challenges. Techniques like fractional flow reserve (FFR), instantaneous wave-free ratio (iFR), and nonhyperemic indices are valuable tools for the precise evaluation of lesion significance. The integration of advanced imaging modalities such as intravascular ultrasound (IVUS) and optical coherence tomography (OCT) enhances these assessments, contributing to personalized management strategies and improved long-term clinical outcomes.

Keywords: ACS, FFR, iFR, LMCA

INTRODUCTION

Left main supplies two-thirds of the myocardial tissue via the left anterior descending artery (LAD) and left circumflex artery (LCx). Large stakes lie in coronary event, postleft main associated acute coronary syndrome (ACS). 3–10% of coronary angiography (CAG) for routine evaluation of angina shows left main involvement. Left main coronary artery (LMCA) disease shows the most difficulties for an adequate angiographic evaluation, especially when intermediate lesions (50–70%).[1] Hence to assess their functional and anatomic significance is important in this setting as they pose a potential diagnostic and therapeutic challenge. This chapter will focus on the assessment of intermediate LMCA lesion, viz. (1) imaging modalities such as intravascular ultrasound (IVUS) and optical coherence tomography (OCT). (2) Percutaneous functional assessment of coronary stenosis: Hyperemic and nonhyperemic indexes.

IMPORTANCE OF LEFT MAIN CORONARY ARTERY IN CARDIAC PHYSIOLOGY

The left main coronary artery typically measures 3–6 mm in diameter and 10–20 mm in length. MI, after left main (LM) plaque rupture, involves the entire left ventricle and the inferior wall of the right ventricle in patients with left dominant anatomy. Complete occlusion of the LMCA, often referred to as a "widow-maker" heart attack, can cause extensive myocardial infarction and is associated with high mortality rates.[2]

Left main stenosis can occur in the ostial (23%), mid-shaft (15%), and distal (61%) segments and depending on the location and severity differ.[3] Variations in the length and bifurcation pattern of the LMCA can influence the presentation and management of coronary artery disease. In 0.03% of patients, the origin of the LMCA is anomalous describing its trajectory between the aorta and the pulmonary artery, a pattern associated with a high risk of sudden death. Anomalous origins, such as the LMCA arising from the right aortic sinus, are rare but clinically significant.[4] In severe cases, LMCA disease can lead to heart failure, arrhythmias, or sudden cardiac death due to the extensive area of myocardium affected. Without revascularization, its prognosis is poor, and the mortality rate can be up to 37% at 3-year follow-up.[4]

SIGNIFICANCE OF LEFT MAIN CORONARY ARTERY INTERMEDIATE LESIONS

Anatomic Assessment (Intravascular Imaging)

The primary intravascular imaging modalities are IVUS and OCT.

Intravascular Ultrasound

Intravascular ultrasound provides detailed visualization of the arterial wall, lumen, and plaque composition, its spread, and classification. IVUS provides information on the calcific burden in the LMCA lesion, which can be used to determine upfront plaque-modification strategies and to assess poststenting complications, such as edge dissection, underexpansion, and stent deformation.[5]

Technical Consideration

Mintz et al.[6] proposed three technical considerations when evaluating LMCA lesion severity. First, the guiding catheter should be disengaged while assessing ostial LMCA stenosis to avoid confusing it with ostial stenosis, and it is important to maintain a coaxial relationship between the IVUS catheter and the LMCA ostium. Second, IVUS is unreliable when imaging of either the LCx or the LAD is done to infer the status of the other vessel tangentially during pullback. Because, either ostial lumen dimension or plaque burden assessment can be misleading. Third, when a pullback is done from LAD or LCx into LMCA, there is a discrepancy between the minimum lumen area (MLA) in the LMCA due to the oblique plane of the IVUS beam when the transducer turns from the daughter vessel with the greatest angle into the LMCA. This will provide an artificially large MLA, but not one that is artificially small; therefore, the smallest MLA is the most accurate.[6]

Evidence

A study by Jasti et al. found that an MLA of <6 mm^2 is associated with a significant reduction in fractional flow reserve (FFR), indicating functionally significant LMCA stenosis.[7] The LITRO study demonstrated that IVUS-guided PCI, resulted in lower rates of adverse cardiac events compared to angiography alone, with a reduction in the composite endpoint of death, myocardial infarction, and target lesion revascularization from 16.0 to 10.0% at 2 years.[8]

Optimization is crucial after LMCA stenting. According to Kang et al.,[9] the optimal poststenting minimal stent area (MSA) should be 8 mm^2 in the LMCA and 7 mm^2 at the level of the point of convergence (POC). This has been linked to increased survival. However, the outcomes of subsequent investigations vary in terms of LMCA MSA. Further insight into the achievable IVUS MSA was provided by a post hoc analysis of the IVUS core laboratory data from the NOBLE trial. The MSA criteria of LMCA (8 mm^2), POC (7 mm^2), LAD ostium (6 mm^2), and LCx ostium (5 mm^2) was not achieved in 3.6%, 0.5%, 5.2%, and 7.6% of patients, respectively. When this "failure to achieve MSA" group was compared to those who achieved satisfactory MSA, there were numerically higher numbers of event rates in the former group: Major adverse cardiac and cerebrovascular events 36.8% versus 20%, death 15.8% versus 5.4%, and repeat revascularization 15.8% versus 11.7%, respectively. None of these were statistically significant due to few event rates and a decreased number of patients who underwent core laboratory analysis.[10] In the EXCEL trial, greater MACE rates (18.2%) were reported in patients who did not achieve post-PCI MSA of 9.8 mm^2 in comparison to those who did (11.5%) at 3-year follow-up.[11] There have been six published IVUS studies assessing LMCA severity, including three with clinical follow-up **(Figs. 1A to C)**.[6]

Optical Coherence Tomography

Technical Consideration

Optical coherence tomography is particularly useful for assessing thin cap fibroatheromas, plaque rupture, plaque erosion, and calcifications. But OCT has a limited penetration depth compared to IVUS, making it less suitable for assessing deep vessel structures and large diameter vessels as LMCA. It also requires blood clearance during imaging, which can be technically challenging for ostial disease.[12]

Evidence

A study by Prati et al.[13] showed that OCT-guided stent implantation resulted in a significant reduction in stent malapposition compared to angiography alone. The LEMON study is the first to assess the role of OCT in LM PCI according to a standardized protocol. A novel OCT criterion called the "LEMON criteria" was established. The stent was divided into two sections, using the carina as the cut-off point. The MSA was then measured in the proximal (upstream carina) and distal (downstream carina) sections. The ratio between MSA and reference MLA was calculated for both sections. The expansion was considered successful if the MSA/reference MLA was ≥80% in both proximal and distal stent

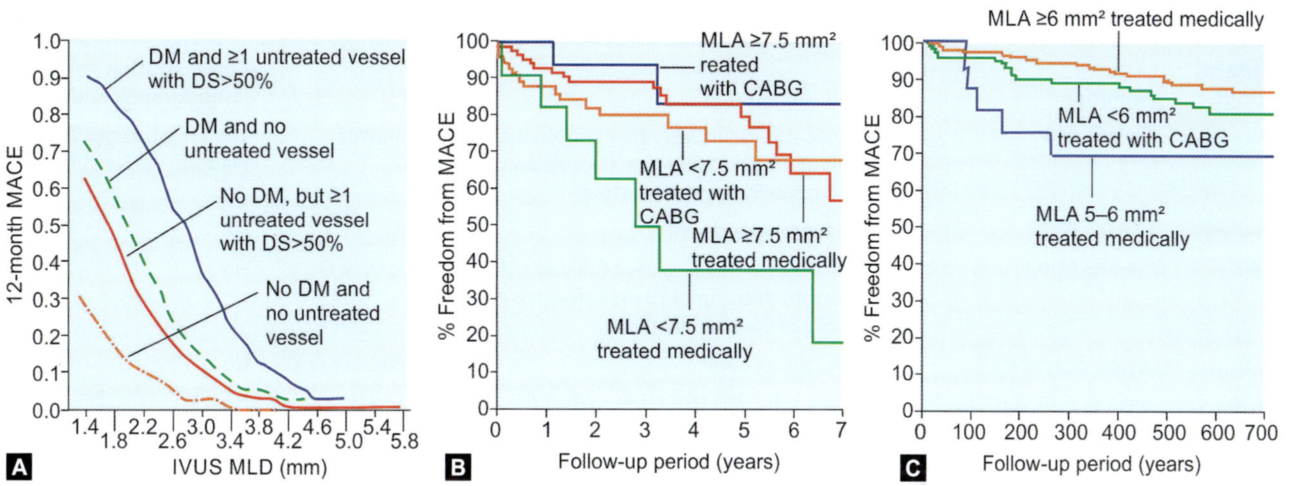

FIGS. 1A TO C: Three studies have related the IVUS minimum lumen area (MLA) in the left main coronary artery to long-term clinical events. Abizaid et al. (A); Fassa et al. (B); and (C) an update of the LITRO Registry in a presentation by de la Torre Hernandez at TCT 2017.
Source: Adapted from Mintz et al. (2018).[6]

sections. The primary endpoint of procedural success was a combination of residual stenosis of <50% by quantitative coronary angiography and thrombolysis in MI-3 flow in all arteries. Adequate stent expansion was achieved in 86% of the cases. The MACE rate at 1 year was 1.4%.[14]

FUNCTIONAL ASSESSMENT (HYPEREMIC AND NONHYPEREMIC INDICES): HYPEREMIC PRESSURE INDICES (FRACTIONAL FLOW RESERVE)

Fractional Flow Reserve

Fractional flow reserve is the ratio between mean distal coronary pressure (P_d) and mean aortic pressure (P_a) during maximal hyperemia gives the functional significance of coronary stenosis. A value less than 0.8 in intermediate lesions represents significant stenosis warranting further intervention.[15]

Technical Consideration

The pressure wire (PW) is advanced distal to the lesion. Pressures must be equalized and measured using a guide catheter that has been partially engaged in the LMCA to prevent a presumed ostial lesion from affecting the measurement. It is always a better option to measure FFR by placing the PW in both branches of the LMCA. For logical reasons, some operators warrant using IV adenosine infusion (140 µg/kg) rather than intracoronary adenosine, as the guide catheter needs to be disengaged for accurate FFR measurement in LMCA disease. In the presence of downstream stenosis, it is essential to treat the distal lesion before making any decisions based on FFR.[15]

Evidence

Several key studies have established the role of FFR in managing LMCA disease. The DEFER study demonstrated the safety of deferring revascularization for lesions with an FFR >0.75, showing favorable long-term outcomes.[16] The FAME trial found that FFR-guided PCI reduced major adverse cardiac events (MACE) compared to angiography-guided PCI, highlighting the importance of functional assessment.[17] The IRIS-FFR registry confirmed that patients with LMCA lesions and an FFR >0.80 had similar long-term outcomes whether revascularization was deferred or performed.[18] Lastly, a study by Jasti et al. compared IVUS-guided to FFR-guided PCI in unprotected LMCA disease, finding excellent outcomes with both but emphasizing FFR's superior functional assessment.[7] Together, these studies support FFR as a reliable tool for guiding revascularization decisions in LMCA disease, reducing unnecessary interventions, and improving patient outcomes.

NONHYPEREMIC PRESSURE INDICES INSTANTANEOUS WAVE-FREE RATIO, DIASTOLIC PRESSURE RATIO, DIASTOLIC HYPEREMIA-FREE RATIO, RESTING FULL-CYCLE RATIO, CONSTANT RESISTANCE RATIO

These indices (detailed in **Table 1**) offer the advantage of not requiring the induction of hyperemia, thereby avoiding the

TABLE 1: Definitions of nonhyperemic pressure ratios.

Type of NHPR	Definition	Calculation period	Device	Coregistration (angiography and IVUS)
iFR	Average P_d/P_a	Diastolic sub-cycle (wave-free period) that begins at the point 25% into diastole and ends 5 ms before end of diastole	PW: OmniWire	Yes (for IntraSight 7 Platform via SyncVision)
Resting	Average P_d/P_a	Whole cardiac cycle	PW/PMC	NA
dPR	Average P_d/P_a	Whole diastole that begins at the nadir of the dicrotic notch until 50 ms before the upstroke of the next heartbeat	PW: OptoWire Deux	No
RFR	Lowest filtered P_d/P_a	Whole cardiac cycle	PW: PressureWire X	No
DFR	Average P_d/P_a (on 5 beats)	Diastolic sub-cycle that begins when the P_a, is less than the mean P_a, and there is a down-sloping P_a	PW: Comet II	No
^{dPR}micro	Average P_d/P_a (on 5 beats)	Diastolic point within diastole halfway between the peak of one waveform and the peak of the next waveform	PMC: Navvus I	No
cRR	Average P_d/P_a	Diastolic sub-cycle (wave-free period) was identified by calculating the time derivative of P_d/P_a, and finding the longest period when it equals zero	PMC: TruePhysio	No

Note: For PWs the sensor is just proximal to the radiopaque part.

(cRR: constant resistance ratio; DFR: diastolic hyperemia-free ratio; dPR: diastolic pressure ratio; iFR: instantaneous wave-free ratio; IVUS: intravascular ultrasound; NA: not applicable; NHPR: nonhyperemic pressure ratio; P_a: aortic pressure; P_d: distal coronary pressure; PMC: pressure microcatheter; PW: pressure wire; RFR: resting full-cycle ratio)

Source: Adapted from Vergni et al. (2024).[19]

side effects associated with hyperemic indices, such as chest pain and dyspnea as well as shorter procedure times.

Instantaneous Wave-free Ratio

The instantaneous wave-free ratio (iFR) is the most widely investigated of all nonhyperemic pressure ratios (NHPRs) and has a value of 0.89 matched best with an FFR ≤ 0.80 **(Fig. 2)**.

Evidence

Several key studies have validated the use of iFR in assessing LMCA disease. The study by Warisawa et al.[20] found that iFR-guided decision-making was noninferior to FFR, with similar clinical outcomes such as death, myocardial infarction, and revascularization rates. The ADVISE II study showed a strong correlation between iFR and FFR, demonstrating similar diagnostic accuracy and predictive value for adverse cardiac events with an area under the ROC curve of 0.90.[21] In the SYNTAX II study, iFR-guided PCI led to improved outcomes compared to angiography-guided PCI, with fewer adverse events and better long-term survival rates.[22] The iLITRO-EPIC 07 study concluded that iFR could safely guide the decision to defer or proceed with revascularization in intermediate LMCA stenosis, with favorable short- and long-term outcomes.[23] Collectively, these studies support the use of iFR as a reliable, nonhyperemic alternative to FFR for evaluating and managing LMCA lesions, providing similar efficacy and improved patient comfort. Though FFR and iFR can guide the decision to revascularize or defer LM lesions; if there are discordant results, performing IVUS and deferring the LM lesion can be considered only when the MLA is above 6 mm^2. However, there is 25–30% discordance between FFR and iFR in LMCA attributing to a larger volume of myocardium affected by these lesions, and the consequent and proportionate increase in the hyperemic flow across the stenotic segments. **Flowchart 1** gives an approach to intermediate LMCA lesions with respect to imaging-guided or physiology-guided cutoffs and alternatives for intermediate results in preliminary test **(Tables 2 and 3)**.[24]

RESTING P_D/P_A

Resting P_d/P_a is evaluated throughout the cardiac cycle, which provides higher microvascular resistance and consequently a lower pressure gradient and potentially lower sensitivity than the diastolic wave-free period of iFR. However, its diagnostic accuracy was high (93.0%) when compared with that of iFR (n = 627).[26] The VERIFY2 study

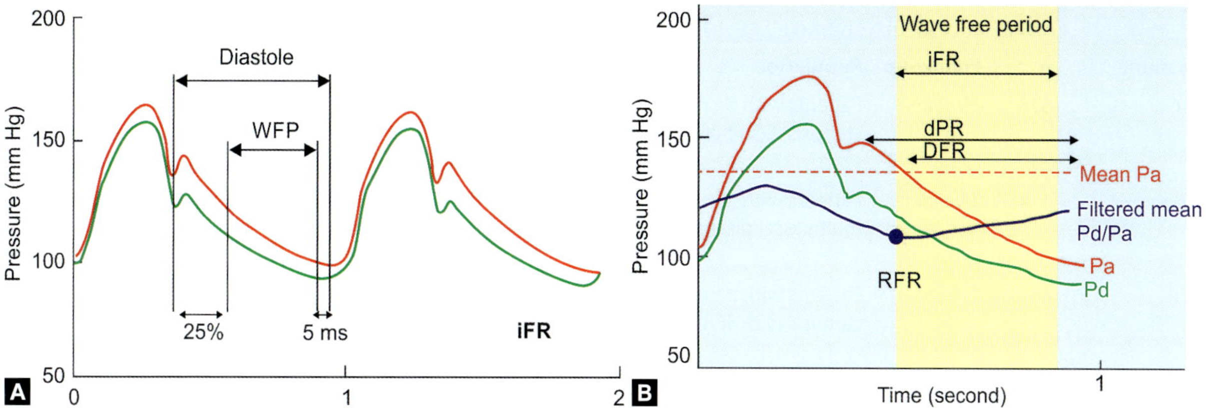

FIG. 2: Commercially available nonhyperemic pressure ratios.[25]

(dPR: diastolic pressure ratio; DFR: diastolic hyperemia free ratio; iFR: instantaneous wave free ratio; RFR: resting full cycle ratio; WFP: wave free period)

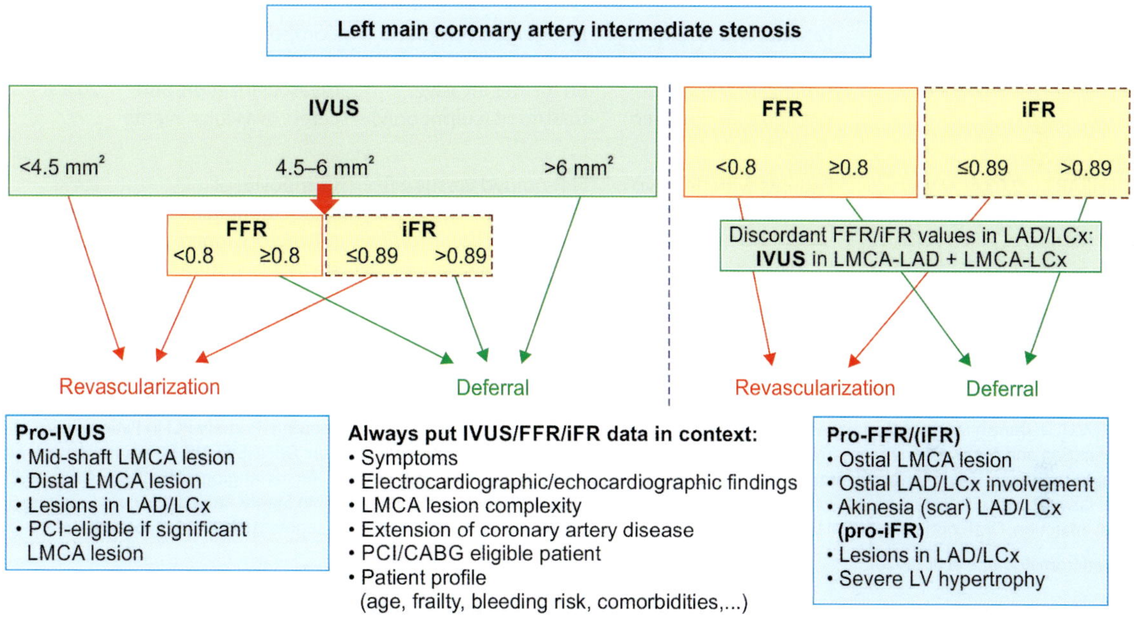

FLOWCHART 1: Alternatives and integrated approach to the assessment of the intermediate left main coronary artery (LMCA) disease. Intravascular ultrasound (IVUS) and fractional flow reserve (FFR) are well established, whereas instantaneous wave-free ratio (iFR) could require more additional data.

(CABG: coronary artery bypass grafting; LAD: left anterior descending artery; LCx: left circumflex artery; LV: left ventricle; PCI: percutaneous coronary intervention)

Source: Adapted from de la Torre Hernandez et al. (2011).[8]

demonstrated a strong correlation between resting P_d/P_a and FFR, showing similar diagnostic performance and clinical outcomes for intermediate LMCA stenoses.[27]

DIASTOLIC PRESSURE RATIO (PRESSURE WIRE)

Diagnostic accuracy was approximately 97.0% in a study by Svanerud et al.[28] (n = 197). In the study by Kang et al.,[18] a sample of 435 patients showed similar vessel-related events at 5 years for negative diastolic pressure ratio (dPR) (7.9%), iFR (8.0%), and FFR (7.7%) values. The CONTRAST study found that the DPR had high diagnostic accuracy and provided outcomes comparable to iFR in guiding revascularization decisions for LMCA lesions.[26]

RESTING FULL-CYCLE RATIO

The RFR is calculated over the whole cardiac cycle. It was detected outside diastole in 12.2% of cases and consequently, according to the authors, lesions of potential significance might be missed by NHPR measured only during diastole. The VALIDATE-RFR study confirmed that RFR-guided decision-making resulted in comparable patient outcomes

TABLE 2: Major randomized controlled trials using wire-based physiological assessment.

Study name	*n*	Follow-up	Population	Comparison	Primary endpoint	Result	*p* value
DEFER	325	15 years	Patients with de novo stenosis (DS >50%)	Deferral with FFR ≥ 0.75 versus performed PCI with FFR ≥ 0.75	MI	2.2% versus 10.0%	0.033
FAME	1,005	5 years	Patients with multivessel disease	FFR-guided versus angiography-guided PCI	Composite of death, MI, or revascularization	28.0% versus 31.0%	0.31
FAME II	888	5 years	Patients with de novo stenosis with FFR ≤ 0.80	FFR-guided PCI plus OMT versus OMT alone	Composite of death, MI, or urgent revascularization	13.9% versus 27.0%	<0.001
DANAMI-3-PRIMULTI	627	1 year	Patients with STEMI with ≥1 clinically significant stenosis in the noninfarct-related vessel	FFR-guided complete revascularization versus no further invasive treatment (culprit only)	Composite of death, nonfatal MI, or ischemia-driven revascularization	13.0% versus 22.0%	0.004
Compare-Acute	885	1 year	Patients with STEMI with ≥1 clinically significant stenosis in the noninfarct-related vessel	FFR-guided complete revascularization versus no further invasive treatment (culprit only)	Composite of death, nonfatal MI, revascularization, and cerebrovascular events	7.8% versus 20.5%	<0.001
iFR SWEDEHEART	2,037	2 years	Patients with de novo stenosis (DS 40–70%)	FFR-guided versus iFR-guided PCI	Composite of death, nonfatal MI, or unplanned revascularization	8.4% versus 8.7%	0.93
DEFINE-FLAIR	2,492	2 years	Patients with de novo stenosis (DS 40–80%)	FFR-guided versus iFR-guided PCI	Composite of death, nonfatal MI, or unplanned revascularization	10.5% versus 11.8%	0.25

(DANAMI-3-PRIMULTI: Danish Study of Optimal Acute Treatment of Patients with ST-Elevation Myocardial Infarction–Primary PCI in Patients with ST-Elevation Myocardial Infarction and Multivessel Disease: Treatment of Culprit Lesion Only or Complete Revascularization; DEFINE-FLAIR: Functional Lesion Assessment of Intermediate Stenosis to Guide Revascularisation; DS: diameter stenosis; FAME: Fractional Flow Reserve Versus Angiography for Multivessel Evaluation; FFR: fractional flow reserve; iFR: instantaneous wave-free ratio; iFR SWEDEHEART: Evaluation of iFR versus FFR in Stable Angina or Acute Coronary Syndrome; MI: myocardial infarction; OMT: optimal medical therapy; PCI: percutaneous coronary intervention; STEMI: ST segment elevated myocardial infarction)

Source: Adapted from Kogame et al. (2020).[25]

TABLE 3: Advantages and limitations of physiological assessment in the catheterization laboratory.

Wire-based physiological assessment			
Hyperemic index	**NHPR**		
FFR	**iFR**	**Novel NHPRs (DFR, dPR, RFR)**	**P_d/P_a**
Advantages			
• Evidence for outcomes up to 15 years (vs. angiography-guided PCI, OMT alone) • Well validated with noninvasive functional tests in various clinical settings • Cost-effectiveness was demonstrated against angiography-guided PCI • Available with all pressure wires	• Evidence for outcomes up to 2 years (vs. FFR-guided PCI) • Validated with noninvasive functional tests in several clinical settings • Well validated with FFR in various clinical settings • Hyperemia independent • Quicker than FFR • Ability with potential to assess serial lesions • Coregistration with angiography available	• Validated with FFR and iFR in limited clinical settings (retrospective) • Hyperemia independent • Quicker than FFR	• Validated with FFR and iFR in limited clinical settings • Hyperemia independent • Quicker than FFR • Available with all pressure wires

Continued

Continued

Wire-based physiological assessment			
Hyperemic index	**NHPR**		
FFR	**iFR**	**Novel NHPRs (DFR, dPR, RFR)**	**P_d/P_a**
Limitations			
• Hyperemia required (additional cost and hyperemic agent–related side effect) • Pressure wire required (additional cost and wire-related complication) • Precise acquisition of coronary pressure required • Prolonged procedure	• Pressure wire required (additional cost and wire-related complication) • Precise acquisition of coronary pressure required • Proprietary and the software of specific vendor required	• No evidence for outcomes • Validation data with noninvasive functional tests are limited • Pressure wire required (additional cost and wire-related complication) • Precise acquisition of coronary pressure required • Proprietary and the software of specific vendor required • No coregistration with angiography available	• No evidence for outcomes • Validation data with noninvasive functional tests are limited • Pressure wire required (additional cost and wire-related complication) • Precise acquisition of coronary pressure required • Susceptible to miscalculation from pressure-wire drift • No coregistration with angiography available

(DFR: diastolic hyperemia-free ratio; dPR: diastolic pressure ratio; IVUS: intravascular ultrasound; NHPR: nonhyperemic pressure ratio; P_a: aortic pressure; P_d: distal coronary pressure)

Source: Adapted from Kogame et al. (2020).[25]

to FFR-guided strategies, including similar rates of death, myocardial infarction, and revascularization.[28,29]

DIASTOLIC HYPEREMIA-FREE RATIO

Diagnostic accuracy was 97.6% in the study by Johnson et al.[26] ($n = 833$). In 926 patients, deferred lesion failure (cardiac death, MI, repeated revascularization) after 3 years was similar for negative diastolic hyperemia-free ratio (DFR) (6.8%), iFR (6.9%), dPR (6.9%), RFR (7.1%), and FFR (5.9%).

The PRESERVE-LM study showed that DFR accurately predicted adverse cardiac events and guided revascularization, improving patient outcomes.[30]

The iFR is defined as the average P_d/P_a during the wave-free period (WFP) (*pink shaded area*). (A) The WFP was calculated beginning 25% of the way into diastole and ending 5 ms before the end of diastole. (B) Diastolic pressure ratio (dPR) is defined as the average P_d/P_a during the entire diastole. DFR is defined as the average P_d/P_a during P_a less than mean P_a with a negative slope. The resting full-cycle ratio (RFR) is defined as the lowest filtered mean P_d/P_a during the entire cardiac cycle.

DIASTOLIC PRESSURE RATIO MEASURED USING A MICROCATHETER (^{dPR}MICRO)

In a study by Arashi et al. ($n = 161$), ^{dPR}micro showed a mean bias of –0.028 and a diagnostic accuracy of 82.2% compared with PW iFR; this reduced value compared with the other NHPRs may have been influenced by the cross-sectional area at the lesion site of Navvus PMC, which is larger than the PW (and also compared with TruePhysio PMC) and this may have overestimated the stenoses. Data are only available in the setting of post-PCI: ^{dPR}micro ≤0.89 was associated with significantly higher cardiac mortality at 2 years in 735 patients (of note due to the limited number of events, receiver operating characteristics analysis was not able to identify an optimal cutoff value and therefore the authors deliberately took the accepted ischemic threshold of 0.89). The study concluded that DPR measured with a microcatheter provided similar diagnostic accuracy and clinical outcomes to FFR, offering a less invasive assessment method.[31]

These studies collectively support the use of resting P_d/P_a, dPR, and DFR as reliable alternatives to FFR for evaluating and managing LMCA lesions. However, larger data and validation studies are awaited.

CONCLUSION

The physiological assessment of intermediate LMCA lesions is crucial for guiding treatment decisions and optimizing patient outcomes. Techniques such as FFR, iFR, and other nonhyperemic indices like resting P_d/P_a and dPR have proven to be valuable tools in this regard. These methods allow for precise evaluation of lesion significance, minimizing unnecessary interventions while ensuring that patients who do need revascularization receive appropriate care. The integration of advanced imaging modalities, including IVUS and OCT, further enhances the accuracy of these assessments by providing detailed anatomical insights. Collectively, the use of these physiological and imaging techniques contributes to a more personalized and effective management strategy for patients with intermediate LMCA lesions, ultimately improving long-term clinical outcomes.[32]

ONLINE REFERENCES

Please scan the QR code provided at the end of the table of contents for References of this chapter.

CHAPTER 149

Management of Thrombus-containing Coronary Lesions

Ajit Desai, Vishal Gavali

ABSTRACT

Thrombus-containing lesions are seen in over 90% of patients presenting with ST-segment elevation myocardial infarction (STEMI), and massive intracoronary thrombus is seen in about 16% of patients. Thrombus is a major deterrent to successful outcomes due to distal embolization, slow flow and no reflow, as well as increased infarct size. Antiplatelets and anticoagulation including the use of glycoprotein (GP) IIb/IIIa inhibitors form the cornerstone of therapy. Interventionists must be well versed with various strategies to manage intracoronary thrombus including the use of manual and mechanical aspiration catheters as well as embolic protection devices (EPDs). Advanced therapies to manage thrombus like excimer laser coronary angioplasty (ELCA) are also available to combat thrombotic lesions. Recent studies also show the efficacy of intracoronary thrombolysis. Drug-eluting stents are currently the standard of care, but the option of deferred stenting should be considered in case of large thrombus burden and ectatic vessels. We present a modified algorithm in conclusion to individualize therapy for the management of thrombus burden.

Keywords: STEMI, intracoronary thrombus, GP IIb/IIIa inhibitors, ELCA

INTRODUCTION

Thrombus is the hallmark of unstable atherosclerotic plaques which leads to acute coronary syndrome. Angiographic evidence of thrombus can be seen in 91.6% of patients presenting with an ST-segment elevation myocardial infarction (STEMI), whereas massive intracoronary thrombus has been reported in 16.4% of patients.[1,2] Despite the advancements in antiplatelet medications, anticoagulant regimens, and percutaneous coronary intervention (PCI), massive thrombus remains a formidable obstacle to successful revascularization. It can lead to increased rates of major adverse cardiovascular events (MACE), no reflow, stent thrombosis, recurrent MI, and death.[3]

PATHOPHYSIOLOGY OF THROMBUS

A thrombus-containing lesion develops when the fibrous cap of an atherosclerotic plaque undergoes structural defects such as disruption or erosion. Plaques vulnerable to disruption or erosion have thin fibrous caps and large lipid cores which are infiltrated with lipid-filled macrophages (foam cells).[4] The shoulder region of a plaque is more prone to disruption. The contact of the disrupted, exposed, and highly thrombogenic subendothelial matrix with the circulating platelets and white blood cells activates the coagulation cascade. The resultant platelet adhesion and aggregation lead to white (platelet-rich) thrombus formation.

The concomitant release of tissue factor from the arterial injury site activates the extrinsic coagulation cascade which leads to the generation of thrombin, which converts fibrinogen to fibrin. This leads to the formation of red (erythrocyte-rich) thrombus which contains erythrocytes, platelets, fibrin, and inflammatory cells and is denser and progressively tougher to disrupt.[5] These constituents determine the level of stability and "aggressiveness" of the thrombus encountered during the intervention.

Furthermore, activated platelets release agents that promote vasoconstriction and aggregation such as serotonin, adenosine diphosphate, thromboxane A2, oxygen-derived free radicals, endothelin, and platelet-activating factor. As the thrombus accumulates, the distal vessel is often accompanied by dynamic vasoconstriction which contributes to the clinical ischemic events.[6]

DETECTION OF THROMBUS-CONTAINING LESION

Various modalities are available to diagnose coronary thrombus. Coronary angiography remains the practical "gold standard" for the recognition of thrombus, which shows the classic findings of haziness or reduced contrast density, persistent staining, irregular lesion contour, "filling defect," or a smooth convex meniscus at the site of a total thrombotic occlusion **(Figs. 1A and B)**. When a thrombus is suspected but not apparent angiographically, the more sensitive techniques for its detection may be utilized, including angioscopy, intravascular ultrasound, or optical coherence tomography **(Figs. 2A to C)**.

GRADING OF THROMBOTIC BURDEN

Angiographically, thrombotic lesions are graded using the thrombolysis in myocardial infarction (TIMI) scale which uses a score ranging from grade 0 (no thrombus) to grade 5 (large thrombus with complete occlusion). Additional classifications have been suggested as outlined in **Box 1**. The factors favoring the formation of a large thrombus burden are listed in **Box 2**.

Following are angiographic morphologic features that suggest the presence of "high-burden thrombus formation":[9]

- A cutoff pattern of occlusion
- Accumulated thrombus proximal to the occlusion
- A reference lumen diameter of the IRA of >4.0 mm

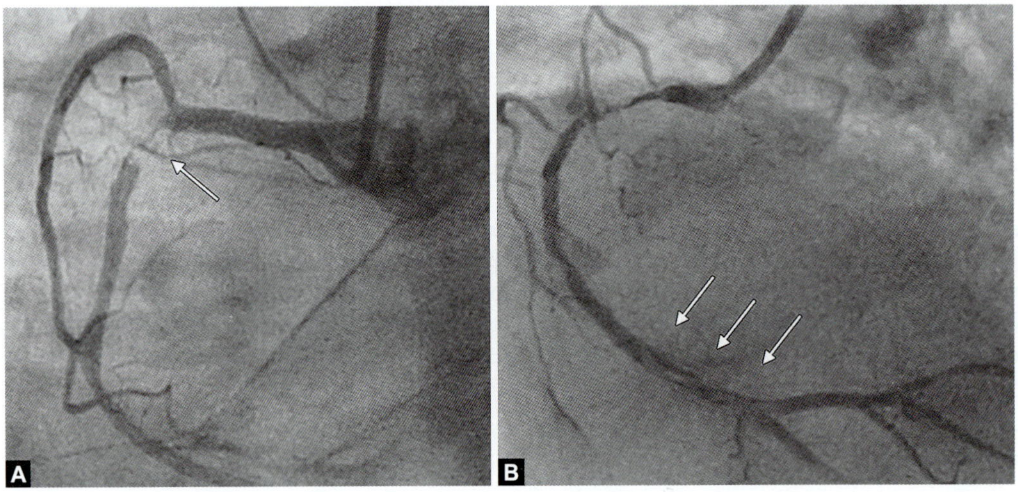

FIGS. 1A AND B: (A) Angiography of right coronary artery showing haziness with irregular filling defect in the proximal vessel representing a thrombotic lesion (arrow); (B) Angiography of RCA with a long linear thrombus in the distal RCA (arrows).
(RCA: right coronary artery)

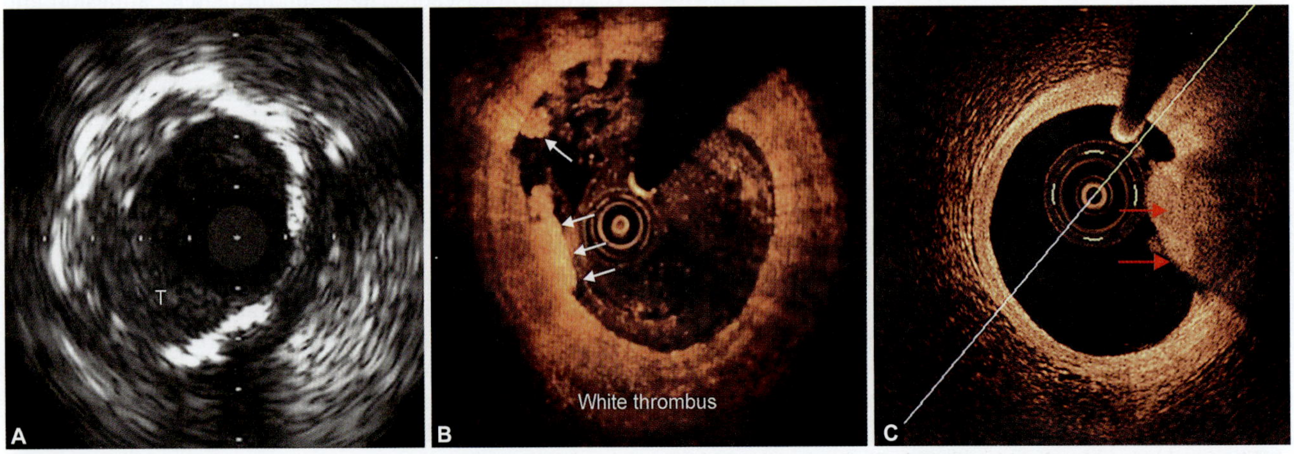

FIGS. 2A TO C: (A) IVUS image showing a calcified, thrombotic lesion (marked T); (B) OCT image showing white thrombus (arrows); (C) OCT image showing a red thrombus (red arrows).
(IVUS: intravascular ultrasound; OCT: optical coherence tomography)

BOX 1 TIMI scale.[7]

- *Grade 0*: No angiographic characteristics of thrombus
- *Grade 1*: Possible thrombus—angiographic features include decreased density of contrast, haziness, irregular lesion contour, or a smooth, convex meniscus at the site of total occlusion suggestive but not diagnostic of thrombus
- *Grade 2*: Definite thrombus present in multiple angiographic views—irregular lesion contour with a significant filling defect. The thrombus's greatest dimension is <1/2 vessel diameter
- *Grade 3*: Definite thrombus in multiple views with greatest dimension >1/2 but <2 vessel diameters
- *Grade 4*: Definite large thrombus with greatest dimension >2 vessel diameters
- *Grade 5*: Complete thrombotic occlusion of the vessel—a convex margin that stains with contrast and persists for several cardiac cycles

Grade 5 reclassification:[1]

Intervention-based: The occlusion is crossed with a guidewire or small balloon. Once the antegrade flow is restored, the culprit thrombus undergoes re-stratification:

- Small thrombus, grades 1–3
- Large thrombus, grade 4

Thrombus grading by a two-category scale:[8]

- Low thrombus grade corresponds to TIMI thrombus grades 1–3
- High thrombus grade corresponds to TIMI thrombus grades 4–5

(TIMI: thrombolysis in myocardial infarction)

- An incomplete obstruction with an angiographic thrombus with the greatest linear dimension more than three times the reference lumen diameter
- The presence of a floating thrombus proximal to the lesion
- A persistent dye stasis distal to the occlusion

BOX 2 Factors favoring large thrombus burden.

Patient-related factors:

- Hypercoagulability
- Hyperglycemia
- Hyperhomocysteinemia
- Heparin-induced thrombocytopenia and thrombosis (HITT)
- Vasculitis
- Increased WBCs
- Prothrombotic states
- Smoking
- *Substance abuse*: Cocaine and methamphetamine
- Male sex

Myocardial infarction-related factors:

- Late presentation (>12 hours) after the onset of chest pain
- Established Q wave MI with continuous chest pain and ischemia
- Cardiogenic shock
- Failed thrombolytics

Vessel-related factors:

- Slow or stagnant antegrade coronary or SVGs flow
- Large anatomical size increases thrombus formation and accumulation in native coronary vessels and SVGs
- *Morphology*: Ectasia and aneurysm

PCI-related factors:

- Triggering of the plaque and thrombus with guidewire, balloon, or stent—the "angry clot" phenomenon
- Inadequate anticoagulation during intervention
- Inadequate stent apposition to the vessel wall lack of or premature cessation or abrupt termination of antiplatelet therapy

Lesion-related factors:

- Acute plaque rupture and complex morphology

MANAGEMENT OF INTRACORONARY THROMBUS

In the presence of a small thrombus burden (grades 1-2), the recommended PCI strategy includes standard pharmacotherapy and stenting. In the presence of a significant thrombus burden (grades 3-5), the management strategies are significantly challenging including pharmacotherapy and mechanical approaches.

Pharmacotherapy

The mainstay of pharmacotherapy includes antiplatelet agents which include aspirin, GP IIb/IIIa platelet receptor antagonists, $P2Y_{12}$ inhibitors (clopidogrel, prasugrel, ticagrelor, and cangrelor), as well as heparin and anticoagulants. The reduction in the thrombotic burden can be achieved with the pharmacological agents before the initiation of PCI, with improved results and reduced risk of distal thrombotic embolization.

- Chronic aspirin therapy has been shown to decrease the thrombotic burden before stent deployment.
- Heparin reduces clot formation and repeals platelet contractile forces.[10]
- Glycoprotein IIb/IIIa receptor antagonists reduce platelet aggregate size as well as improve access to the platelet-rich clot's fibrin.[11]

However, these agents are less useful in the presence of well-formed, active, unstable, or high-grade thrombus, for example, revascularization of old degenerated saphenous vein grafts (SVGs) with large thrombus burden. Slow-flow and no-reflow phenomena occur due to severe microvascular obstruction due to thrombus. While this is best prevented, the strategies used to treat it include manual aspiration catheters (given below), autohemoperfusion, and intracoronary pharmacological agents **(Tables 1 and 2)**.[11]

Although GPIs have demonstrated effectiveness in the context of primary PCI, high bleeding rates remain a major concern. A meta-analysis involving 10,123 patients who underwent primary PCI showed that the use of GP IIb/IIIa

TABLE 1: Pharmacological properties of P2Y12 inhibition.

	Clopidogrel (Thienopyridine)	Prasugrel (Thienopyridine)	Ticagrelor (Triazolopyrimidine)	Cangrelor (Adenosine analogue)
Prodrug	Yes	Yes	No	No
Receptor blockade	Irreversible	Irreversible	Reversible	Reversible
Dose	600 mg LD; 75 mg OD, PO	60 mg LD; 10 mg OD, PO	180 mg LD; 90 mg BD, PO	30 µg/kg bolus; 4 µg/kg/min infusion during PCI
Onset of action	2–8 hours	30 minutes to 4 hours	30 minutes to 4 hours	3–5 minutes

TABLE 2: Pharmacological properties of GP IIb/IIIa inhibitors.[12]

	Abciximab	Eptifibatide	Tirofiban
Type	Chimeric monoclonal antibody	Cyclic heptapeptide	Non-peptide derivative of tyrosine
MW (Da)	47,600	832	495
Receptor binding	Noncompetitive	Competitive	Competitive
GP IIb/IIIa specificity	Nonspecific	Specific	Specific
Antigenicity	Present	Absent	Absent
Plasma half-life	10–30 minutes	2.5 hours	2 hours
Recovery of platelet function	Slow (24–48 hours)	Fast (4 hours)	Fast (4–8 hours)
Thrombocytopenia risk	High (5%)	Low (1%)	Low (1%)
PCI dosing	*Bolus*: 250 µg/kg *Infusion*: 0.125 µg/kg/min (12 hours)	*Bolus*: 180 µg/kg plus 180 µg/kg (after 10 minutes) *Infusion*: 2 µg/kg/min (12–24 hours)	*Bolus*: 25 µg/kg *Infusion*: 0.15 µg/kg/min (up to 18 hours)
Renal adjustment	No	Dose was reduced to half in Cr Cl < 50 mL/min	Dose was reduced to half in Cr Cl < 30 mL/min

inhibitors reduced the incidence of nonfatal MI at 30 days from 8.3% to 5.1% ($p < 0.001$). However, this benefit came with a significant increase in the risk of minor bleeding (3% vs. 1.7%; $p < 0.001$) and thrombocytopenia (0.8% vs. 0.04%; $p = 0.004$).[13]

Intracoronary Thrombolytic Therapy

Intracoronary thrombolytic therapy results in a higher concentration of the thrombolytic agent delivered to the site of the thrombus and has been proven effective. Small studies of using thrombolytic agents as an adjunct to primary PCI showed good results with large thrombus burdens, with improved myocardial blood flow and no increase in major bleeding.[14] The first randomized control study DISSOLUTION Study[15] studied the use of intracoronary urokinase versus saline solution via a microcatheter and showed that the urokinase group had a high incidence of TIMI grade 3 flow, myocardial blush grade, and ST segment resolution. However, McCartney et al.[16] showed that the use of alteplase in a dose of 10 or 20 mg did not reduce the microvascular obstruction or the major adverse cardiac events compared to a placebo group.

Studies have shown that intracoronary tenecteplase[17] or alteplase can improve the TIMI flow and myocardial blush grade with reduced in-hospital mortality and no increase in bleeding risks. The use of intracoronary tenecteplase was evaluated in a study of 9 patients with STEMI and a large thrombus burden where one-fifth of the dose of tenecteplase was given intracoronary and four-fifths was given intravenously followed by a heparin infusion for 24 hours to maintain activated partial thromboplastin time (APTT) 1.5–2 times normal. Check angiography was done in all patients at 4 hours and showed that all patients showed recanalized coronary artery except one patient who needed stenting for a residual lesion. No patients had in-hospital mortality, stroke, or major bleeding. This study showed the feasibility of the use of intracoronary thrombolysis as a means to obviate stenting in patients with large thrombus burdens or ectatic vessels.[17]

When a huge thrombus burden is documented on coronary angiogram, lytic therapy by intracoronary routes could be administered through the guiding catheter or via a microcatheter or using the thrombus aspiration catheter. A ClearWay (Atrium Medical, Hudson, NH) is a low-profile, rapid-exchange therapeutic infusion catheter that can be used for localized delivery of thrombolytic agents into the thrombus via a microporous balloon.

Thrombectomy Devices

Thrombectomy devices aim at reducing the intracoronary thrombus burden. They are classified into mechanical or manual devices.

Manual Thrombus Aspiration

Manual thrombus aspiration of the infarct-related vessel is a useful method of reducing the thrombus burden and improving the microvascular flow rapidly. The catheters are usually 5–7 Fr in size, user-friendly, flexible, with a hydrophilic coating and have a low crossing profile. They are advanced over the guidewire. The distal end is passed up to or across the thrombus and the proximal end is attached to a continued suction. The catheter is passed through the thrombus in order to retrieve as much as possible. Commonly used devices are Export AP (Medtronic, USA) or Thrombuster (Kaneka Corp, Japan). **Table 3** lists the commonly used aspiration catheters in clinical practice **(Figs. 3A to C)**.

The REMEDIA (Randomized Evaluation of the Effect of Mechanical Reduction of Distal Embolization by Thrombus Aspiration in Primary and Rescue Angioplasty) trial[19] found that manual aspiration was associated with improved ST resolution, better myocardial blush grade, and a reduction in no-reflow and distal embolization events. However, these benefits did not translate into a significant clinical advantage.

In the TAPAS study, 1,071 STEMI patients were randomized 1:1 prior to coronary angiography to either thrombus aspiration using the 6 Fr Export catheter (Medtronic, California, USA) or conventional primary PCI.[10] This single-center, prospective, unblinded trial utilized antithrombotic therapy with heparin and aspirin, and 93% of patients also received GP IIb/IIIa inhibitors. Authors have concluded that

TABLE 3: Commonly used aspiration catheters.[18]

Manufacturer	Device trade name	Minimal guiding catheter size (Fr)	Catheter length (cm)	Preloaded delivery stylet	Availability	Distal aspiration lumen (mm^2)	Specific feature
Medtronic	Export XT	6	140	No	EU, US	0.85	Largest trial dataset
Medtronic	Export AP	6	140	No	EU, US	1.08	Largest trial dataset
Medtronic	Export Advance	6	140	Yes	EU	1.19	Buddy wire compatible
Medtronic	Diver CE	6	145	No	EU, US	1.01	Side-holes version available
Vascular Solutions	Pronto V3	6	140	No	US	0.93	Specific tip design
Vascular Solutions	Pronto V4	6–8	138	No	US, EU	1.24	Large aspiration lumen
Vascular Solutions	Pronto LP	6	140	Yes	US	0.69	Low profile for small vessels
Boston Scientific	Fetch 2	6	135	No	US	0.79	N/A
Maquet	Thrombuster II/Xpress-Way	6	140	No	EU	0.69	N/A
Spectranetics	QuickCat	6	145	Yes	US	0.60	N/A
Terumo	Priority One	6, 7	140	Yes	EU	0.85	N/A
STENTYS	Eliminate	6, 7	145	Yes	EU	0.79	Very oblique aspiration lumen
STENTYS	STENTYS AC	6	140	Yes	EU	0.95	Large aspiration lumen
Qualimed Innovative	Pollux	5, 6	136	Yes	EU	0.53	Large aspiration lumen
Merit Medical Systems	ASAP AC Kit	6	140	No	EU, US	1.24	N/A

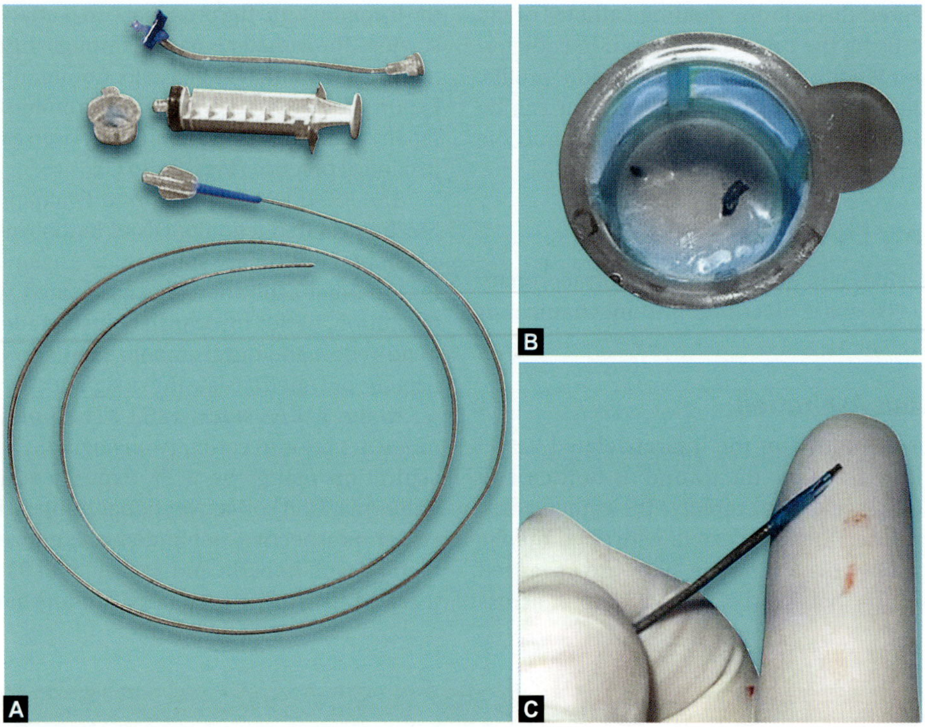

FIGS. 3A TO C: Manual thrombus aspiration catheter.

thrombus aspiration is feasible in a large majority of STEMI patients and results in better reperfusion at the myocardial level.[20]

However, the TASTE (Thrombus Aspiration during STEMI)[21] and TOTAL (ThrOmbecTomy with PCI versus PCI Alone)[22] study did not show the benefit of routine thrombus aspiration in all patients with STEMI. These trials did not improve the myocardial salvage or MACE rates and could lead to an increase in infarct size.

Based on the above studies, the European Society of Cardiology (ESC) guidelines 2017 do not recommend routine use of thrombus aspiration in primary PCI [Class III recommendation, level of evidence (LOE) A], but in patients with a large residual thrombus burden after opening a vessel with a guidewire or balloon, a bailout thrombus aspiration may be considered (Class IIb, LOE C).[23]

The manual aspiration catheters have some limitations including difficult delivery to tortuous vessels and distal coronary vessels, risk of dissection/perforation in case guidewire is not in the true lumen, requirement of multiple runs in large thrombus burdens, inadequate clot extraction due to small holes and low aspiration negative pressure and distal embolization. **Table 4** enlists the brief summary of previous manual thrombus aspiration trials.[24]

Mechanical Thrombectomy Devices

- The AngioJet Rheolytic thrombectomy (AngioJet, Possis/Medrad, Minneapolis, Minnesota, US) uses high-velocity saline jets that dissolve the thrombus and travel backward at high speed to create a negative-pressure zone (venturi effect) leading to suction of the thrombus. The JETSTENT (Comparison of AngioJet Rheolytic Thrombectomy Before Direct Infarct Artery Stenting with Direct Stenting Alone in Patients with Acute Myocardial Infarction) trial evaluated 501 patients with STEMI and did not find significant differences between mechanical thrombectomy and direct stenting **(Figs. 4A and B)**.[25]
- X-Sizer (ev3, Plymouth, Minnesota, US) consists of a helical cutter enclosed within a protective housing, attached to a dual-bore catheter shaft containing guide-wire and vacuum extraction lumens. The X-Tract AMI[26] (X-Sizer for Treatment of Thrombus and Atherosclerosis in Coronary Interventions Trial in Acute Myocardial Infarction) study showed improvement in TIMI 3 flow and MBG postprocedure. The X-Sizer in acute MI for negligible embolization and optimal ST resolution (X-AMINE ST) trial included 201 patients with STEMI and showed an improved ST-segment resolution and reduced distal embolization and no-reflow rates, but it did not demonstrate any significant clinical benefit at 1 and 6 months **(Figs. 5A and B)**.[27]
- *ELCA*: The pulsed-wave ultraviolet-wavelength excimer laser (Spectranetics, Colorado Springs, Colorado, US) has been successfully applied in patients with acute myocardial infarction (AMI). The excimer laser light interacts favorably with several components of the occluding thrombus. Laser-generated acoustic shock waves can separate thrombus from the vessel wall,

TABLE 4: Brief summary of previous manual thrombus aspiration.

RCT and year	Total sample size	TA device/catheter	Findings
REMEDIA (2005)	100	Diver CE catheter	TA improves MBG (2) and STR (68.0% and 44.9% versus 58.0% and 36.7%, respectively) with OR 2.6 [(95% CI, 1.2–5.9); $p = 0.020$] and OR 2.4 [(95% CI, 1.1–5.3); $p = 0.034$], respectively. TA is feasible and improves the angiographic and ECG criteria of myocardial reperfusion compared to PCI alone
EXPIRA (2009)	175	Export catheter	TA improved MBG (2) and STR (88% vs. 60%; $p = 0.001$; and 64% vs. 39%; $p = 0.001$). TA significantly reduced infarct size at 3 months, and lower cardiac death was observed at 9 months
TAPAS (2008)	1,071	Export catheter	• MBG 0 or 1 was reported in 17.1% (TA with PCI) versus 26.3% (PCI alone) ($p < 0.001$) • Cardiac death at 1 year was 3.6% versus 6.7% in TA versus PCI alone [HR 1.93; (95% CI 1.11–3.37); $p = 0.020$]
TASTE (2014)	7,244	Multiple catheters	Death from any cause occurred in 2.8% (TA group) versus 3.0% (PCI group) [HR 0.94; (95% CI 0.72–1.22); $p = 0.63$]. Routine TA before PCI had no effect on 30-day mortality compared to PCI alone. There was no reduction in death from any cause or composite of death, MI, or stent thrombosis at 1 year
TOTAL (2015)	10,732	Export catheter	• Primary outcome occurred in 6.9% (TA group) vs 7.0% in PCI-only group [HR 0.99; (95% CI 0.85–1.15); $p = 0.86$] with no reduction in CV death, recurrent MI, cardiogenic shock, or heart failure within 180 days • Primary outcome at 1 year occurred in 8% of each group [HR 1.00 (95% CI 0.87–1.15); $p = 0.99$]. CV death at 1 year was reported as 4% in each group [HR 0.93; (95% CI 0.76–1.14); $p = 0.48$]

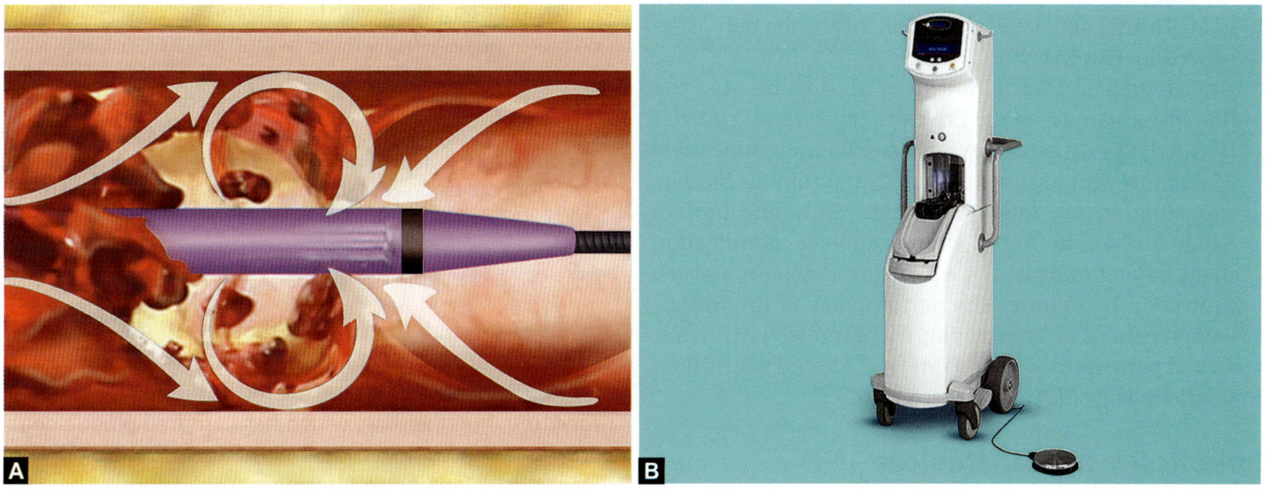

FIGS. 4A AND B: AngioJet Rheolytic thrombectomy. (A) AngioJet catheter with venturi effect for thrombosuction; (B) AngioJet console.

dissolve clots, vaporize procoagulant mediators, dissolve fibrin fibers, and suppress platelet aggregation.

The CARMEL (Cohort of Acute Revascularization of Myocardial Infarction with Excimer Laser) multicenter registry[28] enrolled 151 patients and showed that TIMI flow grade was significantly increased after ELCA, with an improvement in angiographic stenosis.

- *CAT RX*: CAT RX mechanical thrombectomy system, utilizing the Indigo CAT RX Aspiration System (Penumbra Inc., Alameda, CA, US), is designed for continuous aspiration with a larger port and lumen compared to manual aspiration catheters. The CHEETAH (Sustained Mechanical Aspiration Thrombectomy for High Thrombus Burden Coronary Vessel Occlusion) study assessed the safety of continuous mechanical thrombectomy prior to PCI in patients with TIMI thrombus grades 4 and 5 AMI. Conducted between August 2019 and December 2020 across 25 hospitals in the United States,

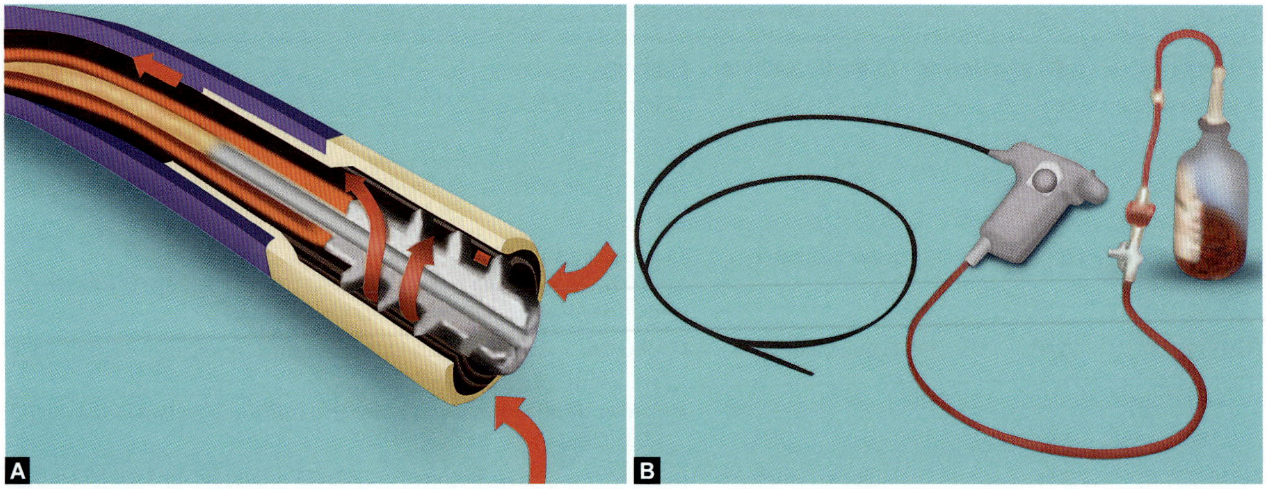

FIGS. 5A AND B: X-sizer system. (A) Helical cutter inside the inner lumen of the catheter. (B) Handheld module.

this single-arm registry enrolled 400 patients. The study demonstrated that sustained mechanical thrombectomy is both feasible and safe for selected patients with a high thrombus burden, as evidenced by the low rate of adverse cardiovascular events. The primary endpoint, which included cardiovascular death, recurrent MI, cardiogenic shock, and NYHA class IV heart failure, was observed in just 3.60% of patients (95% CI, 2.0–6.0%). Additionally, the study reported an impressive final myocardial blush grade (MBG) of 3 in 99.75% of patients by the end of the procedure **(Box 3)**.[23]

- *EnVast stent retrieval*: Spirito et al. documented the first in-human use of the EnVast stent retrieval catheter (formerly known as the NeVa device). Their study included 61 patients with AMI and a significant thrombus burden, reporting strong safety outcomes. Only one patient experienced side-branch embolization, a complication that was later mitigated by employing a vacuum-assisted aspiration technique. The performance of the EnVast catheter alone, before stenting, was impressive, with only 10% of patients exhibiting TIMI flow < 3, and nearly one-quarter having MBG < 2 **(Figs. 6A to C)**.[29]

BOX 3 Optimal technique for manual thrombectomy.[23]

- Start aspiration prior to crossing lesion
- Ensure adequate guide support to reach target lesion with aspiration catheter
- If aspiration slows, change aspiration syringe as syringe can lose suction quickly
- If suction stops suddenly during aspiration despite changing syringe, remove aspiration catheter and flush outside body as tip may be obstructed with large thrombus
- Ensure guide engagement with coronary ostium when removing thrombectomy catheter to avoid losing thrombus which could embolism to cerebral vasculature and cause stroke
- Aspirate guide catheter after thrombectomy to remove air or residual thrombus. Thrombus embolized down noninfarct territory can be catastrophic
- If unable to cross lesion with thrombectomy catheter, consider small diameter balloon dilation and then re-attempt

Embolic Protection Devices

Embolic protection devices aim at capturing the debris liberated during PCI and decrease distal embolization. EPDs can be divided into three distinct types based on their mechanism of operation: Distal occlusion aspiration devices, distal filters, and proximal occlusion aspiration devices **(Table 5)**.

Distal Embolic Filters

Distal embolic filters are devices with a filter bag mounted at the distal end of a coronary guidewire. The device is advanced through the guide catheter with the filter bag in a collapsed state, typically using a delivery sheath (3.2 Fr), and is deployed 2.5–3.0 cm distal to the lesion. After the procedure, the filter bag, which has captured plaque debris, is retrieved using a retrieval catheter (4.2–4.9 Fr). These devices are effective in filtering particles larger than 100–110 µm while maintaining antegrade perfusion. However, their limitations include the potential passage of smaller particles, limited capture efficiency, and complications associated with the advancement, deployment, and retrieval of the filters. Examples of distal embolic filters include the Spider RX (ev3; MedNova, Abbott, Abbott Park, IL, USA), the FilterWire (Boston Scientific, Boston, MA, USA), and the Interceptor (Medtronic, Santa Rosa, CA, USA). Despite their design, randomized studies have not demonstrated a significant benefit of these devices in terms of improved

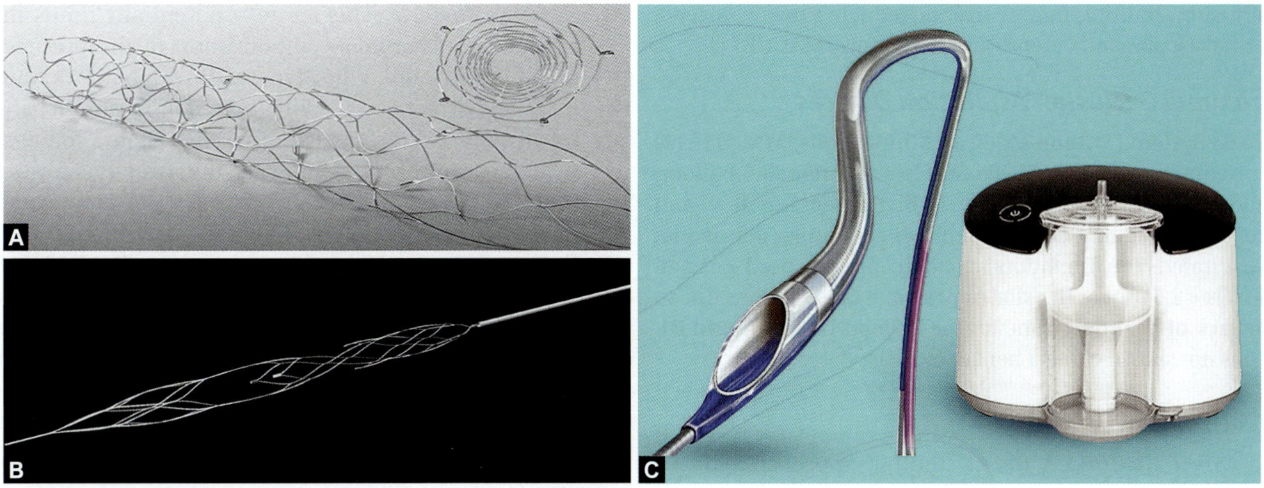

FIGS. 6A TO C: Emerging thrombectomy tool technologies with new designs. (A) Solitaire™ device stent retriever (Medtronic); (B) enVast™ stent retriever (Vesalio); (C) CAT RX powered by Penumbra ENGINE.[24]

TABLE 5: Embolic protection devices (EPDs).

EPD	Used in vessel size	Guide catheter	Crossing profile	Comments
Proximal balloon: Proxis (Velocimed, Maple Grove, MN, US)	3–5 mm	7 Fr	None	*Advantages*: • Establish protection before crossing the lesion • Side branch protection • Complete recovery of debris and vasoactive mediators • Unlimited debris removal • Compatible with conventional guidewire *Disadvantage*: • Myocardial ischemia during balloon occlusion
Distal occlusion balloon: • PurcuSurge guidewire (Medtronic) • TriActiv (Kensey Nash Corp.)	3–6 mm	6 FR 7.8 FR	2.1 Fr 2.8 Fr	*Advantage*: • Can capture debris <100 µm and soluble vasoactive mediators with unlimited debris capture *Disadvantages*: • Aspiration may not remove all particles • Risk of embolization inside branch • Choice of guidewire limited • Risk of myocardial ischemia during balloon occlusion
Distal embolic filters: • FilterWire EZ (Boston Scientific) • Spider RX (Abbott) • Interceptor Plus (Medtronic)	2.5–5.5 mm 3–6 mm 2.5–5.5 mm	6 FR	3.2 Fr 2.7 Fr	*Advantages*: • Maintain antegrade perfusion • Can capture debris > 100 µm *Disadvantages*: • Unable to filter mediators • Capacity of bag limited • Risk of distal embolization during wiring and lesion crossing • No side branch protection • Choice of guidewire not met except Spider RX for which conventional guidewire of 0.014 inch can be used

perfusion, limiting infarct size, or reducing major adverse cardiovascular and cerebrovascular events (MACCE).[30]

Proximal Occlusion Aspiration Devices

Proxis System (St Jude Medical, Minneapolis, MN, USA) is a proximal occlusion device that has an inflatable balloon that is inflated proximally, occluding antegrade flow, and creating a stagnant column of blood containing debris that is aspirated. The limitation is that it cannot be used in small vessels < 2.5 mm or in ostial or proximal target lesions due to the lack of a landing zone for the balloon **(Figs. 7A and B)**. It has not shown clinical benefit in trials.[31]

Stenting Strategies

- *Direct stenting*: A direct stenting approach reduces the incidence of distal embolization by reducing the manipulation and hardware across the thrombus and by trapping the thrombus behind the stent. The disadvantages include underestimation of vessel size, inadequate stent expansion, late stent malapposition, failure to cross the lesion, or inadequate stent expansion in calcified or tortuous vessels. A meta-analysis of five small single-center trials showed improved outcomes with direct stenting as evidenced by a significant improvement of ST resolution and reduction of in-hospital cardiac death.[32] Direct stenting with or without thrombus aspiration might be applied safely in selected patients with AMI with low thrombus grade.
- *Covered stent*: Covered stents are made up of a bare metal stent (BMS) platform covered with a fine mesh that can trap the thrombus and prevent distal embolization. There are two types of stents which have been evaluated in the past: MGuard (InspireMD) and STENTYS (STENTYS SA). MASTER I trial[33] demonstrated the benefit of MGuard in terms of complete ST-segment resolution and lower 1-year mortality, but MASTER II trial[34] that aimed to recruit 1,114 patients was terminated early due to a high rate of stent dislodgement (3.87%). The APPOSITION V trial was stopped prematurely because the noninferiority standard was not met.[35]
- *Deferred stenting*: This strategy potentially limits the risk of distal coronary embolization in the presence of a high thrombus burden. Antithrombotic therapy including prolonged GP IIb/IIIa inhibitors and heparin intravenously can be given for 24–48 hours followed by angiography and PCI in case the thrombus burden reduces. The DEFER STEMI trial[36] showed significantly lower rates of no reflow/slow flow and higher TIMI flow grade in the deferred stenting group. The DANAMI 3-DEFER trial[37] deferred stenting for 48 hours but did not reduce the outcome of all-cause death, heart failure, myocardial infarction, or repeat revascularization compared to conventional PCI over 42 months follow-up.

In conclusion, deferred stenting is not recommended as the routine strategy in primary PCI.

SPECIAL CLINICAL SITUATIONS

- *Stent thrombosis*: Early (<30 days after PCI), late (>30 days after PCI), and very late (>12 months after PCI) stent thromboses are devastating clinical conditions that significantly impact outcomes. Stent thrombosis presents as nonfatal and fatal acute MI, often with marked hemodynamic instability. Primary PCI, including imaging, additional stenting with or without thrombectomy, is effective in restoring vessel patency, but reocclusion and restenosis are frequent. Usually, pharmacotherapy and manual thrombus aspiration catheters are sufficient for small or medium thrombus burdens but mechanical thrombectomy may be required in case of large thrombus burdens.[38]
- *Multivessel coronary thrombosis*: Patients with simultaneous multivessel thrombosis are an uncommon occurrence but frequently present as acute coronary syndrome with hemodynamic compromise. The mechanisms include thrombotic embolization from left heart clots or tumors or acute thrombosis of a single vessel leading to cardiogenic shock, reduced coronary perfusion pressure, and thrombus formation on other pre-existing lesions.[39]

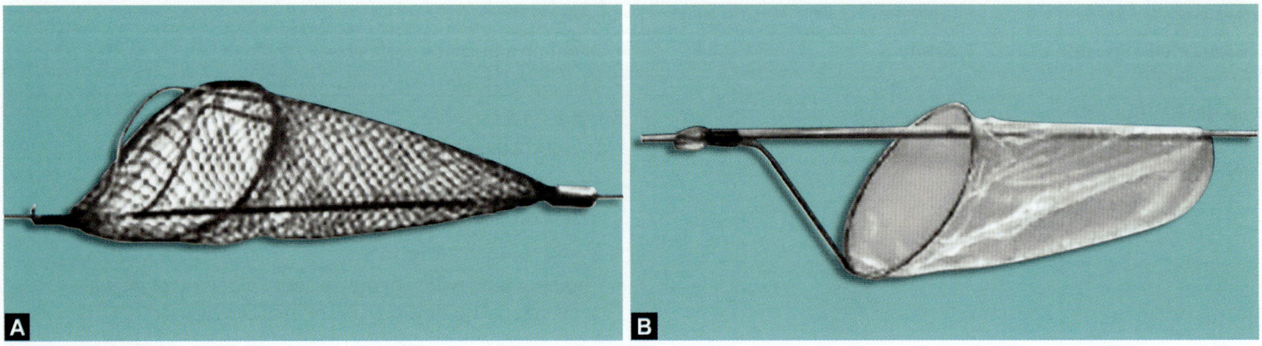

FIGS. 7A AND B: Distal embolic filters. (A) Spider RX; (B) FilterWire.

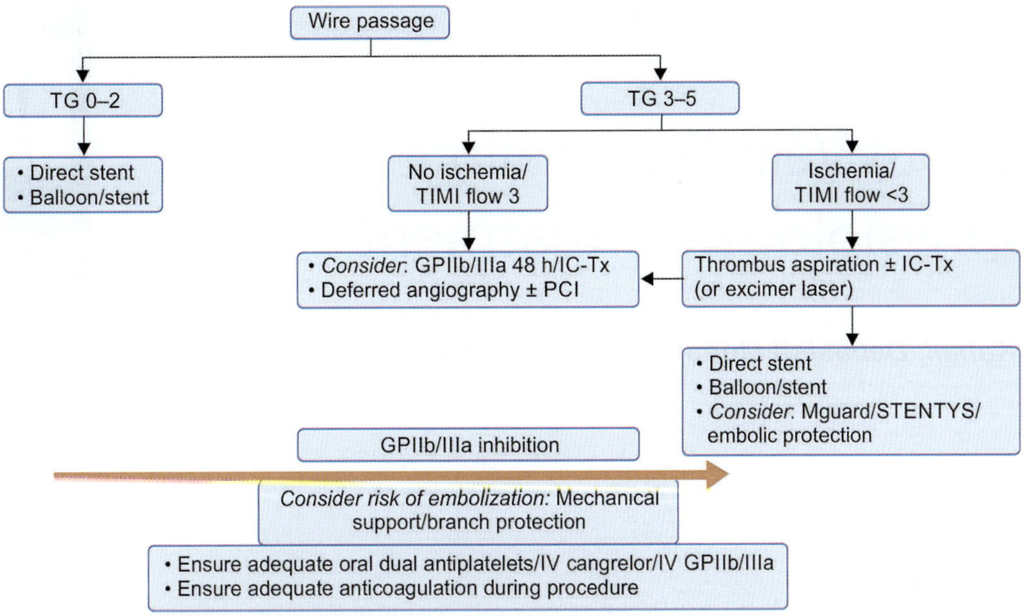

FLOWCHART 1: Algorithm for primary PCI in the presence of large thrombus burden.[40]
(GP: glycoprotein; IC-Tx: intracoronary thrombolysis; PCI: percutaneous coronary intervention; TG: thrombus grade; TIMI: thrombolysis in myocardial infarction)

CONCLUSION

Large thrombus burdens can be a significant deterrent to successful primary PCI in STEMI due to distal embolization, no-reflow, slow-flow, or poor myocardial blush grade and increased infarct size. The therapy includes potent dual antiplatelet agents and effective anticoagulation including the use of GP IIb/IIIa inhibitors. In case of a small thrombus burden, direct stenting can be considered. When there is a larger thrombus burden, the use of manual aspiration catheters or ELCA should be considered. In case of no antegrade flow and persistent or extensive thrombus, mechanical thrombectomy using AngioJet, CAT RX, or excimer laser should be considered. In spite of these maneuvers, if the thrombus persists, stenting should be deferred with the use of intracoronary thrombolysis, intravenous heparin, and/or GP IIb/IIIa inhibitors for 24–48 hours **(Flowchart 1)**. Drug-eluting stents are the stents of choice at present. In conclusion, although each patient requires an individualized strategy to manage thrombotic burden, the outcomes are hinged on the thrombus management and restoration of flow to the microvasculature.

ONLINE REFERENCES

Please scan the QR code provided at the end of the table of contents for References of this chapter.

CHAPTER 150

Saphenous Vein Graft Failure: Pathophysiology to Treatment

Dhiman Kahali, Debasish Mohapatra, Padma Madhab Bisoi

ABSTRACT

René Favaloro revolutionized coronary artery bypass surgery with the use of the great saphenous vein, despite its higher failure rate compared to arterial grafts. Saphenous vein grafts (SVGs) experience notable failure rates due to factors like acute thrombosis, intimal hyperplasia, and accelerated atherosclerosis. Acute thrombosis occurs due to endothelial cell damage during harvesting, while intimal hyperplasia involves the adaptation of vascular smooth muscle cells to arterial pressure. Accelerated atherosclerosis in the neointima layer can lead to late SVG failure. Preventing SVG failure involves optimal target vessel selection, careful graft harvesting, and appropriate pharmacotherapy. Effective management of SVG failure often requires reintervention, typically through percutaneous coronary intervention (PCI) rather than redo coronary artery bypass grafting (CABG). Strategies like embolic protection devices (EPDs), drug-eluting stents (DES), and managing intermediate SVG lesions with medical therapy are crucial for improving outcomes.

Keywords: SVG failure, post-CABG, pathophysiology of graft failure

INTRODUCTION

In the early 20th century, surgical treatments for angina and prevention of death included sympathectomy and pericardial abrasion, aimed at creating collateral circulation. René Favaloro, an Argentine cardiac surgeon, revolutionized coronary artery bypass surgery using the great saphenous vein (GSV). While the GSV is a readily available conduit, it has a higher failure rate compared to arterial grafts due to its need to adapt to arterial blood pressure.

Endothelial cells (ECs) and vascular smooth muscle cells (VSMCs) are sensitive to changes in shear stress and pressure, respectively, necessitating vein arterialization for graft longevity. However, excessive intimal hyperplasia (IH) can lead to graft failure or accelerated atherosclerosis.

Saphenous vein grafts (SVGs) have notable failure rates, with 3–12% occluding before discharge, 8–25% failing at 1 year, and only 50–60% remaining patent after a decade.[1]

PATHOPHYSIOLOGY OF SAPHENOUS VEIN GRAFT FAILURE

Different mechanisms of SVG failure are shown in **Table 1**.

TABLE 1: Different mechanisms of SVG failure.

Mechanism	Acute thrombosis	Intimal hyperplasia	Accelerated atherosclerosis
Timeline	During first week to 1 month	1 month to 1 year	After 1 year—late SVG failure
Attributing factors	• *Technical*: Graft trauma during harvesting, anastomotic deficiencies • *Conduit related*: Conduit size mismatch or preexisting graft pathology • *Extrinsic factors*: Hypercoagulability causing acute thrombosis, mechanical forces	• Arterialization • Platelet activation • Endothelial cell activation • Cytokines (IL-1, IL-6) • Growth factors (PDGF, TGF-β) • Smooth muscle cell (SMC) proliferation and migration	• Local inflammation • Infiltration of foam cells • Accelerated lipid uptake

Acute Thrombosis

The earliest form of SVG failure is acute thrombosis. This begins during vein harvesting, where ischemia, mechanical forces, pH changes, and exposure to oxidizing radicals damage ECs and VSMCs, sometimes exposing the extracellular matrix (ECM) to the vessel lumen. The damaged ECs initiate a prothrombotic response, including the activation of adhesion molecules and a reduction in antithrombotic agents like nitric oxide (NO) and prostacyclin. This leads to platelet and leukocyte activation, with platelets adhering to the ECM or activated ECs and releasing thrombogenic factors such as platelet-derived growth factor (PDGF), transforming growth factor-β, fibrinogen, fibronectin, and von Willebrand factor. Mechanical stress and ischemia-reperfusion injury during harvesting and storage result in endothelial denudation and SMC damage, exposing the ECM and triggering the extrinsic coagulation cascade. Reduced NO and prostacyclin levels cause vasoconstriction and stasis, further promoting fibrin accumulation and thrombus formation.

Intimal Hyperplasia

The next step in the vein's adaptation to its new environment involves activation, phenotypic switching, and migration of VSMCs from the medial to the intimal layer, a process known as IH. In its physiological state, IH stabilizes the intimal layer to withstand arterial pressure and shear stress, a process termed "arterialization" of the saphenous vein (SV). Although IH usually leads to mild lumen reduction without causing significant early stenosis, it can also lead to graft failure.

Intimal hyperplasia begins with paracrine interactions between ECs and VSMCs. Normally, ECs secrete homeostatic molecules like NO to keep VSMCs quiescent and regulate the medial layer tone. However, EC dysfunction disrupts these interactions, leading to VSMC phenotypic switching and synthetic activity. Further intimal thickening occurs through the secretion of ECM components such as elastin, collagen, glycoproteins, and proteoglycans. Additionally, highly proliferative adventitial fibroblasts migrate to the intima, differentiate into myofibroblasts, and contribute to the thickening **(Fig. 1)**.

Accelerated Atherosclerosis

The neointima layer in veins implanted into the arterial circulation is prone to atheroma plaque formation. In veins, some foam cells in the atheroma originate from undifferentiated VSMCs, unlike in arteries where they typically come from macrophages. The atheroma plaque capsule in veins is softer and more prone to rupture and thrombosis.

Intimal hyperplasia sets the stage for atherosclerosis development, leading to late SVG failure. SVG atherosclerosis progresses faster than native coronary artery atherosclerosis and is typically concentric and diffuse, with a poorly defined or absent fibrous cap, making it more rupture-prone. Atherosclerotic changes can appear as early as 1 year after coronary artery bypass grafting (CABG), initially characterized by foam cell accumulation. Between 2 and 5 years postsurgery, a necrotic core develops, forming intermediate SVG lesions. This necrotic core may expand through intraplaque hemorrhage from leaky neoangiogenic vessels, potentially leading to plaque rupture, thrombus formation, and SVG occlusion **(Figs. 2 and 3)**.[2]

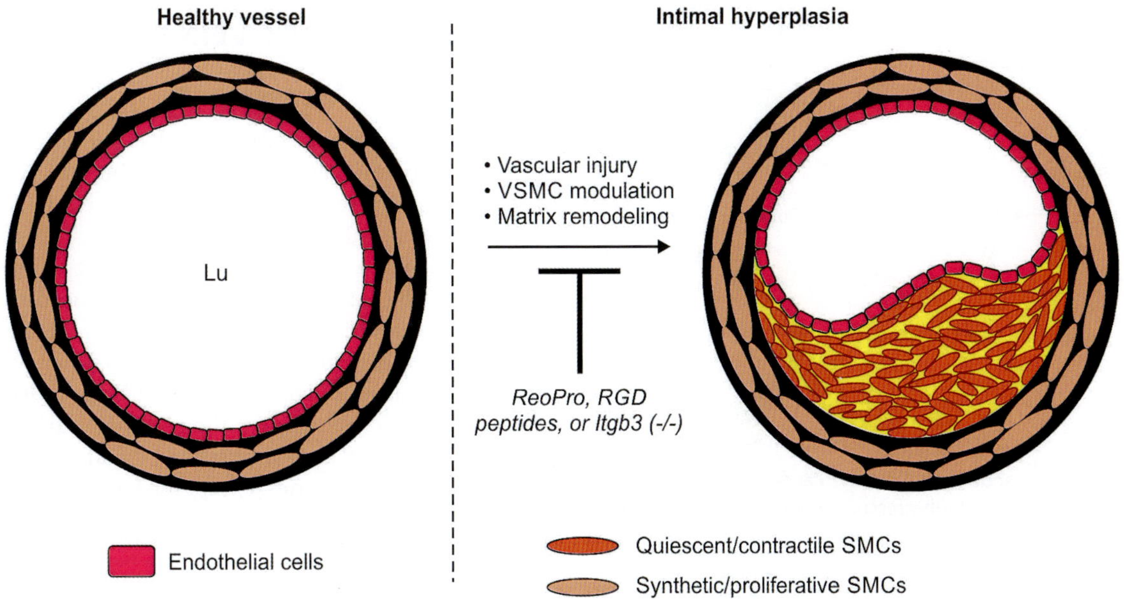

FIG. 1: Difference between intimal hyperplasia and healthy vessel.

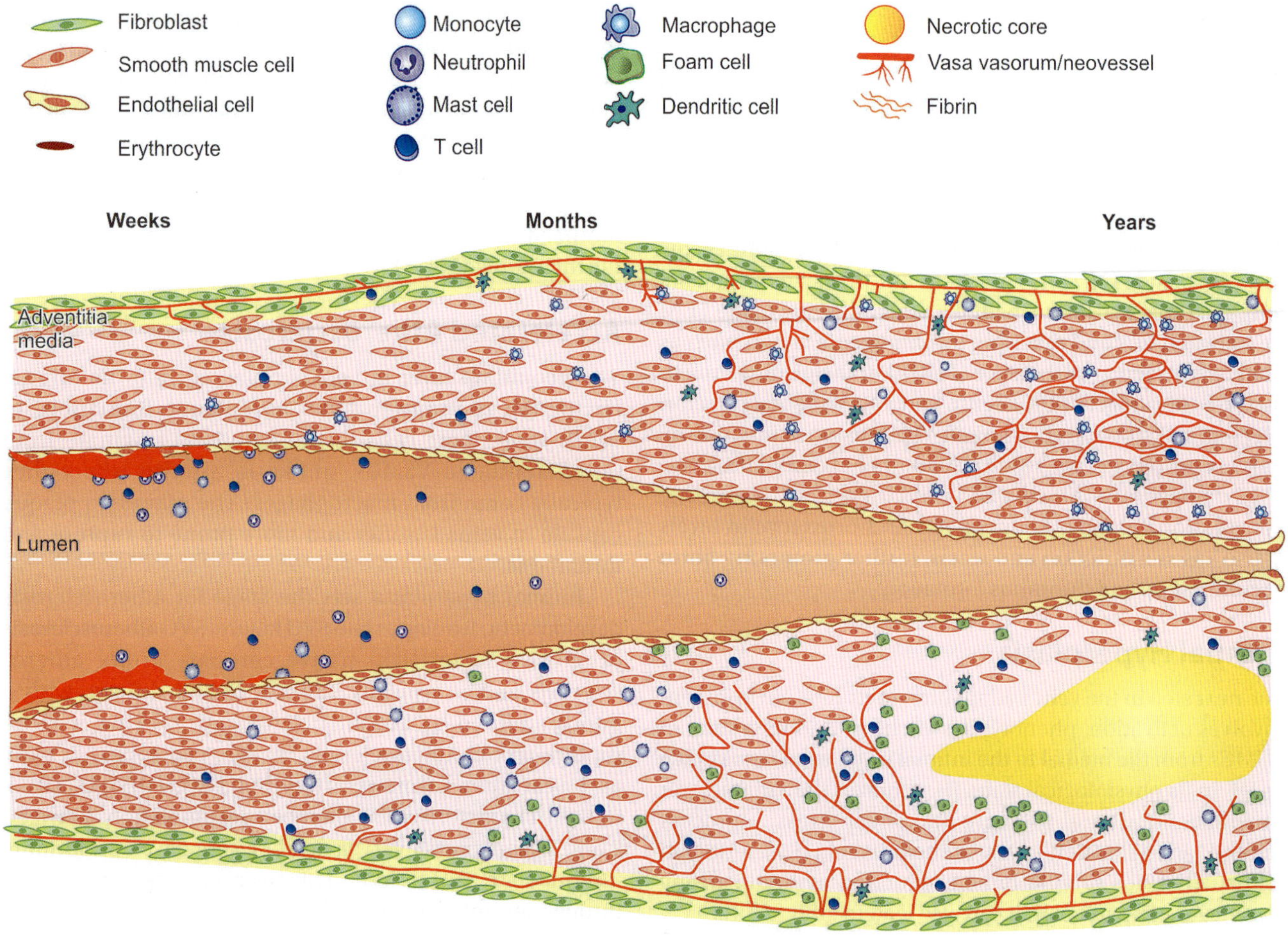

FIG. 2: The process of vein graft remodeling as it occurs under atherosclerotic conditions. Typically, macrophages in the vessel wall engulf lipids and become foam cells. Subsequently, a necrotic core is formed by dying cells and cholesterol depositions. Hypoxia in the vessel wall induces the growth of plaque neovessels.[2]

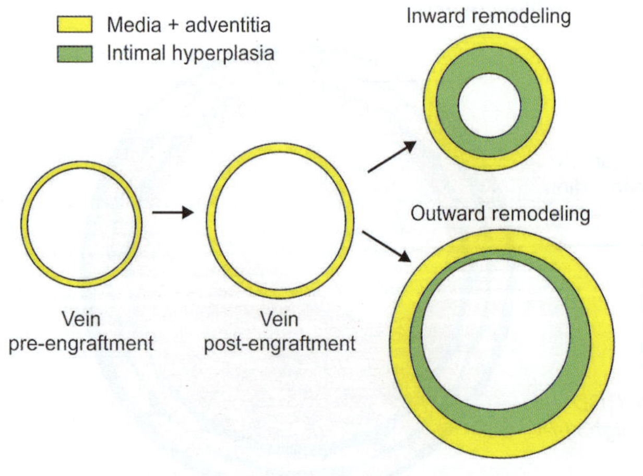

FIG. 3: Vein graft remodeling. Damage caused by graft handling and distension during the high-pressure check for leakage as well as implantation in the high blood pressure surrounding of the arterial circulation results in distention of the venous graft. Depending on local and systemic influences like inflammatory factors, this can result in inward remodeling characterized by IH and a reduced lumen or outward remodeling characterized by moderate IH and an increased lumen.

PREVENTION OF VEIN GRAFT FAILURE

Target Vessel Assessment

Optimal anastomosis sites are disease-free coronary segments. Proximal anastomoses yield better SVG patency due to larger vessel size, minimal size discrepancy, and improved runoff. Long-term graft patency is significantly influenced by the target vessel diameter: at 10 years, SVG patency is 88% in vessels >2.0 mm compared to 55% in vessels ≤2.0 mm, with 80% patency in SVGs to the LAD.[1]

Target vessel quality also impacts graft patency. SVGs to diffusely diseased, calcified arteries with poor distal runoff show higher occlusion rates. The PRAGUE-4 trial reported the lowest patency rates for grafts to collateralized, totally occluded coronary arteries, except the LAD.[3] SVG occlusion risk is higher for grafts to the RCA or circumflex compared to the LAD.

Grafting nonhemodynamically significant lesions can lead to early IMA or SVG failure due to competitive flow. *Botman et al.*[4] found a higher 12-month occlusion rate for SVGs to native vessels with FFR > 0.75 compared to <0.75

(20% vs. 5.9%). *Toth et al.*[5] reported lower graft occlusion rates at 36 months in patients who underwent FFR-guided CABG compared to angiography-guided CABG (5% vs. 21%, $p = 0.031$).

Graft Harvesting

The no-touch technique, where the SVG is harvested with its surrounding tissue intact, preserves vasa vasorum and nerves, avoids distention, and results in better blood flow and pressure tolerance during off-pump CABG. This method may reduce IH and slow atherosclerosis progression, improving short- and long-term patency. Endoscopic vein harvesting (EVH) reduces wound complications but may affect graft patency, as seen in the *ROOBY trial*.[6] However, the *REGROUP trial*[7] found no significant difference in major adverse cardiac events (MACE) between EVH and open harvesting when performed by experienced operators. Proper storage solutions and careful handling of the SVG are crucial to maintaining endothelial integrity and graft patency. Sequential grafting offers revascularization of multiple targets but carries a risk if proximal occlusion occurs. Routine intraoperative flow measurement is recommended to ensure graft quality and identify potential issues.

Pharmacotherapy

The American Heart Association (AHA) recommends aspirin (81–162 mg) and clopidogrel (75 mg) for 1-year post-off-pump CABG to reduce graft occlusion (class I, level A). For on-pump CABG, combination therapy may be considered, but its benefits are less certain (class IIb, level A). DAPT with ticagrelor or prasugrel and aspirin is preferred over clopidogrel and aspirin in acute coronary syndrome (ACS) patients undergoing CABG (class IIa, level B).[8] The European guidelines recommend DAPT resumption in ACS patients post-CABG for up to 12 months, provided there is no need for oral anticoagulation (class I, level B).[9] The *COMPASS trial*[10] substudy found no significant reduction in 1-year SVG failure with rivaroxaban plus aspirin compared to aspirin alone. However, the combination reduced major adverse events.

Statins are crucial for SVG patency. The *ACTIVE trial* showed no difference in SVG occlusion between low- and high-dose atorvastatin. The AHA recommends initiating statin therapy in the preoperative period and resuming it early postoperatively (class I, level A). High-intensity statin therapy (atorvastatin 40–80 mg or rosuvastatin 20–40 mg) is advised for all post-CABG patients under 75 years of age. For those, intolerant to high-intensity statins or at higher risk for drug interactions, moderate-intensity statins are recommended (class I, level A).[8]

Ezetimibe and PCSK9 inhibitors like alirocumab also show benefit in patients with previous CABG (subgroup analysis of IMPROVE-IT trial).[11] Icosapent ethyl, an omega-3 fatty acid, has shown to reduce ischemic events, supporting its use in patients with elevated triglycerides post-CABG (subgroup analysis of REDUCE-IT trial) **(Table 2)**.[12]

MANAGEMENT OF SAPHENOUS VEIN GRAFT FAILURE

Patients often require reintervention after CABG due to graft lesion development or progression of native atherosclerosis. SVG lesions are typically treated with percutaneous coronary intervention (PCI), which is limited by distal embolization and no-reflow during the acute phase, as well as high restenosis and disease progression rates during follow-up.

Choice of Revascularization Modality and Target Vessel

Redo CABG is rarely performed because it involves higher risks and mortality compared to initial CABG. PCI is generally preferred over redo CABG for revascularization in patients with previous CABG, except in cases where PCI is unsuitable, such as with extensively diseased or occluded grafts. Factors favoring redo CABG include reduced ejection fraction, failure of multiple SVGs, and late SVG stenosis. Factors favoring PCI include poor grafting targets, advanced age, ACS, and other comorbidities.

Strategy for Saphenous Vein Graft Percutaneous Coronary Intervention

Percutaneous coronary intervention can target either the culprit SVG or the corresponding native vessel. Observational studies suggest better outcomes with native vessel PCI. The 2018 ESC/EACTS guidelines prefer PCI

TABLE 2: Different strategies to prevent saphenous vein graft failure.

Presurgical	Surgical	Postsurgical
Appropriately selected target vessel (>2 mm diameter with significant stenoses)	Buffered solutions for graft storage	Dual antiplatelet therapy
Grafting of functionally significant lesions only	No-touch technique for graft harvesting	High-intensity statin
Grafting of vessels with good distal targets	Intraoperative graft flow measurement	
Disease-free coronary segment at the anastomosis	Perioperative aspirin administration (81–325 mg)	

to a native vessel over SVG PCI.[9] However, native vessel recanalization can be challenging due to complex lesions, often requiring specialized equipment and expertise. A staged revascularization strategy is sometimes proposed: Treat the culprit SVG lesion first, followed by PCI of the native artery later. The PROCTOR is the first RCT evaluating clinical outcomes of native vessel PCI versus SVG PCI.[13] Continued flow through the SVG after PCI of the native artery can cause stent thrombosis. SVG occlusion with coiling or an Amplatzer vascular plug is often performed to prevent this.[14]

Periprocedural Pharmacotherapy

Saphenous vein graft lesions have a high plaque burden, leading to a higher incidence of no-reflow during PCI compared to native coronary arteries. Strategies to prevent no-reflow and periprocedural myocardial infarction (MI) are critical, as patients with no-reflow have higher long-term risks of MI and death. Intragraft adenosine, nitroprusside, and calcium channel blockers are used to prevent and treat no-reflow. The VAPOR trial showed intragraft verapamil significantly reduced no-reflow rates compared to placebo.[15] Pretreatment with intragraft nicardipine has been effective in reducing no-reflow and in-hospital MACE, making it a preferred vasodilator due to its prolonged action and minimal hypotensive effects. Vasodilators can serve as adjuncts or substitutes for embolic protection devices (EPDs) if EPD use is not feasible.

Glycoprotein IIb/IIIa inhibitors are associated with higher mortality in SVG PCI and are not recommended for routine use **(Flowchart 1)**.[16]

Embolic Protection Devices

Embolic protection devices are the primary strategy evaluated in RCTs to prevent no-reflow during PCI for SVG lesions. The FIRE RCT showed noninferiority of the FilterWire to the GuardWire with respect to 30-day MACE rates.[17] Similarly, the SPIDER RCT found comparable outcomes between the SpiderFX, FilterWire, and GuardWire.[18] The 2018 ESC/EACTS guidelines downgraded the use of EPDs in SVG PCI to class IIa, level of evidence B.[9] Despite ACCF/AHA/SCAI guidelines recommending EPDs, their usage is low (21% in the United States) due to technical challenges, risk of distal vessel injury, and additional time and cost.

Excimer Laser Coronary Angioplasty

Excimer laser coronary angioplasty (ELCA) may reduce distal embolization by vaporizing thrombus and plaque but carries risks of vessel dissection and perforation. The *CORAL trial* indicated no significant difference in no-reflow rates between ELCA without EPDs and EPD use in the SAFER trial.[19] A case-control study suggested ELCA might reduce microvascular obstruction and type IVa MI compared to EPDs, though randomized trials are lacking. ELCA is FDA-approved for multifocal, thrombotic SVG lesions, but no guidelines recommend its use.

Direct Stenting and Stent Size

Direct stenting can trap debris and reduce distal embolization. Aggressive stent expansion in SVG lesions has been associated with higher MI incidence and similar target vessel revascularization (TVR) rates. Direct stenting has shown lower creatine kinase-MB release and target lesion revascularization (TLR) at 1 year compared to conventional angioplasty. A DIVA trial substudy found that stent-only approaches were associated with lower stent thrombosis and target vessel MI rates than stent-balloon strategies. Undersized stents have been used to minimize distal embolization, showing reduced creatine kinase-MB elevation post-PCI with similar 1-year TLR and TVR rates[20] **(Fig. 4)**.

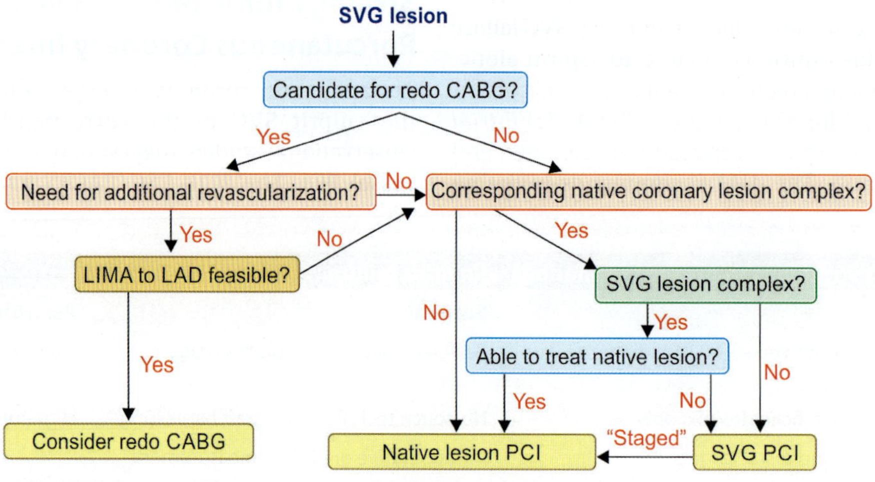

FLOWCHART 1: Stepwise management strategies of SVG lesion.

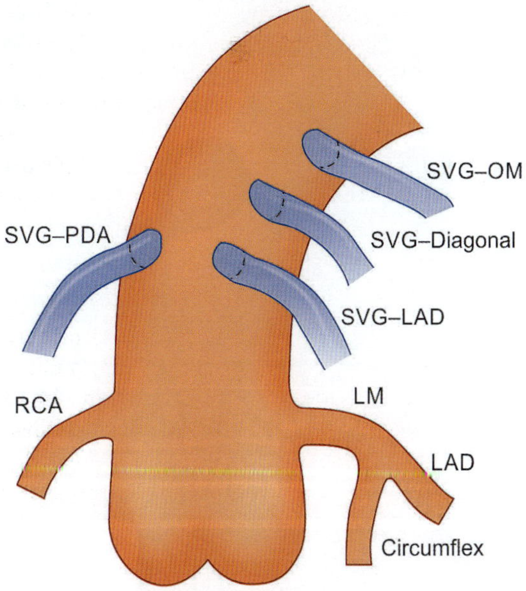

FIG. 4: Usual location of the saphenous vein graft proximal anastomoses.

(LAD: left anterior descending artery; LM: left main; OM: obtuse marginal; PDA: posterior descending artery; RCA: right coronary artery; SVG: saphenous vein graft)

MANAGEMENT OF EARLY POST CORONARY ARTERY BYPASS GRAFTING SAPHENOUS VEIN GRAFT FAILURE

Early Saphenous Vein Graft Failure

Approximately 3–12% of SVGs fail before hospital discharge due to acute graft thrombosis, anastomotic stenosis, graft kinking, overstretching, or postoperative spasm.[21] Routine post-CABG coronary angiography reveals defects in 12% of grafts, often corrected by minor adjustments, open chest PCI, or surgical revision. Clinically significant early graft failure, associated with high mortality (~15%), requires urgent surgical revision or PCI.

Diagnosis and Differentiation

Differentiating between early graft failure and type 5 MI related to native coronary arteries is challenging. Electrocardiography and imaging are not reliable, necessitating coronary angiography. Elevated perioperative cardiac troponin I can indicate early graft failure, with suggested cutoffs at >45× and >70× the upper reference limit at 12 and 24 hours postsurgery, respectively.[21] Emergent coronary angiography is recommended for patients with acute myocardial ischemia, unexplained hemodynamic compromise, low cardiac output syndrome, recurrent ventricular arrhythmias, significant ischemic ECG changes, new ischemic wall motion abnormalities, or large troponin I elevations. PCI is indicated in postoperative cardiogenic shock but carries a risk of perforation at anastomotic sites. Redo CABG is preferred if PCI is unsuitable, especially in severe ischemia cases involving the LAD territory or multiple graft occlusions.

Individualized Treatment

The decision between PCI and redo CABG should be individualized based on multidisciplinary heart team evaluation, considering revascularization feasibility, the area at risk, comorbidities, and clinical status.

TREATMENT OF INTERMEDIATE SAPHENOUS VEIN GRAFT LESIONS (FIGS. 5A TO E)

Intermediate SVG lesions (30–60% diameter stenosis) are common (21–34%) in post-CABG patients and progress rapidly to severe lesions or occlusion, often leading to ACS.

VELETI Studies

The VELETI pilot study randomized 57 patients with intermediate SVG lesions to paclitaxel-eluting stent placement or no stenting, showing a trend toward lower MACE and TLR rates in the stented group after 5 years.[22] However, the VELETI II trial, with 125 patients, found no significant difference in MACE rates between drug-eluting stents (DES) and medically treated patients after a median follow-up of 3.4 years, likely due to late restenosis.[23]

Current Treatment

Patients with intermediate SVG lesions are managed medically, focusing on diabetes control, smoking cessation, and aggressive lipid lowering. Despite achieving mean LDL levels <70 mg/dL in VELETI II, high SVG failure rates suggest the need for stricter lipid control.

MANAGEMENT OF ACUTE AND CHRONIC TOTAL SAPHENOUS VEIN GRAFT OCCLUSIONS

Acute Saphenous Vein Graft Occlusions

Percutaneous coronary intervention of acutely occluded SVGs has poor outcomes. Large cohort studies have shown lower rates of achieving Thrombolysis in Myocardial Infarction (TIMI) III flow in occluded SVGs compared to native vessels (70.2% vs. 95%, $p = 0.03$, and 80.7% vs. 93.6%, $p = 0.0001$) and higher in-hospital mortality rates for SVG PCI.[24] Despite the suboptimal outcomes of SVG PCI, recanalizing the native vessel can be technically challenging and carries risks. Therefore, a staged revascularization strategy is often considered.

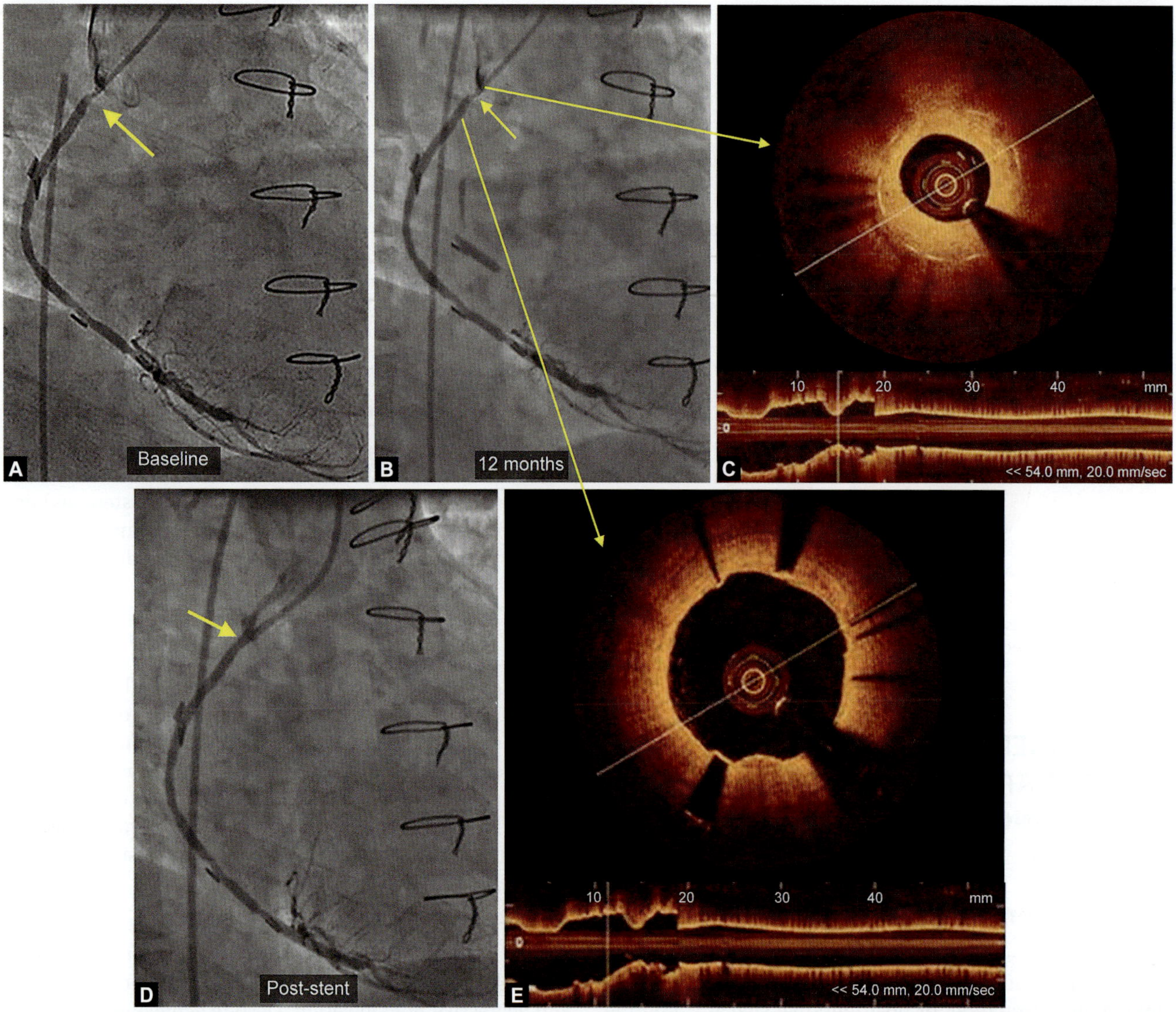

FIGS. 5A TO E: (A and B) Example of in-stent restenosis of an ostial saphenous vein graft lesion 12 months after stenting. (C and E) Optical coherence tomography demonstrated that restenosis was due to neointimal hyperplasia. (D) After repeat stent implantation, SVG patency was restored.

Chronic Total Occlusions

Percutaneous coronary intervention for chronic total occlusion (CTO) of SVGs generally has low success rates and high repeat revascularization rates, leading the ACCF/AHA/SCAI 2011 guidelines to classify it as harmful (class III, level of evidence C).[25] However, in selected cases where no other options are available, PCI of SVG CTOs can provide clinical benefits. In a study of 28 SVG CTO PCIs in 27 patients, the technical success rate was 79%, with two intraprocedural Q-wave MIs (7%). After an average follow-up of 596 ± 429 days, 81% of patients who had successful PCI experienced angina relief, with an acceptable TVR rate of 9.5%.[26]

Retrograde Conduits

Chronically occluded SVGs can be used as retrograde conduits for revascularizing native vessel CTOs. A recent study found that the technical success rates (77% for occluded vs. 87% for patent SVGs, $p = 0.11$) and in-hospital MACE rates (6.4% vs. 8.4%, $p = 0.1$) were similar when using occluded SVGs compared to patent SVGs for retrograde crossing.[27]

CONCLUSION

Saphenous vein grafts are commonly used in CABG, but they have high failure rates necessitating frequent interventions. SVG PCI is complex and carries a higher risk of complications and restenosis compared to native coronary artery PCI. Effective management includes using EPDs to prevent distal embolization and deploying DES if long-term antiplatelet therapy is feasible. When possible, PCI of native coronary arteries is preferred. SVG failure is multifactorial, with occlusion rates around 11% within the first-year post-CABG. Surgical technique and graft construction are critical for optimizing patency. Preventative strategies should focus on antithrombotic and lipid-lowering therapies, and new approaches, such as external stenting of SVGs, are under investigation to further improve outcomes.

ONLINE REFERENCES

Please scan the QR code provided at the end of the table of contents for References of this chapter.

CHAPTER

151

Chronic Total Occlusion: When to and When not to Revascularize

Prathap Kumar N, Manu R, Blessvin Jino

ABSTRACT

The concept to revascularize or not a chronic total occlusion (CTO) is indeed a challenge for the interventionist. When compared to non-CTO lesions, CTO intervention is technically complex, associated with lower rates of success and higher chance of complications. Available evidence from large registries and randomized trials is conflicting and still not sufficient to make definite conclusions. The decision-making process for such cases hence requires proper evaluation of clinical, anatomical, and technical factors.

Keywords: Chronic total occlusion, percutaneous coronary interventions, collateral circulation

INTRODUCTION

Chronic total occlusion (CTO) of a coronary artery is defined as a total occlusion of an epicardial coronary artery, with no antegrade flow beyond the lesion with a duration of at least or >3 months. CTO occurs when an initial ACS event that went unrecognized or not treated or due to a gradual course of luminal narrowing induces the formation of coronary collaterals maintaining the myocardial viability distal to the occlusion. Compared to non-CTO obstructive disease, symptoms of CTO are often different. Exertional dyspnea and fatigue are more common and typical angina is less frequent. The CTO incidence is around 15–20% in patients with CAD and even more common, almost 50%, in post-CABG patients. Patients with CTO are often elder and usually have associated comorbid conditions (smoking, hypertension, diabetes, dyslipidemia, peripheral vascular disease, and previous infarction), which confer an adverse prognosis. The simultaneous presence of a CTO on a nonculprit artery in a case of ACS-STEMI (around 10% of cases) has adverse effects on both short-term and long-term prognosis, particularly if the CTO is supplied by collaterals from culprit vessel. The most frequent site of CTO is the RCA, followed by the LAD, and rarely, the circumflex. CTO is more frequent following CABG both on the native vessel resulting from flow competition and on the grafts. Treatment is quite rare, despite the relative frequency of CTO detection. Medical therapy is considered in majority of cases and only a minority is offered revascularization, that too surgical and rarely percutaneous, in patients with multiple CTO or multivessel disease. Only 15–30% of CTOs are managed percutaneously and among all angioplasties only 5% are being performed for CTOs. This may be due to complexity in technical procedures coupled with high-risk profile and also for want of definite evidence of the benefits of CTO intervention so far.

CHANCE OF SUCCESS

The CTO recanalization success rate is now around 85–90% in CTO specialized centers and around 60–80% in worldwide registers because of the improvement in CTO toolkit materials and the technical advancement achieved by the operators, especially in a retrograde approach.[1] Based on the anatomical and clinical parameters of the lesion and patient respectively, some scores have been published (J-CTO, Euro-CTO CASTLE, PROGRESS-CTO, RECHARGE), which help in predicting the chance of success and risk involved, facilitate in planning the procedure accordingly, and selecting more complex cases for an expert CTO operator. Various techniques are recommended now (antegrade, antegrade dissection and re-entry, and retrograde), which must be used either alone or in combination with each other by the operator based on the characteristics of each CTO. The retrograde approach has significantly improved the success rate but at the cost of a higher chance of complications. The success probability of CTO PCI is lower than that of PCI for nonobstructive lesions, even if complex. A recent study[2] published success rates of 74% and 98%, respectively, for CTO PCI when compared to non-CTO PCI, including complex cases. PCI CTOs are also associated with a higher chance of coronary perforations (3.5% vs. 2%, $p = 0.04$) and cardiac tamponade (0.8% vs. 0.1%, $p = 0.001$), with no significant mortality differences (1.2% vs. 1.5%, $p = 0.51$) and occurrence of major adverse cardiac events (MACE) (4.1% vs. 5%, $p = 0.4$). Native vessel CTO or ISR CTO is associated with similar rates of success and complications. Based on the lesion-wise location, data have found that CTOs of the circumflex carry a higher chance of procedure failure and lower chance of success and is an independent predictor of failure, maybe due to the paucity of collaterals and greater tortuosity of this vessel.

Finally, to increase the success rate of CTO PCI, imaging-based techniques are recommended, such as CT scan and IVUS, for identifying the proximal cap and crossing of the lesion and for stent deployment (IVUS).

CHANCE OF COMPLICATIONS

Simultaneous with the increased rate of success, a decrease in the occurrence of complications during procedures has been noted during the last few years and is currently estimated to be around 3% in expert hands but a rate still higher than that of non-CTO lesion procedures. The common complications encountered are coronary perforation, pericardial effusion and tamponade, side branch occlusion and periprocedural infarction, access site problems, need for emergency CABG, renal damage, stroke, and rarely skin damage from radiation. Mortality risk is marginally lower than 1%.

IS CHRONIC TOTAL OCCLUSION INTERVENTION WORTH CONSIDERING?

Even though technically feasible, the indication of any procedure is based on careful assessment of the cost-benefit ratio. Being a complex procedure requiring lots of dedicated hardware and long procedure time, CTO PCI is economically expensive and associated with significant risks. Therefore, expected benefits should be proportionate to justify the CTO procedure. In this regard, literature data are not equivocal and provide contradictory results mainly between randomized and observational studies, with the former showing less benefit than expected and the latter revealing much more positive results, may be due to possible enrolment bias. The negative results of the randomized studies, reducing their reliability, may be due to low patient enrolment, the higher crossover rates between treatment arms, the short duration follow-up, the improper patient selection, the patient mixing in the treatment of CTOs and non-CTO vessels, including low risk or relatively asymptomatic patients, the nonuniform search for ischemia, and muscle viability before treatment. Instead, observational studies, including some important registers, have provided much more beneficial outcome for CTO PCI. Observational studies benefited from the advantage of a large number of patients, including the long duration analysis (even >10 years),[3] which reveals how the procedural benefits (mortality reduction—both cardiac and total, infarction risk, and future interventions) become manifest only 3 years later from procedure onset, far beyond the randomized trials' study duration. However, registries and observational studies will not take into account the correctness of the subject selection who are much "healthier" and younger than those managed medically.

CHRONIC TOTAL OCCLUSION RANDOMIZED CONTROLLED TRIALS

Six CTO RCT trials, including nearly 1,892 patients, have been conducted during the last decade: EXPLORE, EURO-CTO, REVASC, DECISION-CTO, IMPACTOR-CTO, and COMET-CTO.

1. *EXPLORE trial*:[4] This trial randomized 304 STEMI patients and CTO of a nonculprit vessel to either CTO PCI or OMT. Follow-up after 4 months revealed a 77% success rate and two study groups showed no significant difference on ejection fraction (EF) or LV end-diastolic volume (EDV), except patients with LAD CTO artery who showed revascularization benefit.
2. *REVASC*:[5] This trial randomized 205 chronic stable coronary artery disease patients to either CTO PCI or OMT. Follow-up after 12 months revealed 89% success rate, and two study groups showed no significant differences on the primary end point (MRI-assessed wall thickening in CTO territory) or the secondary endpoint regarding left ventricle functional indices, but showed a significant MACE reduction, because of decreased future reinterventions.
3. *EURO-CTO*:[6] This trial randomized 396 symptomatic CTO patients to either OMT or CTO PCI. Follow-up after 12 months revealed a success rate of 87% with no major differences in MACE (secondary endpoint) but significant enhancement in the quality of life and less angina incidence (primary endpoints) in the CTO PCI group. In this trial, only symptomatic patients were included and viability demonstration was required in case of regional myocardial dysfunctions and all non-CTO lesions were revascularized before randomization.
4. *IMPACTOR-CTO*:[7] This trial randomized 72 RCA-isolated CTOs to either CTO PCI versus OMT. Follow-up after 12 months revealed an 83% procedural success rate. Study revealed significant reduction of stress MRI-based myocardial ischemia (primary endpoint), quality of life, and improvement of the 6-minute walking test

(secondary endpoints), after revascularization, and MACE showed no difference.

5. *DECISION-CTO*:[8] This trial randomized 815 patients with stable angina, silent ischemia, non-STEMI ACS patients to either CTO PCI or OMT. Follow-up after 4 years showed a 91% procedural success rate with no major differences in the primary endpoint (total mortality, CVA, MI, or revascularization). The fact is that nearly 20% of the OMT group underwent PCI, any additional significant non-CTO lesions were revascularized after randomization, expected enrolment was slower and terminated before reaching the estimated subject number initially proposed, myocardial viability assessment was not included in the inclusion criteria, and finally majority of the patients were not that symptomatic.
6. *COMET-CTO*:[9] This trial randomized 100 CTO patients with stable angina or ischemia or viability in akinetic CTO area to either CTO PCI or OMT. Follow-up showed a 94% procedural success rate with significant enhancement in the quality of life (primary endpoint) in the PCI group and no major differences in MACE, reintervention, and total mortality.

In summary, based on an analysis of randomized trials, it emerges that CTO PCI confers symptomatic benefit and enhances the quality of life but the prognostic indices show only a neutral effect. Evidence-based medicine warrants more randomized studies in future to strongly establish the benefit of these procedures, avoiding the limitations previously mentioned.

BENEFITS OF CHRONIC TOTAL OCCLUSION PERCUTANEOUS CORONARY INTERVENTION

On Total Mortality

A meta-analysis[10] of 14 studies regarding total mortality between OMT and CTO PCI showed PCI benefit in 12 studies and only two showed possible advantage by OMT. Medically treated CTO patients have significantly increased mortality than those who were revascularized (RR 1.99; $p = 0.0002$). But there is discordance between randomized and observational studies; the former shows nonsignificant improvement in mortality (RR 1.41; $p = 0.27$) and the latter significantly showed benefit by PCI (RR 2.09; $p = 0.0003$). But the fact is that no randomized studies were conducted to evaluate the procedure's mortality effect.

On Cardiac Mortality

The same meta-analysis[10] revealed an advantage for interventional therapy, which had significantly less mortality risk when compared to OMT (RR 2.36; $p < 0.00001$). The discordance between randomized and observational studies is shown again with the former showing no difference (RR 1.57; $p = 0.27$) and the latter showing significant beneficial effect for CTO PCI (RR 2.42; $p < 0.00001$).

On Major Adverse Cardiac Events

In the same Li's metanalysis,[10] the CTO PCI decreased the MACE risk in contrast to OMT (RR 1.25; $p = 0.03$), and between randomized (RR 1.38; $p = 0.33$) and observational studies (RR 1.25; $p = 0.0004$), no major differences were noted.

On Myocardial Infarction Risk

The same meta-analysis showed that there was no significant rise in MI in OMT compared to CTO PCI. Disparity again exists between observational studies and RCT in which the former showed significantly higher chance of MI without PCI (RR 2.04; $p = 0.002$) and the latter showed nonsignificant benefit of OMT (RR 0.73; $p = 0.21$).

On Symptoms

Randomized trials (IMPACTOR-CTO, EURO-CTO, COMET-CTO) unequivocally revealed that CTO PCI helped in both reducing the symptoms and enhancing the quality of life. The contradictory outcome, seen in DECISION-CTO, is mainly due to the already mentioned shortcomings in applied methodology (subjects with few symptoms, revascularizing non-CTO lesions after randomization, not assessing viability). While selecting patients for CTO PCI, it is useful to assess who can probably obtain the maximum symptomatic benefit after the procedure. OPEN-AP score[11] was recently validated by including seven clinical factors (angina frequency, requirement of nitroglycerine, antiangina drugs number, dyspnea on exertion, more than one CTO, procedure indication for symptoms or not, and patient health questionnaire result), which predict the improvement in symptomatic outcome by PCI. So, ultimately patients who benefit maximally from CTO PCI are the ones who are most symptomatic, including those who have depression.

On Ventricular Function

A meta-analysis,[12] comprising 34 studies, revealed an improvement in LVEF of 4.44% ($p < 0.01$) and a decrease of LV EDV of 6.14 mL/m^2 ($p < 0.01$) following CTO PCI. But the EXPLORE trial,[4] the only RCT, revealed no enhancement in LV function except in the subgroup of subjects with LAD CTO. A different effect based on vessel revascularized was also noted in a trial by Choi et al.[13] in which LAD and circumflex CTO revascularization, but not RCA CTO, resulted in improvement in LVEF.

On Arrhythmic and Sudden Death Risk

A meta-analysis of six studies[14] assessing the chance of occurrence of ventricular fibrillation/ventricular tachycardia

(VT) or suggested defibrillator therapy in the presence of CTO noted that CTO was related with a high chance of arrhythmic events by 1.68-fold (RR 1.68; $p < 0.05$), especially if the infarction was due to CTO. Recurrence of arrhythmia after ablation is also more associated with CTO. Whether opening CTO can reduce this risk is not yet clear and no randomized study has specifically addressed this question. On the other hand, if the infarction is not due to a CTO involved vessel, CTO revascularization won't affect the future risk of arrhythmia (2% vs. 4%; $p = 0.198$).

EFFECT OF CHRONIC TOTAL OCCLUSION PERCUTANEOUS CORONARY INTERVENTION IN DIABETIC AND ELDERLY PATIENTS

Diabetes is recognized as a risk factor for developing a CTO and diabetes prevalence in CTO patients is around 40%. CTO PCI in these diabetic patients is more complex, mainly because the vessels will be calcific and of smaller diameter with high plaque burden resulting in a lower success rate. The meager data on the matter, mainly observational, proved the advantage of revascularization, particularly surgery over medical therapy.[15]

Chronic total occlusion PCI in patients over 75 years of age compared to younger subjects have a less success rate, increased MACE rate, and mortality.[16] Some observational studies, however, show a positive effect on mortality, even in elderly, who had successful CTO revascularization.

EFFECT OF CHRONIC TOTAL OCCLUSION PERCUTANEOUS CORONARY INTERVENTION BASED ON THE ARTERY SITE OF THE OCCLUSION

In the study by Yoneda et al.[17] and in the one already mentioned by Park et al.,[3] only the revascularization of LAD CTO and not LCX or RCA CTO improves mortality. In Gong et al. data,[18] there was no major change in MACE incidence in relation to the vessel revascularized as well as in Canadian registry,[19] where no survival differences were observed based on lesion site.

ROLE OF COLLATERALS

Patients with CTO usually have (80–90%) homo- and/or heterocoronary collateral circulation. Well-developed collaterals will maintain muscle viability but are usually inadequate to maintain sufficient blood flow during stress. The adequate collateral presence is considered safe against future adverse events. So, in the presence of good collateral circulation, CTO patients are usually considered for medical management rather than for revascularization in order to avoid procedural complications. But one observational study,[20] including 738 CTO cases with adequate collaterals, revealed that in contrast to medical management, revascularization (either percutaneous or surgical) decreases the risk of cardiac mortality and MACE. So good collaterals, if present, alone are not a hindrance for CTO revascularization.

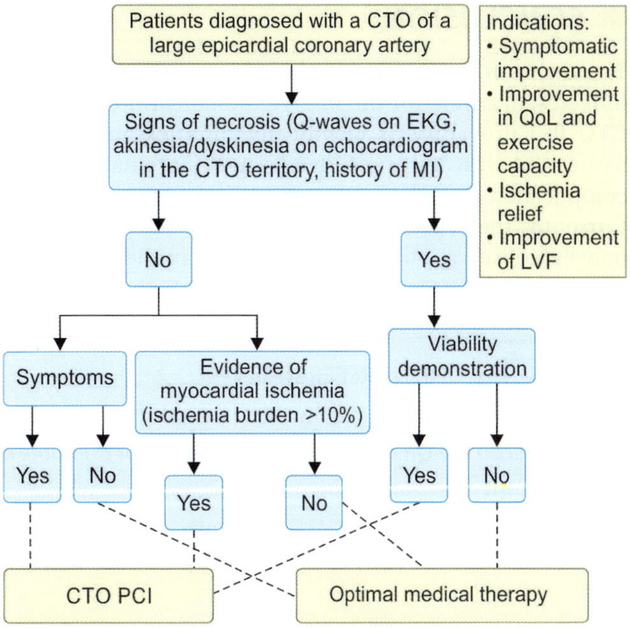

FLOWCHART 1: Diagnostic and therapeutic workup in patients presenting with a chronic total occlusion.

Source: Ricottini E, Coletti F, Nusca A, et al. Coronary chronic total occlusion revascularization: when, who and how? J Clin Med. 2024;13:1943.

DIAGNOSTIC APPROACH

The decision of CTO revascularization should be based on the presence of significant symptoms, including atypical presentations, and their extent has to be evaluated. If symptoms are not present, the ischemic presence and extent caused by the occlusion has to be evaluated. The assessment of myocardial viability is essential in the presence of akinesia or scarring. The method of choice to assess viability or ischemia (SPECT, PET, stress echo-dobutamine, and MRI) is based on experience and local availability, although magnetic resonance imaging is preferred **(Flowchart 1)**.

CONCLUSION

The decision regarding to revascularize a CTO or not is indeed a dilemma for the interventional cardiologist. The CTO PCI procedure is technically complex, more often associated with less success rate and marginally higher complication rate when compared to nonocclusive lesions. Currently, the available data, with significant discordance between observational and randomized studies results, is not sufficient to make a definite final decision regarding the role of the CTO PCI. Hence, it is mandatory to evaluate the clinical parameters (symptoms, LV function, age, comorbid illness, ischemia presence, and extent and viability), anatomical factors (lesion complexity, success probability, and complications risk), and procedural details (center experience and the operator expertise) in the decision algorithm.

ONLINE REFERENCES

Please scan the QR code provided at the end of the table of contents for References of this chapter.

CHAPTER

152

Is Chronic Total Occlusion Opening Worthy: Current Status and Evidence

Dilip Kumar, Abhinay Tibdewal

ABSTRACT

Chronic total occlusions (CTOs) are routinely diagnosed in both asymptomatic and symptomatic patients as well as in the form of a nonculprit lesion in acute coronary syndromes. The main objective of a CTO revascularization should be to alleviate effort-related cardiac symptoms; with a subjective evaluation of symptoms and a patient centric heart team approach. After initial evaluation, several imaging modalities may be used to assess myocardial viability to guide revascularization. Patients with a significant area of viable and ischemic myocardium are usually symptomatic and are most likely to derive the maximum benefit from CTO recanalization whereas on the other hand minor degrees of ischemia or nonviable myocardium generally respond well to optimal medical therapy (OMT).

While the success and safety of CTO interventions has remarkably improved over the years, the average complication rate remains at 3%. The dilemma of the prognostic value of a successful CTO revascularization remains a topic of debate. While meta-analyses have demonstrated a mortality benefit associated with CTO-PCI compared to OMT alone, this evidence is driven by observational data and is not concurred by the randomized controlled trials. As there is lack of data showing mortality and myocardial infarction benefit, current coronary revascularization guidelines recommend CTO-PCI, mainly to improve symptoms and quality of life.

Keywords: CTO, asymptomatic, symptomatic, lesion, therapy, complications

INTRODUCTION

The *definition* of chronic total occlusion (CTO) according to the CTO Academic Research Consortium (CTO-ARC) is an occlusion of an epicardial coronary artery without antegrade flow through the lesion and with a probable or definite duration of ≥3 months, based on angiographic criteria such as a thrombolysis in myocardial infarction (TIMI) grade 0 flow through the lesion with no evidence of a thrombus, no staining at the proximal cap, and the presence of mature collaterals.[1]

The main features of a CTO being an occlusion with no antegrade flow through the lesion with an assumed or reported span of ≥3 months. Bridging collaterals may antegradely fill the target vessel as long as there is absence of antegrade flow through the lesion. Functional occlusions, stated as those with TIMI grade 1 antegrade flow through a critically narrowed but patent lumen, even if not evident on angiography; may not be defined as CTOs.

Lesions <3 months duration have a higher likelihood of acute procedural success compared with older lesions, knowing the clinical history is ideal but very rarely does one come across definitive documented evidence of a previous angiogram demonstrating a total occlusion.

Literature review demonstrates that series of patients who underwent conventional invasive coronary angiography (ICA) reported the presence of at least one CTO in 15–20% of cases.[2,3]

ANATOMY

The histopathology of a normal coronary artery consists of intimal, medial, and adventitial layers. Nevertheless, distinguishing the different layers of the vessel wall may be difficult in a chronically occluded vessel even by intravascular imaging because of considerable architectural disarray. Clinically, it is highly worthwhile to differentiate between the occlusive plaque (composed of the previous true lumen now occupied by atherosclerotic plaque and organized thrombus) and what lies outside it (media and adventitia). Plaque or atherosclerosis is an intimal pathology that is bounded by the internal elastic lamina.[4,5]

PATIENT PROFILE AND SPECTRUM OF PRESENTATION (FIG. 1)

The CTOs may be diagnosed in various clinical scenarios, such as acute coronary syndromes, during an evaluation for chest pain, as a result of documented ischemia using different imaging modalities or incidentally, and during a preoperative evaluation before surgical valve replacement or vascular surgery. While patients with exertional angina or equivalents have a recommended diagnostic and therapeutic protocol to be followed, asymptomatic patients must be treated with caution based on further workup which is generally not accessible to the treating physician at index presentation.[2,3]

All patients discovered with a CTO on angiogram should be critically evaluated as per the clinical scenario including demographics, built, and coexisting conditions such as significant concomitant valvular heart disease, large aortic aneurysms, respiratory illnesses, and chronic debilitating diseases, cognition, etc. The clinical profile of the patient should concur with technical considerations; with a patient centric Heart team approach to make an informed decision between optimal medical therapy (OMT) or revascularization, and in the latter group, between percutaneous coronary intervention (PCI) and surgery.

Patients with CTO are frail, elderly, with higher incidence of diabetes and with a more severely impaired left ventricular (LV) ejection fraction.[3] A cohort of patients may present with ACS, including ST-segment elevation myocardial infarction (STEMI). In the scenario of type 1 myocardial infarction, with either a plaque rupture or erosion in the culprit artery supplying collateral flow to another coronary artery with a CTO, prognosis is poor because of the double injury due to sudden interruption of collateral flow from the culprit artery to the CTO territory, hence making it a state of double jeopardy.[3]

Almost a third of patients who are resuscitated post a cardiac arrest have a CTO identified on the angiogram.[6] Complete revascularization in patients with acute coronary syndrome complicated by cardiogenic shock beyond the infarct-related artery especially with a coexisting CTO has been a subject of debate and discussion. Initially, the SHOCK trial recommended that patients in this complex setting

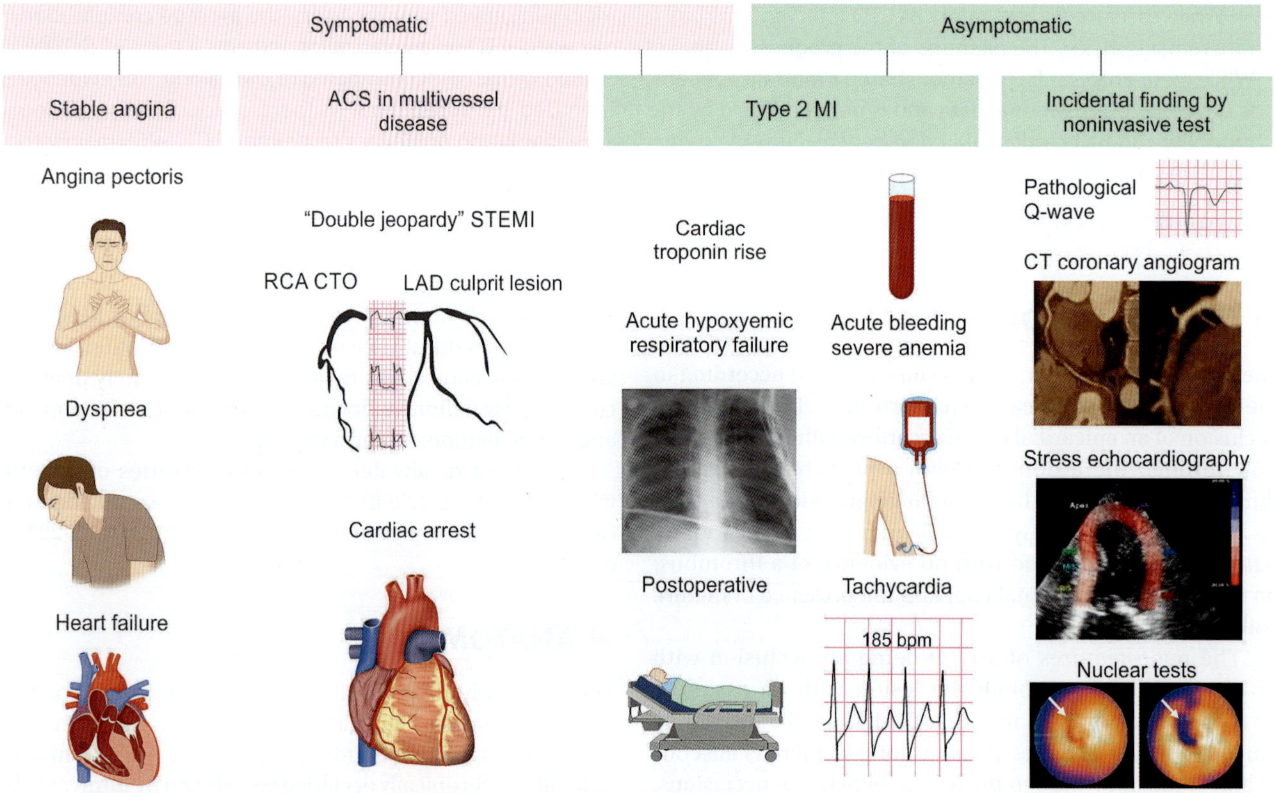

FIG. 1: Clinical presentation of patients with coronary chronic total occlusion.

Source: Galassi AR, Vadalà G, Werner GS, et al. Evaluation and management of patients with coronary chronic total occlusions considered for revascularisation. A clinical consensus statement of the European Association of Percutaneous Cardiovascular Interventions (EAPCI) of the ESC, the European Association of Cardiovascular Imaging (EACVI) of the ESC, and the ESC Working Group on Cardiovascular Surgery. EuroIntervention. 2024;20(3):e174-84.

should undergo complete revascularization but this theory was challenged by other trials.[7,8]

It is well documented that a CTO lesion is commonly diagnosed in cardiogenic shock and associated with high mortality.[9] Hence, the presence of a CTO was not included as an exclusion criterion in CULPRIT-SHOCK, which differentiates it from all other STEMI trials without cardiogenic shock. This permitted the inclusion of a more practical cohort of patients generally seen in daily clinical practice. Exclusion of CTO lesions would have led to a significant selection bias and a lower-risk cohort and hence it was suggested to intervene on the CTO lesions also.

Nevertheless, the CTO interventions were required to be technically easier, with a contrast limit of 300 cm^3 for the overall immediate revascularization. No other complex or retrograde interventional approaches were recommended. The presence of a minimum of one CTO lesion was documented in 22.4% in the culprit-lesion-only arm and in 24.0% in the immediate multivessel PCI arm. In CULPRIT-SHOCK, immediate CTO recanalization was attempted in approximately 50% of patients in the immediate multivessel PCI group and was successful in roughly one-third of attempts. The results for the primary study endpoint were consistent for CTO presence or absence, as shown in the predefined subgroup analysis (p for interaction = 0.26). Thus, neither a CTO intervention nor the presence of a CTO determined the final end result for both treatment strategies.[9] Whereas, there is convincing evidence supporting complete revascularization for STEMI without cardiogenic shock and multivessel disease; these trials were not specifically targeted for patients with CTO lesions in nonculprit arteries.[10]

Patients with non-STEMI-ACS also need immediate revascularization of the culprit artery, with the added dilemma of ruling out the CTO as the underlying reason of the acute event. Apart from clinical clues, the absence of contrast staining, which is pathognomonic of fresh thrombotic occlusions, and the demonstration of well-developed collaterals toward the distal segment of the CTO normally allow a distinction between acute and chronic coronary occlusions.[11]

A common but interesting cohort of patients with type 2 MI (i.e., MI secondary to ischemia due to either increased oxygen demand or decreased supply) present with increased troponin levels, ECG changes and/or regional wall motion abnormalities, with or without symptoms. Treatment in such cases should focus on the acute trigger disrupting a previously stable situation with no immediate need of an urgent or emergent CTO revascularization, but with consideration of it at a later stage.[12]

APPROACH TO THE PATIENT WITH CHRONIC TOTAL OCCLUSION (FLOWCHART 1)

The main objective or indication of a CTO revascularization is relief of effort-related symptoms which are not limited to angina only; dyspnea is at least as frequently seen, and

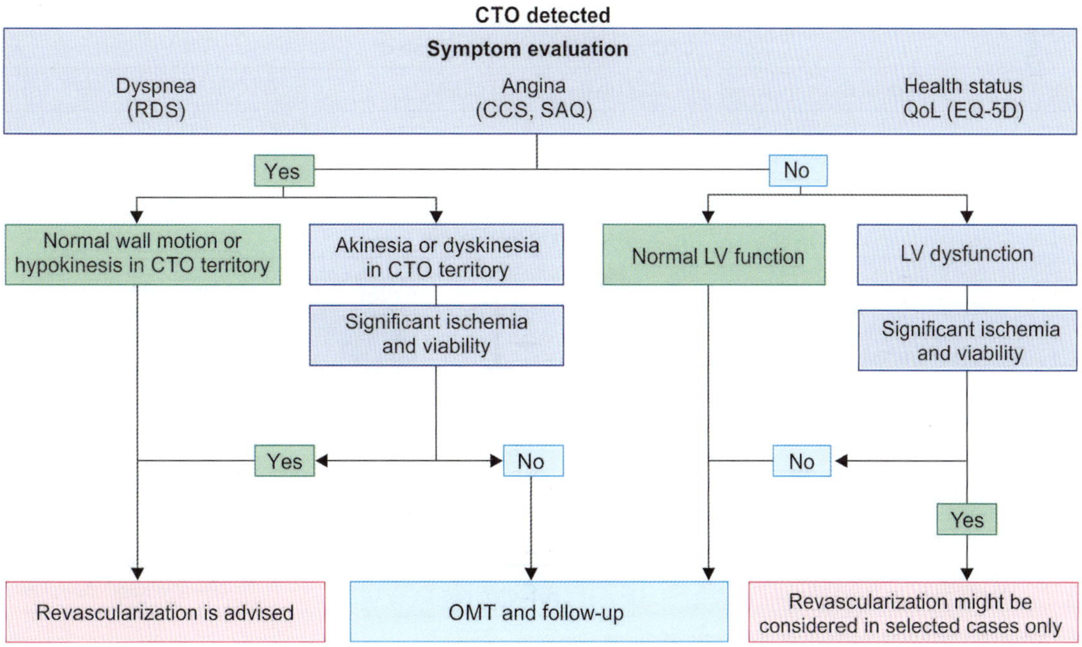

FLOWCHART 1: Approach to clinical decision making in a patient with a chronic total occlusion.

Source: Galassi AR, Vadalà G, Werner GS, et al. Evaluation and management of patients with coronary chronic total occlusions considered for revascularisation. A clinical consensus statement of the European Association of Percutaneous Cardiovascular Interventions (EAPCI) of the ESC, the European Association of Cardiovascular Imaging (EACVI) of the ESC, and the ESC Working Group on Cardiovascular Surgery. EuroIntervention. 2024;20(3):e174-84.

patients report significant improvement in symptoms after successful recanalization.[12] The evaluation of effort or exercise-related symptoms can be fairly performed using tools such as the modified Seattle Angina Questionnaire (SAQ),[13] the EuroQol quality-of-life 5-dimensional score (EQ-5D),[14] or Rose Dyspnea Scale (RDS).[15]

After initial evaluation, different imaging modalities may be used to prove myocardial viability. In case a stress test is not feasible or locally unavailable, a bicycle or treadmill exercise tolerance test might be done to determine the patient's true functional capacity, the severity of exercise-induced angina and/or dyspnea, and their reproducibility compared to the patient's history.

Some patients may have silent ischemia in the CTO territory as well. In this cohort, collaterals commonly avert regional myocardial dysfunction or MI, but their functional capacity to enhance myocardial blood flow to the CTO territory during exercise may be limited. Typically, fractional flow reserve (FFR) assessed distal to a CTO is usually below 0.5.[16,17] In asymptomatic patients with LV dysfunction, the assessment of inducible ischemia/viability may have a prognostic value and might be considered during follow-up to guide coronary revascularization in selected cases only.[18]

In patients with ventricular tachyarrhythmias at presentation, the presence of a coronary CTO is independently associated with higher midterm all-cause mortality.[19] Additionally, in patients with ischemic cardiomyopathy and an implantable cardioverter defibrillator for secondary prevention of sudden cardiac death, the demonstration of an angiographically documented CTO is an independent predictor of appropriate ICD therapy.[20]

The revascularization of a CTO segment should only be recommended if the myocardial segments supplied by it are viable and ischemic upon pharmacological stress or exercise.

Patients with a significant area of viable and ischemic myocardium are usually symptomatic and are most likely to have the maximum benefit from CTO revascularization whereas on the other hand minor degrees of ischemia generally respond well to OMT.[21]

Moreover, patients with significant ischemic burden reduction and no residual ischemia after CTO-PCI have lower rates of all-cause death and nonfatal myocardial infarction as compared with those with significant residual perfusion defect. Further, long-term symptomatic relief was associated with normalization of hyperemic myocardial blood flow levels after CTO-PCI.

Stress cardiac magnetic resonance imaging perfusion, using a gadolinium-based contrast agent and pharmacological vasodilation, is recommended as standard practice for detecting ischemia and viability, presenting accurate data regarding myocardial fibrosis and scarring. Naturally, after successful revascularization, myocardial contractility recovery of those segments supplied by the CTO vessel is likely if transmurality of late gadolinium enhancement (LGE) is <25%, while it is very unlikely if LGE is >75%. Unfortunately, for segments in the intermediate range, the predictive accuracy of LGE transmurality is limited; this aspect might explain why successful CTO-PCI of a dysfunctional but viable myocardium does not lead to the expected LV function recovery in all patients **(Flowchart 2 and Table 1)**.[22,23]

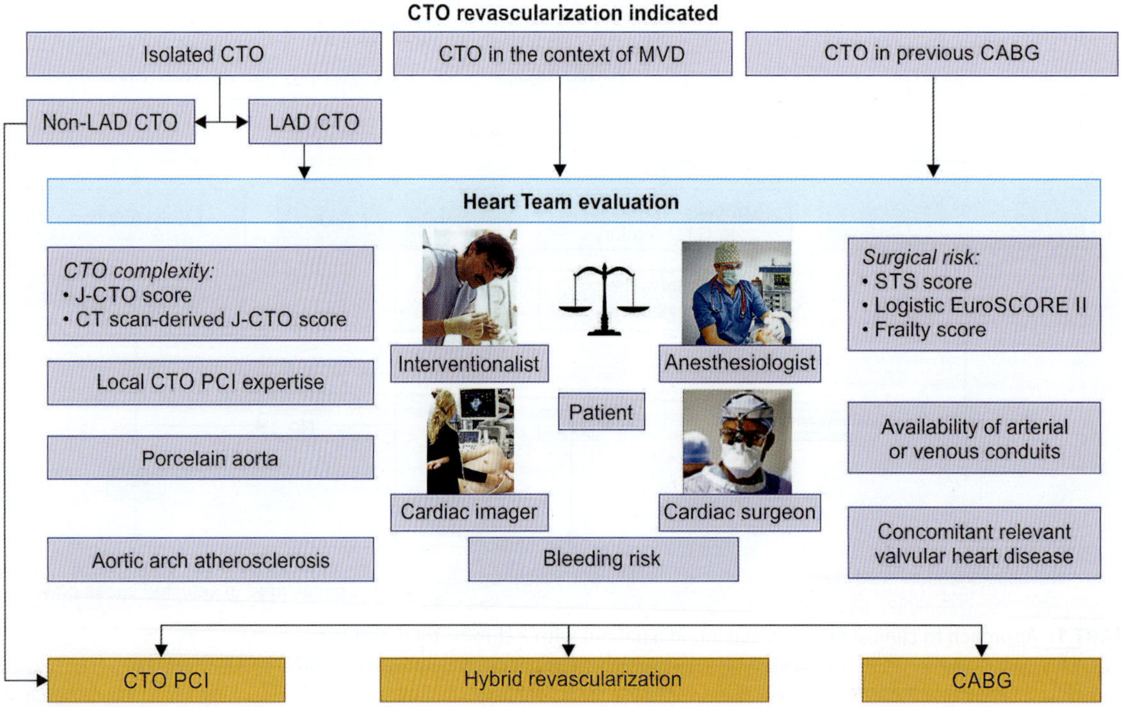

FLOWCHART 2: Approach to strategy of revascularization.

TABLE 1: Expert panel statements for evaluation and management of patients with chronic total occlusion.

	Evidence available
The CTO recanalization success rate has dramatically increased (85–90%), provided that expert operators are offered the full availability of dedicated interventional tools	*RCTs and registries:* Uncontroversial
Frequency and severity of complications is higher (1–3%) compared with most PCI procedures in CCS. This requires careful consideration of the benefit and risk balance before embarking upon CTO recanalization or moving to recanalization modalities (ADR, retrograde) that pose higher complication risks	*Registries and meta-analyses:* Uncontroversial
A specific consent form listing the differences with other PCI procedures (duration, double access, lack of certainty of success, and slightly higher risk of complications) should be submitted to patients and discussed with the main operator before the procedure	Expert consensus
Ad hoc CTO-PCI (i.e., during the same diagnostic angiogram) is discouraged. CTO-PCI should be started only after having ensured that sufficient time is available, experienced operators are present and a well-defined strategy has been developed. The treating physicians will have the opportunity to review indications, perform additional tests if needed, and inform the patient and his family, leaving enough time for decision-making	Expert consensus
The complexity of CTO procedures can be graded, and the most complex (stumpless, ostial, very calcified, or long and tortuous, and previously failed) should be reserved for dedicated operators or performed with proctorship	Expert consensus
The presence of a CTO during ACS (especially STEMI) increases the risk that the patient develops cardiogenic shock, but attempts at recanalization in the acute phase should be discouraged	Randomized trials
Complete revascularization appears beneficial in STEMI, and with less compelling evidence, in NSTEMI. CTO-PCI during primary angioplasty should be discouraged	Randomized trial[11] Expert consensus on timing and modalities of CTO treatment
In CCS patients with multivessel disease with clinical or anatomical preference for PCI over CABG, the timing of CTO-PCI and the sequence of treatment of non-CTO and CTO lesions deserve careful consideration	Expert consensus
Symptoms of angina or dyspnea likely caused by the persistence of a CTO and resistant to medical therapy should be the main driver of CTO recanalization	Randomized trials and registries
Myocardial revascularization decision, in the context of left main/multivessel disease, including CTO lesions, is optimized by a Heart Team approach	ESC and ACC guidelines on myocardial revascularization
Current evidence does not support the use of CTO-PCI to improve prognosis (reduce mortality and incidence of myocardial infarction). Randomized trials have limitations in terms of sample size, patient selection bias and trial design, and it is worth noting the opposite results in large, nationwide, long-term registries comparing patients who had successful or failed CTO with those patients undergoing revascularization or left under medical treatment	Consensus that the conflicting evidence from randomized trials and large registries is still insufficient to draw firm conclusions
Current evidence is still not sufficient to draw firm conclusions on the use of CTO-PCI to improve left ventricular function	Evidence from meta-analyses and registries was not confirmed in a randomized trial
The assessment of inducible ischemia and viability in the CTO territory is advisable in case of LV dysfunction. MRI, if available, should be preferred over nuclear tests and stress echocardiography for viability assessment	Expert consensus

REVIEW OF LITERATURE

The EUROCTO trial demonstrated that PCI was effective at improving some measures of health status. This multicenter, unblinded study randomized 396 patients 2:1 to CTO-PCI plus OMT or OMT alone. The final success rate for PCI was 87%. The retrograde approach was used in 36%. There was no procedural mortality.

For the primary efficacy endpoint at 12 months, the angina frequency score ($p = 0.003$) and the quality-of-life score ($p = 0.007$) had improved for PCI compared with OMT (intention to treat). There was no improvement in the other domains (physical limitation, angina stability, and treatment satisfaction) for PCI compared with OMT. For the primary safety endpoint at 3 years, cardiovascular death or myocardial infarction occurred in 5.0% of the PCI group versus 2.9% of the OMT group ($p = 0.32$).[24]

A distinction in favor of CTO-PCI was only seen when analyzing the composite of mortality, nonfatal myocardial infarction, and ischemia-driven target revascularization

(21.2% vs. 11.0%; $p = 0.008$). Interestingly, this distinction was mainly marked by a higher rate of target vessel revascularization in the OMT alone group (16.8% vs. 3.5%; $p < 0.001$).

In patients with chronic stable angina as a result of the CTO, PCI improved few but not all measures of health status such as angina frequency and quality of life (QoL). There was a higher frequency of complete relief from angina in the PCI group. Major adverse cardiovascular and cerebrovascular events were low and similar between treatment groups at 12 months. At 3 years, cardiovascular death or myocardial infarction was similar between treatment groups, while major adverse cardiovascular and cerebrovascular events were lower in the PCI group versus OMT. This was majorly led by a reduction in ischemia-driven revascularization in the PCI group.[24]

In the DECISION-CTO trial, patients were randomized to CTO-PCI + OMT ($n = 417$) or OMT ($n = 398$). The trial had to be stopped early due to slow enrollment. The results of this trial indicate that routine CTO-PCI + OMT is not superior to OMT alone in reducing cardiovascular outcomes among patients with at least one CTO. During a median follow-up of 4.0 years, the incidence of the composite of death, myocardial infarction, stroke, and target vessel revascularization was similar between the two study groups. One limitation is the high rate of crossover of nearly 20%. Although negative, this is a landmark trial for the field of CTO-PCI. It is one of the first to systematically compare the two therapies. DECISION-CTO does not refute the findings of the EuroCTO trial, and symptom improvement remains the main indication for CTO-PCI.[25]

On the contrary to EuroCTO, which enrolled patients after revascularization of non-CTO lesions, many patients in DECISION-CTO had multivessel coronary artery disease at the time of enrollment, and many of them in both groups underwent revascularization of non-CTO lesions. It is unascertained if the patients remained symptomatic after revascularization of those non-CTO lesions.[25]

EXPLORE was another CTO-PCI trial that focused on patients with STEMI undergoing primary PCI with a coexistent CTO, and showed no improvement in LV function with CTO-PCI. At 4 months, cardiac MRI showed no difference between the two groups in LV ejection fraction and LV end-diastolic volume (the primary endpoints of the study).[26]

Likewise the REVASC trial (a randomized trial to assess regional left ventricular function after stent implantation in chronic total occlusion) in patients with a stable coronary artery disease and a CTO randomly assigned 205 patients to CTO-PCI and no CTO-PCI. At 6 months, cardiac MRI showed no difference between the two groups in segmental wall thickening in the CTO territory and regional and global LV function, as well.[27]

A meta-analysis conducted on >28,000 patients, showed the correlation of successful CTO-PCI with improved long-term survival when compared with procedural failure (OR 0.52, 95% CI 0.43–0.63). Another meta-analysis, conducted on 2,243 patients with successful CTO-PCI, found a LVEF definite increase, with 4.4 percentage points over baseline comparison in absolute terms ($p < 0.01$), as also a reduction in negative ventricular remodeling.[28,29]

Clinical advantage of successful CTO-PCI was found also in large registries. In the OPEN-CTO registry,[1] which enrolled 1,000 patients, investigators reported in the group of successful CTO revascularization a statistically significant improvement in SAQ from 49.4 ± 0.9 to 75.0 ± 0.7 ($p < 0.01$), and after adjusting for baseline differences, the mean group difference in SAQ between successful and unsuccessful CTO-PCI was 10.8 (95% CI 6.3–15.3; $p < 0.001$). At 1 year, the unadjusted MACCE rate was lower in patients with successful index CTO-PCI compared to patients with unsuccessful CTO-PCI (9.4% vs. 14.6%; $p = 0.04$).[30]

In a study conducted by Obedinskiy et al. (IMPACTOR-CTO trial) 94 patients with isolated right coronary artery CTO were randomly assigned to either CTO-PCI or non-CTO-PCI at a single center. The results revealed that CTO-PCI led to a greater reduction in ischemia and improvements in 6-minute walk distance and QoL, as assessed by the SF-36 health survey.[31]

The ISCHEMIA-CTO trial was conducted to assess the effect of CTO-PCI in patients with a CTO lesion and target vessel diameter ≥2.5 mm, and myocardial ischemia in the concerned territory. Initially, all patients were subjected to OMT for at least for 3 months and non-CTO lesions were managed according to guidelines. Thereafter, prior to randomization; myocardial ischemia and QoL is evaluated. Patients are classified into two cohorts based on their SAQ score and randomized to either OMT alone or OMT and CTO-PCI. Cohort A is defined as Low-or asymptomatic patients with a QoL score >60 and/or CCS class <2, and >10% ischemia in the left ventricle. Cohort B is symptomatic patients with a QoL score <60 or CCS class angina >1 and at least ischemia in 5% of the left ventricle. The primary endpoint in cohort A is a composite of major adverse cardiac and cerebral events, hospitalization for heart failure and malignant ventricular arrhythmias. The primary endpoint in cohort B is difference in QoL 6 months after randomization.

The primary aims of the above CTO-trial were to investigate: (1) The outcome of PCI versus OMT of CTO lesions in patients with significant myocardial ischemia (≥10%) without significant symptoms, and (2) The outcome of PCI versus OMT of CTO lesions in patients with symptoms and at least mild myocardial ischemia (≥5%). The main hypothesis is that CTO-PCI has prognostic and symptomatic benefits given sufficient burden of ischemia. Hence, the current trial attempts to address the impact of CTO-PCI on symptomatic and/or prognostic indication.

This trial is designed to study if CTO-PCI improves QoL and MACCE. Both positive and negative results of the trial will affect future guidelines and recommendations on how to treat patients with CTO.[32]

The NOBLE-CTO trial aims to study all-cause mortality and QoL in patients who underwent either PCI-CTO or OMT as the initial strategy (NCT03392415).[33] ORBITA-CTO will evaluate PCI-CTO versus placebo procedure and their influence on relieving symptoms of angina in patients with a previous 3-months OMT (NCT05142215).[34] Simultaneously, studies investigating the effects of recanalization in patients with comorbidities are underway. CTO-HF trial (NCT05632653) will evaluate if PCI-CTO improves survival and HF-related rehospitalizations compared to OMT, whereas the CTO-ARRHYTHMIA (NCT04542460) study aims to assess the incidence of arrhythmias and the impact of PCI and OMT on them in CTO patients.[35]

Probably the aforementioned studies will provide further information of the benefits of PCI-CTO, identify particular cohorts in the greatest need of revascularization, and influence future guidelines and recommendations.

CONCLUSION

Whereas the success and safety of recanalizing CTOs has significantly improved in the last decade, the mean in-hospital complication rate remains at 3%, with high periprocedural myocardial infarction rates and significant additional financial burden. The question of the prognostic value of CTO remains a topic of debate and is determined by study design. While meta-analyses have demonstrated a mortality benefit associated with CTO-PCI compared to OMT alone, this evidence is driven by observational data and is not concurred by the randomized controlled trials. More randomized controlled trials, of adequate sample size, are needed to shed further light on this dilemma. As there is lack of data showing mortality and myocardial infarction benefit, current coronary revascularization guidelines recommend CTO-PCI, mainly to improve symptoms and QoL.

Symptom assessment must be comprehended carefully. Symptoms being subjective are difficult to assess, with differences arising from both the patient and healthcare professionals in the reporting and evaluation of their character and severity. Moreover, the tools for assessing symptoms after an intervention in clinical practice may be more nuanced and patient-specific to those used in research. Addressing some of these issues is important to guide future guidelines and clinical practice. The validation of more original, modern, and customized methods of recording patient symptoms may help to improve the quality of the data. App-based solutions which record daily symptom frequency and severity could potentially yield high-quality, patient-specific data, particularly when incorporated with other metrics such as the burden of antianginal medications. Such approaches may deliver a greater statistical power to detect differences in treatment effects and may address some of the issues associated with symptom data.

In the present day, it would be prudent that the indications for CTO-PCI must be carefully considered in the knowledge that more data from placebo-controlled trials are needed to truly inform practice.

ONLINE REFERENCES

Please scan the QR code provided at the end of the table of contents for References of this chapter.

CHAPTER

153

Chronic Total Occlusion Revascularization: Indications and Techniques

Sridhar Kasturi

ABSTRACT

The CTO lesions are seen in about 25–30% of patients who are undergoing routine angiographic evaluation. PCI of CTO requires special interventional skills to make it more successful with low complication rate. As these procedures are high-risk challenging procedures, there is an increased risk related to radiation, contrast, and access site bleeding. Utilization of advancements in techniques and equipment, CTO algorithms, and heart team approach make it even more successful program.

Keywords: CTO, lesions, PCI, angiographic, evaluation, procedure

INTRODUCTION

Despite the development of significant collaterals, normal coronary flow is observed in <10% of patients with CTO lesions which contributes to increased MACE, arrhythmias, and death. Successful PCI reduces cardiovascular symptoms, improves left ventricular function, and reduction in ventricular arrhythmia related events. CTO-PCI can be recommended to patient who are symptomatic despite taking optical medications and the risks of the procedure are outweighed by the expected benefit.[1]

The CTO-PCI is a high-cost interventional procedure due to usage of more hard ware, prolonged Cath lab hours, high access-related complications, and CIN leading to prolonged hospital stay compared to non-CTO-PCI. It is associated with increased complications compared with non-CTO-PCI, especially coronary perforation, myocardial infarction, emergency CABG, and death related to cardiac and noncardiac death. The risk of PCI is even higher with advanced age, greater CTO lesion complexity, and in certain cases, such as in patients with prior CABG, severe LV dysfunction, and with comorbidities. Before doing PCI, evaluate for anticipated complications, success rate, the specific risks of the approach, and possible improvement of the clinical outcome.[2]

SCORING OF CHRONIC TOTAL OCCLUSION

It is recommended to implement available scoring tools for the proper selection of the case to provide objective assessments of the anatomic and clinical complexity of a CTO prior to PCI planning.[3] In general, most available CTO-PCI scores take into account one or more of the following angiographic characteristics: (1) Proximal cap morphology, (2) Occlusion length, (3) Presence of tortuosity and/or calcium, (4) Quality of the distal vessel, and (5) Characteristics of the collateral circulation **(Table 1)**.

ANGIOGRAPHIC VIEWS FOR CHRONIC TOTAL OCCLUSION STRATEGY AND PLANNING

It is essential to acquire angiographic images through dual injections to assess proximal cap, CTO segment length, tortuosity and calcification, wide field nonmagnification angiographic images involving all segments, and branches of coronaries, without panning, and the angiography run should be long enough to allow accurate assessment of collateral channels for precise planning of CTO procedure

TABLE 1: Scoring of chronic total occlusion.

Study	Characteristics assessed	Score
J-CTO	• Blunt stump	1
	• Length >20 mm	1
	• Intralesion bending >45°	1
	• Mild-severe calcification	1
	• Previous CTO failure	1
RECHARGE	• Blunt stump	1
	• Length >20 mm	1
	• Intralesion bending >45°	1
	• Visible calcification in the CTO segment	1
	• Bypassed on the CTO target vessel	1
	• Diseased distal landing zone	1
CL	• Blunt stump	1
	• Length >20 mm	1.5
	• Non-LAD	1
	• Severe calcification	2
	• Previous CABG or MI	1.5
CASTLE	• Blunt or no stump	1
	• Length >20 mm	1
	• Severe/unseen tortuosity	1
	• Age >70 years	1
	• Previous CABG	1
PROGRESS CTO	• Ambiguous proximal cap	1
	• Circumflex target vessel	1
	• Moderate/Severe proximal tortuosity	
	• Lack of interventional collateral vessels	

strategies.[4] All angiographic images must be interpreted carefully for CTO body anatomy, presence of disease, and tortuosity in the vessel segments proximal and distal to CTO body, bifurcation at the distal landing zone, and visible and usable interventional collaterals. Moreover, assess proximal cap—blunt or tapered, and ambiguous or unambiguous, presence of side branch at the proximal cap, and length of the CTO segment <20 mm or >20 mm for deciding proper PCI strategy **(Flowcharts 1 and 2)**.

GUIDEWIRES FOR CHRONIC TOTAL OCCLUSION

Guidewires play a huge role for successful PCI of CTO and it is essential to keep all the necessary guidewires in the Cath lab to run successful CTO program.[5] Operator should be familiar with different features of guidewire for selecting proper guidewire to make it highly successful with low complication rate, and the characters of the guidewires that influence the selection are: (1) Torque, (2) Tip durability, (3) Tactile feedback, (4) Penetration power, (5) Trackability, (6) Support, (7) Crossing, (8) Flexibility, and (9) Prolapsing **(Flowchart 3)**.

There are several methods for advancing the guidewire in the true-to-true lumen technique. In the sliding technique, using tapered polymer guidewires with soft tips, slight rotational movements, and cautious advances are used to cross the lesion.[6] If the sliding technique is initially unsuccessful or not progressing the wire movement once entering the proximal fibrous cap, then proceeding to controlled drilling technique is typically the next wire handling technique. The drilling technique, performed when

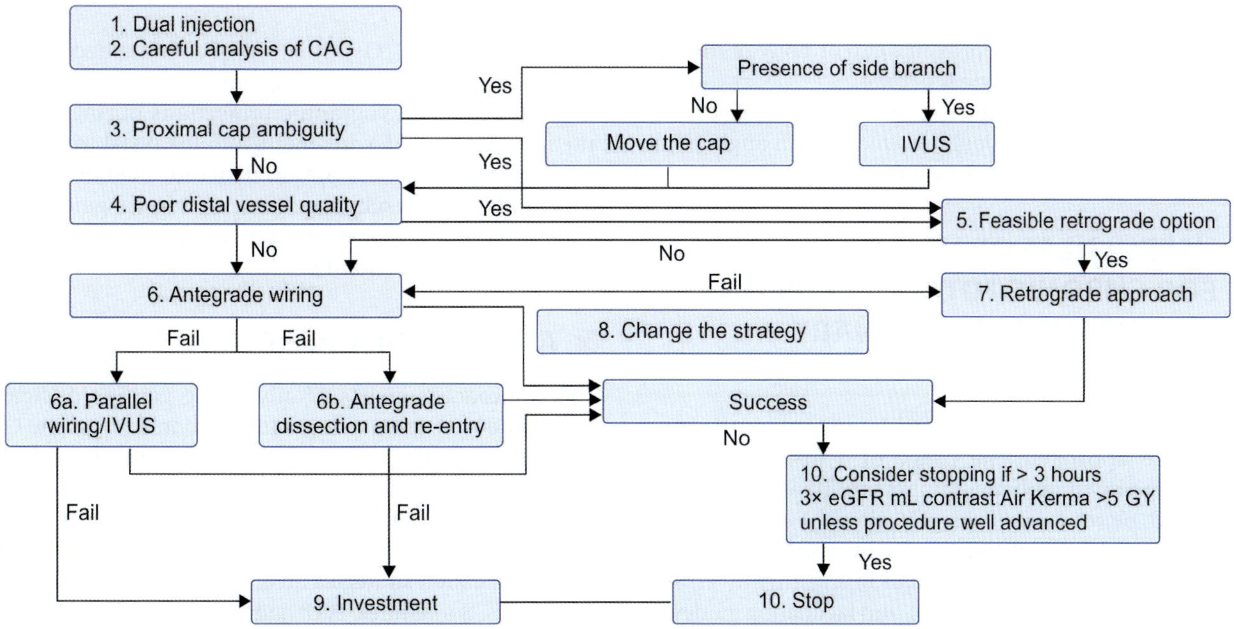

FLOWCHART 1: Chronic total occlusion global algorithm.

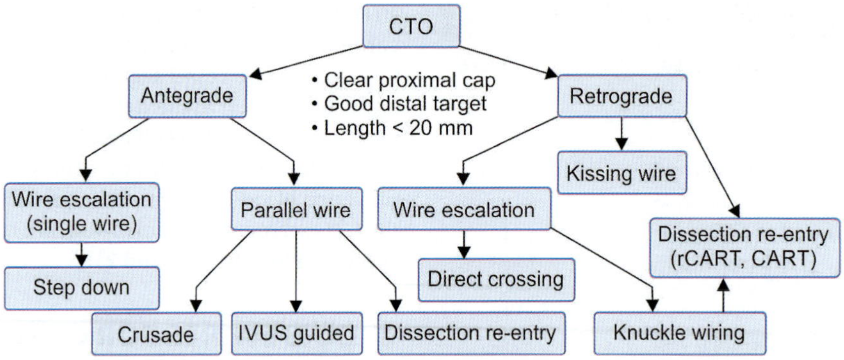

FLOWCHART 2: The hybrid algorithm for chronic total occlusion percutaneous coronary intervention initial approaches.

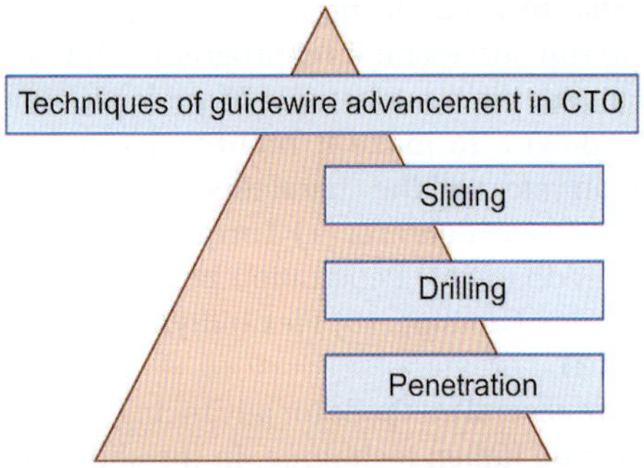

FLOWCHART 3: Techniques of guidewire advancement in chronic total occlusion.

there are harder caps, consists of advancing the guidewire by relatively quick 90° clockwise and counterclockwise rotation of the tip of stiffer guidewire. But some operators will prefer to rotate the wire in the same direction. In some instances, especially in the presence of a blunt cap or more calcified resistant cap drilling with even with the stiffest load tip is ineffective in crossing the proximal cap or body of the CTO where penetration technique is helpful.

Penetration technique—Careful pushing of stiff guidewires without rotational movements with angiography or IVUS image guidance for true lumen tracking.

USEFULNESS OF MICROCATHETERS FOR CHRONIC TOTAL OCCLUSION-PERCUTANEOUS CORONARY INTERVENTION

While performing CTO-PCI with an antegrade or a retrograde approach, the usage of a microcatheter is crucial for providing better support to the CTO wire with enhanced penetration force.[7] It allows easy guidewire exchanges and protects the proximal vessel from stiff CTO guidewire-induced injuries without losing already crossed segment with previous guidewires, and facilitating guidewire maneuvering to side branches (in case of bifurcations in ostial circumflex CTOs). It is well recommended to check guidewire tip position with frequent contralateral injections and orthogonal angiographic projections during crossing attempts. If the guidewire enters into the distal true lumen, the microcatheter is then advanced over it, and the dedicated CTO guidewire is exchanged for a workhorse guidewire to minimize the risk of distal vessel perforation (i.e., wire de-escalation strategy) **(Box 1)**.

BOX 1 Selection of microcatheter based on the purpose of usage.

- Wire support and wire exchange—Fine cross/Caravel/Turnpike LP
- Contrast tip injection and micro channel dilatation—Corsair/Caravel
- Collateral crossing—Epicardial-caravel, straight septal—Corsair/Turnpike, tortuous septal—Caravel.
- Subintimal tracking in ADR—Corsair or Turnpike
- Ballon uncrossable lesions—Tornus or Turnpike gold
- Parallel wiring—Dual lumen catheters (sasuke/twin pass/crusade)
- Proximal cap puncture with side branch—Dual lumen catheter
- Distal vessel perforation management with glue or gel form or fat embolization—Fine cross or Prograte
- Closure of coronary AV fistula with micro coils—Prograte
- Side branch access in bifurcation lesions—Dual lumen Catheters/Ventura or Supercross

ANTEGRADE APPROACH

This approach consists of advancing various dedicated CTO guidewires in an antegrade direction to cross the CTO lesion through the occluded plaque (true-to-true) lesion by using various guidewire manipulations such as sliding, drilling, and penetration. It can be performed by using single or dual lumen microcatheters support with the help of wire escalation strategies involving single or parallel wires techniques. Sometimes, IVUS guided proximal cap puncture or parallel wire technique are also being used to cross CTO body more meticulously and precisely. Initially, polymer jacketed tapered guidewires with a low-penetration force soft-tip (Fielder XT) are used with sliding technique to track visible or invisible microchannels. If these manipulations are not successful, then drilling technique using with 90° rotations of guidewires with intermediate tip load (Gaia 2nd–3rd or Pilot 200) should be used, still unsuccessful in crossing, further attempts should be tried with high penetration force guidewires with greater tip load (Conquest Pro 9–12 or Hornet 10–14). In general, when the proximal cap is blunt, guidewires with intermediate penetration force are used initially instead of wires with low tip load with less penetration force **(Fig. 1)**. After proximal cap puncture with stiff wire, exchanging to less penetrating guidewires is advisable to reduce complications but more penetrating wires may be required for crossing calcific segments.

Finally, in the push and torque technique (penetration technique) the operator advances and rotates the guide wire until the hardest portion of the plaque is reached and then redirects it to a softer part. If during the wiring escalation technique, the guidewire accidentally reaches the subintimal space, it is possible to proceed with the dissection and re-entry technique. Sometimes, the guidewire can be left in the subintimal space as a reference, and a second guidewire advanced through the plaque (parallel guidewire technique).

Antegrade approach is the initial choice and most commonly used choice for the majority of PCI of CTO and it will provide excellent results in carefully selected with suitable anatomy **(Fig. 2)**.[8] Preprocedural predictors of primary antegrade wiring success: Occlusion length <20 mm, proximal cap with tapered tip without ambiguity, and good distal vessel quality without significant disease.

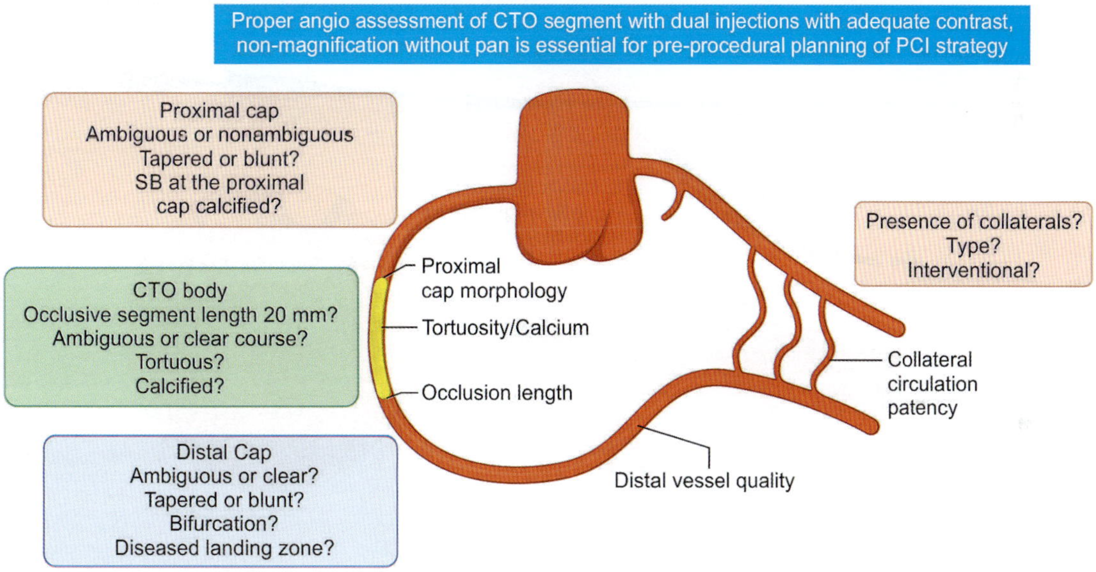

FIG. 1: Dual injection for proper assessment of chronic total occlusion segment.

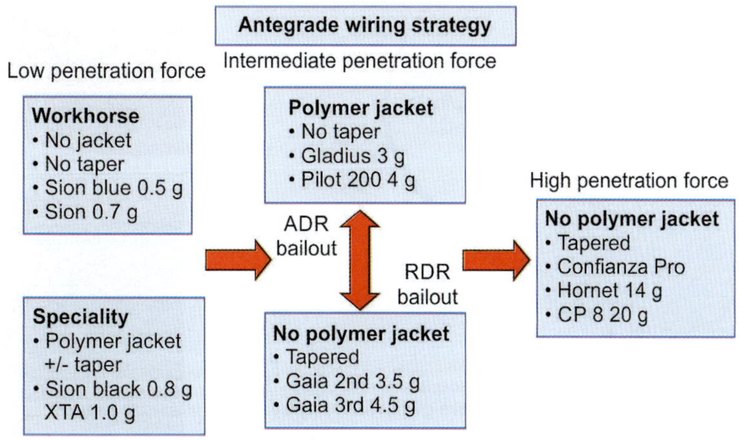

FIG. 2: Antegrade wiring strategy.

As the CTO lesions have wide anatomic variability, failure of guidewire crossing in the antegrade direction were not uncommon. Perforation, dissection, subintimal hematoma, contrast, prolonged irradiation, and operator fatigue are the nightmares during antegrade attempt for CTO wire crossing.

Antegrade Dissection and Re-entry

It remains an important technique for complex CTO lesion subsets where there are limited or poor retrograde options. It is very limited in challenging technical CTO scenarios and cost of the antegrade dissection and re-entry (ADR) devices like CrossBoss and Stingray balloon is very high.[9] ADR has higher perforation rate and increased subintimal space with IMH compared to the retrograde approach. Hence, opt for antegrade wire escalation and restrict it to patients with easy anatomies without interventional collaterals. ADR for complex anatomical lesions should be done in specialized CTO centers with operators having more experience in performing such procedure **(Fig. 3)**. Different re-entry techniques in ADR are as follows:

- Device-based re-entry techniques
  - Stingray LP-based re-entry
  - Recross
- Wire-based re-entry techniques
  - Subintimal tracking and re-entry—STAR
  - Mini-STAR
  - Limited antegrade subintimal tracking and re-entry—LAST
  - Antegrade fenestration and re-entry

The ADR is suitable to patients with diffuse disease and calcium free re-entry zone, distal right coronary artery (RCA) re-entry zone, wire position <0.5 mm from true lumen, absence of bifurcation at distal cap, lack of large intramural hematoma, good retrograde filling, and ease of delivery of the Stingray catheter to the re-entry zone **(Fig. 4)**.[10]

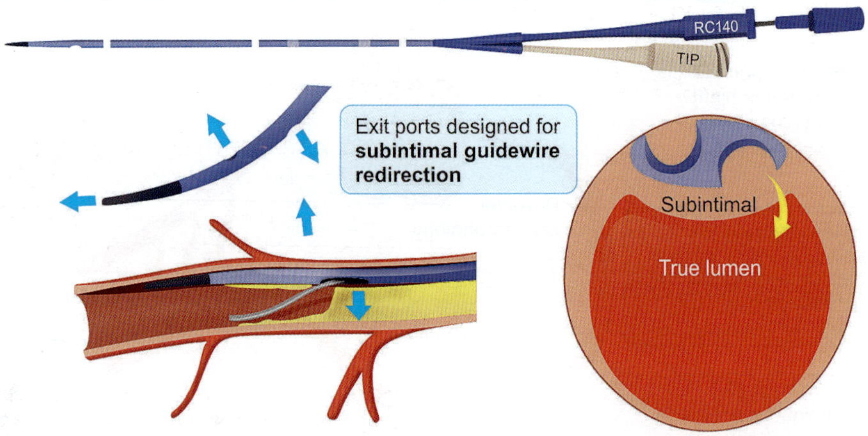

FIG. 3: Recross microcatheter.

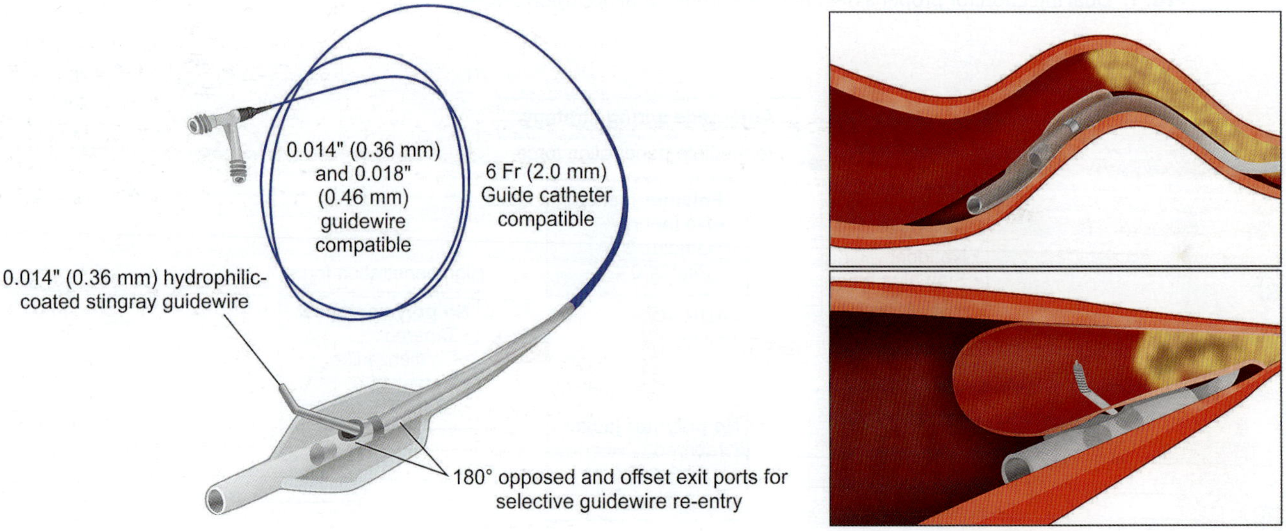

FIG. 4: Stingray balloon.

The ADR to make it more successful requires control of hematoma, small knuckles, and selection of the proper guidewires. ADR is a technique that can be used to increase success and improve safety especially when other options such as retrograde CTO-PCI are not feasible or high risk.

Knuckle Technique

Technique involves forward push is on the looped wire itself rather than the tip itself.[5] Knuckle wiring (and subsequent ADR) has not been the priority method due to rapid extension of the extra plaque space with IMH especially from the antegrade side, requirement of longer stent length, side branch loss, and vessel trauma **(Fig. 5)**.

Polymer jacketed wires are very useful to cross CTO body with knuckle technique (Fielder XT, Gladius Mongo, and Pilot 200) to navigate tortuous anatomy with severe stenotic lesions, and lesions with severe calcification and deemed safer than comparable nonpolymer jacketed wires with similar tip load. Knuckling can improve case efficiency, solve ambiguity, and allow investment/bailout the situation **(Fig. 6)**.

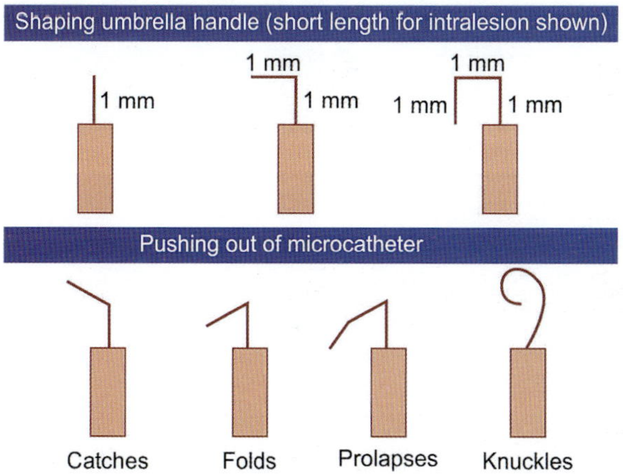

FIG. 5: Shaping umbrella handle.

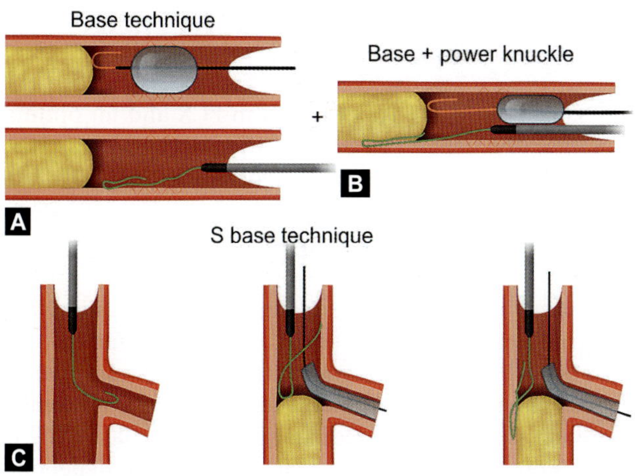

FIGS. 6A TO C: Balloon base technique.

Guidewires with soft tips may not dig in and catch to start knuckle and jacketed tips may slip off and not catch but sometimes, wires with stiff tips required to catch (e.g., Confianza) to initiate knuckles. The stiffer the wire (tip or body), the larger the knuckle and even some soft-tipped wires have stiffer bodies. Guidewires with more stiffness are harder to fold but due to more radial strength they are easier to push forward and less likely collapse, especially in calcified vessels. On the contrary, soft wires are easier to fold but because of less radial strength they are collapsible with less push force and small knuckles can go outside the side branches so be careful about distal perforations with small loops in small side branches. Because of force distribution, usually knuckles will not penetrate out the side of vessels and they are constrained by the vessel architecture, any knuckle that starts in the vessel will stay in vessel. It is safer to start the knuckle with catch before the cap and push through main segment, avoid entering into small side branches, and look for dyssynchronous movement with vessel. Large knuckles with more radial strength can travel segment CTO but the can create large subintimal space.

The use of a guide catheter extension within the proximal CTO to prevent inflow, avoiding extensive dissection beyond the distal cap with knuckled wires, and/or using the CrossBoss close to the landing zone, all help reduce hematoma formation.[11] Usually, it is recommended to do routine aspiration of hematoma from the end hole of the Stingray balloon prior to attempting the puncture **(Fig. 7)**.

Case 1: Antegrade Wire Escalation with Hybrid Approach (Figs. 8 to 11)

A 58-year-old male known hypertensive and diabetic, H/o PTCA (2013) was presented with ACS—Unstable angina. *CAG:* Mid CTO filling from LAD collaterals.

LCA engaged with EBU—3.5-7 Fr guiding catheter, CTO was crossed using Corsair with retrograde approach via septal collaterals from LAD. Initially, unable to cross the lesion with Sion blue with microcatheter support, Then Sion blue changed to 0.014" Fielder XT-R wire. After multiple attempts of careful negotiation through septal collaterals, Fielder XT-R was placed near the bifurcation of the distal LCX.

Check angiography with Corsair. Sion blue wire failed to cross the lesion even after multiple attempts of careful

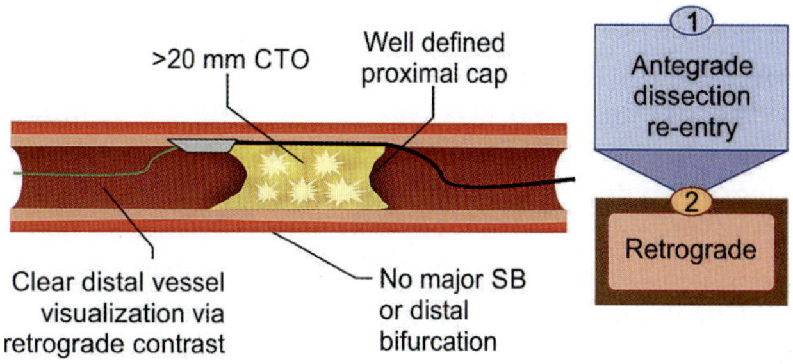

FIG. 7: Antegrade versus retrograde.

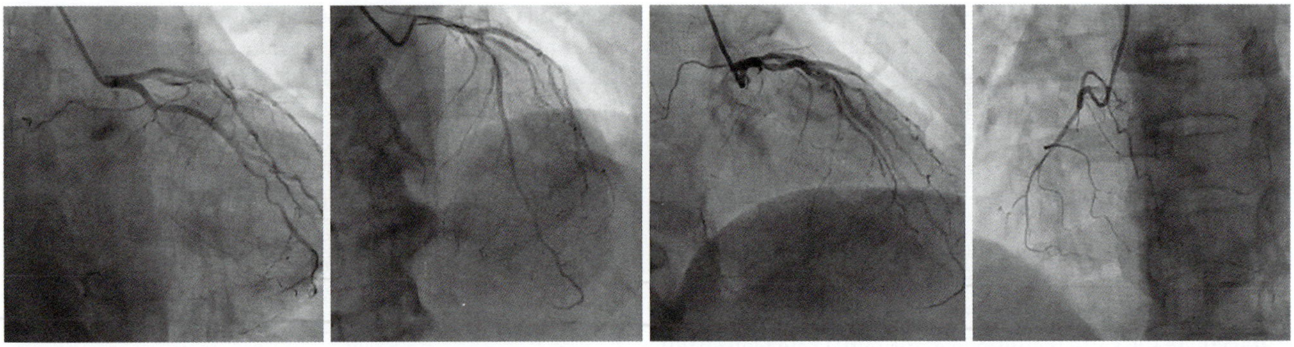

FIG. 8: Coronary angiography-chronic total occlusion.

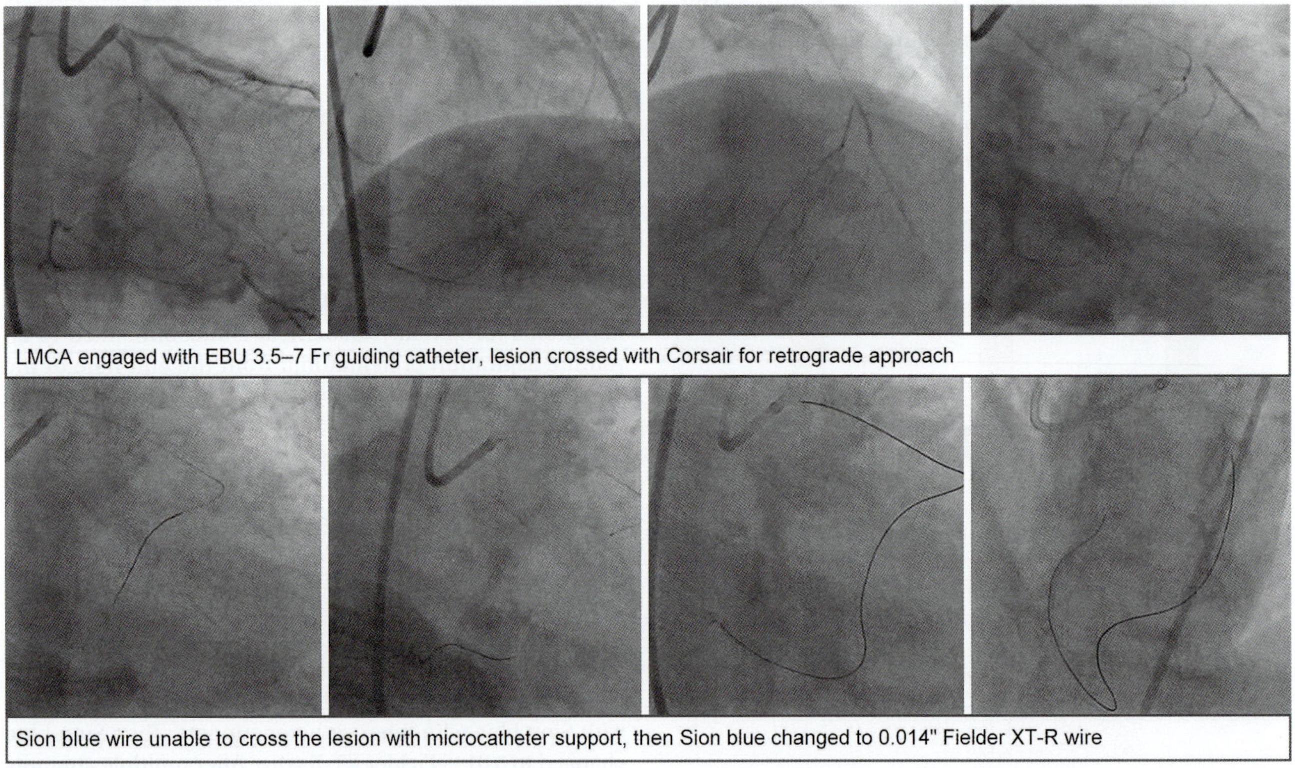

FIG. 9: Wire escalation from Sion blue to Fielder XT-R wire.

manipulations using Corsair through antegrade approach, then Sion blue exchanged with Fielder XT-R wire and the lesion was crossed with Corsair support. Finally, Fielder XT changed to Sion blue, and serial predilatations of CTO was carried out with 1.5 × 10 mm and 2.5 × 15 mm balloons. Subsequently, distal LCX was stented with 2.5 × 48 mm Xience Xpedition Stent and Proximal LCX with 3.0 × 48 mm Xience Xpedition Stent with overlap of 2–3 mm of stent struts. Poststenting IVUS showed under expansion, hence postdilatation was done with 3.5 × 12 mm NC Trek.

Check angiography showed pinching of OM branch, hence it was crossed with Sion blue wire for KBD of LCX bifurcation. Kissing was performed with 2.5 × 15 mm in OM and 3.0 × 12 mm NC Trek balloon in LCX and for optimal dilatation of pinched OM branch. The final result was good with TIMI 3 flow with no complications.

RETROGRADE APPROACH

It is mainly used in complex anatomical settings or when antegrade methods have failed for CTO segments with presence of good usable interventional collaterals with a success rate of 70–90%. The essential step in the retrograde approach is to cross the collaterals without damaging or perforation.[12] Coronary collaterals are classified depending on the anatomy of the coronary tree and the specific

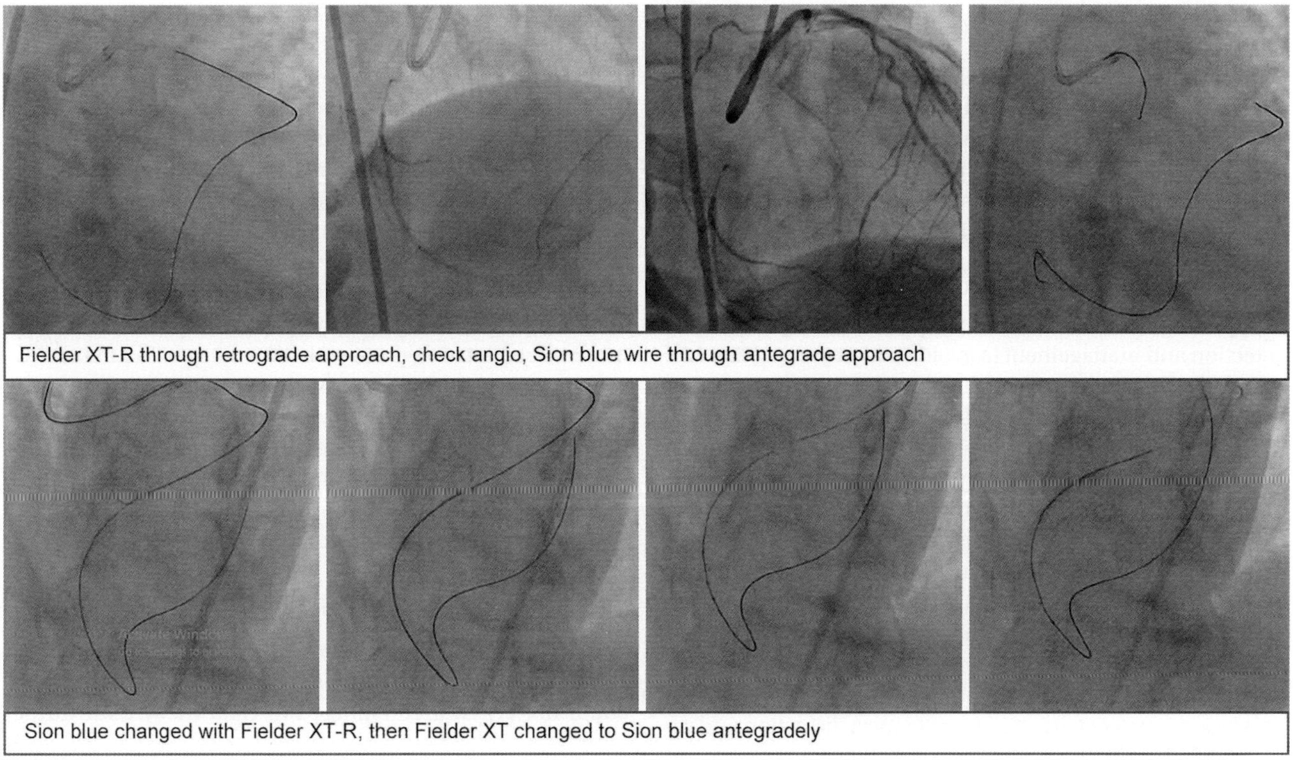

FIG. 10: Retrograde crossing with Fielder XT-R and changed to Sion blue.

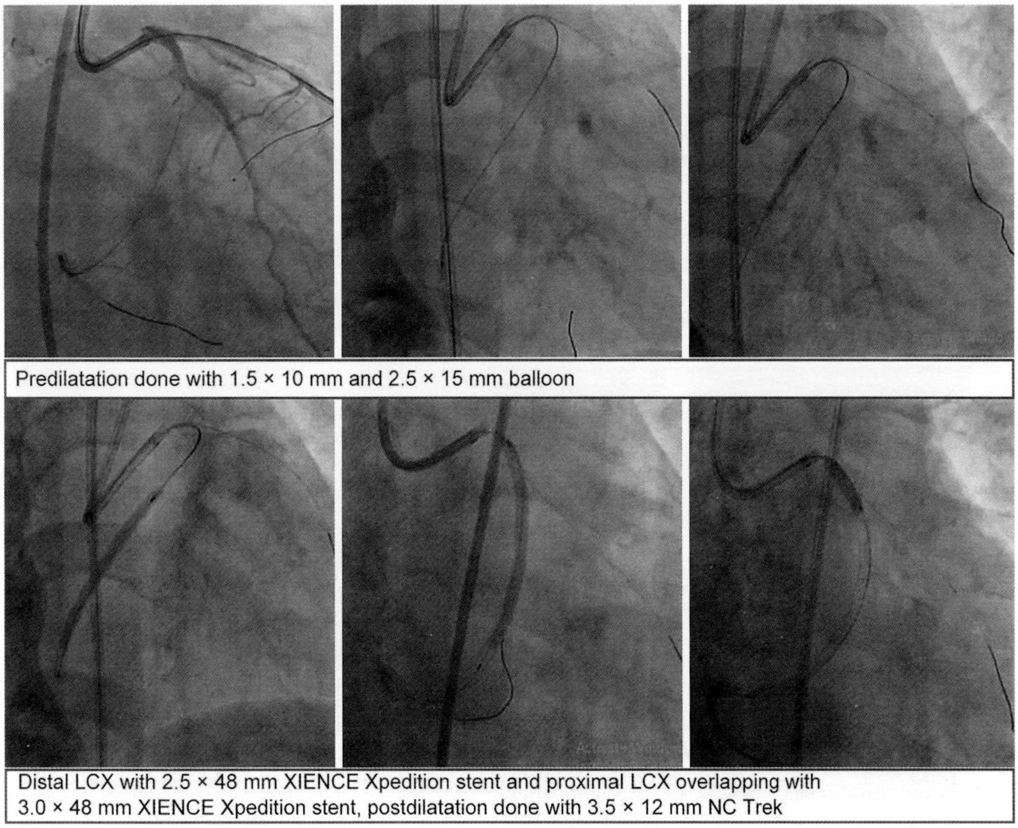

FIG. 11: Angioplasty of left circumflex.

occlusion: Epicardial or septal, contralateral, or ipsilateral. For postbypass patients, the bypass grafts itself can be used as a conduit to tackle the CTO using a retrograde approach. As the passage of guidewires and microcatheters through the collateral channels is not without risk hence careful assessment for choosing good collateral is one of the essential key steps for the successful procedure. One of the most threatening complications of CTO-PCI is coronary perforation, which may occur while crossing collaterals which is more often seen with epicardial collaterals compared to septal and venous graft conduits which requires early detection and management to avoid sudden events **(Fig. 12)**.

After crossing the collaterals with guidewire (usually soft dedicated guidewires such as Fielder XT-R, Sion, Sion Black, and SUOH 03) and with microcatheter, then pass the guidewire with microcatheter support in a retrogradely through the CTO body, from the distal cap to the proximal cap. In general, the distal CTO cap is softer than the proximal cap because it is exposed to lower pressure bed. This makes an easier passage of guidewires through the distal CTO cap. In the RWE technique, as well in the AWE technique, guidewires with higher penetration power are progressively inserted into the distal cap. In the case of failure of the true lumen to true lumen retrograde approach, or when a long lesion is present, it is necessary to use a dissection and re-entry technique such as the reverse controlled antegrade and retrograde tracking. With this technique the subintimal space is reached with an antegrade guidewire that is subsequently expanded with a balloon in order to permit the advancement of the retrograde guidewire from the subintimal space back to the true lumen **(Table 2)**.

Case 2: Optical Coherence Tomography Guided Chronic Total Occlusion of Left Anterior Descending-CrossBoss Technique (Fig. 13)

A 60-year-old male, known hypertensive and diabetic, presented with recent ACS, unstable angina. 2D echo—normal LV function, EF—58%. CAG—CTO of LAD, distal LAD filling retrogradely, and OM1 99% lesion.

Route—RFA, Guide XB—3.5 and JR 3.5–7 Fr, antegrade approach was planned with CrossBoss technique using Fielder XT wire. Initially, Sion wire was used to place CrossBoss tip at the CTO proximal cap, then Fielder XT wire was used to cross the lesion with CrossBoss using rapid rotational movements in the clockwise and alternating with anticlockwise direction. When CrossBoss entered side branches, it was redirected by Fielder wire manipulations after withdrawing it into the LAD and finally entire CTO segment was crossed from true-to-true lumen. Predilatation done with 2.0 × 10 mm Tazuna and 2.5 × 12 mm maverick balloons. Mid LAD stenting done with 3.0 × 38 mm PROMUS element, proximal LAD stenting done with 3.0 × 16 mm PROMUS element, the final result was good with TIMI 3 flow with no complications. If CrossBoss did not enter true lumen, the subintimal crossing with re-entry with Stingray balloon was the option.

Case 3 (Figs. 14 and 15)

The ADR of CTO of proximal RCA with Stingray. Initially, it was attempted with Pilot 150 using Corsair support but could not cross, then changed to Gaia III wire for further

TABLE 2: Antegrade dissection and re-entry versus retrograde dissection re-entry—anatomical challenges.

	ADR	RETRO
Ambiguous CAP	–	+
Bifurcation	–	+
Relevant side branches	–	+
Epicardial	+	–
Ca^+ at the re-entry side	–	+
Disease distal target	–	+

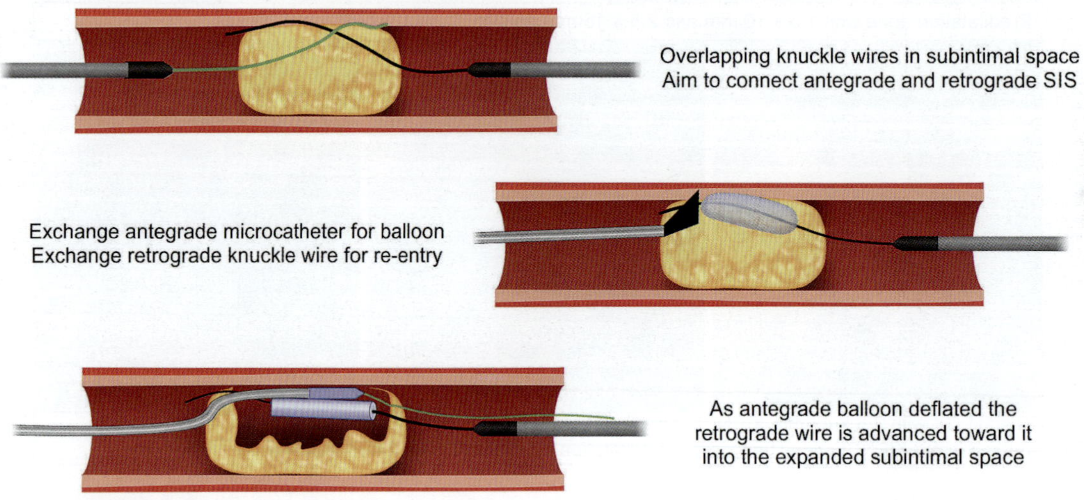

FIG. 12: Retrograde dissection re-entry.

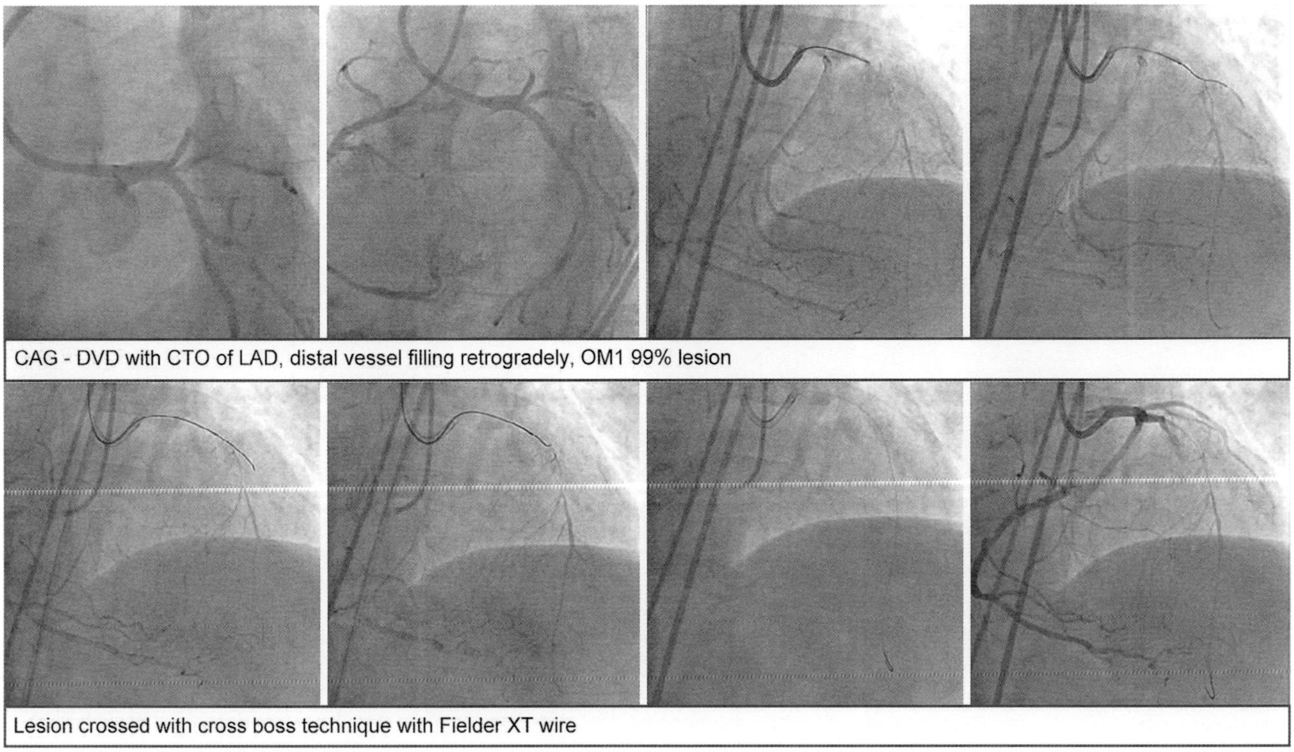

FIG. 13: Coronary angiography followed lesion crossed with CrossBoss technique.

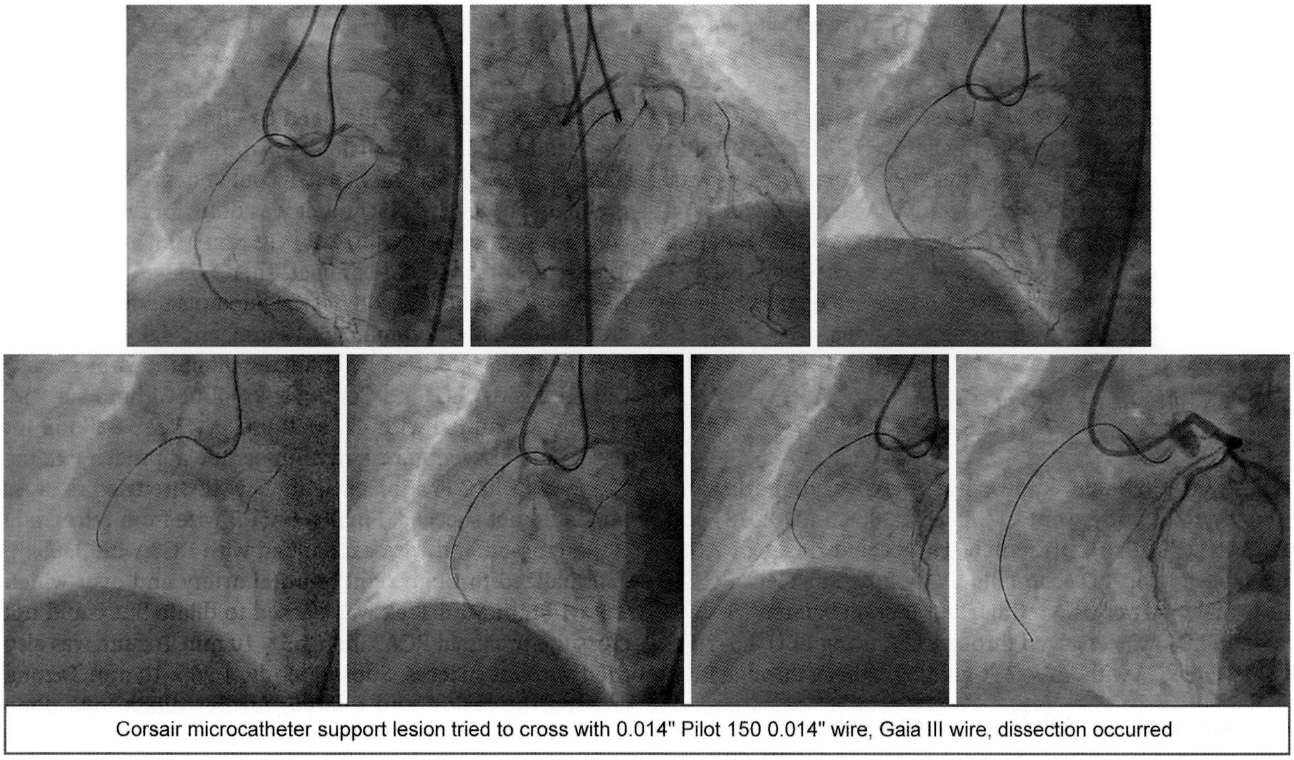

FIG. 14: Dissection re-entry technique.

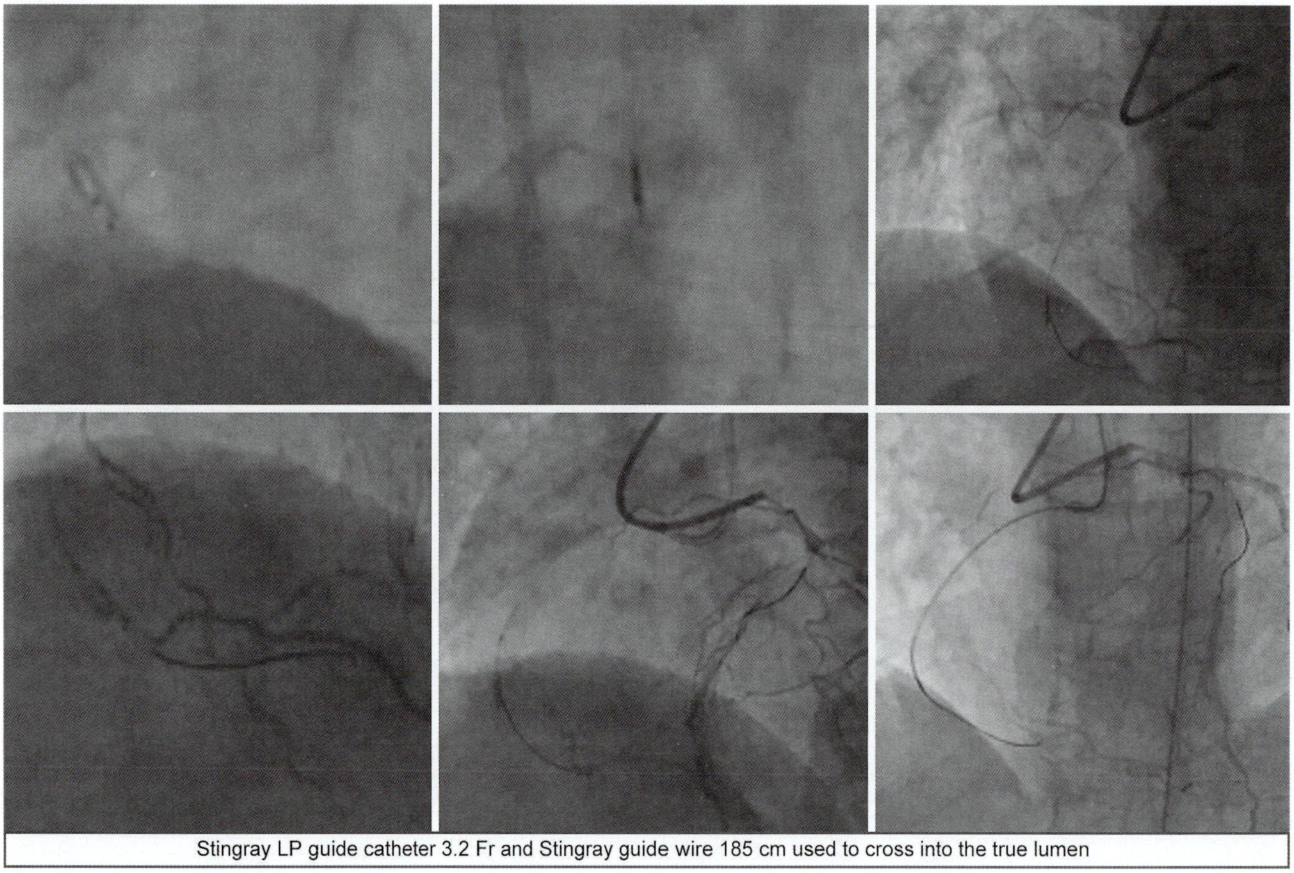

FIG. 15: Chronic total occlusion segment crossed with Stingray.

negotiation which resulted in dissection. Stingray LP guide catheter and 3.2 Fr and Stingray guidewire 185 cm used to cross into the true lumen. Then distal RCA stenting done with 2.5 × 38 mm PROMUS premier, mid RCA stenting with 3.0 × 32 mm PROMUS premier, and Ostio-proximal RCA stenting with 3.0 × 20 mm PROMUS premier. Postdilated with 3.0 × 12 mm and 3.5 × 12 mm NC Trek balloon. The final result was good with TIMI 3 flow with no complications.

Retrograde

Case 4 (Fig. 16)

A 66-year-old male, known hypertensive, diabetic, and hypothyroid, underwent PTCA (LCX-2008, LAD-2018) and POBA (LCX 2018), presented with recent onset of ACS-unstable angina. 2D echo-mild LV dysfunction. *CAG:* RCA—Proximal total occlusion with failed attempt before.

The LCA was engaged through LFA using EBU 3.5-7 Fr-guide, and RCA with AL1—7 Fr-guiding catheter through RFA.

Retrograde Approach (Figs. 17 and 18)

Septal collateral crossing was done using SUOH 03 wire with fine cross support and it was placed in distal RCA, then crossing of distal cap of CTO segment was attempted with Fielder-XT, Gaia, and Fielder FC. Finally, Conquest Pro was used to penetrate distal cap which was able to reach middle of the CTO segment and it could not progress further, then antegrade wire placement was done for reverse CART which was attempted with 2.0 × 12 mm Mini Trek Balloon inflations but could not connect. Then IVUS-guided reverse CART was planned. Further serial attempts of dissection re-entry using 2.5 × 12 mm, 3.0 × 12 mm, and 4.0 × 12 mm NC Trek Balloons and tried by changing different wires namely Gaia II, Fielder FC, and Conquest Pro, but without success. Finally, attempted with 4.0 × 12 mm NC Trek Balloon for retrograde dissection re-entry. Antegrade approach guiding changed to JR 7 Fr, Corsair with Gaia II wire tried to cross but could not succeed. Finally, Gaia II wire from retrograde route crossed and wire exchanged with RG3 with 330 cm, externalized through right femoral artery and over which 2.5 × 15 mm Mini Trek was passed to dilate but could not cross the proximal RCA. Then 1.5 × 10 mm Tazuna was also tried without success. Subsequently, 1.25 × 10 mm Tazuna crossed the lesion and dilated, further dilatations done with 1.5 × 10 mm Tazuna, but failed to cross with 2.5 × 12 mm Mini Trek Balloon.

Then Guidezilla support was given to 2.5 × 12 mm NC Trek to cross and dilated, then distal RCA stented with 2.5 ×

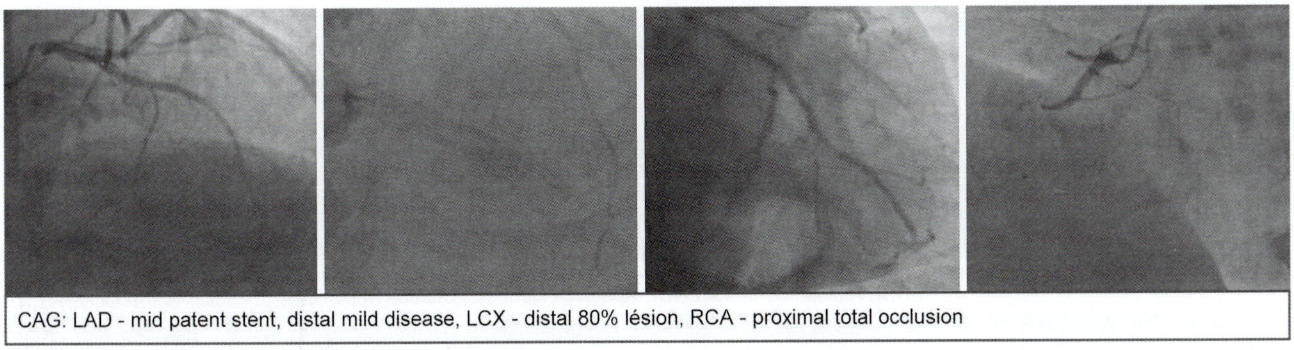

FIG. 16: Chronic total occlusion of right coronary artery.

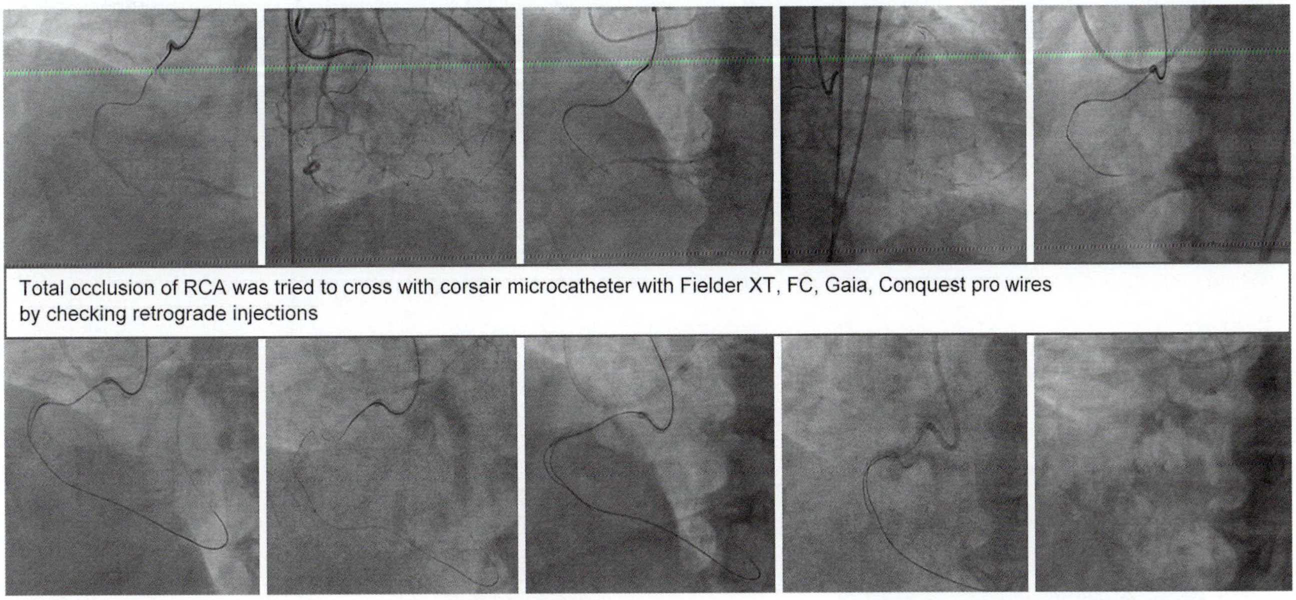

FIG. 17: Chronic total occlusion segment tried to cross with wire escalation technique.

Note: Retrograde approach fine cross on SUOH 03 wire was placed in distal RCA, tried to cross with Fielder XT, Gaia, Fielder FC, Conquest Pro but could not cross then through antegrade approach 2.0 × 12 mm Mini Trek Balloon was dilated up to 16 atms for dissection retrograde reentry. Then IVUS tried to see position of wires but could not cross. Then further dilatation with 2.5 × 12 mm and 3.0 × 12 mm NC Trek Balloon and tried with Gaia II, Fielder FC, Conquest Pro, but could not cross. Then again 4.0 × 12 mm NC Trek Balloon dilated to for retrograde dissection reentry. Finally, retrograde route Gaia II wire crossed and wire exchanged with RG3 with 330 cm externalized through right femoral and over which 2.5 × 12 mm Mini Trek Balloon was not crossing. then with Guidezilla support 2.5 × 2 mm NC Trek Balloon was crossed and dilated.

33 mm XIENCE Alpine, mid RCA with 3.0 × 38 mm XIENCE Xpedition, and proximal RCA with 3.5 × 33 mm XIENCE Xpedition stent. Finally, 3.5 × 28 mm XIENCE Xpedition stent was placed in the ostio-proximal RCA. The IVUS showed malapposition of the proximal portion of the stent which was rectified with 5.0 × 12 mm NC inflations. Further optimization of the proximal to distal RCA stent was performed with high pressure inflations of 3.0 × 15 mm NC Trek. Final result was good without any complications.

USEFULNESS OF INTRAVASCULAR ULTRASOUND IN CHRONIC TOTAL OCCLUSION INTERVENTIONS—ANTEGRADE APPROACH OF CHRONIC TOTAL OCCLUSION (FIGS. 19 TO 23)

Assessing the proximal cap with IVUS requires 7 or 8 French catheter to allow at least two guidewires and IVUS catheter.

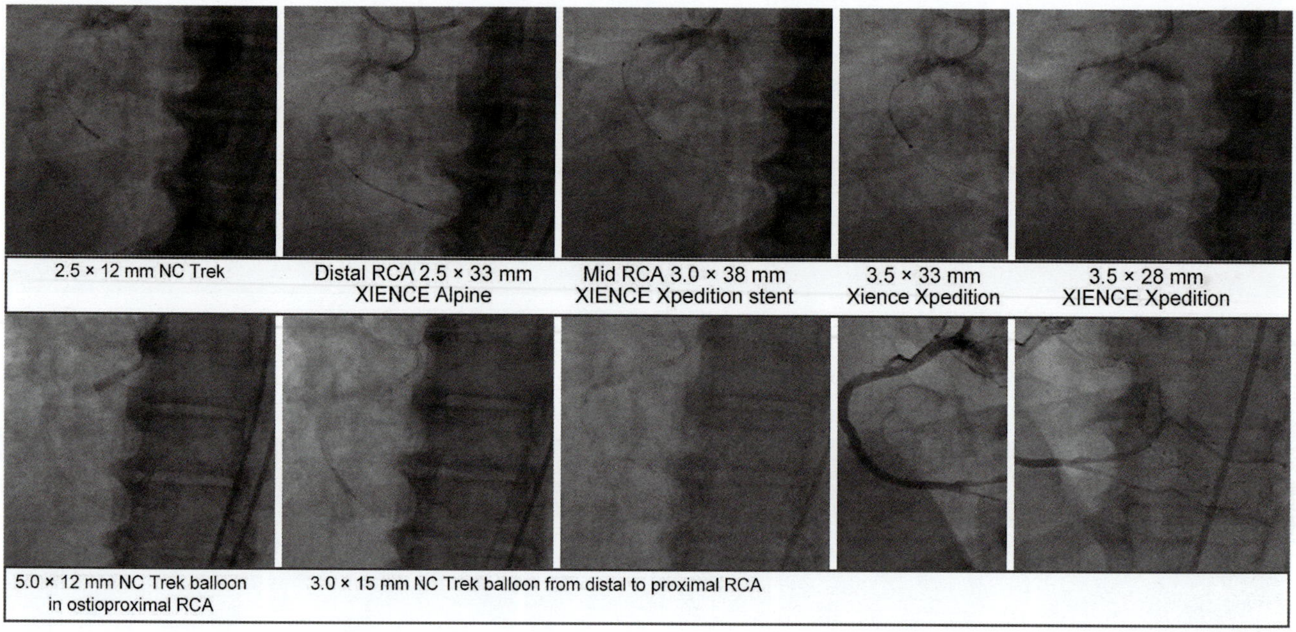

FIG. 18: Angioplasty of the CTO segment.

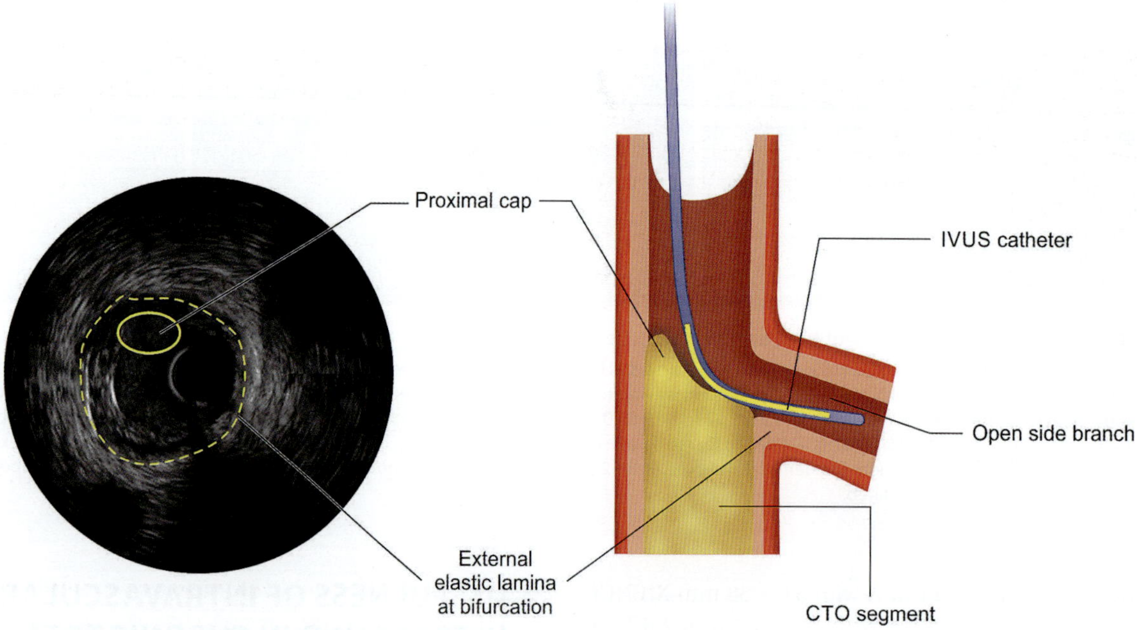

FIG. 19: Use of intravascular ultrasound to resolve proximal cap ambiguity.

Prefer automatic followed by manual pullback from side branch to visualize proximal cap, and minimize antegrade injections to prevent hematoma progression.

The IVUS in SB at the site of CTO is helpful for antegrade puncture of proximal blunt cap by confirming guidewire location, intimal versus subintima. IVUS-guided re-entry from subintimal space during antegrade dissection and reentry after parallel wire failure and when no retrograde option is possible. IVUS is also helpful after STAR with long subintimal segment, by advancing IVUS in false lumen and try to re-enter intima with stiffer wire by showing an example of a procedure.[10]

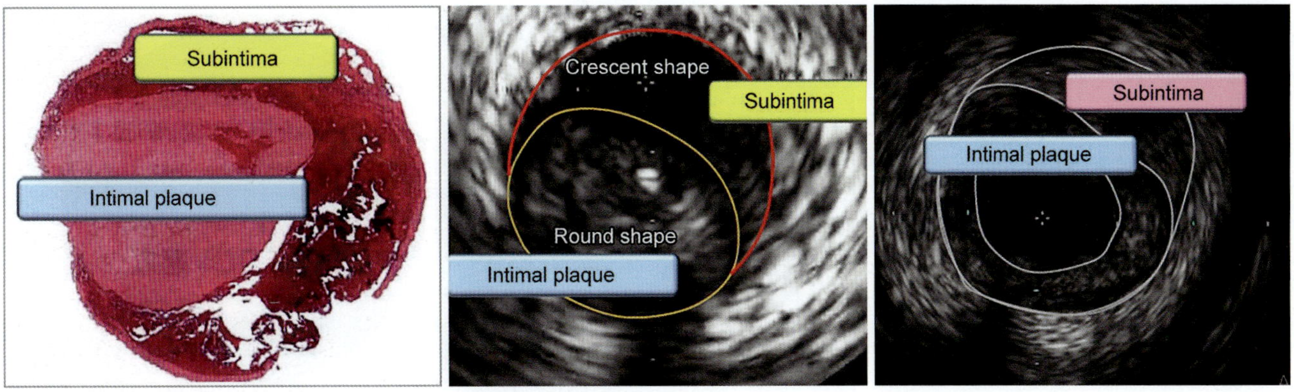

FIG. 20: Important intravascular ultrasound findings in chronic total occlusion-percutaneous coronary intervention.

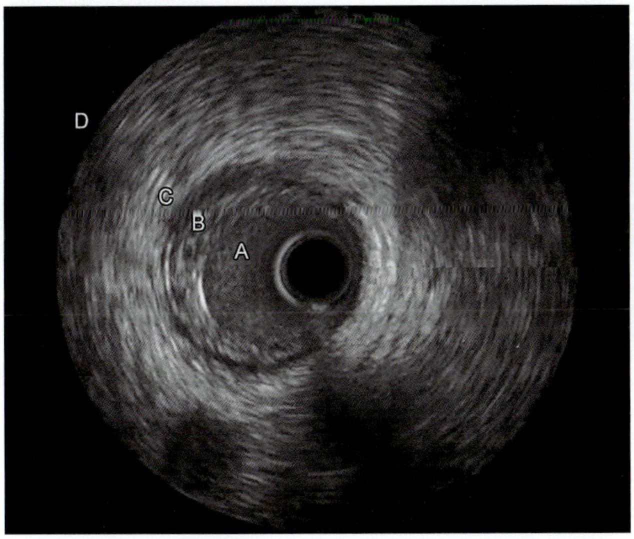

FIG. 21: Identifying the location of guidewire using intravascular ultrasound. Intravascular ultrasound identifies location of a guidewire—anywhere within the three layers of the target vessel (A—Intima, B—Media, C—Adventitia), or D—outside of the vessel (i.e., in the pericardial space).

Source: Sumitsuji S, Inoue K, Ochiai M, et al. Fundamental wire technique and current standard strategy of percutaneous intervention for chronic total occlusion with histopathological insights. JACC Cardiovasc Interv. 2011;4(9):941-51.

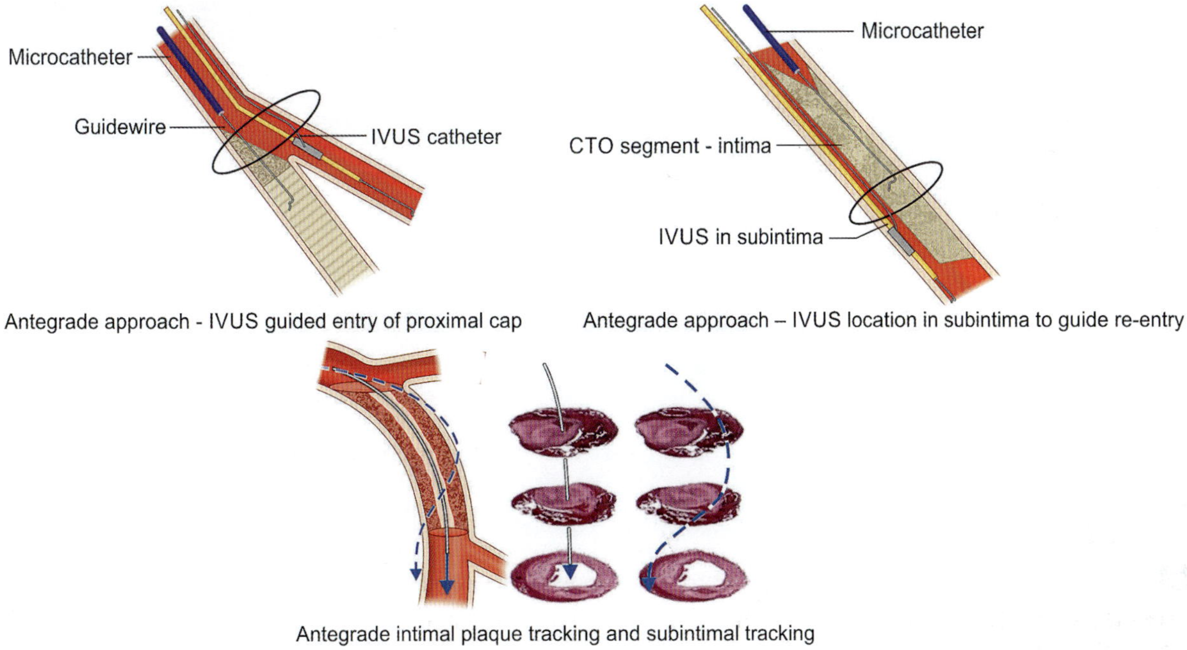

FIG. 22: Intravascular ultrasound guided antegrade approach.

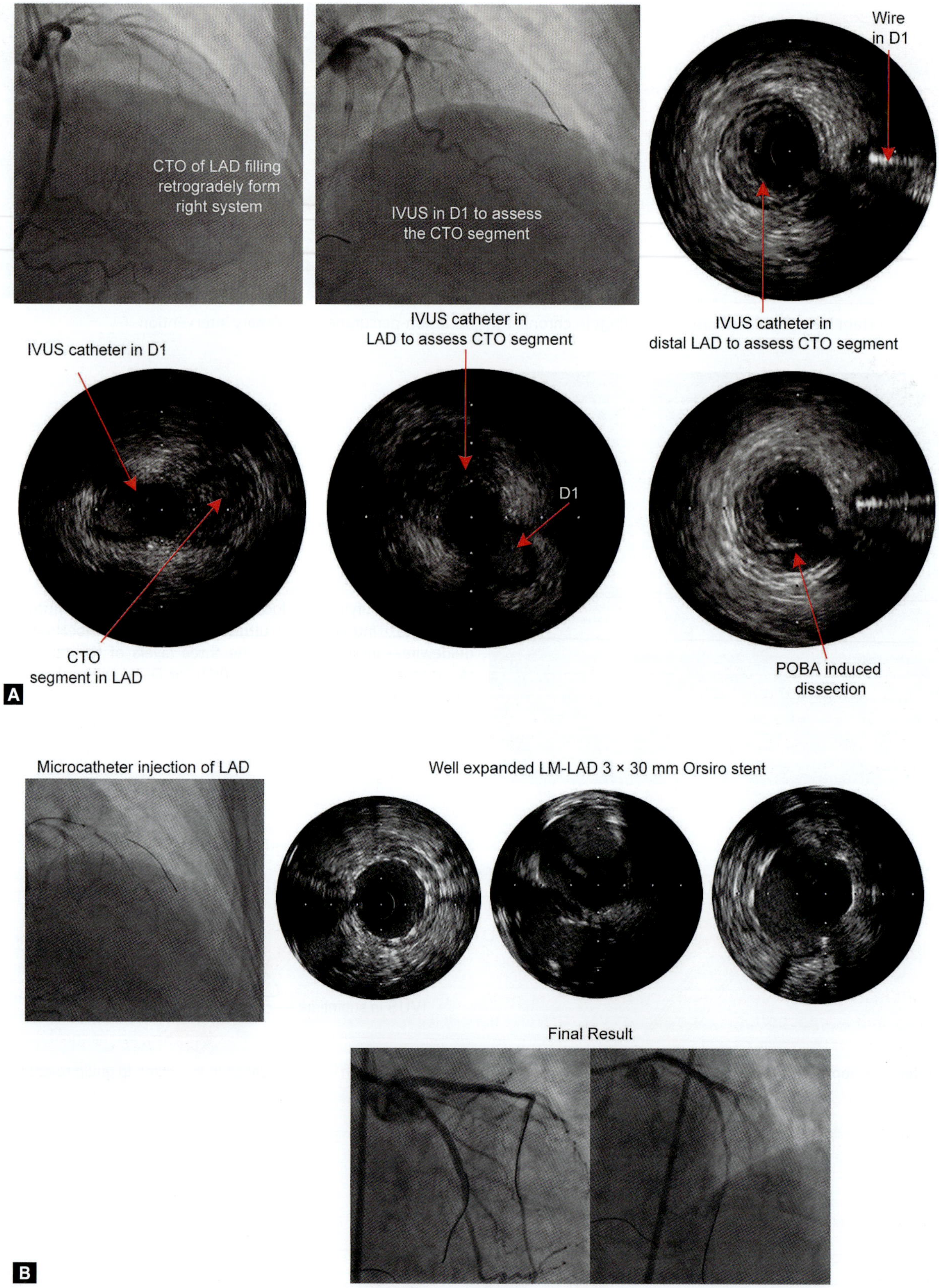

FIGS. 23A AND B: (A) Case example of intravascular ultrasound guided chronic total occlusion of left anterior descending; (B) Angioplasty of chronic total occlusion of left anterior descending.

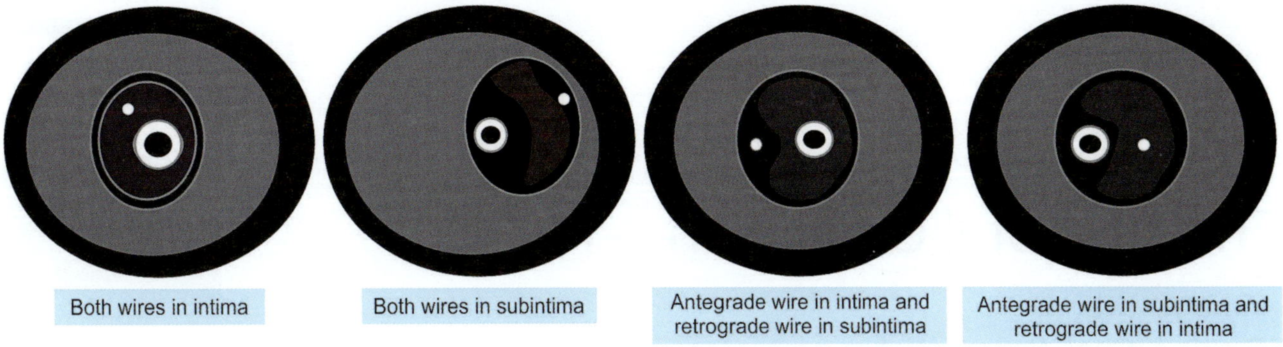

FIG. 24: IVUS identifies location of antegrade and retrograde wires during retrograde PCI.

INTRAVASCULAR ULTRASOUND IN RETROGRADE APPROACH OF CHRONIC TOTAL OCCLUSION (FIG. 24)

The IVUS is very useful to clarify retrograde wire location and the exact point of re-entry in reverse CART it is very useful for balloon sizing and to understand where it is possible to try to make the connection between antegrade and retrograde wires, and permits to optimize stent sizing and expansion in complex coronary reconstruction.

The IVUS identifies location of antegrade and retrograde wires during retrograde PCI. It is also helpful in identifying dissection planes in distal bifurcations, eliminates the need for antegrade injections prior to stenting thereby reduces risk of propagation of iatrogenic dissection distally or retrograde in the aortic wall (ostial RCA CTO) and reduces the risk of CIN by reducing the volume of contrast particularly in diabetics, elderly, and in patients with low GFR.

Uncrossable Lesions

For critical or uncrossable fibro-calcific lesions, it is essential to use thin profile balloons, rotational or LASER for plaque modification to allow further balloon dilatations and stenting. In some instances, uncrossable lesions may be managed with grenadoplasty, Carlino (contrast injection), or subintimal crossing. Moreover, it may require maneuvers involving balloon anchoring, guide extension catheter, and usage of special microcatheters such as Turnpike Gold or Tornus.

Minimize Radiation Risk

The PCI of CTO procedures may lead to high exposure to radiation of both the patient and operating Cath staff which may result in increased radiation hazards and exposure can be reduced using low fluoroscopy frame rates (6–7.5 frames per second) and less use of cine angiography. It is essential to take all the necessary steps to reduce exposure to radiation while managing the procedures.

Procedural Anticoagulation

Periprocedural anticoagulation, an initial bolus of intravenous unfractionated heparin (100 IU/kg) is usually administered. The activated clotting time is then monitored every 30 minutes and top up boluses of unfractionated heparin are subsequently administered to maintain an activated clotting time of around 300–350 seconds.

CONCLUSION

Antegrade approach is the initial and most commonly used choice for the majority of PCI of CTO, and it will provide excellent results if carefully selected with suitable anatomy. Retrograde technique is mainly used in complex anatomical settings or when antegrade methods have failed for CTO segments with presence of good usable interventional collaterals with a success rate of 70–90%. ADR technique (wire based or device based) remains an important technique for complex CTO lesion subsets where there are limited or poor retrograde options.

ONLINE REFERENCES

Please scan the QR code provided at the end of the table of contents for References of this chapter.

CHAPTER

154

Chronic Total Occlusion—Toolkit

Pravin K Goel, Saurav Mishra

ABSTRACT

Chronic total occlusions (CTOs) represent the "final frontier" of coronary interventions. Notwithstanding the modest technical success of CTO-PCI, most of the earlier observational data demonstrated a clear survival benefit free of major cardiovascular events (MACE) in patients undergoing successful CTO revascularization provided if, specific criterions for patient selection, objective evidence of inducible ischemia, myocardial viability, and favorable cost-risk-benefit analysis are met. Recent advancements in the contemporary interventional tools along with top-notched operator expertise have significantly raised success rates, making these procedures more effective, predictable, and safe. Before embarking onto CTO-PCI, one should be familiar and equipped with certain specialized hardware beginning from vascular sheath, guiding catheter, coronary CTO wires, microcatheter, lowest profile semicompliant balloons, antegrade dissection re-entry systems, and hardware facilitating retrograde approach. In addition, to provide continued safety certain paraphernalia that assists in complication management, namely, coronary microcoil, glue, and covered stents too form an integral inclusion in a CTO toolkit.

Keywords: Chronic total occlusion, revascularization, CTO wires, microcatheters, low-profile balloons, guide extension catheter, antegrade dissection reentry, retrograde approach, microcoils, covered stent

INTRODUCTION

Chronic total occlusion (CTO) is defined as a complete luminal obstruction (TIMI flow grade 0) of a native coronary artery for a duration of ≥3 months or a newly documented occlusion not attributable to a similarly recent ischemic event.[1] SYNTAX trial showed that chronically occluded coronary arteries were frequently left untreated. Even during CABG, only 69% of the CTO segments received bypass grafting and complete revascularization was achieved in 49.6%. On the other hand, CTO percutaneous coronary intervention (PCI) success rates above 85% have been achieved.[2] PCI in CTO has evolved considerably with new techniques, equipment, and trained personnel.[3,4] Herein, we explore various CTO-specific hardware essential for successful intervention of a CTO.

CTO HISTOPATHOLOGY AND ITS APPLIED ANATOMY

Most fundamentally, a CTO comprises of four histoanatomical components, namely, proximal cap, body, distal cap, and collaterals. Proximal cap is predominantly comprised of dense fibrosis marked by proteoglycan-enriched extracellular matrix deposition interspersed with calcific atherosclerotic plaque.[3] Tapered tip occlusions containing areas of luminal recanalization with microchannels and loosely packed fibrous tissue often require engagement of leader channel by a floppy tapered tip hydrophilic wire followed by wire tip-load escalation, if required. Blunt proximal cap, on the other hand is typically composed of densely packed collagen necessitating the use of upfront hard penetrating tip wire followed by de-escalation. Microvascular channels are small bridging channels, 160–230 μm in diameter and are configured as corkscrew or acutely angulated fragmented tubular structures that do not traverse the full length of occlusion. Often, they are navigated using hydrophilic coated tapered tip floppy wire. Retrograde collateral channels, mostly are of thin caliber and tortuous which need a low-entry profile, super floppy, hydrophilic tipped wire inside a tapered, hydrophilic sheathed braided microcatheter.[5]

ESSENTIAL CTO-PCI TOOLBOX

Specialized hardware required for CTO revascularization can be classified into the following subcategories:

- *Equipment for providing adequate support and improving delivery of CTO-specific hardware*:
    - Peripheral vascular sheaths
    - Guiding catheters
    - Guide catheter (GC) extension
- *Equipment to facilitate CTO crossing and delivery of CTO-specific hardware*:
    - CTO guidewires
    - Microcatheters
    - Antegrade dissection reentry system
- *Equipment for lesion bed preparation*:
    - Low-profile semicompliant balloon
    - Excimer laser
    - Atherectomy
- *Equipment for poststenting optimization*:
    - High-pressure noncompliant balloon
    - Intravascular imaging:
        - OCT
        - IVUS
- *Equipment specific for retrograde CTO-PCI approach*:
    - Guidewire for collateral surfing
    - Long-length microcatheters
    - Exchange length (300 cm) coronary guidewire
    - Coronary snare
- *Equipment for management of complications*:
    - Coronary microcoil
    - Vascular glue
    - Covered stent

Peripheral Vascular Sheath

Obtaining two arterial accesses is the established norm in most CTO-PCI procedures. It varies from bifemoral, radio-femoral to biradial arterial access depending on operator's choice. Rarely, distal radial and ulnar artery access can also be integrated in the above options depending on operator expertise and patency of the arterial circulation of concerned hand. Left radial cannulation is, however, discouraged so as to leave at least one free arterial graft option. Sheath length recommended for radial access is 11 cm whereas that for femoral access is 45–55 cm. Long large-bore femoral sheaths provide more room for equipment and better tactile feedback and wire manipulation.

Often multiple hardware combinations are needed to facilitate CTO crossing which requires the presence of large caliber guiding catheters (7F or 8F). Glidesheath Slender® (Terumo medical corp, New Jersey, USA) uses a thin-wall technology reducing the outer diameter of the sheath by one Fr size while maintaining larger innerdiameter so that 7F GC can used via radial route. Compatible permutations of various hardware combination as per the size of guiding catheter are:

- *6F GC*:
    - Two balloons
    - One stent with one balloon
    - Finecross® MG microcatheter with anchor/trap balloon
    - Finecross® MG microcatheter with IVUS catheter
    - Stingray™ LP OTW reentry system without trap balloon
    - CrossBoss™ catheter
    - 1.25 and 1.50 mm rotational atherectomy burr
- *7F GC*:
    - Two stents
    - Three balloons
    - Dual-lumen microcatheter with anchor/trap balloon
    - Dual-lumen microcatheter with IVUS catheter
    - Corsair® Pro microcatheter with anchor/trap balloon
    - Corsair® Pro microcatheter with IVUS catheter
    - Stingray™ LP OTW reentry system with trap balloon
    - Corsair® Pro microcatheter with CrossBoss™ catheter
    - 1.75-mm rotational atherectomy burr
- *8F GC*:
    - Three stents
    - Conventional Stingray™ OTW reentry system with trap balloon
    - Dual-lumen microcatheter and IVUS catheter with anchor/trap balloon
    - Corsair® Pro microcatheter and IVUS catheter with anchor/trap balloon
    - 2.00- and 2.15-mm rotational atherectomy burr

Guiding Catheter

An ideal GC for CTO-PCI should provide coaxial engagement, good back-up support, atraumatic tip, and a large lumen to accommodate multiple devices simultaneously.[5] GC with side holes are frequently necessary during CTO-PCI procedures, especially when using a large bore GC to engage the right coronary artery (RCA) to allow for perfusion during a snug engagement of the ostium. However, while performing retrograde CTO-PCI one should avoid using side-hole antegrade GC as it often poses difficulty during externalization of wire. Owing to anatomic orientation, a GC from the right radial artery (RA) access usually provides better support for left coronary artery (LCA), whereas a GC from the left RA access provides better support for RCA. Most commonly used GC for CTO-PCI are:

- *For LCA*:
    - EBU (Medtronic, Minneapolis, MN, USA)
    - XBU (Cordis corporation, NJ, USA)
    - Voda left and CLS curve (Boston Scientific, Natick, MA, USA)

- *For RCA*:
  - Amplatz left and right catheter (AL, SAL, AR)
  - ECR (Medtronic, Minneapolis, MN, USA)
  - Judkins right
  - Hockey stick catheter

Sheathless GC systems [Sheathless Eaucath system (ASAHI Intecc Co Ltd, AIC, JPN), Railway® sheathless access system (Cordis corporation, Santa Clara, CA, USA)] allow the passage of large-bore catheters with smaller overall diameters at the arterial insertion site, as there is no need for a sheath. The sheathless approach to radial access avoids the added mechanical stretching of the vascular sheath that is usually on the order of 1–2F larger than the catheter that is passing within it. Techniques that are commonly used to enhance GC support during CTO PCI are:

- Guide catheter deep intubation in the coronary artery tree.
- Large-bore GCs
- Buddy and anchoring wire techniques.
- Anchoring balloon technique.
- Mother and child GCs technique.

Guide Catheter Extension

The introduction of extension catheters has increased the success rate of lesion crossing by improving GC support. The initial, HeartRail® II (Terumo medical corp, New Jersey, USA) catheter had relatively limited clinical utility due to its limited flexibility and relatively short length of the "child" catheter extending beyond the GC's tip. More recently, the GuideLiner® V3 (Teleflex, Wayne, US), Guidezilla™ (Boston Scientific, Natick, MA, USA), Telescope™ (Medtronic, Minneapolis, MN, USA), and GuidePlus™ II (Nipro corporation, Osaka, JPN) catheters were developed as a rapid exchange "mother and child" system with the advantage of safe deep engagement in the distal vessel. Another innovation in guide extension led to the development of TrapLiner® (Teleflex, Wayne, US) catheter containing an integrated trapping balloon that traps 0.014" guidewire against inner wall of guide to facilitate convenient microcatheter and wire exchanges.

CORONARY GUIDEWIRES FOR CTO-PCI

Guidewires provide the primary interface between hands of the CTO operator and the coronary arteries. Wire manipulation and experience of tactile feedback are important operator skills to master for a successful CTO-PCI. As CTO-PCI-specific guide wires induce perforations more frequently than spring tip guide wires used in non-CTO-PCI, they need different style of wire handling skills.[6] **Table 1** summarizes the properties of various commonly used CTO guidewires. Multiple coronary guide wires with different characteristics are frequently needed to achieve various functions during the CTO-PCI procedure such as:

Microchannels Probing and Crossing

Steerability is the ability and responsiveness of the wire tip to navigate vessels while torquability is the response of the wire to turning by the operator. This property is important in drilling strategy where wire is rotated in a controlled manner to search for path of least resistance. Steerability is achieved by single core wires where force transmission is not dampened by the terminal coil and some specially designed wires capable of torque transmission (dual or composite core). Compound core designs **(Figs. 1A and B)** with double spring coil winds over solid and twisted core have been introduced in the Sion® and Gaia® series of guidewires (ASAHI Intecc, Nagoya, Japan) **(Figs. 2B to E)**. They have increased rotational rigidity with low bend stiffness which is key to crossing microchannels and tapered proximal caps. Recently introduced Gaia Next® series is designed for intentional wiring with 1:1 torque response and flexibility with preshaped uncoated distal 1 mm microcone tip for directional control within the CTO body with increased antitrapping power in tough lesions.

Wires can be coated in polymers to make them more hydrophilic or hydrophobic. Hydrophobic coatings are usually made of silicone and repel water to reduce friction offering good tactile feedback. Hydrophilic coatings attract water, and the coating becomes a gel when wet making the wires more slippery which reduces friction and increases trackability.[7] FIELDER® (ASAHI Intecc, Nagoya, Japan) and FIGHTER® (Boston Scientific, Natick, MA, USA) hydrophilic wires with a tapered polymer jacket are known for their use in recent CTOs (<1 year), for picking up microchannels **(Figs. 2A and D)**. These wires have slightly more lateral support than a work-horse PCI wire. However, FIELDER wires can slide between plaque creating a dissection. These wires also can cause perforation because of less tactile feedback for tissue resistance.

Collateral Circulation Crossing for Retrograde CTO-PCI Techniques

For retrograde use, the basic requirement is that the wire should be longer, with lowest tip load and very low friction with a hydrophilic/polymer jacket coating. At the same time, wire should have improved torque transmission to enable it to negotiate the collaterals (composite/dual core technology). The classic wire is SUOH® 3 with a tip load of 0.3 g. It has a dual-core preshaped tip which leads to precise torque response and flexibility and also contributes to shape retention at the tip. However for selecting branches within the collateral, Sion is a better choice with 1:1 torque control. Other wires that are used for collateral surfing are FIELDER® XT-R, Sion Blue® and Sion® black.

Wires used for externalization should be longer (at least 300 cm long), but at the same time thinner (so that it does not injure the collaterals while passing balloon catheters and other hardware) and have enough lateral support to

TABLE 1: Characteristics of commonly used CTO wires.

Properties of guidewires								
Wire	**Core**	**Tip**	**Tip coat**	**Tip dia (inches)**	**Tip load (g)**	**Polymer coating**	**Radiopaque length (mm)**	**Comments**
Sion Blue	High tensile steel	Dual-core coil, 200 min	Hydrophilic	0.014	0.5	No	30	Lowest tip load
Sion Black	High tensile steel	Dual-core coil, 200 min	Hydrophilic	0.014	0.8	Yes, 200 mm	30	Dual-core, polymer coated
Gaia First	Stainless steel	Composite core, Microcone tip	Hydrophilic	0.010	1.7 2.0 (next)	No	150	Torqueable wire, main feature is composite coil with a central core wire, wrapped by six acetone wires, with spring coil in periphery
Gaia Second	Stainless steel	Composite core, Microcone tip	Hydrophilic	0.011	3.5 4.0 (next)	No	150	
Gaia Third	Stainless steel	Composite core, Microcone tip	Hydrophilic	0.012	4.5 6.0 (next)	No	150	
Whisper MS	High tensile steel (Durasteel)	45 mm coil	Hydrophilic	0.014	1	Yes, 290 mm	30	
PILOT 150	High tensile steel (Durasteel)	45 mm coil	Hydrophilic	0.014	3	Yes, 290 mm	30	
PILOT 200	High tensile steel (Durasteel)	45 mm coil	Hydrophilic	0.014	4	Yes, 290 mm	30	
FIELDER FC	Stainless steel	110 mm spring coil	Hydrophilic	0.014	0.8	Yes, 220 mm	30	
FIELDER XT	Stainless steel	110 mm spring coil	Hydrophilic	0.009	0.8	Yes, 220 mm	160	
FIELDER XT-R	Stainless steel	Composite coil, 160 mm	Hydrophilic	0.010	0.6	Yes, 170 mm	160	FIELDER family but composite coil
FIELDER XT-A	Stainless steel	Composite coil, 160 mm	Hydrophilic	0.010	1	Yes, 170 mm	160	FIELDER family but composite coil
Gladius EX		Composite core	Hydrophilic	0.014	3	Yes	150	
Choice PT	Unibody stainless steel	No coil	Hydrophilic	0.014	2	Yes, 380 mm	350	
PT Graphix	Unibody stainless steel	No coil	Hydrophilic	0.014	2	Yes	30	

Continued

Continued

Properties of guidewires

Wire	Core	Tip	Tip coat	Tip dia	Tip load (g)	Polymer coating	Radiopaque length (mm)	Comments
Cross IT 100	Stainless steel	300 mm coil	Hydrophilic	0.0105	2	No	30	
Cross IT 200	Stainless steel	300 mm coil	Hydrophilic	0.0105	5	No	30	
Cross IT 300	Stainless steel	300 mm coil	Hydrophilic	0.0105	6	No	30	
Cross IT 400	Stainless steel	300 mm coil	Hydrophilic	0.0105	9	No	30	
MIRACLEBROS 3	Stainless steel	110 mm spring coil	Hydrophobic	0.014	4	No	110	
MIRACLEBROS 4.5	Stainless steel	110 mm spring coil	Hydrophobic	0.014	4	No	110	
MIRACLEBROS 6	Stainless steel	110 mm spring coil	Hydrophobic	0.014	9	No	110	
MIRACLEBROS 12	Stainless steel	110 mm spring coil	Hydrophobic	0.014	13	No	110	
Conquest 9	Stainless steel	200 mm coil	Hydrophobic	0.009	9	No	200	
Conquest 12	Stainless steel	200 mm coil	Hydrophobic	0.009	12	No	200	
Conquest Pro 9	Stainless steel	200 mm coil	Hydrophilic	0.009	9	No	200	Distal most 1 mm of tip is uncoated
Conquest Pro 12	Stainless steel	200 mm coil	Hydrophilic	0.009	12	No	200	Distal most 1 mm of tip is uncoated
Conquest Pro 8-20	Stainless steel	200 mm coil	Hydrophilic	0.008	20	No	200	Highest penetrating wire
RG3	Stainless steel	80 mm platinum coil	Hydrophilic	0.010	3	No	30	For externalization

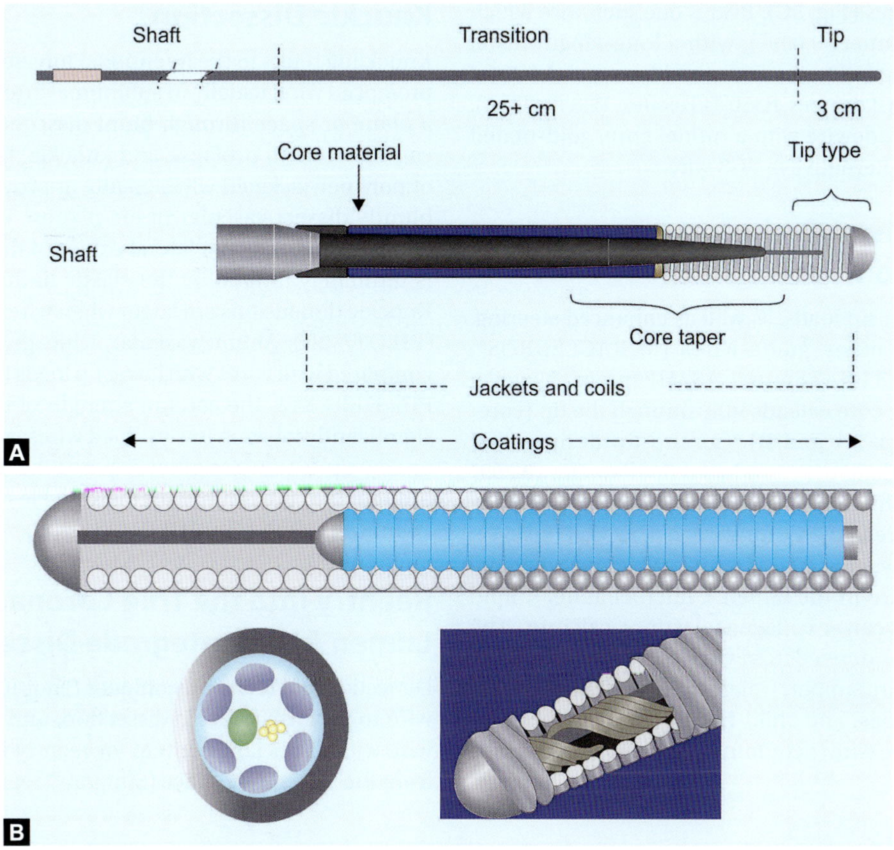

FIGS. 1A AND B: Structural design of a regular PTCA guidewire (A). A compound wire tip construction containing two concentric spring-coil elements plus two shaping elements (Sion® wire, ASAHI Intecc, Nagoya, Japan) (B).

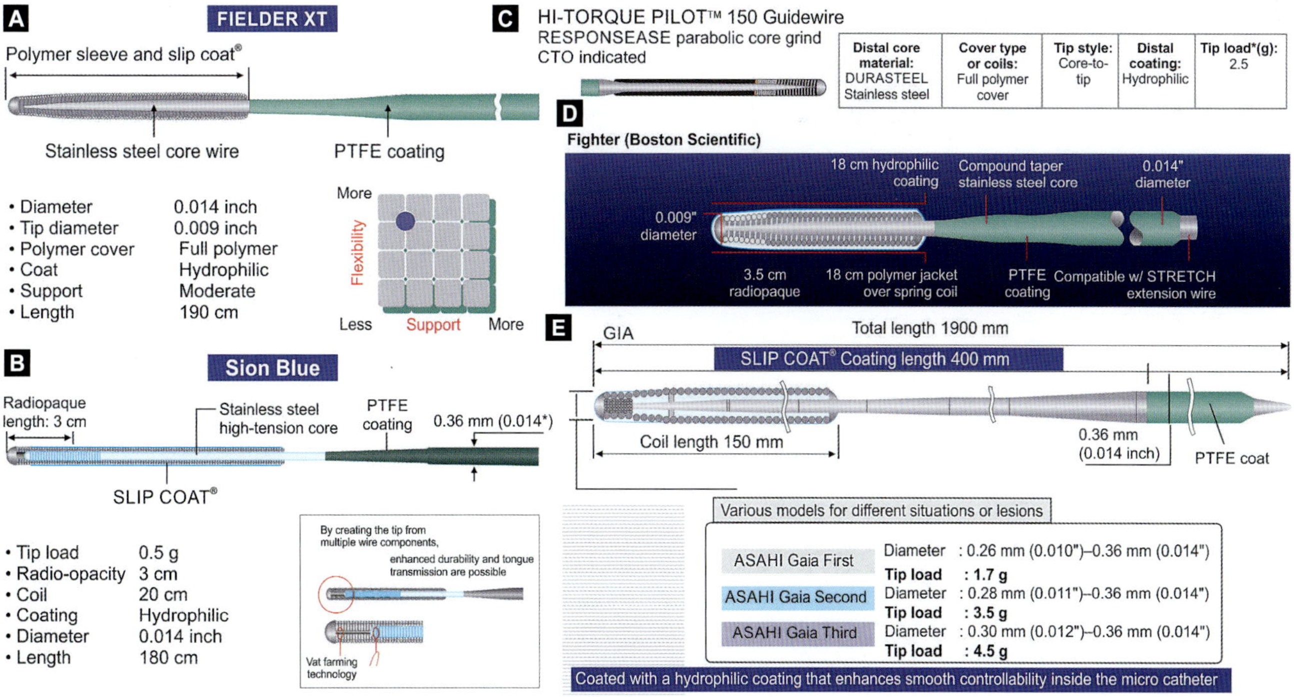

FIGS. 2A TO E: Constructional design of some commonly used CTO wires (A: FIELDER® XT, B: Sion® Blue; C: PILOT™ 150; D: FIGHTER®; E: Gaia®).

enable these passages **(Fig. 3C)**. RG3 is one such wire which is 330 cm long, thinner (0.009"), with a long-length distal hydrophilic coating (170 cm) and provides a good lateral support to deliver PCI devices. R350™ (Teleflex, Wayne, USA), a 0.013", 350 cm guidewire with a nitinol core, gold-plated tungsten coil is an alternative to RG3 wire.

Proximal or Distal Occlusion Cap Penetration

The need for greater tip loads, as well as enhanced steering, has given rise to many guide-wires (MIRACLEBROS®, Conquest® Pro, ULTIMATEbros®; ASAHI Intecc, Nagoya, Japan) in which the core extends fully through the tip (core-to-tip design) **(Figs. 3A and B)**. Core-to-tip designs that combine a high tip load with a reduced tip diameter (0.009" or 0.010") provide increased "penetrating power" which is the ability of the wire to pierce forward in a directed fashion. Stiffness/tissue resistance offered by a CTO increases in the following order: wire in the lumen < microchannel < lipid plaque < proteoglycan < collagen/elastin < calcium. The penetrating power is derived from various factors such as tip load, tapered tip, wire support (microcatheter/OTW balloon, anchoring techniques, and child-in-mother catheter), and lateral support of the wire (determines trackability of a device over the wire).[8]

Knuckle Dissection

Knuckling refers to the intentional forceful advancement of a prolapsed wire, usually in subintimal arterial tissue, to create a plane or space through blunt dissection. While any wire can be made to prolapse and knuckle, the slippery surface of polymer-jacketed wires greatly improves their capacity to bluntly dissect vascular tissue planes. The diameter of the knuckle (and thus the lateral extent of the dissection plane) is ultimately limited by the elastic limits of the adventitia. Knuckle dimensions are larger when wires with high tip loads (PILOT™ 200; Abbott vascular, Chicago, IL, USA) are used compared with wires with lower tip loads (PILOT™ 50, or even FIELDER® XT). The column strength of transitional cores is significantly lower in low tip-load wires; advancing a knuckle on low tip-load wires often requires the microcatheter to be brought into proximity with the knuckle in order to reinforce column strength **(Fig. 2C)**.

Reentry into the True Coronary Artery Lumen After Antegrade Dissection

Dissection and reentry techniques require a polymer-jacketed wire to perform knuckle dissection, and a nonjacketed stiff wire with a specially bent tip for reentry into the true lumen from the subintimal space (Stingray™ reentry system; Boston

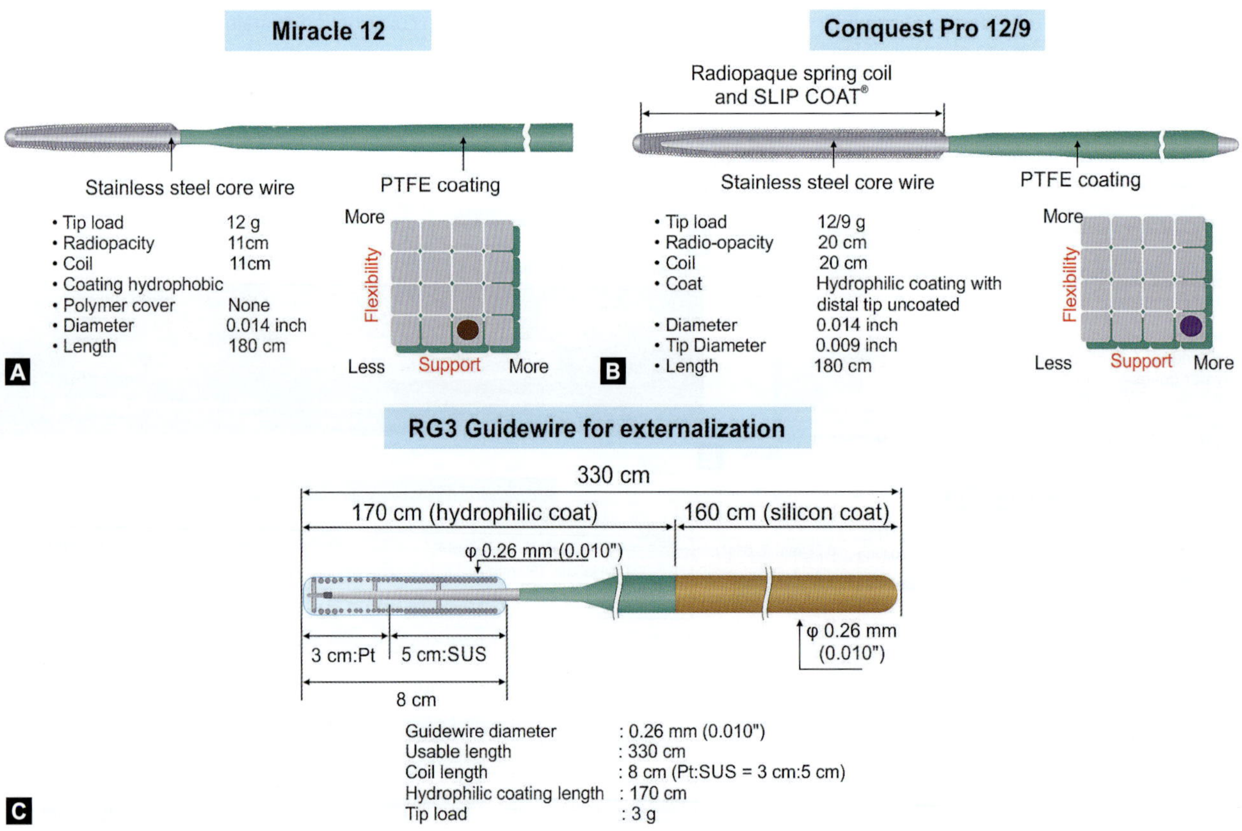

FIGS. 3A TO C: Constructional design of some commonly used CTO wires (A: MIRACLEBROS®; B: Conquest® Pro; C: RG3®).

Scientific, Natick, MA, USA) followed by wire exchange to low-tip load, hydrophilic wire to prevent perforation.

MICROCATHETERS

Microcatheters assists in performing invasive endovascular procedures by serving a broad range of functions in these complex vessel anatomies, namely, bifurcation, ostial lesion, calcification, and CTOs. The selection of microcatheter is also influenced by conditions such as vessel anatomy (irregularity, tortuosity, angulations, bifurcations, epicardial, or septal collaterals), lesion location (distal, mid, or proximal), lesion morphology [anomalous ostial lesion, recent total occlusions (RTOs), etc.], CTO crossing strategy (antegrade vs. retrograde), and guidewire to balloon crossability issues.

Single lumen microcatheters (SLM) are standard microcatheters intended to provide support to enable placement of guidewires in the vessel **(Fig. 4A)**. They are simple to handle and allow wire reshaping or wire exchange without losing the vessel entry. They improve the guidewires penetration ability and could prevent wire tip prolapse/plop. These microcatheters can also be maneuvered through a tortuous arterial segment proximal to the lesion by providing extra support to the guidewire. They can also be used to visualize the distal vessel by injecting contrast medium (tip injection). Dual lumen microcatheters (DLM) have two lumens to facilitate precise and independent handling of two different guidewires **(Fig. 4B)**. One lumen consists of the rapid delivery system which has a distal port at the distal end of the catheter and the other lumen is OTW with distal end opening slightly proximal to the distal tip by a centimeter or so and runs the whole length of the catheter with proximal end at the proximal hub of the catheter. Angulated tip microcatheters have a specific degree of short length bend at the tip. This eases out the wiring of side-branch in bifurcation lesions. It also helps in negotiating extreme bends and proximal tortuosity in vessels having nonaorto ostial critical lesions at the bend. Steerable angulated tip microcatheters [SwiftNINJA™ microcatheter (Merit Medical, West Jordan, UT, USA) and Venture deflectable catheter (Teleflex, Wayne, USA)] additionally enable the successful superselective cannulation and wiring of tortuous branches.

For better penetration and pushability, short-tapered tip is required (like FineCross™ MG). The microcatheter further helps in step down to a regular workhorse wire after crossing the CTO. During CTO-PCI, while treating critically stenosed vessels with a bend trajectory, the operator at times finds that the wire is crossed but it is difficult to cross the lesion with a balloon. Thus, initially improving wire support is at times helpful which is done with a microcatheter. In these situations, a Tornus® microcatheter which moves forward with corkscrew action of up to 20 counter-clockwise turns, could work by crossing the lesion. Microcatheters are also handy in dealing with RTOs. For example, a total occlusion which is 30-day old, regular guidewire (like Sion™ wire) may not be stiff enough to maneuver through the lesion. Whereas the same wire in a microcatheter in such a situation increases wire support and assists lesion crossing. Moreover, it can also be exchanged for a hydrophilic polymer jacketed wire with increased tip load (e.g., PILOT 150 or PILOT 200) if the workhorse wire fails to cross the RTO lesion.[9]

For crossability of long narrow channels like septal collaterals, microcatheter with a long-tapered tip is beneficial (like Caravel™ or Corsair®/Corsair® Pro). For treating

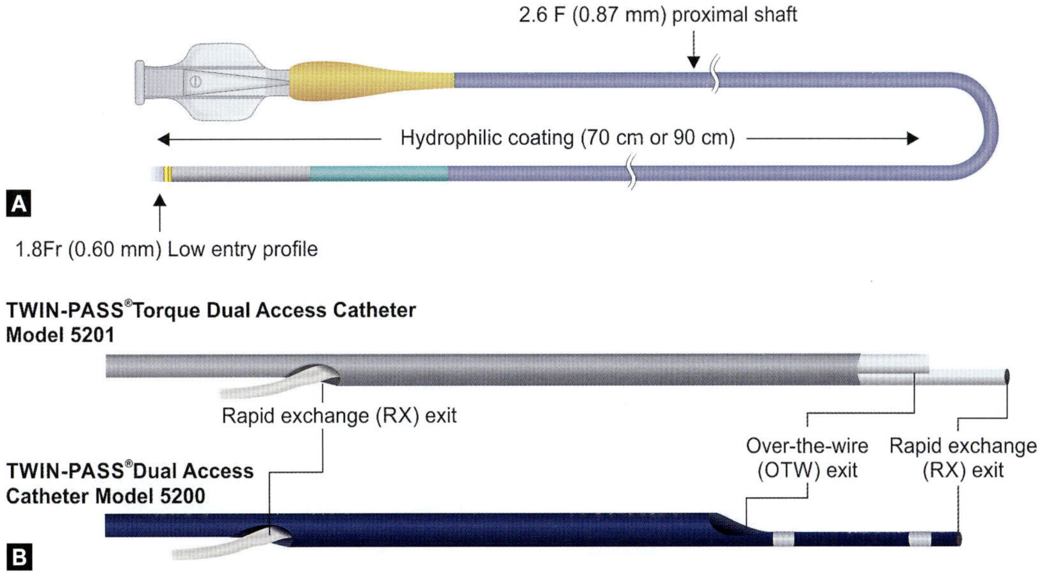

FIGS. 4A AND B: (A) Single lumen microcatheter (FineCross™ MG microcatheter) profile. (B) Dual lumen microcatheter (Twin-Pass Dual® Access microcatheter) profile.

epicardial vessels, operators prefer flexible and tapered tip (like FineCross™ MG) that does not damage the vessels. Often during the intervention, the channels have to be stretched and dilated for facilitating the passage of microcatheters through tortuous path and thus need prevention of recoiling which cannot be achieved by microcatheter with short-tapered tip (e.g., FineCross™ MG). Caravel™ or Corsair® microcatheter can be used to circumvent these vessels and dilate the channels en route. While crossing the collateral, microcatheters can also be used to inject contrast to visualize the finer channels. For CTO operators another challenging part is the point when reentry is very tough and sometimes may obstruct balloon from crossing over. Thus, instead of using a small low-profile semicompliant balloon, stiffer microcatheters like Corsair® can be used to dilating the false channel produced by wire dissection into the subintimal space and create a passage for wire exchange.

ANTEGRADE DISSECTION REENTRY SYSTEM

The BridgePoint System (BridgePoint medical Inc, Minneapolis, MN, USA) induces a controlled subintimal dissection for subsequent reentry in the true lumen. The system has two components—CrossBoss™ catheter and Stingray™ CTO reentry system. The CrossBoss™ catheter is actually a metallic OTW microcatheter with a soft nonpenetrating round tip, used to safely traverse the subintimal expanse across a CTO **(Fig. 5A)**. It has a 2.3F shaft profile, 3F rounded atraumatic distal tip which tracks via fast spin technique, rotating in either direction or is advanced without a wire. Contrary to coronary guide wire loop and hydrodissections, the CrossBoss™ catheter induces a single subintimal track with a small subintimal space that provides good back up support for the reentry into the true lumen at or beyond the distal CTO cap. Once the entire length of occlusion is traversed, CrossBoss is exchanged over a 0.014" guidewire with StingRay™ balloon. It is a very useful tool for intimal crossing of in-stent restenosis (ISR) CTOs. The Stingray™ CTO reentry system includes a balloon catheter and a guide wire, which are designed to accurately target and reenter the true lumen from the subintimal space **(Fig. 5B)**. The balloon catheter has a 2.9F shaft profile, compatible with 6F GC and 0.014" guidewire. The self-orienting balloon at the tip has a flat shape, 0.014" crossing profile, and two offset exist ports opposite to each other with a radio-opaque marker just distal to the port (to mark its orientation toward the true lumen) for Stingray™ CTO reentry guidewire. When inflated this balloon assumes a flat shape and allows orientation of the penetrating wire (Stingray wire) toward the true lumen, radio-opaque markers denominating the two exist ports. The port which is oriented toward the true lumen is chosen to pass the stingray wire which is a tapered wire with a high penetrating force. Once it enters into true lumen the whole apparatus is removed and the channel created used to pass a regular penetrating CTO wire and cross into the true lumen.

LOW-PROFILE DEDICATED CTO BALLOONS

The CTO lesions even after successful wiring are often difficult to cross using workhorse PTCA balloons. Dedicated CTO balloons with tiny tip and crossing profiles, proprietary balloon coating, and puncture resistant design are therefore required for lesion dilatation.[10] CTO balloons often have a single central or proximal marker to help reducing the crossing profile. Low-profile balloons are also required to cross previously deployed stent struts during a bifurcation PCI. Various such CTO-specific balloons available are:

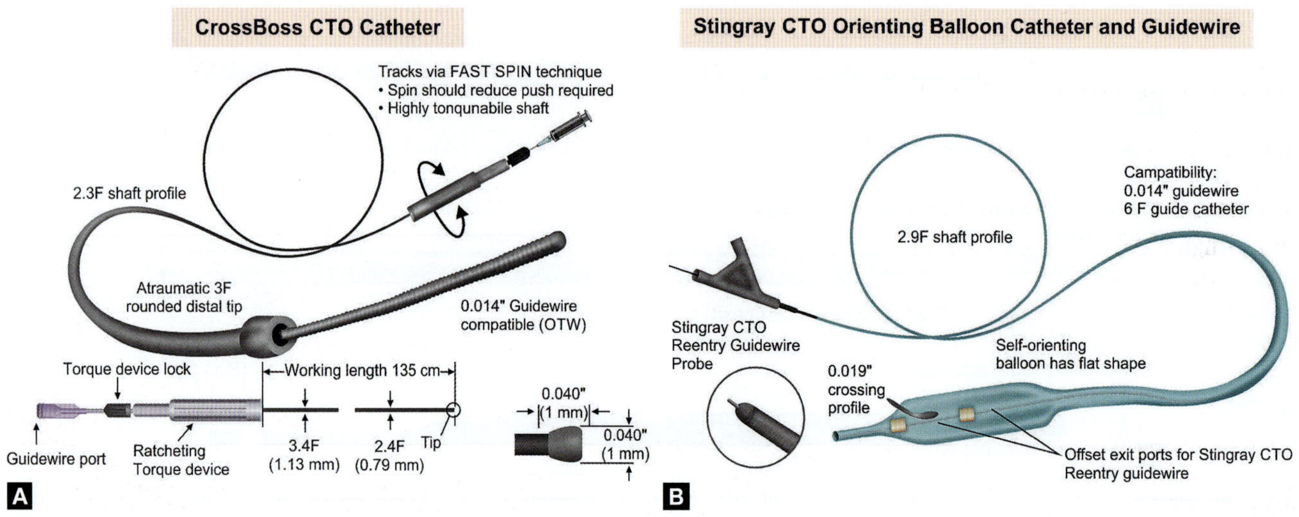

FIGS. 5A AND B: Constructional design of antegrade dissection and reentry system (A: CrossBoss™ catheter; B: Stingray™ re-entry system).

- *Across CTO balloon (Acrostak, Geneva, CH)*: The short tip (ST) model of this balloon sacrifices increased ability to maneuver through torturous vessels in order to provide the increase puncture power and push of its ultrasturdy tip. Over-the-wire (OTW) variant allows for application of increased force and improved pushability.
- *NIC® Nano 0.85-mm CTO balloon (SIS medical, Frauenfeld, CH)*: It has a low-crossing profile (0.0195"), high rated burst pressure (RBP) of 23 atm and a low compliance (0.85 mm at 10 atm and 1.00 mm at 23 atm) making it ideal for use in CTO-PCI.
- Mozec™ CTO (Meril Life Sciences, Vapi, Gujrat, IND)
- *Alveo™ HP 0.75-mm CTO balloon (Brosmed medical, Guangdong, CHN)*: With an ultralow-tip profile of 0.0156", crossing profile of 0.0184" and RBP of 20 atm, it is the world's smallest balloon catheter specifically designed for crossing complex tortuous anatomy and CTOs.

Excimer Laser

Excimer laser coronary atherectomy (ELCA, Spectranetics, Colorado, USA)) is indicated for occluded SVG, calcified lesions, balloon uncrossable CTOs, stent underexpansion, ISR, and ostial lesions. It is increasingly being used in CTO-PCI to facilitate modification of the proximal CTO cap to allow penetration with a wire.[11]

Atherectomy (Rotational or Orbital)

The CTO often contains varying degree of calcification which may pose difficulties in passage of devices. Rotational (Rotablator; Boston Scientific, Natick, MA, USA) or orbital atherectomy (Diamondback 360®; Cardiovascular systems Inc, Minnesota, USA) modifies the intimal calcified plaque by differential ablation and creates the passage diameter enabling the delivery of devices across CTO body.

High-pressure Noncompliant Balloon

Noncompliant balloon is needed for plaque modification and lesion preparation of fibrocalcific lesions as well as poststent optimization to achieve a satisfactory minimal luminal area after CTO-PCI. OPN® NC balloon (SIS medical, Frauenfeld, CH) is one such example with a twin-layer balloon construction with virtually zero dog-boning effect, super high RBP (35 atm), long-tapered tip design for a better crossability, better crossing profile (0.028" of 2.0 mm balloon) than scoring and cutting balloons and lowest linear compliance curve up to over 40 atm.

Intravascular Imaging

Intravascular ultrasound (IVUS) should be utilized to define the ambiguity of the proximal cap, facilitate the reentry into the true lumen, limit the dissection plane, and confirm the distal positioning of the guidewire in the true lumen during retrograde CTO-PCI approach, in addition to stent sizing and optimization. In blunt proximal cap CTOs, identification of true lumen and antegrade puncture of CTO cap should be assisted by manual dynamic IVUS imaging using a catheter placed in adjacent side branch just proximal to CTO's proximal cap.

Optical coherence imaging (OCT) use in CTO-PCI is largely restricted to estimation of vessel size and poststenting optimization. The use of contrast or colloid flush often results in enhancements of dissection planes thereby, limiting the use of OCT.

EQUIPMENT SPECIFIC FOR RETROGRADE CTO-PCI APPROACH

Retrograde approach toolbox includes 7F and 8F systems, long-length support catheters (Corsiar®Pro 150, Caravel®150), guide extension catheters, wires for collateral surfing (Suoh® 3, Sion® Black, FIELDER® XT-R), wires for reverse CART (MIRACLEBROS®, Conquest®Pro, ULTIMATEbros®), wires for externalization (RG3, R350™), 2-cc Luer Lock Syringes for microcatheter contrast tip injection, ≥9F compatible push-pull Y-connectors (OKAY®II Y-connector; Nipro corporation, Osaka, JPN), and dedicated trapping balloon (TRAPPER™ exchange device; Boston Scientific, Natick, MA, USA).

Wire externalization of the retrograde guide wire allows access to both ends of the coronary guide wire and provides excellent support for coronary equipment delivery. Guide extension catheter can be used to facilitate the externalization of wire into antegrade GC. A snare device may be required to capture and exteriorize the wire. The retrograde wire can be pinned in the antegrade GC by an inflated coronary angioplasty balloon. The rail provided by the pinned retrograde coronary wire facilitates the advancement of the retrograde microcatheter to the antegrade GC. Placement of the retrograde microcatheter tip in the antegrade GC provides a platform for wire exchange to a longer wire for externalization from the antegrade homeostatic valve.[12]

EQUIPMENT FOR MANAGING COMPLICATIONS

Vascular perforations can be managed by:

- *Coils and injectable material*: Coils and injectable material are used for an end branch wire perforation. 0.014" coils are detachable, more expensive than pushable coils, and more difficult to deploy; whereas 0.018" coils are widely available and easier to deliver by simple push technique using special microcatheters (Progreat®; Terumo Interventional systems, Japan). Patient's own-clotted blood or fat tissue can be injected in a small branch to seal a wire-induced perforation.

- *Covered or graft stents*: As of now, two coronary covered stents are commercially available in India—Graftmaster® RX (Abbott vascular, Chicago, IL, USA) and PK Papyrus™ (Biotronik, Berlin, Germany). The Graftmaster® RX consists of two stainless steel stents with a middle layer of PTFE. It is bulky and difficult to deliver; hence excellent GC support is important. PK Papyrus™ covered coronary stent system is manufactured by covering the prokinetic energy ultrathin strut, amorphous silicon carbide coated cob alt chromium stent with an electrospun polymeric matrix composed of siloxane-based polyurethane. It may be postdilated more liberally as compared to Graftmaster® RX stent. PK Papyrus™ is easier to deliver compared to Graftmaster® RX **(Fig. 6)**.

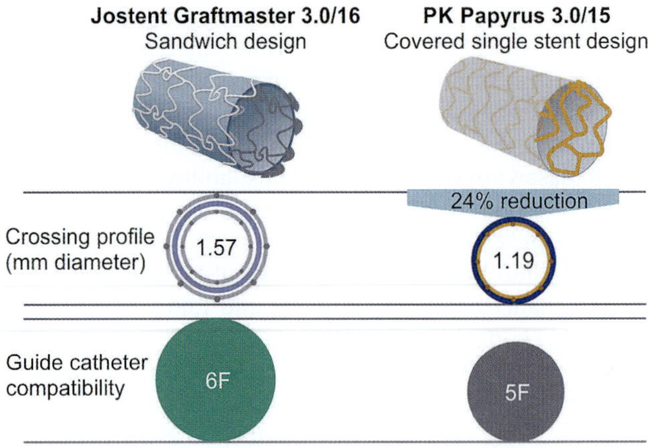

FIG. 6: Commonly available covered stent grafts for coronary artery perforation.

CONCLUSION

Ensuring availability of above discussed hardware is integral to successfully attempting a percutaneous CTO revascularization procedure failing which one cannot achieve CTO-PCI procedural success rates in excess of 90%. Through this chapter, we have attempted to summarize the salient features and clinical applications of various hardware essentials in performing CTO-PCI which constitute a "CTO-toolkit".

ONLINE REFERENCES

Please scan the QR code provided at the end of the table of contents for References of this chapter.

CHAPTER

155

In-stent Restenosis: Mechanism and Diagnostic and Therapeutic Options

KN Srinivasan, I Sathyamurthy

ABSTRACT

In-stent restenosis (ISR) remains a significant complication following percutaneous coronary intervention (PCI), despite advancements in stent technology. While the incidence of ISR has decreased with the introduction of second-generation drug-eluting stents (DES), it still accounts for 5–10% of all PCI procedures today.[1] Accurate assessment of ISR mechanism is achieved with intravascular imaging (IVI) compared to traditional coronary angiography.

The management of ISR is complex and varies based on several factors, including the type of initial stent used and the characteristics of the restenotic lesion. The risk of major adverse cardiovascular events (MACE) is higher with PCI for ISR compared to PCI for de novo lesions, with a median follow-up period of around 30 months.[2]

Two primary treatment options for ISR are drug-coated balloon (DCB) and DES. The choice between DCB and DES should be personalized based on the stent type that caused the ISR and patient-specific factors.[3]

Keywords: In-stent restenosis, intravascular imaging, drug-coated stent, drug-coated balloon

INTRODUCTION

Following balloon angioplasty (BA), there is a significant risk of myocardial infarction (MI) due to immediate vessel closure from dissection, thrombosis, and elastic recoil. This prompted the development of the metallic stent by Sigwart in 1987. However, the introduction of stents brought new challenges, including complications such as in-stent restenosis (ISR), late stent thrombosis (LST), and bleeding due to long-term dual antiplatelet therapy (DAPT).

To address these issues, extensive research in the stent strut thickness, connecting strut, polymer coating, and cytotoxic drug has gone a long way and paved the way to newer second-generation and third-generation drug-eluting stents (DES).

DEFINITION OF IN-STENT RESTENOSIS

Traditionally, restenosis in the context of stent implantation has been defined as a reduction of ≥50% in the lumen diameter within the stented segment or within 5 mm proximal and distal to the stent edges.[4] However, with the advent of intravascular imaging (IVI) modalities such as intravascular ultrasound (IVUS), ISR is now defined more precisely as a reduction of ≥75% in cross-sectional area within the stented segment.[5]

In-stent restenosis can manifest as silent or with symptoms such as angina or heart failure. The majority of ISR cases present as chronic coronary syndrome, characterized by stable angina or with exertional symptoms. However, in approximately 10% of patients, ISR can lead to acute MI.[6] IVUS has also revealed acute plaque rupture and stent thrombosis in patients with ISR, possibly due to neoatherosclerosis.

The incidence of ISR has significantly decreased with the advent of second-generation DES to 5–10% from >30% with bare metal stents (BMS).[6] Determining the exact incidence of ISR is challenging due to multiple factors such as stent type, comorbid risk factors, and lesion complexity. In patients with diabetes, the incidence of ISR with second-generation DES is reported to be 8.7%, compared to 5.7% in nondiabetic individuals.[7] Traditionally, the female gender has been considered a risk factor for ISR due to smaller vessel size and the lack of estrogen after menopause. However, according to a study by Yuan et al. using optical coherence tomography (OCT) imaging, men exhibited significantly more thin-cap fibroatheroma (TCFA) and in-stent neoatherosclerosis (ISNA) compared to women.[8]

CLASSIFICATION OF IN-STENT RESTENOSIS

The angiographic classification of ISR following BMS was proposed by Mehran et al.[9] **(Fig. 1)** based on the length (≤10 mm total, >10 mm diffuse), location (within or beyond stent borders), and severity of the restenosis (occlusion or not).

This comprises four groups namely: type I focal, type II diffuse—within the stent, type III diffuse—within and beyond the stent, and type IV occlusive. But ISR following DES is predominantly focal in nature and this classification may not be fully relevant. Moreover, it does not give any information about the pathology of ISR.

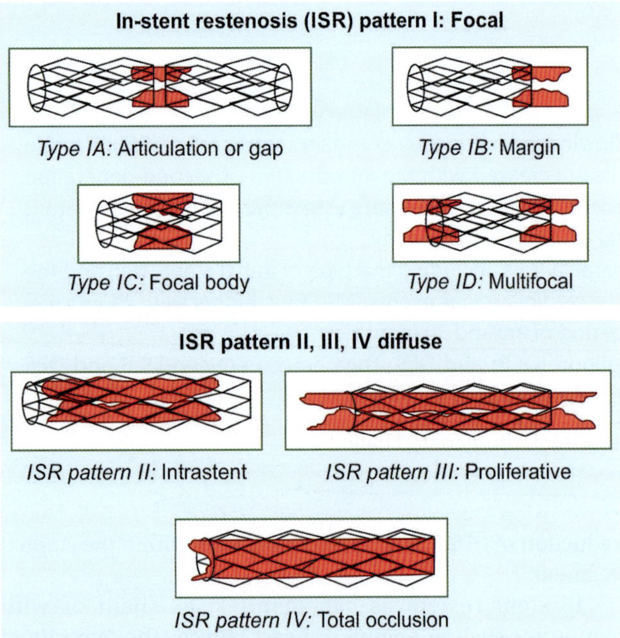

FIG. 1: The classification of ISR proposed by Mehran et al.
Source: Habib Samady, William F Fearon, Alan C Yeung, Spencer B. King III: Interventional Cardiology 2nd edition.

Several classifications for ISR using IVI have been proposed. Shlofmitz et al. **(Table 1)** categorized ISR based on the mechanism, dividing it into five groups considering restenosis length and minimum luminal area in IVUS.[10] Kang et al.[11] and Gonzalo et al.[12] have also proposed IVUS- and OCT-based classifications, respectively.

Additionally, the Society for Cardiovascular Angiography and Interventions (SCAI) has suggested a classification focusing on the time interval and mechanism of ISR, distinguishing early, late, and very late types.[13] These classifications serve to guide treatment options and optimize outcomes in patients with ISR.

MECHANISM OF IN-STENT RESTENOSIS

The mechanisms underlying ISR can be categorized into stent factors, intrastent factors, and extrastent factors, each contributing differently depending on whether the stent used is BMS or DES **(Fig. 2)**. Stent factors associated with ISR include underexpansion **(Fig. 3)**, undersizing **(Fig. 4)**, stent fracture (1–8% incidence),[14] vessel calcification, and geographic miss. Intrastent factors include neointimal hyperplasia **(Fig. 5)**, neoatherosclerosis, calcification, and thrombus. Extrastent factors include multiple stent layers **(Figs. 6A and B)**, vessel calcification, and calcific nodule.

COMPARISON OF BMS-ISR VERSUS DES-ISR

Angiographically, BMS-ISR typically exhibits a diffuse pattern of restenosis, while DES-ISR more commonly presents as focal restenosis **(Figs. 7A and B)**. BMS-ISR shows maximum late lumen loss (LLL) within 6–8 months after stent placement, whereas DES-ISR can experience LLL over a longer period, up to 5 years. Pathophysiologically, BMS-ISR is predominantly driven by neointimal hyperplasia, whereas DES-ISR is characterized by neoatherosclerosis,

TABLE 1: The classification of ISR proposed by Waksman et al.

Type	Definition		Therapeutic guidance
I	Mechanical	Stent underexpansion (type IA)	• High-pressure balloon, ELCA, or IVL • Underexpansion must be treated prior to further stent implantation
		Stent fracture (type IB)	DES
II	Biologic	Neointimal hyperplasia (type IIA)	Balloon, DCB, DES, or VBT
		Neoatherosclerosis, noncalcified (type IIB)	DCB or DES
		Neoatherosclerosis, calcified (type IIC)	Scoring balloon, ELCA, OA, or RA prior to DES
III	*Mixed pattern*: Combined mechanical and biologic etiology		High-pressure NC balloon with DCB, DES, or VBT
IV	Chronic total occlusion		DCB or DES; VBT for multiple layers, CABG as needed
V	More than 2 layers of stent		Balloon, DCB, VBT, or CABG

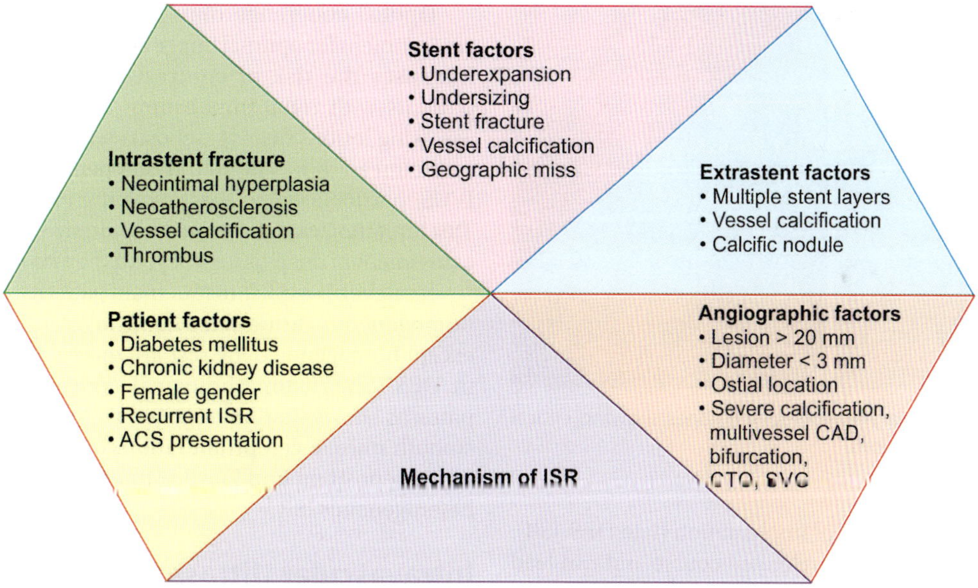

FIG. 2: Factors contributing to ISR.

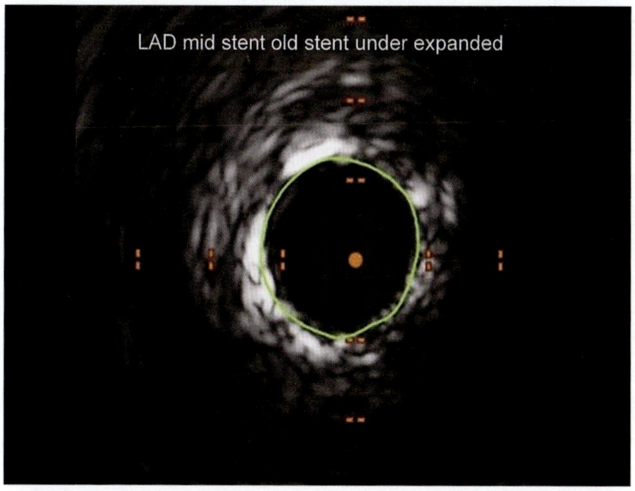

FIG. 3: Intravascular ultrasound image showing stent under expansion.

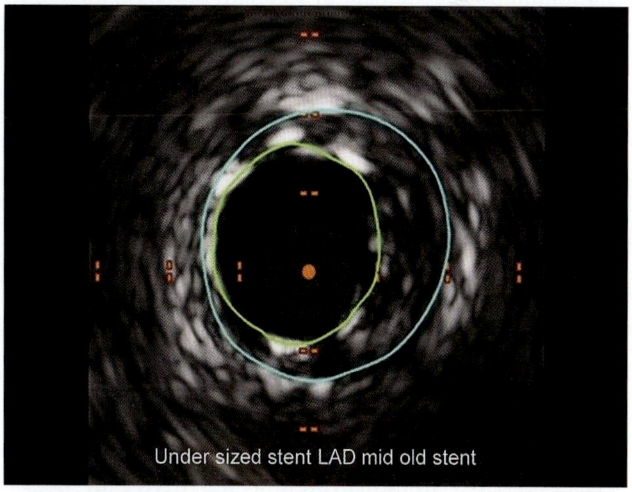

FIG. 4: Optical coherence tomography image showing undersizing of the stent.

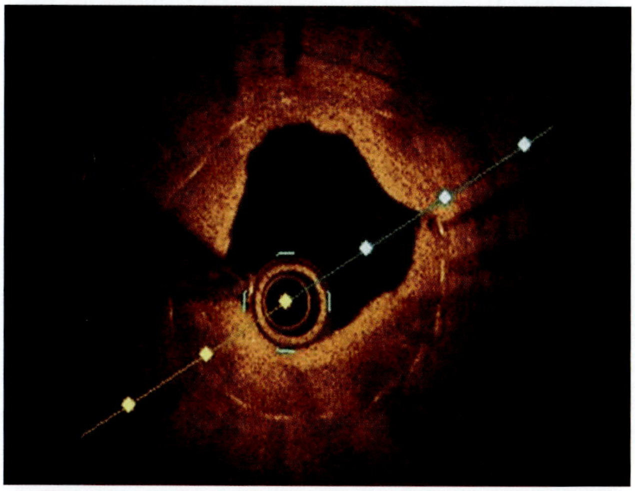

FIG. 5: Optical coherence tomography image showing neointimal hyperplasia.

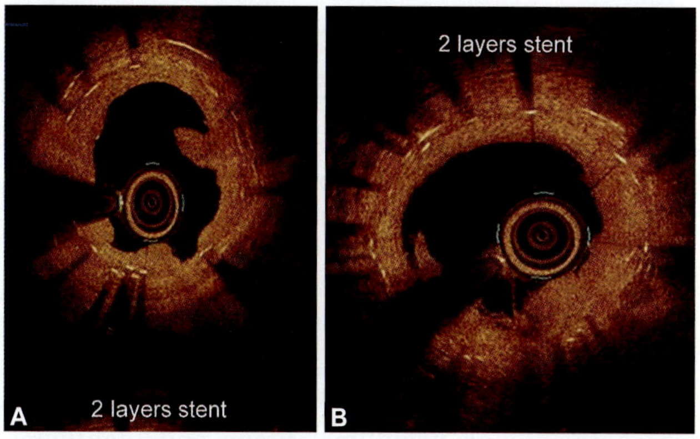

FIGS. 6A AND B: Optical coherence tomography images showing multiple stent layers.

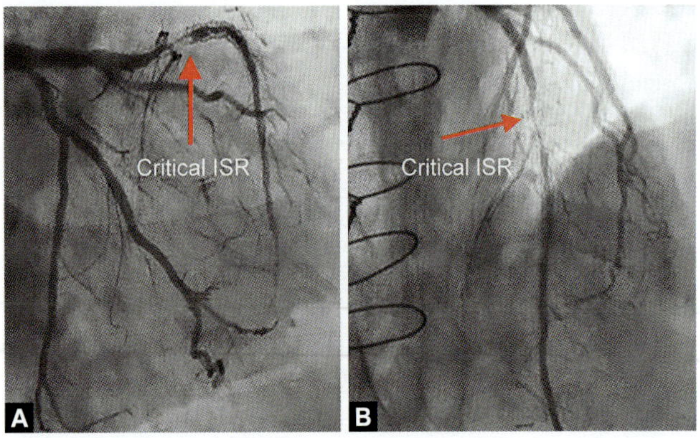

FIGS. 7A AND B: Coronary angiographic images showing critical in-stent restenosis (ISR) lesions.

particularly seen after 1 year of implantation (late DES-ISR). This condition often has an accelerated course and can lead to more complex lesions.[15]

On IVUS, BMS-ISR lesion showed neointimal hyperplasia as a dominant mechanism in 69% and underexpansion in 14% and both in 8%, as against neoatherosclerosis in 59%, stent underexpansion in 18% and both in 16% with DES-ISR.[16] With second-generation DES-ISR, both the mechanisms play a predominant role in causing restenosis.

Optical coherence tomography imaging has further detailed the presence and progression of neoatherosclerosis in DES.

COMPUTED TOMOGRAPHY–CORONARY ANGIOGRAM FOR DIAGNOSIS

In a study conducted by Elwany et al. involving 102 patients with chest pain postpercutaneous coronary intervention (PCI), CT-CAG demonstrated a sensitivity of 86.3% in excluding ISR compared to conventional coronary angiography.[17]

INTRAVASCULAR IMAGING FOR IN-STENT RESTENOSIS

More than conventional coronary angiography, IVI gives accurate information about the mechanism of ISR. Accordingly, guidelines recommend the use of IVI for ISR assessment with a Class IIa, Level B recommendation.[18]

Optical Coherence Tomography

Optical coherence tomography offers superior spatial resolution compared to IVUS, making it highly effective for characterizing neointimal tissue and identifying neoatherosclerosis within ISR lesions. However, OCT also poses specific challenges that impact its clinical utility.

Optical coherence tomography requires a blood-free environment for optimal image acquisition. This requirement increases the risk of contrast-induced nephropathy in patients with renal impairment and poses difficulties in assessing lesions near vessel ostia where blood flow is more pronounced. It has limited tissue penetration compared to IVUS, particularly in cases involving multiple stent layers. This limitation can affect the accurate sizing of the vessel and assessment of deep tissues beyond the stent struts.

It categorizes ISR into four main patterns: Heterogeneous, homogeneous, attenuated, and layered.[12] Among these, except homogenous, the rest are more commonly observed in DES-ISR. Histopathological analysis of OCT-defined patterns shows that homogeneous ISR typically consists of smooth muscle cell proliferation. In contrast, a mixture of fibrin deposition and loose connective tissue characterizes heterogeneous ISR.[19]

Intravascular Ultrasound

Though the limitation of OCT can be overcome with IVUS, tissue penetration is less with IVUS. Hence, a detailed tissue characterization is not feasible. Vessel sizing with IVUS is much better, as it delineates external elastic lamina (EEL). IVUS demonstrates neointimal hyperplasia, neoatherosclerosis, stent under expansion, stent undersizing, and vessel calcification.[16]

MANAGEMENT OF IN-STENT RESTENOSIS

Assessing the clinical significance of ISR is crucial before initiating treatment and functional assessment plays a key role in this evaluation. It can help to determine the hemodynamic significance of ISR lesions and guide decision-making regarding the need for revascularization. However, when fractional flow reserve (FFR) is ≥0.8, deferring revascularization in ISR was associated with comparable outcomes over 36 months to patients with de novo coronary stenosis.[20] Compared to de novo lesions, FFR in ISR lesions may not be decreased despite angiographically similar level of stenosis, due to the morphologic difference.[21] Effective treatment aims to achieve optimal acute gain (difference in minimal luminal diameter (MLD) pre- and immediate postprocedure) and minimize LLL (change in MLD from immediate postprocedure to follow-up angiography).

Drug-eluting Stents

Drug-eluting stent implantations have shown superiority over BA in treating ISR in both meta-analysis and head-to-head trials. It is important to treat the underexpanded stent optimally before implanting a new DES. Treating with the same DES (homo DES) versus different antiproliferative DES (hetero DES) has shown varied results in trials and meta-analysis.

The Drug-Eluting Stents for In-Stent Restenosis 2 study (ISAR-DESIRE 2)[22] did not show any superiority with hetero DES or homo DES. On the contrary, Restenosis Intra-Stent: Balloon Angioplasty Versus Drug-Eluting Stent (RIBS-III)[23] study showed the superiority of hetero DES over homo DES strategy. In general, treating with hetero DES is preferred over the homo DES due to possible drug resistance.

Drug-coated Balloons

Drug-coated balloons (DCB) deliver an active lipophilic drug and excipient to the vessel wall upon inflation, without leaving an additional stent layer behind. This can be beneficial in patients with multiple stent layers, large side branches, or stent maldeployment, where implanting another stent may be challenging or undesirable. Compared to DES, DCB treatment requires a shorter duration of DAPT, reducing the risk of bleeding complications in patients with high bleeding risk. Both paclitaxel-coated and sirolimus-coated DCBs have demonstrated effectiveness in treating ISR lesions.

Paclitaxel-coated DCBs are lipophilic and have shown superiority over plain BA and even BMS therapy in randomized controlled trials (RCTs). They have been compared favorably with DES in terms of reducing target lesion revascularization (TLR) rates.

Sirolimus-coated DCBs have also proven effective in treating ISR. However, direct comparative RCTs are limited. In a small-randomized trial, sirolimus DCB was compared with paclitaxel DCB and reported similar 6-month angiographic and 12-month clinical outcomes.[24] Thus, superiority between the two types of DCBs or over DES cannot be concluded based on current evidence.

Proper lesion preparation is crucial before DCB use as the balloon itself is bulky and may not adequately track complex ISR lesions without prior modification. Techniques such as using cutting balloons or scoring balloons to prepare the lesion have been shown to improve outcomes, as demonstrated in trials such as ISR-DESIRE 4.[25]

In the context of treating ISR, there are considerations regarding the choice between DCB and DES. Kheifets et al. reported higher rates of recurrence and MACE with DCB compared to DES in their single-center experience.[26] However, after adjusting for variables, the overall outcomes were found to be comparable between DCB and DES. In a meta-analysis comparing DES with paclitaxel DCB, DES was shown to be more effective in reducing TLR at the 3-year mark.[27] Additionally, DES resulted in less residual stenosis compared to DCB, and this benefit persisted over a longer follow-up period. In the RIBS-V trial, involving 189 BMS-ISR patients, the *DES-EES* arm was compared to DCB and was found to have acceptable outcomes in terms of binary restenosis (4.7% vs. 9.5%, $p = 22$) and TVR (2% vs. 6%, $p = 0.17$).[28] Similarly, DCB was compared to EES-DES in *DES-ISR* patients in the DARE trial. About 278 patients were randomized to receive either DCB or EES and were found to have similar outcomes (both primary and secondary endpoints).[29] It was a noninferior trial. Similarly, EES was compared to zotarolimus-eluting stent in the RESTENT trial.[30] It randomized 304 DES-ISR patients to EES and ZES and was found to have similar angiographic LLL at 9 months follow-up (0.40% vs. 0.45%, $p = 0.54$) and comparable MACE at the end of 3 years (15.8% vs. 22.6%, $p = 0.28$).

ADJUNCTIVE THERAPY

The use of cutting or scoring balloons in the treatment of ISR helps in preparing the lesion for DEB or DES implantation. Their blade penetrates the plaque and helps to anchor the balloon, minimizing the "watermelon seeding effect" risk. Isolated use of these balloons in ISR treatment may not be sufficient as they cannot inhibit neointimal proliferation.

Plain BA was compared with scoring BA prior to DCB use in DES-ISR in the ISAR DESIRE 4 trial.[25] Scoring BA group had significantly lower in-stent diameter stenosis compared to plain BA. The 1-year TLR was lower in scoring BA but was statistically not significant.[31] Small IVUS studies have supported the clinical utility of cutting balloons in achieving larger lumen gains and favorable angiographic results compared to plain BA.[31,32]

INTRAVASCULAR BRACHYTHERAPY

Intravascular brachytherapy (IVBT) delivers localized radiation to prevent neointimal hyperplasia. Though there were trials with IVBT in BMS-ISR, there is no RCT with IVBT in DES-ISR. Observational studies have shown that IVBT may have a role in recurrent ISR.[33] It is almost obsolete in most centers because of lack of evidence.

ABLATIVE THERAPY

Rotational Atherectomy

A debulking procedure such as RA has been studied with BMS-ISR therapy in RCT but not so with DES-ISR therapy. However, it is still useful in lesion preparation before DES or DCB implantation. It should be considered a high-risk procedure as there is a risk of burr entrapment within the ISR lesion and risk of perforation.

Excimer Laser Coronary Atherectomy

Excimer laser coronary atherectomy is a debulking technique that uses a laser to ablate the tissue. There is no RCT data available with ELCA in DES-ISR therapy. It may be useful in selected cases as a bailout strategy, especially with severe calcification with recurrent ISR.[34]

INTRAVASCULAR LITHOTRIPSY

Intravascular lithotripsy uses localized pulsatile sound waves to circumferentially modify the calcium. Its use in ISR has only limited data and is mostly off-label. Many observational studies have shown its use in ISR cases with severe circumferential calcium. It is more user-friendly and less dependent on operator experience.[35]

CORONARY ARTERY BYPASS GRAFTING SURGERY

Coronary artery bypass grafting (CABG) surgery is a reasonable option in selected patients with ISR. There is no randomized data available comparing CABG versus DES in ISR therapy. However, CABG may be considered in patients with ISR of the left main stent (LMS), recalcitrant ISR in a major vessel, associated multivessel disease, and ISR localized in the LAD ostium.

SPECIAL SCENARIOS

Recurrent In-stent Restenosis

Restenosis that occurs after the initial treatment of ISR is termed recurrent ISR and constitutes approximately 20% of all ISR cases. This form of restenosis typically involves multiple layers of stents, necessitating a strategic approach that avoids repeated stent implantation. Options such as DCB or IVBT are preferred in these cases.

Before initiating treatment, the exact mechanism of recurrent ISR should be determined using IVI techniques. This helps in identifying issues such as stent underexpansion or fractures. Stent underexpansion should be corrected to optimize outcomes, while stent fractures may necessitate additional stent placement.

The use of DCB in recurrent ISR cases involving more than two stent layers has been associated with poorer outcomes compared to cases involving one or two layers. For instance, in a study by Yabushita et al., the 1-year risk of TLR was 14.5% in the one-stent layer group, 14.9% in the two-stent layer group, and notably higher at 41.2% in the three-stent layer group.[36]

Although IVBT is considered a superior modality for treating recurrent ISR, meta-analyses have indicated a 25% risk of TVR at 2 years of follow-up.

In cases of recurrent ISR involving critical arteries, CABG surgery should be considered as a viable treatment option.

In-stent Restenosis Chronic Total Occlusion

In the Mehran classification of ISR,[9] type IV denotes total occlusion occurring after stent placement. When treating ISR with CTO-PCI, outcomes have varied across studies. Some research indicates that outcomes are comparable between ISR CTO-PCI and de novo CTO-PCI procedures. However, other studies have highlighted that ISR CTO-PCI can pose a higher risk compared to de novo CTO-PCI due to factors such as increased procedural complexity and potential complications.

The presence of an old stent provides a roadmap for advancing wires during the intervention, aiding in navigating through the occluded segment. ISR CTO-PCI is considered as a high-risk procedure primarily due to the technical challenges involved, the complexity of the lesion, and the potential for complications during and after the intervention.

DUAL ANTIPLATELET THERAPY AFTER IN-STENT RESTENOSIS-PERCUTANEOUS CORONARY INTERVENTION

Duration of DAPT following ISR-PCI should be tailored based on the clinical presentation of ISR. Generally, the duration of DAPT is shorter following DCB treatment compared to DES implantation.

Recent studies, including a substudy of the PRODIGY trial, have suggested the potential benefits of a longer duration of DAPT (24 months) following ISR-PCI compared to a shorter duration (6 months).[37] However, these findings need validation in larger RCTs to establish definitive guidelines.

CONCLUSION

Despite recent advancements in managing coronary artery disease, including improvements in stent design and delivery technology, ISR-PCI still constitutes a significant proportion of all PCI procedures, accounting for approximately one tenth of cases. Effective preparation of the treatment site before addressing ISR, particularly utilizing IVI such as IVUS or OCT, is crucial. Factors such as lesion characteristics (stent malapposition or calcification) and patient-specific factors should be carefully evaluated and addressed before deciding between DES or DCB. However, managing risk factors and promoting lifestyle modifications remain paramount in optimizing long-term outcomes for these patients.

ONLINE REFERENCES

Please scan the QR code provided at the end of the table of contents for References of this chapter.

CHAPTER

156

Imaging and Management of In-stent Restenosis

Nitin K Kabra

ABSTRACT

Long-term stent-related events remain the Achilles heel of percutaneous coronary intervention (PCI). In-stent restenosis (ISR) accounts for 10% of all PCI procedures in contemporary practice. Repeat PCI may be deferred in patients with ISR and fractional flow reserve (FFR) > 0.75. Intracoronary imaging modalities, such as intravascular ultrasound (IVUS) or optical coherence tomography (OCT), should be routinely used to guide the treatment of ISR. Balloon angioplasty (BA) is still used for cases with focal ISR where the risk of recurrence is deemed to be low. High-pressure BA has an important role in treating drug-eluting stent (DES)-ISR due to under-expansion. Plain BA as well as cutting or scoring balloon are valuable in lesion preparation prior to repeat DES or drug-coated balloon (DCB). Repeat stenting with second-generation DES leads to the best outcomes. DCB is preferable when an additional stent layering is to be avoided, or the risk of bleeding is high. Recurrent ISR after failure of two DES layers is an indication of vascular brachytherapy (VBT). Atherectomy procedures [rotational atherectomy (RA), excimer laser coronary atherectomy (ELCA), and intravascular lithotripsy (IVL)] are indicated for pretreatment of underexpanded stents and calcific ISR. Coronary artery bypass graft (CABG) surgery is preferred to repeat PCI in the left main coronary artery (LMCA) ISR or multivessel disease.

Keywords: ISR, DES, PCI, IVUS, OCT, stent under expansion, stent fracture, neointimal hyperplasia, neoatherosclerosis, minimum stent area, minimum lumen area, cutting or scoring balloon, balloon angioplasty, DCB, VBT, RA, ELCA, IVL

INTRODUCTION

In-stent restenosis (ISR) is a new disease entity, which has emerged after treatment for coronary stenosis with stent implantation became commonplace. A gradual reduction of ≥50% diameter [in the presence of ischemic symptoms or abnormal fractional flow reserve (FFR)] or ≥70% diameter (in the absence of ischemic symptoms) within or 5 mm adjacent to a previously stented vessel segment is termed as ISR. Rates of ISR with drug-eluting stents (DESs) range from 3 to 20%. They are also associated with an increase in late and very late stent restenosis (3% per year), approximately one-half of the patients presenting >2 years after the original stent implantation. Real-world registries show a higher rate of ISR when compared to the reports from randomized trials. Target lesion-related events arising from the stent site may ultimately occur in more than one-half of all patients.[1] ISR accounts for 10% of percutaneous coronary intervention (PCI) procedures in contemporary practice. Among 542,112 patients who underwent ISR PCI, 51.8% presented with unstable angina, 18.7% with NSTEMI, and 8.5% with STEMI. Stable angina was the presentation in 15.1% of patients.[2] Patients presenting with ISR had a greater burden of cardiovascular and noncardiovascular comorbidities.

IMAGING

Coronary Angiography

The diagnosis of ISR is made on angiography. It also tells us about the severity and pattern of ISR. Based on the morphologic pattern, Mehran et al.[3] classified bare metal stent (BMS)-ISR into four types **(Table 1),** which were associated with prognostic and therapeutic implications—increasing target lesion revascularization (TLR) rate with increasing ISR grade. But angiography, being a two-dimensional lumenogram of coronary arteries, has inherent limitations in the assessment of vessel diameter, vessel wall, plaque characteristics, optimal stent expansion and apposition, making it a poor tool for guiding treatment of ISR.

TABLE 1: Mehran classification (angiographic) of ISR.

Mehran classification	Incidence	TLR rate
Type I: Focal—lesions <10 mm in length • *Type IA*: Lesions placed at stent gap • *Type IB*: Stent body • *Type IC*: Stent edges • *Type ID*: Multifocal	42%	19%
Type II: Diffuse—lesions >10 mm intrastent	21%	35%
Type III: Proliferative—lesions >10 mm, extending beyond the stent margins	30%	50%
Type IV: Occlusive—complete vessel occlusion, TIMI flow grade 0	7%	83%

TABLE 2: Waksman classification for DES-ISR.

Type I	Mechanical	Type IA	Stent under expansion
		Type IB	Stent fracture
Type II	Biological	Type IIA	Neointimal hyperplasia
		Type IIB	Noncalcific neoatherosclerosis
		Type IIC	Calcific neoatherosclerosis
Type III	Mixed	Combined mechanical and biological causes	
Type IV	CTO	Chronic total occlusion	
Type V	Multilayer	>2 layers of stent	

Stent Enhancement

StentBoost (Philips), ClearStent (Siemens), and StentViz (GE) are enhanced fluoroscopic imaging techniques useful for the detection of inadequate stent expansion, stent fracture and can be easily and quickly performed in the Cath lab.

Intravascular Imaging

Newer intravascular imaging modalities such as intravascular ultrasound (IVUS) and optical coherence tomography (OCT) provide high-resolution cross-sectional images of coronary arteries and a better delineation of the underlying substrate of ISR (Waksman's classification) helping to differentiate between mechanical problems such as stent underexpansion and strut fractures or biological causes such as neoatherosclerosis and neointimal hyperplasia (NIH).[4] Assessing the main underlying cause of ISR is critical for guiding its optimal treatment. ISR lesion morphology is also predictive of future events **(Table 2)**.

Intravascular Ultrasound

Intravascular ultrasound is an invasive intravascular imaging modality, which uses an ultrasound-tipped catheter (2.9–3.5 F) to generate real-time 360° cross-sectional monochrome grayscale images from reflected ultrasound waves by the vessel walls. The typical axial resolution for commonly used systems is approximately 80–100 µm and lateral resolution is approximately 200–250 µm, whereas tissue penetration is approximately 6–12 mm.[5] Echogenic structures such as fibrous tissue and calcifications produce brighter signals, whereas echo-lucent structures such as lipid collections generate low-intensity signals. Tissue characterization by IVUS radiofrequency data [RFD or virtual histology (VH)] analysis can provide valuable information on the pathogenesis of restenosis by assessing plaque composition.

There is heterogeneity in reporting of IVUS results in stent studies and there are no standard guidelines. The maximum and minimum stent diameters and cross-sectional areas are measured at multiple segments within the stent and similarly for the lumen. In proximal and distal reference segments, external elastic membrane, lumen, and plaque and media (external elastic membrane minus lumen) cross-sectional area and plaque burden (plaque and media divided by external elastic membrane) are measured. The area, maximum thickness, volume, and percentage volume of NIH are calculated.

An IVUS minimum lumen area < 4.0 mm^2 is generally accepted to indicate significant luminal narrowing.

A minimum stent area (MSA) ≤ 5.5 mm^2 **(Fig. 1)** on IVUS is defined as stent underexpansion by the European Association of PCI, whereas many DES-ISR studies have defined stent underexpansion as MSA < 5 mm^2.[6,7]

Neointimal hyperplasia remains the main mechanism of ISR in both BMS and DES **(Fig. 2)** stent underexpansion was the underlying etiology of ISR in 21% of cases, and NIH in 88% of cases in a study of 76 lesions with DES-ISR.[8] However, stent underexpansion as a mechanism of ISR was greater in DES-ISR than BMS-ISR, in an IVUS study of 298 ISR lesions. Stent fracture was seen only in DES-ISR.[9]

In another study (Nordic IVUS study) of 209 patients (DES $n = 121$ and BMS $n = 88$) with ISR, stent underexpansion was present in 58.7% of DES-ISR patients compared to 37.7% of BMS-ISR patients ($p = 0.008$).[6]

In a cohort of 393 patients who underwent left main coronary artery (LMCA) stenting, the rate of ISR was much higher (24.1% vs. 5.4%) in patients with stent underexpansion compared to those without.[7]

In a prospective, multicenter registry of 8,582 patients undergoing PCI with DESs (ADAPT-DES) which evaluated 10 stent expansion indices for their association with lesion-specific 2-year clinically driven TLR found that stent/vessel area at the MSA site <38.9% was superior to traditional measures of stent expansion in predicting 2-year major adverse cardiac events (MACE), driven mainly by the difference in clinically driven TLR.[10]

Based on IVUS findings, Kang et al.[7] classified DES-ISR into focal (luminal narrowing 10 mm in length), multifocal

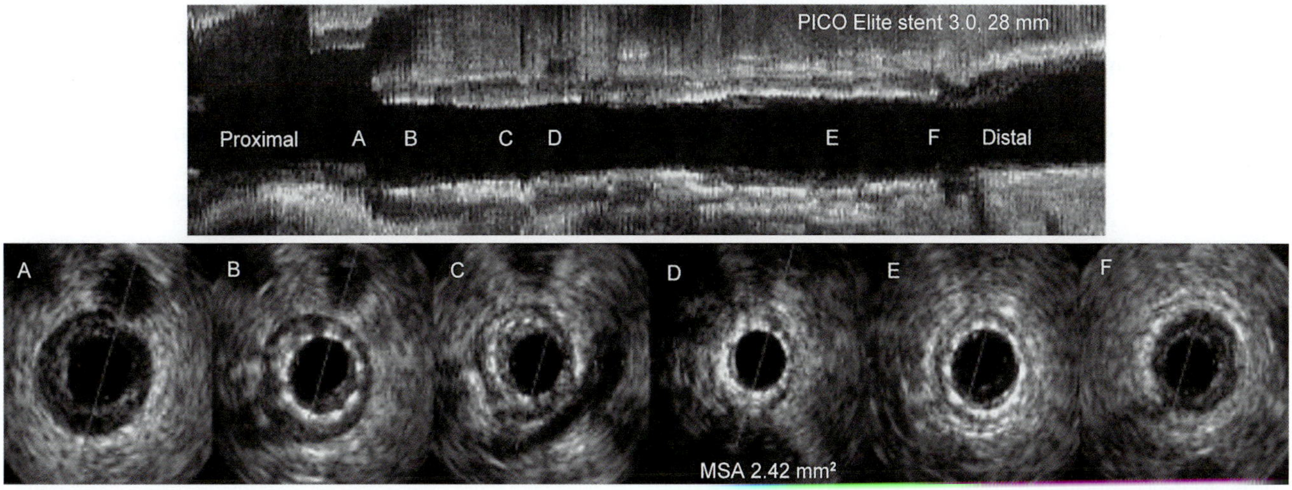

FIG. 1: Intravascular ultrasound (IVUS) findings of in-stent restenosis (ISR) lesion with stent underexpansion.
Source: Adapted from Lee et al. (2023) under CC BY License.[17]

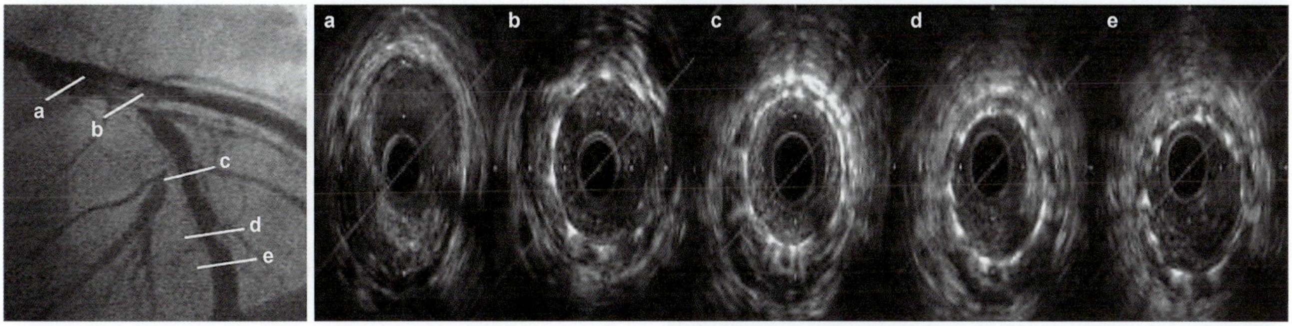

FIG. 2: In-stent restenosis (ISR) lesion of LAD with normally expanded stent and large plaque burden.
Source: Adapted from Lee et al. (2023) under CC BY Licencse.[17]

(>1 focal lesion), or diffuse (luminal narrowing >10 mm in length), seen in 47%, 12%, and 41% of DES-ISR, respectively.

Optical Coherence Tomography

Intravascular OCT, which is an infrared light-based imaging modality, provides high-resolution images of coronary arteries with a 10–20 µm spatial resolution, nearly 10 times higher than that of IVUS. Greater signal-to-noise ratio and the ability to differentiate plaque components such as lipid-rich plaque, fibrous cap thickness, macrophage accumulation, and intraluminal thrombus with high sensitivity and specificity (optical biopsy), enables evaluation of plaque vulnerability in vivo, although its limited tissue penetration usually precludes a comprehensive analysis of the total plaque burden. OCT is the only technique allowing accurate measurements of the thickness of the fibrous cap, a classical marker of plaque vulnerability, and readily detects thin cap fibroatheromas (defined as fibrous cap thickness at the thinnest part <65 µm and an angle of lipidic tissue >180°).

The term **neoatherosclerosis** refers to newly formed lipid-laden or calcified neointima within stents. Gonzalo et al.[11] reported in 2009 that OCT can depict various patterns of neointima within stents with restenosis, which was not provided by IVUS or other imaging modalities **(Table 3)**.

In a study to evaluate differences between early and late-presenting restenosis in second-generation DES using OCT, MSA <4.0 mm^2 (stent underexpansion) and heterogeneous NIH were more prevalent in early ISR, whereas neoatherosclerosis trended toward being more frequent for late ISR (28.9% vs. 15.8%).[12]

In a study of 50 DES-ISR lesions, OCT findings indicating in-stent neoatherosclerosis were frequently identified in patients with DES-ISR, especially late DES-ISR. 52% had at least 1 in-stent thin-cap fibroatheroma (TCFA)—containing neointima. 90% had lipidic neointima and 58% had thrombi. The intimal rupture was seen in 58% of patients and neovascularization in 60%. 18% of lesions had uncovered stent struts.[13]

Advantages of Optical Coherence Tomography

- High-resolution imaging, the capacity to distinguish lipid-containing plaque, and the visualization of coronary artery microstructure. A meticulous evaluation of atherosclerosis.

TABLE 3: Patterns of neointima as depicted by optical coherence tomography in in-stent restenosis.

Homogenous **(Fig. 3)**	High signal tissue composed of smooth muscle cells in a proteoglycan and collagen-rich matrix—fibrous plaque
Heterogenous	Focal bright spots inside low backscattering tissue—neoatherosclerotic plaque or proteoglycan-rich neointimal tissue
Layered	Concentric layers with different tissue properties—high-intensity layer near the lumen and low-intensity layer away from the lumen
Lipid laden **(Fig. 4A)**	Signal-poor region with diffuse border with an overlying signal-rich layer (fibrous cap). The stent strut not visualized due to signal attenuation
Calcific **(Fig. 4B)**	Signal-poor region with a sharp border
Macrophage accumulation	Signal-rich punctate regions that change from frame to frame

Source: Adapted from Gonzalo et al. (2009) under CC BY License.[11]

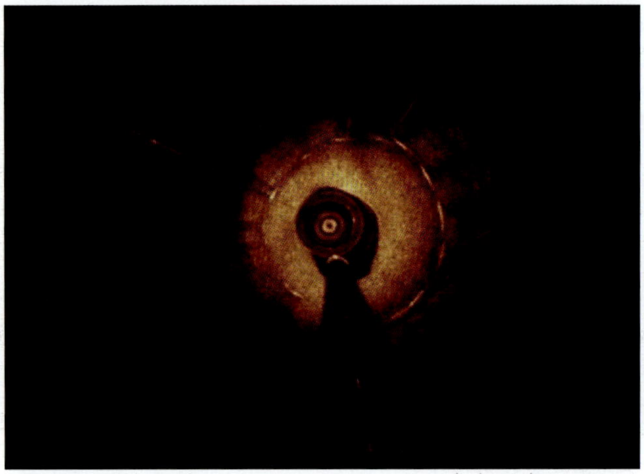

FIG. 3: Optical coherence tomography image of in-stent restenosis showing homogeneous neointima (smooth muscle cells and extracellular matrix).

Source: Adapted from Lee et al. (2023) under CC BY license.[17]

- OCT can depict various patterns of neointima within stents with restenosis, which was not provided by IVUS or other imaging modalities.
- Three-dimensional reconstruction of the implanted stent structure
- Superior to IVUS in the detection of neointimal rupture and thrombi. OCT is superior to IVUS in the detection of even minor degrees of malapposition, tissue prolapse, residual thrombus, and edge dissections

Disadvantages of Optical Coherence Tomography

- Limited penetration depth—inability to visualize the entire thickness of vessel wall, hence vessel remodeling and plaque burden
- Need to clear blood from vessel lumen during image acquisition—difficult to image ostial lesions and severe stenosis
- Extra contrast usage

Newer Imaging Modalities

Dual source computed tomography angiography (DSCTA) has high diagnostic accuracy in detecting ISR, especially for stent diameters of >3 mm, and may be appropriate tools for further evaluation of ISR in the future.[14]

Multimodal approaches utilizing dual probe hybrid catheters [IVUS-OCT, near-infrared spectroscopy (NIRS)-IVUS, OCT-NIRS, OCT-near-infrared fluorescence (NIRF) molecular imaging] will provide a comprehensive visualization of plaque morphology and composition allowing for detection of high risk, vulnerable lesions, thus guiding optimal intervention decisions.[15]

TREATMENT/MANAGEMENT

The treatment of DES-ISR needs to be individualized based on lesion and patient characteristics.

Several studies have indicated that asymptomatic patients with moderate disease severity ISR are unlikely to benefit from routine reintervention. Prospective studies have shown that deferring revascularization in patients with ISR and FFR of over 0.75 is safe and appropriate.[16]

Assessing the underlying substrate of ISR may be critical for guidance and optimization of repeated interventions. Recent large trials which included ISR lesions have reported superior clinical outcomes and lower stent failure rates with intravascular imaging-guided PCI, compared with angiography-guided PCI.[17]

In the RIBS-III study, IVUS was used to guide revascularization in 38.0% of the patients with DES-ISR and was associated with a larger acute gain (1.55 ± 0.6 mm vs. 1.35 ± 0.6 mm, $p < 0.01$) and minimum lumen diameter at 9-month follow-up (1.89 ± 0.8 mm vs. 1.68 ± 0.7 mm; $p < 0.01$); however, it did not reduce the incidence of TLR at 2 years.[18]

In the iOPEN-ISR registry, 1,522 patients with ISR were treated with either IVUS (65.9%) or angiography alone guidance (34.1%). Q wave myocardial infarction (0.3% vs. 1.6%; $p = 0.010$) and target vessel revascularization

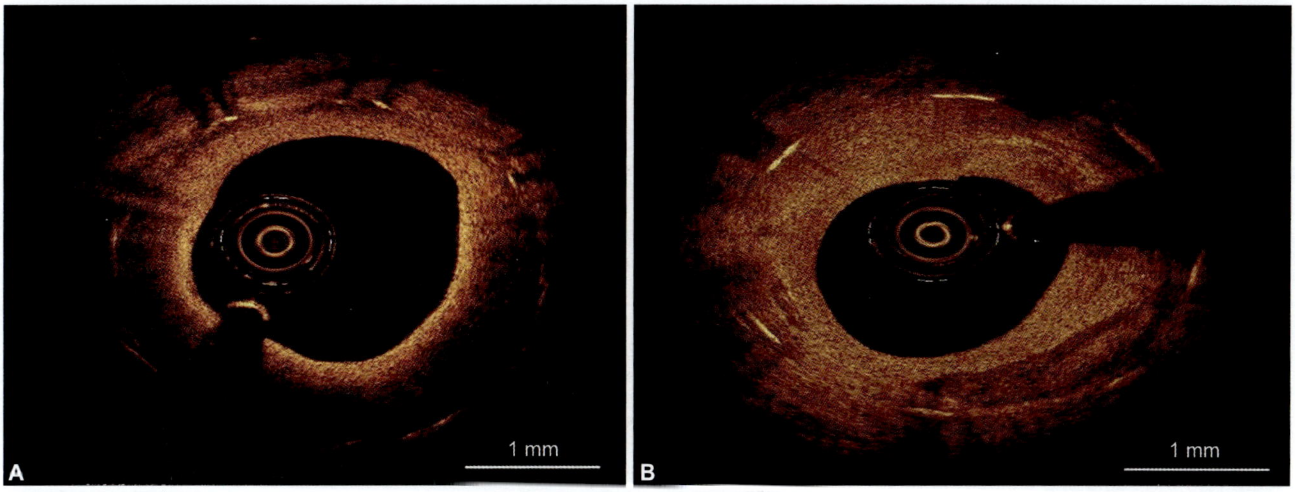

FIGS. 4A AND B: Optical coherence tomography defined neoatherosclerosis. (A) Lipid-laden neointima showing signal-poor region with an overlying signal-rich band corresponding to the fibrous cap. (B) In-stent calcification showing signal poor region with a clear border.
Source: Adapted from Yonetsu et al. (2023) under CC By license.[49]

(14.5% vs. 19.2%; $p = 0.021$) occurred less often in the IVUS than in the angiography cohort at 1 year that was maintained at 2 and 3 years. IVUS guidance was independently associated with a reduced incidence of MACE at 1-year follow-up, in multivariate analysis.[19]

The results of a subanalysis on complex coronary artery disease of the OCTIVUS trial comparing IVUS with OCT for guiding PCI showed that in the setting of ISR, OCT may be associated with improved 2-year clinical outcomes compared with IVUS.[20]

The 2018 ESC/EACTS guidelines recommend the use of OCT and/or IVUS for the detection of stent-related mechanical issues leading to restenosis (Class IIa indication, level of evidence C).

Plain Old Balloon Angioplasty

Plain old balloon angioplasty (POBA) using short balloons with incremental upsizing results in significant improvement in acute angiographic results but is associated with ISR recurrence in up to 50% of patients, mainly due to tissue reintrusion. Balloon slippage can lead to edge dissection and suboptimal results, which can be avoided by using short, low-profile balloons.[21] POBA alone is not routinely recommended for the treatment of ISR. It is used for lesion preparation prior to the use of other therapies. *Super high-pressure balloons (OPN NC)* capable of inflation pressures ranging from 35 to 55 atm may have a role in the treatment of DES-ISR due to stent underexpansion.

Repeat Stenting

Repeat stenting is a common, highly effective strategy in the treatment of ISR with cost reductions in the long term, but with the drawback that another layer of stent is implanted. It is particularly appropriate for cases in which ISR is characterized by focal patterns with distributions predominantly outside the stent (i.e., margins), late ISR due to diffuse neoatherosclerosis, ISR due to fracture of the previous stent, and ISR not located in vessels with small reference vessel diameters. It should be avoided when the primary mechanism of ISR is underexpansion and in recurrent ISR with multiple metallic layers (onion skinning effect).

Bare Metal Stent

There have been no large, randomized trials to evaluate the role of BMS in DES-ISR, and they should not be used as the primary option.[22]

Drug-eluting Stent

In the homo-DES strategy of repeat stenting, a DES with the same antiproliferative agent is used, whereas in the hetero-DES (switch strategy) a DES with a different antiproliferative agent is used which may overcome the issue of drug resistance.[23]

Several large-scale studies, including ISAR-DESIRE[24] and RIBS-II,[25] have shown that the use of DES significantly decreased restenosis rates, reduced neointimal proliferation as seen on IVUS imaging, and improved clinical outcomes compared to balloon angioplasty (BA) in patients with DES-ISR.

Second-generation everolimus-eluting stents showed better angiographic (significantly larger minimum lumen diameter and a lower percentage of diameter stenosis) and clinical outcomes [significant reduction in target vessel revascularization (8% vs. 16%; $p = 0.035$)] at 1 year which were maintained at 3 years than drug-coated balloon (DCB), for treatment of DES-ISR in the RIBS IV trial.[26]

Large studies comparing the potential value of implanting a hetero-DES with a different Limus drug have not been performed. RIBS-III study[18] which was a nonrandomized trial, and a meta-analysis of several observational studies had shown superior outcomes with the hetero-DES strategy but ISAR DESIRE-2,[27] the only randomized trial, did not show a benefit to the hetero-DES strategy for the treatment of sirolimus-eluting stent ISR. Paclitaxel DESs are no longer available, thus limiting the applicability of the hetero DES strategy.

The rates of early recurrent ISR after repeat stenting with DES for ISR are higher compared with those observed after the treatment of de novo lesions. The long-term safety of repeat DES for ISR remains unproven. 5-year landmark analyses of the ISAR-DESIRE 3 trial showed an excess of death (9.3% vs. 20.9%; $p = 0.028$) and cardiac death (5.8% vs. 13.6%; $p = 0.047$) associated with DES compared with DCB. These serious findings call for further data about very long-term clinical outcomes following the treatment of DES-ISR with contemporary DESs.[28]

Drug-coated Balloons

Drug-coated balloons provide antiproliferative therapy without the need for an additional metallic layer. They are rapid-exchange semi-compliant balloon catheters coated with paclitaxel, sirolimus, or biolimus on their surface along with an excipient or carrier that facilitates its transfer to the vessel wall to inhibit neointimal proliferation.

Several trials (ISAR DESIRE 3,[28] RIBS IV,[29] DARE,[30] BIOLUX-RCT[31]) and meta-analyses (DAEDALUS)[32] have demonstrated DCBs to be effective and safe in the treatment of ISR, with outcomes superior to plain BA and similar to repeat first-generation DES implantation but inferior to new generation DES (RIBs IV and RIBS V trials).[33,34]

When compared to POBA in the ISAR-DESIRE 3 trial comprising 402 patients with DES-ISR, DCB reduced MACE at 1 year (23.5% vs. 46.2%; $p < 0.0001$) driven predominantly by lower TLR and this was maintained at 3 and 10 years. Similar positive results have also been shown in the trials by Habara et al.[35] and in the PEPCAD-DES[36] and AGENT-IDE[37] trials.

Drug-coated balloons proved to be noninferior to DES in terms of 6-month angiographic and 1-year clinical outcomes in the DARE (PEB vs. PES) and BIOLUX (PCB vs. PES) trials. The ISAR-DESIRE 3 trial which also compared DCB therapy to 1st generation DES (PES) revealed that DCB application was noninferior to DES placement [diameter stenosis (PEB vs. PES): 38.0% vs. 37.4% (p for noninferiority = 0.011)]. PEPCAD China ISR[38] also showed similar results.

DAEDALUS individual patient data meta-analysis,[32] in which 1,976 patients undergoing DCB angioplasty or DES implantation in all 10 available randomized trials were compared at long-term follow-up (3 years) in the setting of DES-ISR, TLR was significantly higher after DCB angioplasty compared with repeat DES implantation (20.3% vs. 13.4%; HR 1.58; 95% CI 1.16–2.13), but the primary safety endpoint was numerically lower (9.5% vs. 13.3%; HR 0.69; 95% CI 0.47–1.00).

Use of DCB is preferred in patients at high bleeding risk who cannot tolerate dual antiplatelet therapy (DAPT), multilayer ISR, ISR involving major side branch to avoid jailing, ISR of BMS and less aggressive pattern of ISR (e.g., focal) with good lumen expansion after balloon dilatation.

Bioresorbable Vascular Scaffolds

In an observational study comparing bioresorbable vascular scaffold implantation with DCB angioplasty or DES implantation for ISR, DES was associated with reduced TLR at 6–9 months.[39]

Brachytherapy

Delivery of strontium-90 β-radiation locally within the stent decreases neointimal proliferation and was commonly employed for BMS-ISR in the past. No randomized trial has studied the use of vascular brachytherapy (VBT) in DES-ISR. Observational analysis has suggested that IVBT may have a role in recurrent ISR, especially in lesions with multiple layers of the stent. With three or more stent layers, the 3-year target lesion failure rate exceeds 50%. VBT may be repeated after 12 months. Patients undergoing VBT have to be on lifelong antiplatelet therapy.[40]

Combined Interventional Strategies

Adequate lesion preparation plays a pivotal role in the treatment of ISR. Combined strategies using novel devices such as cutting or scoring balloons or debulking devices such as excimer laser coronary atherectomy (ELCA) and intravascular lithotripsy (IVL) before DCB angioplasty or repeat DES implantation have shown promising results for the treatment of ISR.

Cutting/Scoring Balloons

By incising neointimal tissue, these balloons allow better tissue extrusion and achieve better anchoring during angioplasty, resulting in the use of fewer balloons, lesser balloon slippage, and lesser additional stenting. They may be considered in the presence of significant tissue and when balloon migration is of particular concern.

Even though cutting/scoring balloons results in better acute angiographic outcomes in ISR when compared with POBA, randomized studies have failed to show the superiority of cutting balloons in preventing MACE and recurrent ISR.[41]

Restenosis cutting balloon evaluation (RESCUT) trial, the largest randomized trial to date to compare cutting BA to POBA in the treatment of ISR, failed to show improvement in angiographic stenosis or the rate of clinical events during its 7-month follow-up.

Lesion preparation with a scoring balloon followed by paclitaxel-coated BA in 252 patients with DES-ISR showed significantly lower rates of in-segment diameter percentage stenosis at 6–8 months of angiographic follow-up but did not show any significant reduction in MACE in the ISAR-DESIRE 4 trial.[26]

A paclitaxel-coated scoring balloon has shown promising results in a small trial and more studies are needed for this promising approach. A cutting or scoring balloon may allow for better penetration of the drug through the incisions in the plaque.[42]

Atherectomy

Repeat stent underexpansion in patients with underexpansion of the first stent is associated with a higher risk of myocardial infarction (9.7% vs. 1.9%; $p = 0.046$) and TLR (32.4% vs. 13.3%; $p = 0.010$) at 2-year follow-up.[43] Off-label use of debulking techniques, such as rotational atherectomy (RA), orbital atherectomy, excimer laser, or IVL, may be considered in these settings.

Excimer Laser Coronary Atherectomy

Small observational studies but no randomized trials have studied ELCA, which uses ultraviolet energy to vaporize and break plaques. It may have an adjunctive role in lesion preparation, particularly for recurrent ISR in the setting of severe calcification.[44]

Rotational Atherectomy

No randomized trial has studied the use of RA in DES-ISR. Adjuvant RA for lesion preparation in diffuse, severely obstructive, and recurrent ISR before DCB or repeat DES may be helpful, keeping in mind the high risk of burr entrapment.[45]

Stentablation/Rotastenting

Ablation of metal by RA in severely underexpanded and undilatable stents has been reported but carries a high risk of device entrapment and vessel perforation and safer alternatives are now available.[46]

Intravascular Lithotripsy

Uses shockwaves delivered locally by a specific catheter to create fractures within intimal and medial calcium facilitating subsequent stent expansion. Limited data is available on this technique, and it is regarded as off-label use. It could be particularly useful in DES-ISR due to calcium-mediated undilatable stent underexpansion or calcified NIH.[47]

Coronary Artery Bypass Graft

Coronary artery bypass graft for ISR showed superior outcomes to PCI in some studies.[48]

It may be a reasonable option in patients with:

- ISR of the left main stem (LMS)
- Recalcitrant ISR in a major vessel
- Associated multivessel disease
- ISR located in the ostial LAD

Medical Therapy

Oral sirolimus administered before reintervention has been shown to prevent recurrent ISR, but adverse effects and lack of long-term outcomes data preclude its use in routine practice. No drugs have been shown to halt the progression of established ISR in large clinical trials.

Dual antiplatelet therapy for 1 year and intense lipid-lowering therapy and treatment of other cardiovascular risk factors similar to those undergoing PCI for de novo coronary artery disease.

CONCLUSION

Intravascular imaging-guided PCI leads to superior clinical outcomes in patients with DES-ISR. Current data suggests that repeat stenting with second-generation DESs is most likely to lead to the best angiographic and clinical outcomes in DES-ISR. In situations where repeat stenting is not preferable, DCB therapy seems to be a reasonably effective alternative.

ONLINE REFERENCES

Please scan the QR code provided at the end of the table of contents for References of this chapter.

CHAPTER

157

Contemporary Coronary Drug-eluting Stents versus Drug-coated Balloons Update 2024

Panchanan Sahoo, Sateesh Reddy

ABSTRACT

Contemporary drug-eluting stents (DES) are the gold standard for treatment of obstructive coronary artery disease all over the globe. Two important complications of DES are stent thrombosis (ST) and in-stent restenosis (ISR). The medical community all over the world and treating cardiologists fighting untiringly over the last two decades to decrease coronary metal load and stent use speak loud of the slogan "nothing left behind." Although bioresorbable stent use was not successful, contemporary drug-coated balloons (DCB) have shown a promising result and great success in replacing DES not only in the majority of ISR but many cases of de novo coronary obstruction. The present update will give a deep insight into contemporary DES and DCB and draw attention of the medical fraternity through this update to restrict stent use and choose DCB in many cases, which previously had no option but to use DES.

Keywords: Drug-eluting stent, drug-coated/eluting balloon (DCB/DEB), bare metal stent (BMS), target lesion/vessel revascularization (TLR/TVR), main branch (MB), side branch (SB)

INTRODUCTION

Percutaneous coronary intervention (PCI) for obstructive coronary artery disease (CAD) has evolved for almost 40 years since invention of percutaneous transluminal coronary angioplasty (PTCA) by Andreas Gruentzig in 1977. Drug-eluting stent (DES) in present world is the gold standard for catheter-based coronary intervention for obstructive CAD.[1,2] The scope of PTCA has expanded enormously from discrete SVD in the early years, to double, multivessel stenting and even LMCA, complex coronary lesions, and CTO in contemporary world of nonsurgical coronary intervention.

The recoil, dissection, and neointimal formation of vessel after plain balloon angioplasty (POBA) result in acute vessel closure and failure of PCI procedure as high as 40% cases. The use of BMS has been associated with one-third incidence of in-stent restenosis (ISR).[3] Neointimal accumulation remained problematic, resulting in development of ISR in 20–30% of cases.[4] DES an exciting medical technique that reduced ISR to 5–15% with first-generation DES and even lower incidence with second-generation DES. Stent technology has undergone several refinements since discovery by Julio Palmaz between 1978 and 1980. DES was first invented in 2003 and very fast took over the market with a lot of enthusiasm and popularized with refinements year after year. Technology advancements and an improved understanding of the mechanism of ISR have led to the evolution of second-generation DES with thinner struts and greater degrees of early reendothelialization compared to their first-generation counterparts.[5] Even though DES has incrementally improved outcomes after PCI, delayed reendothelialization and stent thrombosis (ST) remain important bottleneck in the success path of PCI. To decrease metal load and with newer concept of nothing left behind, an innovative bioresorbable scaffold with the ABSORB STUDY came to the market. Several stents of this new third generation of DES have been developed over recent years using biodegradable polymers; most of these new stents also use cobalt–chromium or platinum–chromium platforms (allowing ultrathin struts) and many have only abluminal polymer distribution **(Figs. 1A to C and Flowchart 1)**.

BIORESORBABLE STENTS

The ABSORB II study was the first randomized controlled trial (RCT) comparing ABSORB revision 1.1 with XIENCE PRIME.[6]

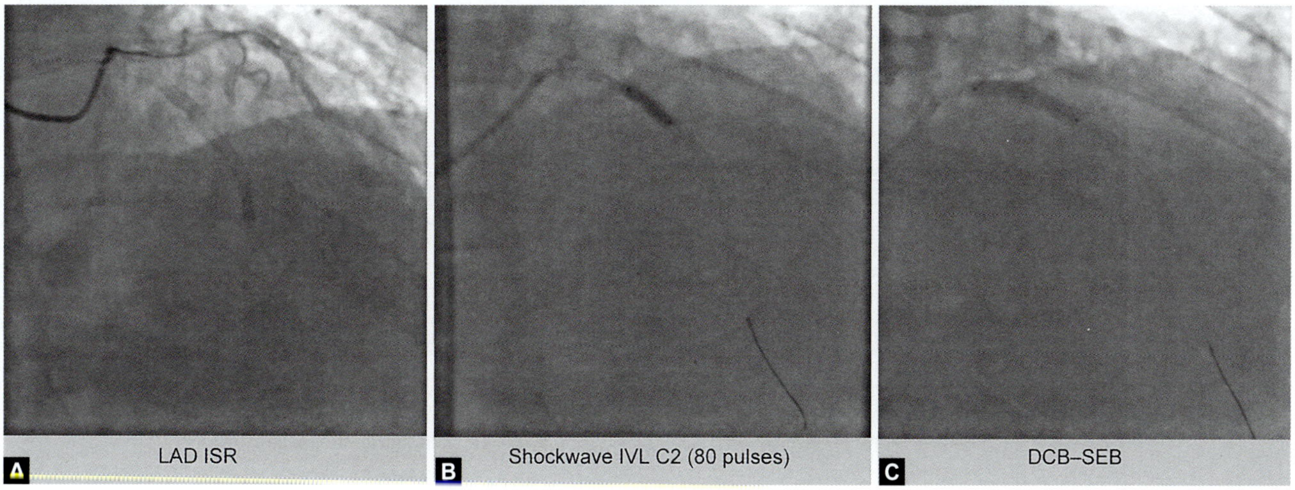

FIGS. 1A TO C: 62/M ISR treated with NCB, IVL, and DCB.

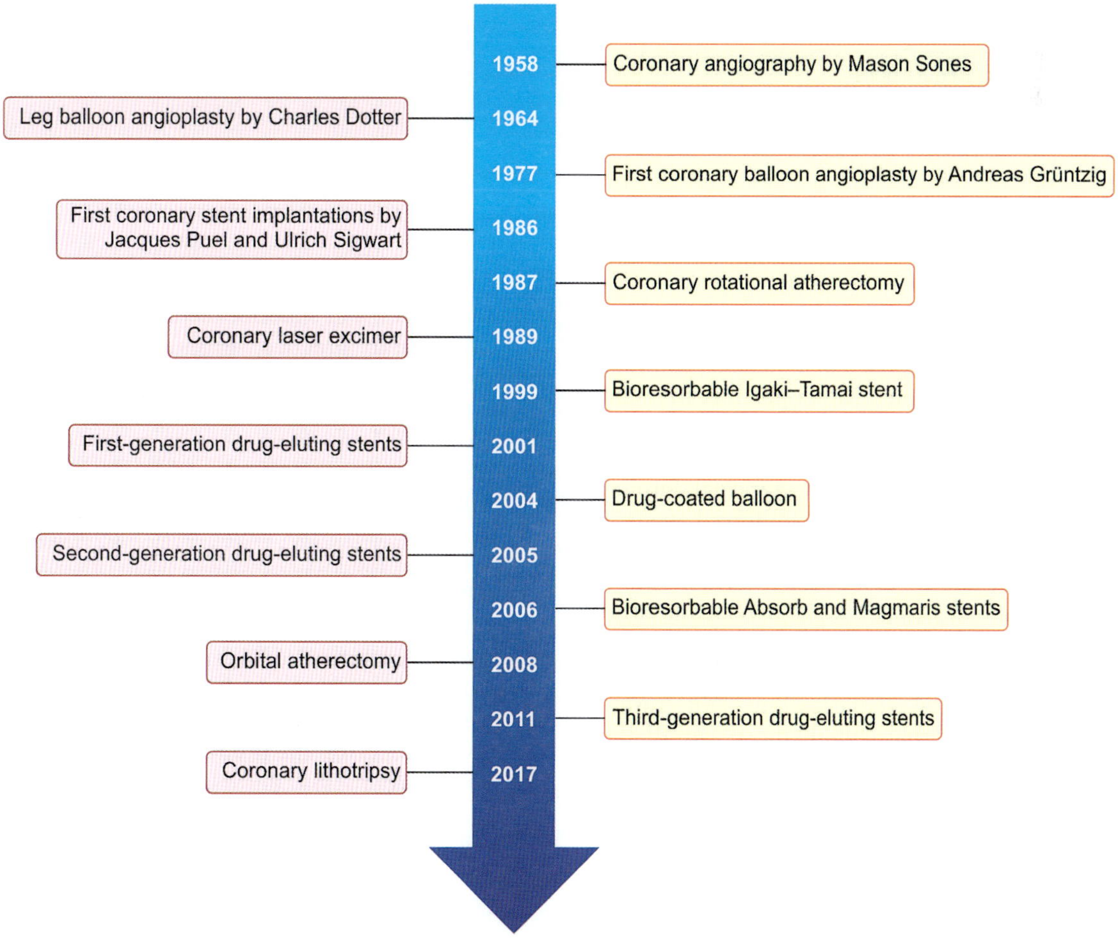

FLOWCHART 1: Evolution of stent.

With the unique mission of no metal, nothing left behind concept to remove metal and polymer from stent, drug-coated/eluting balloon (DEB/DCB) came with successful studies in 2007/2008 **(Flowchart 2)**.

Drug-eluting stents are composed of metallic stents, polymer-based drug delivery platform, and pharmacological agents, immune-suppressant, and/or antiproliferative compounds such as paclitaxel and sirolimus.

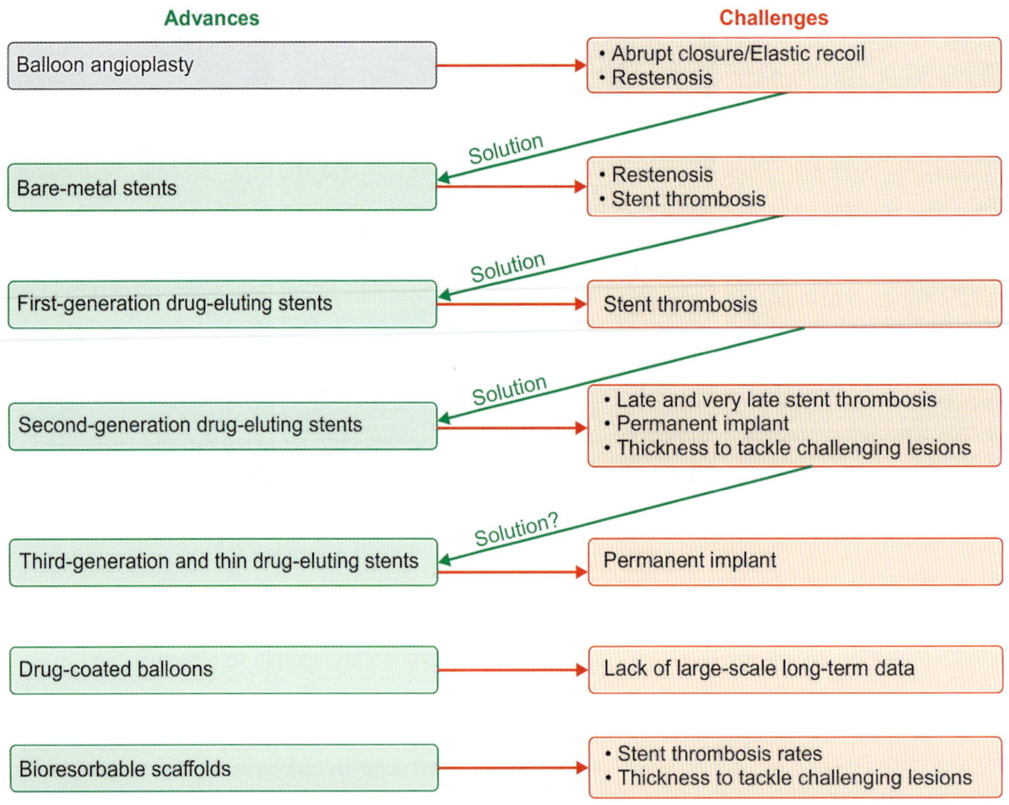

FLOWCHART 2: Advances in stent technology and challenges.

First-generation Drug-eluting Stent

First-generation stents comprised of a metallic, commonly stainless steel platform, coated with a polymer that elutes inflammatory and/or antiproliferative therapeutic agents sirolimus or paclitaxel. Paclitaxel is bacteriostatic and only at higher doses above 100 ng/g it is bactericidal. Sirolimus was originally used as rapamycin, an antifungal agent. The mechanism of action stems from the impedance of cell cycle progression by blocking G1 to S phase transition, thereby suppressing neointimal formation. The RAVEL and SIRIUS trials demonstrated that elution of cytostatic compounds from a stent could effectively reduce the rate of ISR and improve target vessel revascularization (TVR) rates in patients undergoing PCI, particularly those with diabetes with unstable plaque. First-generation DES successfully combated elastic recoil and decreased ISR due to neointimal formation. The problem of ST encountered initially was decreased by the use of dual antiplatelet therapy (DAPT), but the problem of late and very late ST leading to high rates of MI was a constant fatal complication to tackle.

Second-generation Drug-eluting Stent

Second-generation DES offer numerous improvements over their first-generation counterparts. Second-generation devices have decreased strut thickness, improved flexibility/deliverability, enhanced polymer biocompatibility/drug-elution profiles, and superior reendothelialization kinetics. In contemporary practice, second-generation devices are now the predominant coronary stents implanted worldwide. They include paclitaxel, everolimus, and zotarolimus.

- *Paclitaxel*: Taxus Element is an advancement in older PES design. Taxus element used a unique polymer which could release, thus could elute maximum drug within 12 weeks. The Work Horse trial, a noninferiority trial, compared the Taxus Element with Taxus Express. The PERSEUS small vessel trial was a superiority trial which compared element with older BMS control.
- *Everolimus*: It is a second-generation stent that belongs to sirolimus derivative, which is also a cell cycle inhibitor.[7] Everolimus was designed to inhibit SMC proliferation in vitro. Its cytostatic properties rendered it potentially valuable against ISR. The SPIRIT FIRST trial demonstrated similar results with EES versus BMS in de novo coronary lesions. After SPIRIT I came subsequently SPIRIT II and then SPIRIT III, comparing XIENCE V and TAXUS EXPRESS which demonstrated a decrease in major adverse cardiac events (MACE) and improvement in late-lumen loss (LLL). The landmark EXCELLENT trial, the last second-generation trial showed equivalent efficacy of EES to SES. Besides Promus Element stent although had a similar drug and polymer profile offered superior deliverability, thus noninferior compared to the XIENCE and PROMUS.

- *Zotarolimus*: ENDEAVOR I to ENDEAVOR IV showed decreased ISR, decreased ST, and increased vascular healing.[8] Zotarolimus-eluting stent (ZES) uses zotarolimus, an immunosuppressive drug with excellent lipophilic properties eluted over thinner strut cobalt-chromium platform and superior polymer for rapid drug elution and negligible local dispersion, resulting in improved reendothelialization compared to PES and SES. The ENDEAVOR I–IV showed improvement in stent quality. The ENDEAVOR III showed greater LLL and ISR compared to SES (11.7% vs. 4.5%) but paradoxically lower MACE (0.3 vs. 3.5%). The ENDEAVOR IV compared ZES with PES. The ENDEAVOR RESOLUTE is a further stent refinement. The NEWER RESOLUTE INTEGRITY DES uses the same drug but a novel polymer with superior deliverability. The RESOLUTE All-Comer trial compared the Resolute system with Xience V and demonstrated noninferiority of the Resolute system.

Third-generation Drug-eluting Stent

Several new, third-generation DES have been developed over recent years. Along with biodegradable polymers, these new stents use cobalt–chromium or platinum–chromium platforms (allowing ultrathin struts) and several have only abluminal polymer distribution.[9]

Summary of Drug-eluting Stent

First-generation SESs and PESs provided major advances in the treatment of obstructive CAD with marked reductions in ISR. Second-generation stents appear to be safe and efficacious in relation to trackability and deliverability and provide a modest improvement in outcomes compared with their first-generation counterparts. Third-generation stents are further refinement in stent technology, better deliverability and trackability, and less ISR and ST.

DRUG-ELUTING BALLOONS: SHOULD WE USE THEM MORE

Evolution of Drug-eluting Balloon

Drug-eluting balloon is a remarkable treatment method for ISR which can deliver both antiproliferative and anti-inflammatory agents to restenotic vessel segment and does not need extra metal layers of BMS/DES. Although RCTs have compared the clinical efficacy of DES and DEBs so far, treatment of ISR is a field of debate. In 1990, the first concept came that the local delivery of paclitaxel inhibits neointimal proliferation. Following this, in1999, Speck et al. reported even short exposure to paclitaxel was effective in inhibiting tissue proliferation in higher concentrations **(Fig. 2)**.[10,11]

Technology in the Manufacture of Drug-eluting Balloon

Various types of DEB available are noncompliant, semicompliant, and special balloons. These DEBs are coated with antiproliferative drugs that will get released in tunica intima of vessel wall following balloon inflation. The core materials used for DCB preparation include nylon, polyamides, polyvinyl chloride, polypropylene, polyethylene terephthalate, and cross-linked polyethylene. Once DCB is prepared, coating of the active antiproliferative substances such as paclitaxel and sirolimus should be done. Various methods for this coating include dipping, spraying, micropipetting, and drug-coated nanoparticles. In the TRANSFORM I (TReAtmeNt) study on Small Coronary Vessels Magic Touch by nanoparticle technology of a sirolimus-coated balloon failed to achieve noninferior against the SeQuent Please Neo PCB angiographically. The effectiveness of DCB depends on how effectively the drug is transferred to the vessel wall for which biocompatible excipients such as urea, iopromide, shellac, and butyryl trihexyl citrate are used to cover balloons for efficient transfer to the vessel wall. Inflammation and microvascular obstruction are the key challenges faced when there is a loss of particulate covering the DCB to the distal vessel. The balloon catheter is designed to have adequate flexibility, is thin-walled, and has high mechanical strength for effective DEB delivery to target lesion site**(Fig. 3 and Table 1)**.[12,13]

Drug-eluting Balloon Properties

The following properties are essential for the functioning of DEB:
- *Deliverability*: The ability of the balloon to deliver to the lesion site by crossing the calcified, tortuous, and distal lesions
- *Trackability*: The ability of the balloon to curve while translated within the vessel wall
- *Crossability*: The ability of the balloon to pass through a stenotic segment of vessel

Drug-eluting balloon use is beneficial for (1) small vessel de novo disease, (2) large vessel disease, (3) ISR, (4) bifurcation lesions, and (5) patients of higher bleeding risk as there is a shorter duration of DAPT in comparison with DES.

Indication and Limitation of Drug-eluting Balloon

Indications of DEB are ISR and small vessel and large vessel de novo lesions.

Recoil and limitations: Focal vessel wall necrosis is an important limitation.

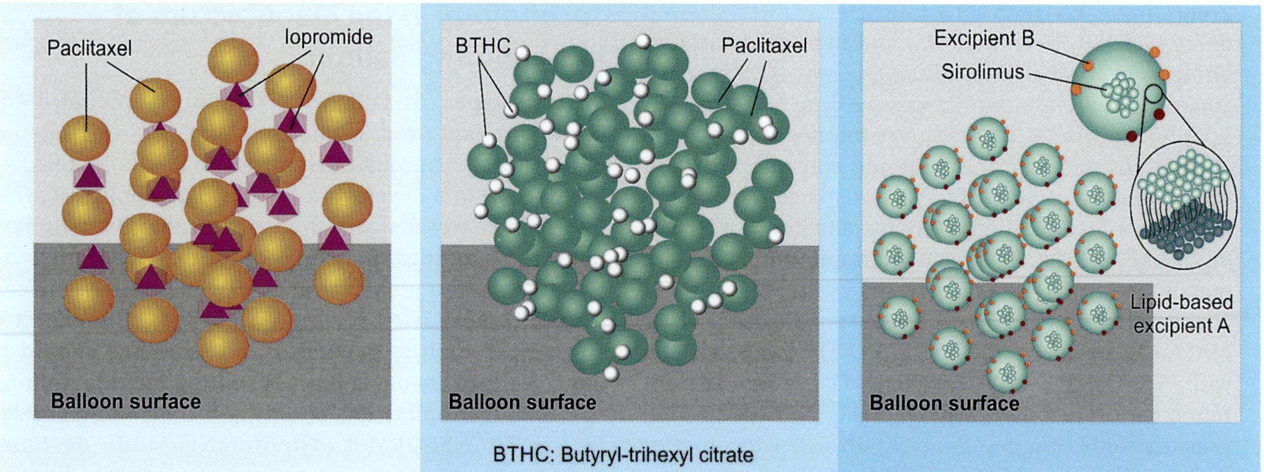

First-generation DCB

Crystalline coating

Efficacy	±
Safety	–
Drug	PTX
Coating homogeneity	–
Particulate formation	+

Second-generation DCB

Noncrystalline coating (Hybrid/Amorphous)

Efficacy	+
Safety	+
Drug	PTX
Coating homogeneity	+
Particulate formation	–

Third-generation DCB

Nanoencapsulation Microcrystalline Coating

Efficacy	?
Safety	?
Drug	SIR
Coating homogeneity	++
Particulate formation	?

FIG. 2: Comparison between different generations of DEB.

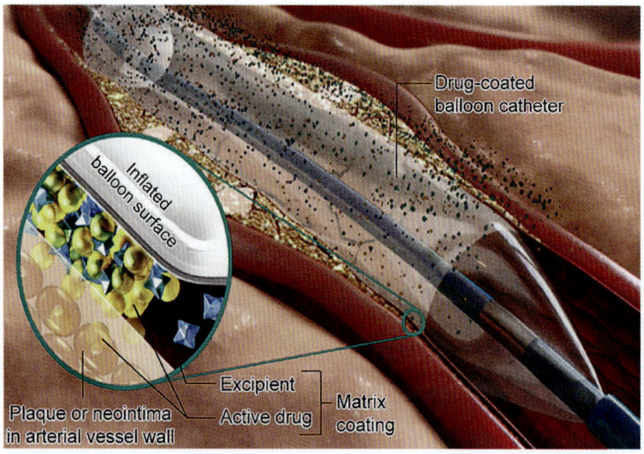

FIG. 3: DCB mechanism of action.

Lesion Preparation and Drug-coated Balloon Delivery

The lesion preparation before DEB delivery plays an important role in the efficient functionality and results of DEB. It results in homogenous drug delivery to the intimal vessel wall, achieving sufficient lumen gain and identifying the lesions at risk of closure. Inadequate lesion preparation before DCB application was an independent predictor of target lesion revascularization (TLR). In case of simple lesions, lesion preparation with a semicompliant or noncompliant balloon is used, with a balloon-to-vessel ratio of 0.8–1.0, with an inflation pressure higher than nominal. For lesion modification, cutting or scoring balloons are used. In complex, calcified lesions, the use of adjunctive intracoronary imaging and therapies including rota ablation, excimer laser atherectomy, and intravascular lithotripsy (IVL) may be considered. Recently, using of DCBs with intravascular brachytherapy has appeared promising for lengthening the ISR-free interval. The lesion-crossing nature of current-generation DCBs is better than that of first-generation DCBs. The success rate of the DCB delivery after adequate predilation is higher for the simple and proximal lesions in comparison to distal lesions, tortuous vessels, and heavily calcified vessel. The latter lesions have high chance of DEB delivery failure. Once the lesion is prepared, one should check for the angiographic criteria for adequate predilation before the DCB is delivered. The results are considered optimal if the balloon is fully inflated at nominal pressure, absence of flow-limiting dissection, TIMI flow grade is III, and residual stenosis ≤ 30%. If adequate predilation results are not obtained, bailout implantation with second- or third-generation DES is recommended. After the successful

TABLE 1: DES versus DEB.

	DES	DEB
Platform of drug delivery	Stent scaffolding	Balloon
Retention	Polymer based	Embedded imprinted
Drug dose	Low: <100–200 mg	High: 300–600 mg
Release kinetics	Slow and controlled	Fast release
Distribution	Strut-based vascular penetration	Balloon surface homogenous distribution
Advantages	Mechanical support	Leave no implant
	Abluminal trapping	Large surface area
	Less drug spillage into the circulation	Less drug localization in the vessel wall
	Proven efficacy in many indications	Accessible to complex lesions and long segments
	No acute recoil tackled dissection	May not require prolonged DAPT

predilation and angiographic results are achieved, DCB should be loaded carefully over the wire as it may shed the drug when touched or after contact with liquid. The lesion should be covered at least 2 mm proximally and distally, followed by sufficient inflation time of at least 30 seconds to allow adequate drug transfer. Attention should be paid to minimizing the transit time to the lesion to avoid excessive drug loss during delivery. Recently, Colombo et al. proposed that in the absence of major dissection distal to aortic coronary pressure ratio (Pd/Pa) values > 0.90 in the main vessel and side branch (SB) support a DCB-only approach.[14,15]

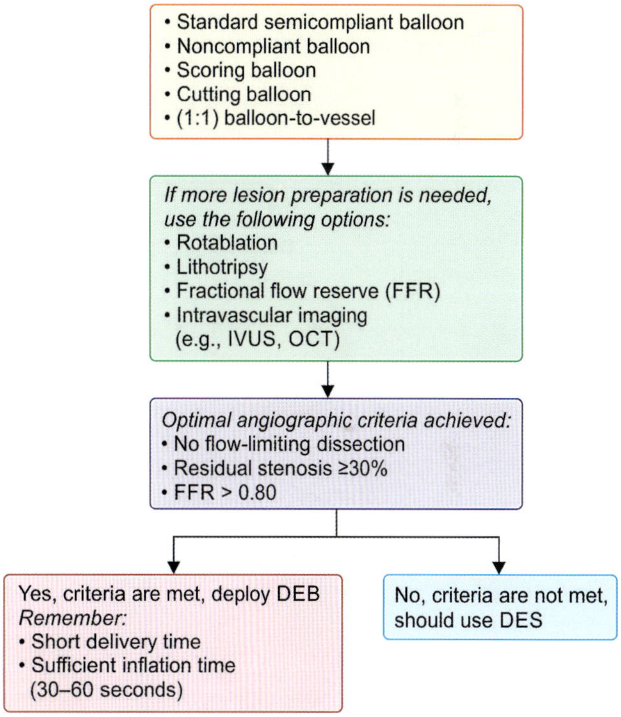

FLOWCHART 3: Algorithm showing DCB treatment.

DRUG-COATED BALLOON-ONLY TREATMENT ALGORITHM ACCORDING TO THE INTERNATIONAL DRUG-COATED BALLOON CONSENSUS GROUP (FLOWCHART 3)

PCB use for ISR: The incidence of ISR is more worrisome for the treating cardiologist as mentioned earlier with the use of BMS to third-generation DES. Various complex mechanisms such as neointimal proliferation, neoatherosclerosis, vascular remodeling, insufficient expansion of the stent, or stent strut fracture result in ISR. To decrease the metal load inside the epicardial coronaries and decrease the incidence of ISR, DEBs are safe and efficient and there is leave no metal behind strategy with the use of DEB. With favorable evidence, the 2014 European guidelines reemphasized in 2023 advocated the use of DCB as Class I (Level of evidence A) recommendation for the treatment of coronary ISR. Various trials have been conducted to see the effectiveness of DEB over DES in use for ISR. The PACCOCATH ISR was the first RCT that showed significantly better angiographic results using PCB compared to uncoated balloons, with less in-segment LLL of 0.03 ± 0.48 versus 0.74 ± 0.86 mm for uncoated balloons ($p = 0.002$), and reduced incidence of ISR at 6 months with DAPT recommendation for only 4 weeks after DCB. Even long-term follow-up results were lower than MACE, mainly driven by the reduction of TLR. This DAPT duration of 4 weeks and better angiographic results with low incidence of ISR has further attracted interventional cardiologists for the use of DEB-only strategy for ISR and high-bleeding-risk patients.[5,16] The RIBS IV [Restenosis Intrastent of DES: Drug-eluting Balloon vs. Everolimus-eluting Stent (EES)] which studies the advantage of EES over PCB showed a significant advantage of EES over PCB for the treatment of DES-ISR. DARE (Drug-eluting balloon for ISR) and RESTORE (The Treatment of DES REstenosis Using DES versus DCB for Preventing recurrent ISR) show the noninferiority of the PCB against second-generation DES. In comparison to DES, DCBs offer delivery of antiproliferative medication to the ISR lesion without additional deployment of metal, with acceptable angiographic and clinical outcomes and a shorter duration of DAPT therapy; thus, if available, DCBs should be preferred over DES for the treatment of ISR **(Fig. 4 and Flowchart 4)**.[17,18]

SVD: It (vessels size < 2.75 mm) has been shown to have higher rates of restenosis regardless of the type of intervention. Earlier PICCOLETO study was prematurely stopped due to increased MACE. Subsequent studies such as BELLO, BASKET SMALL 2, and RESTORE SVD showed noninferiority of DCB compared to DES **(Flowchart 5)**.

Bifurcation lesions: PCI in bifurcation lesion has been considered complex and challenging and a matter of debate. Old PEPCAD V study used DCB in SB and BMS in MB PEPCAD V and BIOLUX 1 showed favorable results using PCBs to treat SB lesions, whereas PEPCAD-BIF showed PCB-only strategy for bifurcation lesions safe and feasible versus POBA.[19]

The "L-sandwich" strategy implants a stent in the SB shaft so that the acute gain of the diameter can be similar to the two-stent technique and can cover dissection. The "L-sandwich" strategy reserves a 3–5 mm stent-free area at the SB ostium to avoid stent overlapping and stent deformation **(Figs. 5A to H and Flowchart 6)**.[20]

LVD: There is limited data on the use of DCB in large vessel disease, whatever data available from nonrandomized trials. Comparable study reports between PCB and second-generation DES at 5 years available from SPARTAN drug-coated study reports.[21,22]

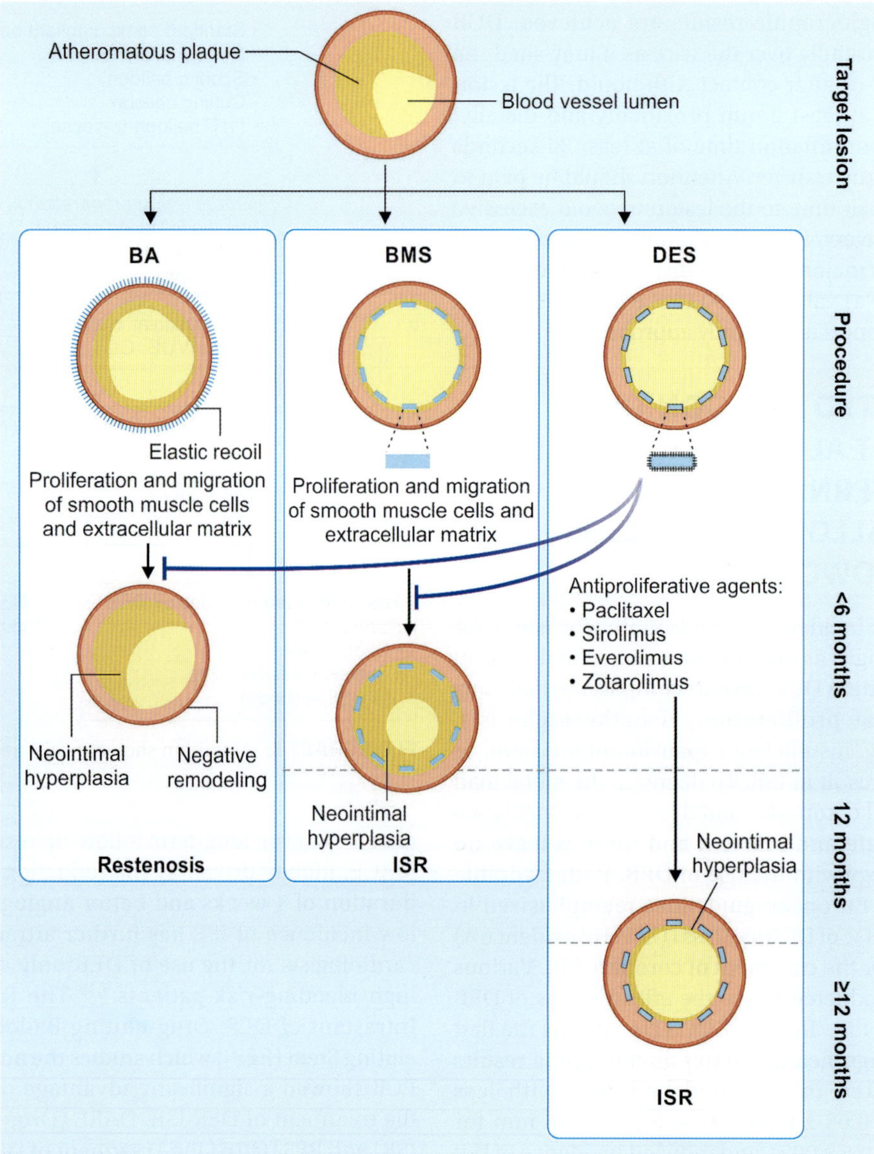

FIG. 4: Mechanism of ISR in BA, BMS, and DES.

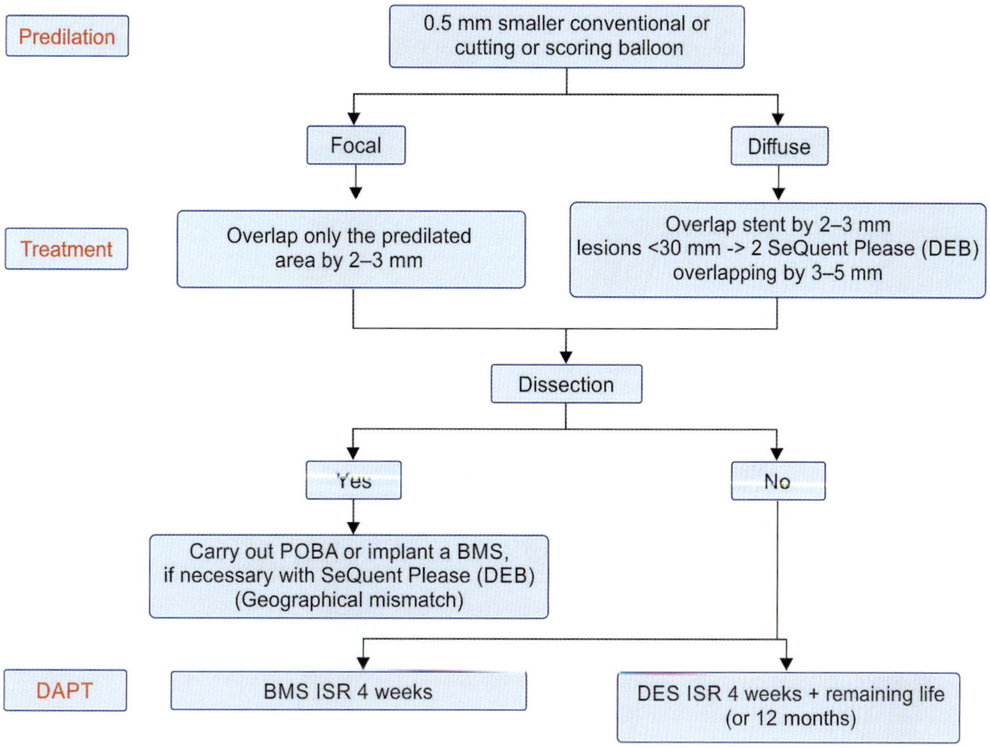

FLOWCHART 4: Treatment of ISR by German (ESC) Consensus Group.

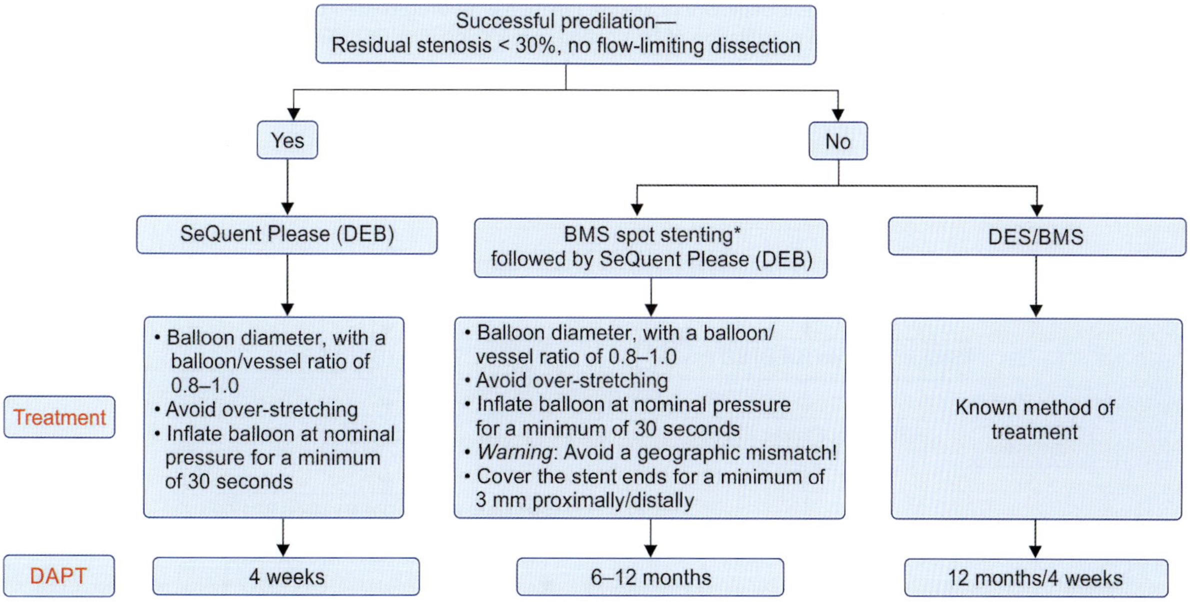

* Small vessel disease is a real challenge for revascularization. As per latest clinical trials and evidences DEB is preferred to decrease metal load and shorten DAPT therapy over DES.

FLOWCHART 5: Treatment of SVD by German (ESC) Consensus Group.

ACUTE CORONARY SYNDROME

The first study evaluating PCB angioplasty was the PAPPA study which demonstrated encouraging clinical results. Recently THE PEPCAD NSTEMI and REVELATION (DCB vs. DES in Acute MI) trials demonstrated DCB-only strategy was noninferior to DES treatment in NSTEMI.[23,24]

Diabetes mellitus: Patients with diabetes have worse clinical outcomes following PCI and CABG. A subgroup analysis of

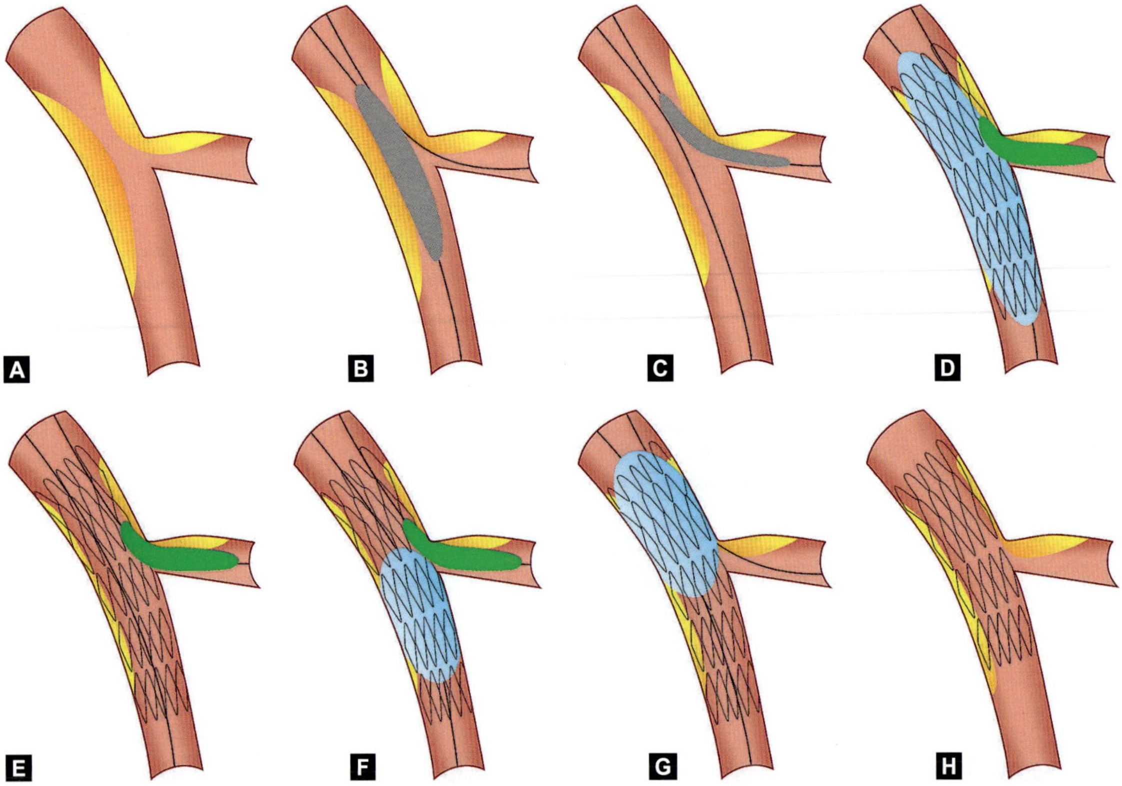

FIGS. 5A TO H: Schematic image depicting the key steps of the hybrid technique: (A) Coronary bifurcation lesion; (B) Preparation for main branch; (C) Preparation for side branch; (D) Stent deployment kissing inflation with drug-coated balloon (DCB); (E) Persistent inflation of DCB when removing stent balloon; (F) Balloon postdilation of bifurcation core kissing with DCB; (G) Proximal optimization technique; and (H) Final results.

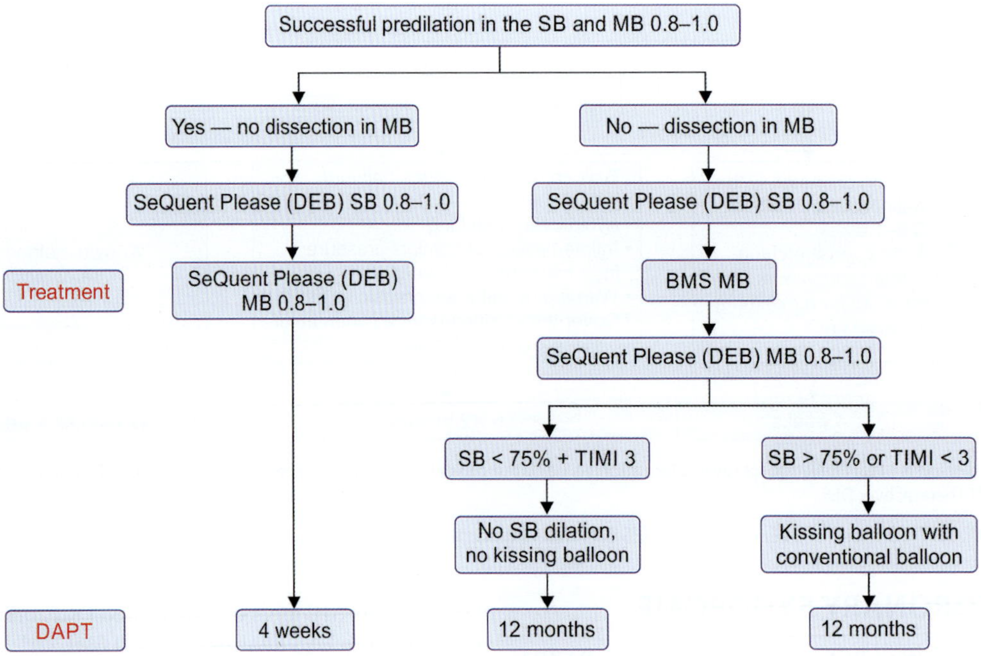

FLOWCHART 6: Treatment of Bifurcation Stenosis by German (ESC) Consensus Group.

the BELLO randomized trial demonstrated superiority of PCB with a better MACE rate in diabetes with SVD.[25]

HBR: DCB angioplasty has been considered the choice of PCI in recent years while thinking of reducing DAPT duration. DAPT duration has been reduced as short as 4 months in cases of high bleeding risk. DCB is preferred over DES angioplasty in ACS patients including STEMI and NSTEMI with de novo coronary and complex coronary lesions such as bifurcation disease, SVD, CTOs, LMCA lesions, long lesions, and MVD. The DCB International Consensus Group recommends 4 weeks of DAPT therapy for de novo coronary lesions **(Flowchart 7)**.[26,27]

LIMUS-COATED BALLOON STUDIES

Limus-based DCB were investigated in the TRANSFORM 1 trial. SCB failed to show noninferiority in net lumen gain at 6 months compared to PCB. The ongoing TRANSFORM 2 trial will compare SEB with current generation EES.[28,29]

CONCLUSION

The concept of the "leave nothing behind" strategy has grown with the advent and research on PCBs. After ESC Class I LOE A recommendation of DCBs for the treatment of ISR, there is growing interest in the use of the technology in diabetes, SVD, long diffuse disease, bifurcation lesions, high bleeding risk, ACS, and complex coronary interventions as these patients may potentially benefit from a DCB-only approach. The decrease in DAPT duration to 4 weeks following DCB has brought new enthusiasm among interventional cardiologists for expeditious DCB use for multifarious indications. The future directions of DES and DCB in 2024 can be imagined for an efficient utilization of robotic PCI and artificial intelligence.

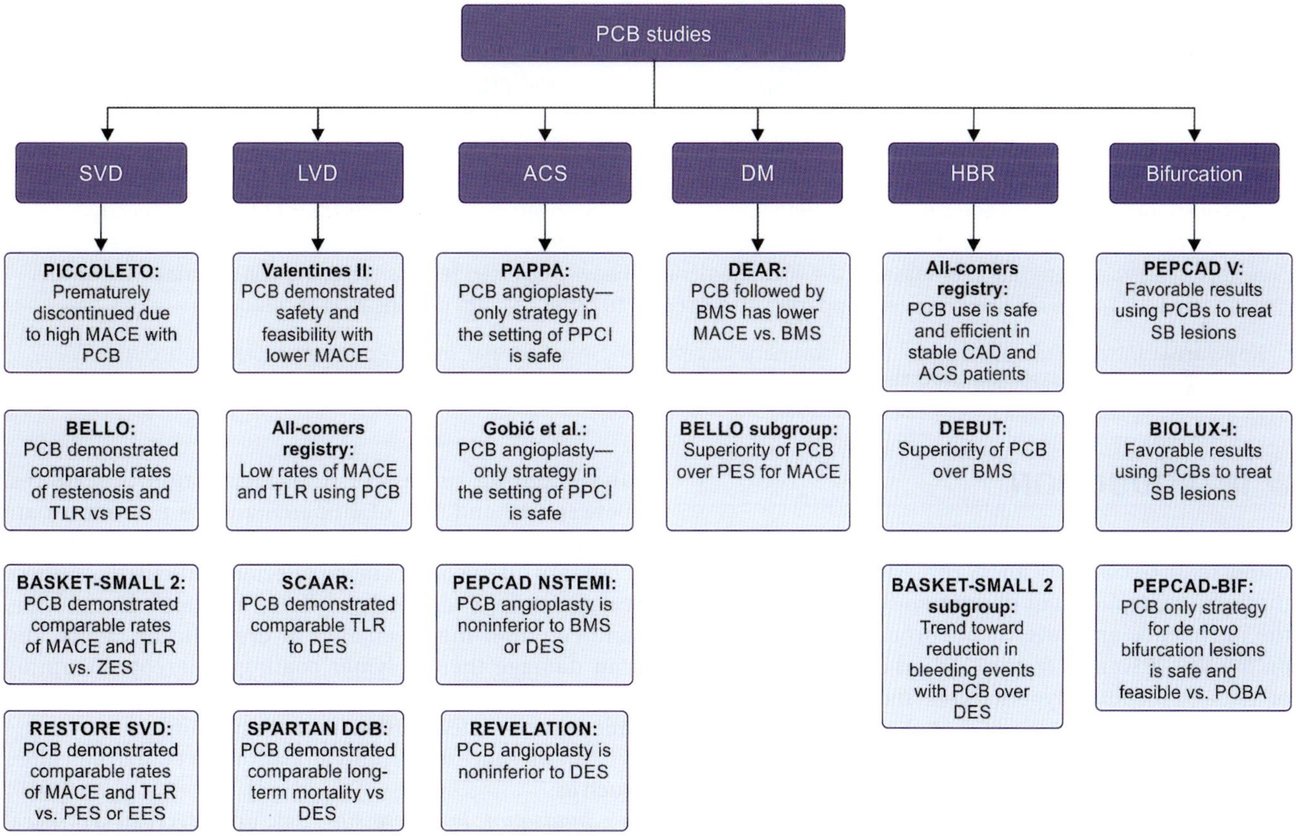

FLOWCHART 7: PCB studies.

ONLINE REFERENCES

Please scan the QR code provided at the end of the table of contents for References of this chapter.

CHAPTER

158

Intravascular Lithotripsy: When and How

Debdatta Bhattacharyya, Saurabh Dhumale

ABSTRACT

Intravascular lithotripsy (IVL) has emerged as a ground-breaking technique in the management of calcified coronary artery disease, addressing the significant challenges posed by vascular calcification during percutaneous coronary interventions (PCI). Traditional methods, such as high-pressure balloons and atherectomy devices, often fail to adequately modify calcified lesions, leading to suboptimal stent deployment and increased procedural complications. IVL, borrowing from extracorporeal shockwave lithotripsy principles, offers a novel approach by delivering pulsatile acoustic pressure waves to disrupt calcified deposits with minimal risk of vessel injury. This technology enhances lesion preparation and enables optimal stent expansion, leading to improved procedural outcomes. Clinical trials, particularly the disrupt CAD series, have demonstrated the efficacy and safety of IVL, with low rates of major adverse cardiac events (MACE) and high success rates even in complex lesion subsets. Despite the high cost and slightly larger profile of IVL devices, its simplicity and promising results make it a preferred alternative in the management of heavily calcified lesions. Ongoing clinical trials will further delineate IVL's role in routine practice, comparing its outcomes to other calcium modification techniques.

Keywords: Intravascular lithotripsy (IVL), coronary calcification, intravascular imaging, intravascular ultrasound (IVUS), optical coherence tomography (OCT)

INTRODUCTION

Percutaneous coronary intervention (PCI) remains the cornerstone of coronary artery revascularization, primarily through the deployment of drug-eluting stents. However, the prevalence and severity of coronary calcification are on the rise, driven by factors such as age, increasing rates of diabetes mellitus, hypertension, and renal insufficiency. This calcification poses significant challenges to traditional revascularization techniques, often complicating procedural execution and long-term outcomes due to issues like stent under-expansion leading to increased risks of restenosis and stent thrombosis together with the devastating complication of coronary perforation.

CHALLENGES POSED BY VASCULAR CALCIFICATION

Vascular calcification significantly diminishes arterial compliance, which can severely impact both the immediate and enduring success of revascularization procedures. Between 18 and 50% of all percutaneous procedures are complicated by the presence of calcified lesions, with coronary interventions being affected particularly.[1,2] These calcifications hinder device delivery, impair stent expansion, and can alter the mechanics of drug-eluting stents, and can damage their polymer coatings, thereby disrupting drug delivery and elution dynamics. (insert pic: electron micrograph of stent pushed through calcium)

The presence of calcium can lead to procedural difficulties such as:

- *Inadequate lesion crossing:* Calcium can create a physical barrier, preventing the passage of balloons and stents.
- *Under-expansion of stents:* Incomplete stent expansion due to calcium impedes proper apposition, leading to suboptimal outcomes **(Figs. 1A and B)**.
- *Increased risk of stent thrombosis:* Poorly expanded stents are prone to thrombus formation, which can result in acute or late stent thrombosis **(Fig. 2)**.
- *Increased risk of in-stent restenosis:* Calcium can obscure angiographic assessment of lesion, making it challenging

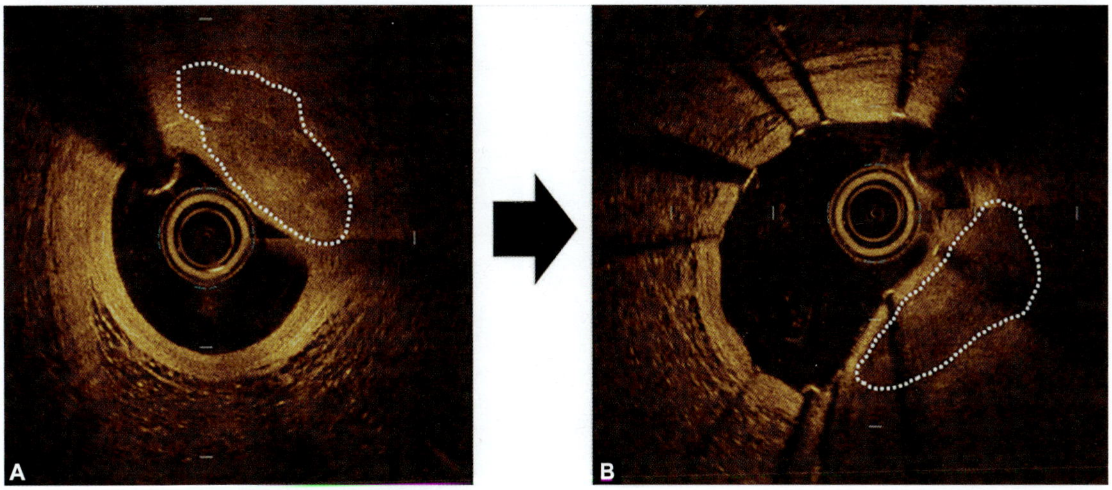

FIGS. 1A AND B: (A) Optical coherence tomography image showing thick calcific plaque, (B) resulting in under-expanded stent due to said calcific plaque.[3]

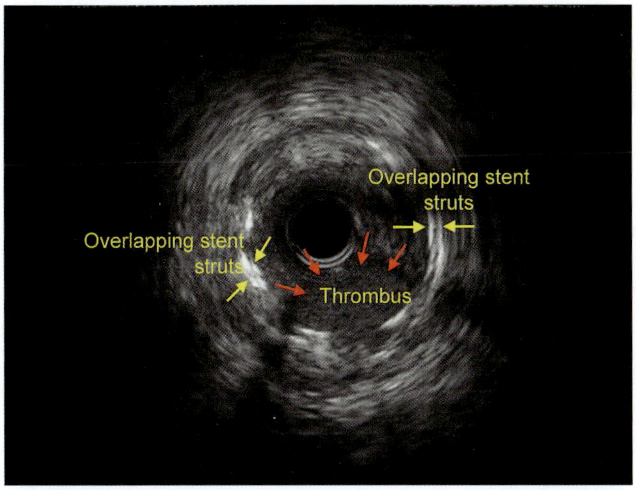

FIG. 2: Intravascular ultrasound image corresponding to the stenosis shows a thrombus at the site of stent overlap and under-expansion.

to accurately assess the extent and severity of the lesion, resulting in undersized and under-expanded stents, leading to increased rates of early and late ISR **(Figs. 3A to C)**.

Until recently, traditional arsenal for tackling calcification included, high-pressure noncompliant balloon catheters (OPN-NC), cutting and scoring balloons, and various atheroablative technologies such as rotational, orbital, and laser atherectomy, faces significant limitations. These methods quite often fail to sufficiently modify the calcium or might induce severe complications such as coronary dissection, slow flow phenomena, myocardial infarction, and even vessel perforation due to barotrauma **(Figs. 4 to 6)**.

INTRODUCTION TO INTRAVASCULAR LITHOTRIPSY

Intravascular lithotripsy (IVL) has been introduced as a transformative approach to address these challenges. Borrowing principles from the extracorporeal shockwave lithotripsy are used to treat kidney stones, IVL adapts these for vascular application. This innovative technique utilizes a balloon catheter embedded with lithotripsy emitters that emit pulsatile acoustic pressure waves. These waves are directed circumferentially, allowing for a targeted and localized disruption of calcific deposits without extensive damage to surrounding tissues.

The effectiveness and safety of IVL have been demonstrated across numerous studies, including the Disrupt CAD series (I–IV), which have shown promising results in treating severely calcified coronary and peripheral arterial stenoses. These studies have not only highlighted the high rates of procedural success, but also provided insights into the mechanisms through which IVL modifies vascular calcium, enhancing lesion preparation, and optimizing outcomes for stent deployment.

This introduction sets the stage for a detailed examination of IVL's mechanisms, its clinical applications, and the potential it holds to revolutionize the treatment of calcified arterial lesions in diverse patient populations.

PRINCIPLES OF INTRAVASCULAR LITHOTRIPSY

Unlike cutting/scoring and noncompliant balloons that depend on inducing barotrauma, IVL relies on the creation of circumferential, pulsatile pressure waves. These waves are

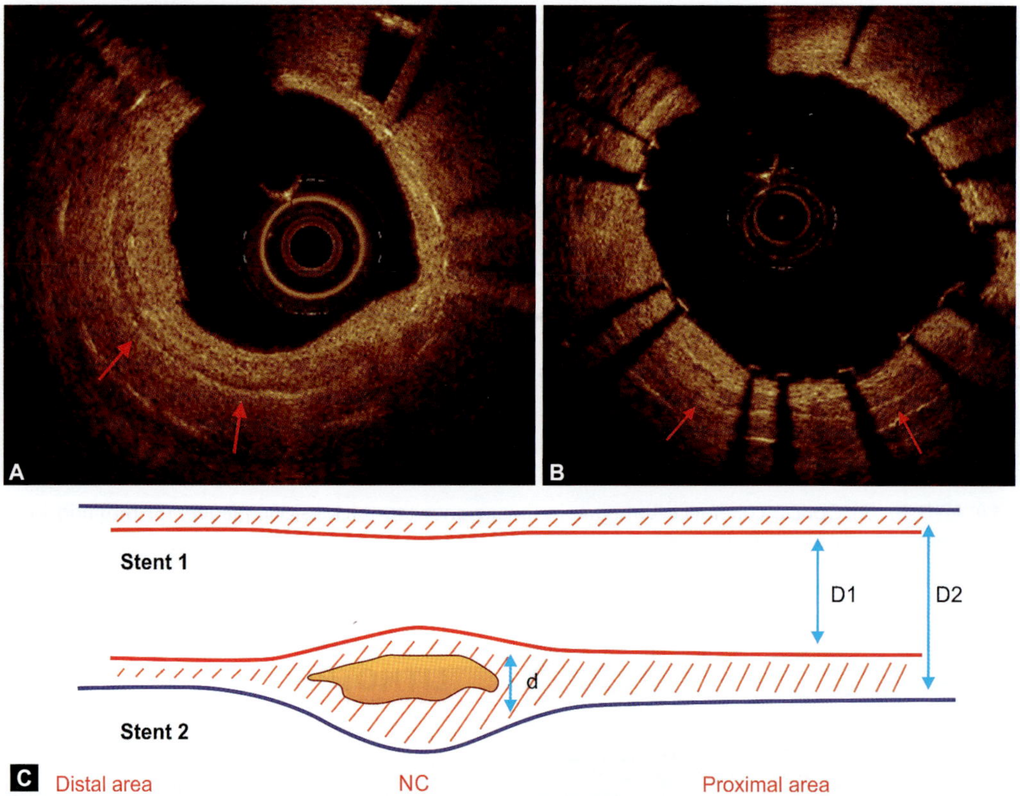

FIGS. 3A TO C: A case of in-stent restenosis with neointimal calcification, indicated by a red arrows, is shown in optical coherence tomography (OCT) images before (A) and after (B) a stent-in-stent implantation. (C) Offers a schematic detailing how neointimal calcification (NC) affects stent expansion, with "D" representing the stent diameter and "d" the distance between stents. These images and schematic highlight the complexities of treating restenosis complicated by calcification and demonstrate the value of OCT in planning and confirming successful interventions.[4]

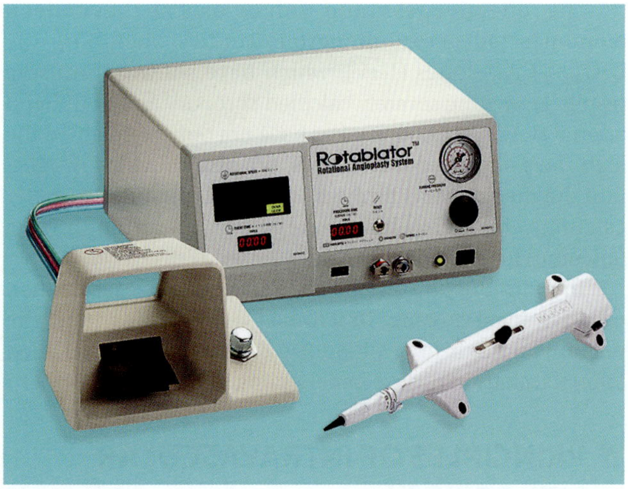

FIG. 4: Rotablator™ rotational atherectomy system, from Boston Scientific.

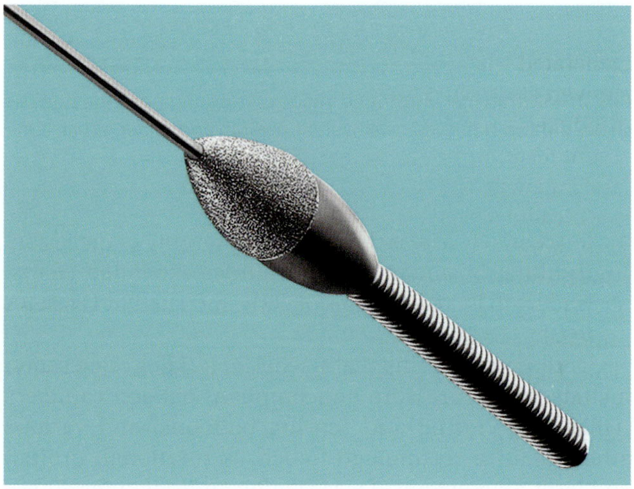

FIG. 5: Burr of Rotablator™ rotational atherectomy system, from Boston Scientific.

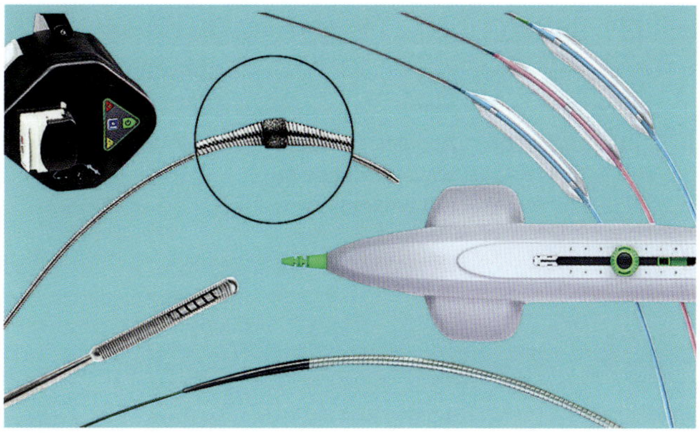

FIG. 6: Diamondback 360 Precision™ orbital atherectomy system (OAS).

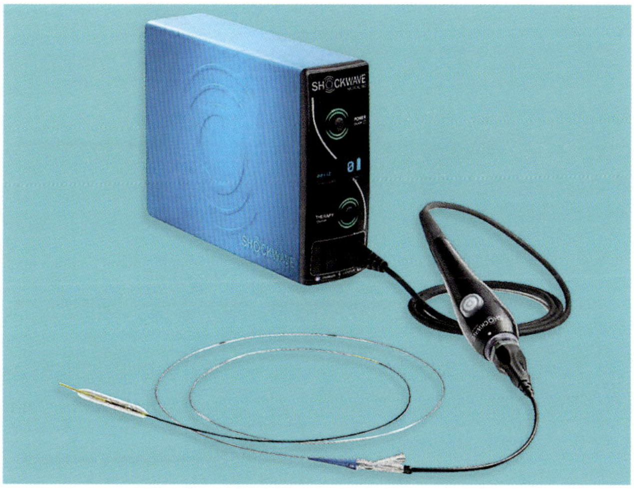

FIG. 7: Shockwave intravascular lithotripsy system.

generated when two lithotripsy emitters within the balloon convert electrical pulses into mechanical energy. This action produces a sonic pressure wave with a force equivalent to about 50 atmospheres (atm). These waves effectively target and fragment both superficial and deep calcium in the vessel wall, leading to the creation of microfractures. Consequently, this increases vessel compliance, aiding in subsequent effective vessel expansion by balloons and stents. The design of IVL ensures that calcium fragments remain in place, minimizing the risk of vessel trauma in noncalcified tissues. This feature also reduces potential complications such as slow-flow or no-reflow that can occur from embolized microparticles in distal vessels **(Fig. 7)**.

INTRAVASCULAR IMAGING-BASED CASE SELECTION FOR INTRAVASCULAR LITHOTRIPSY

Understanding the location, thickness, and distribution of calcification is crucial for selecting the most effective lesion preparation strategy. Traditional coronary angiography, although commonly used, has a low sensitivity for detecting calcification. It fails to identify calcified lesions in about half of the cases and does not provide a reliable assessment of the extent of the calcification, such as its length, thickness, and arc of the calcification.

In contrast, intravascular imaging techniques such as intravascular ultrasound (IVUS) and optical coherence tomography (OCT) offer more precise evaluations. They both are reliable tools for qualitative and quantitative assessments of vascular calcium. IVUS facilitates the identification of the presence, length, and angle of calcium, characterized by a sharp white border with acoustic shadowing. However, this acoustic shadowing limits its capacity to measure the thickness of calcium. On the other hand, OCT provides a more detailed view of calcium's extent, defined as signal-poor regions with sharp, circumscribed borders, and enables quantitative volumetric analyses based on the arc, length, and thickness of the calcification. Despite its detailed imaging capabilities, OCT's lower penetration depth compared to IVUS means it may not as effectively detect deeper calcifications.

The comparative features of the currently available calcium modification technologies highlight that IVL is ideally suited for thick, plate-like calcium (>0.5 mm in thickness, 5 mm in length, and >180° in circumference) which can be either superficial or deep within the vessel wall. Recent OCT analyses have shown that up to 77% of calcified nodules can be effectively modified by IVL, leading to symmetric stent expansion. However, differentiating between calcified nodules that are amenable to IVL and those that are not remains a challenge **(Table 1)**.

INTRAVASCULAR LITHOTRIPSY PROCEDURE STEPS

1. Start with intravascular imaging, see weather OCT/IVUS catheter is able to pass freely through the lesion.
2. If imaging catheter does not pass, then opt for atherectomy (rotational/orbital) prior to IVL.
3. After imaging, determine the appropriate balloon size, using a 1:1 ratio relative to the reference vessel diameter (RVD), or select the largest suitable balloon when the vessel diameter exceeds 4.0 mm.
4. Set up the IVL balloon following prescribed preparation methods, making sure there are no air bubbles in the catheter system.
5. Position the balloon precisely at the lesion site after adequate predilatation.
6. If the balloon is unable to cross the lesion despite of bed preparation, use mother and child catheter technique.
7. Inflate the balloon to a pressure of 4 atm and administer an initial cycle of 10 pulses.
8. After inflation, deflate the balloon completely.
9. Pause for a minimum of 10 seconds to allow for adequate distal blood flow.

TABLE 1: Various coronary calcium modification system and their suitable use scenarios.

Feature	IVL	RA	OA	ELCA	Noncompliant and specialty balloons
Mechanism of action	Acoustic pressure waves induced by electrical energy	Atheroablation	Atheroablation	Acoustic pressure waves induced by ultraviolet light	Barotrauma
Suitable for (imaging defined calcium extent)					
Superficial calcification	+		+	+	+
Deep calcification	+		+/–	+	+/–
Concentric calcification	+	+	+	+/–	+/–
Eccentric calcification	+	+/–	+/–	+	–
Calcified nodules	+/–	+	+	–	–

10. Repeat steps 4–7 as necessary, adjusting the balloon's position as required for optimal treatment. With every balloon inflation and delivery of pulses, watch whether balloon waist disappears, signifying cracks in the calcium.
11. Once you are done with delivering the pulses, increase the pressure to 6 atm, which is the nominal pressure for the balloon.

INTRAVASCULAR LITHOTRIPSY BALLOON SIZING AND EMITTER ALIGNMENT

The IVL employs acoustic emitters, aligned in sequence along the balloon's length. These emitters are set up as diametrically opposite pairs (180° from each other), emitting spherical energy profiles that mirror each other symmetrically along the edge of the balloon. This configuration results in signature patterns of peak acoustic pressures that corresponds to the emitters' placements along the IVL catheter **(Fig. 8)**. When activated, these paired emitters generate acoustic pressure waves that spread circumferentially and transmurally, effectively disrupting vascular calcium. A posthoc analysis from the Disrupt PAD II study, focusing on the Shockwave Lithoplasty DISRUPT trial for peripheral artery disease, underscored the significance of precise IVL catheter sizing and emitter alignment. This study revealed that optimal IVL technique crucially affects 12-month primary patency rates when utilized as a standalone therapy in treating superficial femoral and popliteal arterial segments. Properly sizing the IVL balloon relative to the RVD and ensuring accurate alignment are vital. The study defined optimal balloon sizing as having a ratio of the IVL balloon to RVD of at least 1:1. A therapeutic miss, which compromises treatment efficacy, occurs when lithotripsy does not fully cover overlap segments or the extremities of the lesion.

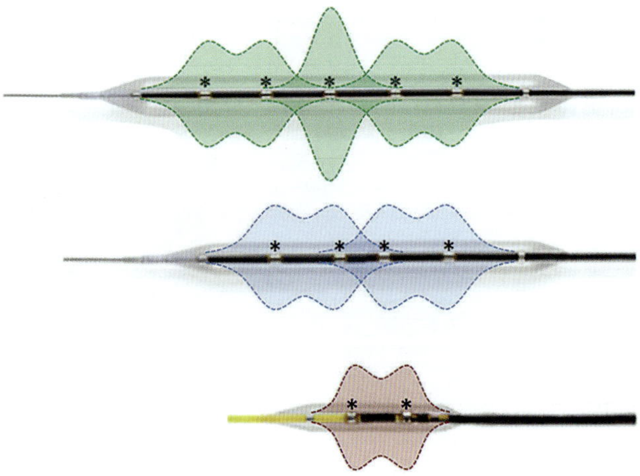

FIG. 8: Acoustic peak pressure aligns with emitter location.[5]

This meticulous approach to IVL application significantly boosts the 12-month primary patency and diminishes the need for subsequent interventions on the target lesion. Notably, no increase in adverse events was reported even when the IVL balloon size slightly exceeded the RVD. Following these insights, the Shockwave M5 and S4 IVL catheters (peripheral) recommend a sizing guideline of 1.1:1 relative to the RVD for optimal coverage, particularly for lengthy lesions. For the Shockwave C2 and C2+ (coronary) IVL catheter, a 1:1 sizing ratio is advised. These guidelines are designed to maximize therapeutic effectiveness and safety across varying vessel dimensions, and have been derived from experiences from both peripheral and coronary lithoplasty.

CASE EXAMPLES

Case 1 (Figs. 9A and B)

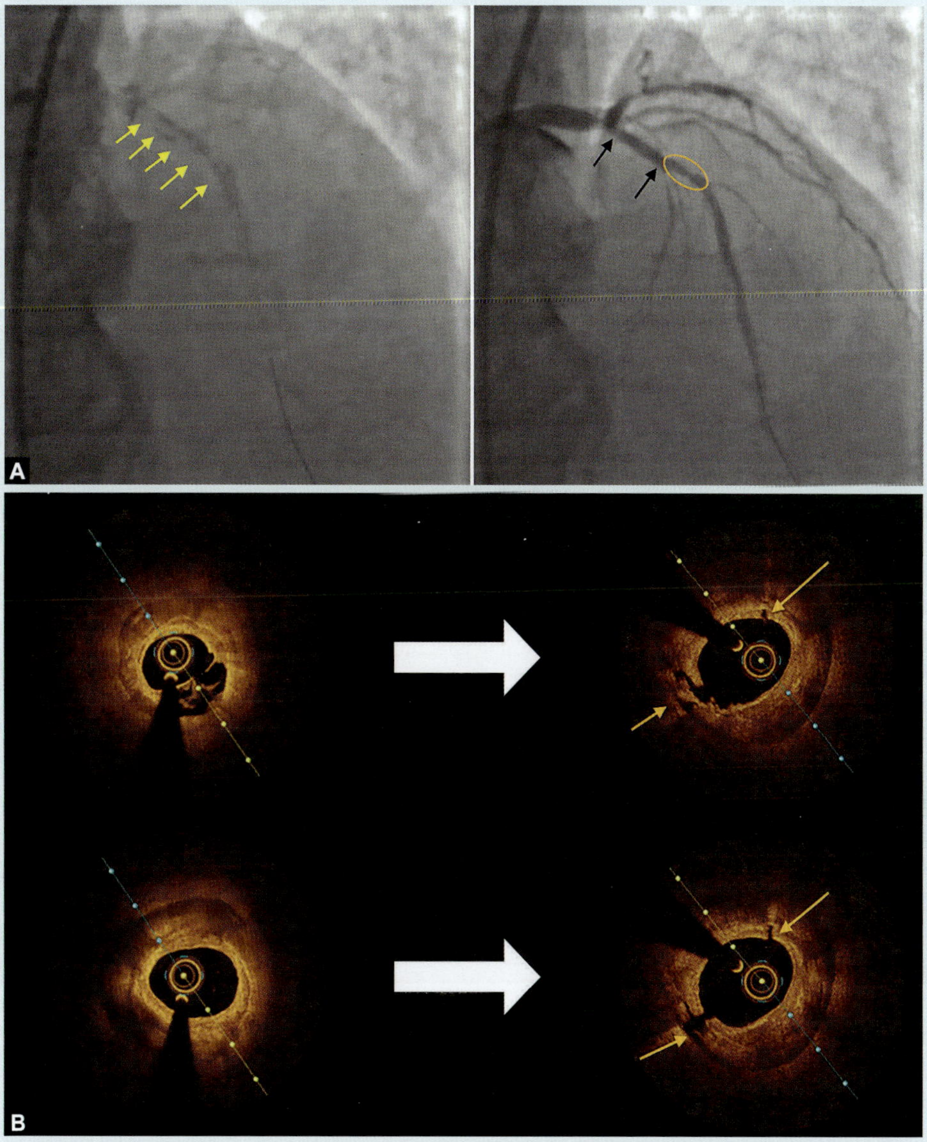

FIGS. 9A AND B: A 74-year-old male patient, who has a history of diabetes and hypertension, presented with unstable angina. His medical background includes anemia due to gastric antral vascular ectasia (GAVE) and a previous percutaneous transluminal coronary angioplasty (PTCA) to the left anterior descending (LAD) artery in 2010. The current evaluation revealed severe diffuse vascular disease (DVD) with heavy calcification. His ejection fraction (EF) was assessed at 50%, indicating a moderate reduction in heart function. Figure (A) Shows "Tram-Track" angiographic calcification with corresponding narrowing of the lumen, while (B) reveals preintravascular lithotripsy (IVL) versus post-IVL optical coherence tomography (OCT) images and subsequent cracks delivered in calcium.

CASE EXAMPLES

Case 2 (Figs. 10A to C)

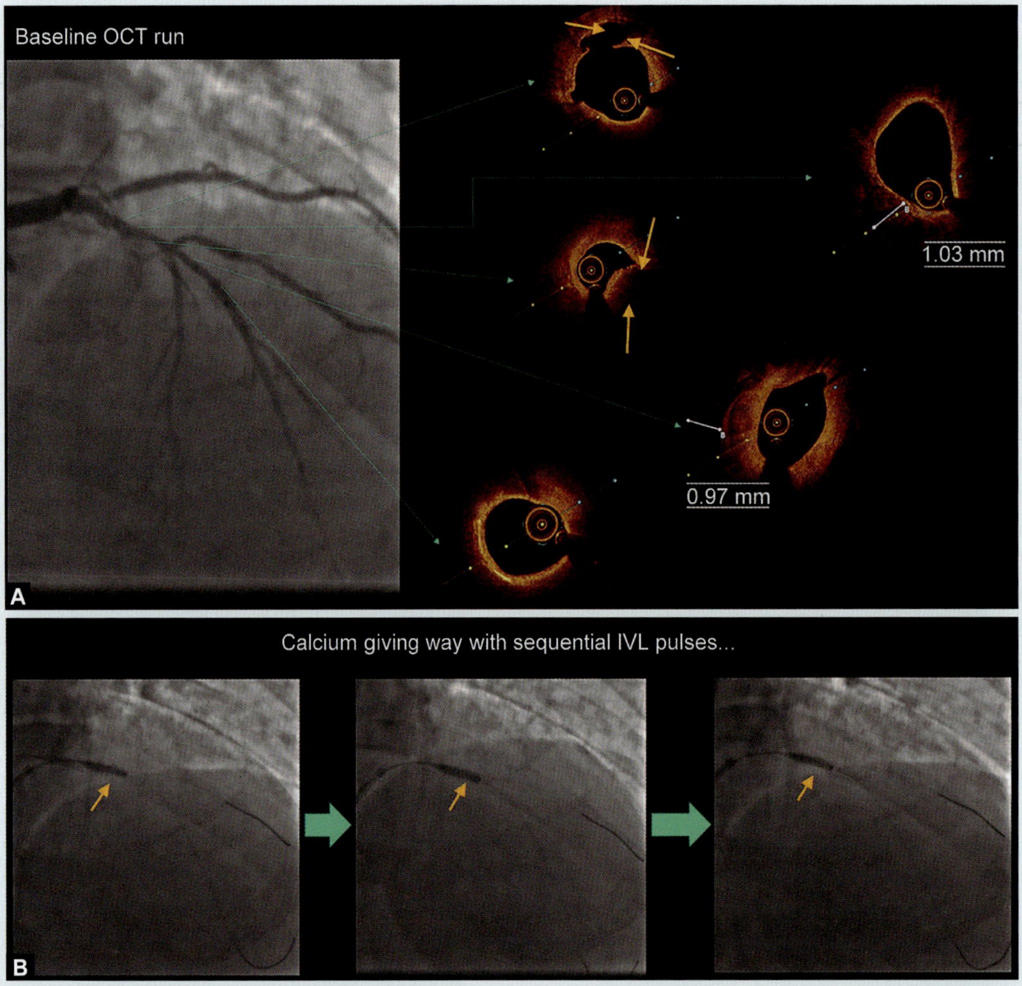

Continued

Continued

Case 2 (Figs. 10A to C)

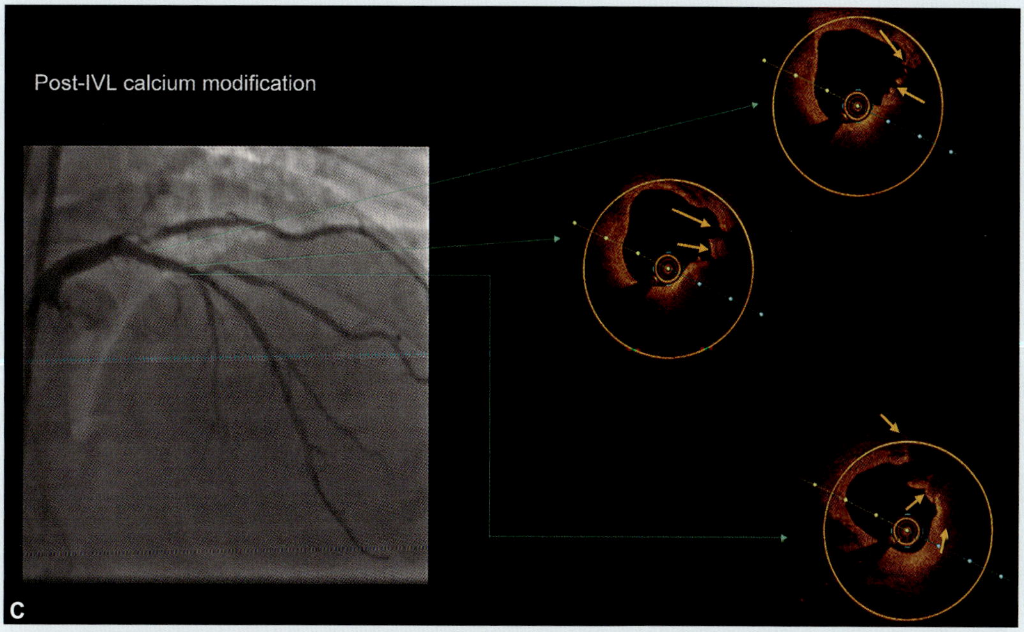

FIGS. 10A TO C: A 57-year-old hypertensive, nondiabetic gentleman had an episode of sudden severe chest pain a week prior to presenting in the outpatient department. He was treated at an outside hospital where he underwent angiography and was referred to us for revascularization. On presentation, patient complained of chronic coronary syndrome (CCS) class III angina and New York Heart Association (NYHA) class II shortness of breath. On examination, he had stable hemodynamics, cardiovascular examination was insignificant with no signs of heart failure. (A) Shows preintravascular lithotripsy (IVL) OCT and various findings including calcium nodule, while (B) shows calcific nodule giving way with sequential pulse cycles of IVL. Finally, (C) shows post-IVL modification and sinking of calcific nodule.

REAL WORLD EVIDENCE

The pooled individual patient data analysis from the four Disrupt CAD studies (I–IV)[6] offers a comprehensive evaluation of IVL for preparing severely calcified coronary arteries prior to stent implantation, making it the most extensive systematic assessment to date. The major findings from this analysis indicate that IVL is safe, demonstrating relatively low rates of in-hospital and 30-day MACE given the complexity of the lesions undergoing PCI. Additionally, IVL proves effective in achieving high procedural success rates across a variety of subgroups, although factors such as prior myocardial infarction, bifurcation target lesions, and longer lesion lengths are associated with increased MACE rates and reduced procedural success.

Despite the initial learning curve in the use of IVL among multiple operators and centers, the device's safety was consistently demonstrated through the series. Indeed, the observed MACE rates, which were low compared to previous studies, were largely driven by the incidence of periprocedural non-Q-wave myocardial infarction. The low event rates were further supported by independent adjudication of patient-level data, adding credibility to these findings. Furthermore, these favorable outcomes were achieved despite the fact that 97% of all target lesions treated were classified as severely calcified by an independent angiographic core laboratory.

The pooled analysis also highlighted the significant length of target lesions and calcified vessel segments treated, which are among the longest reported for any PCI trial. This aspect underscores the challenge of the cases handled and the effectiveness of IVL in managing them without leading to vessel perforation, abrupt coronary closure, or no-reflow events—common complications associated with atheroablative technologies. The very low rates of serious angiographic complications align with IVL's mechanism of action, which involves circumferential and longitudinal multiplane calcium fracture in situ. This method of delivering acoustic energy is not affected by wire bias or device size, unlike other atheroablative technologies.

The recently published 1-year follow-up from the large-scale single-arm Disrupt CAD III study[7] has demonstrated acceptably low rates of adverse clinical events, particularly ID-TLR and ST, with only a single isolated ST event beyond 30 days. This experience suggests that the beneficial impact of IVL on lesion calcium modification and subsequent stent expansion is sustained to at least 1 year.

Beyond these controlled environments of DISRUPT CAD studies, numerous case series and reports have expanded the scope of IVL's application, illustrating its utility across a broader spectrum of complex patient conditions and lesion types. These include cases that were either excluded or underrepresented in the initial studies, such as unprotected left main lesions, ST-elevation myocardial infarction, chronic total occlusions, saphenous vein grafts, eccentrically calcified lesions, and nodular calcifications. This extensive real-world application highlights IVL's versatility and robustness in addressing challenging coronary interventions.

CHALLENGES AND FUTURE ADVANCES

Currently, the adoption of IVL faces typical challenges associated with new technologies, notably its higher costs relative to traditional calcium modification technologies. To assess whether the superior performance of IVL can justify these higher initial expenses, comprehensive cost-effectiveness analyses are necessary. These analyses should consider not only the direct costs of the device but also indirect costs, including those associated with the use of additional balloons and stents, potential complications, repeat interventions, and extended hospital stays.

Another limitation of IVL is its slightly larger crossing profile, which ranges from 0.044" to 0.047", compared to the 0.033" to 0.035" profiles of conventional balloons. This larger size can hinder the deliverability of the technology, particularly in tightly calcified lesions. Until advancements are made to reduce the IVL balloon's profile, adjunctive technologies such as rotational atherectomy (RA) or orbital atherectomy (OA) continue to play a crucial role in preparing these challenging lesions. These ongoing limitations highlight the need for further technological refinements and cost assessments to fully integrate IVL into routine clinical practice for treating calcified coronary artery disease.

CONCLUSION

The IVL offers significant potential for achieving optimal stent expansion, and its simplicity might make IVL a preferred choice over more complex atheroablative technologies. Despite its advantages, dedicated comparative clinical trial data is currently lacking, underscoring a gap in direct evidence comparisons with established methods. The cardiovascular community is keenly anticipating the results of several dedicated randomized trials that are expected to provide deeper insights. Notable among these are the RAINBOW trial, comparing IVL with RA; the BALI trial, contrasting IVL with conventional balloons; the ROLLERCOASTER trial, and the one evaluating IVL against RA and excimer laser coronary angioplasty (ELCA). These studies are crucial for validating IVL's clinical efficacy and operational advantages in a broader spectrum of interventional cardiology.

ONLINE REFERENCES

Please scan the QR code provided at the end of the table of contents for References of this chapter.

CHAPTER 159

Orbital Atherectomy for Calcified Coronary Stenosis: Basics and Beyond

Rohan Naik, Shabbir Ali Shaik, PC Rath

ABSTRACT

Orbital atherectomy (OA) is a valuable tool available to us for the treatment of severely calcified coronary lesions. Diamondback 360® orbital atherectomy system consists of 1.25 mm diamond-coated eccentrically mounted crown that abrades calcified plaque and facilitates stent delivery and stent expansion. It is studied in various randomized and nonrandomized studies and has shown good procedural success and less major adverse cardiac and cerebrovascular events (MACCE) events.

Keywords: Orbital atherectomy (OA), major adverse cardiac events (MACE), in-stent restenosis (ISR), percutaneous coronary intervention (PCI), major adverse cardiac and cerebrovascular events (MACCE), optical coherence tomography (OCT), rotational atherectomy (RA)

INTRODUCTION

The presence of coronary calcification is broadly known to have a negative effect on clinical outcomes in percutaneous coronary intervention (PCI) due to two main reasons: (1) Inability to deliver a stent and (2) inability to achieve adequate stent expansion. When significant coronary calcium is present, there is a lower likelihood of procedural success and an increased risk of periprocedural complications. Specifically, there is an increased risk of major adverse cardiac events (MACE) associated with stent under expansion, stent thrombosis, and in-stent restenosis (ISR). Stent under expansion is one of the strongest predictors of stent thrombosis and ISR.[1] Orbital atherectomy (OA) modifies the calcified plaques and is a good tool in the management of severe coronary calcium.

INDICATION

The primary indication for OA is to facilitate stent delivery in patients with coronary artery disease who are acceptable candidates for angioplasty or stenting of severely calcified *de novo* coronary artery lesions. Atherectomy (orbital or rotational) is a reasonable choice for balloon uncrossable calcified lesions requiring calcium modification.[2,3] Additionally, atherectomy, which was traditionally utilized as a bailout technique for uncrossable lesions, is now being viewed differently as an upfront approach for treating severely calcified lesions as well as for calcified lesions that fail to expand with a balloon-sized 1:1 to the vessel. In these situations, atherectomy allows adequate lesion preparation, which in turn results in better stent deliverability, increased overall stent expansion, and the achievement of maximal luminal gain.[4-7]

MECHANISM OF ACTION

Orbital atherectomy is performed using the Diamondback 360® orbital atherectomy system (Cardiovascular Systems, Inc., Saint Paul, MN, USA), which utilizes a 1.25 mm diamond-coated eccentrically mounted crown that abrades calcified plaque via a mechanism of differential sanding as it encounters the lesion **(Fig. 1)**. The combined effects of differential sanding and centrifugal, pulsatile forces allow preferential abrasion of calcified plaque while healthy tissue flexes away from the crown, thereby minimizing injury *to the medial layer of the vessel.* Simplistically, calcium is engaged while healthy tissue is pushed away. The result is increased vessel luminal diameter, calcium fractures, and improved vessel compliance, all of which are vital to achieving maximal stent expansion and successful PCI of calcified lesions. The entire crown surface is diamond-coated and engineered

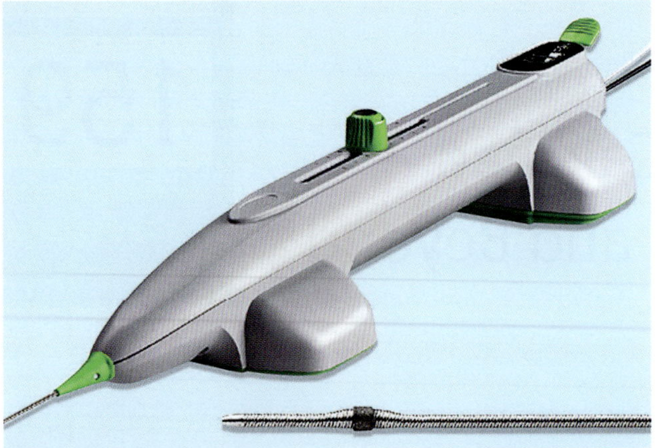

FIG. 1: Diamondback 360® coronary orbital atherectomy system (OAS) device. Coronary OAS device handle and 1.25 mm classic crown.

to allow ablation to be performed bidirectionally (unlike rotational atherectomy). [4,8]

The mechanism is unique in that the crown spins in orbit exerting centrifugal forces while preserving continuous blood flow in the coronary artery throughout the procedure. This property of the orbital atherectomy device, along with the small debris size (approximately 2.04 μm) being smaller than the size of a RBC, may be associated with a lower occurrence of no-reflow and development of transient heart block requiring transvenous pacing.

The characteristic finding seen in intravascular imaging such as OCT is the appearance of a smooth, concave vessel lumen with some interspersed calcium fractures.[9,10]

DEVICE DESCRIPTION, COMPONENTS, AND FUNCTIONING

The Diamondback 360® orbital atherectomy system consists of a drive shaft with the 1.25 mm diamond-coated crown or burr that is advanced over a 0.012" ViperWire Advance coronary guide wire, which has a 0.014" tip. Saline and ViperSlide lubricant (containing egg yolk phospholipids and soybean oil) should be infused continuously during atherectomy to reduce friction between the driveshaft and the ViperWire guide wire, and to reduce thermal injury to the target vessel, which can be a potential cause of restenosis.[4] While the use of RotaGlide lubricating fluid is not mandatory, the use of ViperSlide lubricant is mandatory. Therefore, OA cannot be performed in patients with an allergy to any of the components of the lubricating fluid.

Typically, a 6F guide catheter can be used. The arterial access site may be the femoral artery or the radial artery. The ViperWire is a moderately stiff, stainless-steel wire with a radiopaque distal spring tip. The wire tip is relatively user-friendly, which could be used for primary wiring of the vessel. Commonly, a 0.014" workhorse coronary guide wire is used to first navigate the vessel due to its increased safety and better torque ability, and this wire is then exchanged for the ViperWire using an exchange catheter or microcatheter.

The device is advanced maintaining a distance of at least 5 mm between the tip of the device and the proximal portion of the spring tip to avoid damage and fracture of the ViperWire.[3-5,9] The crown is positioned approximately 5 mm proximal to the lesion. OA is then performed at low speed, with the device advanced gradually at a target speed of 1–3 mm/sec. Ensure 1:1 motion between the advancer knob and the crown as seen via fluoroscopy.

The device has two speed settings: (1) Low speed (80,000 rpm) and (2) high speed (120,000 rpm). The degree of luminal gain achieved is via the speed setting of the burr as well as the rate at which the device is advanced across the lesion, i.e., the traverse speed. As mentioned, therapy is first performed with the device set to low speed and advanced at the target speed. If increased luminal gain is required, this can be achieved by slowing down the traverse speed to 1 mm/sec, and by increasing the device speed, provided the vessel measures >3 mm. High speed should be avoided in smaller vessels. All coronary OA is performed with a 1.25 mm burr. A burr orbit or vessel diameter >2 mm can be achieved by performing OA at high speed (120,000 rpm) with a traverse speed of 1 mm/sec. All initial passes should be performed at low speed, with high speed being used only if additional luminal gain is desired or to assist with lesion crossing in difficult densely calcified lesions, provided the vessel measures >3 mm in diameter and does not have significant tortuosity (risk of perforation).[3-5,9] Once a gentle forward run has been completed, perform a similar backward run. It is important to note that a pecking motion should not be performed, as is performed with rotational atherectomy (RA). Additionally, OA should be performed from healthy-to-healthy segment and care should be taken not to stop atherectomy while within the lesion.

The feedback provided by the device is auditory and tactile.[4,5,9] The operator must pay close attention to the pitch created by the advancing burr coming in contact with and traversing the lesion, as well as the tactile feedback felt at the travel knob while doing so. When the burr first encounters a calcified lesion, a loud pitch is heard from the device handle and increased resistance is felt at the travel knob. As the lesion is successfully modified and traversed, there is less of an audible pitch change and a lack of travel resistance suggesting that maximal lesion modification for that speed has been achieved. At this point, if the vessel is ≥3 mm, the speed can be increased for additional luminal gain. A combination of audible and tactile feedback is used to signal the endpoint for treatment.[4,5,9] The GlideAssist feature, with the device orbiting at 5,000 rpm, is used to assist with device advancement and removal. This allows for use of the device by a single operator.

TIPS AND TRICKS

The tips and tricks are as follows:

- Although occurrence of transient heart block is less common with OA, transient conduction disturbances may occur when a dominant RCA or left circumflex artery is treated. Prophylactic aminophylline (250 mg IV administered ≥20 minutes prior to atherectomy) or a temporary transvenous pacemaker can be considered.
- Nitroglycerin can be administered (via guide or device side tubing) prior to initiation of atherectomy and intermittently during treatment to minimize slow flow and no-reflow.
- A 6F guide catheter or larger can be used routinely; however, if a guide extension is required, a 7F system becomes necessary.
- Start at 80,000 rpm in all vessels.
- Maintain 1:1 motion between the burr and advancer knob. If 1:1 motion is lost, stop the burr, pull back the knob and burr, and attempt to reengage the lesion with gentle forward motion.
- Avoid pecking motion of burr and do not use excessive force.
- OA is a time-dependent therapy. Ideal technique involves gentle forward and backward motion with a traverse speed of 1–3 mm/sec for optimal luminal gain.
- Each treatment should not exceed 30 seconds. The device will deliver an audible alert at 25 seconds, and the burr will power off at 30 seconds. When the alert is heard, the burr should be withdrawn to a healthy area of the vessel. Theoretically, burr entrapment should be less common with OA owing to its bidirectional burr function.
- Allow a rest time between treatments, which is at least as long as the treatment period.
- OA of stented segments is usually not recommended. If atherectomy of a segment distal to a stent is required, this can be done in conjunction with a guide extension catheter used to shield the stent.
- OA may provide superior debulking in large caliber vessels such as the left main coronary artery.
- Due to its construction and orbital burr motion, a 1.25 mm burr can treat a lumen which is >1.25 mm. Remember, the goal of OA is to produce sufficient debulking of intimal and medial calcium with production of calcium fractures, thereby facilitating stent delivery and allowing optimal stent expansion.
- The ideal technique to treat aorto-ostial lesions with OA (provided the lesion can be crossed with a wire) is to advance the burr beyond the lesion using GlideAssist and treat at low speed in a retrograde direction. Ensure the guide catheter is coaxial to prevent aorto-ostial dissections. More controlled burr motion can be achieved by advancing the nose cone of the device into the lesion keeping the crown 0.5 mm from the lesion. As with standard practice, it is important to engage the lesion before escalating device speed to prevent an unconstrained burr orbit in the ostium. In the hands of less experienced operators, RA may be preferred for the treatment of aorto-ostial lesions.
- The number of runs correlates with the amount of luminal gain achieved. More than 5 minutes of atherectomy time should not be performed with a single crown.

CLINICAL DATA

In 2008, the first-in-human study of OA including 50 patients was performed across two centers in India.[11] This was the Safety and Feasibility of Orbital Atherectomy for the Treatment of Calcified Coronary Lesions (ORBIT-I) study,[11] which was a prospective, nonrandomized study in which patients with *de novo* calcified coronary lesions underwent OA followed by stent placement. This study demonstrated an excellent procedural success rate of 94% and device success rate of 98%. The cumulative MACE rate was 4% while inhospital (related to 2 MIs), 6% at 30 days, 8% at 6 months, and 18.2% at 3 years. There were six dissections and one perforation which occurred. Of note, only 18.4% of patients were treated with the currently used 1.25 mm burr.

The pivotal Evaluate the Safety and Efficacy of OAS in Treating Severely Calcified Coronary Lesions (ORBIT-II) study[12] was a prospective, nonrandomized, multicenter study, which enrolled 443 patients in the United States (US). The primary efficacy endpoint of residual stenosis <50% after OA and stent placement without inhospital MACE was higher than the performance goal (88.9% vs. 82%). Stent delivery occurred successfully in 97.7% of cases. Low rates of inhospital MI (0.7%), cardiac death (0.2%), and target vessel revascularization (0.7%) occurred. The safety endpoint of freedom from 30-day MACE was 89.6% (CI 86.7–92.5%), which was greater than the predefined cutoff of 83%. Therefore, the primary safety and efficacy endpoints were met by a significant margin. This led to device approval in the US in 2013. At 3-year follow-up, the cumulative MACE rate was 23.5% (6.7% cardiac death, 11.2% MI, and target vessel revascularization 10.2%). Of note, the ORBIT-I and II trials excluded patients with unprotected left main disease and left ventricular systolic dysfunction with ejection fraction ≤25%, and chronic kidney disease (unless on hemodialysis). Since these studies seemed to have excluded a population of patients frequently encountered in clinical practice, further data was sought.

The real-world multicenter all-comer observational registry comprising 458 patients across 3 centers was used to investigate the outcomes of OA.[13] This study allowed for the evaluation of patients who had been previously excluded, including those with acute coronary syndrome. At 1-year follow-up, the rate of MACCE was 12.6%, death occurred in 4%, and target vessel revascularization in 7.5% of patients. The complication rate was low with dissection, perforation, and slow flow/no-reflow occurring in <1% of cases. This study demonstrated the safety and efficacy of OA in this complex, all-comer patient population.

The largest ever PCI trial involving 2,000 patients with severe calcific coronary disease (ECLIPSE; NCT03108456) is a randomized (1:1), prospective, multicenter trial evaluating two different vessel preparation strategies—conventional balloon angioplasty versus routine OA of severely calcified lesions prior to stent implantation.[14] This study will evaluate the role of routine lesion preparation utilizing OA and is expected to have results reported later this year.

COMPLICATIONS

The possible complications associated with OA include dissection, perforation, and slow flow/no-reflow.[5,9,11,15-17] These are known to occur in increased frequency with atherectomy. Complication rates are commonly reported based on the incidence seen in the ORBIT-II Trial.[12] Dissection occurred in 2.3% cases, perforation occurred in 0.9% cases, and slow flow/no-reflow occurred in 0.2% cases. Abrupt vessel closure occurred in 0.9% of cases. Real-world multicenter registries have shown even lower rates of complications. Bradycardia and heart block occur infrequently with OA. Burr entrapment is also less common.

ORBITAL ATHERECTOMY COMPARED WITH ROTATIONAL ATHERECTOMY

Orbital atherectomy is a relatively newer technology having been first performed in 2008 while RA has been performed for over three decades. Both atherectomy devices perform effective calcium and lesion modification and have been shown to have similar outcomes. This is largely based on retrospective studies showing similar short-term outcomes, outcomes at 30 days and at 1 year.[18-20] Data regarding the degree of calcium debulking has been somewhat conflicting. Initial studies suggested that OA produced deeper tissue modification and lacunae as seen on OCT.[10] Additionally, OA was found to produce more calcified plaque modification as well as noncalcified plaque modification in vessels with larger luminal area, while in vessels with smaller luminal areas, the degree of lesion modification was similar with both techniques.[21] Despite the initial larger luminal gain achieved with OA, the final luminal area achieved following stent implantation remained similar using both techniques.[21] More recently, a single-center prospective randomized clinical trial involving 100 patients was performed to assess the safety and efficacy of OCT-guided PCI using OA versus RA.[18] In this study, using RA resulted in a greater stent expansion and larger maximum atherectomy area but procedural outcomes and clinical events remained similar between the two groups. A trend toward more slow flow and no-reflow following RA was noted but did not reach statistical significance due to study power. Additionally, vascular healing was sufficient in both groups as assessed by OCT performed at 8 months.

Each of the above studies has limitations. The initial study showing more effective calcium modification with OA may have been influenced by selection bias with relatively less severely calcified lesions having been treated with OA.[22] The more recent randomized trial discussed earlier showing greater stent area being achieved with RA has also been discussed in terms of the treated lesions not having sufficiently severe stenosis as is often encountered in clinical practice considering preintervention imaging with a 2.7F OCT catheter was possible in all these cases. Additionally, contrary to routine practice where atherectomy is usually done upfront, in this study, the majority had predebulking of lesions performed with balloons including scoring and cutting balloons.[23]

In summary, a particular atherectomy device may have an advantage in a particular situation and should be used as such in these situations, but broadly speaking based on the available data (and the lack of randomized data), the clinical and safety outcomes associated with both devices appear similar.

SPECIAL SITUATIONS WHERE ORBITAL ATHERECTOMY OR ROTATIONAL ATHERECTOMY MAY BE PREFERRED BASED ON EXPERT CONSENSUS

The special situations where orbital atherectomy or rotational atherectomy may be preferred based on expert consensus are as follows:

- If radial access is necessary, OA can be used through a 6F system while being able to treat larger lumen vessels by adjusting device speed (120,000 rpm) and traverse speed, without having to upsize the guide catheter.
- For treatment of aorto-ostial disease, although OA can be successfully used, anecdotally RA offers better control and may be the preferred choice.
- Significantly angulated and tortuous vessels pose challenges for both techniques but may be better suited to RA. Note that this is anecdotal, and both techniques have been successfully used in these situations.
- For treatment through stents and ISR, RA is feasible and has been performed. Although small studies exist, routine OA through stents is not recommended. An even better option would be to consider alternate strategies such as laser atherectomy or intravascular lithotripsy.
- In a patient with a prohibitive egg allergy, RA can still be performed without RotaGlide; however, ViperSlide (which also contains egg yolk) use is compulsory during OA.
- In patients with severe LV dysfunction, OA may offer the advantage of allowing continuous flow throughout the treatment period and being possibly associated with less slow flow/no-reflow, which may be poorly tolerated in this situation.
- If treatment of the last remaining coronary artery is required in a patient with prior myocardial infarctions or

CTOs in whom the development of slow flow or no-reflow may be catastrophic, OA may be preferred.
- The single burr size and lesser wire bias associated with OA make it attractive for the treatment of longer lesions and calcified nodules, although either device may be used.

NOVEL SECOND-GENERATION MICRO CROWN ORBITAL ATHERECTOMY

Like the original classic crown, the OAS Micro Crown uses an orbiting, diamond-coated crown to reduce luminal plaque burden **(Figs. 2A and B)**. The same design principles and mechanism of action of the OAS Classic Crown apply to the OAS Micro Crown. The two primary design objectives for the OAS Micro Crown design were: (1) To enhance its ability to traverse tighter lesions and (2) to produce an orbit similar to that of the Classic Crown device but at lower speeds (low and high speeds of 50/80 versus 80/120 krpm), thereby reducing the potential for thermal injury.[24]

The size of diamond-coated crown is 1.25 mm for both devices, but the diamond-coated distal tip allows the novel second-generation Micro Crown OAS **(Fig. 2A)** to more easily traverse a 0.5 mm diameter channel, representing a 60% reduction in the minimum lesion size the device is able to treat compared with previous Classic Crown device **(Fig. 2B)**.

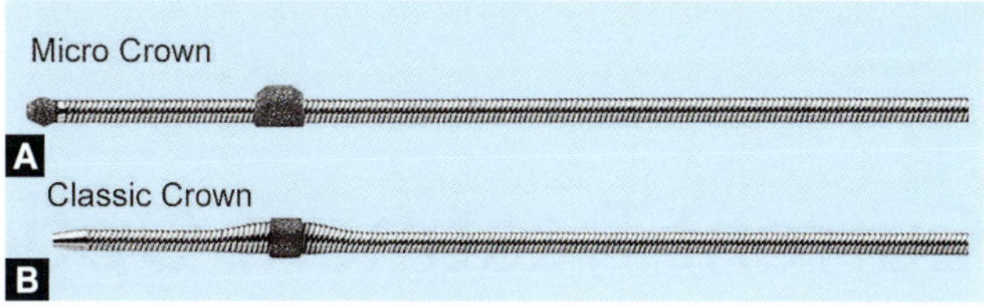

FIGS. 2A AND B: The Diamondback 360® Micro Crown and Classic Crown orbital atherectomy system.

CONCLUSION

The presence of coronary artery calcification is known to worsen clinical outcomes associated with PCI. It is of the utmost importance that severe coronary calcium should be accurately detected and appropriately treated to produce a successful and durable coronary intervention. OA is an important lesion preparation tool available to us to achieve this goal.

ONLINE REFERENCES

Please scan the QR code provided at the end of the table of contents for References of this chapter.

CHAPTER

160

Current Treatment Options for Refractory Angina

Tarun Kumar, Abhishek Kumawat, Karthikeyan R

ABSTRACT

Refractory angina (RA) presents a challenging clinical scenario characterized by persistent chest pain despite optimal medical therapy and revascularization. Key strategies for treatment of RA include enhanced medical therapy, novel antianginal agents, and advanced revascularization techniques. This chapter summarizes recent evidence and expert consensus to guide clinicians in navigating the complexities of RA management effectively.

Keywords: Angina, refractory, EECP, CAD

INTRODUCTION

Conventionally, angina is treated with antianginal medications, CABG, and percutaneous coronary intervention (PCI).[1,2] ECS (2019) defined refractory angina (RA) as "Refractory angina refers to long lasting symptoms (>3 months) due to established reversible ischemia in the presence of obstructive coronary artery disease (CAD), which cannot be controlled by escalating medical therapy with the use of second- and third-line pharmacological agents, bypass grafting, or stenting including PCI of chronic total coronary occlusion."[3] This definition does not include nonobstructive CAD, which is an important cause of RA. Recurrent angina causes recurrent hospital admissions and poor quality of life (QoL).

Many treatment options are available but have a low level of evidence in their favor. There are many reasons to defer further revascularization in patients with CAD, e.g., anatomic complexity of CAD and unsuitable anatomy such as CTO, lack of graft material, multiple restenosis, diffuse vein graft disease, poor LV function, poor distal targets, severe chronic extracardiac diseases, and advanced age.[4,5]

In this chapter, we discuss recent advances and recommendations on therapy for RA.

NONINVASIVE THERAPIES FOR PATIENTS WITH REFRACTORY ANGINA

Optimal medical therapy is important for management of patients with RA. Despite optimal use of guideline-directed anti-ischemic therapies and myocardial revascularization, many patients with stable CAD continue to experience disabling symptoms, often categorized as having limited treatment options.[6]

Exercise training improves physiological outcomes, such as a reduced rate-pressure product and enhanced fitness, leading to a lower angina threshold. Cardiac rehabilitation is effective in lowering cardiovascular mortality by 26% and rehospitalization rates by 18%.[6]

Refractory angina may be prevalent in 5–10% of stable CAD patients. Many emerging therapeutics may be suitable and efficacious to improve QoL in RA.

NOVEL THERAPEUTIC TECHNOLOGIES IN REFRACTORY ANGINA[7]

Treatments Addressing Myocardial Perfusion

Several treatments addressing myocardial perfusion **(Table 1)** beyond PCI, surgical revascularization, or antianginal drugs have been developed.

Enhanced External Counterpulsation

Enhanced external counterpulsation (EECP) works physiologically in a similar fashion as intra-aortic balloon pulsation (IABP); it enhances diastolic coronary blood flow and decreases ventricular wall tension during active

TABLE 1: Treatment addressing myocardial perfusion.

Type of therapy	Safety	Recommendation
EECP	Mild equipment-related side effects including paresthesia, skin abrasion or ecchymosis, bruises, leg or waist pain	ACC/AHA: IIB/B ESC: IIB/B
Transmyocardial laser revascularization	Postprocedural myocardial infarction, heart failure, cardiac tamponade, and death	ACC/AHA: IIb/B ESC: III/A
Coronary sinus reducer	Device migration, coronary sinus perforation, access site bleeding	ACC/AHA: NA ESC: IIB/B
Extracorporeal shockwave myocardial revascularization	No side effects	NA (ESC guidelines stating that more data are needed before establishing a potential recommendation)
Gene/cell therapy	Catheter-induced ventricular tachycardia during mapping, postprocedural myocardial infarction during cell mobilization and collection, access site bleeding	NA (currently only for research purposes)

counterpulsation. Appropriately timed air pressure applied to lower legs, thighs, and then upper thighs creates diastolic augmentation (44%) of aortic pressure.[8] Observational studies in patients with RA reported that significant angina improvement occurred with 35 treatments (1-hour sessions) over a 2-month period.[9] Animal studies on EECP suggested the development of collateral circulation and autoregulatory increases in endothelial vasoactive factors, including vascular endothelial growth factor (VEGF), NO, and fibroblast growth factor-2 (FGF2).[10] There are reductions in inflammatory markers and oxidative stress, improvement in metabolic profile (e.g., 1% drop in HbA1c), and decreases in systolic blood pressure, likely also related to increases in vasoactive factors. In a meta-analysis of 18 observational studies with a total of 1,768 patients treated with EECP, 85% had improvement in ≥1 angina class.[11] Another study found that immediately post-EECP, reduction in severe angina was from 89 to 25%, with improvement in 1 CCS angina class in 78% of patients.[12]

Current recommendations for EECP in RA are ACC/AHA (2023): IIB/B and ESC/EHA (2019): IIB/B **(Figs. 1A and B)**.

Cardiac Shockwave Therapy

In extracorporeal shockwave myocardial revascularization (ESMR) therapy, low-energy shockwaves are delivered by a generator system accompanied by ultrasound imaging to target the myocardial ischemic area of interest. It is a noninvasive treatment (usually 9 sessions of 1,000 shocks each) that promotes blood flow to tissues by inducing local vasodilatation and neoangiogenesis by stimulating angiogenic pathways from the shockwave mechanical transduction. ESMR stimulates NO synthesis and release, VEGF upregulation, stimulation of bone marrow cell differentiation into endothelial cells, and an increase in endothelial progenitor cells.[13] ESMR is safe with no side effects, associated with reductions in hospitalization and improvement in symptoms, angina, QoL, and myocardial function as shown in two open-label studies.[14,15] A meta-analysis of 39 small studies showed consistent benefits on angina relief and QoL parameters, but improvements in exercise time were modest.[16] ESMR is currently available in many European countries but not in the United States.

Coronary Sinus Reducer

The coronary sinus reducer (CSR) is a balloon-expandable, hourglass-shaped stent that is made up of stainless steel. It creates a controlled stenosis of the coronary sinus.[17,18] Narrow coronary sinus restricts drainage from the venous blood flow from the left circulation; it creates a trans-sinus pressure gradient that results in the redistribution of coronary arterial blood flow to underperfused myocardium.[19] Subepicardial arteries normally constrict in response to stress, thereby redirecting blood supply to the subendocardium and this process can be theoretically reversed with the CSR.[19] In the phase II double-blind, sham-controlled COSIRA trial (Coronary Sinus Reducer for Treatment of Refractory Angina), patients treated with CSR had a significant improvement in angina class and QoL ($p = 0.003$), Seattle Angina Questionnaire scores ($p = 0.03$), and exercise time. ORBITA-COSMIC (2024)[20] a double-blind, randomized, placebo-controlled trial conducted in the UK, showed no improvement in transmural myocardial perfusion, but the CSR did improve angina compared to placebo. The potential side effects of CSR are tamponade and stent embolization. The current recommendation for CSR for RA is ESC/EHA 2019: Class IIB/B **(Fig. 2)**.

Transmyocardial Laser Revascularization

Reptilian hearts lack coronary blood vessels and instead have myocardial fenestrations that facilitate the delivery of

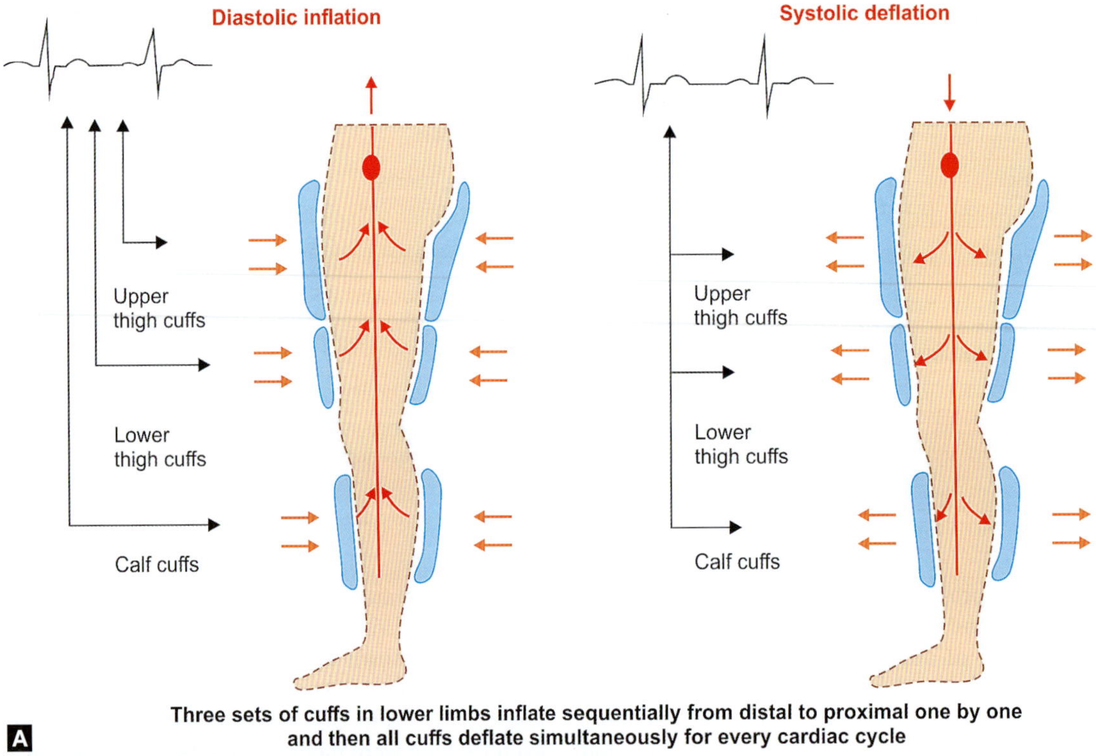

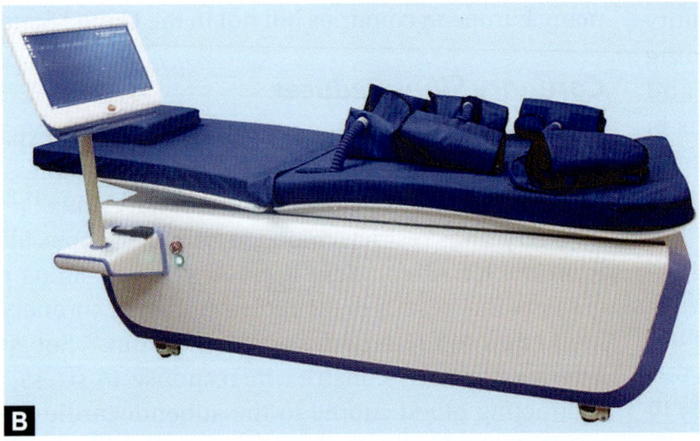

FIGS. 1A AND B: Enhanced external counterpulsation.

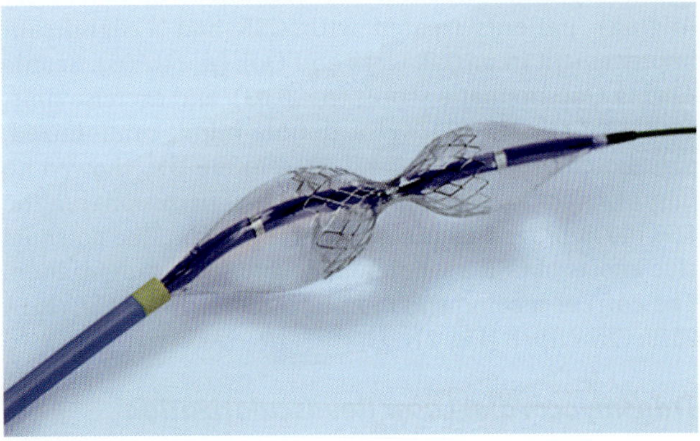

FIG. 2: Coronary sinus reducer device.

oxygenated blood. Transmural channels, typically 1 mm in diameter, can be created in ischemic myocardium using either surgical (epicardial) or percutaneous (endocardial) laser ablation. The US Food and Drug Administration (FDA) has approved transmyocardial laser revascularization (TMLR) for RA, where laser energy is used to create channels in the myocardium, allowing blood from the ventricle to enter.

Randomized trials evaluating the role of TMLR versus medical management in angina treatment included six trials with blinded endpoint assessment using exercise tolerance tests (ETT). Five trials demonstrated statistical improvements in angina frequency and ETT performance, while one trial showed a benefit in angina frequency but not in ETT performance.[21] In these studies, the 1-year mortality

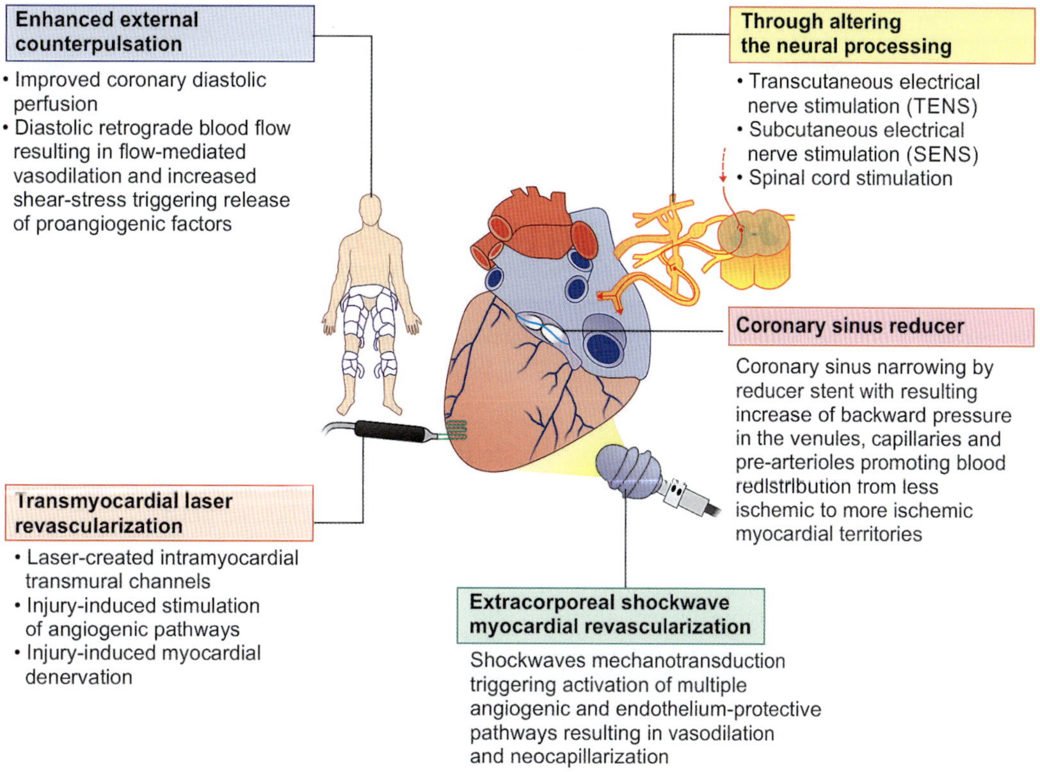

FIG. 3: Summary of new therapeutic nonpharmacological treatment approaches to refractory angina and their proposed mechanism of action.

rate was 2–16%, with an average of 9% with TMLR and 8% in the control groups.[22,23]

Direct TMLR was approved by FDA on the basis of several RCTs, but the largest randomized trial that compared percutaneous TMLR with a blinded sham-control group showed no benefit in angina reduction or exercise time and an increase in morbidity **(Table 1)**.[24]

In 2012, ACC/AHA stable ischemic heart disease gave a class IIb recommendation to TMLR, but based on the above study, it is no longer warranted **(Fig. 3)**.

Treatment Addressing Neural Processing

Neuromodulation for Refractory Angina

Neuromodulation modulates a pain signal at any point of its transmission. It can be done permanently using chemical or mechanical methods or intermittently using electrical methods. Examples are spinal cord stimulation (SCS), subcutaneous electrical nerve stimulation (SENS), and cardiac sympathectomy.

Spinal Cord Stimulation

Spinal cord stimulation was the preferred method by the European Society of Cardiology study group. However, it is not frequently used now. In SCS, a multipolar electrode is surgically inserted in the epidural space, typically between the C7 and T4 vertebrae, where cardiac sympathetic fibers synapse with sensory neurons of the spinal cord. In addition to an analgesic effect, SCS can alter sympathetic tone, which may also reduce angina.[25] In one randomized trial, SCS versus CABG in 104 patients with angina and multivessel CAD showed similar relief in angina; however, patients undergoing CABG had a reduction in objective ischemia on ETT ($p = 0.005$) and better maximum workload ($p = 0.02$).[26]

Cardiac Sympathectomy

Cardiac sympathectomy of the left stellate ganglion has been performed for ventricular arrhythmia storm. No large case series has been published in patients with RA, and hence there is no recommendation for cervical sympathectomy in patients with RA.

Transcutaneous Electrical Nerve Stimulation

Transcutaneous electrical nerve stimulation (TENS) exploits low-intensity electrical currents, applied by means of chest electrodes, to stimulate large diameter afferent fibers. This may result in afferent pain signal suppression, translating into pain quality modulation with patients referring replacement of pain with a vibrating sensation.[27,28]

Improved exercise capacity, reduced incidence of angina, and decreased nitrate usage with TENS were initially reported.[29]

TABLE 2: Treatment addressing neural processing.

Type of therapy	Safety	Recommendation
Transcutaneous electrical nerve stimulation	No side effects	ACC/AHA: NA ESC: IIb/C
Subcutaneous electrical nerve stimulation	No side effects	NA
Spinal cord stimulation	Hardware-related (lead migration, device failure, lead fracture) and biological complications (infection and pain over the implant site, dural puncture headache, dural infection, and neurological damage)	ACC/AHA: IIb/B ESC: IIb/B
Cervical sympathectomy	Vasovagal reactions (hypotensive response) and anesthetic vascular injection, frozen shoulder, access site bleeding, surgical complications	NA

Subcutaneous Electrical Nerve Stimulation

Subcutaneous electrical nerve stimulation is commonly used in noncardiac chronic pain disorders. Its application for RA is recent, with limited clinical data. In SENS, peripheral subcutaneous multipolar electrodes are implanted in the parasternal area where patients typically feel angina, stimulating subcutaneous nerve terminations. The electrode is tunneled to a pulse generator generally implanted in the upper abdomen. The use of the subcutaneous route over the anterior chest wall is technically easier and quicker, and may avoid most of the SCS implantation drawbacks, with no need for antithrombotic withdrawal during the procedure.

In the pilot study of seven patients undergoing SENS implantation, the procedure had 100% feasibility. All patients presented improvement in exercise capacity and QoL, and no major periprocedural adverse events were observed **(Table 2)**.[30]

Biologic Approaches

Protein or Genetic Approaches

The use of biological agents to stimulate myocardial angiogenesis has been the subject of intense research over the last years. Intracoronary or intramyocardial delivery of angiogenetic factors led to the development of genetically modified plasmid or viral vectors. In trials, angiogenetic factors chiefly included were VEGF and fibroblast growth factor.

Administering proangiogenic protein directly into coronary arteries or through intracoronary injection was the initial angiogenic method tested in patients with RA. While showing promising outcomes in trials such as VIVA and FIRST, gene therapy and stem cell therapy offer a more durable and effective approach for treating RA compared to protein therapy.[31]

Initial trials on single gene transfer therapy did not show any significant benefit; AdVEGF-165 KAT trial[32] showed slight improvement in perfusion ($p < 0.05$) but no improvement in total exercise time, and AdVEGF (NORTHERN trial)[33] showed no benefit on both perfusion and total exercise time.

Newer advances in vector techniques, e.g., XC001 is a novel replication-deficient recombinant Ad5 vector designed to transfer VEGF DNA into myocardial cells; it will splice in three isoforms of VEGF, which closely resembles the physiologic form of human VEGF.

The EXACT trial[34] (Epicardial Delivery of XC001 Gene Therapy for Refractory Angina Coronary Treatment) assessed the safety and preliminary efficacy of XC001 in patients with no option RA. This results in higher 100× levels of angiogenesis than vectors expressing single isoform of VEGF. It is a promising treatment for RA, and the study drug was safe and well tolerated. There were exploratory improvements in exercise duration and ischemic burden, and these parameters were sustained for up to 12 months. This product is currently in phase II trials.

Cell Therapy

The underperfused myocardium is an ideal target for angiogenic stem cell therapy. Multiple preclinical and clinical trials have established the role of bone marrow-derived stem cells to stimulate and enhance perfusion in both myocardial and peripheral tissues.

Autologous CD34+ bone marrow-derived endothelial progenitor cells demonstrated the highest in vivo angiogenetic properties. Multiple RCTs on CD34+ cell therapy for RA have demonstrated improvement in exercise capacity on treadmill, lower frequency of angina throughout a 3–12-month period, and significant decrease in all-cause mortality in 24 months.[35-38]

The US **FDA** granted **regenerative medicine advanced therapy (RMAT)** designation to a late-stage **CD34+ cell therapy program** for the treatment of **RA**.

CONCLUSION

Refractory angina management requires a multifaceted approach that combines optimized medical therapy with judicious use of revascularization techniques and emerging novel therapeutic options. Many promising approaches include EECP, shockwave therapy, neuromodulation, CSR, and gene and angiogenic cell therapies. Ongoing research into novel antianginal agents underscores the dynamic nature of this field **(Flowchart 1)**.

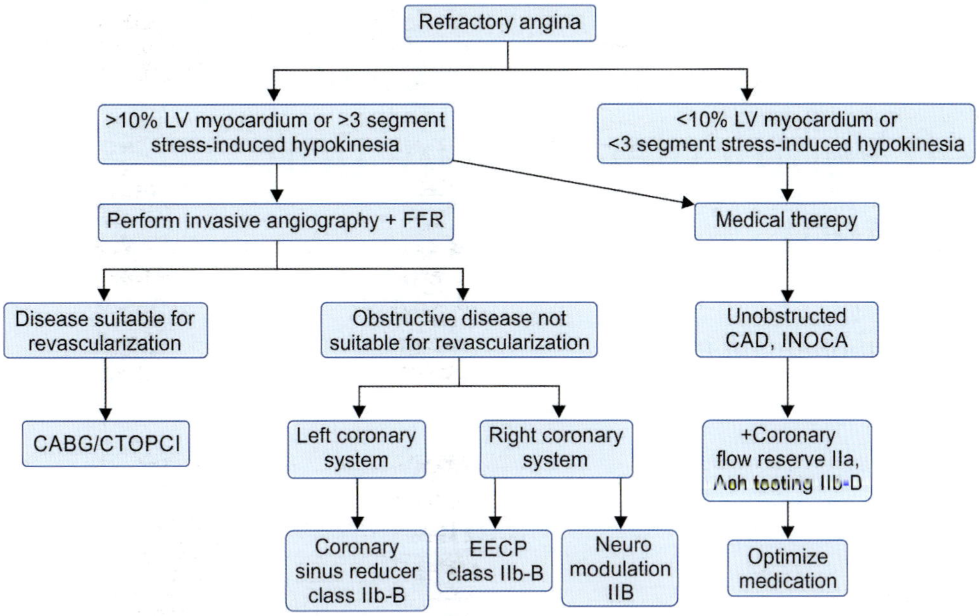

FLOWCHART 1: Take-home table.

Courtesy: Derived from ECC/EHA 2019 stable ischemic heart disease.

ONLINE REFERENCES

Please scan the QR code provided at the end of the table of contents for References of this chapter.

CHAPTER 161

Multivessel Coronary Artery Disease with Left Ventricular Dysfunction: Management

Saroj Mandal, Shubhanshu Pal

ABSTRACT

Ischemic heart disease, often caused by obstructive coronary artery disease, is the most common cause of left ventricular (LV) dysfunction and subsequent heart failure. A study found that 71.4% of patients with heart failure and reduced ejection fraction had multivessel coronary artery disease. This review aims to summarize management strategies for patients with multivessel disease and LV dysfunction.

Keywords: Ischemic heart disease, obstructive coronary artery disease, ventricular dysfunction, multivessel

INTRODUCTION

Ischemic heart disease, most often resulting from obstructive coronary artery disease (CAD), is the most frequent cause of LV systolic dysfunction and subsequent heart failure.[1,2] In this regard, the term ischemic cardiomyopathy is generally used to identify patients with significant LV systolic dysfunction coexisting with/thought to be caused by severe CAD [i.e., significant left-main or multivessel CAD with/without prior myocardial infarction (MI)].[3]

A study published in the Journal of American Heart Association found that among patients with heart failure and reduced ejection fraction (HFrEF), presence of triple vessel coronary artery disease was present in 14% and 17.3% in the patient group of LVEF 10–35% and 36–49% respectively.[4] In another study, among patients with LVEF < 40% and established coronary artery disease, triple vessel disease was found in 47.2% and double vessel disease was found in 24.2% cases.[5] Overall presence of coronary artery disease led to higher in-hospital mortality among patients with HFrEF according to another study.[6]

This review is an attempt to summarize the management strategies of patients of multivessel disease and LV dysfunction which broadly incorporates the following:

- Treatment of obstructive CAD
- Management of symptoms
- Long-term therapy for CAD
- Special therapy for complications—cardiac and noncardiac

TREATMENT OF OBSTRUCTIVE CORONARY ARTERY DISEASE

The LV systolic dysfunction in background of CAD is due to combination of irreversible MI and reversible hibernating myocardium. The prospect of reversing hibernation has underpinned the rationale for revascularization of ischemic cardiomyopathy. But it is highly debated whether revascularization improves prognosis or systolic function.

PRETREATMENT EVALUATION

With advent of newer pharmacotherapy, optimal medical therapy (OMT) has changed the paradigm of management of patients with CAD and LVSD. However, revascularization has the potential to reverse or slow down the effect of ischemia on myocardium and prevent recurrent MI. Especially in the background of progressive CAD intervention becomes utmost important and it is characterized by the following:

- Decrease in LVEF >5–10%
- New ventricular arrhythmia
- New and unexplained angina/dyspnea
- Worsening angina/angina equivalent

However, revascularization may not be safe/effective in certain conditions, e.g., severe HF, advanced comorbid conditions such as CKD, diffuse CAD, or irreversible myocardial injury. Thus, clinical evaluation for determination of risks and benefits of PCI/CABG/OMT alone is important.

CLINICAL EVALUATION

Proper history, physical examination, laboratory testing, and imaging is necessary. These findings will help in determining risks of revascularization, particularly with CABG.

SURGICAL RISK ESTIMATION

Surgical risk estimation includes general assessment, risk score estimates, and finally determination of overall surgical risk. 30-day mortality is often assessed by STS (Society of Thoracic Surgeons) Score or the EuroSCORE II. However, these scores are particularly not validated for patients with LV systolic dysfunction, thus they may underestimate the actual risk.

VIABILITY ASSESSMENT

Dysfunctional myocardium is considered viable if:

- Regional dysfunction improves after revascularization by at least one point (akinesis to hypokinesis or hypokinesis to normal)—Regional viability.
- Overall EF increases significantly (>5%)—Global viability.

Various imaging modalities can be used to assess viability of myocardium, e.g.,

- *Thallium myocardial uptake:* At rest and at 4 hours and 24 hours after injection is assessed. An uptake ≥50% at rest or after redistribution implies viability. Technetium can also be used in this purpose.
- *Low-dose dobutamine echocardiography:* Improvement in regional contraction with low-dose dobutamine infusion (<10 μg/kg/min) is called myocardial contractile reserve. A subsequent decline in contraction at higher dose reflects ischemia. This biphasic response is highly predictive of myocardial viability.
- *PET scan:* It assesses metabolic uptake of glucose analogue tracer, i.e., the metabolic viability. Also, the perfusion is assessed by N or Rb tracer. A mismatch between the two implies viability, whereas if there is decline in both the uptake, it suggests irreversible injury. PET has highest sensitivity (~90%) but the lowest specificity (~58%) for viability assessment.
- *Cardiac MRI:* Late myocardial hyperenhancement 10 minutes after gadolinium injection is sign of myocardial scarring and it highly predicts nonviability when it involves >50% of the transmural thickness. Whereas, involvement of <25% of myocardial thickness predicts viability.

In the chronic ischemic setting, revascularization for ischemic LV dysfunction is beneficial regardless of viability testing and regardless of improvement in EF as revascularization improves symptom status, HF, and mortality. It also prevents further deterioration of LV function and further MI, preserve infarct border integrity, and reduce arrhythmogenesis. However, viability may be used to guide specifics of segmental revascularization (e.g., one may not choose to revascularize nonviable RCA territory).

WHAT DO THE TRIALS SAY?

The *PROTECT 2 study*[7] reported an absolute increase in LVEF of 13.2% due to reverse remodeling, which was more frequent in those with more extensive revascularization and was associated with fewer MACE and improved symptoms.

STICH (Surgical Treatment for Ischemic Heart Failure) *trial*[8] was the first RCT for this aspect and it revealed that, in selected patients, surgical revascularization was associated with 3-fold excess of death in first few weeks, but at long-term follow-up of 10 years (*STICHES trial*),[9] survival benefit was apparent. In a substudy of the STICH trial, it was shown that patients with viable myocardium who underwent CABG had higher 10 years survival than those assigned to OMT alone, whereas patients without viability also showed nonsignificant higher survival in CABG arm than those assigned to medical therapy alone. This suggests that the presence or absence of viability did not affect the benefit of CABG.

REVIVED-BCIS2 trial[10] was the first RCT for safety and efficacy of PCI in ICMP. 700 patients (mean age 70 years) with severe LV systolic dysfunction (mean EF 28%) with extensive CAD (Median British Cardiovascular Intervention Society Jeopardy Score 10) and evidence of hibernation in at least four myocardial segments that could be revascularized were randomized to PCI or OMT alone. Event rate in PCI group was identical to OMT group in a median follow-up of 3.4 years. This lack of benefit was consistent across all prespecified subgroups, regardless of whether there was complete or incomplete revascularization. But Kansas City Cardiomyopathy Questionnaire Summary Score (KCCQ) significantly improved in the PCI group in the first 6 and 12 months, which was not sustained in the 24 months follow-up. Although EF improved in both groups and an improvement of >4.7% was associated with reduction of death and CHF. In summary, PCI did not achieve the primary endpoint in this trial, but it was associated with an improvement in quality of life, reduced rate of spontaneous MI, and a trend for reduced need of AICD termination of ventricular arrhythmias **(Table 1)**.

PPAR-2 trial,[11] the only trial of viability-guided management, randomized patients with respect to FDG-PET guided therapy or standard care. At the end of 1 year, primary endpoints were similar in both the groups. Although, because of high prevalence of protocol deviation limits, the external validity and clinical translation of this study.

WHAT IS THERE IN GUIDELINES?

According to the 2018 ESC guideline of myocardial revascularization,[13] in patients with LV dysfunction and

TABLE 1: Characteristics of studies of revascularization in LV systolic dysfunction.[12]

Trial acronym	Heart	PARR-2	STICH	REVIVED-BCIS2
Number of patients enrolled	138	430	1,212	700
Primary outcome	All-cause mortality	Cardiovascular death, MI, hospital admission due to cardiac cause	All-cause mortality	Al cause mortality hospitalization for HF
Secondary outcome		Time to primary outcome. Time to cardiovascular death	Cardiovascular death, death by any cause, hospitalization for cardiovascular cause	LVEF at 6 and 12 months, quality of life scores, New York Heart Association class, Canadian Cardiovascular Society class, cardiovascular death, MI, unplanned revascularization, change in NT-proBNP, major bleeding, health resource use
Inclusion criteria	Heart failure ≥6 weeks on diuretics with history of MI, LVEF ≤35%, ≥5 viable segments with reduced contractility	LVEF ≤35%, suspect for CAD based on coronary angiogram, previous revascularization, previous MI, positive stress perfusion imaging	LVEF ≤35%, CAD deemed suitable for revascularization	LVEF ≤35%, extensive coronary artery disease (British Cardiovascular Intervention Society jeopardy score of ≥6) viability in at least four dysfunctional myocardial segments amenable to revascularization with PCI
Exclusion criteria	Recent acute coronary syndrome or stroke, revascularization required for angina or valve surgery, ventricular arrhythmias requiring device therapy. Life-limiting comorbidity	Patents with final revascularization strategy decision already made, fluorodeoxyglucose viability info already known, recent (<4 weeks) MI, unsuitable for revascularization, emergency revascularization, surgery for valvular heart disease needed, severe comorbidities	Aortic disease needing surgery; cardiogenic shock within 72 hours of randomization planned PCI; recent MI causing left ventricular dysfunction; history of >1 past CABG; life expectancy <3 years for noncardiac causes; likely poor treatment adherence; previous heart, kidney, liver, or lung transplantation	MI in the 4 weeks before randomization, acute decompensated HF, or sustained ventricular arrhythmias within 72 hours before randomization, value disease requiring imminent intervention, glomerular filtration rate <25 mL/min (unless on dialysis)
LVEF at enrollment	24%	27%	28%	27%
Imaging technique allowed	Stress echo, PET, SPECT	PET	Stress echo, SPECT	Stress echo, cardiac magnetic resonance, SPECT/PET
Revascularization technique	CABO (*n* = 30) and PCI (*n* = 15)	CABG (*n* = 71, 68%) and PCI (*n* = 33, 32%)	CABG	PCI
Median follow-up	59 months	5 years	STICH: 4.7 years	
			STICH long term 9.8 years	41 months
Outcome	No significant benefit of revascularization over OMT	No significant difference between PET-guided and standard strategies	No benefit of revascularization over OMT at 5 years At 10 years CABG was associated with a lower all-cause mortality than OMT [072 (95% CI 0 64–0 82); *p* <0.001]	No significant benefit of revascularization over OMT quality-of-life scores at 6 and 12 months appeared to favor the PCI group, but the difference had diminished at 24 months
Pitfalls	Underpowered, smaller enrollment than planned (138 out of 800 planned patients)	Low protocol adherence (24% did not adhere to PET findings)	Significant crossover (17% of medical therapy group underwent CABG), small sample, no left man disease in medical therapy alone group	Relatively underpowered, largely paucisymptomatic patients (97% with no or mild angina and 73% with mild dyspnea)

multivessel disease, CABG has class I recommendation. In case of double vessel disease, PCI has got IIa indication, and in case of triple vessel disease PCI has got IIa recommendation based on discussion with Heart team regarding coronary anatomy, expected completeness of revascularization, and comorbidities. Also noninvasive assessment of myocardial viability has been given class IIb recommendation in this guideline.

The 2021 ACC/AHA/SCAI guideline,[14] CABG has been given class I recommendation for this subgroup of patients for survival benefit. For patients not suitable for CABG, GDMT with or without PCI has been suggested. But no recommendation for PCI has been given.

In summary, the age of the patient, comorbidities, relationship between myocardial viable segments, and coronaries suitable for revascularization, feasibility of complete revascularization—all should be taken into consideration while deciding the strategy of revascularization **(Fig. 1)**.[15]

MANAGEMENT OF SYMPTOMS

Treatment for Angina

In patients with LV systolic dysfunction, proper decongestion of patient can relieve anginal symptoms as well. In many cases medical therapy of angina is the only solution because of the following factors:

- Coronaries unsuitable for revascularization, e.g., diffuse coronary disease.
- Several attempts of PCI/CABG, which may limit further benefit or preclude further attempts.
- Lack of vascular conduit for CABG.
- Severely impaired LVEF.
- Comorbidities (Age, CVA, advanced CKD, complications of diabetes, etc.)

β-blockers have antianginal effects, and also they reduce mortality. So in patients who can tolerate lower BP, initial optimization of β-blocker therapy is first goal.

If optimal β-blocker therapy does not treat the anginal symptoms and patient can still tolerate lowering BP, increasing dose of ARNI/ACEi/ARB should be the next goal. In the next step the second line medications of HFrEF can be initiated (e.g., hydralazine-isosorbide dinitrite).

In case of refractory angina despite optimization of heart failure therapy, further antianginal therapies are warranted and the choice generally depends on the blood pressure. For patients with lower BP, ranolazine or trimetazidine can be used. Whereas in hypertensive patients, second generation dihydropyridine calcium channel blockers (e.g., amlodipine, felodipine) can be initiated. Non-DHP CCBs should be avoided in ICMP patients.

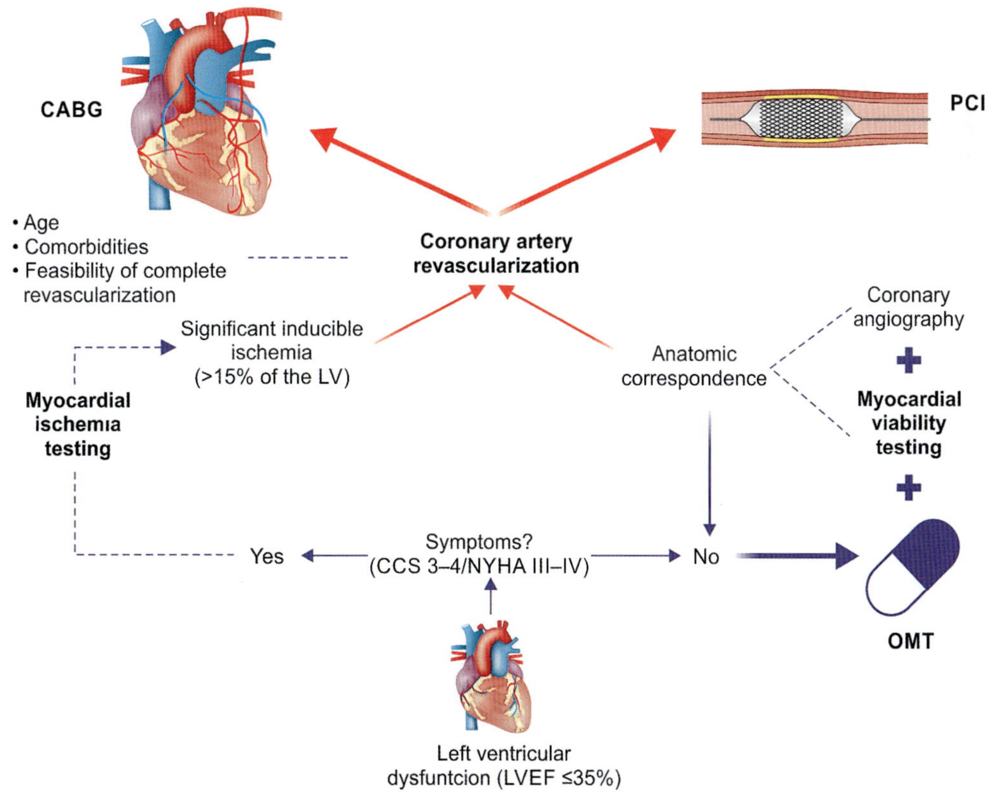

FIG. 1: Therapeutic-diagnostic algorithm for left ventricular dysfunction.[15]

Ranolazine

Ranolazine exerts antianginal effect by inhibiting late inward Na channels, partial inhibition of fatty acid oxidation. It also has favorable glycometabolic and antiarrhythmic effects.

Trimetazidine

It acts by improving metabolic efficiency of ischemic myocardium by shifting the metabolism from fatty acid oxidation to glucose oxidation. Also, it is postulated that this drug can alter mitochondrial calcium metabolism and have cytoprotective effects.

Nicorandil

Nicorandil is a potassium channel opener and thus an arterial and venous dilator. It mimics the mechanisms of ischemic preconditioning and protect the myocardium from subsequent attacks.

Ivabradin

Ivabradin inhibits sinus node pacemaker current and thus lower the heart rate. It has shown to increase exercise capacity and reduce anginal frequence.

Other options that have been tried in refractory angina are perhexiline, allopurinol, endothelin receptor blockers, fasudil, testosterone, stem cell therapy, and therapeutic angiogenesis.

Nonpharmacologic Therapies

Five nonpharmacological therapies that have been tried in refractory angina are—External counterpulsation, spinal cord stimulation, transmyocardial laser revascularization, coronary sinus reducer, and apheresis.

External Counterpulsation

It increases arterial blood pressure and retrograde aortic blood flow during diastole. It was evaluated in MUST-EECP trial and found to have increased exercise tolerance and decrease in anginal episodes.

Spinal Cord Stimulation

Spinal cord stimulation at T1–T2 level have been tried. It may have the effect by suppressing the capacity of intrinsic cardiac neurons to generate activity during ischemia and reducing sympathetic activity or redistribution of myocardial blood flow.

Transmyocardial Laser Revascularization

It uses laser ablation to create transmural channels in the ischemic myocardium in order to restore perfusion.

Coronary Sinus Reducer

It is an hourglass shaped metal mesh that is placed in coronary sinus to produce a stenosis and increasing pressure in the myocardial bed. This causes redistribution of blood flow to the underperfused segments. It has been tried in COSIRA trial and recently concluded ORBITA-COSMIC trial.

Treatment for Heart Failure

The management of heart failure part is similar to the other types of HFrEF. Typically diuretics are used to relieve congestion. The four pillars namely, ARNI/ACEi/ARB, SGLT-2 inhibitor, β-blocker and MRA should be initiated and up titrated to maximal tolerated dose. These medications reduce mortality and also reduce hospitalization. In selected cases ICD/CRT can be beneficial.

LONG-TERM THERAPIES FOR CORONARY ARTERY DISEASE

Lifestyle Changes

Strict diet control, weight reduction, physical activity, and smoking cessation have paramount importance in the long-term management of CAD. Cardiac rehabilitation programs can be beneficial for them as well.

Antiplatelet Therapy

Long-term aspirin therapy is recommended for all patients of this group. For those, who have history of GI bleed, clopidogrel is a reasonable alternative. For those patients having ACS or PCI recently, a P2Y12 inhibitor should be added.

Anticoagulant

In stable CAD with multivessel disease, patients with low bleeding risk can be started with rivaroxaban 2.5 mg orally once daily according to the findings of COMPASS trial. Other indications of anticoagulation remains AF or venous thromboembolic disease.

Statins

High intensity statins should be used in all cases for lowering LDL cholesterol below target levels. If LDL remains high despite high intensity statins, intensification with ezetimibe and PCSK9 inhibitors should be strongly considered.

The importance of addressing the comorbidities associated with CAD is very crucial for long-term management. Also, colchicine is coming up recently as a tool for secondary prevention in CAD.

SPECIAL THERAPIES FOR COMPLICATIONS

Cardiac Complications

Additional management is warranted in patients with complications of ICMP.

- *Advanced heart failure*—It may require mechanical circulatory support or cardiac transplant.
- *Valve disease*—Most commonly these patients have associated mitral valve disease. Proper assessment of

valve function should be assessed beforehand, so that it can be addressed while fixing the coronaries.

- *Arrhythmia*—Proper pharmacologic and device therapy, if necessary should be implemented.
- *LV aneurysm*—Patients of ICMP may develop ventricular aneurysm or pseudoaneurysm. This also should be imaged properly, so that corrective surgery can be done during revascularization.

Noncardiac Complications

Among the noncardiac complications, most important is the renal impairment in form of cardiorenal syndrome. However, chronic heart failure can have multisystem effects and that should be dealt properly for comprehensive patient care.

CONCLUSION

The management of patients with multivessel coronary artery disease and left ventricular systolic dysfunction primarily depends on the presentation of the patient. In the background of stable CAD, the role and significance of revascularization is somewhat reduced by the recent progress in pharmacotherapy. Ensuring optimal heart failure therapy should be of utmost priority in every patient. On the other hand, Coronary Revascularization is extremely important in the background of ACS and in selected patients as detailed in this review. Management of these patients are best carried out in the presence of a dedicated 'HEART TEAM' as timely intervention both from interventionist and cardiovascular surgeon is extremely crucial to prevent mortality and symptom-free survival of the patient.

ONLINE REFERENCES

Please scan the QR code provided at the end of the table of contents for References of this chapter.

CHAPTER 162

Nonmetal Coronary Interventions: DCB and BRS

Rishi Sethi, Monika Bhandari

ABSTRACT

Globally, CAD burden is high due to complex lesions. Advancements in stent technology and experienced operators can improve complex PCI results, but repeat revascularization risk remains. Bioabsorbable stents and DCB could help, but further research is needed.

Keywords: CAD, lesions, improvement, DCB

INTRODUCTION

Percutaneous coronary intervention (PCI) or coronary angioplasty has evolved a lot ever since Andreas Gruentzig performed the first successful coronary angioplasty treatment on September 16, 1977 with the use of a balloon.[1] PCI is now an effective solution in many patients with atherosclerotic coronary artery disease (CAD) presenting with acute myocardial infarction or stable angina. In the initial days, plain old balloon angioplasty (POBA) was used but it was associated with acute vessel recoil and acute closure (30–40%) following PCI and restenosis in intermediate to long-term follow.[2] Further research in this field led to the invention of a bare-metal stent (BMS) that addressed the immediate acute vessel closure enhancing the procedural success of PCI but the problem of restenosis remains unaffected.[3,4] Drug-eluting stents (DES) platforms were then introduced and significant advances in the drug, its polymer coating and the drug delivery with better stent strut designs found an effective way to minimize the restenosis to <3%.[5] Thereafter PCI became an alternative mode of coronary revascularization to many complex lesion subsets such as bifurcation, chronic total occlusion, long and diffuse disease, and left main as well apart from simple coronary lesions. Currently, PCI is also used as a complimentary revascularization solutions to the subjects who are otherwise candidates for surgical revascularization through coronary artery bypass graft (CABG).

However, despite technical advancements and improved medical therapy [dual antiplatelet therapy (DAPT)], stent thrombosis (ST) especially late and very late remain a concern, even with the latest generation of DES.[6,7] According to recent reports, a stent failure rate of up to 2% per annum is seen especially in complex and long lesions.[8,9] The persistence of metallic platforms, leaving the vessel "caged" and impairing its vasomotor functions after stent implantation is an important reason behind this. In addition, though lesser than BMS, ISR remains an Achilles' heel, occurring in 3–20% of patients with newer generation DES and is best available DAPT.[10] Moreover, in young patients, leaving permanent metal material within the coronary arteries may be a hindrance for CABG if the need arises in future. Therefore, there is always room for newer technologies that can overcome the shortcomings of available DES.

WHY WE NEED METAL FREE PCI: CHALLENGES OF DES?

- *Need for pronged DAPT*: After DES implantation although decreases the chances of ISR, the patient needs prolonged DAPT up to 12 months till the stent is completely endothelialized to prevent ST. Although with a better stent platform and the use of biocompatible or biodegradable polymer shorter duration of DAPT is possible still it is preferable to give at least 6 months of DAPT. DAPT use can lead to hemorrhagic complications which result in increased morbidity and mortality, especially in the elderly and those with prior history of hemorrhage and bleeding diathesis. In addition, patients taking anticoagulants for various reasons are also at heightened risk of major bleeding complications due to the combined use of DAPT, so its use needs to be shortened. Similarly, in patients requiring major surgery, DAPT needs to be stopped which makes them vulnerable to ST and its sequelae.[11]

- *Adverse effects of permanent metal in coronaries*: Another potential limitation of DES is the persistence of metallic foreign bodies and often a durable polymer within coronaries. Either of them may result in vascular inflammation, and neoatherosclerosis which may lead to ISR and late ST.[12] On the other hand metallic stents also impair the physiological vasomotor function of the vessel and impair the phenomenon of late luminal enlargement and if placed in the distal coronary segment, the potential for grafting within this stented segment is lost. There are also issues with using DES in small vessels as chances of restenosis are higher with small-diameter stents.[12] Another major challenge is PCI of bifurcation lesions where despite advancement in stent technology clinical outcomes may be unsatisfactory, especially in the side branch (SB). Studies reveal that although ISR incidence in the main branch is reduced from up to 40–60% to 2.5%, repeat revascularizations for restenosis at the SB ostium remain an obstinate problem. The incidence of ST is also high occurring in up to 4.4% of patients after bifurcation PCI as compared to only 1.4% of patients with nonbifurcation lesions. The majority of trials which studied bifurcation PCI demonstrate a higher risk of subacute ST with dedicated two-stent techniques.[13] Lastly, the presence of diffuse coronary lesions is again a challenge as a longer stent increases the odds of ST.

THE NEED FOR METAL-FREE CORONARY INTERVENTION

Bioabsorbable/biodegradable stents with no permanent metal in coronaries represent an attractive alternative revascularization modality. This is because they provide temporary vessel scaffolding avoiding the potential long-term complications of metallic stents.[14,15] This technology offers several potential advantages, which may such as restoration of vasomotion, facilitating repeat procedures, and cardiac imaging with MRI if the need arises. Moreover, complications such as stent-strut fracture and delayed allergy to the polymer which although not common but troublesome would not be there.[16] Additionally, there are chances of late lumen gain if the artery is not splinted (positive remodeling).[17] Thus in many respects, a temporary metallic scaffold which dissolves after fulfilling its role, is preferable over a permanent intracoronary metallic prosthesis.

Drug-coated balloon (DCB) catheters on the other hand are made up of regular semicompliant balloons and a matrix coating applied to the surface of the balloon comprised of two elements—a lipophilic active drug and a spacer which increases the solubility of the active drug facilitating its transfer from the balloon surface to the vessel wall. DCBs are a worthy substitute for stent implantation functioning by delivering an antiproliferative drug into the vessel wall with the release of the drug in a more even distribution through single balloon inflation. Studies have shown a minimum of one month of DAPT is safe with this metal-free technology.[18] Thus it can be helpful in situations where DAPT needs to be shortened and places where stent implantation even bioabsorbable stents or scaffolds (BRS) should be avoided such as small vessels, diffuse lesions, and SBs involving bifurcations.

BIOABSORBABLE STENTS OR SCAFFOLDS

Development of biodegradable stents was first started in the 1990s. The principle concept of these stents is to provide a temporary scaffold of polymers or metals coated with an antiproliferative drug or gene restoring vessel patency and permitting positive arterial remodeling. The polymeric stents are more flexible than metal and various polymeric materials which are used include polyglycolic acid (PGA), poly-L-lactic acid (PLLA), polycaprolactone (PCL), and poly (D, L-lactide) copolymer (PDLLA). The time for degradation of polymeric stents ranges from 6 months to over 24 months.[19] On the other hand, magnesium alloy is the most commonly used alloy for metal base BRS. Histological animal studies demonstrate complete biodegradation of the alloy within 56 days of implantation. This is replaced by neointimal hyperplasia and calcium deposition which is less marked than after conventional stents.[20,21]

Polymeric BRS

- *Igaki-Tamai stent*: This self-expanding and springy stent marketed by Kyoto Medical Planning Co Ltd, Kyoto, Japan is made up of high molecular weight PLLA polymer. It has a strut thickness of 170 µm with 24% stent strut surface/vessel coverage. Tamai et al. reported the first-in-man series of 25 stents in 2000. An acceptable rate of restenosis and TVR (6.7%: 1/15 patients) with no deaths or MI was seen after the initial 6-month angiographic and intravascular ultrasound (IVUS) follow-up.[22] There was no significant stent recoil and negative vessel remodeling on long-term follow-up but there were two cases of a definite stent scaffold thrombosis and a 50% major adverse cardiac events (MACE) rate.[23]
- *REVA stent:* This is a tyrosine-derived polycarbonate polymer biodegradable stent (REVA Medical) that

encompasses elements that slide open and then lock into place preventing its deformation on expansion thus virtually eliminating recoil. This stent is radio-opaque with high radial strength and uses standard balloons for deployment. There was a normal healing response at 28 days on histological evaluation in porcine-stented arteries with no acute or chronic inflammation. Modification of the stent resorption rate should be done according to the specific needs (coronaries, vulnerable plaques, diabetic lesions, and drug delivery). The REVA Endovascular Study Of a Bioresorba Coronary Stent (RESORB) enrolled 30 patients in a nonrandomized manner and assessed MACEs at 30 days and after a follow-up period of 5 years. The lesion treated had average diameter stenosis (DS) of 70% and there was a good acute luminal gain [MLD (mm) of 0.88 ± 0.39 preimplant and 2.76 ± 0.36 postimplant]. Moreover, the device also successfully prevented negative remodeling.[24]

- *The bioabsorbable everolimus-eluting stent or BVS (Abbott Vascular, CA, US)*: It is made up of two polymers [PLLA semicrystalline polymer coated with poly-D, L-lactide (PDLLA)]. Both these polymers fully biodegrade within approximately 18 months. The crossing profile of the stent is 1.4 mm with a strut thickness of 150 µm. ABSORB Study was a multicenter, open-label, nonrandomized, single-arm study of 30 patients done to assess its feasibility and efficacy. The lesions treated were discrete de novo lesions (8 mm long) in a single coronary artery. The patients were followed at 6 months and 12 months to assess MACEs and ST angiographically as well as imaging [IVUS or optical coherence tomography (OCT)].[25] The MACE rate at 12 months was 3.3% with no late stent thromboses and in-stent late loss was 0.44 mm angiographically which was mainly due to a mild reduction of the stent area (–11.8%) by IVUS. Intimal hyperplasia was nonsignificant. On OCT imaging, the presence of a thin layer of intimal coverage on almost all of the struts was reassuring but 7% of 671 struts in 13 stents investigated showed malapposition at follow-up. Late-acquired malapposition was seen in seven of the 25 patients by IVUS, with a reduction in the stent area suggesting chronic stent recoil.[25] The acute recoil of the was studied by Tanimoto et al., in 27 selected patients from the ABSORB study and compared with an equal number of patients using the metallic everolimus-eluting cobalt-chromium stent in the SPITIT I and II trials. No significant difference was seen in acute absolute recoil in both groups (0.20 vs. 0.13 mm), implying that BVS stents have as good radial strength as their metallic counterparts.[26]

Metallic BRS

- *Magnesium stents*: This is a balloon-expandable, tubular and slotted BMS carved by laser from a tube of a biodegradable magnesium alloy and rare earth elements.[21] It has two radio-opaque markers at either end for visibility. The stent has an open mesh design ideal for side-branch access with large cells. It has got low-elastic recoil (<8%), with minimum shortening after inflation (<5%). Degradation rates of stents range from 60 to 90 days. The PROGRESS-AMS (Clinical Performance and Angiographic Results of Coronary Stenting with Absorbable Metal Stents) trial studied Biotronik's magnesium stent in 63 patients. Patients had a de novo lesion in a single coronary artery with a lesion length of 13 mm or less and reference diameter between 3.0 and 3.5 mm.[20] The primary endpoints of the trial were cardiac death, nonfatal myocardial infarction, or clinically driven target lesion revascularization (TLR) occurred in 15 patients (24%) at 4 months follow-up. At the 1-year follow-up, there was no stent and no deaths. At 1 year, the TLR rate was 45% and elastic recoil was 7%. The mechanisms for late loss as seen on IVUS were neointimal formation, the decrease in external elastic membrane volume and an increase in volume outside the originally encircled stent with no substantial changes in the original plaque volume.
- *Iron-based BRS*: Iron-based BRS have high radial strength and are highly biocompatible but their main limitation is a longer corrosion period and clearance from the vessel. It has shown similar efficacy and safety profiles to current-generation everolimus DES in preclinical porcine models.[27]

Combination Stents

Tacrolimus-eluting cobalt-chromium polymer stent: Tacrolimus-eluting stent, Mahoroba™, has been developed (Kaneka Corporation), combining a thin, flexible cobalt-chromium alloy coated with a PDLA polymer incorporating tacrolimus.[28] It has balloon-expandable struts with a thickness of 75 µm with the polymer on the abluminal side composed of tacrolimus 0.94 µg/mm^2 and degradation of the matrix in 9 months. In a porcine model, this stent demonstrated early endothelialization and reduction of neointimal thickening up to 90 days after implantation.[29]

INITIAL EXPERIENCE WITH BRS

The Absorb BRS was the first biodegradable stent approved for use by the US Food and Drug Administration (US FDA). The approval came based on several large, multicenter, randomized controlled trials (The ABSORB II, ABSORB III, ABSORB CHINA, ABSORB JAPAN, TROFI II, and EVERBIO III trials).[30-35] These trials compared ABSORB to a contemporary cobalt–chromium everolimus-eluting stent (CoCr-EES). The results of all trials demonstrated similar performance characteristics and safety profiles of both devices but increased rates of scaffold thrombosis at 1 year was demonstrated in subsequent analyses in the absorb cohort.[36,37] This trend continued at 3 years follow-up,[38] with increased ischemia-driven TLR in the ABSORB cohort. After 3 years of follow-up, the adverse events stabilized and were comparable to CoCr-EES at 5 years during which there was complete scaffold dissolution.[39] Due to the increased rate of ST the stent was withdrawn from the US market in 2018.

LESSONS LEARNT FROM ABSORB FAILURE

Although the results of the absorb trials led to its withdrawal, the program provided some valuable lessons, in particular in BRS deployment techniques.

- *Deployment technique*: Smaller substudies showed that optimal deployment techniques reduce inadequate vessel sizing, malposition, and scaffold underexpansion reducing the rates of scaffold thrombosis, and the "PSP" technique (predilation, proper sizing, and postdilation) also emerged.[40]
- *Imaging*: The vessel sizing should essentially be done using imaging. Accurate vessel sizing for BRS implantation can be done only with OCT. Imaging also helps in better understanding modes of scaffold thrombosis.[40]
- *Strut thickness and design*: There are solid- and fluid-mechanical alterations after ABSORB deployment due to the bulky strut design of the ABSORB BVS which induces excessive mechanical loading over the arterial circumference and recirculation zones around the strut surface. The thicker struts trigger the development of greater neointimal hyperplasia and late lumen loss (LLL) over time compared to contemporary metal DES due to increased circumferential stress and low endothelial shear stress even though the stress is temporary.[40]
- *Vessel size*: BRS should be avoided in vessels with a reference vessel diameter (RVD) of <2.5 mm and >3.75 mm. In smaller vessels, there are increased rates of BVS scaffold thrombosis (up to fourfold). When deployed in vessels with RVD < 2.25 mm, there was an increased rate of device thrombosis (4.6% vs. 1.5%) and TLF (12.9% vs. 8.3 %) compared to metallic DES.[30] On the other hand use of BRS in large vessels (>3.75 mm) caused under expansion or scaffold fracture.[41]
- *Lesion anatomy*: Inferior outcomes have been demonstrated in small-scale studies and clinical trials in complex lesions such as in-stent restenosis, bifurcation PCI, ostial lesions, and severely calcified lesions.[42-44]

ADVANCEMENT IN BRS TECHNOLOGY: REGAINED INTEREST AND HOPE

Higher strut thickness was one of the main culprits behind the increased rate of scaffold thrombosis with early-generation BRS. But to prevent vessel recoil strut thickness (>150 µm) was required at the cost of longer resorption times. Apart from this, thicker struts led to polymer dismantling and scaffold discontinuity.

With advancements in BRS technology and through innovations in stent design, reductions in strut thickness have been achieved with some BRS (MeRes100, Meril Life Science, Gujrat, India; Mirage, Manli Cardiology, Singapore; MAGNITUDE, DEFIANCE and APTITUDE BRS Amaranth Medical, Mountain View, CA, USA; Firesorb, MicroPort, Shanghai, China). Future BRS with thinner have better crossing profiles and deliverability. Moreover, the chances of scaffold thrombosis are also less due to reduced shear stress at the vessel wall, resulting in less turbulent blood flow, improved endothelization, and less thrombus formation.[45] Periprocedural myocardial infarction and restenosis rates are also reduced with thinner struts.[46,47] Through this advancement in stent and strut design, lower-profile scaffolds have been made possible without sacrificing radial strength.

DEFIANCE BRS has the thinnest struts of 85 µm. The *APTITUDE BRS* (115 µm) already showed better healing properties than ABSORB BRS in porcine arteries. The *RENACENT II* study (n = 60) has demonstrated the safety and efficacy of APTITUDE BRS in humans with a high clinical (98%) and procedural success (100%). The angiographic LLL was only 0.3 mm at 24 months. The *RENACENT III* evaluated *MANGITUDE BRS* (98 µm, in patients with CAD with myocardial ischemia). It showed 97% device and procedural success with an acceptable LLL of 0.28 mm. At 2-year data demonstrated the safety and efficacy of the device at 2 years. There was no scaffold thrombosis, and 97% of struts were endothelized at 2 years with a luminal gain of 1.6 ± 0.3 mm following BRS implantation. So, despite the minimal strut thickness its performance was similar to its thicker congeners (AMPLITUDE and FORTITUDE). Amaranth Medical Inc, USA altered the properties of PLLA by heating and extrusion called "postprocessing" producing ultrahigh molecular weight PLLA polymers which have superior tensile strength (10 times higher elongation at break) and refractoriness to fracture during expansion (such as postdilatation) compared to conventional PLLA and similar to metallic stents.[48]

Many newer BRS have resorption times less than that of ABSORB (around 3 years). This will be advantageous in shortening the duration of dual antiplatelet and early restoration of vasomotion. *Magmaris* BRS has the shortest elution time of 9–12 months and has shown high rates of vasomotion (80%) at 6 months in the BIOSOLVE II study.[49] The large BIOSOLVE IV trial (n = 1,024) has also established the safety and efficacy of Magmaris BRS in the broad patient population with low scaffold thrombosis (0.5%) at 1 year.[50]

Currently, *MeRes100* is approved for clinical use in India while five (*ABSORB, DESolve, ART Pure, Fantom, and Magmaris*) are CE-approved for use under clinical trials. The European Association of PCI (EAPCI) in conjunction with the European Society of Cardiology (ESC) has laid down a structured framework for evaluation of newer BRS in future. They recommend a follow-up period in trials well beyond the expected resorption time of the BRS. The extended follow-up will aid in the demonstration of the long-term safety of the device and will allow assessment for vessel patency, neointimal growth, and residual inflammation after resorption of the device.[48] Results of several ongoing trials on better innovative techniques are awaited. These innovations might lead to improved outcomes compared to early-generation devices.

DRUG-COATED BALLOON

Drug-coated balloon is a novel technology based on fast homogenous transfer of antiproliferative drugs into the vessel wall by single inflation. The basic concept of DCB is rapid healing of the vessel wall owing to the fast release of the drug. The full exposure of drugs to smooth muscle cells in a short duration results in a sustained effect in the first hours to days after angioplasty. DCB is a semicompliant angioplasty balloon which is coated with an antiproliferative agent and transiently releases drug within 30–60 seconds unlike the long-term drug release of DES.[51]

Technical Aspects

It was demonstrated from initial experimental work that a rapid drug uptake by the tissue and drug persistence in the vessel wall to compensate for a short contact time is the main prerequisite for nonstent-based approaches for local drug delivery. After initial experiments with a variety of different coatings on balloon catheters taxane compounds such as asprotaxel and paclitaxel were investigated finally. Moving ahead, the combination of a highly lipophilic drug and a specific coating matrix was finally tested in a small first-in-human trial of coronary ISR, in which a significantly lower incidence of restenosis was demonstrated.[52]

Thereafter, sirolimus and its derivatives were also investigated for use in DCBs. However "limus" substances had poorer transfer rate compared with paclitaxel and reversible binding to rapamycin receptor. Several approaches have been developed to solve the sirolimus drug delivery system. One is the liquid formulation in a porous balloon and the SABRE (Sirolimus Angioplasty Balloon for Coronary In-Stent Restenosis) trial was studied with sirolimus in a liquid formulation delivered by a porous balloon for coronary ISR.[53] But a crystalline sirolimus coating with butylated hydroxytoluene as an excipient showed up to 50% drug persistence at 1 month and a clinical randomized trial using this formulation in DES ISR showed comparable in-segment LLL between the paclitaxel- and the sirolimus-coated balloon groups after 6 months with no difference in clinical events at 12 months.[54,55]

Importance of Lesion Preparation for DEB Success

The lesion should be adequately prepared to gain the proper benefits of DCB. For simple lesion dilatation using a semicompliant or a noncompliant balloon with a 1:1 balloon-to-artery ratio is adequate. However, in difficult balloon negotiation or underfilled or undersized vessels, serial dilatation starting from smaller balloon size and reassessing after administering vasodilatation should be done. In cases where the lesion does not open with a standard semicompliant or noncompliant balloon, high pressure noncompliant or scoring, or cutting balloon should be used, especially while dealing with ISR patients. In more difficult lesions, adjunctive therapy such as rota-ablation, orbital atherectomy, laser, or lithotripsy can be employed.[52]

Characteristics of adequately prepared lesion:

- Correct vessel size balloon inflates fully
- ≤30% residual stenosis
- TIMI (thrombolysis in myocardial infarction) flow grade 3
- Absence of a flow-limiting dissection (type A and B dissections are acceptable)

A properly engaged guide catheter with good guide support is paramount to ensure that DCB reaches the target lesion in one attempt. It should be of correct vessel size and inflated for a prolonged duration and should be handled carefully.

Current Indications of DEB

- *Small coronary vessels:* The interventional treatment of coronary arteries is defined as lesions in vessels ≤2.5 mm in diameter usually account for 30–50% of total coronary procedures. The PEPCAD I study was the first RCT which assessed the DCB (SeQuent Please) in small vessels. It consisted of 114 patients with lesions <2.8 mm.[56] At 6 months, the in-segment LLL was 0.16 ± 0.38 mm compared to 0.62 ± 0.73 mm with BMS. The rate of MACE at 12 months was 6.1% vs 37.5%, out of 15% mainly due to target TLR.[57] BELLO trial included 182 patients with lesions < 2.8 mm randomized to two either an In.Pact Falcon balloon and the TAXUS DES. After 6 months of follow-up, LLL was significantly lower in the DCB-arm than in the DES-arm (0.08 ± 0.38 mm vs. 0.29 ± 0.44 mm; $p = 0.001$) which translated into reduction in MACE at 3 years of follow-up.[58,59] In the SeQuent SVD Registry of 479 patients with de novo lesions of small RVD (≥ 2.0 mm and ≤ 2.75 mm), TLR and MACE rates were lower with DCB at 9 months (4.7% and 3.6%, respectively).[60] BASKET-SMALL 2 trial also showed noninferiority of DCB for treatment of native small coronary vessel disease with similar event rates at 12 months.[61]
- *Coronary in-stent-restenosis*: A large meta-analysis of RCTs demonstrated DCBs equivalent to DES in reducing revascularization for BMS ISR, but were somewhat less efficacious in DES ISR. Patients with multiple previous stent layers are the most suitable candidates for DCB use as it will protect relevant SBs emerging from the stent

with ISR, and those who are candidates for shorter DAPT because of high bleeding risk.[62] Based on this, current guidelines on myocardial revascularization recommend the use of DEB for ISR treatment (Class I, Level of Evidence: A).[63]

- *Bifurcation disease*: Coronary bifurcation PCI is still challenging due to unsatisfactory angiographic clinical outcomes, mostly in the SB. Even with the use of the latest generation DES, there remains the risk of restenosis risk, especially if more complex techniques are used. Due to this reason provisional bifurcation approach is preferred over the dedicated two-stent strategy. The DEBUT study (n = 117) categorized patients into three arms—(1) DCB pretreatment + BMS; (2) BMS + uncoated balloon; and (3) paclitaxel DES + uncoated balloon. Although good results were achieved with the DCB + BMS arm, it was not superior to BMS, mainly because of good results of the POBA-treated SB in both BMS and DES arms.[64] In the multicentric BABILON RCT MACE and TLR rates were higher in the DCB group than the DES group (17.3% vs. 7.1%; p = 0.105 and 15.4% vs. 3.6%; p = 0.045) because of greater and nonsignificant LLL with DCB pretreatment and BMS implantation in MB showed.[65] The multicentric PEPCAD BIF RCT compared the DCB-only strategy with POBA in 64 patients with coronary bifurcation lesions. There was significantly lower restenosis with the DCB strategy (6% in the DCB-only group vs. 26% in the POBA group, p = 0.045). The results implied that the DCB-only strategy can be used for bifurcation lesions with acceptable angiographic results after careful lesion preparation.[66]
- *High bleeding risk*: Bleeding events after PCI lead to increased mortality as well as ischemic events like non-fatal MI.[66] DCBs can be preferred over stents in patients who are at high bleeding risk such as frail elderly patients, patients on anticoagulants, or patients having chronic kidney disease or those with bleeding diathesis. Although DAPT duration can be shortened with the latest generation of DES, it can be stopped in case of severe life-threatening bleeding much earlier after DCB than after DES as there is no risk of ST. The recommended duration of DAPT after the only strategy in de novo vessels is 4 weeks based on expert opinion, with good results in recent clinical trials for stable patients.[67] RCTs and registry data of 1,500 patients have shown no incidence of acute or subacute thrombosis after a DCB-only treatment.[68] Some studies have reported an acute thrombosis risk of only 0.2% after DEB-only PCI.[69] Thus in high bleeding risk patients (previous life-threatening bleeding or upcoming major surgery) only the DCB strategy can be employed because of the low thrombotic risk with them.
- *Diffuse coronary lesions*: Stent length is an independent predictor of TLF.[70] PCI using ≥60-mm overlapping DES has demonstrated high TLR rates of up to 24%. Studies have shown that PCI of coronary lesions >25 mm in length, the DCB outcomes (DES used as bailout) were comparable to DES only approach. Thus, DCB alone using DES as a bailout to limit stent length in vessels with diffuse disease can be an alternative and useful approach.[71]

CONCLUSION

The burden of CAD is globally high with a lot of patients having complex lesions such as bifurcations, ISR, and diffuse coronary stenosis involving small vessels. However, with the advancement in stent technology and experienced operators, good results can be obtained in complex PCI also. However, the risk of repeat revascularization is still troublesome. The availability of BRS and DCB in certain special scenarios would be helpful in this regard. However, we need further research and advancement in these technologies for desired outcomes.

ONLINE REFERENCES

Please scan the QR code provided at the end of the table of contents for References of this chapter.

CHAPTER

163

Metal Less Percutaneous Coronary Interventions: Future of Angioplasty

Mahesh Nalin Kumar, Joyal J Kandathil, Arya Subhadra, Ashwin Mahesh

ABSTRACT

Coronary artery stents have become the most common therapeutic intervention in medicine, used in over 90% of treatments. Technological advances have improved the efficacy and long-term safety of second- and third-generation devices, reducing restenosis rates. Drug-eluting stents release antiproliferative drugs from polymer coatings on the stent surface, reducing restenosis and requiring fewer revascularizations. However, metallic DES still has limitations, and treatments guided by intravascular imaging are crucial for maximizing the advantages of current stent technology.

Keywords: Coronary artery stents, treatments, technology, efficacy safety, drugs

INTRODUCTION

The biggest advancement in the field of percutaneous coronary intervention (PCI) since balloon angioplasty is the use of coronary artery stents. Nowadays, stents are used in >90% of treatments, which makes this method one of the most often used therapeutic interventions in medicine.

The last three decades have seen tremendous technological advances that have improved the efficacy of drug-eluting stents (DES) use and the long-term safety of second- and third-generation devices, resulting in a rapid and reproducible decrease in restenosis.[1,2] Antiproliferative drugs could be carefully released from polymer coatings on the stent surface, thanks to DES. With the use of these devices, the rate of restenosis was effectively reduced, and <5% of the target lesion required recurrent revascularization. The many versions of newer-generation drug delivery systems (DES), many of which claimed to have unique polymers, strut designs, or antiproliferative drug properties, all lead to a plateau in the relative advantages.[3-5] Improved medical care, sophisticated implantation methods, and intravascular imaging guidance have all contributed to the successful development of coronary artery stents and the related therapeutic advantages.

Metallic DES is still unable to meet a few requirements, nevertheless. In actuality, almost half of the bad events that follow PCI are linked to stents, not the underlying condition getting worse. Treatments guided by intravascular imaging seem to hold the key to maximizing the advantages of current stent technology.[6]

Fully bioresorbable scaffolds (BRSs), composed of both naturally occurring and synthetic biodegradable polymers, undergo bioresorption leading to the restoration of cyclic pulsatility and vasoregulation. They are intended to offer mechanical support and drug delivery similar to metallic DES early (within 6–12 months) after PCI. Young acute coronary syndromes, in-stent restenosis, unjailing coated side branches, and avoiding a permanent "full metal jacket" are among the conditions for which BRSs may be particularly beneficial. However, it is crucial.

POTENTIAL ADVANTAGES AND DRAWBACKS OF BIORESORBABLE SCAFFOLDS[7]

Reduction in Very Late Events with Vascular Bioresorbable Scaffolds

- Restoration of cyclic pulsatility and normal vasomotion
- Normalization of shear stress and cyclic strain
- Restoration of normal vessel curvature
- Reduced risk of very late polymer reactions
- Avoidance/resolution of stent malapposition
- Avoidance/resolution of late strut fractures
- Reduced neoatherosclerosis

- Unjailing of side branches
- Formation of a (neomedia) cap over lipid-rich plaque
- Plaque regression

Advantages of Vascular Bioresorbable Scaffolds

- Unjails covered side branches, restoring access
- Avoids full metal jacket, restoring late bypass surgery options
- Allows treatment of in-stent restenosis without necessitating a permanent additional metal layer
- Facilitates noninvasive imaging follow-up without artifacts
- Addresses physician's and patient's desires to avoid a permanent implant

Disadvantages of First-generation Vascular Bioresorbable Scaffolds

- Some devices require cold storage and specific deployment techniques
- Thicker/wider struts with larger crossing profile (more difficult to deliver)
- Greater attention to procedural technique required
- Greater risks of acute strut fracture compared with metallic DES
- Intraluminal scaffold dismantling
- Higher early rates of scaffold thrombosis and TVMI, particularly in small vessels **(Fig. 1)**

PHASES OF BIORESORBABLE SCAFFOLD FUNCTIONALITY

Refer to **Figures 2 and 3**.

LESSONS FROM FIRST GENERATION BIORESORBABLE SCAFFOLD

The first commercially available advanced vascular BRS, in the initial clinical trial (ABSORB Cohort A) involving 30 patients reported low major adverse cardiovascular events (MACE) over 2–5 years, demonstrating noninferiority to the best DES. However, subsequent modifications (BRS version 1.1) aimed at improving structural integrity resulted in increased MACE rates at 12 months and beyond, raising concerns about safety.[9,10] The safety profile of BRS was further questioned in subsequent trials and registries, such as GHOST-EU and ABSORB-II, showing higher rates of scaffold thrombosis.[11,12] Several limitations of first-generation BRS such as due to material low ductility, tensile strength, and elongation-to-break. Mechanical stress causing scaffold damage, discontinuity, and malapposition, which further heightens the risk of adverse events.[13] Procedural factors, such as inadequate vessel sizing and malapposition during implantation, play significant roles in scaffold thrombosis risk. Optimal predilatation, accurate sizing, and postdilatation (PSP) strategies have been suggested to reduce adverse events, with imaging guidance crucial for precise implantation and follow-up assessment.[14] Diabetic patients may have increased scaffold restenosis rates, and specific lesion types such as bifurcation and heavily calcified lesions may require more aggressive preparation.[15] Advanced imaging techniques like optical coherence tomography help in assessing vessel injury and neointimal hyperplasia, influencing strut embedment. Understanding these factors is vital for optimizing BRS implantation strategies and monitoring patient outcomes effectively.[16]

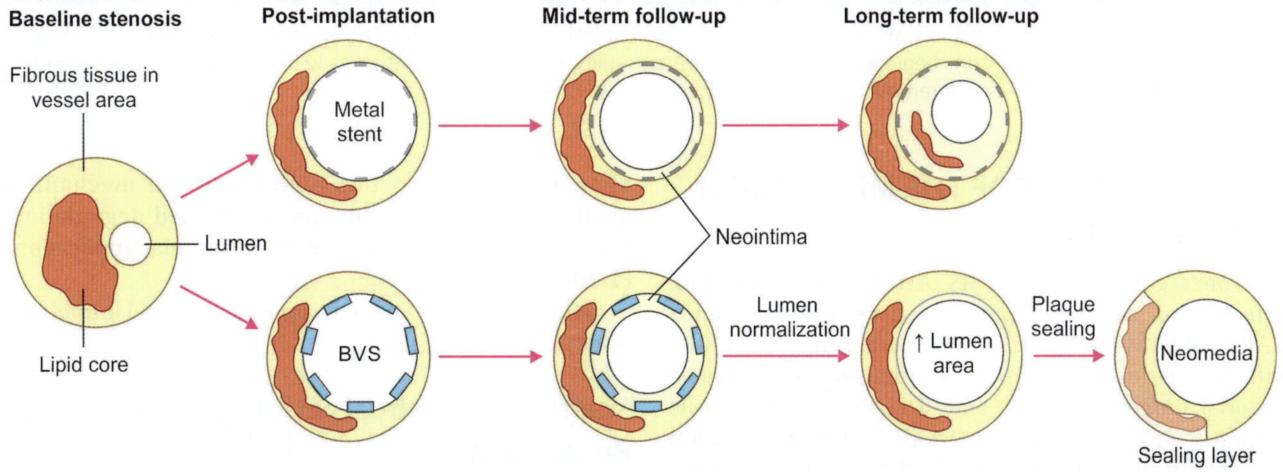

FIG. 1: Differences in vascular healing between bare metal stent and bioresorbable vascular scaffolds. Optical coherence tomography at 6–12 months and 2–5 years after absorb implantation shows absorption of struts and endothelial layer formation and by formation of a connective tissue neo media after strut resorption. Bare metal stent leads to constraint of vessel leading to neoatherosclerosis.[7]

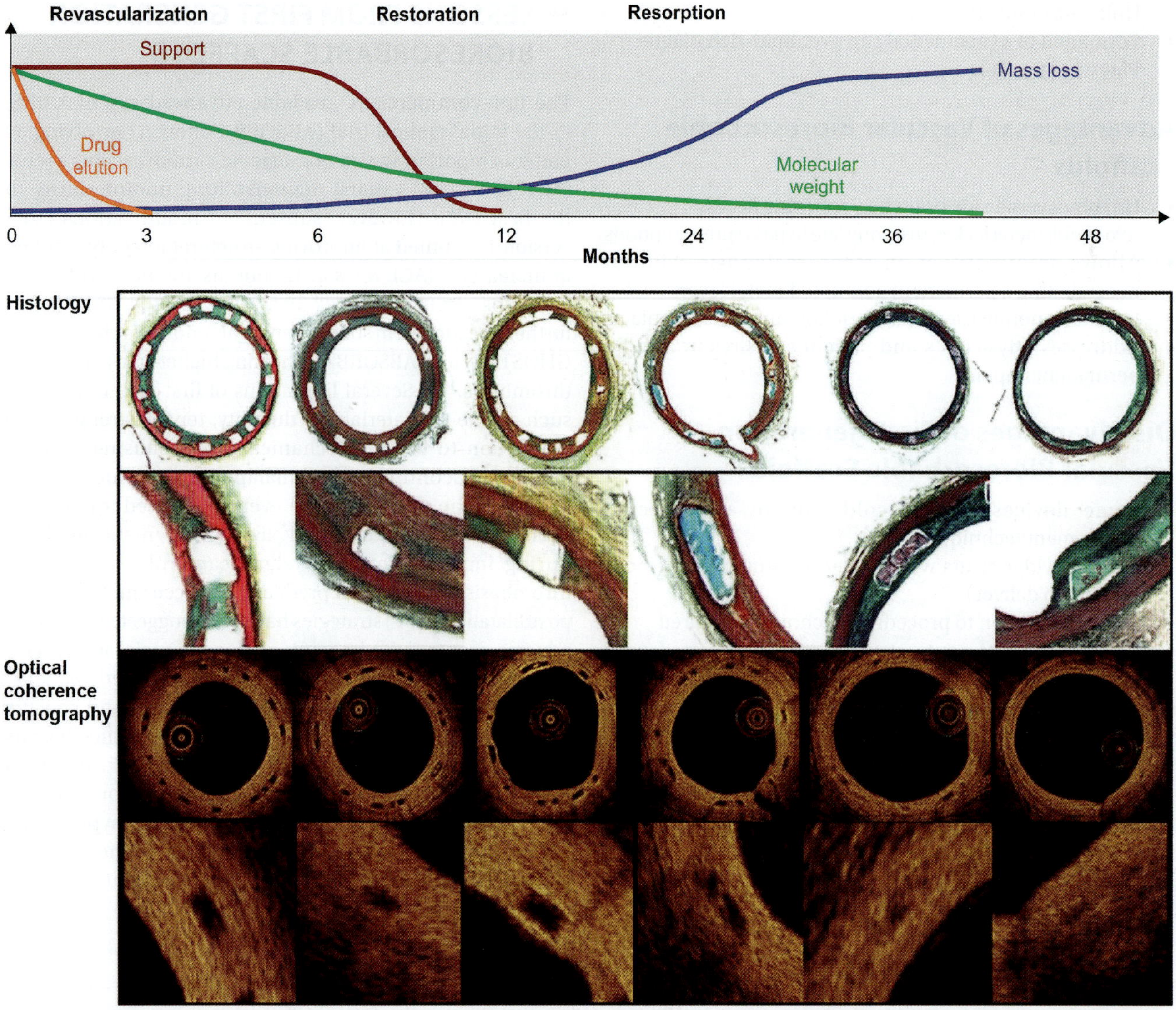

FIG. 2: Three phases of bioresorbable scaffolds functionality: (1) Mechanical support and drug delivery immediate phase at ≈6 months, (2) The restoration phase where struts begin to disappear and cyclic pulsatility and vasomotion return at 12 months, and (3) Total resorption leading to return of adaptive vascular remodeling responses by 24 months.[7]

IMPROVEMENT OF THE MECHANICAL PROPERTIES

The next generation of BRS ArterioSorb BRS from Arterius Ltd. has decreased strut thickness to 95 μm.[17] HARTSORBTM by HARTLON, is another innovative BRS with 90-m struts.[18] Magnesium, a promising bioresorbable material, outperforms PLLA and PDLLA in terms of tensile strength and elongation at break. These magnesium alloy-based BRS begin to degrade after around 3 months, eventually changing into an amorphous calcium phosphate phase during the resorption process.[19,20] STENTiT, a new BRS incorporates polymeric microfibers into its support grafts.[17] Each of these developments indicates continuous attempts to develop BRS with enhanced mechanical qualities, biocompatibility, and controlled degradation, improving the field of BRSs for cardiovascular applications **(Table 1)**.

What we learned from the past is that scaffold thrombosis is the Achille heel of BRS.

Scaffold Thrombosis Etiology and Prevention

The BRS was designed to gradually degrade thus restoring vasoreactivity and prevent late ST due to residual metallic stent. But the incidence of ScT led to ultimately withdrawn from the global market on September 14, 2017.

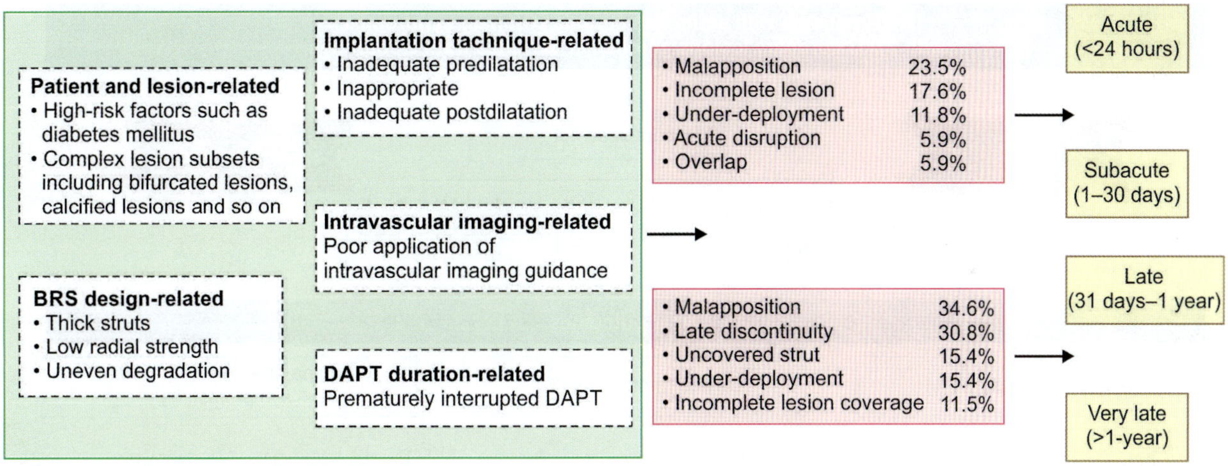

FIG. 3: Differences in vascular healing between metal stents and absorb bioresorbable scaffolds.[8]

TABLE 1: Mechanical properties and degradation time for different polymers and metals.[19]

Materials	Tensile modulus (GPA)	Tensile strength (MPA)	Elongation at break (%)	Degradation time (months)	Radiopacity
PLLA	3.1–3.7	60–70	02-Jun	>24	–
PDLLA	3.1–3.7	45–55	02-Jun	06-Dec	–
Oriented–PLLA	05-Jul	220–260	40–70	>24	–
Pure magnesium	40–45	220–330	20-Feb	03-Dec	+
Pure iron	200–210	170–270	50	>9	+
316 steel	190–200	668	48	Biostable	+
CoCr	210–235	820–1,200	35–55	Biostable	+

Note: The material lacks sufficient (–) and better (+) radiopacity.

(PLLA: poly-L-l actic acid; PDLLA: poly-D-L-lactic acid; CoCr: cobalt chromium)

PATIENT AND LESION CHARACTERISTICS AND INFLUENCE ON OUTCOME (FIG. 4)

Patient-related

For early ST acute myocardial infarction and heart failure where significant contributing factors.[21] Cardiogenic shock causes insufficient coronary perfusion which leads to liver dysfunction and limited drug absorption. Late ST is predisposed by diabetes mellitus and renal failure, with history of malignancy being the strongest predictor (OR 17.5, 95% CI 4.7-65.3) due to prothrombotic phenotype bleeding under DAPT treatment.[8]

Lesion-related

Type B and C lesions, vessel diameters of <2.25 mm and >3.75 mm due to high risk of ScT is in small vessels (<2.25 mm) and scaffold dislocation larger diameter vessels, however, it is safe to implant in well-prepared calcified lesions.

Bioresorbable Scaffold Design on Outcome

The BRSs have thicker struts than contemporary DES 100-150 microns versus 50-80 microns. This hinders endothelialization. In the future the thickness of scaffolds needs to be reduced, thus minimizing coronary flow disturbance; and for better mechanical properties.

Implantation Technique and Influence on Outcome

A meta-analysis of five ABSORB prospective studies showed that the factors which reduced ScT were predilation with a ≥1:1 balloon-to-artery ratio and optimal postdilation.[8]

Sizing of Scaffold

It is preferred to use IVI for BRS implantation. We need to select the appropriate scaffold size. Undersized and malapposed scaffold may collapse into the lumen and hastening the formation of ScT. The 1 year MACE and MI rates also increase when oversized scaffolds in a relatively small vessel.

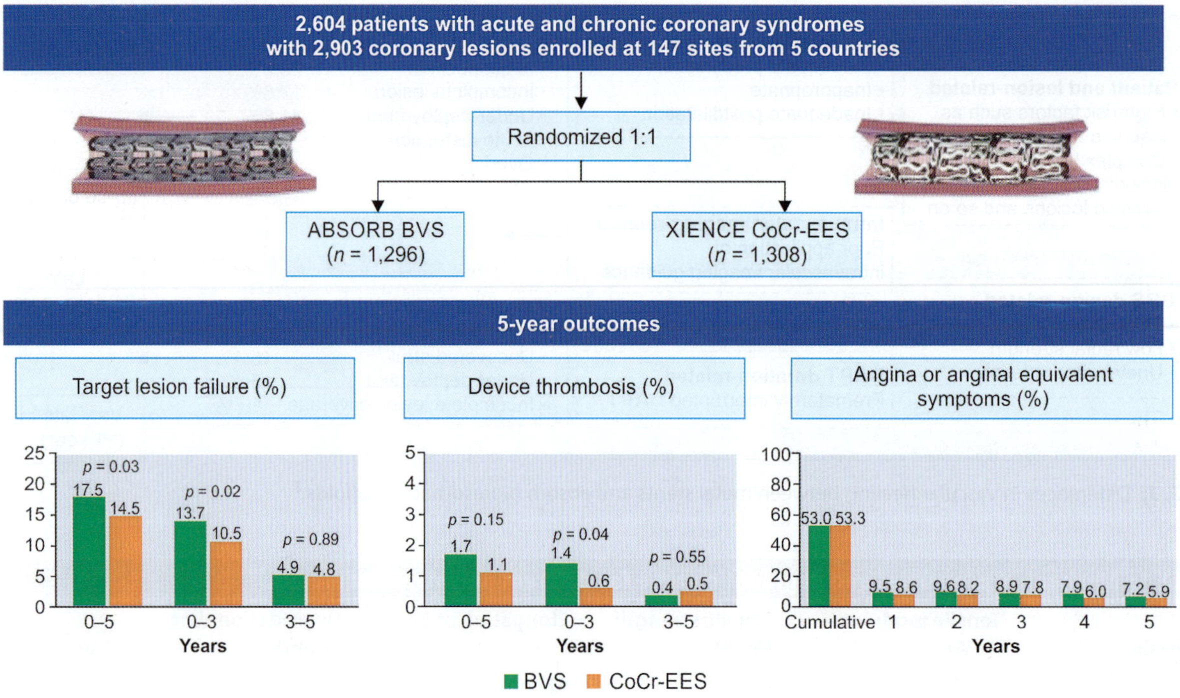

FIG. 4: Five year results from ABSORB IV trial.

Postdilation of Scaffold

Postdilation is also preferably done under IVI with a noncompliant balloon at 16–25 atm, with a nominal diameter up to 0.25–0.50 mm larger than that of the scaffold.

Intravascular Imaging

The IVI is mandatory for implantation and follow-up. OCT is the preferred modality.

Dual Antiplatelet Therapy Duration

Duration of dual antiplatelet therapy (DAPT) should be for 6–12 months, may be longer in complicated lesions:

- Comparison of BRS to metallic DES showed that at 5 year, rates of target lesion failure were higher with BRS than DES (17.5% vs. 14.5%, $p = 0.03$).
- Device thrombosis rates were also higher with BRS than DES at 3-year follow-up and between 3 and 5 years.
- However, rates of angina were at nearly 50% of patients within 5 years and were similar with both devices.[23]

INDIAN SCENARIO

MeRes100 The ®MeRes100 PLLA sirolimus-eluting scaffold, 100 µm thick, features a hybrid cell design and is expected to degrade over 2–3 years. Its structure enables optimal vessel wall conformity, high radial strength, and includes platinum markers for better positioning. Initial MeRes-1 study[24] findings ($n = 108$) showed promising results at 6 and 12 months, reporting low late lumen loss (LLL) and no restenosis. IVUS revealed minimal neointimal hyperplasia, while OCT displayed robust scaffold coverage. Extended outcomes confirmed its efficacy and safety up to 3 years with maintained lumen patency and not very late scaffold thrombosis. The MeRes-1 Extend study (64 patients) reported a 1.61% MACE rate at 2 years with minimal TLR and no scaffold thrombosis. OCT imaging showed consistent flow and excellent strut coverage at 6 months with a low late lumen loss.[25]

DRUG-COATED BALLOONS

In the case of peripheral and coronary artery disease, drug-coated balloons (DCBs) offer a clinical therapy option for local medication delivery without the requirement for a transient or permanent implant.

With relatively little systemic exposure, an effective local drug concentration is reached. A number of DCB characteristics, however, are essential to guaranteeing efficient drug delivery to the intended site. These characteristics include: (1) the shape of the balloon surface; (2) the uniformity of drug distribution along the balloon's surface; (3) drug stability during manufacturing, handling, and storage; (4) the degree of premature loss during transit to the target vessel segment; (5) the capacity to release during balloon expansion; (6) the efficiency of transfer to the vessel wall; and (7) the quantity of particulate material released to the distal circulation **(Fig. 5 and Table 2)**.[26]

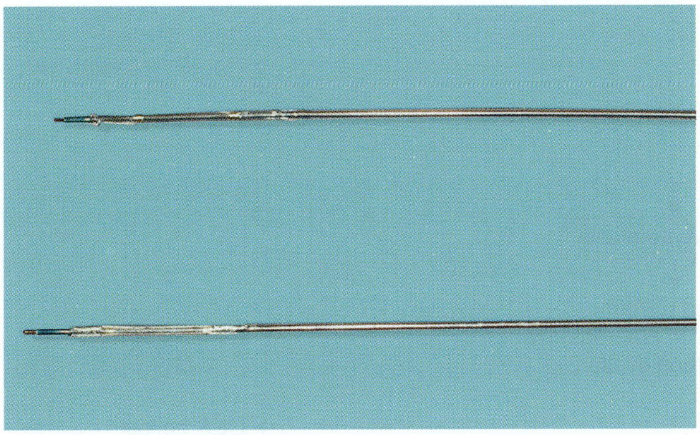

FIG. 5: The balloons were coated with paclitaxel at a concentration of 1.3–3 μg/mm² of balloon surface; they were intended for angioplasty.[27] Approximately 10% of the initial dose of paclitaxel was lost during the catheter's advancement through the guiding catheter and hemostatic and 80% of the dose was released during inflation. <20% of the dosage produced at the target site is immediately absorbed into the vessel wall; the majority is dispersed throughout the blood stream as particulate debris. It was discovered to have produced a notable, dose-dependent, statistically significant decrease in angiographic late lumen loss (LLL) and an equally striking, statistically significant rise in minimal lumen diameter as compared to controls at the 5-week follow-up.[28] At present, the preferred medication is paclitaxel, often administered at a dosage of 2–3.5 μg/mm² balloon surface.[29]

TABLE 2: Drug-coated balloon device.

Device	Additive and substance class	Dose (mg/m²)	Approval	Vessel territory
MOXY™	Polysorbate + sorbitol	2	CE certified and FDA	Peripheral
IN.PACT™ (Admiral, Pacific, Falcon)	Urea	3.5	CE certified and FDA approved	Coronary/ peripheral

CORONARY APPLICATION

In-stent Restenosis

As the standard approach for DES-ISR, DCB treatment avoids many metal layers, minimizes the requirement for prolonged DAPT, permits operation reproducibility, and appears to have a beneficial long-term impact on hard endpoints. Careful lesion preparation ensuring adequate initial lumen gain, including the use of customized balloons, could reduce the negative effects on angiographic results. The first attempts to combine BMS with DCB to produce a novel kind of "polymer free DES" fell short of limus-DES. Patients with coronary small vascular disease (SVD) treated with DCB alone had better long-term results than patients treated with DCB plus BMS in the same segment. Consequently, the "DCB-only" technique was proposed by an expert consensus panel.[30-32]

The highest level of recommendation for the stent in-stent technique and the use of DCB in the treatment of BMS- and DES-ISR (class 1 level A, respectively) is provided by the ESC guidelines for revascularization in both 2014 and 2018.

The Paccocath™ balloon group in the Paccocath in-stent restenosis (ISR)-I trial demonstrated notably superior angiographic outcomes (in-segment late luminal loss 0.74 ± 0.86 mm versus 0.03 ± 0.48; $p = 0.002$) and corresponding 12-month clinical outcomes. The Paccocath ISR-II experiment builds upon the preliminary results of the first ISR trial, which showed that the Paccocath™ balloon catheter's positive benefits persisted for up to 5 years following the intervention.[33]

In contrast to "simple" predilation with a semicompliant balloon, the ISAR-DESIRE 4 trial demonstrated that in patients with DES-ISR, predilation with a scoring balloon prior to use of a DCB was linked with a considerable reduction of diameter stenosis and binary restenosis at follow-up angiography.[34]

By using DCB treatment as the standard approach for DES-ISR, several metal layers are avoided, a shorter course of DAPT is required, the process can be repeated, and long-term hard endpoints appear to benefit. By using specialized balloons and meticulous lesion preparation to ensure adequate initial lumen gain, the negative effects on angiographic results might be minimized **(Flowchart 1)**.

Coronary De Novo Disease

The first attempts to combine BMS with DCB to produce a novel kind of "polymer free DES" fell short of limus-DES. Patients with coronary SVD treated with DCB alone had better long-term results than patients treated with DCB plus BMS in the same segment. Consequently, the "DCB-only" technique was proposed by an expert consensus panel.

The guidelines are based on the basic idea of meticulous lesion preparation with a balloon to vascular ratio of 0.8–1.0. When lesion preparation yields satisfactory results, the operator can proceed with a DCB stand-alone strategy; otherwise, in the event of major dissection (type C or higher), the operator can utilize a stent (or potentially a next-generation scaffold).[35,36]

Femoropopliteal Artery

The use of DCB in femoropopliteal arteries is increasingly the norm. But the class impact does not exist. The applicability of the encouraging results of the coronary Paccocath ISR-I and II trials to peripheral artery restenosis prevention remained uncertain. Immediately after the coronary ISR study was launched, the Thunder and FemPac trials, regarding the effectiveness and tolerance of Paccocath™ paclitaxel-coated balloon catheters in preventing restenosis in the superficial femoral artery.[37]

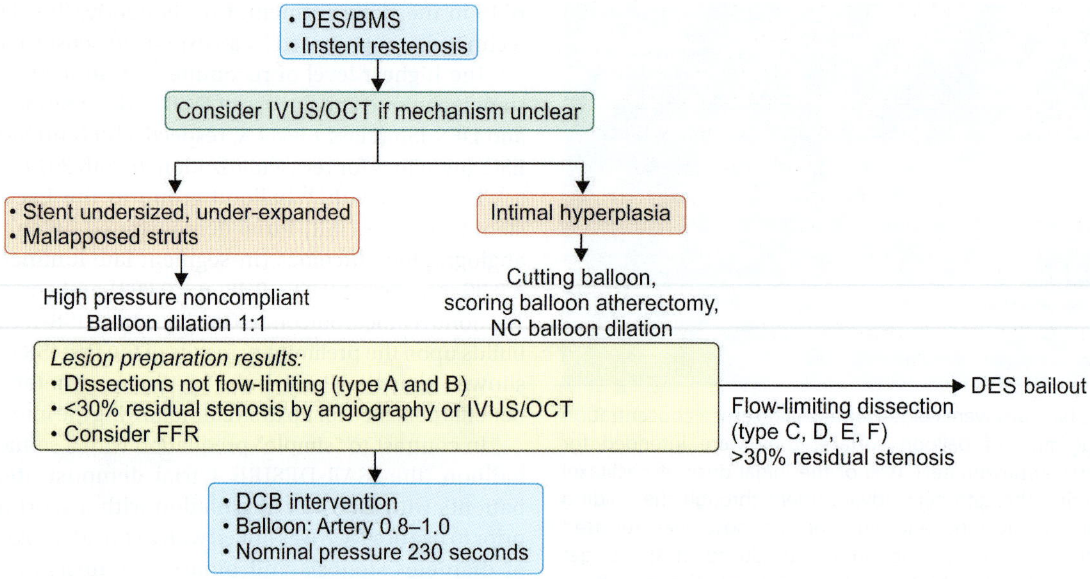

FLOWCHART 1: A primary drug-coated balloon strategy for treatment of in-stent restenosis.

The FemPac trial supported the findings of the Thunder trial by showing that paclitaxel exposure for a brief period of time may be enough to prevent restenosis in injured peripheral arteries. Meanwhile, Thunder's 5-year data demonstrate a persistent benefit of DCB over conventional PTA without any indications of late catch-up. Nevertheless, this long-term analysis only included patients who were available for follow-up and had not previously undergone revascularization, which resulted in an overrepresentation of DCB patients. Regrettably, a higher total number of deaths in this subgroup was misinterpreted for a methodologically flawed meta-analysis as purported proof of a higher long-term mortality rate following DCB. Nevertheless, a meta-analysis revealing higher mortality 2 or more years following therapy with stents or balloons coated with paclitaxel was released in December 2018.[21,38,39]

Compared to standard angioplasty and stent technologies, DCB offer several advantages: (1) the potential for homogeneous drug delivery to the vessel wall; (2) an immediate drug release without the need for a polymer, which can cause chronic inflammation and late thrombosis; (3) the option to use balloon catheters alone or in conjunction with a bare metal stent; (4) the possibility of reducing antiplatelet therapy; and (5) lower restenosis rates in target peripheral (and also coronary) arteries when compared to conventional treatment. In situations like femoropopliteal arteries, where stent insertion is neither desirable nor feasible, DCB can also be used.

The results from randomized controlled coronary clinical trials consistently show that paclitaxel in a matrix of soluble additive coated on balloons reduces neointimal formation, as well as LLL, restenosis, and repeat revascularization in patients with complex coronary artery lesions. It seems that in the coronary circulation, paclitaxel coated balloon angioplasty holds the greatest promise for lesions in which stent deployment is not desirable or technically challenging (e.g., in-stent restenosis, long and distal lesions, very angulated segments, small vessels, or bifurcation lesions).

The treatment of coronary ISR has been recognized as an acceptable indication for DCB (ESC recommendations class 1 level A recommendation) based on data from randomized clinical trials.

A DCB-only angioplasty approach in coronary de novo disease satisfies the criteria of the "leaving nothing behind" principle.

Meanwhile, DCB was on the verge of replacing other treatments for the transfemoral region as the norm. Despite the significant methodological shortcomings in the meta-analysis and the lack of a definite pathomechanism, it has created a great deal of ambiguity, which has prevented many patients from receiving the most appropriate medicine for the peripheral angioplasties.[38,39]

CONCLUSION

Although new generation DES are thought to be the greatest technology available right now for percutaneous intervention and represent the latest revolution in the field, there is still room for improvement, particularly in terms of very long-term clinical outcomes, with these late events likely resulting from the metallic cage's continuous presence.

Akin to metallic DES, BRS have been developed to provide drug delivery and mechanical support. After complete resorption, the vascular structure returns to normal, including expanded vessel wall remodeling and function potentially improving very late clinical outcomes.

The DCB have similar outcome despite the drug used. Adequate data from studies indicate it can be used in DES ISR and hence ESC guidelines class 1 level A recommendation. In coronary de novo disease, DCB emphasizes the concept of "leaving nothing behind". In femoropopliteal arteries it is becoming the current treatment option.

However, the role of BRS and DEB in clinical practice remains investigational and will need further development.

ONLINE REFERENCES

Please scan the QR code provided at the end of the table of contents for References of this chapter.

CHAPTER 164

FFR Angiography versus Catheter-based FFR: Pros, Cons, and Caveats

Prasant Kr Sahoo, Nitish Prasad, Shyam Prasad Sahoo

ABSTRACT

Two primary methods for fractional flow reserve (FFR) measurement are CT angiography-based FFR and catheter-based FFR, each offering distinct advantages and limitations. CT angio-based FFR is a noninvasive approach that uses computational fluid dynamics (CFD) to estimate FFR from angiographic images, streamlining the diagnostic process and reducing patient discomfort. Catheter-based FFR, considered the gold standard, involves direct pressure measurements across coronary lesions using a pressure-sensitive guidewire, providing highly accurate functional assessments. This review compares these two techniques, exploring their clinical applications, advantages, disadvantages, and the current evidence supporting their use. Understanding these methods' comparative effectiveness is crucial for optimizing CAD management and improving patient outcomes.

Keywords: Fractional flow reserve, coronary artery disease, CT angio-based FFR, catheter-based FFR, coronary stenosis, computational fluid dynamics, functional assessment

INTRODUCTION

Fractional flow reserve (FFR) is a crucial diagnostic tool for evaluating the hemodynamic significance of coronary artery stenosis, playing a pivotal role in guiding treatment decisions for patients with coronary artery disease (CAD).[1] FFR is defined as the ratio of the pressure distal to a coronary lesion to the pressure proximal during induced hyperemia, usually achieved through adenosine administration. Clinically, FFR values of ≤0.80 are indicative of significant stenosis, which is associated with an increased risk of adverse cardiac events, including myocardial infarction and mortality.[1] A systematic review involving 78,897 patients revealed that FFR-guided percutaneous coronary intervention (PCI) significantly reduces all-cause mortality and myocardial infarction compared to nonphysiology-guided strategies.[2] Beyond immediate decision-making, FFR also offers valuable prognostic information following PCI. Studies have demonstrated that post-PCI FFR values of ≤0.85 are predictive of target vessel failure.[3] Furthermore, the integration of FFR with coronary flow reserve (CFR) enhances the predictive accuracy for future coronary events.[4]

Accurate FFR measurement is essential for making informed decisions in managing patients with CAD, as it aids in determining the need for revascularization and optimizing treatment strategies.[5] By identifying stenoses that are hemodynamically significant, FFR can reduce unnecessary invasive procedures, thereby improving patient outcomes and ensuring that interventions are appropriately targeted.[5] Traditional methods of assessing coronary stenoses, such as angiography alone, often fall short in predicting the functional significance of a lesion.[6] Angiography provides a visual assessment of the coronary anatomy but does not offer direct information on the physiological impact of a stenosis.[7] FFR fills this gap by providing a quantitative measure of the pressure drop across a lesion during induced hyperemia, which correlates with the potential for myocardial ischemia.

There are two primary approaches for measuring FFR: (1) CT angio-based FFR (FFR-angio) and (2) catheter-based FFR (FFR-wire). CT angio-based FFR represents a noninvasive technique that uses computational fluid dynamics (CFD) to estimate FFR values based on standard coronary angiographic images.[8] This method eliminates the need for additional instrumentation, such as pressure wires, and avoids the administration of hyperemic agents like adenosine.[8] FFR-angio has gained popularity due to its ability to streamline the diagnostic process, potentially reducing procedural time, cost, and patient discomfort while still providing critical information about coronary physiology.[9]

On the other hand, catheter-based FFR (FFR-wire) involves the direct measurement of pressure gradients across coronary stenoses using a pressure-sensitive guidewire.[10] During this procedure, a specialized guidewire is advanced across the stenotic segment of the coronary artery, and pressure measurements are taken proximal and distal to the lesion during hyperemia induced by agents like adenosine.[10] FFR-wire is considered the gold standard for functional lesion assessment, with a wealth of clinical evidence supporting its use in guiding revascularization decisions.[11]

Given the increasing reliance on FFR in the management of CAD, it is essential to understand the comparative effectiveness of the two primary methods—(1) CT FFR-angio and (2) FFR-wire. However, there is a notable lack of literature directly comparing these two approaches. This gap in the current research underscores the need for a comprehensive review. Therefore, this review aims to provide a detailed analysis of both techniques, focusing on their respective advantages, disadvantages, and clinical applications.

CT ANGIOGRAPHY-BASED FFR

CT angio-based FFR represents an advanced noninvasive method for assessing the functional significance of coronary stenosis, utilizing angiographic images to provide crucial diagnostic information.[12-14] Unlike traditional FFR, which relies on pressure wires to measure pressure gradients across a lesion, angio-based FFR employs computational models to estimate FFR values from standard coronary angiograms.[15]

The fundamental principle behind CT angio-based FFR is to use CFD to analyze the blood flow and pressure distribution within the coronary arteries.[15] By processing angiographic images, the method reconstructs the three-dimensional (3D) geometry of the coronary vessels and simulates blood flow under hyperemic conditions. The resulting estimates of pressure gradients provide insights into the hemodynamic significance of coronary stenoses, helping clinicians make informed decisions about the need for intervention.[15]

This innovative technique leverages two angiograms with angles > 25°, combined with independent 3D vessel reconstruction and numerical pressure drop calculations.[16] By doing so, CT angio-based FFR allows interventional cardiologists and researchers to obtain precise anatomical quantifications of one or multiple lesions within the analyzed coronary segment. This approach enables a detailed evaluation of both individual and consecutive lesions, enhancing the ability to determine their functional significance accurately.[16] A study indicated that CT FFR angio exhibited a sensitivity of 91%, a specificity of 100%, and a diagnostic accuracy of 96.8%.[17]

Several angiography-derived FFR methods have been developed to estimate FFR without directly instrumenting the coronary arteries, each offering unique characteristics and varying levels of supporting evidence. These methods generally involve two core components—(1) the creation of a 3D anatomical model of the coronary vessels using at least two angiographic projections and (2) the application of different fluid dynamics computation approaches. It has shown high-diagnostic accuracy (87%) in both small and large validation studies, including successful use in multivessel disease and SYNTAX score reclassification. A recent multicenter trial (FAST-FFR) confirmed its high-diagnostic performance.

VIRTUAL FRACTIONAL FLOW RESERVE

Initially described in the VIRTU-1 study,[18] this method utilizes 3D vessel reconstruction from orthogonal angiographic projections. It combines pressure and flow data with a complex transient CFD analysis, though this approach can be time-consuming. An improved version using pseudotransient steady-state CFD has significantly reduced computation time to approximately 3 minutes while maintaining similar diagnostic accuracy.[19] Virtual FFR (vFFR) has also been used to predict the physiological response to stent placement, showing a mean difference from actual post-PCI FFR of 0.01 ± 0.03.[20]

Quantitative Flow Ratio

Initially developed as FFRQCA, this method involved 3D quantitative coronary angiography and TIMI frame count to estimate volumetric flow rates and calculate FFRQCA.[21] Quantitative flow ratio (QFR), introduced later, simplifies the process by using two angiographic projections and various mathematical equations to derive three values—(1) fixed-QFR (fQFR), (2) contrast-QFR (cQFR), and (3) adenosine-QFR (aQFR). cQFR and aQFR, which are patient-specific, generally show better correlation with FFR than fQFR, avoiding the need for adenosine.[22] QFR has demonstrated high-diagnostic accuracy and agreement with FFR in various studies,[23] and its performance has been validated in different patient populations and conditions, including acute coronary syndrome[24] and in-stent restenosis.[25-27]

SIMPLIFIED MODEL OF FFR CALCULATION

This method provides a simplified approach to FFR calculation without specialized software, using TIMI frame count and simplified fluid dynamics equations based on commercially available 3D models.[28] While it offers fast computation, it may require invasive FFR in a subset of cases.

Cardiovascular Angiographic Analysis Systems for Vessel Fractional Flow Reserve

Cardiovascular angiographic analysis systems (CAAS)-vFFR involves 3D vessel reconstruction and the measurement of resting aortic pressure during angiography, with empirical estimation of hyperemic flow. This method has been validated in various studies, demonstrating high-diagnostic accuracy and good correlation with invasive FFR.[23] It has also shown utility in predicting post-PCI FFR and in patients with left main coronary disease.[29]

The FFR versus FFRCT provides simultaneous calculation of pressure and flow across the entire coronary tree **(Figs. 1A and B)**. In contrast, information pertaining to invasively measured FFR is only available in vessels that have been interrogated with the pressure wire, which is typically decided during invasive coronary angiography at the discretion of the interventionists.[20] While anatomic percentage of stenosis is evaluated at the location of the lesion, invasive FFR is typically measured by positioning the pressure sensor in the distal part of the vessel and then manually pulling the pressure sensor back to the ostium to assess the distribution of abnormal epicardial resistance along the course of the vessel.[20] In both invasive FFR and FFRCT, the distal values in any given vessel reflect the cumulative pressure loss and impact of all disease proximal to the measurement location. Values obtained by both techniques may vary depending on the measurement location within a vessel.

Computational Pressure-flow Dynamics Derived FFR and Coronary Angiography-derived Diastolic Pressure Ratio

The most recent methods, introduced in the FLASH FFR study[30], utilize continuous measurement of aortic pressure and TIMI frame count for resting velocity, with novel computational pressure-flow dynamics (CPFD) to calculate computational pressure-flow dynamics derived FFR (caFFR). This method boasts rapid computation time and high-diagnostic performance.[30] A related index, coronary angiography-derived diastolic pressure ratio (caDPR), operates as a resting physiological index with a cut-off ≤0.89, also showing high-diagnostic accuracy against invasive FFR.[31]

Pros, Cons, and Caveats of CT Angiography-based FFR Methods

Angiography-based FFR methods have emerged as valuable tools in coronary artery assessment, offering various benefits alongside some limitations. One major advantage is their noninvasive nature, reducing the need for additional catheterization. This minimizes patient discomfort and risk associated with invasive procedures. These techniques have demonstrated strong diagnostic performance, with sensitivity and specificity rates often exceeding 90%.[22] They also offer long-term follow-up benefits, as their accuracy has been consistent over extended periods, reinforcing their utility in guiding treatment decisions.[23] For instance, QFR, which has been extensively validated, shows high-diagnostic accuracy with pooled sensitivity of 89% and specificity of 90%.[32] Similarly, CAAS-vFFR offers rapid computation, with a median time of 5 minutes compared to 7 minutes for invasive FFR, facilitating quicker clinical decision-making.[33] Additionally, methods such as QFR have demonstrated broad applicability, with successful testing in diverse populations

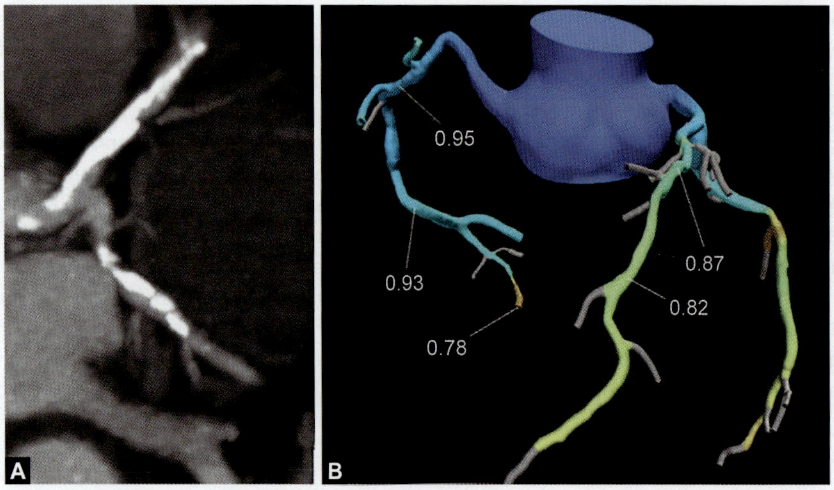

FIGS. 1A AND B: CT angio-based FFR evaluation.

including those with microvascular dysfunction and diabetes, and in conditions such as acute coronary syndrome.[23,34,35]

Despite these advantages, there are several limitations and caveats to consider. Most notably, these techniques still involve some degree of invasiveness and require specialized skills and expertise for accurate interpretation.[36] Some methods, such as those that rely on CFD, can be time-consuming and costly, with procedures often taking over 15 minutes and costs being very high.[36] Additionally, the requirement for intravenous (IV) or intracoronary (IC) adenosine in some techniques can complicate the procedure and limit their applicability.[36] Advanced methods such as vFFR and CAAS-vFFR often require high-quality imaging and advanced technologies, which may not be available in all clinical settings. For example, CAAS-vFFR has been shown to be limited by the quality of images, with only about one-third of routinely acquired images being eligible for analysis.[37,38] Furthermore, many methods, including QFR, are restricted to evaluating a single vessel, which may limit their utility in cases involving complex coronary anatomy such as bifurcations or ostial lesions.[22] Additionally, the accuracy of these methods is dependent on image quality; poor-quality images or motion artifacts can compromise diagnostic performance. The reliability of methods such as simplified model of FFR (FFRsim) and caFFR has been questioned due to their validation in smaller, single-center studies, which may not fully represent broader patient populations.[30,38] Since noninvasive determination of FFR is based on cCTA data, increased image noise, beam-hardening artifacts from metallic devices and especially motion artifacts can influence its quality. Since CT-based FFR research so far has only been performed with stable patients and nonacute cases, its accuracy in patients with acute coronary syndrome remains unknown. Furthermore, the postprocessing steps may be time-consuming and costly. Finally, the model used for fluid dynamics may be inaccurate for patients with changes in the hematocrit or hemoglobin concentration.

Caveats related to these methods include an "uncertainty zone" where methods exhibit reduced reliability, particularly within FFR values ranging from 0.77 to 0.86. In these cases, invasive FFR may still be necessary for accurate assessment.[39] Most methods also struggle with complex lesions such as those at bifurcations, ostia, or within bypass grafts, which can affect their applicability.[39] Furthermore, while these methods are promising, their performance in real-world settings may vary from clinical trial results, highlighting the need for continued evaluation and validation.[38,40]

CLINICAL EVALUATION OF COMPUTED FFR MEASUREMENTS

Two large prospective multicenter studies, the *DISCOVER-FLOW* (Diagnosis of Ischemia-Causing Stenoses Obtained Via Noninvasive Fractional Flow Reserve) and the *DeFACTO* (Determination of Fractional Flow Reserve by Anatomic Computed Tomographic Angiography) evaluated the diagnostic accuracy of CT-based noninvasive FFR measurements. In both studies, noninvasive measurements were compared with invasive FFR. Both studies demonstrated that the diagnostic performance of computed noninvasive FFR was superior for the detection of hemodynamically-relevant coronary stenoses compared to coronary CT angiography alone (DISCOVER-FLOW: Accuracy of 84% vs. 59%), mainly due to a reduction of false-positive findings detected by coronary CT angiography.

Catheter-based FFR

Catheter-based FFR is a diagnostic technique used to assess the functional significance of coronary artery lesions. By measuring pressure differences across a stenosis, FFR provides a quantitative evaluation of how much a lesion impairs blood flow.[10] This technique is widely considered the gold standard for guiding treatment decisions, such as determining the need for PCI.[11] The procedure involves advancing a pressure-sensing guidewire through the coronary artery to obtain pressure measurements at two points—(1) proximal and (2) distal to the lesion.[10]

During coronary catheterization, a catheter is introduced into the femoral or radial artery through a sheath, and a guidewire is advanced to navigate the vascular pathway. FFR involves the use of a pressure wire equipped with a sensor, typically a transducer, at its tip to measure pressure, temperature, and flow across the coronary artery, which helps in assessing the severity of a stenosis. This assessment is conducted under conditions of maximal blood flow, known as hyperemia, which is usually induced by administering agents such as adenosine or papaverine. The pressure measurements are taken as the wire is gradually pulled back across the vessel.[41]

In interpreting FFR results, higher values suggest that the stenosis is not functionally significant, while lower values indicate that the lesion may be causing significant blood flow restriction. Although there is no definitive cut-off value for abnormal FFR, clinical trials generally use a range between 0.75 and 0.80 to determine whether a stenosis is hemodynamically significant **(Fig. 2)**.[42]

Pros, Cons, and Caveats of FFR

The FFR offers several advantages over other techniques used to evaluate narrowed coronary arteries, such as coronary angiography, intravascular ultrasound (IVUS), or CT coronary angiography. One of the key benefits is its ability to account for collateral flow, which can make an anatomical blockage functionally insignificant.[43] Unlike standard angiography, which can sometimes underestimate or overestimate the degree of narrowing by only visualizing the contrast within the vessel, FFR provides a more precise functional assessment of the stenosis. Additionally, FFR is less susceptible to variability between patients compared to other indices of vessel narrowing, ensuring more consistent results across different individuals.[44] Moreover, FFR enables

$$\text{FFR} = \frac{\text{Distal coronary pressure (Pd)}}{\text{Proximal coronary pressure (Pa)}}$$
(During maximum hyperemia)

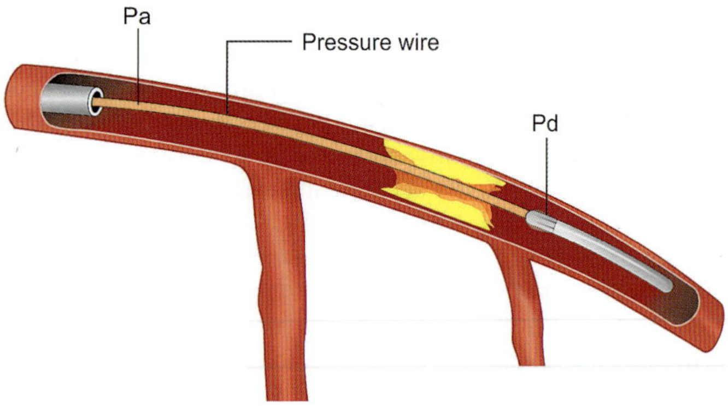

FIG. 2: Principle of catheter-based FFR.

real-time estimation of the impact of a narrowed vessel on blood flow, allowing for immediate therapeutic interventions such as balloon dilatation and stenting during the same procedure.[6]

The FFR is an invasive procedure that requires catheterization of the coronary arteries, which introduces inherent risks such as bleeding, infection, and vascular complications.[45] These potential complications necessitate careful consideration, particularly in patients with higher risk profiles.[45] Additionally, performing FFR requires a high level of skill and expertise. Variations in technique can significantly impact the accuracy of the results, underscoring the importance of proper training and experience for operators.[46] The cost of FFR is another notable disadvantage.

The FFR also has certain caveats that limit its applicability. The technique may be less effective for assessing complex lesions, such as those in bifurcations, ostia, or involving bypass grafts, where the anatomical challenges can affect the accuracy of the measurements.[8] Additionally, the invasive nature of the procedure carries risks beyond the typical complications associated with catheter insertion, including adverse effects from adenosine administration, which further complicates its use. Lastly, FFR requires specialized equipment and facilities, which may not be available in all medical settings, potentially limiting its accessibility and widespread adoption.[10]

CLINICAL STUDIES AND OUTCOMES

Tebaldi et al. (2023) conducted the HALE-BOPP study, a large multicenter prospective analysis of 1,305 patients with 2,422 diseased vessels, to evaluate the long-term outcomes of FFR-guided coronary revascularization. Patients were grouped into angio-revascularized, FFR-revascularized, and FFR-deferred categories. The study found that FFR-deferred vessels had the lowest target vessel failure (TVF) rate at 6%, compared to 7% for FFR-revascularized and 11.7% for angio-revascularized vessels over a median follow-up of 3.6 years. These results confirm that an FFR-based strategy is both safe and effective in improving long-term outcomes.[47]

Hideo-Kajita et al. (2018) conducted a meta-analysis to evaluate the clinical outcomes of complete revascularization (CR) in STEMI patients with multivessel disease (MVD) who did not present with cardiogenic shock. The analysis included nine studies encompassing 3,317 patients and compared the outcomes of CR using either angiography-guided or FFR-guided interventions with those of culprit-only revascularization. The findings demonstrated that CR significantly reduced major adverse cardiovascular events (MACE) (OR 0.49; 95% CI 0.36–0.66; $p < 0.001$), all-cause mortality (OR 0.69; 95% CI 0.48–0.98; $p = 0.04$), and repeat revascularization (OR 0.38; 95% CI 0.28–0.51; $p < 0.001$) at a follow-up period of 12 months or more. Specifically, FFR-guided CR was associated with a reduction in MACE (OR 0.52; 95% CI 0.30–0.90; $p = 0.02$), largely due to a decreased rate of repeat revascularization (OR 0.41; 95% CI 0.21–0.80; $p = 0.009$). These results suggest that CR in STEMI patients with MVD, particularly when guided by FFR, is associated with improved clinical outcomes compared to culprit-only revascularization.[48]

Takahashi et al. (2022) conducted a systematic review and meta-analysis to evaluate the diagnostic performance of computational FFR derived from angiography (Angio-FFR), IVUS-FFR, and optical coherence tomography-FFR (OCT-FFR), using conventional FFR as the gold standard. The study reviewed 49 studies, encompassing 7,010 lesions for angio-FFR, 305 lesions for IVUS-FFR, and 667 lesions for OCT-FFR. The analysis found that all three novel FFR indices demonstrated high-diagnostic accuracy. Specifically, Angio-FFR had a sensitivity of 0.87 (95% CI 0.84–0.89) and a specificity of 0.93 (95% CI 0.91–0.95); IVUS-FFR showed a sensitivity of 0.90 (95% CI 0.84–0.94) and a specificity of 0.95 (95% CI 0.90–0.98); and OCT-FFR had a sensitivity of 0.85 (95% CI 0.78–0.91) and a specificity of 0.93 (95% CI 0.89–0.95). The summary correlation coefficients with conventional FFR were 0.83 (95% CI 0.80–0.85) for angio-FFR, 0.85 (95% CI 0.79–0.91) for IVUS-FFR, and 0.80 (95% CI 0.74–0.86) for OCT-FFR. The study concludes that computational FFR derived from invasive imaging techniques shows clinically acceptable diagnostic performance and supports its use in clinical practice.[49]

A study by Di Serafino et al. (2013) involving 223 patients with stable or unstable angina and intermediate stenosis found that FFR-guided PCI, performed when FFR

and GIIb/IIIa receptor blockers were associated with better preservation of flow through the filter, reduced procedural ischemia, and reduced occurrence of abrupt closure, no reflow, or distal embolization compared to the group with no GIIb/IIIa receptor blockers. A similar benefit was not seen with GuardWire and GIIb/IIIa receptor blockers.[33] The possible explanation for this is that the GIIb/IIIa receptor inhibitors prevent platelet inhibition and deposition on the surface of the filter wire, thereby preventing filter occlusion.

LEFT INTERNAL MAMMARY ARTERY STENTING

Internal mammary artery grafts have shown longer patency rates when compared to other arterial and venous grafts. Arterial grafts are more likely to develop stenosis at distal anastomosis than SVGs. LIMA's severe atherosclerosis is rare and similar to native coronary artery atherosclerosis. In-hospital mortality after arterial graft PCI is identical to SVG PCI and significantly higher than native coronary interventions.[34] The intervention of IMA can be challenging due to the difficulty of cannulating the IMA—which may lead to IMA or subclavian dissection—the length and location of the lesion, the tortuosity of the vessel, which makes device delivery difficult, and slow-flow/no-flow due to the accordion effect.

- The IMA grafts are engaged, preferably in the RAO position. The standard guiding catheters used are IMA and JR. The catheter is advanced over a 0.035" guidewire and then withdrawn with a slight counterclockwise rotation to hook the IMA graft. A long sheath can be used for femoral access to improve the support of the guiding catheter. A shorter length guide (85 or 90 cm) can be used to reach the distal anastomosis. A left radial approach can be taken in case of challenging guide catheter engagement.

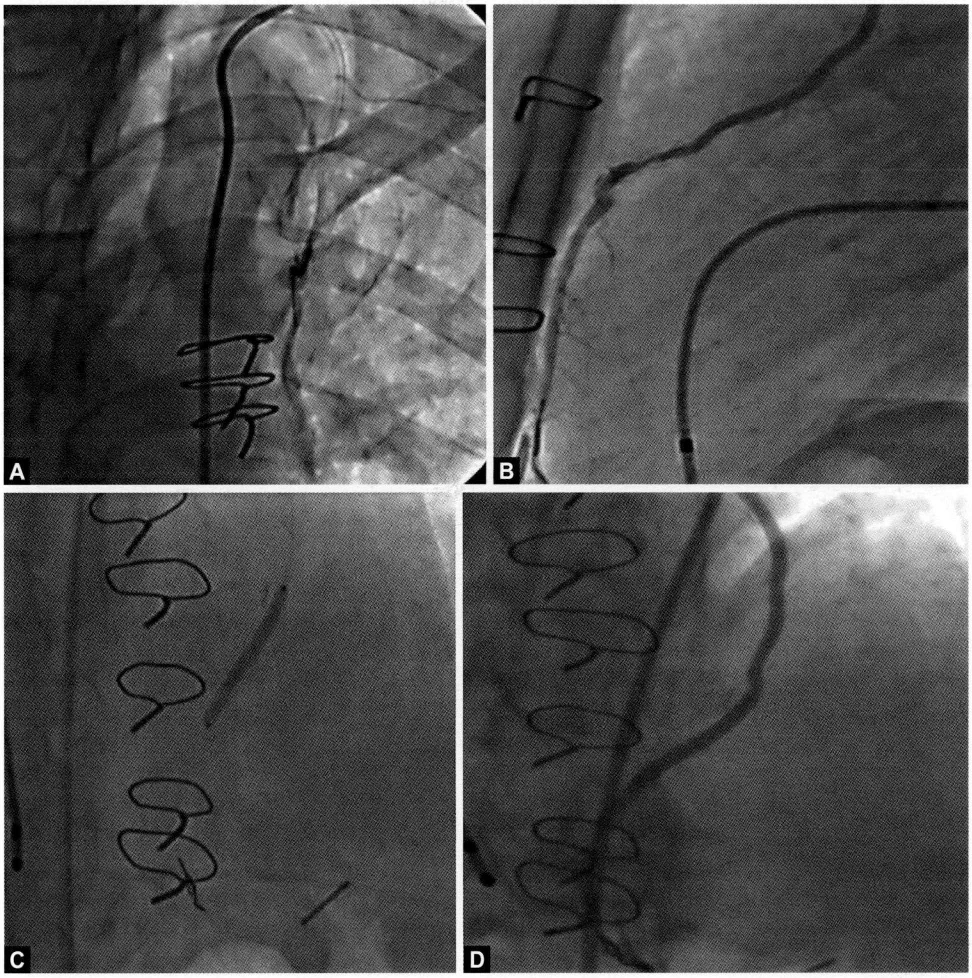

FIGS. 3A TO D: The percutaneous coronary intervention of left internal mammary graft. (A) LIMA hooked with IMA guiding catheter. (B) Angiography of the LIMA showed a tubular lesion with 80% stenosis at the LIMA–LAD anastomotic site. (C) The lesion was predilated with a 2.0 × 15 mm semicompliant balloon, followed by a 3.0 × 28 mm sirolimus-eluting stent (Cypher, Cordis, J&J) deployment. (D) The final angiogram showed TIMI III across LIMA and LAD.

(LIMA: left internal mammary artery; LAD: left anterior descending)

- Experience with balloon angioplasty and stenting of IMA graft is limited. In a retrospective study of 50 patients who underwent PCI to LIMA, 68% of the lesions were located at the LIMA coronary anastomosis site. The restenosis rate was higher if stenting was performed (65% vs. 18%, $p = 0.005$). Event-free survival was 65% in cases of stent implantation, whereas, in cases of pure balloon dilation, it was 100%.[35] In another registry, in-hospital and 1-year clinical outcomes of 174 consecutive patients were studied. Anastomotic lesions were evident in 128 cases (63%), and they were more commonly treated with balloon angioplasty (116/128, 91%), whereas lesions located at the ostium ($n = 16$, 8%) were more frequently treated with stents (11/16, 69%). In hospital, significant complications were scarce, and at 1-year follow-up, target lesion revascularization rates were low (7.4%) and comparable with those of previous reports.[36]
- In case of acute graft failure after LIMA to LAD anastomoses, directly deploying a covered stent may be preferred to avoid anastomotic site avulsion and perforation.[37] However, there is no data on stent longevity in LIMA grafts.
- Device deliverability can be ensured by using more trackable hardware, shorter stents and balloons, buddy wires, guide extensions, etc. **Figures 3A to D** illustrate a case of IMA stenting.

CONCLUSION

Percutaneous coronary intervention of post-CABG patients is technically challenging as both native coronary and bypass grafts have complex lesions. The native coronaries frequently have diffuse, calcified and CTO lesions, while bypass grafts, specifically venous grafts, have diffuse degenerative lesions. It is preferable to perform native coronary artery instead of bypass graft PCI. However, one frequently ended up doing bypass graft angioplasty due to acute clinical presentation. Venous and arterial grafts are associated with engagement difficulties, the challenges posed by tortuous and long vessels and the increased risk of slow-flow and no-reflow phenomena. Optimal results require meticulous planning, appropriate use of various hardware including EPD, and aggressive use of intra-arterial vasodilator therapy. Intravascular imaging can be of use for optimal results after stent implantation. A close follow-up is necessary, as graft vessel PCI is associated with higher MACE rates at short- and long-term follow-ups.

ONLINE REFERENCES

Please scan the QR code provided at the end of the table of contents for References of this chapter.

CHAPTER

166

Myths and Facts about Arterial Coronary Artery Bypass Grafting

OP Yadava

ABSTRACT

Notwithstanding the salutary long-term outcomes of arterial grafts, multiarterial grafting has not seen the traction that it deserves. Various reasons have been put forward, some valid and others just confounders emerging out of unfounded myths associated with arterial myocardial revascularization. This is an attempt to demystify some of these myths, using the Occam's razor technique of parsimony, keeping matters simple and straight.

Keywords: Arterial conduits, CABG, internal mammary artery, radial artery, arterial myocardial revascularization, contraindications

INTRODUCTION

The 1986 seminal paper by Loop et al.[1] from the Cleveland Clinic demonstrated long-term patency of left internal mammary artery (IMA) conduit to left anterior descending (LAD) coronary artery and its salutary effects on 10-year survival over all saphenous vein (SV) revascularization—93.4% vs. 88% for single-vessel coronary artery disease (CAD), 90.0% vs. 79.5% for double vessel CAD, and 82.6% vs. 71% ($p < 0.0001$) for triple vessel CAD, respectively. The resistance of IMA to atherosclerosis derives from its structural, physiological, and molecular characteristics, which make IMA immune from generation of adhesion molecules, transfer of inflammatory cells which induce smooth muscle proliferation, and impervious to lipoprotein permeation; all of which are antecedent to an atherosclerotic plaque. Therefore, LIMA to LAD graft has been touted as the holy grail of coronary artery bypass grafting (CABG) surgery. However, just as all the merits of using arterial conduits are well founded, certain myths about them have also crept in. It is time, therefore, to dispel these myths, which I would like to label as the "Dirty Dozen."

MYTH #1

Internal Mammary Artery is Foolproof

Though the predischarge graft failure rates are higher with the SVs (3–12%), arterial grafts too are prone to early failure due to technical errors, dissection, or acute thrombosis; 1–1.25% of IMA and 3–4% of radial arteries (RAs) fail predischarge. In fact, in the Project of Ex-vivo Vein Graft Engineering via Transfection (PREVENT) IV trial, LIMA-LAD failed in 8.6% of patients on routine surveillance angiography at 12–18 months.[2]

MYTH #2

Saphenous Vein is Down and Out

The SV, with a Class IIa recommendation from the 2018 European guidelines,[3] is the most common used conduit worldwide and accounts for nearly 80% of all grafts in CABG.[4] However, accelerated early failure of SV conduits in CABG has been a matter of concern and research lately. "Surgical technique, pressure distension, storage solutions, and technical support systems, pharmacological agents and therapeutics are the key elements identified in preventing or accelerating graft failure" **(Fig. 1)**.[5] With proper vein harvesting, handling, and storage, patency rates comparable to arterial grafts have been reported. The salutary results of no-touch (NT) SV grafting have been verified in a propensity-matched analysis,[6] randomized controlled trial (RCT),[7] and meta-analysis, wherein it reduced occlusion at 1 year [odds ratio (OR), 0.49; 95% confidence interval (CI) 0.29–0.82, $p = 0.007$].[8]

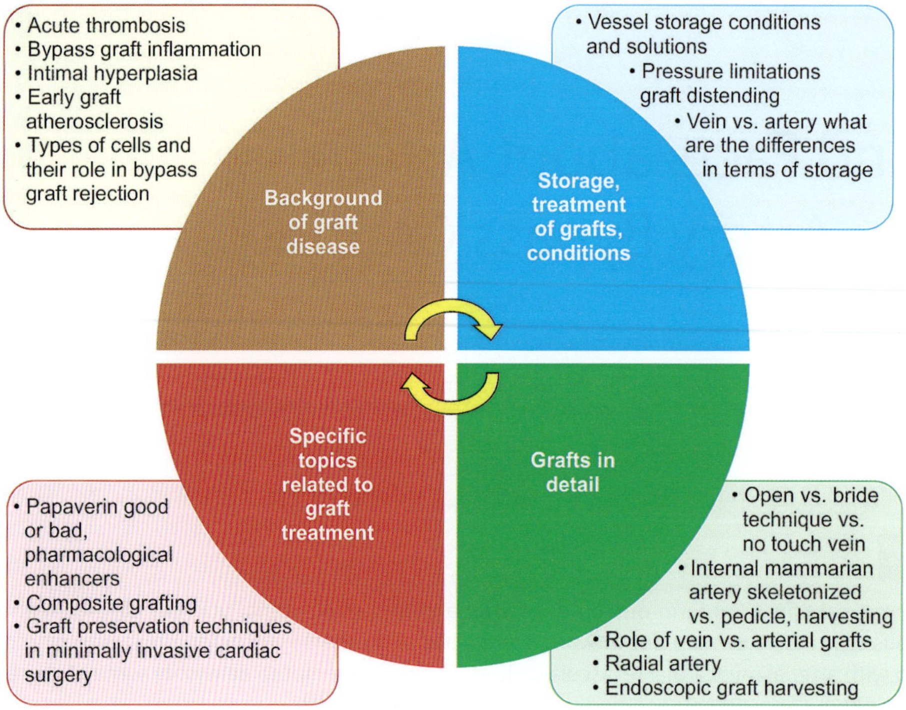

FIG. 1: Overview graft treatment, handling, and related topics.[5]

MYTH #3

There is a Paucity of Arterial Grafts

Nothing can be further from truth than this averment. Besides the two IMAs, there are two RAs, right gastroepiploic artery (RGEA) and even inferior epigastric arteries (IEA), which can be used if there is a paucity of conduits. The RA is currently a mainstream conduit and has been validated on long-term follow-up of 15 years in the Radial Artery Patency and Clinical Outcomes (RAPCO) RCT.[9] Even RGEA has yielded satisfactory midterm to long-term outcomes with the 10-year graft occlusion rate comparable to right IMA (10.3 and 8.4%, respectively; $p = 0.639$) with no statistically significant difference in 15-year survival (52.9% vs. 49.4%; $p = 0.470$) or freedom from major adverse cardiac and cerebrovascular events (MACCE—56.4% vs. 64.6%; $p = 0.364$).[10] However, RGEA and IEAs are technically difficult to harvest and the results have not been uniformly validated, and therefore remain as secondary (only-go-to-in-despair) conduits.

MYTH #4

Internal Mammary Artery Patency to All Coronary Territories is Same

Tatoulis et al. from Melbourne, Australia, demonstrated that LIMA patency was higher when grafted to the LAD (97.1%), compared to the obtuse marginal branch of the circumflex coronary artery (91.7%).[11] Similarly for right IMA, there was a hierarchy of patency for coronary territory grafted [LAD—best; right coronary artery (RCA)/posterior descending artery (PDA)—worst].[11] Differential patency may be influenced by the type of arterial conduit, being highest for RA when grafted to the RCA (80.65%), and for right IMA to the anterolateral territory (92.86%).[12] Therefore, coronary bed and the degree of peripheral run-off, besides the conduit, and other technical factors like size match, kinks, lie, tension, type of anastomosis, and, numero uno, the surgeon—skills and rigor—are important determinants of the patency of grafts.

MYTH #5

Bilateral Internal Mammary Arteries No better than Single Internal Mammary Artery

Though a number of observational studies and meta-analyses have demonstrated better outcomes with the use of bilateral IMAs, the same has not been validated by randomized data. The Arterial Revascularization Therapies (ART) trial was not able to demonstrate any significant difference in all-cause mortality at 10 years in an intention-to-treat analysis of patients undergoing bilateral versus single IMA grafting

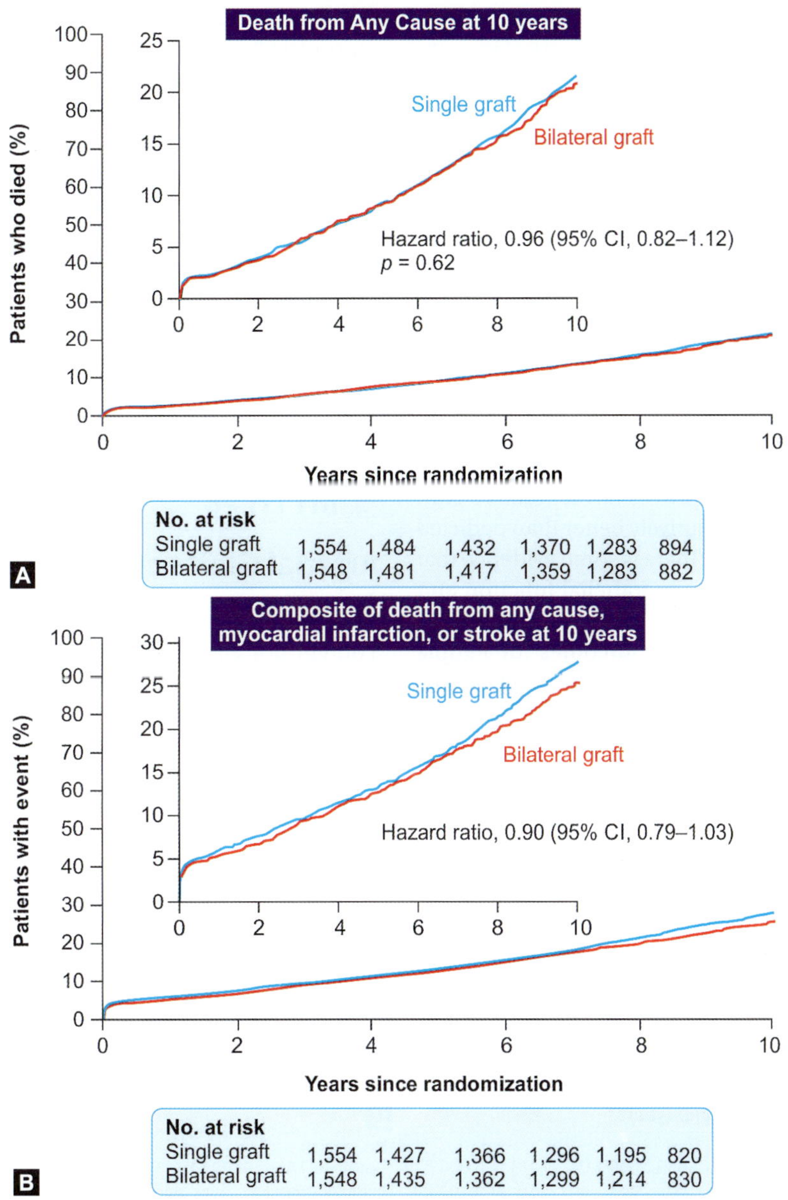

FIGS. 2A AND B: Primary outcome of death from any cause and composite outcome of death from any cause, myocardial infarction, or stroke at 10 years. Hazard ratios use the single-graft group as the reference. Insets show the same data on an enlarged *Y*-axis.[13]
(CI: confidence interval)

(Figs. 2A and B).[13] Notwithstanding a number of structural flaws in the planning and conduct of the trial, in a subsequent as-treated analysis, there were early shoots of advantage for bilateral IMAs over single IMA. Probably, a longer follow-up is needed to appreciate this benefit, as shown by Lytle et al.[14] from Cleveland Clinic in 2004, who demonstrated divergence of survival curves in favor of bilateral IMAs in the second decade postoperatively. A better designed Randomized Comparison of the Clinical Outcome of Single versus Multiple Arterial Grafts (ROMA) trial is currently on to address this conundrum.[15]

MYTH #6

Internal Mammary Artery is Immune to Competitive Flow

Sabik et al.[16] in 2003, in an article in *Annals of Thoracic Surgery*, demonstrated that the unadjusted IMA patency rate at 15 years was 92% and the risk factors associated with IMA occlusion were lesser degree of proximal coronary stenosis ($p < 0.0001$), thereby suggesting that the patency rates of IMA decreased as the coronary competitive flow increased.

The same was also borne out by the PATENCY IV study, with stenosis of <75% of native coronary artery (OR 1.76) and additional graft to diagonal (OR 1.92), each a surrogate of competitive flow, predictive of IMA failure.[2] Needless to mention, muscular arteries, especially RAs, are more susceptible to competitive flow (string sign) and SV performs the best in such situations.

MYTH #7

Skeletonized Internal Mammary Arteries are better than Pedicled Internal Mammary Arteries

The widely held belief that skeletonization of IMA preserves smooth muscle function and improves intraoperative graft size and flow, and therefore is intuitively better than pedicled IMA, has lately been challenged. There is some evidence that skeletonization may compromise endothelial function and structural and functional integrity of these grafts. In a post hoc analysis of the Cardiovascular Outcomes for People using Anticoagulation Strategies (COMPASS) CABG study, IMA occlusion rates at 1 year were higher in the skeletonized group (9.6%) than in the pedicled group (3.9%); and at 3-month follow-up, skeletonized graft was associated with higher rates of MACCE [7.1% vs. 2.1%, adjusted hazard ratio (aHR) 3.19; 95% CI 1.53–6.67; *p*-0.002] and repeat revascularization (5.0% vs. 1.4%, aHR 2.75; 95% CI 1.10–6.88; *p*-0.03).[17] The same was also borne out by the post hoc analysis of ART trial, where at a follow-up of 10 years, even though the primary outcome of mortality was same, the secondary outcomes of major adverse cardiovascular events (MACE) and sternal wound complications were higher with skeletonization **(Figs. 3A to C)**. However, when experience of >50 cases of skeletonization was factored in, there was no difference (HR 1.04; *p*-0.78).[18]

MYTH #8

Arterial Grafts can be Used in All Situations

Though not an absolute contraindication, one should be wary of using bilateral IMAs in morbidly obese (body mass

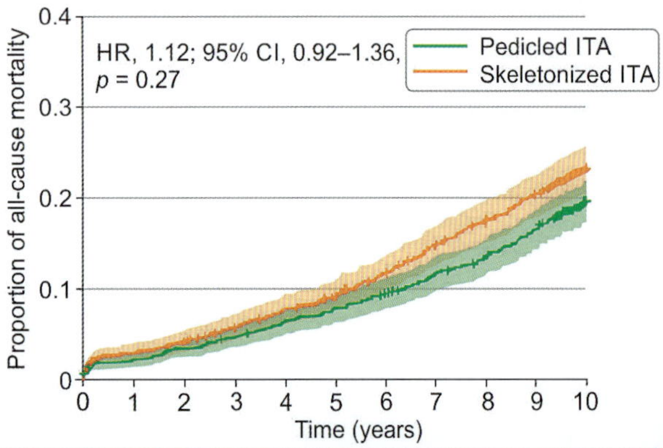

A

No. at risk											
Pedicled ITA	1,166	1,137	1,122	1,105	1,085	1,068	1,047	1,018	996	960	629
Skeletonized ITA	995	964	949	928	907	889	861	826	795	765	552

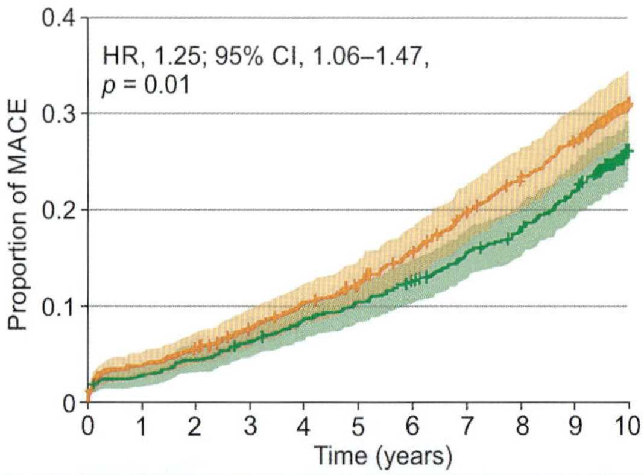

B

No. at risk											
Pedicled ITA	1,166	1,117	1,083,	1047	1,015	986	960	928	900	856	556
Skeletonized ITA	995	932	905	870	828	802	769	727	695	662	466

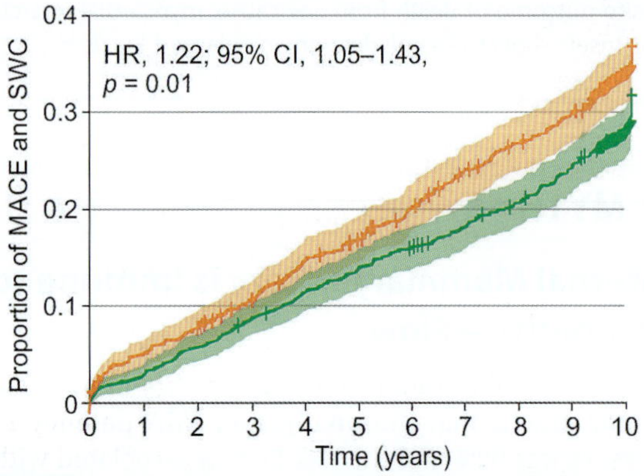

C

No. at risk											
Pedicled ITA	1,166	1,117	1,083	1,047	1,015	986	960	928	900	856	556
Skeletonized ITA	995	932	905	870	828	802	769	727	695	662	466

FIGS. 3A TO C: Kaplan–Meier curves of (A) all-cause mortality, (B) major adverse cardiac events (MACE), and (C) MACE and sternal wound complication (SWC) among the entire cohort.[18]
(HR: hazard ratio; ITA: internal thoracic artery)

BOX 1 Contraindications to the use of radial artery (RA) as a conduit for coronary artery bypass grafting.[20]

When not to use RA:
- History of major arm trauma
- Prior surgery on the arm
- Vasculitis
- Raynaud's syndrome
- Scleroderma
- Advanced chronic kidney disease
- Dialysis
- Angiography via RA access
- Insufficient ulnar artery compensation, evaluated with Allen's test, Barbeau's test, echo-Doppler, Doppler plethysmography
- Mild-to-moderate stenosis of the coronary target vessel, evaluated with visual inspection, quantitative coronary angiography, fractional flow reserve

index > 40 kg/m^2), insulin-dependent diabetes, and severe chronic obstructive airways disease.[13] The former two increase the risk of deep sternal wound infections (DSWI), and the emphysematous lungs may kink pedicled IMA. Even proximal subclavian artery stenosis precludes the use of pedicled IMA,[19] though it may still be used as a free graft. The RA should not be harvested whenever the patency of the palmar arch is compromised. Other contraindications for the use of RA, some of them relative, are listed in **Box 1**.[20]

Gumption dictates that even patients who are hemodynamically or electrically unstable should be deemed unsuitable for arterial grafting, as the urgency may not allow extra time required for arterial conduit harvesting, unless one harvests them on cardiopulmonary bypass.

MYTH #9

All Arterial Grafts are Equal in Efficacy and Patency

Though the territory to which the conduit is grafted matters with the highest patency rate to the LAD, followed by circumflex and RCA, not all arterial conduits perform equally well. Even intuitively speaking, they are not expected to perform equally well because IMA is an elastic artery, while RA and RGEA are muscular arteries. The endothelium of IMA has lesser fenestrations, less intercellular junction permeability, greater elution of nitric oxide from endothelium, and higher production of antithrombin heparin sulfate and tissue plasminogen activator, all of which make it less vulnerable to atherosclerosis. To the contrary, RA is a muscular artery and as a consequence has a thick tunica media. It is prone to smooth muscle cell proliferation and transmigration to the subintimal layer and even spasm and string sign.

Definitely, LIMA-LAD is the gold standard, but right IMA and the RA compete for the status of the best second arterial conduit. Right IMA was found to be inferior to RA in the COMPASS-CABG substudy with a higher rate of graft failure at 26.8% than RA (9.9%, adjusted OR 2.69; *p*-0.008).[21] In the Radial Artery Database International Alliance (RADIAL) study, at the mean angiographic follow-up of 65 ± 29 months, the graft occlusion rate of RA of 9.4% was <13.5% for right IMA.[22] However, there was no difference for any outcomes between IMA and RA, although DSWI was slightly higher with right IMA graft.[23] Even in a retrospective analysis of Society of Thoracic Surgery (STS) national database, even though Schwann et al. found higher 15-year survival with the use of right IMA at 82%, against 57% with the use of RA, on propensity-matched analysis, this difference was negated and both conduits were considered equivalent, especially in institutions with high use of bilateral IMAs.[24]

MYTH #10

Results of Arterial Grafting are Suboptimum in Women

There is a general bias against women in use of multiarterial graft (MAG) strategy, and the use of three arteries was higher in men (10.5% vs. 7.3%, $p = 0.048$).[25] This is notwithstanding the fact that on Cox proportional hazard modeling, there was no difference in the beneficial effects of bilateral IMAs between the sexes, with similar 10-year survival, and female sex was not an independent predictor for late death.[26] ROMA-Women trial is currently ongoing "to rigorously test the MAG hypothesis in women" and the results are keenly awaited.[27]

MYTH #11

Arterial Grafting is Associated with Higher Risks

In a retrospective propensity-matched analysis by Rocha et al., usage of MAG, including triple arterial, was not associated with increased in-hospital mortality (triple arterial—0.8%, vs. two arterial—2.5%; *p*-0.26).[28] Safety of MAG was confirmed even in the elderly,[29] with significantly improved long-term survival [12-year Kaplan–Meier survival after total arterial revascularization (TAR), 50.3%; non-TAR, 43.1%; HR 0.86; 95% CI 0.80–0.93; *p*-0.001].[30]

MYTH #12

Single Inflow LIMA-RIMA "Y" is Not Safe

Safety of both single- and double-inflow composite grafting is well established for left main stenosis, severe left ventricular (LV) hypertrophy, and severe LV dysfunction. LIMA-RA "Y" grafting has been shown to be safe and effective in a 21-year survival analysis by Royse et al.[31] Composite LIMA-RIMA "Y" lends to total arterial, anaortic off-pump surgery which has been shown to provide complete myocardial revascularization with reduced aortic handling and therefore less cognitive impairment and adverse neurological outcomes, while at the same time maintaining the increased survival associated with arterial grafts.[32]

CONCLUSION

A number of apocryphal ambiguities regarding the practice of arterial grafting in CAD have been perpetuated and need to be dispelled. Arterial grafts are truly the holy grail, albeit only when used for appropriate indication, which incidentally far outnumber the contraindications.

ONLINE REFERENCES

Please scan the QR code provided at the end of the table of contents for References of this chapter.

CHAPTER

167

Postcoronary Artery Bypass Grafting Management: Advances

Srinivas Rao Maddury, Kartik Pandurang Jadhav, MS Prashant

ABSTRACT

Postcoronary artery bypass grafting (post-CABG) patients have a range of pathophysiologic derangements, which can be well managed by following guideline-directed and standardized therapy. In recent years there have been multiple innovations and advancements in this specialized post-CABG care, that have improved overall mortality and morbidity. This chapter will highlight the steps in post-CABG care and recent advances.

Keywords: Advances in post-CABG care, post-CABG care, futuristic ICU care

INTRODUCTION

According to some estimates, there are about >400 cardiothoracic surgical centers across India, with >1,150 cardiac surgeons, performing 190,000 coronary artery bypass graftings (CABGs) every year. With the ever-growing need for such specialized procedures, we need more skilled surgical hands, anesthetists, perfusionists, skilled nursing hands, and well-equipped facilities to perform such life-saving procedures. The CABG is faced with the daunting task of managing perioperative events, scenarios, and patterns of pathology which requires training in international standards.

The CABG can be classified into on-pump CABG, off-pump CABG, minimally invasive cardiac surgery (MICS), and totally endoscopic coronary artery bypass (TECAB) surgery. During a CABG surgery, the body is subjected to iatrogenic injury, which leads to patho-physiological derangements. Postsurgical derangement syndromes include systemic inflammatory response syndrome (SIRS), systemic hemodilution, coagulopathy, and cardioplegic arrest. The SIRS in turn leads to capillary leak and systemic vasodilation. The excessive usage of crystalloids along with systemic vasodilation will lead to volume overload. Myocardial depression which usually results in cardiac systolic/diastolic dysfunction can be a consequence of cardioplegia, or dyselectrolytemia during CABG.[1] Managing these post-CABG pathophysiological conditions is a nightmare for any anesthetists, critical care specialists, and intensive care unit (ICU) experts. This chapter tries to cover the latest management guidelines for post-CABG patient care and some promising innovations in this field.

POINTS TO PONDER

1. The systemic changes in a patient during the post-CABG phase include increased sympathetic tone, vasodilation, relative state of coagulopathy, respiratory depression, hypothermia, blood loss, fluid overload, high heart rate, hypertension, excessive pain, hyperglycemia, hypokalemia, myocardial edema, compromised cardiac function, and shivering **(Fig. 1)**.
2. Therefore, following CABG, the patients will be on ventilator, anesthesia, sedation, inotropes, and multiple indwelling catheters for monitoring the vitals.
3. The weaning of the mechanical ventilator, inotropes, and pain management must be carried out in a staged manner.
4. Some patients with poor cardiac function and cardiogenic shock may require an intra-aortic balloon pump (IABP), extracorporeal membrane oxygenation (ECMO), and/or Impella.
5. The monitoring tools at the disposal of post-CABG patients in ICU include two arterial cannulas for arterial pressures, a pulse oximeter to check oxygen levels, Swan Ganz catheter to evaluate wedge pressure, central venous line to read central venous pressures, which will help us to determine cardiac output (CO), arterial blood gas (ABG) analysis, ultrasound/echocardiography to know

the ventricular function, urinary output measurement by Foleys catheter, and temporary pacemaker.

6. There is a state of water and salt overload due to the administration of crystalloid, blood products, and colloid solutions. The early postoperative period has relatively low intravascular volume despite overall increased total body water. This actually requires augmenting preload to achieve the required CO. On the contrary, diuresis is desired during the recovery phase for 24 to 48 hours, which corrects the redistribution of fluid from interstitial space.
7. Duration of CABG surgery is directly associated with the extent of release of inflammatory mediators like cytokines. Therefore, large studies have shown that increased CABG duration is associated with postoperative death, pulmonary, multiorgan failure, reoperation for bleeding, renal, and neurologic complications.[2]
8. Intraoperative traumatic myocardial injury, myocardial ischemia, and ischemia-reperfusion injury were associated with serial troponin I levels, which will predict all-cause 1-year mortality. The threshold for troponin T in one such study fixed the cutoff of >50 times the upper range limit, obtained 12 hours postoperative.[3]

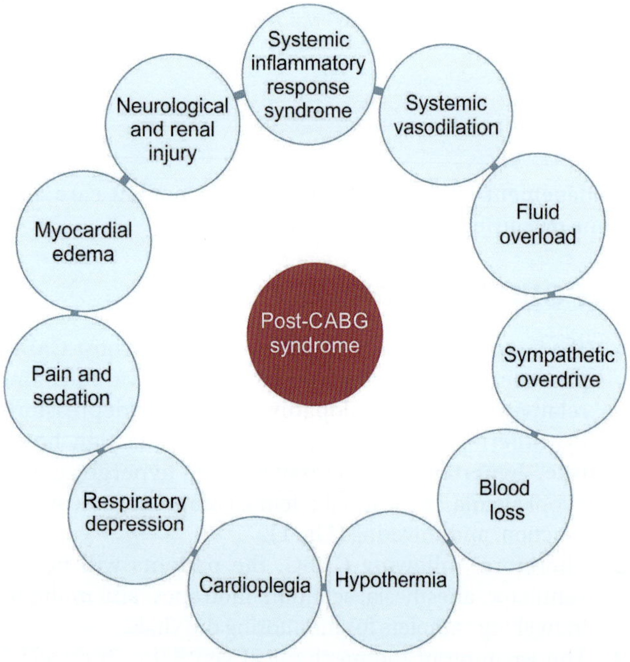

FIG. 1: The pathophysiological derangements noted in post-CABG patients when shifted from OT complex to ICU.

"HANDOFFS" PROCESS

The care during CABG surgery can be further fragmented into superspecialized care units. This superspecialized care includes highly trained staff, who follow efficient ways of safe transfer of patients from one specialized care unit to another. The patients get transferred between specialized care units like ICU to the operating room, floor to the operating room, and then subsequently from the operating room to the ICU, then to rehab centers. This formal and standardized process of communication between the experts in the above perioperative care includes verbal and written communication regarding the patient's status and medical instructions. These terminologies are known as "handoffs". Handoffs include preoperative handoff, intraoperative handoffs, postoperative handoffs, and rehabilitation **(Fig. 2)**. A large systemic review of intraoperative anesthesia handoffs revealed that poor outcome in patients was directly associated with the quality of patient handoffs.[4]

INITIAL STABILIZATION AND RESUSCITATION

The first phase of postoperative "handoffs" includes initial stabilization and resuscitation. Some of the endpoints of resuscitation are mentioned below.

1. Adequate oxygenation delivery (DO_2) is directly proportional to CO and arterial oxygen content (CaO_2). CO in turn is directly proportional to heart rate (HR) and stroke volume (SV). CaO_2 is proportional to hemoglobin (Hgb) concentration, oxyhemoglobin saturation in the artery (SaO_2), and partial pressure of oxygen in an artery (PaO_2).

$$DO_2 = CO \times CaO_2$$

$$DO_2 = [HR \times SV] \times [(1.34 \times Hgb \times SaO_2) + (0.0031 \times PaO_2)]$$

2. The above equation shows that adequate oxygenation can be achieved by maintaining Hgb concentration of >8 g/dL, continuous monitoring of saturation of >90%, maintaining CO >2 L/min, and achieving hemostasis.

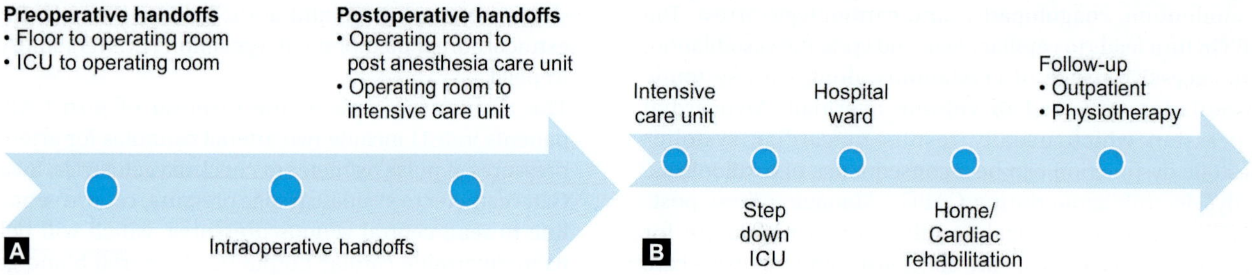

FIGS. 2A AND B: (A) The CABG timeline and (B) the post-CABG timeline.

3. Blood transfusion to maintain Hgb >8 g/dL, mechanical ventilation to maintain SpO_2 of >90%, and by using pulmonary artery catheter (PAC) we can estimate CO and proper fluid management needs to be done according to PAC reading.
4. Adequate hemostasis achieved during the CABG helps to maintain required stroke volume (SV) and in turn CO. First hour loss should not exceed 400 mL and second hour and subsequently 200 mL/h. Re-exploration if 400 mL drain in 1 hour or 200 mL for 2 hours or around 100 mL for 4 hours.
5. Various recommended dosages of statins, beta-blockers, ARB/ACE inhibitors, and antiplatelets in the perioperative period are shown in **Table 1**.[5]

SEDATION

Patients are in a state of sedation when being shifted out of the operation room to the ICU. Most preferred sedatives are short-acting like propofol, dexmedetomidine, ketamine, and midazolam. The latest guidelines in enhanced recovery after cardiac surgery (ERACS) protocols early extubation is essential, and the sedation is to be strategized according to the extubation plan. Each patient requires an individualized plan for each patient, but the protocols help anesthetists, critical care specialists, and ICU experts to plan de-escalation and reallocate the resources as required.

- Dexmedetomidine is routinely used as a sedative, analgesic, and anxiolytic in the ICU. It is an alpha-2 adrenergic agonist and is a sympatholytic that is used during weaning from mechanical ventilation in post-CABG care. A head-to-head comparison with propofol has revealed shorter ICU stay, duration of delirium, reduced incidence of respiratory depression, and lower hospital charges with dexmedetomidine.[6] Some negative points about this drug are its ability to cause hypotension and bradycardia at high infusion rates.
- Propofol is a potent anesthetic agent that is usually used in patients who require prolonged mechanical ventilation or unstable patients. It is a short-acting drug that is given as an IV infusion. It has no analgesic effect; therefore, it is often used in conjunction with opioids.
- Benzodiazepines are routinely avoided in post-CABG patients as continuously delivered agents.

TABLE 1: Various recommendations on statins, beta-blockers, ARB/ACE, and discontinuing antiplatelets before CABG and restarting after CABG.[5]

Elective CABG	When to discontinue before surgery	When to restart the medication
Aspirin	To continue	Within 6 hours (81–325 mg)
Clopidogrel	5 days	Within 24 hours (OPCABG; post PCI, ACS)
Prasugrel	7 days	–
Ticagrelor	7 days	Within 48 hours
Eptifibatide	4 hours	–
Tirofiban	4 hours	–
Abciximab	12 hours	–
High dose statins Atorvastatin 40–80 mg	To continue (Aim 30% drop in LDL; age < 75 years)	To continue
Moderate intensity	To continue (Statin intolerant; age > 75 years)	To continue
Beta-blockers	• All pre-CABG patients • Minimum 24 hours before Sx	• All patients with a history of (H/o) • H/o MI • LV dysfunction
ARB/ACE	• To continue (ACC 2022) • Stop (ESC)	• Restart once stable (ACC 2022) • Stop (ESC)

ANALGESIA

Chest is one of the most important postoperative symptoms that need detailed evaluation as it can suggest either infection, inflammation, or even ischemia **(Flowchart 1)**. In the case of inflammation, opioids were the mainstay of analgesia in the past. Now with the advent of nonopioid medications, opioid analgesia is given judiciously. Also, according to the ERAS protocols postoperative, age-adjusted, multimodal, and opioid-sparing pain management is the ideal strategy. Nonopioid analgesics, opioid usage, regional anesthetic, and local anesthetic techniques constitute multimodal pain management. Inadequate pain management leads to several complications, most prominently pulmonary complications (respiratory splinting secondary to thoracotomy leading to

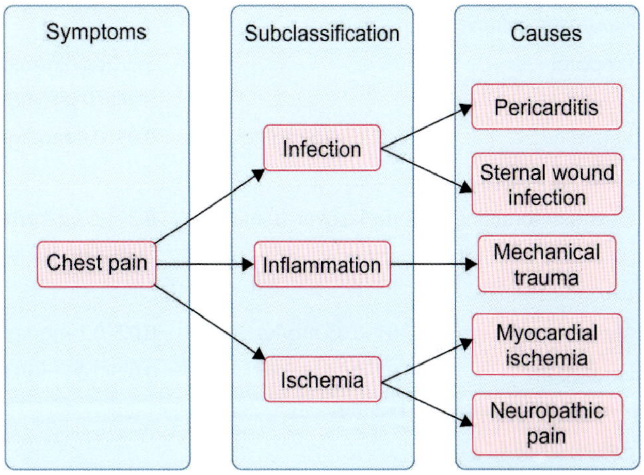

FLOWCHART 1: Various causes of chest pain in post-CABG patients.

pulmonary insufficiency, pulmonary congestion leading to pneumonia), cardiovascular complications (high catecholamines lead to high myocardial oxygen demand and risk of arrhythmias), delirium secondary to acute pain, and persistent pain syndrome **(Tables 2 and 3)**.

Opioids

Opioids are a potent group of analgesics used routinely in ICU. They are associated with prolonged intubation, excessive sedation, postoperative nausea, vomiting, ileus, and respiratory depression.[7] Therefore, all the recent

TABLE 2: Routinely used analgesics in post-CABG patients.

Drugs	Loading dose	Maintenance dose	Onset of action	Subsequent dosing
Opioid analgesics				
Fentanyl	25–100 µg	0.7–10 µg/kg/h	<1 to 2 minutes	30–60 minutes
Morphine sulphate	2–10 mg	2–4 mg every q2h or 2–30 mg/h infusion	5–10 minutes	q4h–Q5h
Methadone	None	IV 2.5–10 mg q12h/q8h Oral 10–40 mg q12h/q6h	IV: 10–20 minutes Oral: 30–60 minutes	IV: q8h Oral: q8h–q12h
Nonopioid analgesics				
Acetaminophen	None	Oral: 325–1,000 mg q4h/q6h IV: 650 mg q4h to 1 g q6h Max: 4 g/day	Oral: 30–60 minutes	q4h–q6h
Ketorolac	30 mg	IV 15–30 mg q6h Max: 120 mg/day	30 minutes	q6h–q4h
Ibuprofen	None	Oral 400 mg q4h IV: 400–800 mg q6h Max: 3 mg/day	30 minutes	q4h–q6h
Gabapentin	None	Oral: 100 mg q8h followed by (f/b) 300–1,200 mg q8h	Variable	
Pregabalin	None	75 mg q24h to q12h f/b 150–300 mg q12h	Variable	

TABLE 3: Routinely used sedatives during post-CABG ICU stay.

Drugs	Loading dose	Maintenance dose	Onset of action	Subsequent dosing
Anesthetic sedative				
Propofol		5–50 µg/kg/min Max: 70 µg/kg/min	1–2 minutes	3–10 minutes
Ketamine	IV: 0.25–0.5 mg/kg	0.05–0.4 mg/kg/h	<1 minute	10–15 minutes
Centrally acting alpha 2 agonist				
Dexmedetomidine	1 µg/kg over 10 minutes	0.2–1.5 µg/kg/h Start with 0.2 and titrate every 30 minutes	5–10 minutes	q1h–q2h
Benzodiazepines				
Midazolam	0.01–0.05 mg/kg	0,02–0.1 mg/kg/h	2–5 minutes	30 minutes
Lorazepam	0.02–0.04 mg/kg (1–2 mg)	0.02–0.06 mg/kg every q2h to q6h	15–20 minutes	q6h–q8h
Antipsychotics				
Haloperidol	0.03–0.15 mg/kg	0.03–0.15 mg/kg every 30 minutes to q6h	5–20 minutes	30 minutes to q6h

protocols include the judicious use of opioids. Usually, sick patients who might require prolonged ventilator are placed in fentanyl infusion which has good analgesia with mild sedation. Another good option for bolus administration is to use IV hydromorphone 0.5 mg when patients are in pain.

Nonopioid Analgesia: Acetaminophen

Acetaminophen administration in post-CABG care is the first-line drug in many ICUs across the world. This drug improves pain scores, is relatively safe, reduces opioid usage, and reduces delirium. Another advantage of acetaminophen is it can be administered from any route (oral, rectal, or IV) with similar potency. Hepatotoxicity is a worry in patients receiving >3 g/day of dosage.

Nonopioid Analgesia: Nonsteroidal Anti-inflammatory Drugs

Use of NSAIDs are very restricted due to the FDA black box warning. The warning on nonsteroidal anti-inflammatory drugs (NSAIDs) is with regards to re-myocardial infarction, cardiac arrests, stroke, pulmonary embolism, reduced transient GFR, and CABG graft thrombosis. Only patients who are refractory to opioid and acetaminophen, an NSAID for a limited duration, in selected patients with good renal function, can be given. Ketorolac 15 mg Q6h for 24 hours can be used.

Nonopioid Analgesia: Ketamine

Ketamine in subanesthetic doses is found to have a good analgesic effect, opioid-sparing effect, no respiratory depression, low incidence of nausea/vomiting, and stable hemodynamics. Ketamine is associated with hallucinations at high doses.

Nonopioid Analgesia: Gabapentinoids

Gabapentinoids are avoided in CABG patients, elderly, and renal dysfunction patients as it is known to cause excessive sedation, respiratory depression, dizziness, and visual disturbances. These side effects magnify when coadministered with opioids. Small doses for limited periods can be used to reduce the opioid dosing.

REGIONAL ANESTHETIC TECHNIQUES

Neuraxial Techniques

Neuraxial techniques include thoracic epidural analgesia (TEA) and intrathecal analgesia (ITA). Metanalysis of TEA in 2023 involving 4,332 cardiac surgical patients. TEA reduces pain effectively, lowers pain scores efficiently, lowers risks of respiratory depression, reduces myocardial infarction, lowers atrial fibrillation or flutter, and lowers cases of delirium, and transfusion noted during various studies. There was a high incidence of hypotension noted during metanalysis. No cases of spinal epidural hematoma (SEH).[8] Intrathecal analgesia (ITA) has been in use for many decades. It reduces post-CABG pain scores and pulmonary complications.[9]

Thoracic Nerve Blocks

Bilateral paravertebral blocks (BVB) and fascial plane thoracic nerve blocks (FPTVB) are specialized nerve blocks that require specialized skills. BVB reduces pain scores, helps early extubation, and decreases ICU and hospital stay.[10] FPTVB includes pectoral nerve block, erector spinae plane, transverse thoracic muscle plane, intercostal nerve block, serratus anterior plane, and parasternal anesthetic infiltration. These are easy to perform, reduce pain scores, reduce opioids, and reduce the dose of propofol or fentanyl.[11]

MANAGEMENT OF MECHANICAL VENTILATOR

- Post CABG imaging in ICU which includes chest X-ray and lung ultrasound. Chest X-ray rules out pneumothorax, pleural effusion, mediastinal effusion, endotracheal tube, vascular line placement, and atelectasis. Similarly, lung ultrasound rules out pneumothorax, atelectasis, pneumonia, pulmonary embolism, and defective diaphragmatic motion.
- Ventilation settings are managed by monitoring arterial Hgb saturation (SpO_2), end-tidal carbon dioxide ($EtCO_2$), and ABG analysis. Titration of ventilator settings is done with a target of SpO_2 being >90%.
- Ideal tidal volume should begin from 6 to 8 mL/kg; target respiratory rate 10–14 breath/min; positive end-expiratory pressure (PEEP) 5–8 H_2O and higher PEEP during pulmonary edema.
- ERAC protocols mandate early extubation within 6 hours. Preoperative and intraoperative strategies are undertaken to reduce the intubation time. These include multimodal pain management, temperature control, proper hemostasis, regulated lung ventilation, fluid balance management, and reducing the use of drugs such as opioids and benzodiazepines, and reversal of neuromuscular blocking. Prolonged intubation with controlled ventilation is associated with increased morbidity, mortality, and higher cost.
- **Table 4** shows fast-track weaning in post-CAG patients.

Inotrope Support

- Selection of appropriate inotrope and vasoactive agent dosing is started to treat ventricular dysfunction and vasoplegia. Inotropes are required in the first 6–12 hours after ICU transfer to avoid ischemia and cardiogenic shock.
- The titration is backed by readings from the arterial line.

Mechanical Circulatory Support

- Post-CABG myocardial dysfunction occurs in about 5–6% of the patients.[12]
- Refractory ventricular dysfunction leading to cardiogenic shock can be managed by temporary mechanical support IABP, ECMO, ventricular assist devices, and Impella.
- The ventricular assist devices are inserted during surgery and continued till LV dysfunction resolution.

TABLE 4: Fast track weaning in post-CABG patients.

Rewarming	• Rewarming done with warm blankets • This is to avoid shivering and increase O_2 consumption, hypocoagulation • Rewarming temperature should be >36°C
Reversing NM block	• After rewarming, NM block is reversed • This reversal is effected with neostigmine, glycopyrolate, or sugammadex • This allows patient to initiate spontaneous respiratory trigger on ventilator
Wean sedation	• Following NM block reversal patient is weaned off the sedation • This weaning process involves reducing infusion rate for sedatives • Make sure patient is fully awake and following commands
Regulate ventilation	• Ventilator settings should be weaned from volume control to pressure support • This should be titrated down till patient breathes spontaneously • Continous monitoring of tida volume is important
Extubation	• Typically extubation should be carried out within 4–6 hours • This is to ensure early mobility • The main criteria for extubation is hemodynamically stable patient

CARDIAC ARREST AND ARRHYTHMIA MANAGEMENT

- The risk of cardiac arrest is highest in the first 6 hours of post-CABG period. Some of the causes for the same are myocardial ischemia, pericardial effusion, large hematoma, arrhythmias, and tension pneumothorax.
- ACLS protocol in post-CABG patients is quite different when compared to other patients. External compressions are not initiated immediately due to the risk of internal damage to grafts and stitched parts of the valve of the sternum. Full-dose adrenaline injection is avoided given the risk of accelerated hypertension leading to suture disruption. Very small doses of adrenaline of 50 µg are given in increasing doses supported by temporary pacing and are used to stimulate the heart. Also, sometimes re-exploration followed by direct cardiac massage by hands is done after thoracotomy. In the case of VT/VF defibrillation is done with a DC shock of 150 Joules.[13]
- Atrial fibrillation is the most common arrhythmia in post-CABG patients. It develops in the first 2–7 days. A combination of medical therapy has proven to reduce the incidence of post-CABG AF. Drugs such as beta-blockers (metoprolol 25 mg OD) and pre-operative administering oral amiodarone at 100 mg twice daily are used **(Flowchart 2)**.

OTHER CONDITIONS

- Proper management of patients with comorbidities such as diabetes with insulin, hypertension with antihypertensives, and chronic kidney disease patients with hemodialysis are to be carried on meticulously as per specialist advice.
- In case of complications like acute stroke in post-CABG patients involves early diagnosis with MRI of the brain

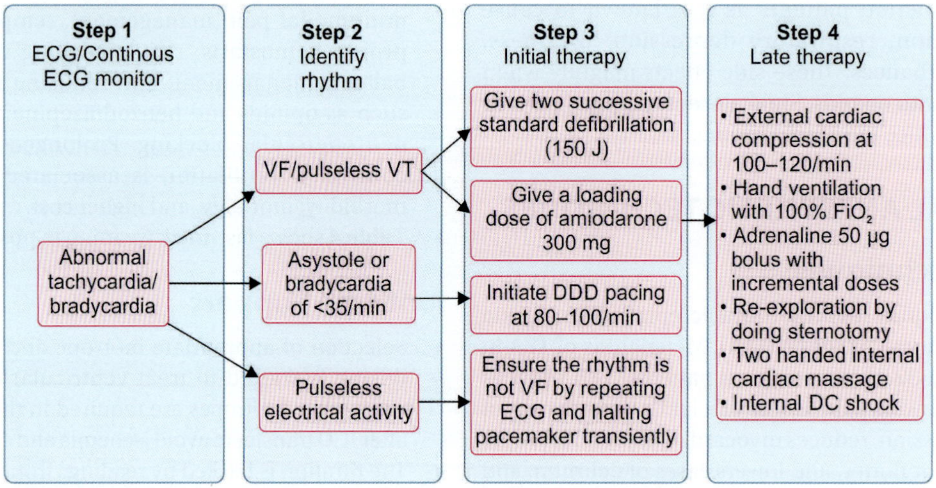

FLOWCHART 2: Abnormal cardiac rhythm and its management strategies.

and treatment with endovascular thrombectomy or intra-arterial thrombolysis.

- Delirium in post-CABG patients is well known and some medications like haloperidol, dexmedetomidine, olanzapine, and quetiapine can be employed in the management of the same.

MEDICAL BREAKTHROUGHS

Artificial Intelligence Application in Intensive Care Unit

When machines are made to mimic human intelligence in analyzing complex data, this process is called artificial intelligence (AI). Patients in cardiac intensive care unit (CICU) is a unique population when compared to medical or surgical ICU. Multiple studies have included machine learning to analyze CICU data sets retrospectively. These studies have mainly studied mortality risk stratification scores.[14] These ML scoring systems have surpassed conventional statistical methods in the ICU.[15] Multiple scores with real-time mortality risk prediction models need to be developed and validated.[16] There is a huge scope of research in this field. Other than the vitals and blood reports, ECG and echo imaging data can also be used in ML algorithms to analyze the deep learning process **(Flowchart 3)**.[17]

Shockwave Therapy in Postcoronary Artery Bypass Grafting Patients

In a pilot study conducted in Austria named CAST-HF trial indicated that applying shock wave therapy (SWT) to the cardiac tissue after CABG produced improved LVEF and physical capacity in the treatment group. This is explained by the cardiac regeneration happening at the site of the application of SWT. This study used a tabletop device named Nonvasiv Medical GmbH, Konstanz, Germany and a sterile single-use applicator releasing electrohydraulic shockwaves (Heart Regeneration Technologies GmbH, Innsbruck, Austria). This applicator was inserted in a sterile plastic cover along with gel and was kept in contact with the myocardium. Around 300 impulses per coronary artery supply territory were applied at an energy flux density of 0.38 mJ/mm^2 and a frequency of 3 Hz. The results showed an 11.3% increase in LVEF in the SWT group and a 6.3% increase in the sham group. Similarly, the 6-minute walk test improvement in the SWT group was 127 m and 43.6 m in the sham group. These results are encouraging and there is tremendous scope to improve on this initial success.[18]

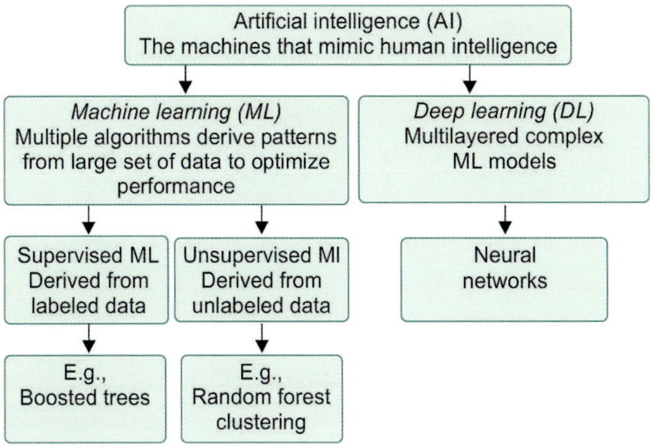

FLOWCHART 3: The structure of artificial intelligence (AI).

Early Diagnosis of Postcoronary Artery Bypass Grafting Atrial Fibrillation

Multiple biomarkers to predict post-CABG AF are in the initial stages of evaluation. One such pilot study conducted showed good predictive value of serum fibroblast growth factor-23 (FGF-23). The study showed that higher levels of FGF-23 levels were able to predict post-CABG AF with a sensitivity of 92.3% and specificity of 87.23%. This pilot study emphasized the presence of comorbid conditions in the preoperative stage leads to post-CABG AF. Better management of such preoperative conditions well before the patient is taken for surgery may lead to better outcomes.[19]

Nano-silver Coated Catheter for Urinary Tract

Post-CABG infections are dreaded complications of retaining an in-dwelling catheter in the urinary tract. Catheter-associated urinary tract infection (UTI) mostly happens due to prolonged retention of the catheter in the bladder. These catheters not only injure the urethra but also promote bacterial migration and subsequently infection. Therefore, newer nanosilver coated catheters have been used in post-CABG patients, and they have shown reduced incidence of UTI. This also in turn reduces antibiotic usage, and hospital stays and fastens rehabilitation.[20]

Early Warning System for Cardiac Arrest

An early warning system for early detection of cardiac arrest is based on remote digital monitoring of post-CABG patients. This involves continuous monitoring of the patient by applying a sensor device to the chest wall of the body and monitoring cardiac rhythm with vital monitoring. These data points about vitals are captured by the temporal convolutional network (TCN). Once data is captured, the data is analyzed in real-time by deep Taylor decomposition (DTD). It analyses patients for ECG rhythm, vitals, and oxygen saturation, and some devices also check perspiration patterns. Based on these factors a risk score is calculated and then a warning is raised in case of score crosses a prescribed cutoff. This revolution and help to detect and manage sudden cardiac deaths in post-CABG patients at home.[21]

Multidepartment Approach

Many studies have shown that CABG affects a patient's physical health, quality of life, physical function, emotional status, and ability to re-enter societal duties. Psychosocial dimensions contribute a lot to the above-mentioned condition. Understanding these factors in a nuanced way will help patients to recover faster. Multiple departments like the department of psychology, neuropsychiatry, health counselors, health educators, pain management experts, social care experts, home nurses, and teleconsultation with doctors can help to contribute to the overall better care for the patient. This combined approach results in improved outcomes.[4]

Continuous Health Education

Some of the studies conducted in the CICU setup have revealed poor knowledge of patients regarding knowledge of CABG and its complications. This incomplete knowledge leads to unmitigated concern, fear of complications, and lack of clarity about the outcomes. This uncertainty affects the overall mental health and recovery. One way of dealing with this lack of knowledge is by nurses posted in the CICU. Development of posters, placards, and booklets about CABG and its outcomes for patients in simple language to understand the condition and mitigate unwarranted fears. The studies have shown to have improved knowledge which has improved their outcomes.[22]

Early Mobilization and Aerobic Exercises

Some of the patients who underwent CABG, develop reduced atelectasis, pleural effusion, nonhealing of wounds, and iatrogenic infections leading to long ICU stays and hospital stays. The major cause of these complications includes prolonged immobilization. Therefore, studies have shown that early immobilization leads to faster recovery. Overall, the length of stay was reduced by 24 hours after initiating early mobilization within 24–48 hours of CABG. This reduced atelectasis, improved oxygen saturation, reduced time on the ventilator, and time on a noninvasive ventilator.[23] Similarly, an RCT involving 40 post-CABG patients was studied and found to have improved recovery with aerobic exercise. Aerobic exercise improves the mean distance walked by 12.91%, whereas it was 11.08% in the control group.[24]

Nanotechnology in Wound Healing

Chronic nonhealing wounds, on the other hand, require additional therapeutic properties, which could be obtained by employing exosomes (Exo) and nanoparticles (NPs) to encourage rapid and superior healing outcomes. The same technology can be used for faster healing of postoperative CABG surgical wounds in the future.[25]

CONCLUSION

The advent of the latest technology and ever ever-evolving field of neo-materials have made it possible to create devices that have revolutionized post-CABG care. The prospects of future ICU care create a hope of prompt, error-free, and automated ICU cubicles for patients. Along with the newer technology, the development of futuristic drugs like nanotech drugs might play a vital role in wound healing and faster repair of CABG wounds.

ONLINE REFERENCES

Please scan the QR code provided at the end of the table of contents for References of this chapter.

SECTION 15

Structural Intervention

Section Outline

CHAPTER

168

Aortic Stenosis: Core Concepts in Diagnosis and Prognosis in Different Cohorts

Satish K Parashar

ABSTRACT

With increasing life expectancy, aortic stenosis (AS) has emerged as one of the most common valvular lesion universally. In view of age-related comorbidities, the assessment of its severity, which if misinterpreted, may have significant prognostic and management issues. Echo-Doppler is the first line of investigation. However, there are several factors impacting the assessment of severity. Since all AS parameters, assessed by Doppler echocardiography, are flow-dependent, hence, evaluation of flow status, such as stroke volume index and aortic flow rate are keys when assessing its severity. Hence, various hemodynamic cohorts of AS, based on flow status have been described. As is not solely a valvular disease but have myocardial, valvular, and vascular components. Among various cohorts, the low-gradient AS subgroups are challenging, particularly in differentiating true-severe AS (where aortic valve intervention is necessary) and pseudo-severe AS (where conservative management is recommended). Various techniques to do so are described, which include dobutamine stress echo, projected aortic valve area (AVA) multidetector CT scan (MDCT), systolic time intervals, etc. This chapter will review only diagnostic approaches and prognostic implications of different AS subtypes.

Keywords: Aortic stenosis, low gradient, flow, dobutamine

INTRODUCTION

Aortic stenosis (AS) is one of the most common valvular lesions world wise, especially in Western population. As such it is strongly age-related, hence, prevalence is expected to rise with age. Since majority of the patients are elderly, hence, AS is no longer a simple valvular heart disease of left ventricular outflow obstruction but is accompanied by other cardiac and comorbid conditions. Because of the significant variations of the disease, identifying patients at high risk and even earlier detection of patients with AS before developing symptomatic severe AS is becoming increasingly important. Over the past decade, challenges due to discrepancies with grading AS severity and the necessity of integrating the valve gradient with flow patterns were recognized when a significant subset of patients were found to have small AVAs suggestive of severe AS with lower gradients despite preserved LVEF. As a result, under the umbrella of severe AS (based on AVA < 1.0 cm^2), a hemodynamic classification of AS was proposed, as described below.

ASSESSMENT OF SEVERITY

Echocardiography, combined with echo-Doppler, continues to be the first line of investigation. Three parameters are usually needed to classify the severity of aortic valve stenosis, in presence of normal LV functions, as shown in **Flowchart 1**.[1,2]

- Peak transvalvular velocity (V_{max})
- Mean pressure gradient (P_{mean})
- Aortic valve area (AVA) by continuity equation method/ indexed to body surface area (BSA)

Based on Doppler principle, the maximum transvalvular velocity needs to be obtained from any acoustic window that provides the highest aortic jet velocity, which is also noted for future follow-up studies. Assessment should always be undertaken when blood pressure (BP) is well under control to minimize the effect of another increased afterload. Low pressure gradient across the aortic valve depends on two main factors: (1) AVA—the smaller the AVA, the higher the pressure gradient and (2) the flow across AV; the lower flow,

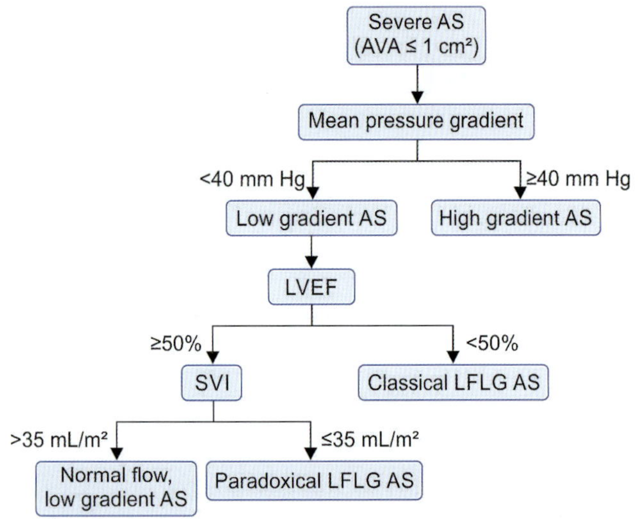

FLOWCHART 1: Severity of aortic stenosis.[4]

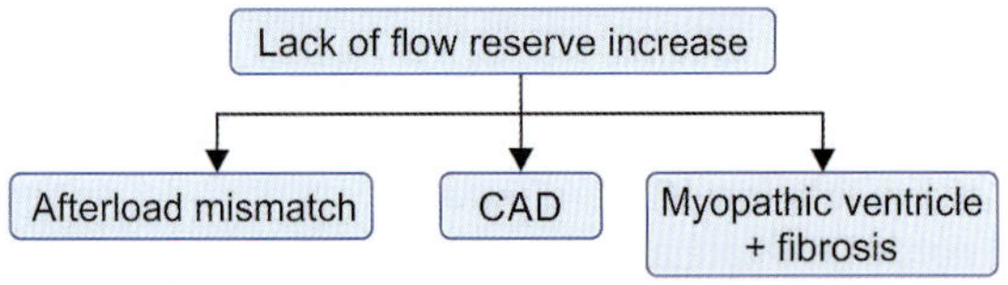

FLOWCHART 2: Possible reasons for low flow reserve.

the lower the pressure gradient. Almost in 35–40% of cases of AS, there is discordance between AVA (<1.0 cm^2) suggesting severe AS, or AVA indexed to BSA (≤0.6 cm^2/m^2) and P_{mean} gradient (<40 mm Hg suggesting nonsevere AS). Most of these patients have a "low flow state" across the aortic valve, which is defined as an indexed stroke volume < 35 mL/m^2. Low flow reserve is multifactorial **(Flowchart 2)**.[3] As there are some fallacies with SVi, hence, some studies suggest that aortic flow rate (FR), which is calculated by dividing the LV-SV by left ventricular ejection time (ET) has a better prognostic value than SVi, both and rest and after exercise[5] However, in another study, Sen et al.[6] seem to challenge this assumption and did not find any prognostic role of aortic FR. As such both SVi and TFR need to be assessed though the later is believed to be more significant.

HEMODYNAMIC COHORTS AND SEVERITY

As mentioned earlier, since all AS parameters, assessed by Doppler echocardiography, are flow-dependent, hence, evaluation of flow status is a key when assessing AS severity. Besides SVi, low flow state is also defined by aortic valve FR of < 200 mL/s. Based on flow pattern, AS can be classified in the following cohorts.

High-gradient (HG Aortic Stenosis)

This is the usual cohort of severe AS, defined as a peak velocity across the AV ≥ 4 m/s and a P_{mean} ≥ 40 mm Hg. AVA is typically ≤ 1.0 cm^2 or ≤0.6 cm^2/m^2. When peak velocity or P_{mean} is lower than above values, then AVA ≤ 1.0 cm^2 is defined as severe AS. However, these parameters are frequently inconsistent with each other since they depend on individual's body habitus, SV, and other coexisting conditions such as hypertension and associated high-flow states such as severe anemia and thyrotoxicosis. As regards body habitus, women normally have lower SV than men and thus the AV gradient is lower in women for a given AVA. Obese patients have higher SV than those with normal weight due to excess adipose tissue. As such an indexed AVA (AVAi) ≤ 0.6 cm^2/m^2 has been used as a criteria for severe AS. Very severe AS is being defined as AV max ≥ 5 m/s or P_{mean} of ≥ 60 mm Hg.

Patients who start out as normal flow high-gradient (HG) severe AS eventually transform into low-flow low-gradient (LFLG) severe AS with reduced LVEF through a number of mechanisms such as reduced capillary density, chronic subendocardial ischemia, interstitial fibrosis, and afterload mismatch.[7]

Low-gradient Aortic Stenosis

Three types of low-gradient severe AS have been described based on the LVEF and the flow state as shown in **Table 1**.

Classical Low-flow Low-gradient AS with Reduced LVEF

It is seen in about 5–10% of all cases of AS and is defined as AV area < 1.0 cm^2, P_{mean} < 40 mm Hg with a stroke volume index < 35 mL/m^2, total FR of < 200 mL/s, and a LVEF of <50%. As regards SV, measuring LVOT diameter (LVOTd) at the annulus or very close to it provides the most accurate measures of SV and AVA, it gives good accuracy and reproducibility. Measuring LVOTd 5 or 10 mm below significantly underestimates these parameters and leads to significant overestimation of the severity of AS and prevalence of low-flow status. At the time of diagnosis, patients who fit this definition typically have other abnormal echo features.[8] Right ventricular dysfunction and atrial fibrillation are one of them.

Diagnostic Approach

- Before proceeding with further evaluation, it is important to exclude any measurement or calculation error, especially pertaining to AVA and ejection fraction, both liable to high technical errors.

TABLE 1: Subclassification of low-gradient AS. AVA is in cm^2.

Type	AVA	Mean gradient	SVi (mL/m^2)	EF
LFLG	<1.0	<40	<35	<50
PLFLG	<1.0	<40	≤35	>50
NFLG	<1.0	<40	>35	>50

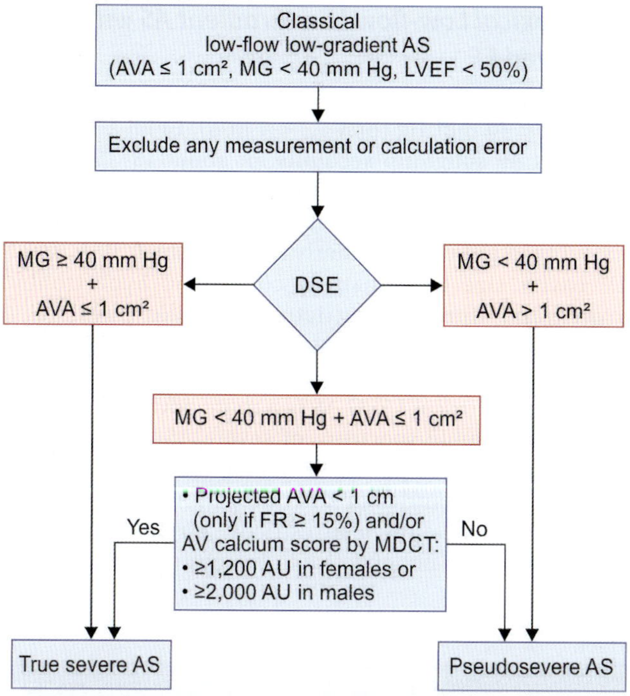

FLOWCHART 3: Diagnostic approach to classical low-flow low-gradient AS.[4]

- Assessment of FR which, if abnormally reduced, then the next step is followed.
- The next recommended steps after TTE is low-dose dobutamine stress echo (DSE), discussed separately below **(Flowchart 3)**.

Low-dose Dobutamine Stress Echocardiography (LDSE)

This helps to assess (1) the presence of contractile reserve, which is referred to as at least 20% increase in LV SV with peak DSE compared with rest (2) differentiate true severe AS (TSAS) from pseudo severe AS (PSAS). In tTSAS, following dobutamine **(Flowcharts 3 and 4)**, there will be no appreciable change in AVA which is fixed due to intrinsic severe valve disease, but by increasing the flow the mean gradient increases. In LV dysfunction, sufficient force is not generated to fully open the aortic valve. As such in PSAS, increasing flow will increase AVA > 1.0 cm^2 or >0.2 cm^2 from baseline, and hence, the mean pressure gradient remains < 40 mm Hg. In cases with reduced LV flow reserve/no contractile reserve, the DSE is regarded as inconclusive, then MDCT is recommended to obtain an aortic valve calcium score. It is suggested that combining MDCT and DSE information is important for clinical decision-making, as it is known that a higher proportion of patients with beneficial outcomes have combined CT and DSE information than when applying DSE or NCCT alone.[9]

DSE and LVEF

Regardless of LVEF, the association between DSE gradients and AS severity assessed by MDCT, demonstrated significant heterogeneity between LVEF subgroups. Aortic valve area displayed uniform optimal cutoff between LVEF subgroups (1.0 cm^2 vs. 0.9 cm^2 vs. 0.8 cm^2, LVEF < 35%, LVEF 35–50%, with the highest accuracy in patients with LVEF < 35%) and not at or below 50%. As such DSE findings are more significant if LVEF is <35%.[10]

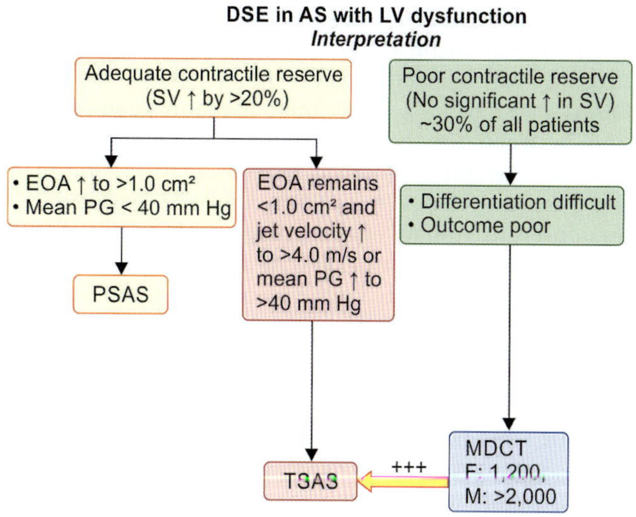

FLOWCHART 4: Interpretation of LDSE.

Multidetector Cardiac Tomography (MDCT)

In some cases, as mentioned earlier, discordant measurements on echocardiography can present diagnostic challenges. MDCT-AV calcium scoring has been shown to be a valuable complementary test for facilitating clinical decision-making. The diagnosis of TSAS is suggested if the MDCT AV calcium score is > 1,200 AU in females or >2,000 AU in males. This sex-related discrepancy is partly explained by a higher fibrosis-calcium ratio in women compared with men. P_{mean} gradient and V_{max} exceeded AVA in diagnosing severe AS adjudicated with MDCT. Hence, discrepancies imply that a diagnosis of severe AS is more likely if we use MDCT-assessed AVC rather than DSE data. This test also has the added benefit of being independent of loading conditions and hemodynamic effects, which are often difficult to standardize. The clinical improvement is highest in patients with concordant DSE and MDCT findings and that combining information from MDCT CS and DSE may better identify patients with beneficial outcomes.[11]

Projected AVA[12]

AVA measured at low FR is not a good prognostic or diagnostic marker for TSAS. There is usually wide variation of flow augmentation with DSE. Hence, another proposed method to differentiate between TSAS and PSAS is projected AVA which is an estimation of how much the AVA would be at a hypothetical value of transvalvular FR (Q) (250 mL/s). Calculating Q by an earlier method involved three measurements namely, LVOT-d, LVOT-VTI, and ET measured from AV Doppler spectrum, at basal and peak dose. The formula was 1,000 × CSA LVOT × LVOT-VTI/ET. To avoid multiple measurements, a simplified method was suggested which included only two simple measurements—CSA_{LVOT} × $Vmean_{LVOT}$ × 100. There is a fairly good correlation between the two methods. If projected AVA is ≤1.0 cm², then the diagnosis of true-severe AS is confirmed and if the projected AVA is >1.0 cm², then AS is considered pseudosevere. Annabi et al.[13] prospectively analyzed DSE criteria in 186 patients with LFLG AS and reduced LV systolic function. The sensitivity for the identification of TSAS was higher with projected AVA (86%) than with standard DSE criteria (63%). **Figures 1 and 2** show a case-based study by one of the methods.[14]

Systolic Time Intervals

This includes assessment of aortic acceleration (AT) and ET and their ratio. Value of AT > 100 ms and AT/ET < 0.35 are indicative of severe AS. Details are not mentioned due to constraint of space.[15]

Paradoxical Low-flow Low-gradient AS with Preserved EF

It is defined as AVA ≤ 1.0 cm², transvalvular mean pressure gradient < 40 mm Hg (or V_{max} < 4 m/s), LVEF ≥ 50%, and SVi. This AS subgroup accounts for about 15–35% of the symptomatic and 5–10% of the asymptomatic severe AS patients. The classic characteristics described with this AS subtype are usually elderly females, small BSA, small LV cavity size with marked concentric hypertrophy, myocardial fibrosis, restrictive diastolic physiology, reduced LV longitudinal systolic function, and increased global LV afterload resulting in reduced SVi (≤35 mL/m²). As such paradoxical LFLG AS is a more advanced stage in the hemodynamic spectrum of severe AS. Other factors associated with this pattern include pulmonary hypertension and right ventricular dysfunction. As these patients often have a left ventricular restrictive physiology pattern, DSE is sometime not effective in increasing flow and may

Parameters at rest

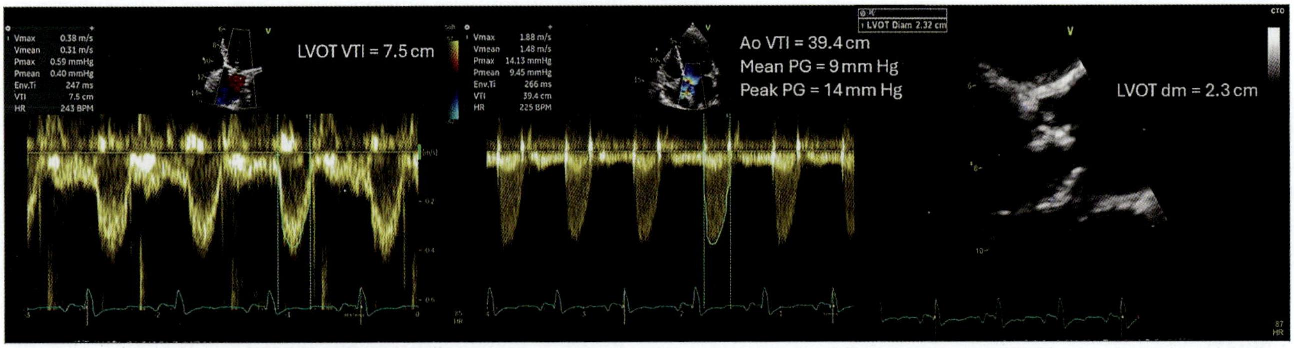

Stroke volume = 0.785 × 2.3 × 2.3 × 7.5 = 31 mL

Flow rate = SV/ET

$$\text{AVA by CE} = \frac{0.785 \times 2.3 \times 2.3 \times 7.5}{39.4} = 0.78\ \text{cm}^2$$

Flow rate = 31/0.26 sec = 119 mL/sec

VTI ratio = 7.5/39.4 = 0.19

FIG. 1: Results of study on a patient with LFLG AS.

At rest	**Low dose DSE**
AVA = 0.78 cm²	AVA = 0.90 cm²
Flow rate = 119 mL/sec	Flow rate = 180 mL/sec

$$\text{AVA (rest)} + \left\{\frac{\text{AVA (dob)} - \text{AVA (rest)}}{\text{Flow rate (dob)} - \text{Flow rate (rest)}}\right\} \times \left(250 - \text{flow rate (rest)}\right) = \boxed{\text{Projected AVA}}$$

$$0.78 + \left\{\frac{0.90 - 0.78}{180 - 119}\right\} \times \left(250 - 119\right) = \boxed{1.03\ \text{cm}^2}$$

FIG. 2: Results of study on a patient with LFLG AS.

be associated with side effects in these patients. In addition, calculating the valvuloarterial impedance (Zva), which reflects the global load the LV is facing, that results from both valvular and vascular loads, may be useful in distinguishing the severity of paradoxical LFLG AS.[16] Zva value of >5.0 mm Hg/mL m^2 is an indicator of severe AS. However, since Zva is a flow-dependent parameter, this index may be less reliable in low-flow states since small changes in stroke volume can produce large changes in Zva. Hence, MDCT will still be an additive diagnostic modality. Around 15% of patients with paradoxical LFLG AS have wild-type transthyretin (ATTR) cardiac amyloidosis, which may result in LV hypertrophy with a small LV cavity.[17]

Normal-flow, Low-gradient (NFLG) AS with Preserved EF

It is defined as AVA area < 1.0 cm^2, P_{mean} < 40 mm Hg, but normal stroke volume index > 35 mL/m^2 and normal LVEF of >50%. Patients with NFLG AS are reported to have less severe disease than the other AS categories with lower BNP and preserved LV longitudinal function. These patients usually have moderate AS. However, in some patients, the increased systolic BP and decreased aortic compliance may substantially decrease the pressure gradient across AV and may lead to an NFLG in a patient with severe AS. However, as mentioned earlier, measurement errors need to be excluded.

LV Strain Imaging

LVEF has been a subject of some controversy in valvular heart diseases especially AS. By the time, EF falls though still within acceptable limits, it is already too late, with irreversible damage established and the "therapeutic window" for intervention missed. Speckle tracking echocardiography is a well-validated technique which enables highly reproducible, angle-independent assessment of regional and global LV systolic function in longitudinal, circumferential, and radial planes. Longitudinal strain is most sensitive in the presence of myocardial disease and well-studied. Routine incorporation of GLS in the evaluation of all patients with moderate-to-severe AS is justifiable, as it predicts exercise capacity, it correlates with the severity, magnitude of LVH, extent of fibrosis, and LVEF, and it predicts MACE and death rate both in symptomatic and asymptomatic patients. Hence, GLS is a robust marker in diagnosis, prognosis, and response to management, when below 16%.[18]

Role of Artificial Intelligence (AI)

It is an upcoming field which will help in early detection of AS, even in asymptomatic stage, differentiate between various phenotypes, high- and low-risk patients, timing if intervention. The AI-ECG model has been effectively utilized by Mayo Group to differentiate between moderate and severe stenosis from USA population. They developed a setup to understand which features of the ECG were used by human intelligence (medical expert) and by an AI model. However, further research in this field will continue to assess its effective role in clinical practice.[19,20]

BRIEF PROGNOSIS OF COHORTS

Among patients with severe AS, those with classical LFLG severe AS hold the worst prognosis with 2-year survival rate of 40–60% with conservative management because the severity of AS is often under-recognized and surgical treatment is delayed. In PARTNER trial, 2-year mortality was reported to be 76%. TAVI is more suitable for these patients. The absence of contractile reserve is also a marker of increased operative mortality but majority of these patients still benefit from AV intervention which is associated with improved survival and symptoms when compared to conservative management. Paradoxical LFLG AS has worse prognosis than HG AS and NFLG AS but better than classical LFLG AS. The likelihood of remaining alive for 3 years without TAVI/AVR has been reported to be about fivefold lower than normal flow state. Symptomatic patients with a PLF-LG severe AS have a markedly impaired survival among those treated medically compared to patients who undergo AV replacement (TAVI or SAVR). A combination of more advanced age, more frequent comorbidities such as hypertension, worse intrinsic myocardial damage, and lesser referral for surgery are reasons for the worse outcome. Among patients undergoing AVR, both classical and paradoxical LFLG AS have higher surgical risk compared with HG AS. The prognosis of NFLG severe AS is similar to that of HG severe AS. On the other hand, patients with LG PSAS have an outcome similar to that of patients without AS.

TECHNICAL CHALLENGES OF ECHOCARDIOGRAPHY

The predominant few challenges are (1) to get an accurate measurement of peak jet velocity and mean pressure gradient across AV by using multiplanar imaging and keeping Doppler beam as parallel to flow as possible (2) underestimation of LVOTd, utilizing continuity equation method. Since the LVOTd is squared in the equation, hence, any little error in measurement of LVOT may result in significant error in AVA assessment and SV calculation. The maximum diameter should be measured close to the annulus and an average of three readings taken. Recommended to Include calcification in above measurements. Thus, the initial step done when echocardiographic measurements show discordance between AVA and gradients is to rule out various measurement errors.

CONCLUSION

LFLG severe AS represents a complex, heterogeneous subset of patients. Identifying these patients can be challenging, before defining various subtypes, it is important to rule out various measurement errors especially, LVEF, LVOT, gradients, etc. As these are flow-related parameters, hence, evaluation of SVi and total AV FR is essential, though FR provides more incremental prognostic value beyond clinical risk factors, LGAS with low-flow state is of particular challenge for clinical decision-making, especially when differentiating TSAS (where intervention will be beneficial) versus PSAS (where conservative medical management is appropriate). In LF/LG AS with reduced LVEF, low-dose DSE is beneficial for the confirmation of AS severity and risk stratification. In the setting of partial or no flow reserve, projected AVA and/or calcium scoring with MDCT have proved useful to determine severity and guide management. The role of MMI and echo is complementary and their positive roles are discussed. The limitation of use of DSE in LVEF > 35% needs to be appreciated.

ONLINE REFERENCES

Please scan the QR code provided at the end of the table of contents for References of this chapter.

CHAPTER

169

Spectrum of Aortic Valve Diseases from Neonates to Elderly and Its Management

Tom Devasia, Monika P Jawanjal, Mukund Prabhu

ABSTRACT

Aortic valve diseases comprise a major spectrum of aortic valve abnormalities that affect individuals across the age from neonates to the elderly. In today's era of transcatheter interventions, the management of aortic valve disease has advanced significantly. Depending on the patient's age and the severity of the condition, the treatment varies from neonates to elderly individuals. This chapter provides a comprehensive overview of aortic valve diseases with a focus on the etiology, anatomical characteristics, clinical presentation, diagnostic modalities, and management strategies across the age-groups from neonates to elderly.

Keywords: Aortic stenosis, bicuspid aortic valve, transcatheter aortic valve replacement

INTRODUCTION

Aortic valve diseases encompass a wide range of structural and functional abnormalities affecting the aortic valve. These conditions can manifest across the entire lifespan, from neonates to the elderly. The spectrum of aortic valve diseases includes aortic stenosis (AS) due to congenital unicuspid or bicuspid aortic valves (BAVs) and aortic regurgitation (AR) resulting from valvular or annular abnormalities. Managing these diverse conditions requires a comprehensive understanding of the etiology, pathophysiology, diagnosis, and appropriate therapeutic interventions. In this chapter, we will explore the spectrum of aortic valve diseases across age-groups and delve into the contemporary management strategies employed to optimize patient outcomes in various aortic valve pathologies.

DEFINING THE AORTIC ROOT

The aortic root is a complex structure that includes the aortic valve leaflets, their attachments, interleaflet trigones, sinuses of Valsalva, sinotubular junction, and the annulus. Each component has distinct microscopic, anatomical, and physiological properties, making the aortic root an intricate unit that channels a large volume of blood with minimal resistance and stress.

In adults, the normal aortic valve area is 3–4 cm^2 and consists of three leaflets: The right, left, and noncoronary cusps, named after the corresponding coronary arteries. Each cusp has three layers of extracellular matrix: Fibrosa (collagen) on the aortic side, spongiosa (proteoglycans) in the middle, and ventricularis (elastin) on the ventricular surface. The cusps are attached to the aortic root in a semilunar pattern, with a thickened nodule at the free margin, called the nodule of Arantius, which acts as a coaptation area for the neighboring leaflets. Calcification of the nodule of Arantius is associated with AR **(Fig. 1)**.

Let us delve deeper into neonatal and pediatric aortic valve diseases. These conditions are distinct from those seen in adults and often have unique etiologies, presentations, and management strategies.

AORTIC VALVE DISEASES IN NEONATES TO ADOLESCENTS

Congenital Aortic Stenosis

Congenital AS, often linked to unicuspid or BAV, is one of the most common valvular anomalies. BAV is the most prevalent congenital heart disease in children, adolescents, and adults, affecting 0.5–2% of the population.[1,2] Congenital AS is three times more common in males and is a progressive condition

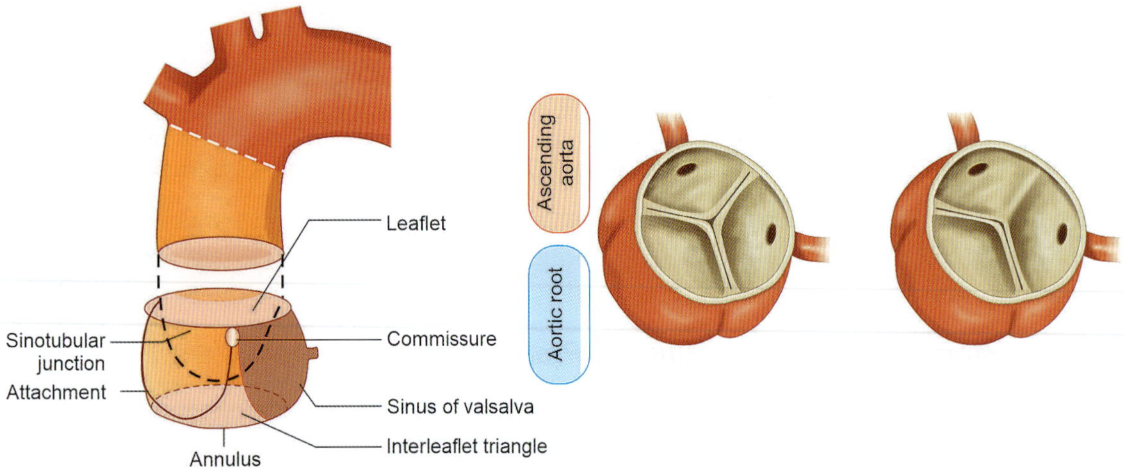

FIG. 1: Anatomy of the aortic root.

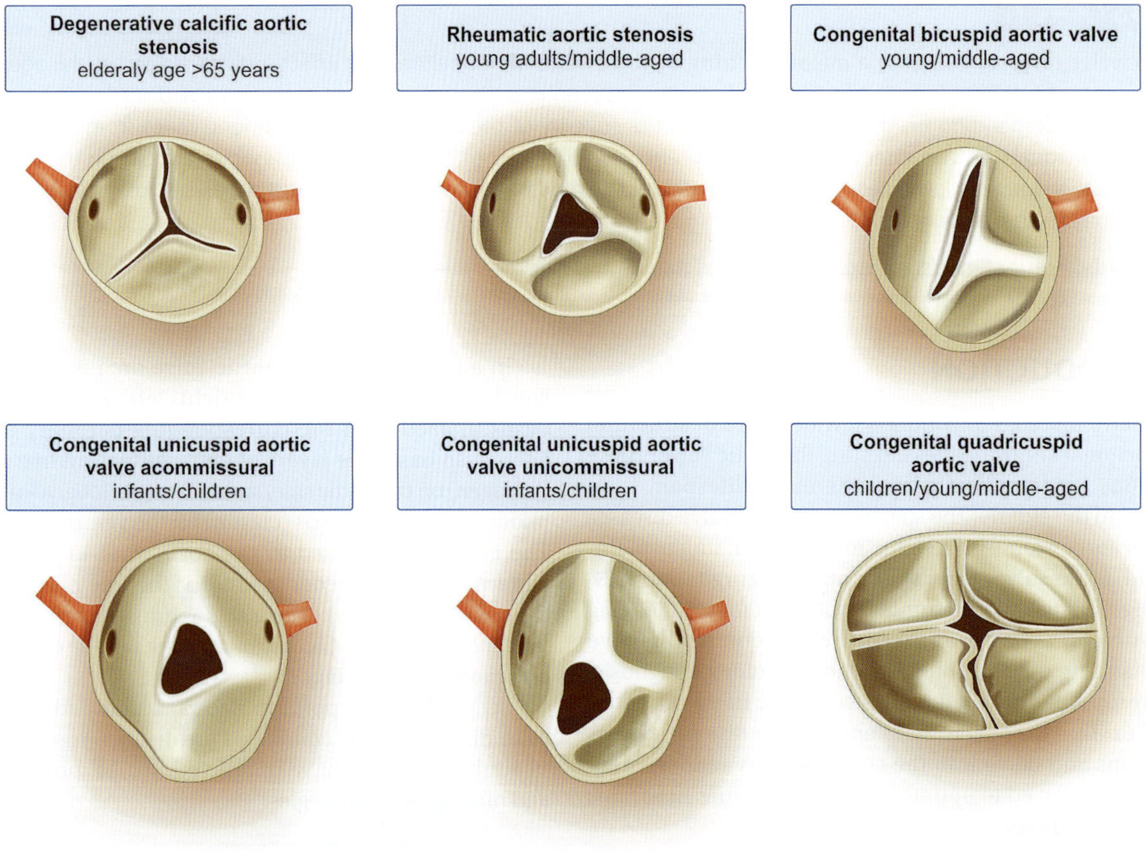

FIG. 2: Spectrum of aortic valve diseases and age of presentation.

that often requires transcatheter or surgical intervention based on severity and symptoms. It can occur as an isolated defect or may be associated with other cardiac defects in about 20% of cases and may also be part of genetic syndromes or connective tissue disorders.

Unicuspid Aortic Valve

The unicuspid aortic valve is a rare congenital anomaly with a single crescent-shaped leaflet. It can be either acommissural, with no lateral attachment to the aorta and a central pinhole orifice due to complete fusion of all three raphes, or unicommissural, with one attachment to the aorta and an eccentric slit-shaped orifice **(Fig. 2)**. The acommissural type often presents at a young age with severe AS.

Bicuspid Aortic Valve

Bicuspid aortic valve (BAV) is the most common congenital valve defect, affecting about 2% of the global population, with a male-to-female ratio of 3:1. It involves two unequal-sized leaflets, where the larger one often has a central ridge called a raphe, formed by fused commissures. BAV is a disorder of valvulogenesis and may be isolated or associated with other cardiac defects, aortopathy, or genetic syndromes like Turner, Williams, and Marfan syndromes, the most common association being coarctation of aorta.[2] Turner's syndrome, in particular, shows a 15–30% occurrence of BAV. The most common genes associated with BAV include *NOTCH1*, *KCJN2*, *GATA6*, *FBN1*, *SMAD6*, and *ACTA2* **(Fig. 3)**.

The presentation of BAV ranges from asymptomatic to severe valvular diseases. In children, it is often asymptomatic, detected by a systolic click and murmur, and commonly diagnosed incidentally or during familial screening. BAV may also be part of complex congenital heart defects like Shone's complex or hypoplastic left heart syndrome (HLHS).[3]

Rarely neonates with BAV present with critical AS, requiring urgent intervention like transcatheter balloon aortic valvuloplasty. Congenital AS is a progressive condition and may require multiple interventions in a lifetime. Recently, BAV has gained attention due to advances in the transcatheter aortic valve interventions and the intricacies involved while treating the patients with BAV. The various clinical presentations of BAV from neonates to the elderly are summarized **Flowchart 1** and **Table 1**.

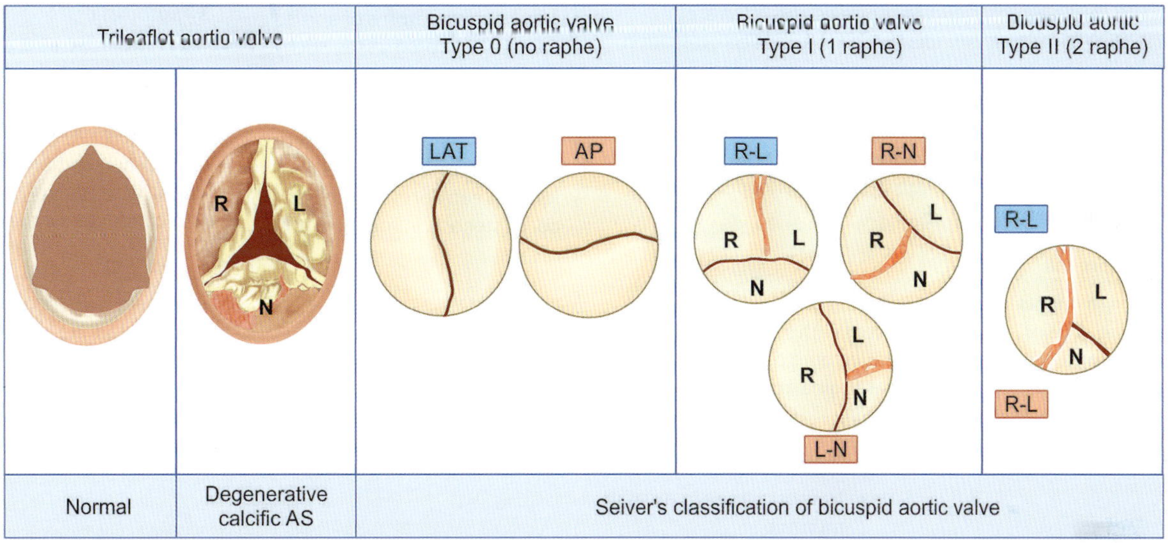

FIG. 3: Seiver's classification of bicuspid aortic valve.

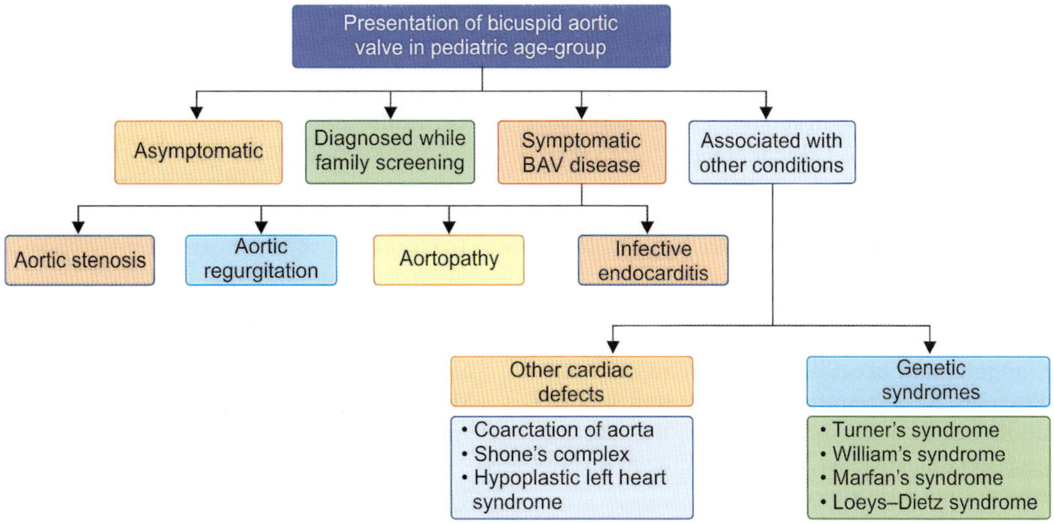

FLOWCHART 1: Presentation of bicuspid aortic valve (BAV) in pediatric age-group.

TABLE 1: Spectrum of clinical presentation of bicuspid aortic valve from neonates to elderly.

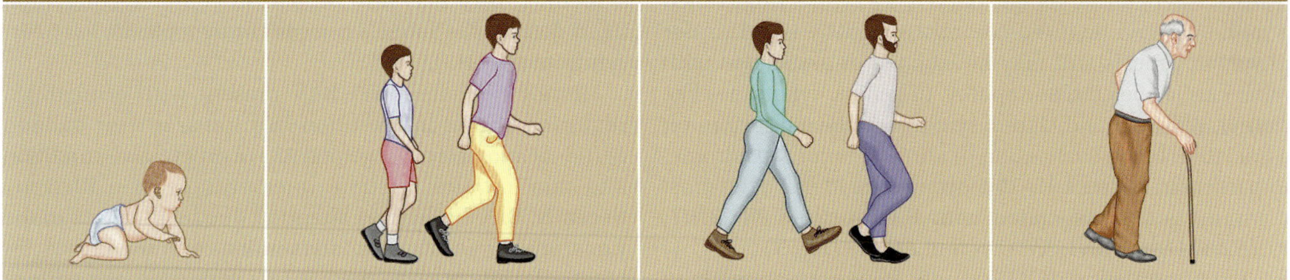

Neonates and infants	**Children and adolescent**	**Adult and middle-aged**	**Elderly**
Aortic stenosis			
• Critical aortic stenosis presents in neonates and with cardiogenic shock, poor perfusion of peripheral organs, cyanosis • In infants, severe aortic stenosis may present as heart failure, breathing difficulty, growth failure	• Children who survive infancy and reach adolescence are rarely symptomatic and often are diagnosed as a routine evaluation due to presence of a click or murmur or as a part of screening • Sometimes as aortic stenosis progresses, children may present with dyspnea, syncope, angina	• In adulthood, many patients may remain asymptomatic • May have symptoms of aortic stenosis as it progresses, such as angina, syncope, or dyspnea • Infective endocarditis • In patients with bicuspid aortic valve, the disease progression leads to early presentation of aortic stenosis in middle age	• In elderly patients, often aortic stenosis is symptomatic • May present as angina, syncope, heart failure, or even sudden cardiac death or infective endocarditis • Conduction abnormalities due to extension of calcium into conduction system
Aortic regurgitation			
Uncommon in infants unless they had prior intervention or surgery	Older children and adolescents may present with severe aortic regurgitation with dyspnea. Fatigue, nocturnal angina, palpitations	May present with progressive symptoms, fatigue, dyspnea, palpitations, nocturnal angina, heart failure	May present with progressive symptoms, fatigue, dyspnea, palpitations, nocturnal angina, heart failure
Endocarditis			
	• Prolonged fever • New or change in existing murmur • Conduction block • Fatigue, weight loss, fever • Heart failure		

Bicuspid aortic valve mainly presents as asymptomatic, AS or AR, aortopathy, or infective endocarditis.

- ***Aortic stenosis*:** In BAV, cusp fusion reduces the effective orifice area, leading to AS. Critical congenital AS can present in neonates with shock, acute heart failure, and poor perfusion, typically after ductus arteriosus closure, requiring urgent intervention like transcatheter balloon aortic valvuloplasty or surgery. AS is a progressive disease and may lead to left ventricular hypertrophy (LVH), growth failure, and exertional symptoms like syncope, angina, and breathing difficulty in children and adolescents often requiring intervention before adulthood. In adults with congenital BAV, the disease progresses faster than degenerative AS, leading to severe symptoms requiring early intervention.
- ***Aortic regurgitation*:** In BAV, AR occurs due to a defect in the coaptation of the aortic cusps. Most of the times AR results after prior aortic interventions, inadequate coaptation due to unequal cusps or active or healed endocarditis, or sometimes due to annuloaortic ectasia due to cystic medial degeneration.[2,4]
- ***Aortopathy*:** BAV is frequently associated with abnormal dilatation or aneurysm of aorta due to cystic medial degeneration. Although aortopathy is common, complications like dissection or rupture are rare unless associated with connective tissue disorders such as Marfan's, Ehlers-Danlos type IV, Loeys-Dietz, or Turner's syndrome.

American College of Cardiology has given the guidelines for sports participation in children with BAV, summarized in **Table 2**.[5]

TABLE 2: Summary of ACC/AHA guidelines for sports participation in patients with bicuspid aortic valve.

Aortic stenosis		Aortic regurgitation		Aortic dilatation	
Symptomatic	Restricted from all competitive sports	**Symptomatic**	Restricted from all competitive sports	Normal ascending aorta and root Z score < 2	No restriction
Asymptomatic		**Asymptomatic**			
Mild	No restriction	Mild	No restriction		
				Z score 2–3.5	Can participate in low-to-moderate static or dynamic sports (Ia, Ib, Ic, IIa, IIb, IIc)
Moderate	Can participate in low to moderate static or dynamic sports (Ia, Ib, IIa)	Moderate (Normal LV function and no progression on echo)	No restriction		
		Severe (normal LV function and no progression on echo)	Can participate in low-intensity sports		
Severe	Can participate in low intensity sports				
				Z score > 3.5	No competitive sports

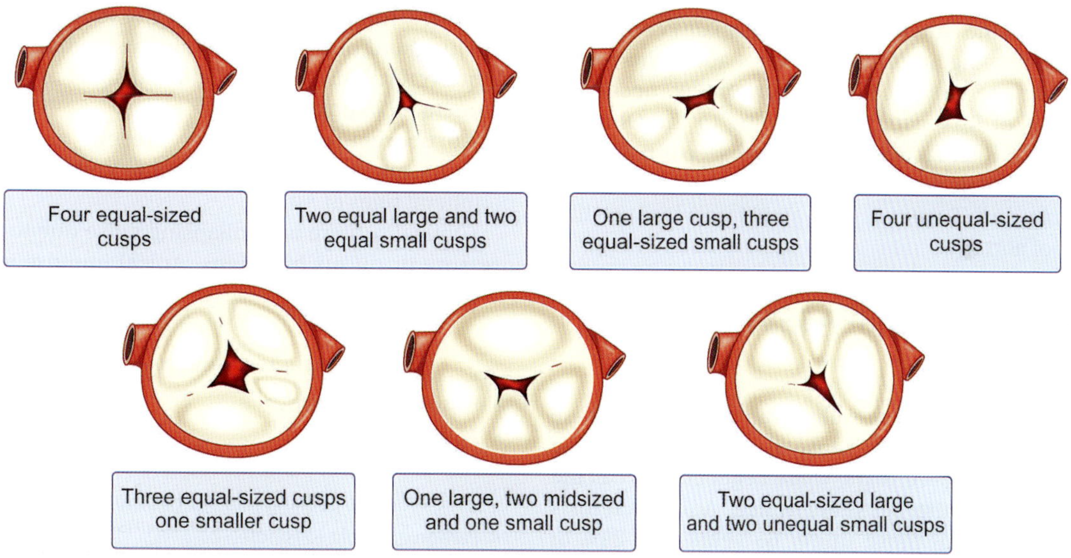

FIG. 4: Hurwitz and Roberts classification of quadricuspid aortic valve.
Courtesy: Yang Liu et al.[8]

- ***Endocarditis:*** Individuals with BAV are at increased risk of endocarditis, which can range from small vegetations to aortic root abscesses. Patients may present with prolonged fever, embolic events, new or changed murmurs, conduction blocks, sepsis, renal failure, heart failure, or acute pulmonary edema due to severe complications like leaflet perforation. Current guidelines recommend endocarditis prophylaxis only for those with a history of endocarditis or prior aortic valve interventions.[6]

Quadricuspid Aortic Valve

Congenital quadricuspid aortic valve (QAV) is a rare cardiac defect, with a prevalence below 0.05%. Hurwitz and Roberts classified QAV into seven subtypes, as shown in **Figure 4**. QAV often leads to AR, primarily due to unequal cusps and progressive fibrosis causing non-coaptation. QAV most commonly presents as an isolated defect and remains asymptomatic for a long time. QAV rarely requires intervention; unless severe AR or endocarditis leads to complications like heart failure or conduction abnormalities. AS is an uncommon presentation with QAV. It seldom presents in neonatal period or infancy and progression to severe symptomatic AR usually occurs in adulthood or middle age.[7] AS is an uncommon presentation with QAV.

AORTIC VALVE DISEASES IN ADULTS AND MIDDLE-AGE POPULATION

In adulthood and middle age, common aortic valve diseases include AS, AR, often due to BAV, rheumatic valvular heart disease or connective tissue disorders, and aortopathy. In patients with BAV, abnormal shear stress leads to leaflet calcification and root dilation, causing AS, AR, or aortic dilatation. As per the natural history data from all studies on BAV, age is the primary determinant of disease progression.[2] AS typically develops from leaflet calcification driven by shear stress, endothelial dysfunction, inflammation, lipoprotein deposition, and fibrosis. Rheumatic heart disease causes AS through inflammation and commissural fusion, leading to leaflet thickening, restricted mobility, and varying degrees of stenosis and regurgitation.[9]

In adults and the elderly with BAV, aortopathy commonly affects the ascending aorta. Though rare, aortic dissection is the most severe complication of aortopathy, occurring in about 0.1% of BAV patients according to the Olmsted County Study.[2] Risk factors for aortic dissection in BAV patients include male sex, hypertension, genetic syndromes like Marfan's and Turner's, and associated lesions like coarctation of aorta.[2]

AORTIC VALVE DISEASES IN THE ELDERLY

Aortic stenosis is the most prevalent valvular heart disease in elderly. BAV is the leading cause of aortic valve disease in individuals aged 50–70 years, while degenerative calcific AS typically occurs after 70 years of age. Aortic sclerosis affects about 1–2% of those under 65 years and 29% of those 65 years and older. Although aortic valve disease can impact all age-groups, it poses distinct challenges in elderly population. In degenerative AS, calcification and degeneration of the body of leaflet are the primary mechanisms of valvular narrowing.[4] Commissural fusion is the hallmark of rheumatic valvular heart disease and is associated with mitral valve disease.[4]

CLINICAL PRESENTATION

Aortic stenosis can manifest with various symptoms, including exertional dyspnea, chest pain, syncope, and progressive heart failure. Elderly patients often present with comorbidities that may complicate diagnosis and management.

Clinically, there is a slow rising late peaking pulse, called as "pulsus parvus et tardus" classically seen in severe calcific AS, best felt, in the carotid arteries **(Fig. 5)**. The apical impulse is usually heaving type, undisplaced, unless associated with concomitant AR. The second heart sound (S2) becomes soft and paradoxical split may be audible. There is a high-pitched, midsystolic, harsh, crescendo-decrescendo murmur, best heard at the second right intercostal space, which may radiate to apex due to Gallavardin phenomenon, or to the carotids.[10] Thrill may be present. The murmur increases on squatting and decreases on sudden standing and Valsalva maneuverer.[10] The classical clinical signs of severe AS are enumerated in **Box 1**.

Aortic regurgitation may present as palpitations, nocturnal angina, dyspnea, and sometimes clinically evident peripheral signs of AR.

Clinically, there is a collapsing pulse due to wide pulse pressure or pulsus bisferiens. Apical impulse is displaced

BOX 1 Clinical signs of severe aortic stenosis (AS).

- Pulsus parvus et tardus
- Apico-carotid delay
- Heaving apical impulse, not displaced
- Long loud late peaking mid systolic murmur
- Paradoxical split S2/single S2
- Low systolic BP with narrow pulse pressure

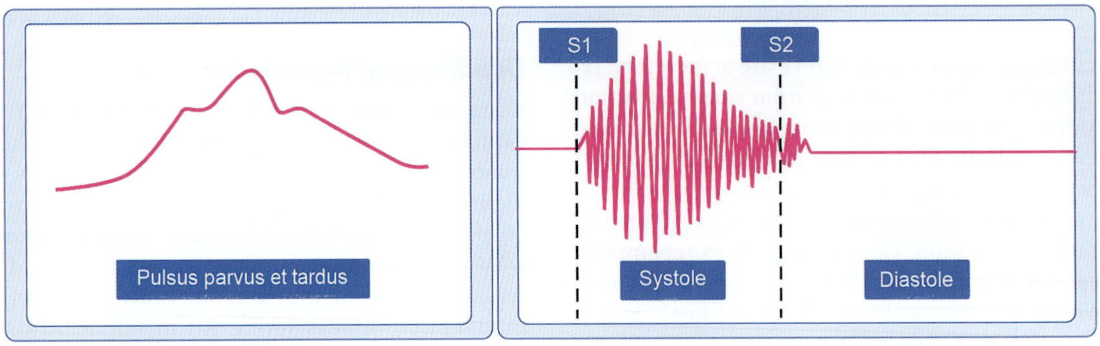

FIG. 5: Pulse and midsystolic murmur in severe calcific aortic stenosis.

due to dilated left ventricle (LV). Peripheral signs of AR may be present. There is a high-pitched blowing early diastolic murmur, best heard in the Erb's area in leaning forward position at the end of expiration. The classical clinical signs of chronic severe AR are enumerated in **Box 2**. Acute severe AR has a catastrophic presentation and the classic clinical signs of severe AR are absent.

BOX 2 Clinical signs of severe aortic regurgitation (AR).

- Hill's sign
- Bisferiens pulse
- Wide pulse pressure with low diastolic pressure
- Peripheral signs of AR (Duroziez murmur—most important)
- Peripheral signs—may be less prominent in LV dysfunction, acute AR other valvular lesions
- Cardiomegaly—dilated hyperdynamic LV
- Length of diastolic murmur—>50% of diastole
- Austin Flint murmur

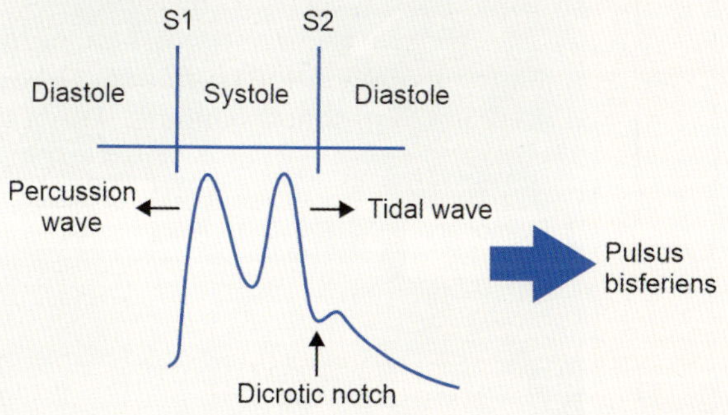

Important causes of AS and AR are enumerated in **Table 3**. As per ACC/AHA guidelines, AS and AR are classified into four stages elaborated in **Table 4**.[5]

TABLE 3: Important causes of AS and AR.

Causes of AS	Causes of AR
Congenital	
• Unicuspid aortic valve • Bicuspid aortic valve, QAV • HLHS • As a part of syndromes, SHONE complex	• Bicuspid aortic valve, QAV • Connective tissue disorders—Marfan syndrome, Loeys–Dietz syndrome, Ehlers–Danlos syndrome • Aortic valve leaflet prolapse, ventricular septal defect • Congenital subaortic membrane
Acquired	
• Rheumatic valvular heart disease • Degenerative calcific AS • Hyperlipoproteinemia II • Ochronosis • Radiation • *Drugs*: Fenfluramine • Chronic kidney disease • Metabolic disorders like Goucher's diseases	• Rheumatic valvular heart disease • Infective endocarditis • Trauma • Degenerative aortic valve disease • Autoimmune diseases like ankylosing spondylosis, rheumatoid arthritis, SLE • *Drugs*: Fenfluramine • Aortopathy, aortic dissection, ascending aortic aneurysm • Annuloaortic ectasia

TABLE 4: Stages of AS and AR as per ACC/AHA 2020 guidelines.[6]

Stages of AS		Stages of AR	
Stage	**Description and definition**	**Stage**	**Description and definition**
A	• At risk of AS • Aortic sclerosis/bicuspid AV • Peak Vmax < 2 m/sec	A	• At risk of AR • Aortic sclerosis/bicuspid AV • Diseases of aortic sinuses or ascending aorta • History of rheumatic fever
B	• Progressive AS • Mild AS • Peak Vmax 2–3.9 m/sec	B	• Progressive AR • Mild-to-moderate AR • Vena contracta < 0.6 cm • Jet width < 65% of LVOT
C	• C1—severe asymptomatic AS with normal LVEF > 50% Vmax > 4 m/sec; mean gradient ≥ 40 mm Hg • C2—severe asymptomatic AS with reduced LVEF < 50% Vmax > 4 m/sec; mean gradient ≥ 40 mm Hg	C	• Severe asymptomatic AR • Vena contracta > 0.6 cm • Jet width > 65% of LVOT • Regurgitant volume > 60 mL/beat • Regurgitant fraction > 50% • EROA > 0.3 cm²

Continued

Continued

Stages of AS		Stages of AR	
Stage	**Description and definition**	**Stage**	**Description and definition**
D	• D1—severe symptomatic AS with normal LVEF > 50% Vmax > 4 m/sec, mean gradient ≥ 40 mm Hg • D2—severe symptomatic as with reduced LVEF < 50% Vmax < 4 m/sec, mean gradient < 40 mm Hg, low flow low gradient AS • D3—severe symptomatic as with normal LVEF > 50% Vmax < 4 m/sec	D	• Severe symptomatic AR • Vena contracta > 0.6 cm • Jet width > 65% of LVOT • Regurgitant volume > 60 mL/beat • Regurgitant fraction > 50% EROA > 0.3 cm^2 • Angiographic grade 3+–4+

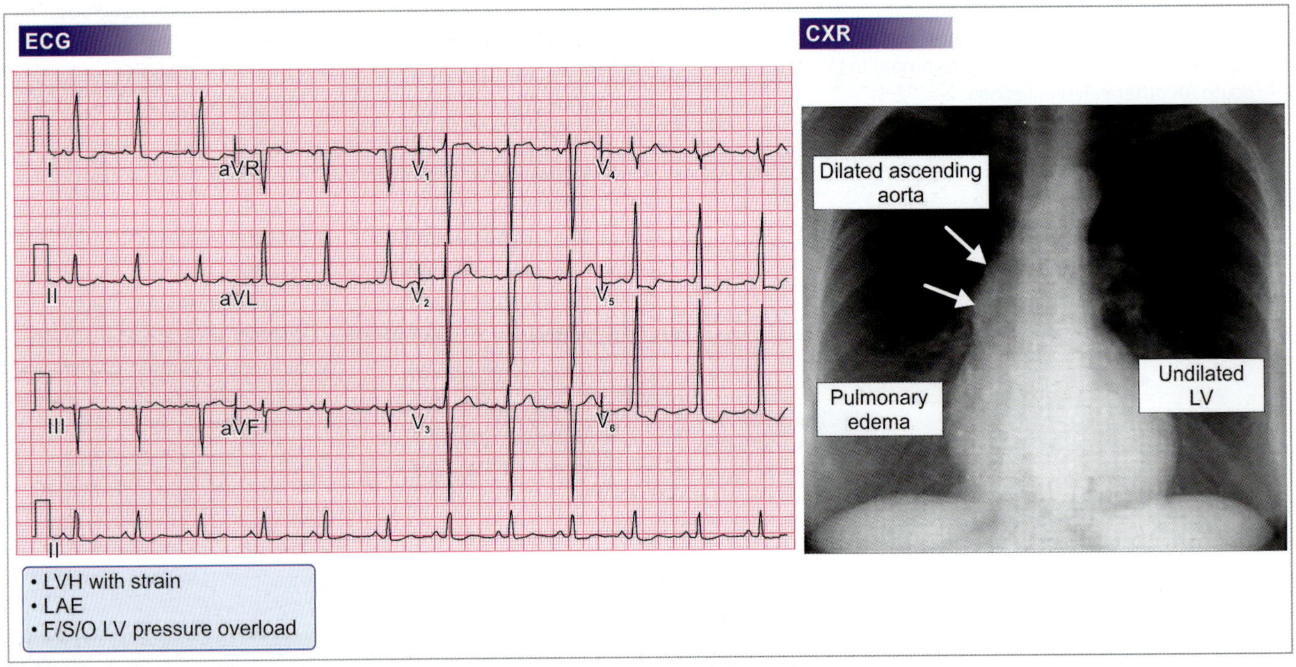

FIG. 6: ECG and CXR in a patient with degenerative severe calcific AS.

INVESTIGATIONS IN AORTIC VALVE DISEASES

Electrocardiography and Chest X-ray in Aortic Valve Diseases

In neonates with congenital severe AS, ECG at birth and in early neonatal period shows right ventricle (RV) dominance. As the age progresses and LV takes over the systemic circulation, by early infancy ECG shows LV forces, by late infancy onwards ECG shows LVH and left atrial enlargement (LAE).[6]

In adulthood, as the disease progresses, ECG shows LVH with strain and LAE. The ECG may vary depending on the extension of calcification into the conduction system. It may present as LVH with strain and LAE, LAHB, IVCD, LBBB, bifascicular or trifascicular block, first-degree AV block, or even complete heart block **(Figs. 6 and 7)**.[7]

In neonates with critical AS, chest X-ray may reveal pulmonary edema and venous congestion. In adults and middle-aged patients, a chest X-ray might show ascending aortic dilatation, pulmonary congestion, and valvular calcification. In elderly patients with severe AS, valvular calcification and signs of pulmonary venous congestion with LVH are commonly evident.[8]

Echocardiography in Aortic Valve Diseases

Echocardiography is an indispensable tool for the diagnosis, evaluation, and guiding the treatment plan in patients with aortic valve disease in any age-group from neonate to elderly.

The fetal echocardiography also has gained importance in the prenatal diagnosis of aortic valve diseases and other congenital heart diseases. In the recent years, prenatal diagnosis of AS has helped in the treatment of congenital AS

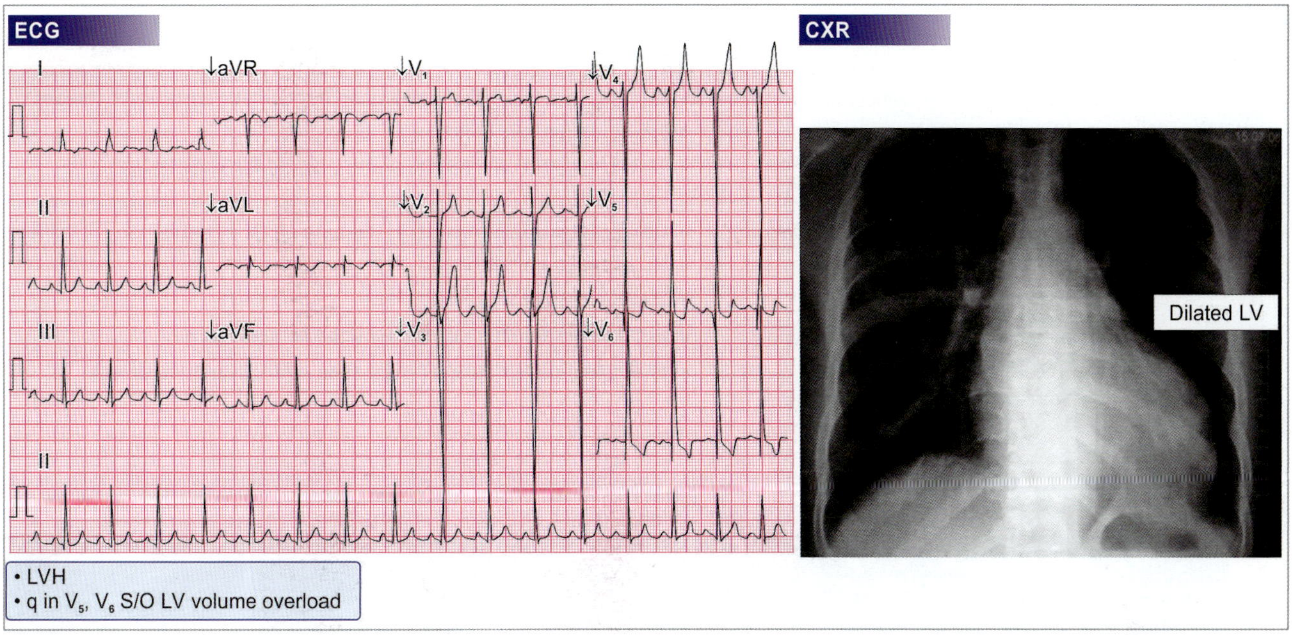

FIG. 7: ECG and CXR in a patient with severe AR.

with fetal cardiac intervention preventing development of HLHS.[9]

Echocardiography provides detailed analysis of morphology, severity, and function of aortic valve and helps in the accurate diagnosis and planning appropriate treatment. **Box 3** enumerates the important parameters to be studied for comprehensive evaluation of aortic valve diseases.

BOX 3 Echocardiographic evaluation of aortic valve disease.

- Evaluation of anatomy, morphological characteristics, calcification of leaflets, and M-mode evaluation
- Assessment of severity of aortic stenosis
- Assessment of associated lesions
- Assessment of systolic and diastolic LV function and strain

Evaluation of Anatomy, Morphological Characteristics, Calcification of Leaflets and M-mode Evaluation

The initial evaluation of aortic valve disease involves parasternal long-axis (PLAX), parasternal short-axis (PSAX), and M-mode echocardiography to assess the anatomy and morphology of the aortic valve and the root. This helps identify number of cusps, calcification, mobility, and the etiology of the disease. **Table 5** outlines key morphological features seen on transthoracic echocardiography (TTE) in PLAX and PSAX views. TTE typically provides a comprehensive assessment of aortic valve diseases, with transesophageal imaging being reserved for patients with suboptimal windows **(Table 5 and Fig. 8)**.[11-13]

TABLE 5: Morphological features seen in parasternal long-axis (PLAX) and parasternal short-axis (PSAX) view in various types of aortic valve diseases.

Aortic valve	PLAX	PSAX
Unicuspid aortic valve	• Systolic doming of a single cusp • No calcification	• Pinhole-shaped (acommissural) or slit-shaped (unicommissural) orifice • In systole rounded free edge is seen • In late diastole single commissural attachment is seen
Bicuspid aortic valve	• Systolic doming of the leaflets • Eccentric closure line on M-mode	• Elliptical systolic orifice • Raphe is not seen in systole • In diastole, raphe may be seen • Calcification of cusp/raphe

Continued

Continued

Aortic valve	PLAX	PSAX
Trileaflet rheumatic aortic valve	• Thickened aortic leaflets with restricted mobility • Associated mitral valve disease	• Commissural fusion is the hallmark of rheumatic aortic valve disease • Triangular systolic orifice • Thickening and calcification of the cusps at the leaflet edges
Trileaflet degenerative calcific aortic valve	• Heavily calcified leaflets predominantly in the body of the leaflet • Reduced systolic opening	• Calcification predominantly in the base and the central body of leaflets • No commissural fusion • Stellate-shaped systolic opening
Quadricuspid aortic valve	• In PLAX, diastolic prolapse of one or the other leaflet • Sometimes changing closure line	• In TTE, the commissural lines form the "X" configuration • In TEE, four distinct cusps can be seen , with coaptation defect

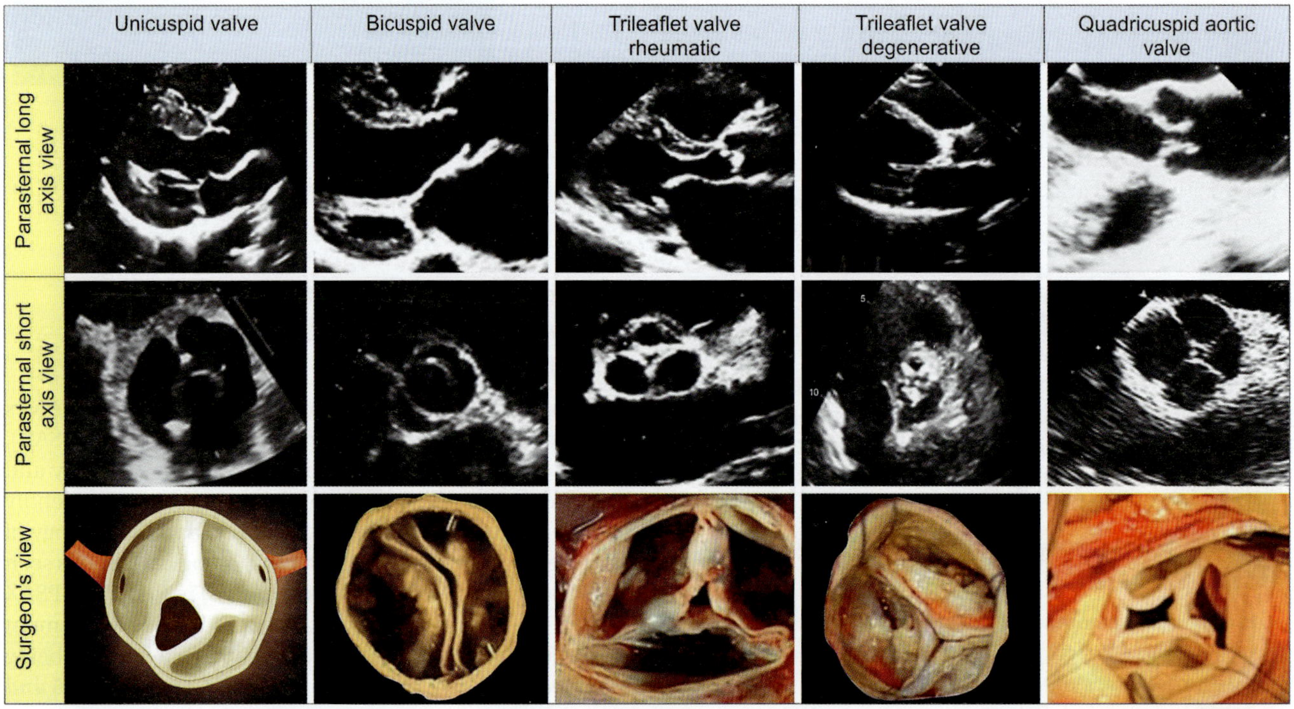

FIG. 8: Various morphologies of aortic valve as seen on transthoracic echocardiography in parasternal long-axis (PLAX) and parasternal short-axis (PSAX) views.

Assessment of Severity

With the recent advancements in transcatheter aortic valve interventions, meticulous assessment of severity of aortic valve diseases and suitability for interventions plays an important role in the management of aortic valve diseases. For patients with renal dysfunction or contrast allergies where CT evaluation is not feasible, 3D-TEE and cardiac MRI are used for aortic valve evaluation and guiding transcatheter aortic valve replacement (TAVR). The important parameters used for assessment of severity of AS are enlisted in the **Table 6**.

Cardiac Computed Tomography and Magnetic Resonance Imaging

Multislice cardiac CT plays an essential role in planning the transcatheter interventions for aortic valve. Cardiac CT accurately assesses the size of the annulus, coronary heights, leaflet length, calcification, and vascular access feasibility. **Figure 9** shows cardiac computed tomography (CT), enface view of aortic valve showing different morphologies. In the patients with contrast allergy or renal dysfunction where CT evaluation is not feasible, 3D TEE and cardiac MRI can be used.[14]

TABLE 6: Important parameters for assessment of aortic stenosis with cutoff values for severe AS.

Parameter	Method/Advantages/Limitations	Cut-off value for Severe AS
Aortic jet velocity	• Measured in the view where the maximum pressure gradient is obtained usually in AP5C or AP3C, rarely right parasternal • Limitation—flow-dependent	4 m/sec
Mean gradient	• Pressure gradient calculated from velocity using the Bernoulli equation • Limitation—flow-dependent	40 mm Hg
Aortic valve area by continuity equation	• LVOT diameter is measured in PLAX view, zoomed image, in midsystole at the base of the LVOT, inner edge to inner edge • Calculated using continuity equation with the help of following parameters: (1) AS jet velocity by CWD; (2) LVOT diameter; (3) LVOT velocity recorded with pulsed Doppler	1 cm^2
Velocity ratio or Dimensionless index	• VR = V (LVOT) ÷ V (AV) • Doppler method • Less variability as compared to continuity equation	0.25
Planimetry area	• TTE/TEE/3D ECHO can be used to measure AVA by planimetry • Difficult with severe valve calcification	1 cm^2

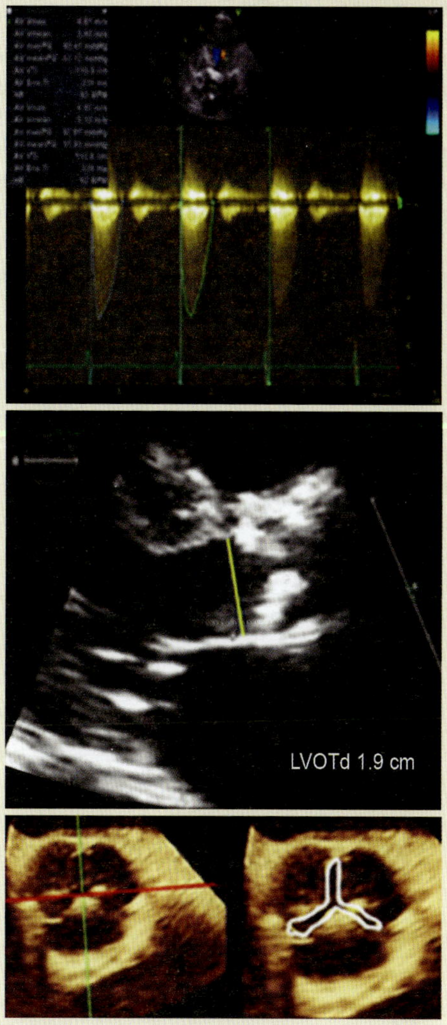

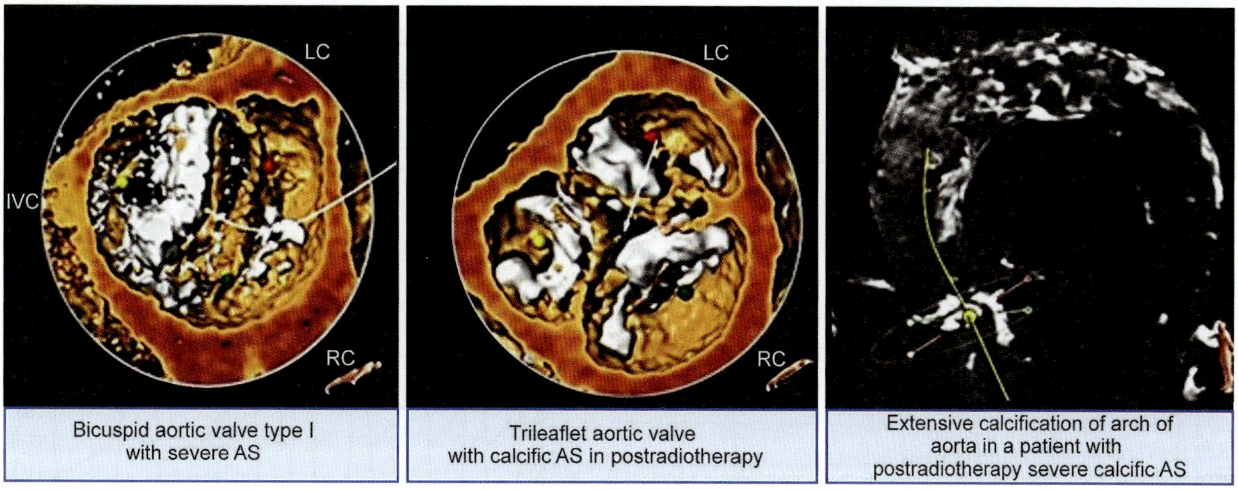

FIG. 9: Bicuspid aortic valve type I with severe AS, severe calcific AS in a patient who has received radiotherapy.

Cardiac Catheterization in Aortic Valve Disease

Invasive cardiac catheterization can accurately assess the severity of aortic valve diseases. In the current era, echocardiography has been instrumental in the assessment of severity of aortic valve diseases; however, it may sometimes overestimate the aortic valve gradients by calculating the peak instantaneous gradient, whereas cardiac catheterization precisely provides peak-to-peak and mean gradients for appropriate decision-making **(Figs. 10A to D)**. In critical AS, the catheter pullback from LV to aorta demonstrates increase in gradient as the catheter across already narrowed aortic valve will causes further obstruction. This is called as "Carabello's sign". Catheterization also differentiates fixed and dynamic LVOT obstruction as shown in **Figures 10 and 11**. Fixed obstruction shows a slow, delayed aortic upstroke, while dynamic obstruction presents a brisk upstroke with a spike-and-dome pattern **(Fig. 10C)**. Premature ventricular contractions (PVCs) also help in differentiating fixed and dynamic LVOT obstruction. In fixed LVOT obstruction, there is increased pulse pressure after PVC, whereas in dynamic LVOT obstruction, there is a decrease in pulse pressure with a significant increase in systolic pressure and the gradient, known as the Brockenbrough–Braunwald–Morrow phenomenon, typical of hypertrophic obstructive cardiomyopathy (HOCM) **(Figs. 11A and B)**.

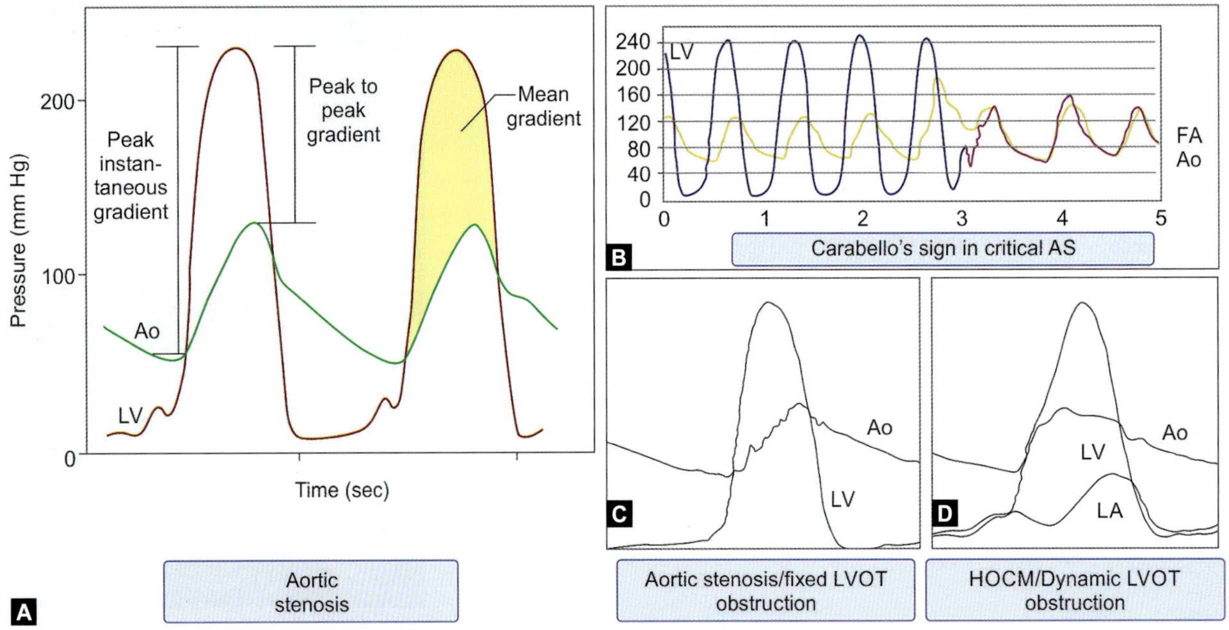

FIGS. 10A TO D: Cardiac catheterization in aortic stenosis.

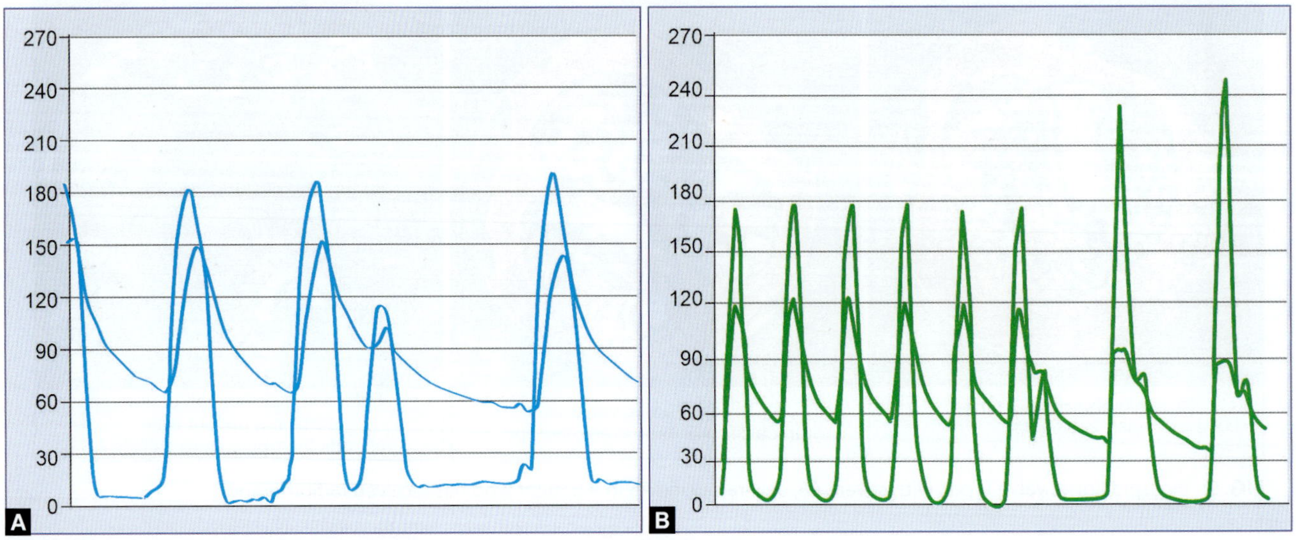

FIGS. 11A AND B: (A) In aortic stenosis/fixed LVOT obstruction, post premature ventricular contraction, there is increase in pulse pressure; and (B) Brockenbrough–Braunwald–Morrow phenomenon in dynamic LVOT obstruction.

MANAGEMENT

Fetal Interventions

Fetal cardiac interventions is an evolving branch. As cardiac development is completed by 8 weeks, most of the congenital heart diseases can be detected by 12th week of gestation. Severe AS in fetus evolves into HLHS, if not treated in the fetal period. Fetal severe AS can lead to severe systolic and diastolic dysfunction of LV and underdevelopment of LV. In the year 2014, Freud et al. first time published the data of fetal aortic valvuloplasty outcomes for severe as evolving into HLHS.[10,15] **Box 4** enumerates the echocardiographic criteria for the diagnosis of fetal AS evolving into HLHS.[15]

BOX 4 **Echocardiographic criteria for the diagnosis of fetal AS evolving into hypoplastic left heart syndrome (HLHS).**

- Narrow aortic jet $>$ 2 m/s
- Dilated dysfunctional left ventricle
- Neodevelopment of mitral regurgitation
- Monophasic mitral inflow Doppler
- PFO shunting left-to-right in a fetus
- Reversal of flow in the aortic arch
- Abnormal pulmonary venous flow pattern
- Endocardial fibroelastosis

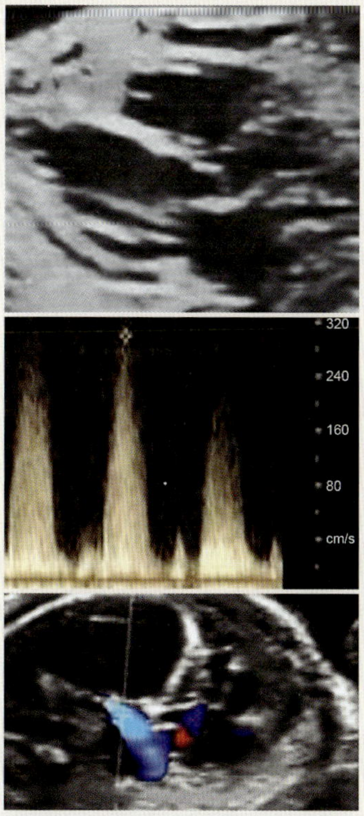

Fetal balloon aortic valvuloplasty is performed using a transapical approach with ultrasound-guided puncture and the coronary wire is advanced into the aorta **(Fig. 12)**. The coronary balloon is advanced and balloon aortic valvuloplasty is performed, which improves the clinical outcomes, allows LV development, and prevents progression to HLHS.[9,15]

Balloon Aortic Valvuloplasty (Fig. 13)

In 1985, Professor Dr Alain Cribier performed the first balloon aortic valvuloplasty for severe AS.[16] Today, this procedure serves as a bridge therapy in patients with severe symptomatic AS who are not candidates for surgical or TAVR, such as young, pregnant, critically ill, or pediatric patients. Balloon aortic valvuloplasty improves hemodynamics and symptoms in patients with severe AS.

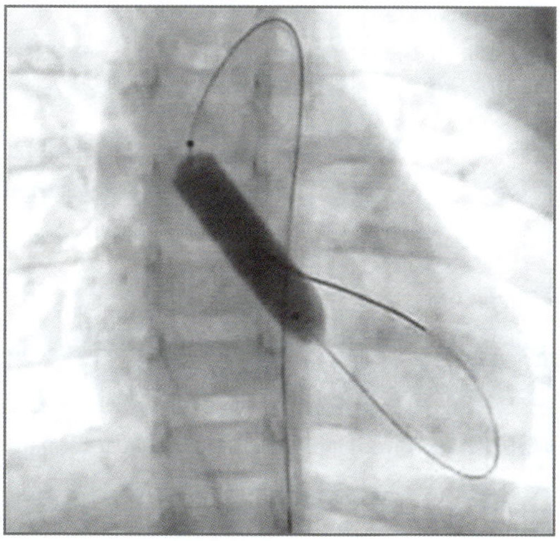

FIG. 13: Balloon aortic valvuloplasty done for severe AS in a 5-year-old child.

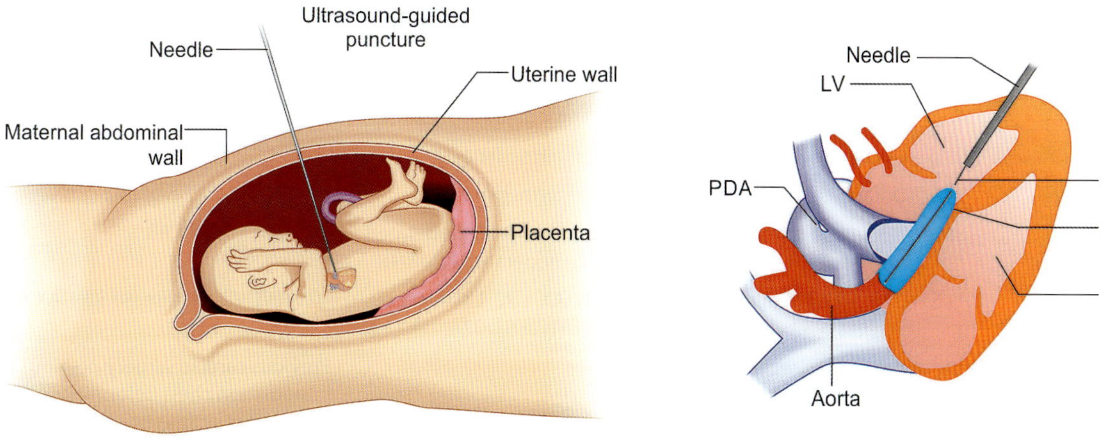

FIG. 12: Diagrammatic representation of fetal cardiac intervention showing balloon aortic valvuloplasty.

The procedure is performed under echocardiographic and fluoroscopic guidance via femoral approach in both pediatric and adult patients. For fetal and neonatal patients, vascular access is selected based on operator's preference and anatomy. An appropriately sized balloon is advanced across the aortic valve and inflated during rapid right ventricular pacing (160–220/min) with hemodynamic monitoring. Invasive and echocardiographic gradients are measured, and AR is assessed echocardiographically or angiographically.[17,18]

Current indications and complications of balloon aortic valvuloplasty are enlisted in **Flowchart 2** and **Box 5**.

BOX 5 Complications of balloon aortic valvuloplasty.

- Vascular site complications
- Acute aortic regurgitation
- Stroke
- Conduction blocks requiring permanent pacemaker implantation
- Myocardial infarction
- Ventricular arrhythmias, rarely death

Surgical Aortic Valve Replacement

Until 1985, surgical aortic valve replacement (SAVR) was the only and the gold standard treatment for symptomatic severe aortic valve disease, before the advent of TAVR. With the evolution of TAVR as a less invasive option in recent years, both SAVR and transfemoral TAVR are now Class I recommendations for severe symptomatic AS, according to ACC/AHA and ESC guidelines. **Table 7** outlines the factors to consider when choosing between SAVR and TAVR with a heart team approach.[19]

Transcatheter Aortic Valve Implantation/Replacement

Transcatheter aortic valve replacement has emerged as a revolutionary treatment for symptomatic severe AS. This minimally invasive procedure has transformed the management of aortic valve diseases, providing new hope for high-risk or inoperable patients. On April 16, 2002, Professor Dr Alain Cribier performed the first TAVR in a patient with critical AS and cardiogenic shock via transvenous access. Over the past 20 years, TAVR has evolved significantly and now has become the standard care for symptomatic severe AS with prohibitive surgical risk.

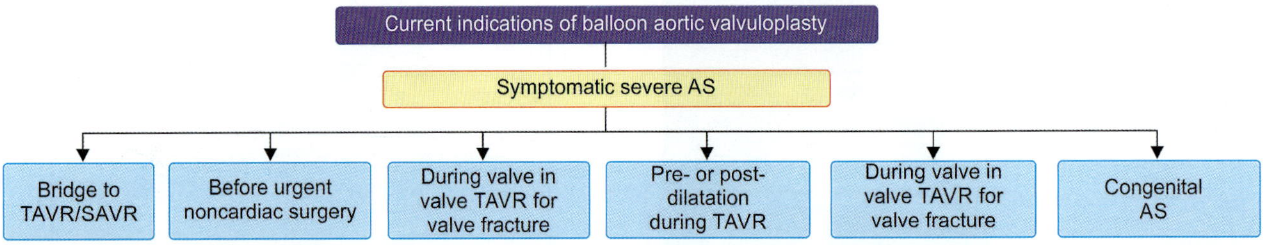

FLOWCHART 2: Current indications of balloon aortic valvuloplasty.[18]

TABLE 7: Factors to be taken into account when deciding SAVR versus TAVR.

	← Favors SAVR		Favors TAVR →
Age	65	75	85
Frailty	Low	Moderate	Severe
Surgical risk	Low	Moderate	Severe
Femoral access	Unfavorable	Intermediate	Favorable
Valve morphology	Unfavorable	Intermediate	Favorable
Associated valve disease	Severe AR severe primary MR/severe TR	Severe secondary MR moderate/severe MS moderate AR/MR/TR	Mild AR/MR/TR
Associated CAD	TVD, SYNTAX > 22, LM disease SYNTAX > 32	TVD, SYNTAX < 22, LM disease SYNTAX < 32	SVD/DVD LM disease SYNTAX < 22
Others	Other aortic disease requiring surgery, active infective endocarditis		Previous cardiac surgery previous chest irradiation chest deformity multiple comorbidities like COPD, CKD

The PARTNER I trial (2010) showed TAVR benefits high-risk severe AS patients, while the PARTNER II trial (2016) found TAVR noninferior to SAVR in intermediate-risk patients. Data from the PARTNER III trial (2019) indicated TAVR is superior to SAVR in low-risk patients regarding death, stroke, and rehospitalization at 1 year.[20-22]

Since its inception, TAVR technology has evolved significantly in terms of indications, safety, vascular accesses like transaxillary, transcaval, and transcarotid approaches. Despite this, the transfemoral approach remains the most widely used, with advanced devices designed primarily for it **(Fig. 14)**. The success of TAVR for severe calcific symptomatic AS is well-documented through clinical trials and real-world studies **(Fig. 15)**.

While the long-term durability of TAVR valves is a subject of ongoing research, they have shown excellent results in the intermediate term, making them a viable option for most patients above 65 years of age. The complications associated with TAVR are enumerated in **Box 6**.

Transcatheter aortic valve replacement has revolutionized the entire management of aortic valve diseases and current trials aim to expand its indications beyond degenerative calcific severe AS **(Fig. 16)**.[23]

With ongoing research and expanding indications, TAVR has the potential to become the standard of care for a broader range of patients with aortic valve diseases. As the field continues to evolve, the collaboration of cardiologists, cardiothoracic surgeons, and electrophysiologists and interdisciplinary teams play a strategic role in providing the best care to patients with aortic valve disease. TAVR is not just a medical advancement; it represents a new era in cardiovascular medicine, offering hope to patients who were once deemed inoperable.

BOX 6 Complications of TAVR.

- Vascular site complications
- Acute aortic regurgitation
- Annular rupture
- Stroke
- Conduction blocks requiring permanent pacemaker implantation
- Myocardial infarction due to coronary occlusion
- Ventricular arrhythmias, rarely death

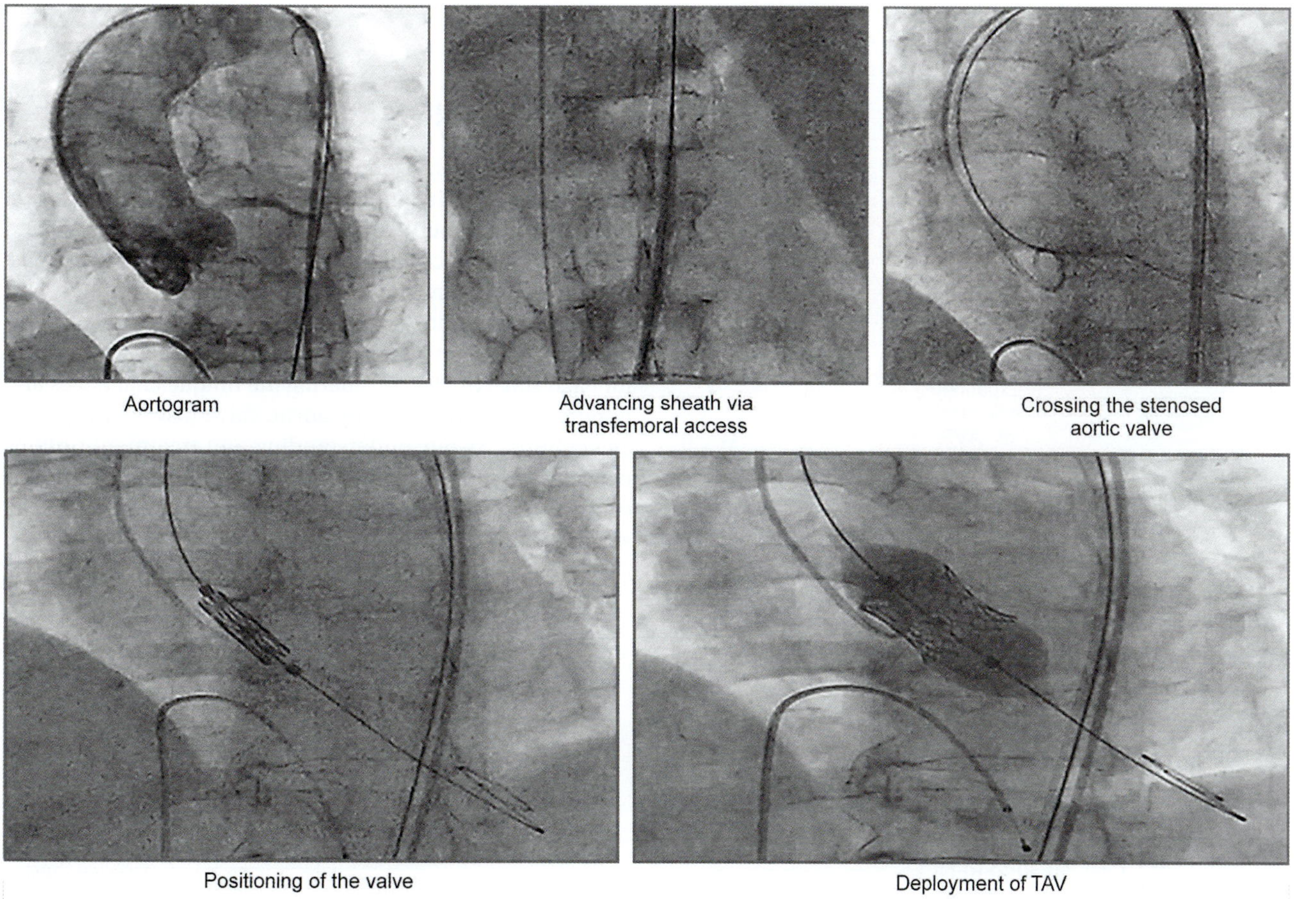

FIG. 14: Steps involved in transfemoral TAVR.

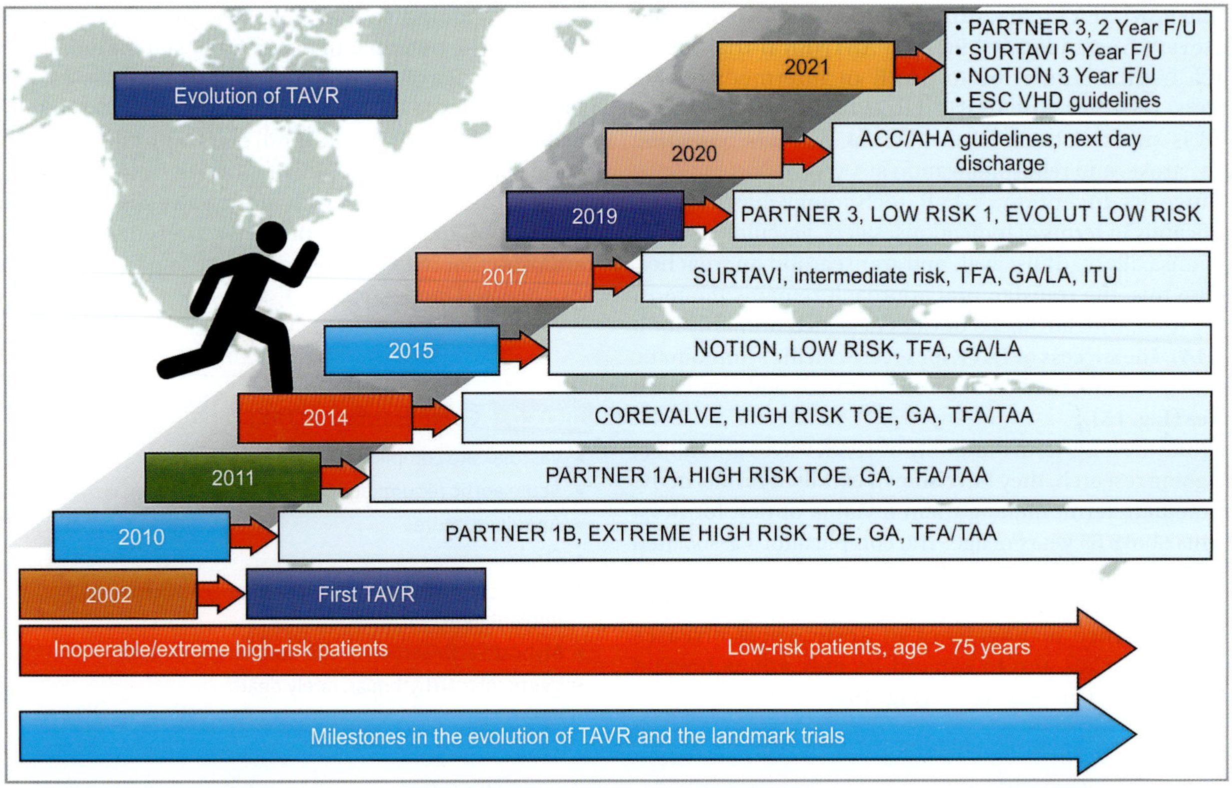

FIG. 15: Timeline of evolution of TAVR and clinical trials.

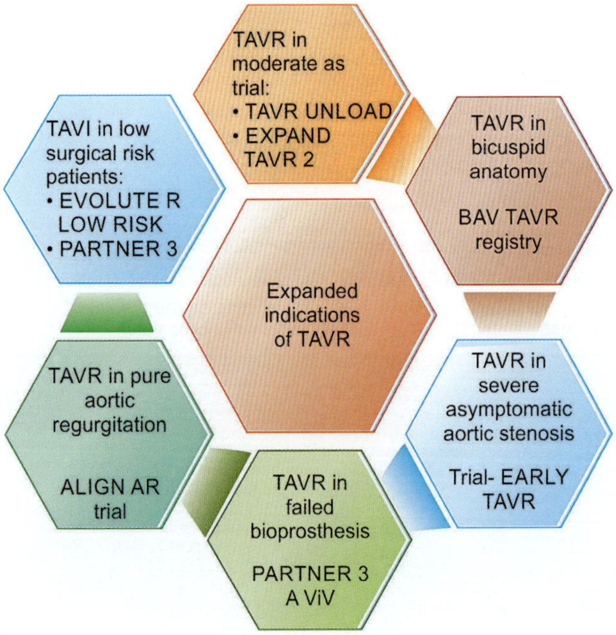

FIG. 16: Expanded indications of TAVR.

CONCLUSION

Aortic valve disease encompasses a broad spectrum of pathologies affecting individuals across their lifespan, from the prenatal period to advanced age. Timely diagnosis and intervention are crucial in optimizing patient outcomes. Advances in diagnostic imaging, surgical techniques, and TAVR have revolutionized the management of aortic valve disease across age groups. Tailored approach is required for each stage of life, considering the unique challenges and opportunities presented by aortic valve disease in various age cohorts. As our understanding and treatment options continue to evolve, the future holds promise for improved care and outcomes for patients with aortic valve disease at all stages of life.

ONLINE REFERENCES

Please scan the QR code provided at the end of the table of contents for References of this chapter.

CHAPTER 170

Transcatheter Aortic Valve Implantation in Degenerated Surgical Aortic Valve: New Hope

Ashish Kumar, Himanshu Dabral, Rajneesh Kapoor

ABSTRACT

Valve-in-valve (ViV) transcatheter aortic valve implantation (TAVI) has become a well-established alternative for managing failed bioprosthetic surgical aortic valves, especially in patients who are considered high risk for undergoing repeat surgical procedures. Although this method is less invasive compared to surgical reoperation, it brings its own set of challenges, including a higher likelihood of valve malposition, prosthesis-patient mismatch (PPM), and the risk of coronary obstruction. Therefore, selecting the right patients and thorough preprocedural planning are crucial to reducing these risks. This chapter presents a detailed review of the key operative considerations during the ViV TAVI procedure, providing valuable insights to help clinicians navigate this complex and evolving field.

Keywords: TAVI, aortic stenosis, valve in valve, bioprosthetic valve, surgical valve deterioration

INTRODUCTION

With increasing popularity of transcatheter aortic valve implantation (TAVI) procedures, there has been a noticeable shift toward the increased use of bioprosthetic valves, gradually replacing mechanical valves in many cases. Despite their growing popularity, bioprosthetic valves are prone to degeneration and eventual failure. This issue becomes particularly pressing as younger patients receive these valves, raising concerns about a possible increase in bioprosthesis failure rates in the future. For patients who are not ideal candidates for traditional surgery, a less invasive reintervention may be necessary. As a result, the number of valve-in-valve (ViV) TAVI procedures is expected to rise significantly. Although current devices and techniques effectively manage many cases of degenerated bioprosthetic valves, ViV TAVI poses specific challenges. These challenges mainly stem from the limited space within the aortic root, which can lead to high residual gradients, severe prosthesis-patient mismatch (PPM), and mechanical complications like coronary obstruction caused by the displacement of the bioprosthetic valve leaflets. This chapter offers an up-to-date analysis of the preprocedural evaluations, procedural methods, and clinical outcomes related to ViV TAVI.

TYPES OF SURGICAL BIOPROSTHETIC AORTIC VALVES

Surgical bioprosthetic heart valves (BHVs) can be classified in number of ways namely:

- *Type of tissue used (porcine vs. bovine pericardium)*: Generally, bovine pericardial valves tend to fail due to stenosis, while porcine valves are more prone to regurgitation.
- *Frame structure (stented, stentless, or sutureless)*: These differences result in distinct fluoroscopic appearances, which are essential for accurate ViV TAVI deployment. Stented valves are the valves most commonly implanted worldwide.
- *Implantation technique (intra-annular vs. supra-annular)*: Recent advancements leading to supra-annular implantation have led to increase in effective orifice size and reduction in the likelihood of severe PPM.
- *Mounting of leaflets on stent post (internal vs. external)*: Models such as Mitroflow (LivaNova) and Trifecta (Abbott) with externally mounted leaflets may enhance hemodynamic performance and lower the risk of significant PPM, but they can also increase the risk of coronary obstruction during ViV TAVI in certain

anatomical scenarios. Looking ahead, innovations in surgical valve design, such as the expandable hinge feature in the INSPIRIS surgical aortic valve (SAV) from Edwards Lifesciences, may support better ViV TAVI outcomes by accommodating larger transcatheter heart valves (THVs) and further reducing the risk of PPM.[1]

MECHANISM OF FAILURE IN SURGICAL BIOPROSTHETIC AORTIC VALVES

Surgical BHVs can fail for various reasons, as identified by the Valve Academic Research Consortium (VARC)-3 criteria.[2]

- Structural valve deterioration (SVD)
- *Non-SVD (NSVD)*:
  - Paravalvular regurgitation
  - PPM
- Valve thrombosis
- Endocarditis

While mechanical valves are more vulnerable to thrombosis, bioprosthetic valves are more likely to experience valve deterioration. SVD involves intrinsic, irreversible changes to the prosthetic valve, including wear and tear, leaflet damage, flail leaflet, leaflet fibrosis, calcification, and strut fractures. These changes often lead to stenosis and/or regurgitation. The European Association of Percutaneous Cardiovascular Interventions (EAPCI), in collaboration with the European Society of Cardiology (ESC) and the European Association for Cardio-Thoracic Surgery (EACTS), has developed a definition of SVD that classifies the condition into different stages based on echocardiographic findings shown in **Table 1**.

Echocardiography (including TEE) helps to diagnose etiology of BHV failure and differentiate between SVD and NSVD in the presence of high transprosthetic gradients as shown in **Table 2**.

INDICATIONS FOR ViV TAVI VERSUS REDO-SAVR

The ViV TAVI is typically recommended for patients with SVD who are considered high or extreme risk for undergoing repeat surgical aortic valve replacement (SAVR). For those at intermediate or low surgical risk, redo-SAVR should be the preferred option unless they present with anatomically challenging conditions, e.g., calcified aortic root, hostile chest. In younger patients, where valve durability is a significant concern, redo-SAVR is often advised due to the uncertain long-term outcomes of ViV TAVI. Additionally, redo-SAVR is recommended for patients with anatomical features that increase the risk of coronary obstruction during ViV TAVI, particularly when the BASILICA procedure (bioprosthetic aortic scallop intentional laceration to prevent coronary artery obstruction) is not feasible or when precise commissural alignment of the THV is required to prevent

TABLE 1: Stages of structural valve deterioration.

	Echocardiographic findings
Stage 0 (no SVD)	Normal valve morphology and function
Stage 1 (morphological SVD)	Intrinsic permanent structural changes to the prosthetic valve (leaflet integrity or structure abnormality, leaflet function abnormality, and strut/frame abnormality)
Stage 2 (moderate hemodynamic SVD)	• Mean transprosthetic gradient ≥ 20 mm Hg and <40 mm Hg • Mean transprosthetic gradient ≥ 10 mm Hg and <20 mm Hg change from baseline • Moderate intraprosthetic aortic regurgitation, new or worsening (>1+/4) from baseline
Stage 3 (severe hemodynamic SVD)	• Mean transprosthetic gradient ≥ 40 mm Hg • Mean transprosthetic gradient ≥ 20 mm Hg change from baseline • Severe intraprosthetic aortic regurgitation, new or worsening (>2+/4) from baseline

TABLE 2: Echocardiographic features to differentiate patient prosthesis mismatch from structural valve degeneration.

Normal function	PPM (NSVD)	SVD
Normal valve structure and motion	Normal valve structure and motion	Abnormal valve structure and motion
Vpeak < 3 m/s, MeanG < 20 mm Hg	Vpeak > 3 m/s, MeanG > 20 mm Hg	Vpeak > 3 m/s, MeanG > 20 mm Hg
EOA > 1 cm^2; DVI ≥ 0.35	EOA > 1 cm^2; DVI 0.25–0.34	EOA variable; DVI < 0.25
EOA within normal range	EOA normal	EOA reduced
EOAi > 0.85 cm^2/m^2	EOAi ≤ 0.85 cm^2/m^2	EOAi ≤ 0.85 cm^2/m^2
Increase in MeanG < 10 mm Hg and decrease in EOA < 0.3 cm^2 during follow-up	Increase in MeanG < 10 mm Hg and decrease in EOA < 0.3 cm^2 during follow-up	Increase in MeanG ≥10 mm Hg and decrease in EOA ≥0.3 cm^2 during follow-up

(DVI: Doppler velocity index; EOA: effective orifice area; EOAi: indexed effective orifice area; MeanG: mean gradient; Vpeak: peak velocity)

obstruction by a split bioprosthetic valve leaflet. Patients with severe PPM and appropriate anatomy may also be considered for ViV TAVI, potentially with additional procedures like balloon valve fracture (BVF).

PROCEDURAL ASPECTS OF ViV TAVI

Evaluating Types and Dimensions of Surgical Valves

Accurately identifying the type of surgical bioprosthesis is essential for evaluating the suitability of ViV TAVI and for detailed procedural planning. Information on the manufacturer, model, and size of the SAV can typically be retrieved from the original operative report. Additionally, imaging techniques such as fluoroscopy and computed tomography (CT) can assist in confirming these details. It is important to note that the manufacturer-labeled size does not correspond to the true internal diameter (ID) of the prosthesis. The stent ID, which measures only the stent frame's diameter, often differs from the true ID, depending on the specific type of stented SAV and the method used to mount the tissue leaflets onto the stent frame.[3] **Figures 1A to C** showing effect of leaflet type and mounting on the stent and true ID of stented SAVs. **Table 3** showing examples of stented SAVs comparing stent ID with true ID.

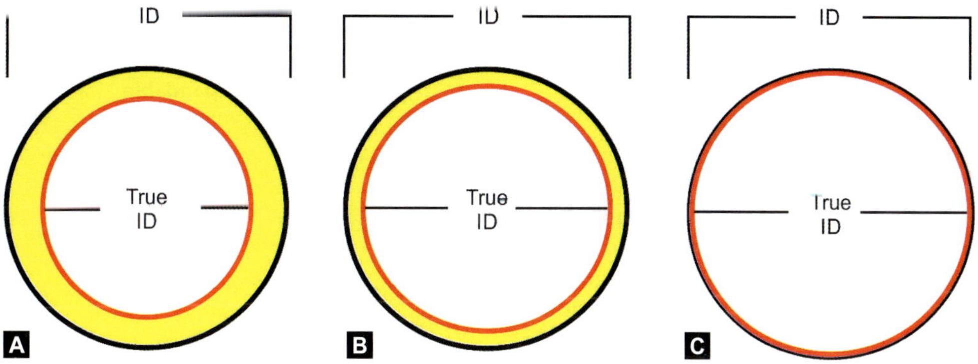

FIGS. 1A TO C: (A) For porcine valves, the true internal diameter (ID) is at least 2 mm smaller than the stent ID. (B) In pericardial valves, where the leaflets are sutured within the stent frame, the true ID is at least 1 mm smaller than the stent ID. (C) For pericardial valves with leaflets sutured outside the stent frame, the true ID matches the stent ID.

TABLE 3: Examples of stented surgical aortic valves where the labeled size, stent, and true internal diameters differ.

Stented SAV name (Manufacturer)	Mosaic (Medtronic)	Magna 3000 (Edwards Lifesciences)	Mitroflow (Liva Nova)
	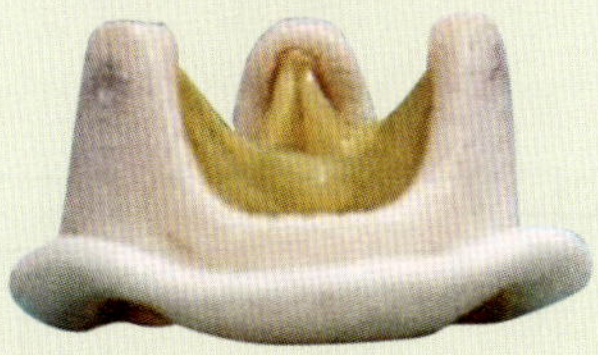	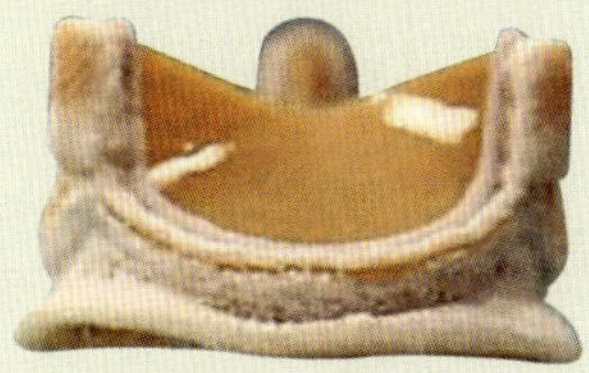	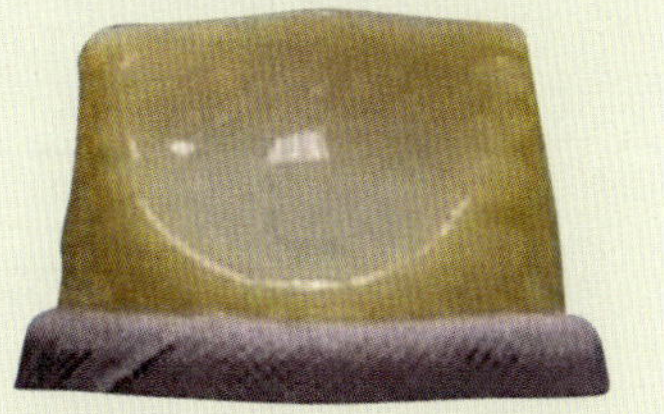
Type of SAV	Porcine valve	Bovine pericardial valve, internally mounted	Bovine pericardial valve, externally mounted
Manufacturer-labeled size	23	23	23
Stent dimension (stent ID)	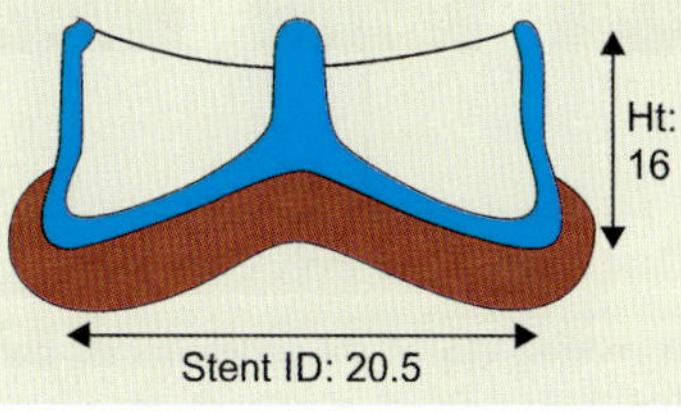	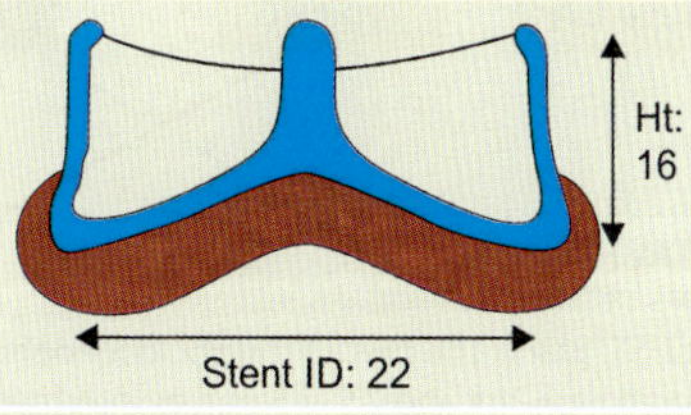	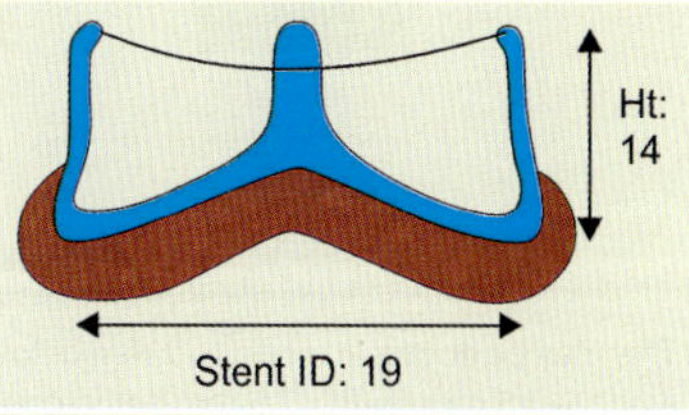
True ID	19	21	19

Evaluating Coronary Obstruction Risk in ViV TAVI

The risk of coronary obstruction is higher in ViV TAVI compared to native TAVI, largely due to the fact that SAV leaflets often extend beyond the aortic root above the sinotubular junction (STJ).[4] During ViV TAVI, these SAV leaflets will become displaced, potentially forming a cylinder-like "neoskirt" that can obstruct coronary flow. To assess the risk of coronary obstruction in ViV TAVI, a multidetector computed tomography (MDCT) scan is essential for measuring the valve-to-coronary (VTC) and valve-to-STJ (VTSTJ) distances. Distances under 3 mm are generally indicative of a higher risk for coronary obstruction. The BASILICA procedure can be utilized to mitigate this risk by splitting the problematic SAV leaflet prior to the TAVI procedure.[5] **Flowchart 1** showing algorithm to determine need for BASILICA in ViV TAVI.

Transcatheter Heart Valve Selection in ViV TAVI

The selection of the type and size of the TAV for implantation in an SAV is influenced by several factors. To prevent TAV migration, a certain degree of oversizing is generally recommended. Recent studies suggest that positioning the TAV at a higher level within the SAV can enhance hemodynamic performance by improving the circularity of the THV and minimizing leaflet pinwheeling (the twisting of the leaflet-free edges due to excessive leaflet redundancy).[6-8] Although balloon predilatation is rarely used in ViV TAVI, postdilatation may be advantageous for optimizing the expansion and circularity of the THV frame. **Table 4** showing considerations for choosing between balloon-expandable and self-expanding TAV implantation in a deteriorating SAV.

Balloon Valve Fracture in ViV TAVI

In patients with severe PPM linked to smaller SAVs, ViV TAVI may not alleviate the existing PPM because the THV is inserted within an already small SAV. In cases where severe PPM exists but with no or mild SVD, ViV TAVI is unlikely to

TABLE 4: Considerations for choosing between balloon-expandable and self-expanding transcatheter aortic valve (TAV) implantation in a deteriorating surgical aortic valve (SAV).

Factors	Balloon-expandable valve preferred	Self-expanding valve preferred
Smaller SAV (true ID < 23 mm)		✓
Need for coronary reaccess	✓	
Pure aortic regurgitation in a stentless SAV	✓	✓
BVF feasible	✓	
BVF not feasible or safe		✓

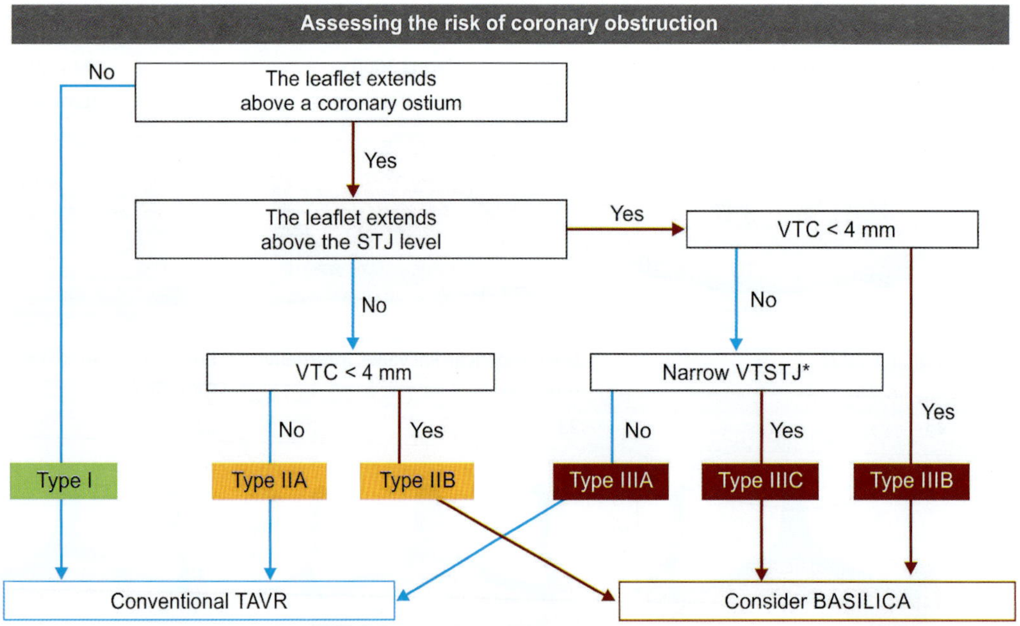

*This may be above, at, or up to 2 mm below the STJ plane. The precise threshold for defining a narrow VTSTJ is still undetermined, but it is currently categorized as <2.5–3.5 mm (with <2.5 mm being considered high-risk and 2.5–3.5 mm as intermediate-risk).

FLOWCHART 1: Suggested algorithm for assessing aortic root anatomy and determining the need for BASILICA in ViV TAVI.

TABLE 5: Potential advantages and disadvantages of balloon valve fracture (BVF) before or after transcatheter aortic valve implantation (TAVI).

	BVF before TAVI	BVF after TAVI
Advantages	• Easier to implant self-expanding valve with less sizing mismatch • Can confirm successful fracture before finalizing TAV size	• Better TAV expansion, especially in balloon-expandable valves • Less risk of acute severe aortic regurgitation
Disadvantages	• Acute severe aortic regurgitation causing hemodynamic collapse • May need to post-dilate to optimize hemodynamics	• TAV migration or embolization • Acute TAV failure from leaflet injury • Unknown effect on TAV durability

provide significant benefits since it does not address the root cause of the PPM. BVF has been suggested as a technique to increase the actual ID of the SAV, allowing for the implantation of a larger or better-expanded THV to enhance hemodynamic performance and potentially reduce the severity of preexisting PPM.[9] This method involves inflating a noncompliant balloon (e.g., Atlas Gold Balloon) within the SAV at high pressure to fracture the stented SAV frame, thereby facilitating better expansion of the implanted TAV or enabling the placement of a larger TAV without risking frame underexpansion. However, not all stented SAVs are suitable for BVF.[10] BVF cannot be performed on sutureless and stentless SAVs; however, in sutureless valves, balloon valve remodeling (BVR) through overexpansion may be possible. BVF should be avoided in patients who have undergone bio-Bentall aortic root replacement with a stented SAV due to the risk of aortic root rupture usually due to disruption along the surgical suture line at the ventriculo-aortic junction. BVF can be carried out either before or after TAVI. **Table 5** showing pros and cons of BVF before and after TAVI.

CLINICAL OUTCOMES AFTER ViV TAVI

Clinical outcomes following ViV TAVI differ in several ways from those seen after conventional TAVR.[11,12] A matched comparison between conventional TAVI and ViV TAVI demonstrated that the ViV group had lower mortality rates, even after accounting for baseline differences. The stented bioprosthetic valve frame provides protection to nearby structures during valve implantation, which reduces the risk of mechanical complications such as annular injury and damage to the aortomitral curtain. Consequently, conduction abnormalities are less frequent, with the rate of pacemaker implantation after ViV TAVI consistently under 10%. Additionally, the stented bioprosthetic valve frame offers strong support for sealing after ViV TAVI, significantly lowering the risk of PVL, provided the previously implanted valve did not already have PVL. However, certain adverse events are more prevalent in ViV TAVI, including residual elevated gradients (particularly in small, stenotic surgical valves), clinical thrombosis, THV malpositioning (especially in regurgitant stentless valves or those with poor fluoroscopic markers), and coronary obstruction.

CONCLUSION

ViV TAVI offers a promising alternative for patients with failing surgical bioprosthetic valves, particularly those at high surgical risk. However, careful preprocedural planning, including evaluation of the surgical valve type, coronary obstruction risk, and THV selection, is crucial for achieving optimal outcomes. Emerging techniques such as BVF and BASILICA are valuable tools in expanding the applicability and success of ViV TAVI in complex cases.

ONLINE REFERENCES

Please scan the QR code provided at the end of the table of contents for References of this chapter.

CHAPTER

171

Transcatheter Aortic Valve Replacement: Status 2024*

Harinder K Bali, Navdeep Singh Sidhu

ABSTRACT

Initially introduced as a treatment option for patients with severe aortic stenosis (AS) who are at prohibitively high risk for surgery, transcatheter aortic valve replacement (TAVR) has come a long way to being a viable and effective option for surgery even in patients of younger age and lower surgical risks. This has caused a paradigm shift in the management of AS patients. Powered by the continuous improvements in the prosthesis designs, increased operator experience, and continued generation of robust clinical data, it is likely to be offered to newer subsets of patients and with newer indications in the very near future. Here we discuss the recent advances in this field and the future outlook.

Keywords: TAVR, TAVI, transcatheter, aortic, valve replacement, aortic stenosis

INTRODUCTION

Since its first clinical use in 2002, the transcatheter aortic valve replacement (TAVR)/transcatheter aortic valve implantation (TAVI) has caused a major shift in the management strategies of patients with symptomatic severe aortic stenosis (AS) and is currently a well-established and approved treatment option in eligible patients. Advancements in prosthesis designs, enhanced operator experience, and growing clinical data have resulted in progressive expansion of its use to include newer subsets of younger and low-risk patients, and in wider clinical situations. This has brought into focus many novel considerations like valve durability, coronary access after TAVR, and redo-TAVR. Here, we discuss the current status of TAVR and future considerations.

CURRENT INDICATIONS

The valvular heart disease guidelines issued by both the American [American College of Cardiology (ACC)/American Heart Association (AHA)][1] and the European [European Society of Cardiology (ESC)/European Association for Cardio-Thoracic Surgery (EACTS)][2] societies advocate stratifying patients with severe AS needing valve replacement into three groups: First group being suitable for surgical aortic valve replacement (SAVR), second being suitable for TAVR, and the third in whom the decision between SAVR and TAVR should be taken on the basis of an individualized approach involving shared decision-making **(Table 1)**. Whereas the ACC/AHA guidelines recommend SAVR for patients < 65 years of age who have a life expectancy of >20 years, the ESC/EACTS guidelines advocate SAVR for patients <75 years of age who have an STS-PROM/EuroSCORE < 4 or for operable patients in whom TAVR is not feasible. According to ESC/EACTS guidelines, the patients selected for TAVR should be older than 75 years or be at high risk (STS-PROM/EuroSCORE > 8), but the ACC/AHA guidelines advocate TAVR for patients > 80 years or with life expectancy < 10 years **(Flowchart 1)**.

AVAILABLE TRANSCATHETER AORTIC VALVE REPLACEMENT DEVICES

With rapid expansion and uptake of TAVR across the world, there has been a constant evolution of TAVR devices, in

*We dedicate this chapter to Professor (Dr) Alain Cribier, the father of transcatheter aortic valve replacement, who passed away unexpectedly on February 16, 2024.

TABLE 1: Clinical decision making and factors affecting the choice between SAVR and TAVR.[3]

	← Favors SAVR	Favors TAVR →	
Age	<65	65–85	>85
Surgical risk	Low	Intermediate	High-prohibitive
Frailty	Low	Moderate	Severe
Valve morphology	Unfavorable	Intermediate	Favorable
Femoral access	Unfavorable	Intermediate	Favorable
Other valve disease	• Severe AR • Severe primary MR • Severe TR	• Severe secondary MR • Moderate/severe MS • Moderate AR/MR/TR	Mild AR/MR/MS/TR
Coronary artery disease	• 3-vessel disease and SYNTAX >22 • LM disease and SYNTAX >32	• 3-vessel disease and SYNTAX ≤22 • LM disease and SYNTAX ≤32	• 1 or 2-vessel disease • LM disease and SYNTAX ≤22
Other factors	• Aortic disease requiring surgery • Septal hypertrophy requiring surgery • Active endocarditis		• Porcelain aorta • Chest deformity • Past cardiac surgery • Past chest radiation • Multiple comorbidities

(AR: aortic regurgitation; LM: left main; MR: mitral regurgitation; MS: mitral stenosis; SAVR: surgical aortic valve replacement; SYNTAX: Synergy Between Percutaneous Coronary Intervention with TAXUS and Cardiac Surgery; TAVR: transcatheter aortic valve replacement; TR: tricuspid regurgitation)

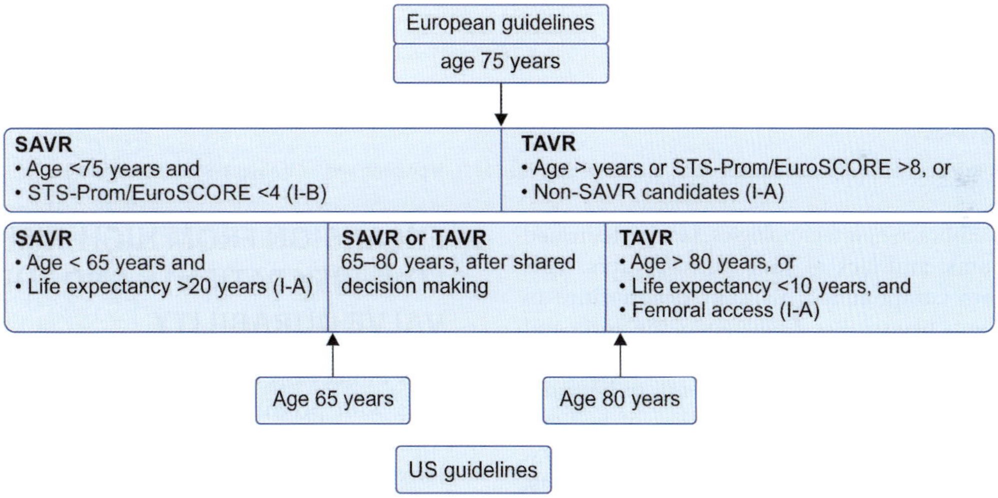

FLOWCHART 1: Comparison of European versus US guidelines for TAVR indications.[4]
(SAVR: surgical aortic valve replacement; STS: Society of Thoracic Surgeons; TAVR: transcatheter aortic valve replacement)

terms of both launch of new devices and improvements in the existing ones. Depending on the mechanism of valve expansion, major TAVR devices currently available **(Table 2)** have been subclassified into self-expanding valves (SEV) and balloon-expanding valves (BEV). The mechanically expanding valves (MEV) devices such as Lotus and Lotus Edge have been withdrawn due to issues with the delivery system.

TRANSCATHETER AORTIC VALVE REPLACEMENT IN INDIA

Like many other developing countries, the uptake and expansion of TAVR in India has been lagging behind many American and European countries, with the first case of TAVR reported in 2011.[6,7] This has probably been related to the high cost of the devices, reluctance among physicians

TABLE 2: Major TAVR devices currently available.[5,6]

Device	Leaflet position	Route	Delivery system outer diameter (F)	R/R
CoreValve[*,†]	SA	Transvascular/transaortic	18	+/+
Evolut Series R[*,†]	SA	Transvascular/transaortic	14, 16	+/+
Evolut PRO[*,†]	SA	Transvascular/transaortic	16	+/+
Evolut PRO+[*,†]	SA	Transvascular	14, 16	+/+
Accurate Neo[*,†]	SA	Transvascular/transapical	18	–/–
Accurate Neo2[*,†]	SA	Transvascular/transapical	14	–/–
Portico[*,†]	IA	Transvascular/transaortic	18, 19	+/+
Navitor[*,†]	IA	Transvascular	14, 15	+/+
Hydra[*,†]	SA	Transvascular	18	+/+
Allegra[*,†]	SA	Transvascular	18	+/+
JenaValve[*]	SA	Transapical	32	+/–
Sapien[†,‡]	IA	Transvascular/transapical/transaortic	22, 24	–/–
Sapien XT[†,‡]	IA	Transvascular/transapical/transaortic	16, 18, 20	–/–
Sapien 3[†,‡]	IA	Transvascular/transapical/transaortic	18, 21	–/–
Sapien 3 Ultra[†,‡]	IA	Transvascular	18	–/–
Sapien 3 Ultra Resilia[‡]	IA	Transvascular	18	–/–
Sapien X4[‡]	IA	Transvascular	18	–/–
MyVal[†,‡]	IA	Transvascular	14	–/+
MyVal Octacor[†,‡]	IA	Transvascular	14	–/+

*Self-expanding valves.
†Currently available in India.
‡Balloon-expanding valves.

(IA: intra-annular; R/R: repositionability and retrievability; features are described as "+" if present, and "–" if absent; SA: supra-annular)

and patients to embrace new technologies, lack of dedicated training programs, and lack of specialized centers. This has been further compounded by many peculiarities of the Indian patients like smaller diameters of the aorta and peripheral vessels, low coronary ostia, higher prevalence of rheumatic valvular disease, higher prevalence of bicuspid aortic valve (BAV), and higher calcification of leaflets, which warrant special attention in terms of feasibility, durability, procedural complications, and long-term results. Nevertheless, the procedure is gaining popularity in the country, and with the approval of an indigenous valve (Myval, Meril Life Sciences, Vapi, Gujarat, India), the cost of the procedure has come down significantly. This is likely to enhance the uptake of this technology in the country as the procedure is still not covered under the government insurance schemes and most of the patients have to pay from their own pockets.[7,8] Myval is available in a wider range of sizes (from 20.0 to 32.0 mm, with an increment of 1.5 mm compared to 3.0 mm in other commercially available valves). Myval has been shown to be noninferior to the contemporary Sapien and Evolut series valves in terms of 30-day primary outcomes in the recently published LANDMARK randomized controlled trial (RCT).[9]

EXPANSION FROM HIGH-RISK TO LOW-RISK PATIENTS AND THE VALVE DURABILITY

After its initial FDA approval for severe symptomatic AS patients with prohibitive risk (in 2011) and with high risk (in 2012), there has been gradual expansion of this attractive treatment option to include patients with newer indications and with lower surgical risk. Increasing clinical evidence resulted in FDA approval in 2015 for "valve-in-valve" (ViV) TAVR for patients with failed surgical bioprosthesis and to include intermediate-risk severe AS subjects (in 2016) and low-risk severe AS subjects (in 2019).[10] Although the current guidelines do not recommend TAVR as the preferred treatment option in patients with low risk, the number of such patients undergoing TAVR is increasing steadily, many times due to patient and/or physician preference. With the increased use of TAVR for patients with intermediate and low risk, many of whom are of younger age, attention has been focused on determining the long-term outcomes of the prosthesis and its durability. Recently, new standardized definitions of bioprosthetic valve dysfunction (BVD) and

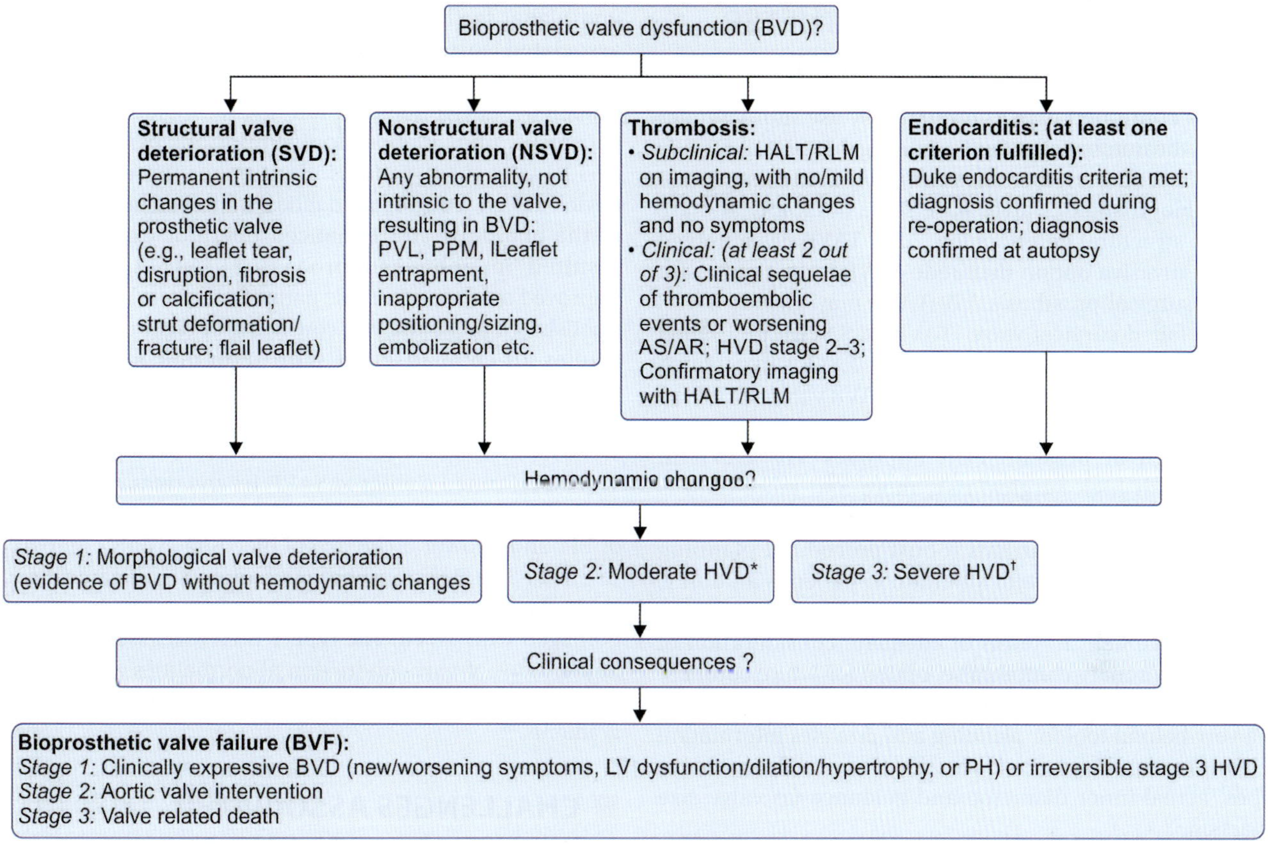

**Moderate HVD*: ≥10 mm Hg increment in mean transvalvular gradient, with mean gradient ≥20 mm Hg and concomitant reduction in effective orifice area ≥0.3 cm^2 or ≥25% and/or reduction in Doppler velocity index (DVI) ≥0.1 or ≥20% from previous echocardiographic evaluation 1–3 months after the procedure, OR new onset or increment of ≥1 grade in intraprosthetic AR with resultant ≥ moderate AR.

†*Severe HVD*: ≥20 mm Hg increment in mean transvalvular gradient, with mean gradient ≥30 mm Hg and concomitant reduction in effective orifice area ≥0.6 cm^2 or ≥50% and/or reduction in DVI ≥0.2 or ≥40% from previous echocardiographic evaluation 1–3 months after the procedure, OR new onset, or increment of ≥2 grades in intraprosthetic AR with resultant severe AR.

FLOWCHART 2: Definitions and staging of bioprosthetic valve dysfunction.[5,11-14]

(AR: aortic regurgitation; AS: aortic stenosis; HALT: hypoattenuated leaflet thickening; HVD: hemodynamic valve deterioration; LV: left ventricle; PH: pulmonary hypertension; PPM: patient–prosthesis mismatch; PVL: paravalvular leak; RLM: reduced leaflet motion)

failure have been developed by the Valve Academic Research Consortium 3 (VARC-3) and the European Association of Percutaneous Cardiovascular Interventions (EAPCI)/ European Association for Cardio-Thoracic Surgery (EACTS) **(Flowchart 2)**.[11-13]

Pooled data from multiple RCTs and registries have demonstrated that except for the first-generation BEVs, the mid-term (7–8 years) durability of TAVR prosthesis is nearly as good as that of SAVR bioprosthesis.[14] There is a lack of data on long-term (10 years and beyond) durability of TAVR prosthesis. The NOTION RCT has recently completed the 10-year follow-up and has shown reassuring results with lack of any important differences in terms of major clinical outcomes between TAVR and SAVR and sustained differences in hemodynamic performance as evaluated by echocardiography in favor of TAVR. However, it is worth acknowledging some important limitations of this study, such as modest sample size (280 patients), advanced age of the patients (mean age 79 years), exclusion of patients with BAVs, and lack of adequate power.[15] Many observational studies have shown good long-term durability of TAVR prosthesis at 10–12 years with low rates of structural valve deterioration (SVD) and bioprosthetic valve failure (BVF).[16,17]

To mitigate the problem of SVD, many innovative approaches have been developed, the major ones being the use of RESILIA tissue (by Edwards Lifesciences) and the DurAVR™ THV system (Anteris Technologies). RESILIA tissue incorporates stable capping of aldehyde moieties to prevent calcium binding and allows dry storage to facilitate leaflet handling and their preservation.[18] The DurAVR™ prosthesis is an innovative biomimetic BEV manufactured using only a single piece of tissue to simulate the anatomical and hemodynamic characteristics of the native aortic valve.[19]

VALVE-IN-VALVE TRANSCATHETER AORTIC VALVE REPLACEMENT

With the continued expansion of TAVR use into younger patients, the number of patients outliving the valve durability and thus needing another valve is steadily increasing, as the current bioprosthetic valves have finite durability and are prone to structural deterioration. Also, TAVR has emerged as a less invasive option than redo-SAVR for patients with a failed surgical prosthesis. ViV TAVR may include TAVR inside a failed surgical valve (TAVR-in-SAVR), in a failed TAVR valve (TAVR-in-TAVR), and in a TAVR valve, which has been previously placed in a failed SAVR valve (TAVR-in-TAVR-in-SAVR).[20]

Although at present, FDA approves ViV TAVR in subjects with high surgical risk, more and more data is being continuously generated for its use in lower-risk patients. ViV TAVR warrants robust procedural planning and execution with careful attention to patient's anatomy, characteristics of previous valve, and planning for long-term management in terms of adequate consideration of the risk of coronary compromise, option for future coronary access, and hemodynamic outcomes. The ViV App (UBQO) is a very helpful tool for planning and provides information relating to the fluoroscopic visualization of different valve types, actual inner diameter, and guidance for valve size selection.[20]

In the absence of a dedicated RCT in this area, the data supporting ViV TAVR has been derived from observational studies and meta-analysis of these studies. A meta-analysis of 11 observational studies consisting of 8,326 patients demonstrated significantly lower 30-day cardiovascular mortality and all-cause mortality and major bleeding in patients undergoing ViV TAVR in comparison to redo-SAVR. Rates of cerebrovascular events, myocardial infarction (MI), and permanent pacemaker implantation (PPI) were similar in both arms. At mid- to long-term follow-up of 6 months to 5 years, ViV TAVR did not differ from redo-SAVR with respect to the rates of cardiovascular mortality, all-cause mortality, and stroke. However, the postimplant transvalvular gradients and the risk of prosthesis–patient mismatch (PPM) were higher in the ViV TAVR arm.[21]

TRANSCATHETER AORTIC VALVE REPLACEMENT FOR BICUSPID AORTIC VALVES

With an estimated prevalence of 1–2% in the general population, BAV is the most common congenital valvular abnormality and is seen in one-third to half of the patients who need aortic valve intervention.[22,23] The pivotal TAVR RCTs excluded patients with BAV, in view of potential anatomic challenges including fused raphe, asymmetrical and higher leaflet calcification, bigger annular sizes, and associated aortopathy in many cases. Early experience with first-generation devices showed poorer in-hospital outcomes, device malposition, higher incidences of PVL, pacemaker implantation, aortic injury, and cerebrovascular accidents in these patients. Continuous improvements in device design, imaging modalities, improved understanding of the anatomy, and enhanced operator expertise have resulted in enhanced procedural success rates and improved outcomes in these patients. Improta et al. recently published a meta-analysis consisting of eight observational studies for comparison of short-term outcomes in TAVR versus SAVR in BAV and nine observational studies for comparing outcomes for type 1 versus non-type 1 BAV stenosis managed with TVAR.[24] It has been shown that TAVR performed similar to SAVR for the rates of mortality, stroke, and acute kidney injury and had a higher incidence of PPI and a lower incidence of bleeding events compared to SAVR. The BAV morphology had no significant impact on 30-day mortality, stroke, and bleeding events in subjects managed with TAVR. The type 1 BAV was associated with higher rates of new conduction abnormalities and PPI, but these patients had mildly lower postprocedure transvalvular gradients.[24]

CHALLENGES ASSOCIATED WITH TRANSCATHETER AORTIC VALVE REPLACEMENT

- *Cerebrovascular events and antithrombotic therapy*: Stroke is one of the most dreaded complications of TAVR, with most events occurring during or within 72 hours of the procedure. The need to prevent this complication stimulated the development of cerebral embolic protection devices such as Sentinel and Emblock.[10] Both devices incorporate the use of filters to prevent the distal embolization of debris during the procedure. The Sentinel device has been evaluated more rigorously and was approved by the FDA in 2017. However, the use of these devices has been compounded by the results of recently published PROTECTED TAVR RCT, which demonstrated no lowering of stroke rates within 72 hours with the routine use of a protection device during TAVR. A reduction in the incidence of secondary outcome of disabling stroke with these devices in this trial needs to be viewed with caution in light of overall negative results.[25] Recent results from the STS/ACC TVT registry have shown a small, borderline significant benefit of these devices in terms of reduction in stroke associated with death or a discharge to a non-home location (a proxy for disabling stroke).[26] In this field, the results of the BHF PROTECT-TAVI study are eagerly awaited.

Another important component for the prevention of cerebrovascular events after TAVR is the use of antithrombotic therapy. The ESC/EACTS 2021 guidelines recommend long-term single antiplatelet therapy (SAPT) (75–100 mg aspirin/day or 75 mg clopidogrel/day) after TAVR in the absence of indication for oral anticoagulants (OAC). In the presence of OAC indication, these guidelines recommend long-term OAC alone. In patients with recent coronary stenting (<3 months), dual antiplatelet therapy (DAPT) with aspirin (75–100 mg/day) and clopidogrel (75 mg/day) is recommended post TAVR for 1–6 months depending on the bleeding risk, followed by lifelong SAPT.[2] According to ACC/AHA 2020 guidelines, SAPT, preferably aspirin, is recommended lifelong for TAVR patients in the absence of indication for OAC. These guidelines also make it reasonable to consider DAPT for 3–6 months after TAVR or the use of vitamin K antagonists (VKAs) for 3 months after TAVR in patients at low bleeding risk and absence of any OAC indication.[1] The patients with atrial fibrillation (AF), venous thromboembolism (VTE), or hypercoagulability should continue OAC after TAVR, with the use of both VKAs and direct oral anticoagulants (DOACs) as per standard dosing and practice guidelines.[1,2]

In a recently published meta-analysis consisting of two RCTs and six observational studies, there was no difference between VKAs and DOACs after TAVR in patients with AF in terms of all-cause mortality, stroke, and major bleeding events; whereas the DOACs were associated with a lower risk of any bleeding.[27]

- *Conduction abnormalities*: Rhythm abnormalities are the result of direct tissue injury during the TAVR procedure, and some patients require PPI after the procedure. A recent meta-analysis has shown that males may be at a higher risk for PPI after TAVR compared to females, probably related to the use of larger prostheses in this subset.[28] Higher rates of conduction abnormalities have been associated with SEVs compared to BEVs, with rates of PPI ranging from 5 to 10% with Sapien valves versus nearly 25% with SEV CoreValve. However, the recent series of Sapien 3 valve is associated with higher PPI rates, likely related to increased radial strength due to addition of an outer skirt for reducing the risk of paravalvular leaks.[29] Recently, some modifications of the TAVR technique have been proposed to mitigate the risk of conduction abnormalities. Sammour et al. described an innovative method of deploying BEVs by decreasing the depth of valve implantation from about 3.2 to about 1.5 mm for the Sapien 3 valve resulting in a reduction of PPI rates at 30 days from 13.1% to 5%.[30] These results led to the adoption of the cusp-overlapping technique during SEV deployment to have a higher implantation position resulting in lower PPI rates.[31]

  It is worth noting that high implantation may theoretically be associated with higher rates of aortic regurgitation (AR) and prosthesis embolization;[32] however, the overall safety of the cusp-overlapping technique is comparable to the conventional method.[33]
- *Coronary access*: With the continued expansion of TAVR in younger and lower risk patients, preservation of coronary access is of paramount importance. Factors unique to TAVR, like the native leaflet displacement, commissural malalignment, and supra-annular platforms, make access to the coronary ostia challenging compared to the SAVR. Modifications in the implantation techniques to improve commissural alignment and leaflet modifications with "bioprosthetic or native aortic scallop intentional laceration to prevent iatrogenic coronary artery obstruction (BASILICA)" have improved the access to coronary ostia after TAVR.[34] The recently published ALIGN-ACCESS and REACCESS-2 studies have demonstrated the positive impact of commissural alignment on coronary access after TAVR.[35,36]

FUTURE CONSIDERATIONS

Transcatheter aortic valve replacement has evolved tremendously over the last two decades and its popularity is likely to keep increasing in the future also with improvements in the prosthesis design, increasing data, and increasing operator experience. Its use is likely to be expanded to newer subsets of patients with newer indications.

Treatment with TAVR in subjects with pure native AR has been associated with increased use of a second valve and residual regurgitation in the initial studies;[37] however, the development of newer dedicated devices like the Trilogy transcatheter heart valve (JenaValve Technology, USA) provides a therapeutic option for high-risk symptomatic AR patients. The recently published results of the ALIGN-AR trial have demonstrated a technical success rate of 95%, with promising short-term clinical and hemodynamic outcomes and the study met the noninferiority margin for primary safety and efficacy outcomes.[38]

Traditionally, aortic valve replacement is advocated for symptomatic severe AS. However, recent data from many observational studies have suggested the detrimental effect of moderate AS on mortality, especially when coupled with left ventricular (LV) dysfunction.[39] This has led to the exploration of the possible use of TAVR in subjects with nonsevere AS with the launch of many RCTs including TAVR UNLOAD, PROGRESS, and Evolut EXPAND TAVR II Pivotal.[10]

Another area of active research is the use of TAVR in asymptomatic severe AS subjects. The guidelines recommend the use of valve replacement in symptomatic severe AS, with consideration for SAVR (IIa) for asymptomatic very severe AS (mean gradient > 60 mm Hg, peak velocity > 5 m/s), LV systolic dysfunction, or markedly increased BNP levels (three times the upper limit of normal) on repeat testing.[2] The publication of RECOVERY and AVATAR trials has challenged this pathway for the management of AS patients. The RECOVERY RCT consisting of 145 asymptomatic severe AS patients, found a lower incidence of composite of operative mortality or cardiovascular death at follow-up in patients undergoing early SAVR in comparison to the conservative arm.[40] The AVATAR RCT of 157 subjects with asymptomatic severe AS demonstrated that early SAVR was associated with lower primary composite endpoint of all-cause death, MI, stroke, or unplanned heart failure hospitalization in comparison to the conservative arm.[41] In this field, the trial of transcatheter intervention, the EARLY TAVR is currently undergoing.[5]

CONCLUSION

Since its inception in 2002, TAVR has matured into an effective and viable alternative to surgery for aortic valve disease and its use continues to expand to include newer indications and newer subsets of patients.

ONLINE REFERENCES

Please scan the QR code provided at the end of the table of contents for References of this chapter.

CHAPTER

172

Transcatheter Aortic Valve Replacement for Aortic Regurgitation: Next Steps and Future Challenges

Raghav R Nagpal, Haresh Mehta

ABSTRACT

Percutaneous treatment of calcified severe aortic stenosis transcatheter aortic valve replacement (TAVR) has gained popularity over the past decade, with improvements in valve technology encouraging wider indications. However, there have been few patients treated with TAVR for pure AR anatomy as an off-label use. With careful planning and execution, TAVR valves can be safely deployed with nonspecialized devices for pure AR anatomy. Although TAVR is widely accepted, long-term study results are needed before it can be widely accepted as a treatment.

Keywords: TAVR, treatment, stenosis, calcified

INTRODUCTION

Over the past decade, percutaneous treatment of calcified severe aortic stenosis has been widely accepted for transcatheter aortic valve replacement (TAVR). Improvements in valve technology have encouraged skilled operators to widen the indication. In some such attempts, there have been few patients treated with TAVR for pure AR anatomy as an off-label use.

The anatomy of patients with pure AR is different than that of calcified aortic stenosis. Therefore, the operators come across unique challenges in using TAVR for these patients.

With careful consideration, planning, and execution, there is now some understanding of how a TAVR valve can be safely deployed with the currently available nondedicated devices for pure AR anatomy. This chapter focuses on planning and execution tips and tricks learned from real-life experiences using TAVR in pure AR anatomy.

CHOICE OF TREATMENT

Surgical aortic valve repair or replacement (SAVR) is the conventional treatment. However, the Euro Heart Survey showed that valve intervention was "underutilized" in approximately 8% of patients because of an elevated risk of perioperative mortality due to advanced age or multiple comorbidities. This rate was even higher in patients with lower LVEF.

As per current guidelines, if patients with isolated severe AR have indications for SAVR and are suitable candidates for surgery, TAVR is a contraindication due to the technical challenges imposed by the absence of anchoring aortic valve calcification. The 2020 ACC/AHA Valvular Heart Disease Guidelines strongly advise against the use of TAVR in patients with isolated severe AR.[1]

CONCERNS USING TRANSCATHETER AORTIC VALVE REPLACEMENT FOR PURE AORTIC REGURGITATION

Transcatheter aortic valve replacement is not encouraged in pure AR because of challenges that could compromise procedural success. The absence of calcification of the aortic annulus and the frequent coexistence of aortic root dilation pose significant difficulties for positioning and anchoring of transcatheter heart valves (THVs). The absence of an anchoring factor (calcium) leads to an increased risk of no or inadequate sealing, causing a significant amount of paravalvular leak and/or embolization **(Box 1)**.

As a practice when planning a transcatheter aortic valve implantation (TAVI) in pure AR patients, one should look to oversize THVs a minimum of 20% to enable valve sealing, since oversizing is the main anchoring mechanism in these patients. With this amount of oversizing, the risk of annular rupture and the need for a pacemaker also increase. Pure

BOX 1 Challenges of TAVR in AR.

- Absence of annular calcium
- Risk of THV embolization or malposition
- Unpredictable positioning and deployment
- Dilated aortic root
- Increased stroke volume
- Large size of aortic annulus

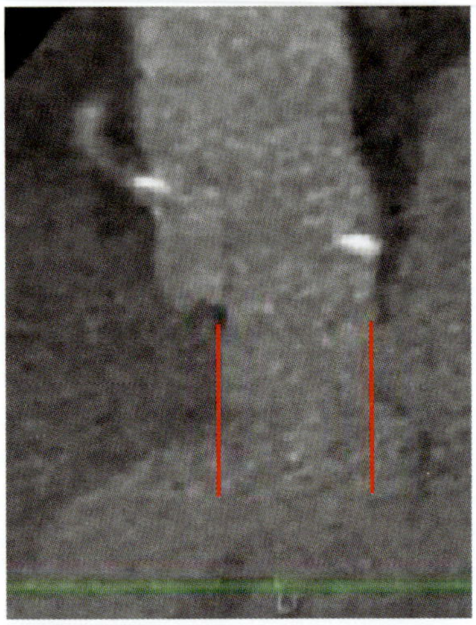

FIG. 1: Tubular anatomy.

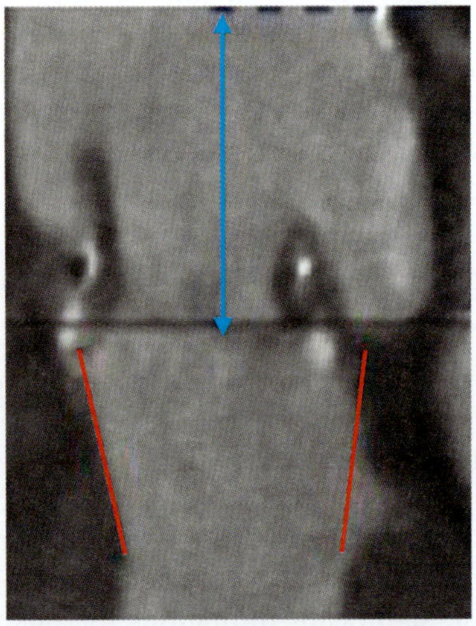

FIG. 2: Flared anatomy.

AR patients have a larger stroke volume combined with increased tissue elasticity, which leads to a suction effect that makes precise valve deployment more challenging. Also, LVOT-aorta morphology is important in these patients for determining the risk of THV embolization and for valve sizing. Tubular and flared LVOTs are at lesser risk of THV embolization than tapered anatomy **(Figs. 1 to 3)**.

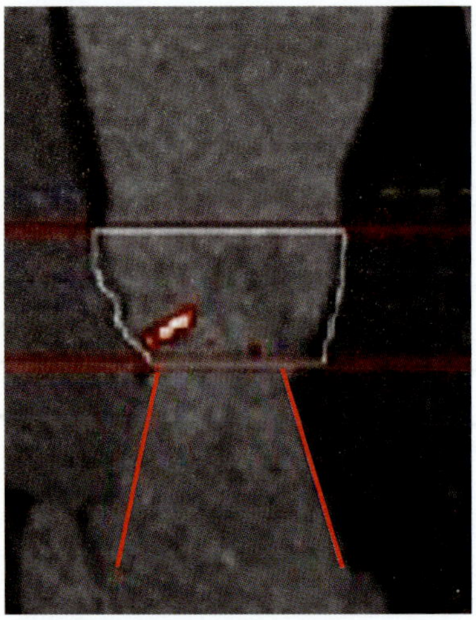

FIG. 3: Tapered anatomy.

LITERATURE FOR TRANSCATHETER AORTIC VALVE IMPLANTATION IN PURE AORTIC REGURGITATION

There is no randomized clinical trial that has compared TAVR with SAVR for the treatment of pure AR or compared specific THVs. The data available today are mostly case reports, single-center experiences, or meta-analyses.

With this data, the literature supports the feasibility of TAVR in patients with pure AR with the currently available devices; however, it comes with several technical challenges and risks of complications are to be managed.

Haddad et al. reported a systematic review and meta-analysis to summarize the available evidence on the use of TAVR in patients with pure AR and compare outcomes between first- and second-generation valves. The main outcome of interest was all-cause mortality at 30 days. A total of 638 patients across 12 studies were included. The mean age ranged from 68 to 84. The Society of Thoracic Surgeons score ranged from 5.4 to 13.1% and EuroSCORE ranged from 18.2 to 33%. The incidence rate of all-cause mortality at 30 days was found to be 11%. All-cause mortality at 30 days for first-generation valves had an incidence rate of 15% compared to 7% in second-generation valves with subgroup interaction analysis ($p = 0.059$). Device success incidence rate in second-generation valves was 92% versus 68% in first-generation valves with $p = 0.001$. TAVI appears to be a feasible treatment choice for pure AR patients at high risk for surgical valve replacement. Second-generation valves show promising results in terms of short-term outcomes.[2]

One of the largest series to date, reported by Yoon et al., included patients treated with first- and second-generation THV and with new-generation devices Evolut R (Medtronic) and SAPIEN 3 (Edwards Lifesciences). This study showed that the use of new-generation devices was associated with improved procedural outcomes. The difference was mainly driven by lower rates of need for a second implant and significant residual AR.[3]

Similar conclusions were yielded by a meta-analysis published by Rawasia et al. The group receiving a new-generation device had lower 30-day mortality [9.1% (6.8–11.7%) vs. 15.3% (10.3–21.1%)] and higher device success rate [92.8% (86.6–97.2%) vs. 75.2% (63.6–85.2%)] compared to the group receiving old-generation devices. Although the outcomes for patients undergoing TAVI for severe AR remain worse when compared with those undergoing TAVI for on-label indications, the difference continues to narrow.[4]

In a recent international, multicenter, observational study that enrolled all consecutive patients with symptomatic severe noncalcified AR undergoing TAVR with the Myval device [balloon expandable valve (BEV)], a total of 113 patients were recruited. The annular area was beyond the recommended range for extra-large sizes in 2.6% of cases, and additional volume was added in 92% (median 4 cc, up to 9 cc). The extra-large sizes were used in 95 patients (84.1%), and the mean oversizing was 17.9 ± 11.0%. The technical success rate was 94.7%; the rate of residual ≥ moderate aortic regurgitation was 8.9%, and the pacemaker rate was 22.2%. There were no cases of annular rupture, cardiac tamponade, or aortic dissection, but in four patients (3.5%) valve embolization occurred. Thirty-day and 1 year mortality were 5.3% and 9.7%, respectively. Technical success was associated with better survival (97.1% vs. 72.7%; $p = 0.012$), and valve embolization was the main determinant of mortality ($p = 0.047$).[5]

The PANTHEON (Performance of Currently Available Transcatheter Aortic Valve Platforms in Inoperable Patients with Pure Aortic Regurgitation of a Native Valve)[6] study retrospectively included patients who underwent TAVR with currently available devices [both self-expanding (SE) and balloon expandable (BE)] for severe AR. Technical and device success rates as well as a composite of all-cause mortality and heart failure rehospitalization at 1 year were evaluated. The rate and clinical consequences of acute transcatheter valve embolization and migration (TVEM) were also considered.

A total of 201 patients were included. Overall technical and device success rates were 83.6% and 76.1%, respectively, and did not differ between SE and BE devices. These figures were mostly due to TVEM occurrence (14.6% vs. 16.1%; $p = 0.47$) and residual moderate or greater aortic regurgitation (9.2% vs. 10.1%; $p = 0.87$). Patients who experienced TVEM compared to those without TVEM had a significantly higher incidence of the composite endpoint at 1 year (25.7% vs. 15.8%; $p = 0.05$).

WHICH DEVICE IS PREFERRED?

Initial data showed poorer outcomes with TAVI in pure AR with higher rates of device embolization, higher mortality, higher rates of second valve implantation, and unacceptable degree of paravalvular leak.

Early experience with first-generation self-expanding valves, which were favored initially because it was thought to facilitate safe anchoring by oversizing without an increased risk for annular disruption, had disappointing results.

The use of second-generation balloon-expandable and self-expanding valves demonstrated improved outcomes in patients; however, higher than acceptable procedural complications and mortality rates were observed.[7]

Currently, both platforms' latest iterations—the self-expanding Evolut R/PRO/PRO+/FX (Medtronic) and the balloon-expandable SAPIEN 3/Ultra (Edwards Lifesciences)/Myval (Meril Lifesciences)—are used for off-label procedures in pure AR. There is no evidence currently comparing the performance of specific new-generation devices.

TIPS AND TRICKS FOR EXECUTING A PURE AORTIC REGURGITATION CASE WITH CURRENTLY AVAILABLE TRANSCATHETER HEART VALVES

Self-expandable Valve

Target a minimum of 25% of valve oversizing. This can be achieved by careful assessment of the cardiac CT, which will give the annulus and the aortic root dimensions.

The deployment must be done using prolonged rapid pacing. Post complete deployment, the pacing rate should be gradually reduced to reduce the risk of embolization due to a sudden increase in cardiac output.

The nature of the valve is to either dive in toward the LVOT or eject out. Target to implant deeper to reduce embolization risk. However, this comes at the cost of increased chances of a permanent pacemaker implantation.

There can be a need for a second valve if there is valve migration during or immediately post deployment. The operator should have a bailout second valve ready. The second valve can be implanted in reference to the first THV at a little higher position. In this technique, the metallic frame of the first THV acts as an anchoring agent for the second THV. This technique should only be used post careful assessment of CT ensuring large sinuses to accommodate two tall frame valves and confirming that there is no risk of formation of a tube graft compromising the coronary perfusion due to sinus sequestration.

Balloon Expandable Valve

The operator will need to consider adding extra volume in the valve balloon to ensure a minimum oversizing of 20–25%. To reduce the risk of valve embolization, consider deploying at a deeper depth toward LVOT, leaving a safe margin for foreshortening and the possibility of postdilation at a safe depth. The above-mentioned use of two valves can be employed in BEVs also. Post complete deployment, the pacing rate must be reduced gradually.

Hybrid

As the rate of second valve implant is higher in a pure AR anatomy, the operator must do a careful assessment of CT pre-case to ensure the best sequence of valve [self-expandable valve (SEV) in BEV or BEV in SEV or BEV in BEV or SEV in SEV] in case a second valve is required. Choosing the right sequence will impact the lifelong management of the patient, especially if needing a coronary intervention.

TRANSCATHETER VALVE EMBOLIZATION AND MIGRATION OCCURRENCE: FROM CAUSES TO BAILOUT STRATEGY

- The common causes of TVEM were THV failure to anchor, malpositioning, excessive manipulation, and inappropriate sizing.
- The SEV embolizes slightly more frequently on the aortic side than the BEV devices, which move more frequently to the left ventricular outflow tract **(Fig. 4)**.

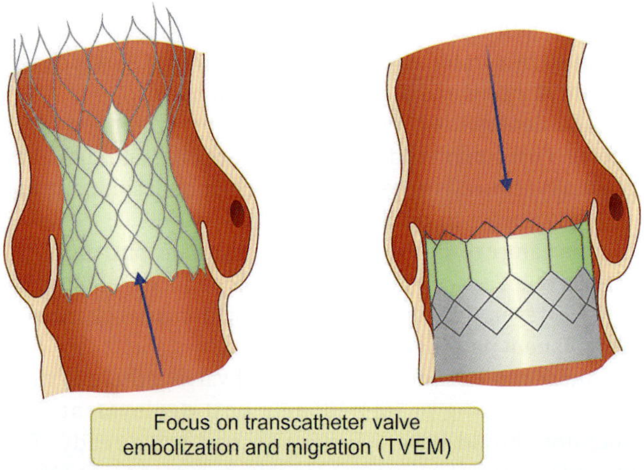

FIG. 4: TVEM: SEV versus BEV.

- Postdilatation is an independent risk factor for TVEM. During postdilatation, the mechanical interaction between the dilated prosthesis and the native valve may not provide a secure anchor at the aortic ring because of the absence of leaflet calcification.
- Bailout strategies for TVEM depending on the degree of valve migration include:
  - Upfront implantation of second valve
  - THV snaring + second valve implantation
  - Repositioning through balloon inflation
  - Conversion to surgery
- Ventricular TVEM is linked to higher surgical conversion and in-hospital mortality.

MANAGING NATIVE VALVE PURE AORTIC REGURGITATION IN THE COMING TIMES

Current commercially available THVs in AR are not an ideal solution, and there is a need for dedicated transcatheter devices designed specifically for AR anatomy, which can ensure a safer and more predictable outcome.

JenaValve (JenaValve Technology) and J-Valve (JC Medical) are two such devices undergoing feasibility studies in the United States.

The JenaValve THV is made up of a self-expanding nitinol stent with a porcine pericardial valve. There is a presence of "locators" attached to the valve frame that clip onto the leaflets upon deployment, facilitating anchoring without relying on annular calcification or the need for oversizing **(Fig. 5)**. The other positive features of this TAVR system are: (1) the supra-annular location of the actual valve, theoretically improving hemodynamics, and (2) the presence of large cells at its aortic end and the possibility of anatomically correct alignment with native sinuses, facilitating coronary access. A potentially negative feature is the lack of a dedicated sealing skirt, which might increase the risk for significant postprocedure PVL. It

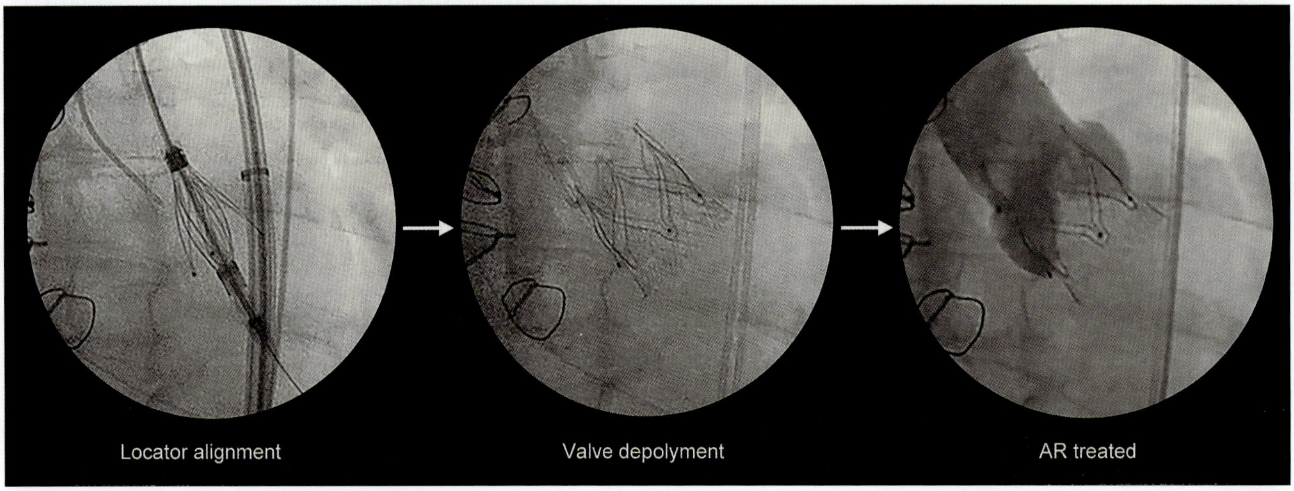

FIG. 5: JenaValve THV anchoring and deployment.

is available in three sizes with a perimeter range of 66–90 mm **(Fig. 6)**.

The initial experience in Europe using the JenaValve THV for pure severe AR was encouraging, with the valve being successfully implanted via a transapical approach in >96% of patients. However, a high mortality of 20% was observed in patients at 1 year follow-up.

With the need for transapical access, a higher risk of mortality was observed in the early generation of JenaValve. The newer JenaValve Trilogy THV transfemoral system was tested initially in patients with severe aortic stenosis with encouraging results[8] and most recently in severe aortic regurgitation patients.

JenaValve Trilogy Heart valve system in high surgical risk patients with symptomatic, severe aortic regurgitation: The ALIGN AR Trial[9] enrolled 180 patients, and the 1 year data was presented at TCT 2023. Baseline CT annulus perimeter was 78.7 ± 8.9 mm, CT annulus area 480.1 ± 101.4 mm^2, with large size valve implanted in 57.2%, medium size in 20%, and small size in 22.8% patients. Technical success was achieved in 95% cases, valve embolization occurred in 2.2%, and aortic dissection in 0.6% cases. Annular rupture, ventricular perforation, or coronary obstruction did not occur in any patient. The new pacemaker implantation rate was about 24%. At 1 year, mean aortic gradient was 4.3 and EOA 2.8 mm^2. At 1 year, 92.2% of the patients had no PVL, 7.8% patients had mild PVL, and 0% had moderate/severe PVL. Positive LV remodeling was seen with a reduction in LVESD from 39.6 to 34.2 mm ($p < 0.0001$) and LVESV from 70.6 to 52.1 mm ($p < 0.0001$). The trial achieved its 30-day safety outcome and 1-year efficacy outcome.

In 2023, J Valve by Genesis Medtech Company was granted breakthrough device designation by the US Food and Drug Administration (FDA). The grant is for the treatment of pure AR and AR-dominant mixed aortic valve disease. Currently, any patient's eligibility for this device must be evaluated by a Heart Team approach to be a high risk for SAVR. It has a transfemoral deployment system and comprises bovine pericardial leaflets, nitinol frame, and fabric skirt to mitigate PVL **(Fig. 7)**. It has U-shaped

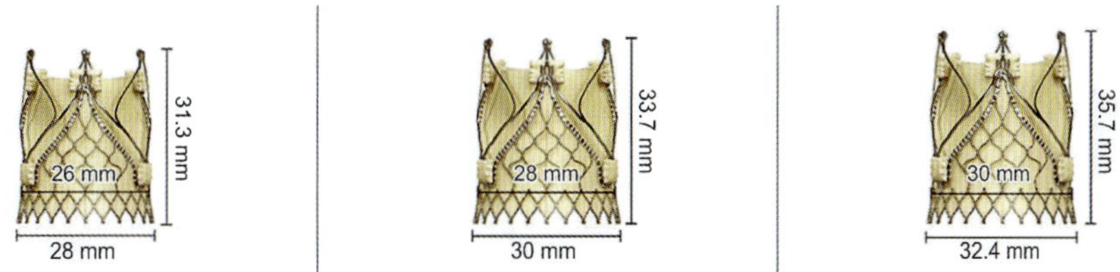

Trilogy-THV-S	Trilogy-THV-M	Trilogy-THV-L
	Annular perimeter range	
66–74 mm	71–79 mm	76–85 mm
	Annular diameter range	
21–23.6 mm	22.6–25.2 mm	24.2–27 mm

FIG. 6: JenaValve trilogy THV sizing.

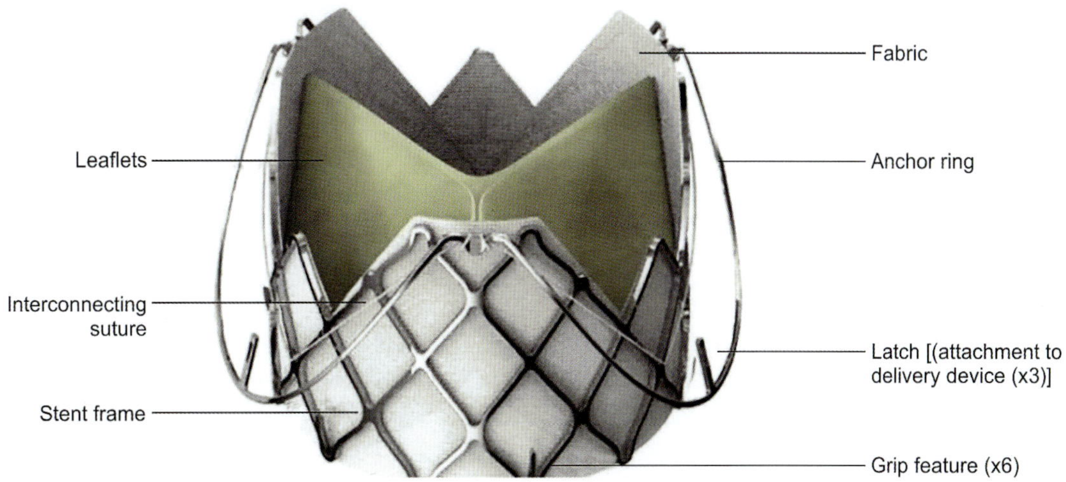

FIG. 7: J valve design.

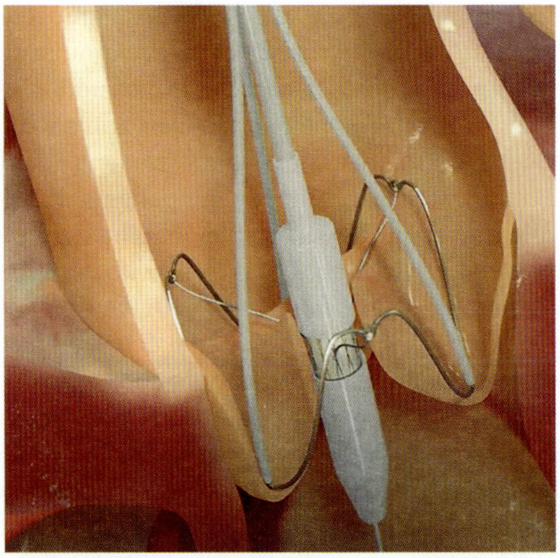

FIG. 8: J valve anchoring.

TABLE 1: J valve sizing.

J-valve TF size (mm)	Annulus diameter (mm)	Annulus perimeter (mm)	Annulus area (mm^2)
22	18–21	57–66	254–346
25	21–24	66–75	346–452
28	24–27	75–85	452–573
31	27–30	85–94	573–707
34	30–33	94–104	707–855

anchor rings that facilitate accurate self-positioning of the replacement aortic valve **(Fig. 8)**. It is available in five valve sizes intended to treat perimeters 57-104 mm **(Table 1)**. The J valve TF EFS study[10] 30-day data of 15 high-risk patients, recently published at CRT 2024, showed 0% valve embolization, 0% residual AR/PVL, 0% need for pacemaker and excellent hemodynamics with mean gradient of 5.57 and EOA 2.91 cm^2 at 30 days. This study excluded patients with congenital unicuspid or bicuspid aortic valve, LVEF < 25%, aortic root diameter > 5 cm, aortic annulus perimeter <57 or >104 mm, previous prosthetic aortic valve, and more than moderate mitral regurgitation. The JOURNEY pivotal trial of J valve is anticipated to begin enrolment in 2024.

With such newer dedicated devices for pure AR, treatment of this challenging anatomy will become more feasible in the coming times. Patients with coexistent aortic root/ascending aorta aortopathy have been excluded from all these feasibility studies and their management remains entirely surgical.

CONCLUSION

Transcatheter aortic valve replacement is a very well-accepted treatment modality for calcified severe aortic stenosis and in combination with mild-to-severe AR. However, in pure AR it is still an off-label use. With the currently available valves, there have been cases performed with optimal results. However, overall rates of valve embolization and pacemaker requirement have been higher than acceptable limits. The new devices show good promise in having a more predictable and safe deployment of a transcatheter valve. However, long-term study results are awaited before it can be approved in various countries and widely accepted as a treatment of choice.

ONLINE REFERENCES

Please scan the QR code provided at the end of the table of contents for References of this chapter.

CHAPTER 173

Transcatheter Aortic Valve Implantation: Recent Advances

Vijay Kumar, Vishal Rastogi, Vivudh Pratap Singh, Avinash Mani, Dhananjay Kumar, Ashok Seth

ABSTRACT

Over the past two decades, transcatheter aortic valve implantation (TAVI) has seen significant advancements, with expanded indications, advanced planning tools, and the concept of lifetime management of aortic stenosis. Advancements in imaging tools, software applications, and artificial intelligence have improved planning and safety. TAVI is now becoming minimalistic, with same-day discharge strategies like PCI.

Keywords: TAVI, PCI, management, aortic stenosis, software, AI

INTRODUCTION

The field of transcatheter aortic valve implantation (TAVI) has seen numerous advancements in the last two decades. Indications of TAVI have expanded. Tools of planning are now more advanced. Customization and better planning of TAVI through the use of newer imaging tools, software applications, and artificial intelligence is coming into practice. Valve sizing and selection is done through consideration of multiple device and patient-related factors. The concept of lifetime management of aortic stenosis is now emphasized in order to help the physician in choosing the first procedure and first valve for the patient, so that there is just a need of one open-heart surgical procedure in the patient's lifetime. Newer innovations are happening very fast in the field of device, leaflet, and procedural hardwares. Procedural practices are today better understood and have enhanced the success and safety of this therapy. TAVI is becoming minimalistic today with same day discharge strategies like PCI. This chapter will discuss different areas of recent advancements in the field of TAVI.

BOX 1 **Expanding indications of transcatheter aortic valve implantation.**

Indication for AS management:

- Asymptomatic severe AS:
  - DANAVR study
  - EASY-AS trial
  - EVoLVeD trial
  - EARLY TAVR trial
- Bicuspid aortic valve:
  - PROGRESS trial
  - TAVR UNLOAD trial
  - EXPAND II trial

Specific indication:

- Young patients
- Bicuspid aortic valve

Other venue:

- Non-TF, nontransthoracic route
- Aortic regurgitation

EXPANDING INDICATIONS OF TRANSCATHETER AORTIC VALVE IMPLANTATION (BOX 1)

It started as a procedure for patient of severe aortic stenosis in cardiogenic shock who was inoperable, and from there on has become the standard of care for patients of severe aortic stenosis with numerous comorbidities and high surgical aortic valve replacement risks. In the last two decades the indications have expanded across low and intermediate surgical risk cohorts. Younger and younger age group patients are undergoing TAVI and is no more restricted for 70 years and above age population. Bicuspid morphology, pure aortic regurgitation, degenerated/failed surgical bioprosthetic valves and rings, failed TAVI valves, aortic roots with small, ultra small, large, and extremely large annulus all can have TAVI with good outcomes and there is data supporting it. The anatomical and procedural challenges have been better understood and defined to make TAVI successful in these patients utilizing newer devices and techniques.[1-3] New-generation devices seem attractive for bicuspid aortic valve stenosis, but sizing algorithms might need to be modified. Timing to proceed with TAVI and procedural safety are crucial in truly asymptomatic patients with severe calcified aortic stenosis. TAVI might complement afterload reduction with medical therapy in patients with heart failure and moderate aortic stenosis. Treatment for pure aortic regurgitation might demand dedicated transcatheter valve designs to secure device anchoring in noncalcified aortic roots.

EMPHASIS ON LIFETIME MANAGEMENT OF AORTIC STENOSIS (FIG. 1)

It is a new concept where focus is shifting from choice of intervention (TAVI vs. SAVR) to a lifetime management of a TAVI patient (often an initial TAVI prosthesis selection). Key factors for first valve selection include hemodynamics and valve durability, easy commissural alignment, and coronary access, possibility of a valve in valve, and lower pacemaker rate. The heart team goal should be to limit the patient to a maximum of one surgery. Expected survival of the patient and valve should be taken into decision making. Likelihood for TAVI as the second valve should be advised. There is now adequate data on 10-year durability of TAVR valves.

TAVI in patients with expected survival over 10 years have unexpected outcomes. Surgical explant data is associated with high mortality and hence it is an important point about not subjecting younger patients into this situation.[4-7]

ADVANCEMENTS IN TOOLS FOR PLANNING TRANSCATHETER AORTIC VALVE IMPLANTATION

New Imaging Modalities

Multi detector multislice CT has been the gold standard imaging tool for planning a TAVI case with the help of dedicated software.[8] 3D TEE is a good tool to do annular sizing and can be used when we want to avoid contrast.[9] A 3D dataset of the aortic annulus is collected. The 3D quantification program is then activated. The three multiplanar reconstruction planes (the aortic short-axis, long-axis, and coronal planes) are aligned during systole, to obtain the three nadirs of the sinuses of Valsalva simultaneously in the short-axis MPR. Rotating the sagittal and coronal planes to identify the hinge points is necessary to measure the diameter of the "true" annulus. The "true" aortic annulus is defined by the blood-tissue interface in the aortic short-axis MPR. Multi-modality cardiovascular imaging approaches such as noncontrast CT, 2D and 3D noncontrast MRA , 2D CMR SSPF, and 2D and 3D TEE imaging with automated software have been used for pre-TAVI workup in

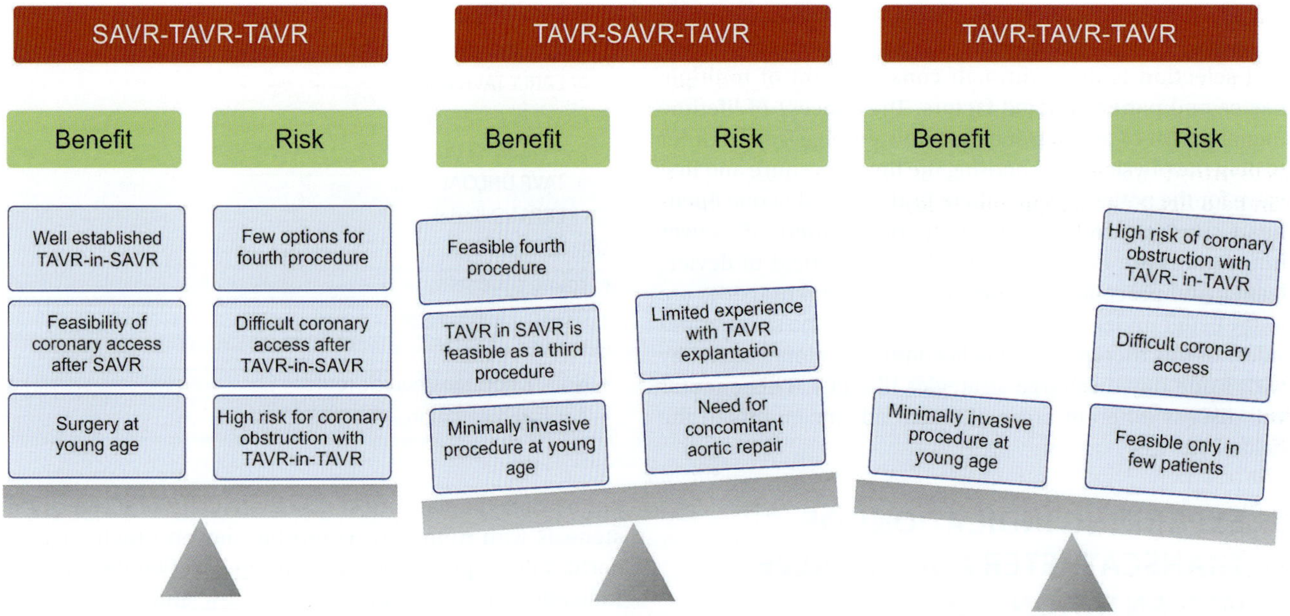

FIG. 1: Potential strategies in lifetime management of severe aortic stenosis in young patients.

Source: Yerasi C, Rogers T, Forrestal BJ, et al. HYPERLINK "https://pubmed.ncbi.nlm.nih.gov/34112453/" Transcatheter versus surgical aortic valve replacement in young, low-risk patients with severe aortic stenosis. JACC Cardiovasc Interv. 2021;14(11):1169-80.

patients with severe kidney dysfunction undergoing TAVI.[10] 3D printing, another recent advancement is a process of bringing 2D digital imagery into something that can be held and felt. The software converts these images generated by CT, MRI, or echocardiography into something that the printer can reasonably format.[11] Patient-specific 3D-printed models have been used for preprocedural device sizing, benchtop prediction of procedural complications, planning for valve-in-valve and bicuspid aortic valve procedures, and more. Therapeutic utility in managing complications like paravalvular leak is excellent.[12] Subclinical leaflet thrombosis, defined by the presence of hypoattenuating leaflet thickening (HALT) and reduced leaflet motion (RLM) are detectable with help of CT and guide best in treating with oral anticoagulants.[13]

Algorithms, Apps, and Tools for Transcatheter Aortic Valve Implantation

Quick THV oversizing calculation apps for native valves, and apps for valve in valve TAVI, and planning for coronary protection are all available on iOS and android platforms. Unlike the past, when operators had to search through literatures to find out case specific information about the surgical valve or ring, identifying them on fluoroscopy, choosing the correct size of the VinV, its positioning and placement strategies, size of postdilation balloon or balloon size for valve fracture is all on the touch screen and click of mouse. All these information searching from literature was difficult but today the smartphone platform have collated vast information on dedicated apps.[14] The app interface allows collation of complex data, especially when it involves thousands of permutations and combinations, and also allows use of data in various formats such as text, images, animation and movie clips, making it a perfect tool to provide guidance on the native valve, valve-in-valve and valve-in-ring procedures. By utilizing the smartphone platform we could collate this complex information in the form of apps, so as to provide information specific to a clinical scenario that can be quickly and simply obtained, and which could be of help in planning and performing the procedures.

Artificial Intelligence in Transcatheter Aortic Valve Implantation

Numerous machine learning platforms and models have been developed for TAVI patient selection, procedural planning, and postimplantation monitoring and will be contributing to optimized outcomes. However, challenges of AI must be addressed to ensure its safe and responsible integration because a publication bias for AI with positive outcomes can be overestimated without its validation and applicability.

Large language platforms (LLMs) in AI like ChatGPT have been looking attractive support tools of the future. Recent publication in JACC intervention showed that ChatGPT selected TAVI and SAVR correctly in all cases but Google BARD did so 70% of the time and suggested SAVR for one TAVI leaning case and TAVI for five SAVR leaning cases. It thus needs a larger language model that is better validated, and the doctors and patients can derive information in safe and secure way.[15,16]

Guidance to Physicians from the Contemporary Guidelines[14-16]

The SAVR is recommended in younger patients who are at low risk for surgery (<75 years and STS PROM Euro score II <4%) or in patients who are operable and unsuitable for transfemoral TAVI (IB). TAVI is recommended in older patients ≥75 years or in those who are at high risk STS-PROM EURO score II >8) or unsuitable for surgery (1A).[17,18]

The 2020 ACC AHA guidelines recommendations for choice of SAVR versus TAVI for patients whom a bioprosthetic AVR is appropriate include SAVR as class IA for symptomatic and asymptomatic severe AS patients and any indication for AVR who are <65 years of age and a life expectancy >20 years (assuming SAVR durability >10 years and TAVR durability <10 years); for 65– 80 years of age and no anatomic contraindication to transfemoral approach, TAVI is recommended after shared decision about the balance between expected patient longevity and valve durability (assuming SAVR + VinV TAVI provide >20 years and TAVI + redo TAVI also provide 20 years of life with functioning prosthesis); lastly for the symptomatic severe AS patients >80 years or for younger patients with life expectancy <10 years and no anatomic contraindication for transfemoral approach, TAVI is preferred over SAVR (presuming that all SAV and TAV have equal durability and plan in a way patient reaches 85 years of age.[19]

CHANGING CONTEMPORARY PROCEDURAL PRACTICES

Choice of Valves and Sizing

Choice of valves and sizing is the key to success of a TAVI procedure. Numerous transcatheter heart valves are now available and that makes valve selection difficult. Most patients are suitable for any valve but in real life patient-related factors and device-related factors influence in selection of valves.[20] Emphasis is on minimizing the complications, implanting valves with good durability, and hemodynamics to every patient who undergoes TAVI.

Vascular Access and Closure

Using pigtail catheter and fluoro-guided puncture techniques have been replaced with ultrasound guided access, using micro puncture needle set helping in a safe access site free from dissections and calcified segments of the femoral artery.[21] Preclose with single ProGlide and a collagen based device has become standard of practice in place of two suture devices thereby minimizing the risk of stenosis of the access vessel.[22] New and more objective and safe closure devices like Manta device is also showing good closure results.[23] Dedicated sheaths for the self-expanding platforms and esheaths of balloon expanding valves have lower profile and better hemostatic valves which cause less trauma to the vessels. The sheath size is getting smaller and smaller. Intravascular lithotripsy has revolutionized TAVI access and today transfemoral TAVI is feasible in 98% of the patients.[24] Transcaval route is an excellent option when no transarterial access site is available. It utilizes the principles of electrosurgery, and the closure is achieved safely and successfully. It has a learning curve to it but can be done easily once learnt.[25]

Newer Concepts in Positioning, Deployment, and Implantation of Devices

The self-expanding valves are now positioned using cuspal overlap view which helps in shallow implantation and lesser pacemaker complications and PVL than the past.[26] Fluoro visible markers are there to help identify depth of implantation. Axial stabilizing arches help in deploying some self-expanding valves at lower pacing rates or even without pacing and are useful in pure aortic regurgitation cases as well.[27] The upper crowns in Acurate neo2 valve are hooks that overlie the native cusps and prevent them from pinching the ostia. Commissural alignment, coronary alignment for future reaccess, and intervention are all kept in mind while navigating the delivery system to the positioning and deployment of valves.[28,29] The balloon expanding valve have got dedicated anchors to hook in pure aortic regurgitation cases and makes deployment more stable.[30]

Coronary Protection

It is important for both native valves as well as when TAVI is planned for valve-in-valve cases. Risk to coronary ostia occlusion is not merely the height of coronaries but there are numerous factors to be investigated, many indices to be measured, and a knowledge of the devices is essential to gauge the risk of occlusion. Parking the stent before implantation was one of the old methods to bail out a coronary occlusion situation by chimney stenting, but today right choice of valves, shorter frames, and large cells dedicated to stay in front of coronary artery access point are used in order to prevent this catastrophe.[31] BASILICA and SHORT cut are some of the techniques where intentional laceration of the coronary occlusion "risk posing leaflet" is done through electrosurgery or mechanical disruption by dedicated wires and then implanting the new valve is done.[32,33] Coronary revisit is need of the present times, when TAVI has shifted to younger population who have a full life ahead.[34,35] There are challenges in these procedures and a learning curve to it involving imaging and the procedural steps lies in.

NEWER INNOVATIONS

Present Generations Transcatheter Heart Valves (Table 1)

They have low profile, easily deliverable catheter systems through femoral artery of small (5–5.5 mm) caliber and

TABLE 1: Current generation of transcatheter heart valves.

New generation valves	Features	Additional features
Evolut R Medtronics	• Supra-annular • Self-expanding valve	• Porcine tissue • Recapturable and repositionable • Sealing skirt • 23, 26, 29, 34 mm
Evolut Pro Medtronics	• Supra-annular • Self-expanding valve	• Porcine tissue • Recapturable and repositionable • 23, 26, 29, 34 mm • Advanced sealing
Evolut Pro plus Medtronics	• Supra-annular • Self-expanding valve	• Recapturable and repositionable • Advanced sealing skirt • 23, 26, 29, 34, 5 mm vessels for access
Evolut Fx Medtronics	• Supra-annular • Self-expanding valve	• Flex catheter • Radio-opaque gold markers for deployment and commissure location, optimized stability layer
Evolut Fx plus Medtronics	• Supra-annular • Self-expanding valve	Facilitate coronary access windows through a modified diamond-shaped frame design which is four times larger than previous iterations of Evolut R

Continued

Continued

New generation valves	Features	Additional features
Acurate neo2 *Boston scientific*	• Supra-annular • Self-expanding valve	• Porcine leaflets, 23/25/27 mm • *Axial stabilization arches:* Provide stability while deployment; useful in pure AR. • *Extra-large cells:* Good for coronary access • *Upper crown:* Supra-annular anchoring and captures native leaflets to provide coronary clearance • Lower crown minimizes protrusion into LVOT so lesser conduction defects • Top-down deployment • I sleeve
Portico Abbott vascular	• Intra-annular leaflet placement • Self-expanding valve Nitinol frame nonflared	• FlexNav delivery system reduces distal profile to be 14F-15F, hydrophilic coating and stability layer, ergonomic proximal handle and can be good for 5 mm, • Large open cells for coronary access • 23, 25, 27, 29 mm • Repositionable and resheathable before full release at 80% deployment.
Navitor Abbott vascular	• Intra-annular • Self-expanding valve	• Three large visible radio-opaque markers • Smart sealing system syncs with cardiac cycle • No rapid pacing needed • Nontapered stent • Stable deployment • Anticalcification • FlexNav system • 23, 25, 27, 29, 35 mm size to cater 30 mm annulus • 5 mm minimum vessel diameter
Hydra SMT	• Supra-annular • Self-expanding valve	• Three tentacle designless metal at outflow • Mid frame high hoop strength, lower frame high radial strength, and low radial strength at outflow for conformability • Large frame cells >15 Fr • Extended sealing skirt • Nonflared inflow part reduces conduction abnormality
Jena and Jena plus Jena valve tech inc	• Supra-annular • Self-expanding valve	• Porcine tissue and Nitinol frame • 23, 25, 27 mm • Three positional feelers allow correct positioning clips the prosthesis to native valve • Dedicated for aortic regurgitation
Trilogy Jena valve tech inc	• Supra-annular • Self-expanding valve	• Porcine tissue • Dedicated for aortic regurgitation • Locator technology allows alignment • Large open cells
J valve JC Medical	• Supra-annular • Self-expanding valve	• Pure aortic regurgitation • U shaped anchor rings • Low profile • Slides to position • Locking mechanism
Venus A and Venus Med tech	Supra-annular	• Three radio-opaque markers • Segmental release • Enhanced radial force for bicuspid valves • Commissural and coronary alignment

Continued

Continued

New generation valves	Features	Additional features
Venus vitae	Balloon expanding valve	• Dry tissue technology • Steerable delivery system • Gold markers • Self adaptive antiparavalvular leak mechanism
Vita flo *microport cardioflow*	Supra-annular	• Bovine tissue • Special decalcification • Hybrid density frames with PET skirts
Taurus one *peijia medical*	• Supra-annular • Self-expanding valve	• Bovine • Cone-shaped inflow • Severe calcified and bicuspid
Sapien 3 *Edward life sciences*	• Intra-annular • Balloon expanding valve	• Bovine tissue, cobalt chromium frame • 20, 23, 26, 29 mm • Sealing skirt • E sheath
Sapien ultra *Edward life sciences*	• Intra-annular • Balloon expanding valve	• 40% tall skirt height and open cell geometry • Short frame height • 20, 23, 26, 29 mm
Sapien x4 *Edward life sciences*	• Intra-annular • Balloon expanding valve	• Advanced calcium blocking technology • Dry tissue storage • 23, 26, 29 mm can be deployed at 16 different diameters in 0.5 mm increments • Can be deployed at 16 different diameters
Myval *Meril life sciences*	• Intra-annular • Balloon expanding valve	• Bovine • Honeycomb like hybrid of open and close cells • 20, 21.5, 23, 24.5, 26, 27.5, 29, 31.5, 32, 20–32.5 mm sizes
Octacor *Meril life sciences*	• Intra-annular • Balloon expanding valve	• Two row hybrid interlaced octagonal cell design • 20–32 mm sizes • Croco dial compass crimping tool for commissural alignment
Siegel MiRus TAVR system	Balloon expanding	• Rhenium super alloy, ultra low-profile 8 Fr, 18 cells 9 cells per row, nickle free, dry porcine, 8 Fr/sheath, no valve foreshortening

best suited for most morphologies and for a wide range of annular sizes.[36,37] The new devices give good hemodynamics, are associated with lesser complication rates, and at par with surgical valves in terms of durability. Future coronary reaccess and interventions through specially dedicated large cells in self-expanding valves have made coronary reaccess easier and safety against coronary ostia occlusion risks. Commissural alignment mechanisms in most of the new generation THVs provide ease for future coronary reaccess. Diamond-shaped large, dedicated cell of Evolut fx and large cells of Acurate neo2 are examples of self-expanding valves which have ease of coronary reaccess. They have better radial strength, are recapturable, repositionable, have adaptive and effective sealing mechanisms and skirts, and very importantly more efficiently decalcified leaflets, e.g., (the Resilia used in sapien ultra and X4 THVs) intended to give a durability of 25 years equivalent to surgical bioprosthetic valves.[38,39] **Table 1** shows the new generation transcatheter heart valves available and some of them are in innovation phase or need more data for approval.

Future Technologies and Iterations in Pipeline

New leaflet technology, premounted devices with dry valve technology, ultra-low profile aortic valve, THVs with shorter frames, large cells for coronary access, commissural alignment mechanisms with intent of coronary protection, and easy future access are all in pipeline.[40] Newer frame material with more radial strength is also in trial phase. An armamentarium of cerebral embolic protection devices is running through trials to see which would provide full safety against stroke.[41,42] Leaflet modification techniques such as BASILICA and SHORT CUT are still to mature and be approved as standard procedures of coronary protection in valve-in-valve cases.[43] Finally, other areas like flow diversion in the ascending aorta, application of intravascular lithotripsy on the calcified leaflets of aortic valve are all new ideas in treatment and management of aortic stenosis without implantation of any valve is also in the pipeline.

COMPLICATION RATES LESSER AND BETTER HANDLED

Complications of TAVI are much less with the present generation of devices and increasing knowledge of the implantation techniques. Valve Academic Research Consortium (VARC) 3 updated their standardized definitions of clinical endpoints for transcatheter and surgical aortic valve clinical trials, including bioprosthetic valve dysfunction and failure, structural complications, conduction disturbances, and repeat hospitalizations, among others.[44] Vascular complications are much less with diminishing sheath size and better delivery systems. Degeneration of valve is less with better leaflet technology. Transfemoral TAVI is today a 98% successful procedure.

Newer Strategies to Predict and Minimize Post-transcatheter Aortic Valve Implantation Conduction Abnormalities (Flowchart 1)

It is very important to predict who are at risk for conduction disturbances as it is an important barrier to early discharge practices in TAVI especially the low risk TAVI patients.[45] Preexisting conduction RBBB is a known variable for the risk of CHB with TAVI but contribution of anatomic features and procedural variables to delayed heart block have been considered to be minor.[46] The EP study registry data emphasizes that complete heart block and left bundle branch block remain lesser than a decade back, but still in today's TAVI practices some require pacemaker implantation or even face mortality down the road in follow-up. Delayed abnormalities and worse outcomes are important. 5–28% of TAVI patients experience AV conduction problems. Baseline RBBB was not predictive of late heart block. New LBBB or baseline preexisting LBBB was not related necessarily to development of CHB during the procedure or after wards. Intraprocedural utility of His bundle recordings by structural cardiologists can be a useful tool to identify patients at risk for AV block. EP predictors of CHB after discharge were HV

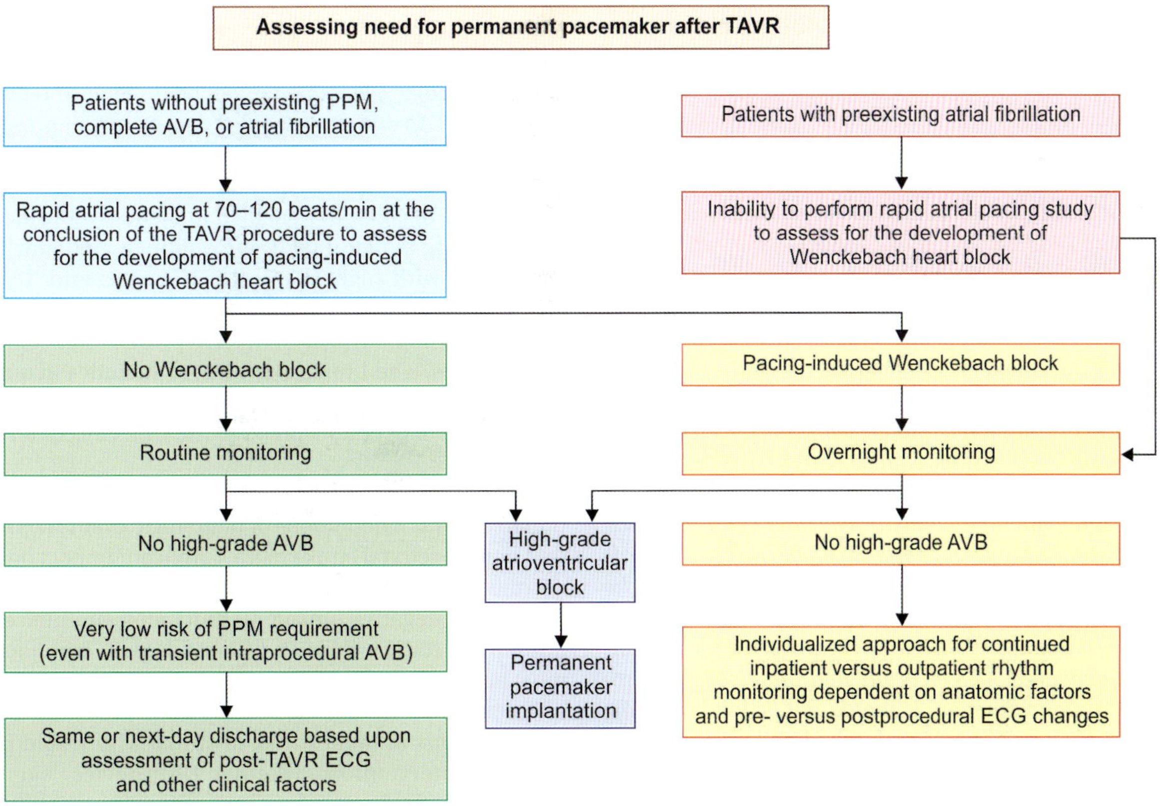

FLOWCHART 1: Conduction abnormality evaluation plan for permanent pacemaker implant.

Source: HYPERLINK "https://www.jacc.org/doi/10.1016/j.jcin.2020.09.063"Sammour Y, HYPERLINK "https://www.jacc.org/doi/10.1016/j.jcin.2020.09.063" Krishnaswamy A, Kumar A, et al. Incidence, predictors, and implications of permanent pacemaker requirement after transcatheter aortic valve replacement. HYPERLINK "https://www.jacc.org/journal/interventions" J Am Coll Cardiol Intv. 2021;14(2):115-34.

interval of 80–90 ms post-TAVI, AH interval, and Wenckebach cycle length. The positive predictive value was fairly low and pacemaker implantation decision cannot be based on these, but negative predictive value was reasonable.[47-51] EP diagnostics will help in patients who have preexisting RBBB and other conduction abnormalities. Clinical implication of new LBBB is still unclear but is linked to bad outcomes and prevents LVEF to improve. Known procedural strategies that reduce the chance of LBBB include optimizing the depth of implantation, measuring membranous septum length, and optimizing valve sizing. Research on monitoring the patients with LBBB and exploring treatment methods such as resynchronization and left bundle branch pacing should be studied.

New Thoughts, Advancements, and Guidance in Pacemaker Implantation after Transcatheter Aortic Valve Implantation

The 2013 guidelines recommended pacemaker implantation as (class I and LOE C) for high degree complete AV block after TAVI, especially with low escape rhythm or it was after a clinical observation of 7 days to assess if it persists or resolves and then do PPI.[52] In 2021 ESC guidelines, PPI has to be done in patients with complete or high degree heart block that persists for 24–48 hours after TAVI and early PPI to be considered if preexisting RBBB developing any further conduction disturbance during or after TAVI (IIa and LOE B).[53] There has been a decrease in the pacemaker implantation rates with new generation supra-annular self-expanding THV by newer procedural optimization techniques, however, conduction disturbances still continue to be an important problem and need permanent pacemaker implantation. *Leadless pacemaker implantation* has become popular in recent years because of lesser risk of infection and no risk of lead dislodgement.[54] However, a 2 years post-TAVI study shows similar safety and efficacy with leadless and transvenous pacemakers. *VVI leadless pacemakers without AV synchrony function have been used more commonly in the patients and have not shown worsening heart failure hospitalizations. Leadless pacemakers can be used in patients with atrial fibrillation and those who do not need AV synchrony, and patients on dialysis who have consumed their large vein access for different ports. It can be used temporarily in selected patients of TAVI who have transient bradycardia and conduction blocks.*

Leadless pacemakers should not be preferred for patients who absolutely need AV synchrony and those patients with normal LV systolic function. It should not be used in young people in whom long-term RV pacing may lead to desynchrony and raise the need of CRT which can be done presently by transvenous route. Transvenous pacing is established, but the leadless pacemakers are currently underdevelopment evolving with latest platforms allowing AV synchrony, CRT, and conduction system pacing features. *Temporary permanent pacemaker (TPPM) is a new concept* being used as a bridge after TAVI. These can be done in patients who have persistent CHB or ≥2:1 AVB or first degree AVB plus new onset LBBB developing during TAVI procedure or within 1 month after TAVI. EXPLOSIVE study and RECOVER study are showing good results and reduce unnecessary permanent pacemaker implantations, lower costs, improve patients quality of life and clinical outcomes.[55-60]

Paravalvular Leak Reduction Measures

Post-TAVI PVL have reduced with the new generation devices having an external skirt and an internal skirt that seals well the crevices. Some newer THVs have adaptive sealing cuffs which are dynamic and provide good sealing minimizing the PVL rate in calcified anatomies. Better optimization techniques of positioning and deployment have also resulted in reduction of this complication. In the past, significant PVL has been associated with longer length of stay, total cost of hospitalization and readmission rates, and adverse outcomes in long-term.[61-63]

Cerebral Protection Systems Evolving to Minimize Stroke (Table 2)

Increased operator experience, advancement in technology, and increasing number of TAVI in low-risk patients are now seen to have reduced incidence of stroke but it still remains a feared complication.[64] Most patients are still elderly and have a huge burden of comorbidities and increased risk of cerebrovascular events and it will be difficult to reduce the risk to <1%.[65] In one study, pooled data from four prospective RCTs evaluating the TriGUARD CEP device-DEFLECT III, REFLECT I, REFLECT II, and the NEURO TAVI REGISTRY without use of CEP have enabled to identify diffusion gated MRI showing a high total lesion volume (>500 mm^3) to be associated with highest rates of ischemic and disabling stroke and a lower rate of complete stroke recovery. This can serve as a strong surrogate marker in pivotal trials comparing CEP devices. The limitations of MRI includes acquisition protocols variations and the expense and logistics, and hence once school of operators prefer to use CEP devices for all the TAVI cases.[66-68]

The other study provides a clinical validation of the updated VARC 3 definitions of neurologic events confirming that periprocedural stroke has a significant impact on 1 year mortality after TAVI with type 1 NeruoARC events.[69] Overall events had negative impact on outcomes and hence every attempt to reduce the risk of neurological complications must be made.

Ideal solution will be to identify some predictors that can mark patients at highest risk of stroke who would benefit from an intervention—whether CEP device, aggressive antithrombotic therapy, or something else to reduce this complication. The PROTECTED TAVR indicated that disabling strokes are less frequent when protection is added to TAVI.[70] Currently, operators need more clinical data before they change their practices as some have doubts on

TABLE 2: Cerebral protection devices: Important features and regulatory status.

	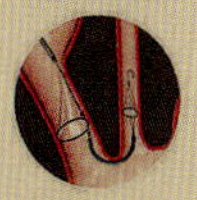 SENTINEL™	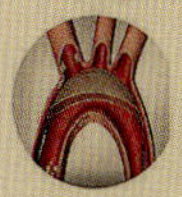 TriGUARD 3™	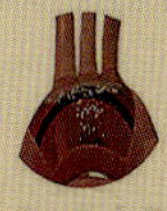 ProtEmbo®	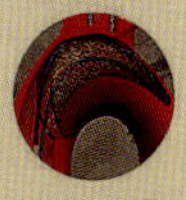 Emblok™	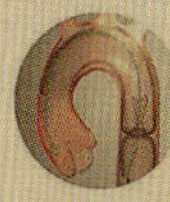 Emboliner™	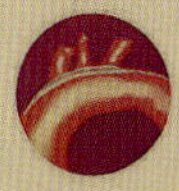 POINT-GUARD™	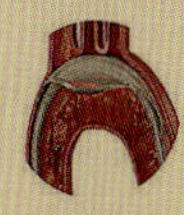 CAPTIS™	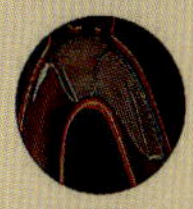 FLOWer™
	SENTINEL™	**TriGUARD 3™**	**ProtEmbo®**	**Emblok™**	**Emboliner™**	**POINT-GUARD™**	**CAPTIS™**	**FLOWer™**
Regulatory status	CE mark, FDA	CE	SIH	SIH	SIH	SIH	FIH	FIH
Cerebral embolic protection	Partial	Complete	Complete	Complete	Complete	Complete	Complete	Complete
Concept	Partial capture	Deflect	Deflect	Capture and removal	Capture and removal	Deflect	Capture and removal	Capture and removal
Pore size	140 µm	115 × 145 µm	60 µm	125 µm	150 µm	105 µm	115 × 145 µm	70 µm
Vascular access	Right radial	Femoral	Left radial	Femoral (contralateral)	Femoral (contralateral)	Femoral (contralateral)	Femoral (ipsilateral)	Femoral (contralateral)
Access size	6 Fr	8 Fr	6 Fr	11 Fr	10 Fr	10 Fr	16 Fr	12 Fr
Heparin coating	No	Yes	Yes	No	Yes	No	No data	No data

(CE mark: European Conformity; Fr: French; FDA: food and drug administration; FIH: first in human; SIH: second in human)

the benefits of CEP devices related to the debate over the clinical data or to the financial impact or both. The ongoing BHF PROTECT trial in UK and the PROTECT trial results combined may address these doubts and the clinical practice could become more uniform.[71]

Cerebral embolic protection devices are categorized as intravascular filter, aortic arch deflectors, and capture and remove devices. Sentinel cerebral protection system belongs to the intravascular filter category and is the only FDA approved device capable of capturing 99% debris but unclear on clinical efficacy. Aortic arch deflectors provide complete cerebral protection for all the three great vessels, deflect the debris, are simpler, have lower profile, and can be used through radial or femoral access. Devices under study in this group are TriGUARD and Prot Embo.[72] Devices that capture and remove debris are more complex, bulkier, and go by femoral access, can sometimes have interaction with the TAVR system. Examples in this group are Emboliner (Emboline), Emblok (Innovative cardiovascular systems), FLOWer (aortic lab and Captis (Filterlex) and Point Guard. Captis is hybrid device having deflector and debris removal abilities.[73-75]

ANTIPLATELETS AND ANTI-COAGULANTS IN TRANSCATHETER AORTIC VALVE IMPLANTATION

Recent data shows dual-antiplatelet therapy to be associated with increased risk for bleeding events, particularly early postprocedure, compared with single-antiplatelet therapy with aspirin.[76] Concerns surrounding the potential for thrombotic complications have raised the possible need of additional OAC for patients with no baseline indications for anticoagulation. Although effective in preventing thrombus formation at the valve level, the bleeding risk has shown to be unacceptably high, and the net benefit of combining antiplatelet and OAC therapy is unproven. For patients with indications for the use of long-term OAC, such as those with atrial fibrillation, the adjunctive use of antiplatelet therapy increases bleeding. Whether direct oral anticoagulant agents achieve better outcomes than vitamin K antagonists remains under investigation.[77-79] Overall, single-antiplatelet therapy and OAC appear to be reasonable strategies in patients without and with indications for concurrent anticoagulation.

MISCELLANEOUS NEW IDEAS AND CONCEPTS

Prioritizing patients out of the waiting list of TAVI with the aid of specially created tools like the SWIFT TAVI algorithm, "*shared decision making (SDM)*" through online interactive decision aids and *minimalistic approach* with "*same day discharge*" are some of the new practices happening fast in USA and European centers of excellence keeping in mind the cost of longer hospitalization, cost of insurance, and also with an aim to make TAVI, a simple structural procedure akin to a PCI.[80-83]

CONCLUSION

Recent advancements in TAVI have revolutionized in the last two decades from time of its inception to the present day practices. There has been effective solutions to the challenges of TAVI seen in the past and appears to have matured enough to become the standard of care for valve replacement in aortic stenosis. There has been an explosion of this procedure around the world surpassing the numbers of surgical aortic valve replacement. Unlike the past, when a high risk surgical AVR patient would go for TAVI, today, a patient who is unfit or high risk for TAVI would be referred for SAVR. This is a paradigm shift in the management of aortic stenosis in last two decades due to advancements in all aspects of the therapy. However, long-term data to support valve-in-valve over surgical replacement through randomized trial is still awaited, a gloomy data on surgical explants of TAVI valves and an insufficient data on transcatheter aortic valve in degenerated TAVI Valve (TAV in TAV), transcatheter aortic valve in TAV in TAV (degenerated TAVI valves twice), should discourage the race to do TAVI in young and very young. It is the role of the physician/heart team to rightly counsel the young patients of aortic stenosis in the paucity of data at this point of time.

ONLINE REFERENCES

Please scan the QR code provided at the end of the table of contents for References of this chapter.

CHAPTER

174

Bicuspid Aortic Valve: Most Frequent, Not Benign Congenital Heart Disease

BS Yadav

ABSTRACT

The bicuspid aortic valve (BAV) is the most common congenital heart disease (CHD). It is a disease of the aortic valve (AV) and aorta. Initially, BAV patients are asymptomatic as the valve function is normal. It is a disease of progression due to the degeneration of these two structures: AV and aorta. It manifests with complications in the third to fifth decades of life; the majority will manifest with AV dysfunction in the form of aortic stenosis (AS) or aortic regurgitation (AR). Aortic degeneration leads to dilatation, aneurysm, or dissection. Approximately 20% may remain asymptomatic till the end. These complications may culminate in heart failure and death. Early diagnosis and timely treatment are essential to save these patients.

Keywords: Bicuspid aortic valve, aortic aneurysm, aortic regurgitation, aortic stenosis, aortic valve surgery, infective endocarditis, transcatheter aortic valve replacement

INTRODUCTION

Four hundred years ago, in his sketches, Leonardo da Vinci described four, three, and two cusps of the aortic valve (AV).[1] He mentioned that the AV works best with three cusps.

As described in various autopsy and echocardiographic studies, the bicuspid aortic valve (BAV) is the most common congenital heart disease (CHD) with an incidence of 0.5–2% in the general population.[1,2] The male–female ratio is 3:1. There is a high risk of developing complications.[3]

The availability of echocardiography (echo) has revolutionized the diagnosis and management of BAV cases. Assessment of both, the AV and aorta, can be done with echo, magnetic resonance imaging (MRI), and CT angio. Early clinical detection and echo surveillance are crucial to intervene at an appropriate time, to prevent fatal outcomes in BAV cases.

BICUSPID AORTIC VALVE—NOT A BENIGN CONDITION

- It begins with an almost normal heart.
- The magnitude of this disease is 2% of the population.
- It is a disease of not only an abnormal number of cusps, but it involves the aorta as well.
- It is a progressive disease that manifests with catastrophic complications and even death.
- It can lead to complications of AV dysfunction (AS, AR, IE) and aortic root dilatation at a much younger age.
- Infective endocarditis (IE), dissection of the aorta, and heart failure are life-threatening conditions.
- Mainly treatment is surgical and sometimes interventional; with treatment, long-term survival is good.
- Only some patients remain normal till the end.
- So, it is no longer a benign condition because it is not a simple two-cusp valve; it can be life-threatening.

GENETICS AND INHERITANCE

The role of genetics, in BAV cusp formation, is incompletely understood and no single gene is found responsible. However, the significant influence of genetics in BAV is supported by the following facts:[4]

- BAV is the result of abnormal valvulogenesis where two cusps fail to separate.
- The inheritance is autosomal dominant.
- BAV can be familial or sporadic.
- 9–17% incidence is observed in first-degree family members of BAV cases.[4]
- BAV is associated with other CHDs that have genetic origin, e.g., Turner's syndrome.

TABLE 1: Significant influence of genetics in BAV is supported by different facts.

CHD	% of BAV cases
CoA	50–70
Aortic arch obstruction	36
VSD	15–30
Turner's syndrome	30
William syndrome	30
Sinus of Valsalva aneurysm	15–20
Loeys–Dietz syndrome	2.5–17

- Genes implicated are q^4, q^{13}, q^{15}, mutation in Notch1 and Tgfb1-4 (in Loeys-Dietz syndrome).[2]

The simultaneous involvement of the valve and aorta may be explained on the basis of the embryogenesis of the heart. Mesodermal tissues form major parts of the heart. Semilunar valves and ascending aorta are developed from the neural crest. Abnormal migration of neural crest tissue may be one of the reasons for the simultaneous involvement of these two structures.[2,4]

ASSOCIATION OF CONGENITAL HEART DISEASES WITH BICUSPID AORTIC VALVE (TABLE 1)

In the genetics of BAV, various theories of pathogenesis are proposed and they are as follows:[3]

- Abnormal neural crest migration
- Absence of nitric oxide synthetase
- Abnormal blood flow pattern with unequal stress on cusps resulting in abnormal development

ANATOMY OF BICUSPID AORTIC VALVE

Normal AV has three cusps, three commissures, three sinuses, and three interleaflet triangles. Cusps are named according to the origin of coronary arteries **(Fig. 1)**:

- Left coronary cusp (LCC)
- Right coronary cusp (RCC)
- Noncoronary cusp (NCC)

The BAV has only two cusps, two commissures, and three sinuses. One cusp has two parts joined by a raphe (an aborted commissure formation). A rare variety of BAV has two cusps, two commissures, and two sinuses.[3]

CLASSIFICATION

There are many types of classifications described for BAV, but the most important is the International Consensus Classification and Nomenclature for congenital BAV.[5] This classification recognizes three types of BAVs.

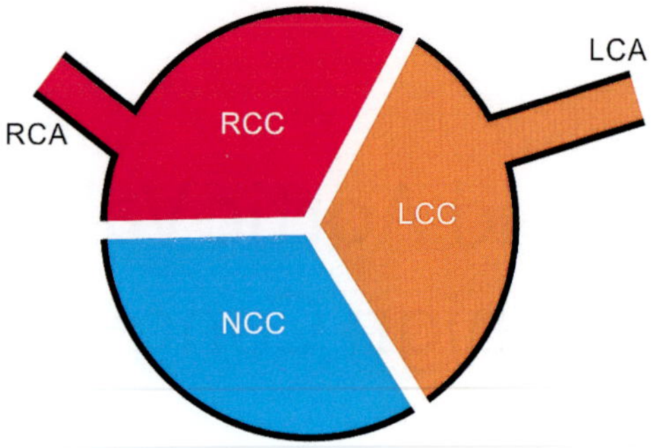

FIG. 1: Normal aortic valve.

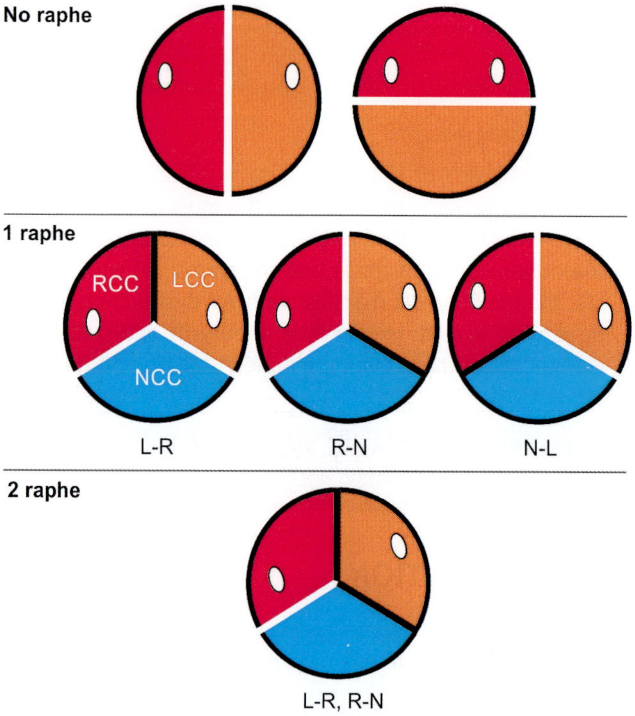

FIG. 2: Two sinuses and fusion type BAV.

1. *Fused type BAV (90–95%)*:
   a. R–L cusp fusion (70–80%)
   b. R–N cusp fusion (20–30%)
   c. L–N cusp fusion (3–6%)
2. *Two sinuses type BAV (5–7%)* **(Fig. 2)**:
   a. Laterolateral type
   b. Anteroposterior type
3. *Partial fusion or forme fruste type* **(Fig. 3)**: This is a recently added type. There is a small raphe with <50% cusp fusion. The number of raphes, symmetry, and presence of coarctation of the aorta (CoA) are additional considerations.

TYPES OF AORTOPATHY[5]

Aortopathy is of two types:

- *Ascending aorta type*: Dilatation beyond STJ. Seen in 70% cases.

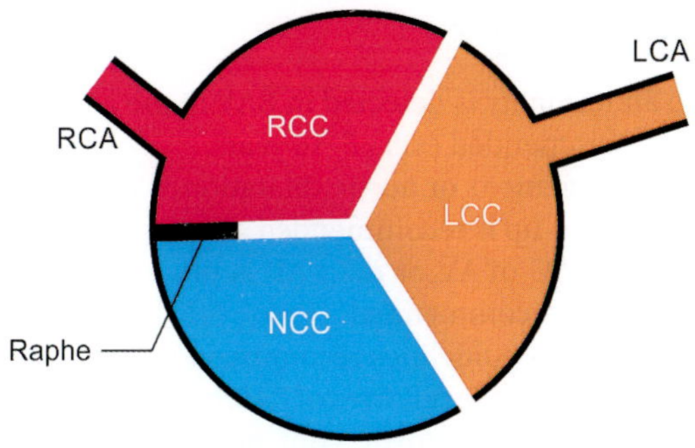

FIG. 3: Partial fusion or forme fruste type BAV.

- *Root type*: More chances of dissection of the aorta. Seen in 30% cases.

CLINICAL PROGNOSTIC SUBSETS[5]

- Typical valvulo-aortopathy is the most common subset with progressive aortic dilatation and BAV dysfunction. Prognosis is better in this subset.
- Complex valvulo-aortopathy is associated with complex CHD, for example, Turner syndrome, CoA, and Loeys-Dietz syndrome. This group has a worse prognosis, accelerates fast, and needs early treatment.
- Undiagnosed or uncomplicated valvuloaortopathy. Being mild and nonprogressive, it is diagnosed at autopsy or incidentally on investigations.

DIAGNOSIS

The BAV becomes symptomatic in adult life. Diagnosis in the initial period is by detection of an aortic ejection click and systolic murmur. Diagnosis is confirmed by echo. Echocardiography is a gold standard diagnostic test for BAV diseases. Echo can demonstrate detailed anatomy of the valve including the number of cusps, closure line, raphe, doming, leaflet redundancy, IE, aorta, and associated CHD, e.g., CoA. Doppler parameters will assess the severity of valvular lesions. Transesophageal echo may be superior in some cases like aortic dissection and IE. Echo results are suboptimal in cases of calcified valves. CT angio and MRI are additional diagnostic tools, which are especially useful in calcified AVs and to assess the entire length of the aorta. CT and MRI have better diagnostic ability. MRI (3D/4D) can precisely demonstrate the movements of the AV and other cardiac structures.[5] Details of sinotubular junction (STJ), ascending aorta, and arch are better defined by CT and cardiac MRI. It is particularly useful in cases of CoA. Cardiac MRI can also give information about the functional anatomy, perfusion, and myocardial viability.[6,7]

NATURAL HISTORY

Bicuspid aortic valve disease is progressive in nature. It starts at birth as an anatomical variation and usually manifests in adult life with complications of valve deformity, infection, and ascending aortic diseases like aneurysm or dissection. These changes are due to the following factors:

- Hemodynamic stress on valve structure and aorta
- Progressive fibrosis and calcification of AV
- Degeneration in the medial wall of the aorta leading to dilatation
- Infection of BAV

In one study, the progression of pressure gradient was observed at the rate of about 18 mm Hg per year in bicuspid aortic stenosis (AS).[8,9] Once an AV gradient of 20 mm Hg or mild AR is detected, yearly follow-up should be done.

COMPLICATIONS

The major complications are:

- Aortic stenosis
- Aortic regurgitation (AR)
- Aortopathy—aortic dilatation, aneurysm, and dissection
- Infective endocarditis

Aortic stenosis of BAV has an incidence of 59–81% and is the most common complication.[5,7] Hemodynamic stress, thickening, fibrosis, and irreversible calcification over the years lead to AV narrowing. BAV AS usually manifests a decade earlier than senile degenerative AS.[8] AS appears at a younger age and progresses faster.

Aortic regurgitation is also common in BAV. Prevalence of AR described is 59% of cases[9] and increases with age, but severe AR is seen in only 20% of cases. Mechanisms leading to AR include the following:

- Redundant valve tissue present in the BAV during abnormal cardiogenesis
- Annuloaortic ectasia
- Aortic root dilatation
- Infective endocarditis
- Postballoon dilatation or post-transcatheter aortic valve replacement (TAVR)

Aortic regurgitation in BAV is rapidly progressive and needs surgical aortic valve replacement (SAVR), as per conventional indications of AR surgery. SAVR in AR is done at the mean age of 46 years as compared to AS where the mean age is 63 years.[9]

Infective endocarditis is a fatal complication. BAV is an important substrate for developing IE. In pathological studies of IE, BAV was present in 25% of cases.[2] IE can complicate into cusp perforation, fistula, or abscess formation. AV conduction blocks and heart failure can also occur. In a study of 408 cases of IE, 12% had BAV.[10] In another study conducted 25 years after the diagnosis of BAV, 26% developed aortic aneurysm.[11,12]

TREATMENT

The ACC/AHA guidelines for BAV lesions recommend following the same guidelines as for tricuspid aortic valve (TAV) stenosis and AR:[11,13]

- Ascending aorta replacement is reasonable with aortic valve replacement (AVR) with an aortic diameter of 4.5 cm or more along with SAVR if SAVR is being planned.
- SAVR and aortic root replacement in asymptomatic or symptomatic cases with aortic root diameter of >5.5 cm.[10]
- If the diameter is >5 cm and the diameter increment is 5 mm/yr or more, SAVR is indicated.
- TAVR may be considered as an alternative in AS.

In BAV AS, AV peak-to-peak systolic gradient (PSG) of 60 mm Hg or PSG of 50 mm Hg with ECG LVH strain pattern in patients who do strenuous work are also the indications for SAVR or TAVR. In BAV, AVR is performed 5–10 years earlier as compared to senile AV disease.[7] In children < 18 years of age, aortic balloon valvotomy is the treatment of choice but recurrence is common. Ross's procedure is also an alternative to SAVR.

Significant AR requires surgery less often as compared to AS (30% vs. 70%). AV repair is an alternative to SAVR in some cases. Aortic dilatation with a diameter of ≥45 mm is seen in 25% of cases at 25 years.[10] CoA is present in 7–10% of BAV cases, whereas 50–70% of CoA have BAV.[5]

Transcatheter aortic valve replacement is now available, as an alternative to surgical AVR. Problems with TAVR include a lower success rate and more complications such as malposition of the device or paravalvular leak. This happens due to raphe calcification and the elliptical shape of the annulus. With new generation TAVR devices, the results are improving and now TAVR is recommended even for medium- to high-risk cases.[12]

No drug treatment is available for BAV disease. Trials are underway for statins to prevent fibrosis in the valve. ACE inhibitors are under trial to prevent aortic root dilatation. Vasodilators are used for AR as a standard treatment. Prophylaxis for IE is recommended in all cases of BAV if there is a risk of bacteremia.

FOLLOW-UP

- If no abnormality is detected in BAV in the aorta, follow-up is recommended every 5–10 years.
- If AV involvement or aortic dilatation is detected, then yearly follow-up is recommended.
- If 20 mm PSG of AV or mild AR is present, then yearly follow-up is recommended.
- The ACC/AHA guidelines recommend routine screening of first-degree close relatives of BAV and aortic dilatation.
- Pregnancy-dilated aortic root of >40 mm should be operated on before pregnancy. If diagnosed during pregnancy, a 4–6-week echo follow-up is advised; there is a high risk of dissection in the third trimester.

CONCLUSION

Bicuspid aortic valve is the most common CHD. It appears as a benign anatomical variant but in the long term, it is no more benign due to its associated complications. It is a progressive disease of two structures, the AV as well as the aortic root and ascending aorta. There is a prominent genetic and familial association. Screening of first-degree relatives of BAV is recommended. Complications occur in adult life, which is in the form of AS, AR, IE, and aortopathy (dilatation, aneurysm, dissection).

Treatment options are effective and lifesaving. They include:

- SAVR or repair of AV
- Bentall procedure, repair of aorta
- Aortic valve balloon valvuloplasty; Ross procedure is done in children
- TAVR is a developing alternative in bicuspid AS

New-generation devices in TAVR are now commonly being used with improving results. Timely detection and proper evaluation of candidates are vital. If applied at the appropriate stage of disease progression, it carries an excellent long-term prognosis.

ONLINE REFERENCES

Please scan the QR code provided at the end of the table of contents for References of this chapter.

CHAPTER

175

Percutaneous Transcatheter Mitral and Tricuspid Valve-in-Valve Implantation

Nandhakumar Vasu, Ajit S Mullasari

ABSTRACT

Transcatheter mitral valve-in-valve (M-ViV) implantation in a failed bioprosthetic degenerated valve has become the standard of care in high-surgical-risk patients. Transseptal access has become the contemporary port for the M-ViV procedure. The transcatheter tricuspid valve-in-valve (T-ViV) procedure, with limited data, shows a promising future. This chapter reviews the indications, procedural technique, and clinical outcomes of mitral and T-ViV procedures.

Keywords: Transcatheter mitral valve replacement, mitral valve-in-valve implantation, tricuspid valve-in-valve implantation, valvular heart disease, left ventricular outflow tract obstruction

INTRODUCTION

Transcatheter valve replacement for valvular heart diseases began from the aortic position. Transcatheter valve replacement for native atrioventricular valves (AVV) is more complex since they have complex anatomy and their relation with vital structures such as the subvalvular apparatus, the conduction system, the coronary sinus, the left circumflex artery, and the right coronary artery (RCA). A degenerated bioprosthetic valve at the mitral or tricuspid position is amenable for transcatheter valve therapy, as the landing zone is optimal for the currently existing balloon-expandable transcatheter aortic valve implant (TAVI) systems of *Meril* and *Edwards*. The native AVV anatomy is modified by the cardiac surgeon while implanting a bioprosthetic valve by excising the native leaflets, reconstructing the irregular annulus plane to a circular landing zone, and partly removing the subvalvular apparatus.

This chapter focuses on transcatheter valve-in-valve therapy using the currently available balloon-expandable TAVI systems at the mitral and tricuspid positions.

TRANSCATHETER MITRAL VALVE-IN-VALVE IMPLANTATION

In 2020, the American College of Cardiology/American Heart Association guideline for the management of patients with valvular heart disease recommended transcatheter valve therapy for failed mitral bioprosthesis with either stenotic or regurgitant physiology in patients with high or prohibitive surgical risk (Class IIa).[1] Surgery is the Class I recommendation for failed mitral bioprosthesis in low- and intermediate-risk patients.

Computerized Tomography Assessment

Three important aspects are assessed in the electrocardiogram (ECG)-gated computerized tomography (CT) before mitral valve-in-valve (M-ViV) implantation. These are (1) valve sizing, (2) prediction of left ventricular outflow tract (LVOT) obstruction, and (3) interatrial septal (IAS) crossing.

Valve Sizing

The sizing of the valve is performed at the landing zone or the sealing zone. In the M-ViV procedure, this is at the sewing ring. The Pie Medical 3-Mensio software is used at our center for CT assessment. Once the annulus plane is defined, the software gives three automatic measurements: (1) Trigone-to-trigone (TT), (2) commissure to commissure (CC), and (3) anteroposterior (AP) diameters **(Fig. 1A)**. All three measurements are the same for a circular sewing ring, whereas they are different and are important in native mitral valve replacement. Three important measurements measured manually are (1) area-derived outer diameter

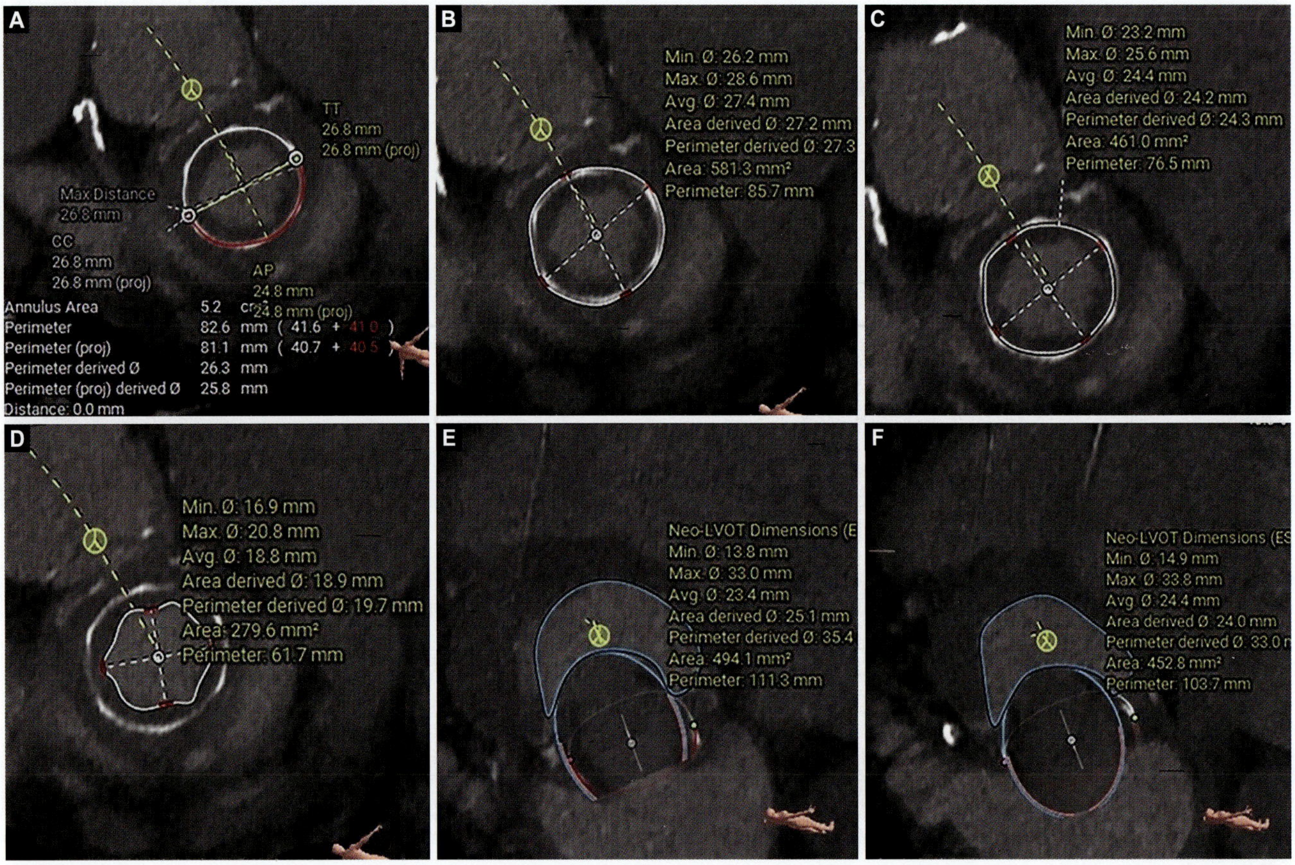

FIGS. 1A TO F: CT assessment for mitral valve-in-valve implantation in a failed 27 mm Biocor valve. (A) 3-Mensio automated measurement shows commissure-to-commissure distance, trigone-to-trigone distance, and the anteroposterior distance. (B) The area-derived outer diameter was 27.2 mm. (C) The area-derived inner diameter was 24.2 mm. (D) The diameter excluding the pannus and the degenerated material was 18.9 mm. (E) The neo-LVOT area after placing a virtual valve at the end-diastole was 494.1 mm^2. (F) The neo-LVOT area at the end of the systole was 452.8 mm^2.

(CT: computerized tomography; LVOT: left ventricular outflow tract)

(Fig. 1B), (2) area-derived inner diameter, which is considered for sizing **(Fig. 1C)**, (3) area-derived CT-measured inner diameter **(Fig. 1D)**. **Figures 1B and C** show the outer and inner area of a 27 mm Biocor valve as 581 mm^2 and 461 mm^2, respectively. The sizing is performed using the inner diameter. The area of 461 mm^2 gives a diameter of 24.2 mm. A 24.5 mm *Meril Myval* is oversized by 2.5%, a 26 mm *Myval* is oversized by 15.4%, and a 27.5 mm *Myval* is 28.9% oversized. For an M-ViV, 5–20% of area oversizing is acceptable as the closing pressure is high compared to the aortic position and there is a risk of atrial embolization if not adequately oversized. A 26 mm *Myval* is the valve of choice in the case in whom the CT is depicted.

Prediction of Left Ventricular Outflow Tract Obstruction

A virtual transcatheter valve is placed inside the bioprosthetic valve and the neo-LVOT area is measured at the end-diastole and end-systole **(Figs. 1E and F)**. The neo-LVOT area <190 mm^2, left ventricular end-diastolic dimension of <48 mm, left ventricle mass index >105 g/m^2, annulus to the septal distance of <17.8 mm, and a relative wall thickness of >0.38 are predictors of LVOT obstruction. Aorto-mitral angle is not a predictor of LVOT obstruction in multivariate analysis.[2]

Interatrial Septal Crossing

There is a dedicated IAS crossing application in the 3-Mensio software. After defining the interatrial septum, the ideal septal puncture point is located with a red cross in the AP projection and in the coplanar view on an imaginary horizontal line drawn at the lowermost point on the mitral sewing ring. The distance of the landing zone from the septal puncture point can be measured. As a rule of thumb, this septal-mitral distance of >35 mm is enough to maneuver the valve delivery system. A simulation of the delivery catheter from the IVC through the septal puncture point into the mitral valve can be created after defining the superior vena cava (SVC) and inferior vena cava (IVC).

Technique of Mitral Valve-in-Valve Implantation

Transseptal and transapical access are the two approaches for a transcatheter M-ViV procedure. In the Valve-in-Valve International Data (VIVID) registry, 64.4% of the patients underwent M-ViV through transapical access, whereas 34.5% underwent transseptal access.[2] Currently, transseptal access is used in almost all patients. The procedure is done with transesophageal echocardiogram (TEE) guidance under general anesthesia. Baseline images of the mechanism of bioprosthetic valve failure is documented. **Figures 2A to C** shows the degenerated torn leaflet leads to a flail leaflet with severe valvular leak as a mechanism of valve failure. A venous access is obtained with ultrasound guidance from one of the common femoral veins preferably on the right side due to ease of working. The venous access is primed with a single ProGlide™ (Abbott) percutaneous vascular closure device and a 9F short sheath is secured. An arterial access is obtained from the contralateral common femoral artery with a 6F short sheath for hemodynamic measurements and real-time monitoring during the procedure.

A 6F pigtail catheter is placed in the noncoronary access through the arterial access for additional guidance during transseptal puncture. The ideal transseptal puncture site is the inferior and posterior part of the fossa ovalis. Fluoroscopically, the transseptal needle should be at an imaginary horizontal line drawn at the lowermost part of the circular mitral sewing ring **(Fig. 2D)**. The TEE probe is positioned so that the ultrasound beam from the probe faces the required puncture site in fluoroscopy **(Fig. 2D)**. The 90° view shows the bicaval view, and the transseptal needle is placed in the inferior part of the septum **(Fig. 2E)**. The X-plane cursor is placed on the needle in the bicaval view, and we can confirm the AP position of the needle **(Fig. 2F)**. If the needle is more anterior, a clockwise torque

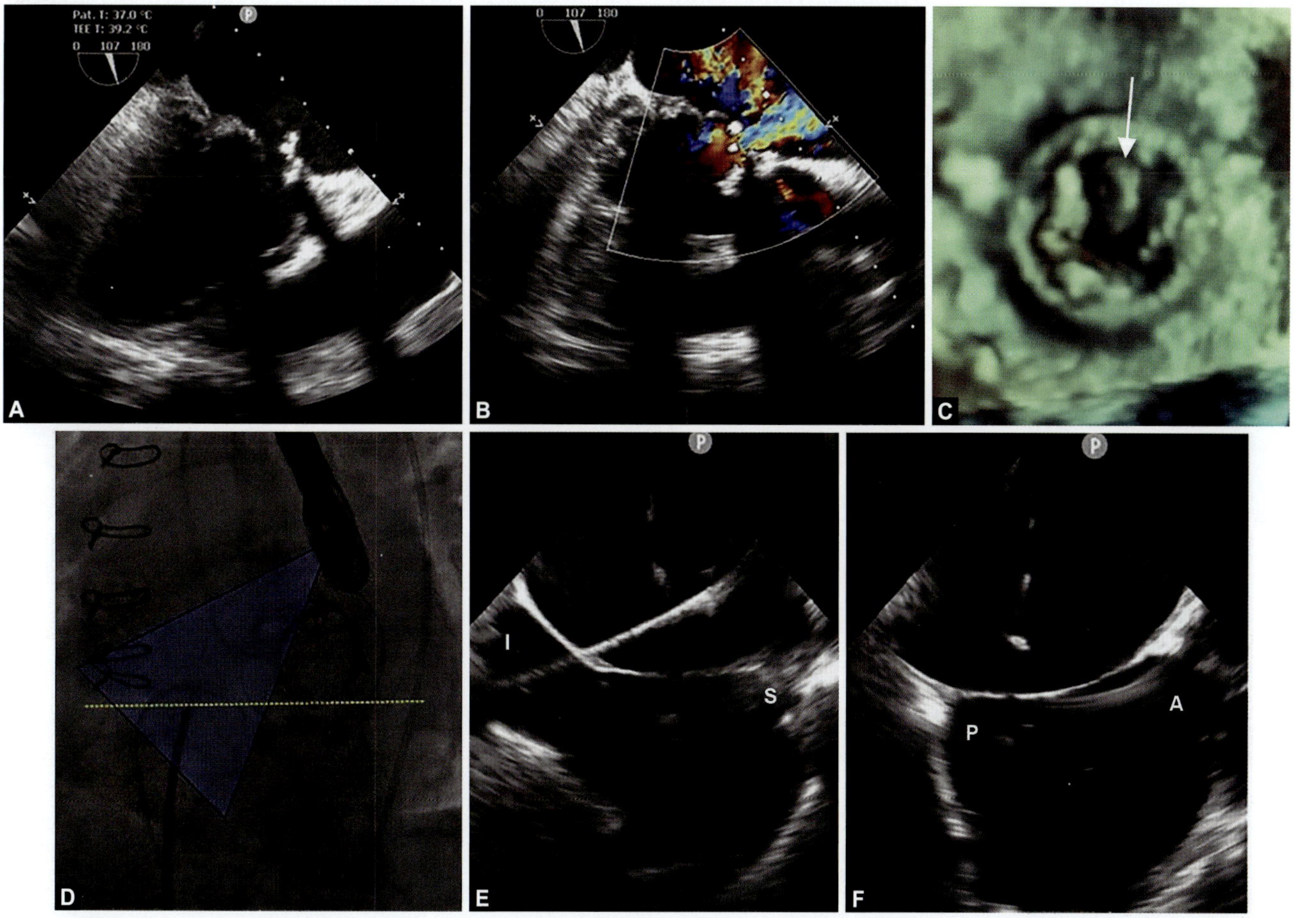

FIGS. 2A TO F: TEE guidance during mitral valve-in-valve implantation. (A) Mid esophageal 100° view shows the thickened, degenerated, and torn leaflet prolapsing into the left atrium during systole. (B) A color Doppler interrogation shows the severe valvular leak through the torn leaflet. (C) A 3D live image of the failed mitral bioprosthesis shows the systolic prolapse of the torn flail segment. (D) Fluoroscopic confirmation of the inferior position during septal puncture was confirmed with an imaginary yellow horizontal line drawn at the bottom of the mitral valve. In fluoroscopy, the TEE transmitter should face the needle (blue triangle) to identify the needle position. (E) TEE bicaval view shows the SVC(S) and IVC(I) and the septal puncture site. (F) The X-plane on the septal puncture site in the bicaval view shows the anteroposterior septum and the posterior puncture site.

(IVC: inferior vena cava; SVC: superior vena cava; TEE: transesophageal echocardiogram)

of the needle brings it posteriorly, and if the needle is too posterior, then a counterclockwise torque drives the needle anteriorly.

We use a BRK (Abbott, St. Jude) series of needles in our center for transseptal puncture. For a normal right atrium (RA), a BRK needle is ideal, whereas for a dilated RA, a BRK-1 needle is required. If the IAS is thick, a unipolar cautery with 40W PureCut energy application over the proximal hub of the needle for a brief period of 3 seconds helps in securing transseptal access into the left atrium (LA). A 0.025" coil spring wire is placed in the LA and an 8.5F steerable Agilis sheath is placed in the LA. A 5F pigtail catheter is taken with a 0.035" J-shaped wire through the Agilis sheath and used to cross the mitral valve. A combined en-face view in the left anterior oblique caudal view and a coplanar view in the right anterior oblique projection is useful for crossing the valve **(Fig. 3A)**. The crossing through the central valve opening rather than perforating the leaflets or paravalvular crossing is confirmed with a real-time 3-D LIVE TEE view **(Fig. 3B)**. A 0.035" × 275 cm extra small SAFARI[2] (3.2 × 2.9 cm) stiff wire is placed in the left ventricle, and the Agilis sheath is removed.

After placing the 14F or 16F expandable sheath, the IAS is dilated with a 12- or 14 mm × 4 cm balloon to facilitate the delivery of a crimped valve **(Figs. 3C and D)**. Flossing of the valve with the same dilated balloon is done with caution to predict the crossing ability of the valve delivery system, especially in a severely stenotic valve **(Fig. 3E)**. This flossing should not be done if any mobile thrombus or degenerated valve material is seen in TEE, as it may produce stroke during flossing. The *Meril Myval* or the *Octacor* valves can be crimped over the balloon from outside and taken through the Python sheath. The valve is positioned with two landmarks in the coplanar view. (1) The distal edge of the transcatheter valve should correspond with the distal edge of the failed bioprosthetic valve post. (2) The middle marker of the balloon should be on the middle of the sewing ring of the bioprosthetic valve **(Fig. 3F)**. The valve is deployed slowly under rapid ventricular pacing over 8–10 seconds **(Fig. 3G)**. In case of increased gradient (mean gradient >10 mm Hg), a postdilatation is done to remodel or fracture the failed bioprosthetic valve frame. The balloon size needed to fracture the bioprosthetic valve frame is 1 mm above the bioprosthetic valve size. An IAS device closure for the iatrogenic atrial septal defect is required in an uncommon scenario of desaturation due to a right to left shunt or with a Qp:Qs ≥ 2:1 which persists after 6 months.

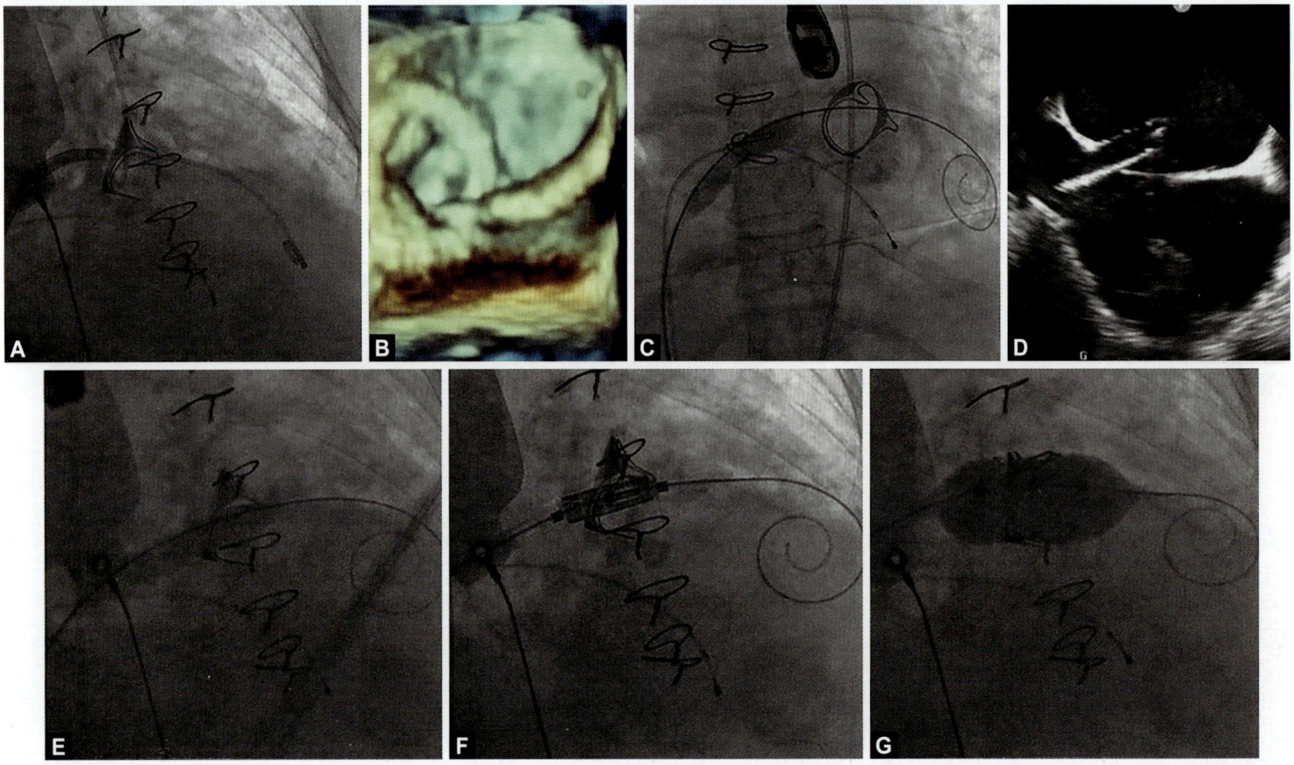

FIGS. 3A TO G: Mitral valve-in-valve implantation using *Meril Myval*. (A) In a cusp overlap view, a pigtail was advanced from an LA Agilis sheath across the mitral bioprosthetic valve into the LV. (B) A 3D live image confirms the pigtail crossing through the center of the valve orifice and rules out the paravalvular crossing. (C) A 14 × 40 mm noncompliant balloon is dilated across the interatrial septum to facilitate the navigation of the transcatheter delivery system. (D) Septal dilatation is shown in TEE bicaval view. (E) Flossing of a degenerated valve with an inflated 14 × 40 mm balloon to predict the difficulty in crossing with a transcatheter valve. (F) A *Meril Myval* is positioned inside the failed mitral bioprosthesis. (G) A completely deployed *Meril Myval* inside the failed mitral bioprosthesis.

(LA: left atrium; LV: left ventricle; TEE: transesophageal echocardiogram)

Clinical Outcomes

The VIVID registry data showed a technical success of 93.5% for M-ViV. The mean gradient after the procedure was >10 mm Hg in 8.2% of the patients and >5 mm Hg in 59.9%. The device embolization, migration, or malposition was noted in 2.4%, and a second transcatheter heart valve was needed in 2.8%. The LVOT was seen in 1.8%.[3] Guerrero et al. prospectively studied the 1-year outcome of M-ViV (n = 30) using Edwards SAPIEN XT and SAPIEN 3 valves. Technical success was achieved in all patients. The all-cause mortality at 30 days was 3.3% and was unchanged at 1 year.[4] The 4-year adjusted survival was 66.7% for M-ViV, emphasizing careful selection of the patients.

TRANSCATHETER TRICUSPID VALVE-IN-VALVE IMPLANTATION

Transcatheter tricuspid valve-in-valve (T-ViV) implantation is indicated in high or prohibitive surgical risk patients with failed bioprosthesis (Class IIa).[1] Surgery is the Class I recommendation for low- or intermediate-surgical-risk patients. However, this guideline should be read cautiously, as the evidence from left-sided bioprosthetic failures mainly drives this recommendation. Repeat tricuspid valve surgeries carry high in-hospital mortality.[5] T-ViV is a safe alternative option for these patients. The limited data available for T-ViV procedures is encouraging.[6]

Computerized Tomography Assessment

The CT assessment for T-ViV is different from M-ViV. There is no dedicated application in the 3-Mensio software. Multiplanar reconstruction with axial, coronal, and sagittal sections is essential in CT analysis.

- Sizing the valve with inner diameter **(Fig. 4A)**, and outer diameter **(Figs. 4B and C)** is to know the size of the failed bioprosthesis. A 5–15% area oversizing is acceptable as the closing pressure on the right side is not as high as at the mitral position.
- Distance between the IVC–right atrial junction to the midpoint of the landing zone (sewing ring of the failed bioprosthesis) in coronal planes.

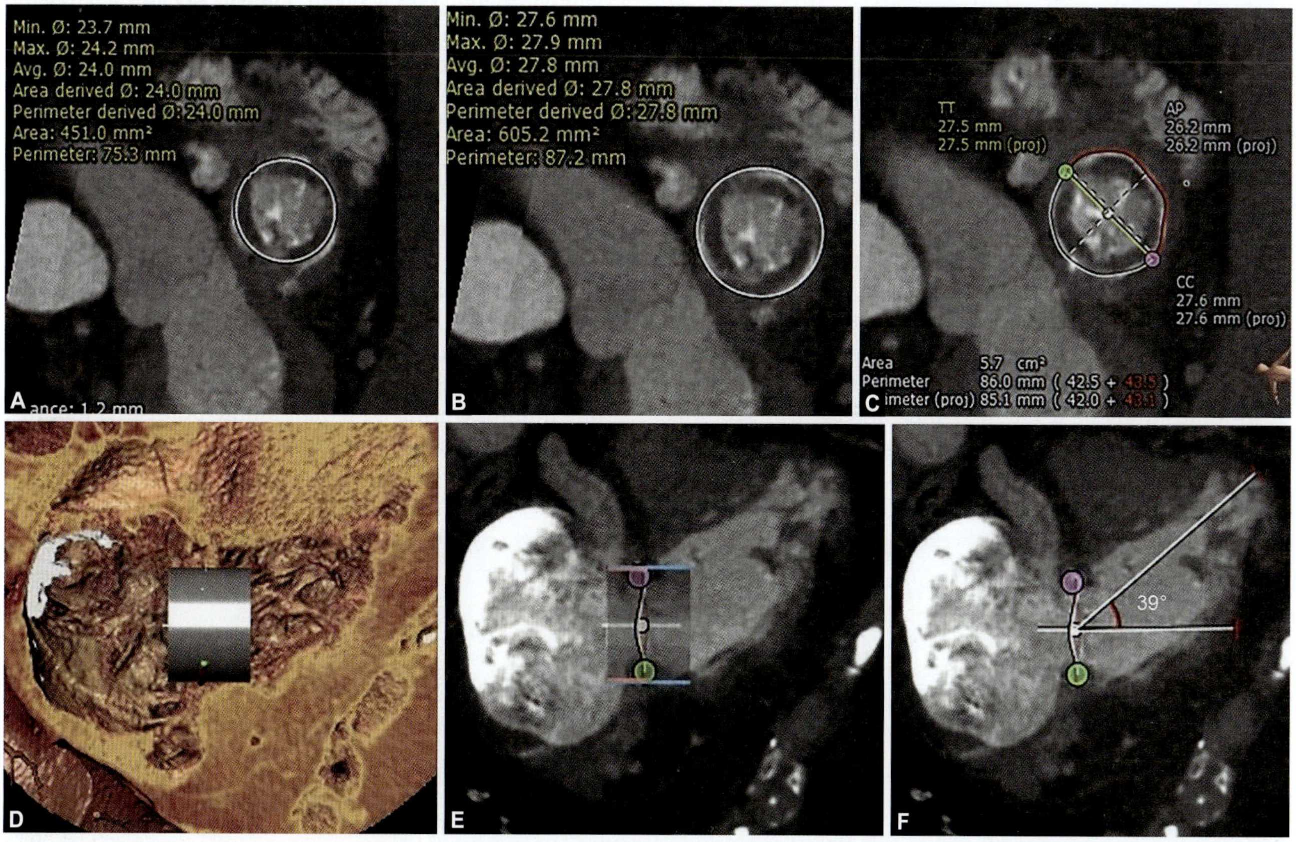

FIGS. 4A TO F: CT assessment of tricuspid valve-in-valve implantation for a 27 mm degenerated Epic valve. (A) The inner area was 451 mm^2 and the area-derived diameter was 24.0 mm. (B) Area-derived outer diameter was 27.8 mm. (C) Off-label use of 3-Mensio mitral valve application for the tricuspid valve annulus sizing. (D and E) Simulation of a virtual 26 mm *Meril Myval* at the tricuspid position using 3-Mensio mitral application. (F) The angle between the valve trajectory and the right ventricle apical axis.

- We measure the angle between the IVC and the bioprosthetic valve trajectory in the right anterior oblique projection.
- The distance between the tricuspid annulus to the RCA. There is a case report of RCA subtotal occlusion after the Edwards Cardioband annuloplasty system, though this is not reported after T-ViV.[7] Given this theoretical possibility, we consider VTC to RCA distance of >4 mm to be safe in T-ViV with valve fracture at our center.
- The angle between the axis of the simulated transcatheter valve and the right ventricle apical axis determines the canting of the valve **(Figs. 4D to F)**.

Technique of Tricuspid Valve-in-Valve Implantation

The procedure can be done under conscious sedation or general anesthesia. TEE and apnea during valve deployment are required during the procedure and are the reasons for general anesthesia. As the tricuspid valve sewing ring is closely related to the conduction system, an intentional fracture of the failed bioprosthetic sewing ring increases the probability of a complete heart block. Rapid ventricular pacing during the valve deployment is at the operators' discretion. Rapid ventricular pacing is preferred in patients with more than mild pulmonary hypertension, as the valve can embolize into the RA. Severe bioprosthetic valvular regurgitation is always associated with high right ventricular pressure, whereas severe valve stenosis is associated with normal or decreased right ventricular pressure. Since the temporary pacing catheter cannot be jailed across the tricuspid valve, the pacing catheter is placed in the left ventricle through one of the common femoral arteries.

Jailing the pacemaker or implantable cardioverter defibrillator (ICD) leads during the T-ViV is not advisable. If lead extraction is possible, the leads are removed followed by implantation of a leadless pacemaker, transvenous coronary sinus pacing, or epicardial pacing, subcutaneous ICD, or implantation of an extravascular ICD. If the leads are nonextractable, after explaining the risks of lead failure and device infection, the leads may be jailed.[8]

One of the common femoral veins, preferably from the right side for operator comfort is chosen as the main access port. The operator crosses the failed bioprosthetic tricuspid valve with a 7F Swan-Ganz balloon-tipped catheter or with a pigtail to avoid chord entangling. Once a 6F pigtail is positioned at the right ventricular apex, a 0.035" × 275 cm extra small SAFARI[2] (3.2 × 2.9 cm) stiff wire is placed through the pigtail and positioned in the right ventricle. The crimped valve over the delivery system is positioned at the landing zone. If the delivery system buckles in the RA, a further push of the delivery system is stopped, and one needs to look for the reasons **(Figs. 5A to C)**. These may be wire bias, noncoaxial system, or severe stenosis.

Once the valve is positioned at the landing zone, the flexion if at all applied during crossing is neutralized to avoid unnecessary tension on the system. In Biocor or Epic valve, as the stent posts are not visible, the position of the valve is entirely based on the sewing ring **(Fig. 6A)**. Once the position is confirmed the slow inflation of the system over 8–10 seconds is performed, till complete deployment **(Figs. 6B and C)**. A pigtail is placed in place of stiff wire and a right ventriculogram is taken. **Figures 6D and E** show the normal functioning of the implanted *Meril Myval* in diastole and systole respectively. A fluoroscopic image of the *Meril Myval* in a coplanar view shows the ventricular flaring **(Fig. 6F)**.

Clinical Outcomes

Among the 156 patients who underwent T-ViV in the VIVID registry, a SAPIEN XT valve could not be advanced across the stenotic bioprosthesis and was retrieved in one patient. In two patients, the valve embolized into the RA or right ventricle. One was a Melody valve and the other one was a SAPIEN valve. Five patients died before the completion of one month. During a median follow-up of 13.3 months, 17 additional patients died.[6] There is an anecdotal report available for T-ViV using *Meril Myval*.[9]

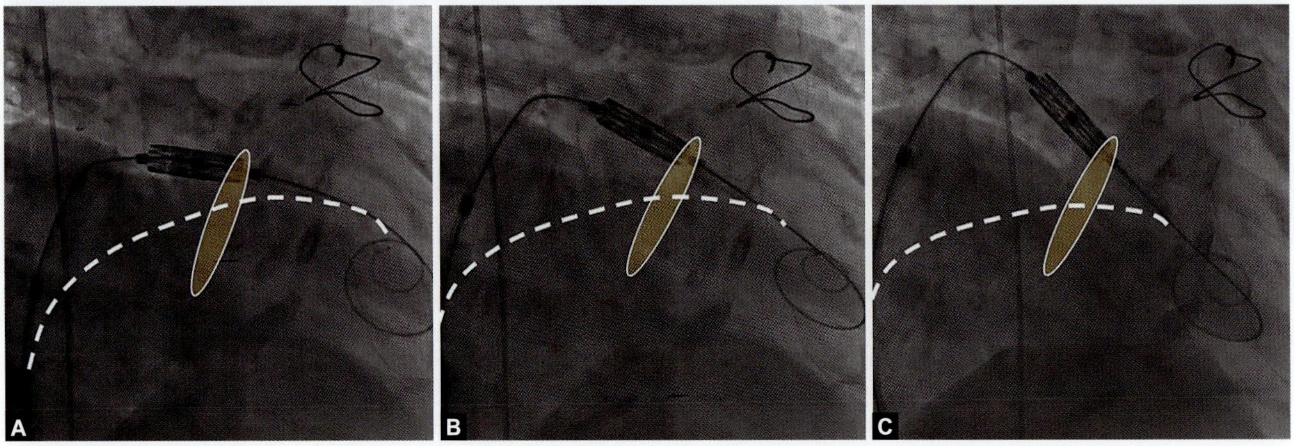

FIGS. 5A TO C: Right atrial buckling of the delivery system. Due to an unfavorable anterolateral wire bias progressive buckling of the delivery system in the right atrium as the operator further pushes is noticed. The dotted white line is the ideal wire position.

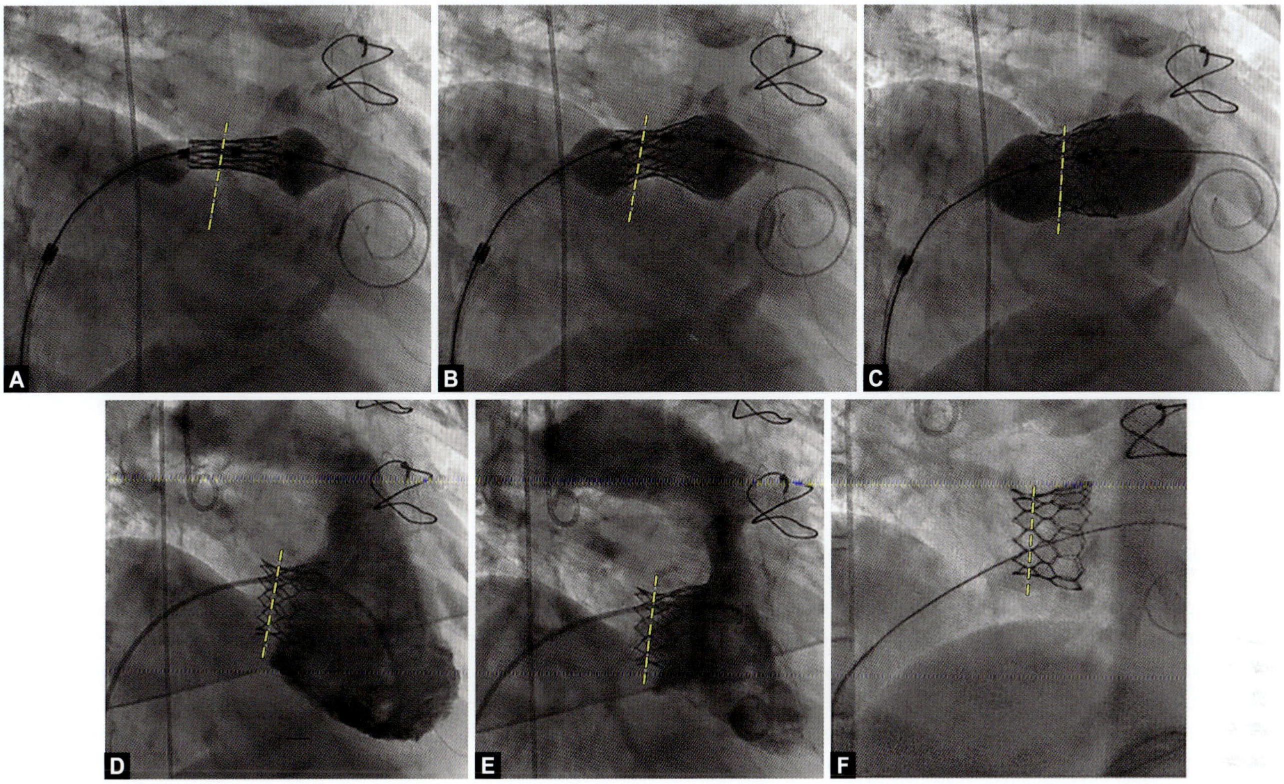

FIGS. 6A TO F: Tricuspid valve-in-valve implantation. (A) A 26 mm *Myval* is positioned with the figure of 8 sewing rings of the degenerated 27 mm Epic valve. (B) The navigator balloon is slowly inflated over 8–10 seconds without rapid ventricular pacing since the right ventricular pressure was normal due to stenotic physiology. (C) Complete deployment of the 26 mm *Myval*. (D and E) A pigtail right ventriculogram during diastole and systole shows the normal functioning of the *Myval*. (F) Fluoroscopic coplanar view confirms the ventricular and atrial flaring of the valve frames. A yellow dotted vertical line in all panels marks the bioprosthetic sewing ring corresponding to the landing zone.

CONCLUSION

Transcatheter M-ViV for a failed bioprosthetic valve is an established treatment modality in high-surgical-risk patients. The transseptal M-ViV procedure recently showed a promising 1-year outcome for intermediate-risk patients.[10] T-ViV is in its early stages though with limited available reports but shows promising outcomes.

ONLINE REFERENCES

Please scan the QR code provided at the end of the table of contents for References of this chapter.

CHAPTER

176

Transcatheter Therapies for Tricuspid Regurgitation: 2024

Rajendra Kumar Jain, Shirisha Reddy Kommareddy

ABSTRACT

Tricuspid regurgitation (TR) is a frequent and complex problem, commonly combined with left-sided heart disease, such as mitral regurgitation. Significant TR is associated with increased mortality if left untreated or recurs after therapy.[1] TR was historically often called the neglected valve and remained undertreated. Understanding that severe TR carries mortality independent of other variables has led to renewed interest in this condition. Newer classification systems for understanding the etiology and mechanism of TR have been proposed. A newly expanded grading system of TR includes massive and torrential TR in addition to previously used mild, moderate, and severe grades.

Surgery was traditionally the treatment option during left-sided valve surgery and had high mortality. Transcatheter therapies have been developed to overcome this and have proven to be effective in improving quality of life. TRI score is a recently developed tool to predict in-hospital mortality for isolated TR surgery and helps in decision-making.

In this chapter, we briefly describe anatomy, classification, grading, and various transcatheter therapies with their mechanisms for reducing TR.

Keywords: Tricuspid valve, tricuspid regurgitation, TRIC valve, transcatheter tricuspid valve replacement

INTRODUCTION

Significant tricuspid regurgitation (TR) affects ~1.6 million people in the United States.[2] TR is caused by pathology involving the tricuspid valve or primary TR and secondary or functional TR. Majority of patients had functional TR. TR leads to progressive right heart failure, RV dysfunction, decreased quality of life, and mortality. TR itself can be a predictor of adverse events independent of TV function, LVEF, PH, and associated left heart disease.[3]

Treatment of TR medically involved diuretics and rhythm control for AF patients. Tricuspid-valve surgery has a class I recommendation only for patients with severe TR at the time of left heart cardiac surgery according to American College of Cardiology guidelines.[4] The 2021 European Society of Cardiology and European Association for Cardio-Thoracic Surgery guidelines also mention surgery as a class I recommendation for symptomatic patients with severe isolated primary TR and without severe right ventricular dysfunction.[5]

Transcatheter therapies for the treatment of severe TR are evolving and can reduce TR severity. Various methods including repair systems to reduce the coaptation gap, annuloplasty, and replacement options are available. The transcatheter edge-to-edge repair (TEER) is the most commonly used device, and other devices are being developed.

ANATOMY

The tricuspid valve complex consists of leaflets, tricuspid annulus (TA), chordae tendineae, papillary muscles, and right atrial and ventricular myocardium. The tricuspid valve usually has three leaflets—septal, anterior, and posterior, as shown in **Figure 1**. The anterior leaflet extends from the anteroseptal commissure to the anterolateral papillary muscle. The septal leaflet is inserted into the fibrous portion of the TA. The posterior leaflet is inserted into the lower RV myocardium and its expansion is limited by the diaphragm; hence, TA dilation occurs predominantly in the anterolateral direction.[6]

There is variation in the number of leaflets. TV has been classified according to the number of leaflets as follows: Type I—three leaflets and type II—two leaflets. One study showed that three leaflets (type I) were seen in only 54% of the patients, four leaflets were seen in 39% of the patients, two leaflet configuration (type II) in 4.5% of the patients, and five leaflets in 2.4% of the patients.[7] Wider coaptation distance, smaller leaflet grasp area, and complex subvalvular anatomy with multiple jets may be some of the problems encountered during intervention with additional leaflets **(Fig. 2)**.

Tricuspid annulus is an elliptical structure and its posteroseptal portion is more apical than the anteroseptal one.

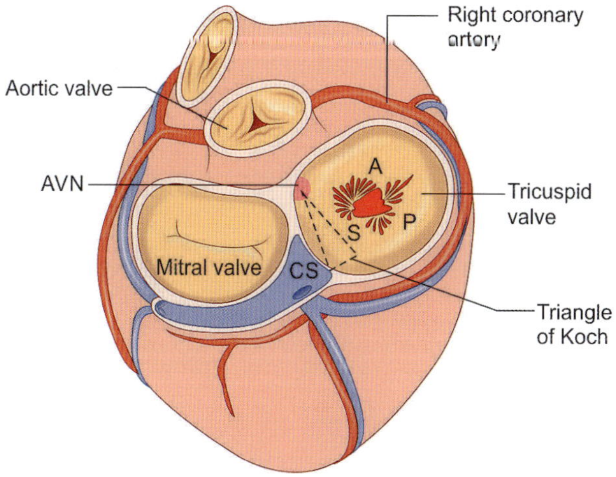

FIG. 1: Anatomy of tricuspid valve and surrounding regions.

The papillary muscles that support the leaflets are multiple and variably subdivided. Each papillary muscle connects to the homolateral leaflet by chordae tendineae. This is unlike LV papillary muscles wherein each supplies both leaflets. This leads to easy expansion of TA leading to functional TR.

Important structures surrounding the TV include the right coronary artery and AV node, which lie close to the TV and can be damaged during procedures as shown in **Figure 1**.

ETIOLOGY AND CLASSIFICATION OF TRICUSPID REGURGITATION

Tricuspid regurgitation has been classified as primary and secondary. Primary TR involves an intrinsic defect of the valve and secondary TR is due to changes in the right atrial and ventricular myocardium leading to TR with a normal valve structure. Cardiac implantable electronic device-related TR is an entity described in the recent classification systems as shown in **Table 1**.

CLINICAL PRESENTATION

Patients present with features of right heart failure like elevated JVP, exercise intolerance, hepatic congestion, ascites, and peripheral edema. Cardiohepatic syndrome (CHS) can occur in late stages. It is divided into two types—types 1 and 2. Type 1 is acute or ischemic and type 2 is chronic or congestive. CHS is often associated with cardiorenal syndromes. Patients who develop these are often unsuitable for intervention due to advanced disease.

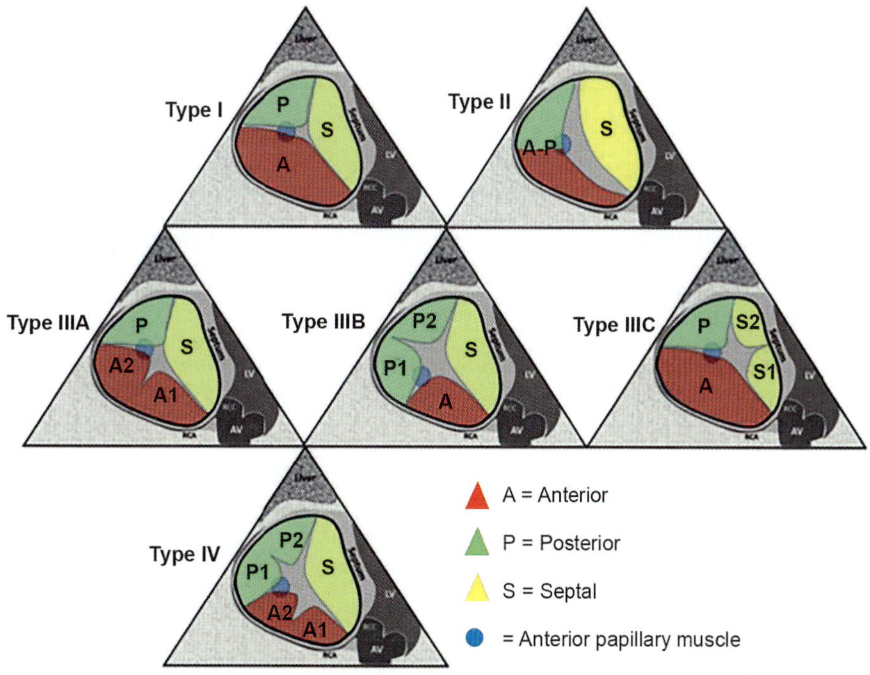

FIG. 2: Type I has three leaflets; type II has two leaflets; type III has four leaflets, further divided as type IIIA (two anterior), IIIB (two posterior), and IIIC (two septal); type IV with more than four leaflets.

Hahn R, Weckbach L, Noack T, et al. Proposal for a Standard Echocardiographic Tricuspid Valve Nomenclature. JACC Cardiovasc Imaging. 2021;14(7):1299-305.

IMAGING

Preprocedural planning is important for assessment of suitability and safety. 2D echo is useful for assessing etiology, severity of TR, RV size and function, LV EF, PH, and other valvular disorders. RV function is assessed by TAPSE, RV GLS, fractional area changes, and 3D EF. Accurate RV function assessment is crucial for determining prognosis. RV–PA coupling refers to the relationship between RV contractility and RV afterload. RV–PA uncoupling occurs when RV contractility cannot increase to match RV afterload, resulting in RV dysfunction and right heart failure. A higher TAPSE/PASP ratio carries a better prognosis.[9]

3D echo, which is becoming increasingly available, helps in better evaluation of the morphology of leaflets and surrounding structures **(Table 2)**.

Transesophageal echocardiogram (TEE) is used to assess TV leaflets, subvalvular apparatus, left-sided structures, and surrounding structures.

TABLE 1: Classification of tricuspid regurgitation.

Primary tricuspid regurgitation	Secondary tricuspid regurgitation	CIED-related tricuspid regurgitation
Congenital • Ebstein anomaly • Atrioventricular canal defects • Tricuspid valve dysplasia	Atrial functional • Normal LV systolic function • Severe atrial dilation • Absence of apical tethering of TV leaflets	CIED-induced leaflet impingement
Myxomatous degeneration	Ventricular functional due to left-sided disease • Left ventricular systolic dysfunction • Aortic valve disease • Mitral valve disease	
Systemic disease • Sarcoidosis • Lupus erythematosus • Rheumatic disease	Primary right ventricular disease • Right ventricular myopathy • RV ischemia • Arrhythmogenic right ventricular cardiomyopathy	
Malignancy • Carcinoid • Tumors involving the right heart	Severe primary pulmonary hypertension	
Infective endocarditis		
Iatrogenic causes • RV biopsy		
Chest wall trauma		
Drug induced		

Source: With permission from Agarwal and Hahn (2023).[8]

TABLE 2: Grading tricuspid regurgitation severity by echocardiography.

	Mild	Moderate	Severe	Massive	Torrential
Structural					
Right ventricle and right atrium size	Usually normal	Normal or mild dilation	Usually dilated	–	–
Inferior vena cava diameter	<2 cm	<2 cm or 2.1–2.5 cm	>2.5 cm	–	–
Qualitative					
Color flow jet area	Small, narrow, central	Moderate central	Large central	–	–
Continuous wave Doppler jet	Faint, often parabolic	Dense, parabolic, or triangular	Dense, often triangular	–	–
Semiquantitative					
Vena contracta width (mm)	<3.0	3.0–6.9	7–13	14–20	≥21
Quantitative					
Effective regurgitant orifice area (mm^2)	<20	20–29	40–59	60–79	≥80
Regurgitant volume (mL/beat)	<15	15–29	45–59	60–74	≥75

Source: With permission from Ambrosino et al. (2024).[10]

Intracardiac imaging (ICE) catheter is introduced via femoral vein and navigated into the heart for obtaining 2D and 3D images. It provides additional benefit during procedures.

CT is useful in patients undergoing intervention. It helps in evaluating TA size and location, coronary anatomy, and identifies fluoroscopy planes. SVC and IVC and their surrounding structures can be studied which is important in procedures like caval valve implantation (CAVI) for sizing and vascular access.

Cardiac MRI is useful for RV function, regurgitant fraction, and volume assessment. Leaflet structure, PH, presence of endocarditis, and fibrosis can be evaluated. Arrhythmias and pacemaker leads can produce artifacts during MRI.

Right heart catheterization is done for assessment of hemodynamics and is done in patients with severe PH. Patients with severe PH are considered high risk for intervention. PVR > 3 W units or PASP > 70 mm Hg are usually excluded.

MANAGEMENT (TABLE 3)

Surgical Therapy

Surgical therapy involves either repair or replacement of the tricuspid valve. It is usually done with left-sided valve surgery. Isolated TR surgery is rare.

Transcatheter Therapy

Transcatheter tricuspid valve repair (TTVr) systems—coaptation device, annuloplasty systems.

Transcatheter tricuspid valve replacement (TTVR) systems—heterotopic or orthotopic valves **(Fig. 3)**.

Coaptation Devices

Coaptation devices aim to reduce TR by increasing leaflet coaptation by cinching leaflets together or by filling the gap with a spacer. TEER has been the most commonly used repair system. It uses two clips to grasp the leaflets and reduce leaflet coaptation gap and thus reduce TR.

MitraClip System

Initially designed for mitral valve, it was used off-label for TR. It is the most common TTVr system used due to familiarity of use in MR patients.[6] It is a cobalt chromium polyester-covered system with two arms to grasp two leaflets. It uses a 24-French delivery system and can be delivered through transfemoral or transjugular access. Newer, MitraClip G4 is available now and allows for independent leaflet capture.

Predictors of the success of MitraClip on TR include, primary TR with valve prolapse or secondary TR with normal leaflets, central/anterolateral jet, coaptation depth < 10 mm, coaptation gap < 7.2 mm, leaflet length > 10 mm, and absence of global RV dysfunction.[12-14]

TABLE 3: Currently available transcatheter TR therapies and related trials.[6,11]

Mechanism		Device	Study/Trial
Coaptation devices	Edge-to-edge repair	MitraClip	
		TriClip	TRILUMINATE
		PASCAL	CLASP TR
		Mistral	
	Spacer devices	FORMA	SPACER
Annuloplasty devices	Direct ring	Cardioband	TRI-REPAIR, TriBAND
		IRIS Millipede ring	
	Indirect ring	TRAIPTA (transatrial intrapericardial tricuspid annuloplasty)	
	Direct suture	TRiAlign	SCOUT
		TriCinch	PREVENT
		PASTA (pledget-assisted suture tricuspid valve annuloplasty)	
TVR devices	Orthotopic valves	NaviGate	
		TriSOL	
		LUX-Valve	
		TriCares	
		EVO-QUE	TRISCEND
		Intrepid	
	Heterotopic valves	Sapien	
		TricValve	TRICUS
		Tricento	

TriClip

It is similar to MitraClip using leaflet grasp method and has a steerable guiding catheter suitable for the right heart. TriClip G4 has been developed for TR with four different clip sizes.

TRILUMINATE study done in 85 patients with moderate or greater TR. TR was reduced to moderate or less in 60% and at least one grade reduction in 85%.[15]

PASCAL Device

It can be used for both mitral and tricuspid valves. It has a central spacer and arms to grasp leaflets. Spacer fills the regurgitant orifice and reduces TR.[16]

The CLASP TR trial done in 34 patients showed procedural success in 85%, and 70% patients had at least two TR grade reduction at 30 days. Improvement was noted in echo parameters, specifically the PISA, EROA, and vena contracta width.[17]

The FORMA Spacer Device

FORMA spacer device is a foam-filled polymer balloon that provides a surface for native leaflets to coapt.[18] It is delivered from the left subclavian vein through a rail anchored at the septal portion of the RV apex.[19] The rail is also anchored to the subclavian vein. This was studied in 29 patients. The device was implanted in 27 patients and explanted in 2 patients, one due to migration and the other due to infection.[20] 31% MAE occurred at 30-day follow-up. Improvement in TR and echo (EROA, vena contracta width) parameters is shown. The device is depicted in **Figure 4**.[18]

Some of the emerging coaptation devices are Mistral Device, CroíValve, and Cerclage-TR block **(Fig. 5)**.

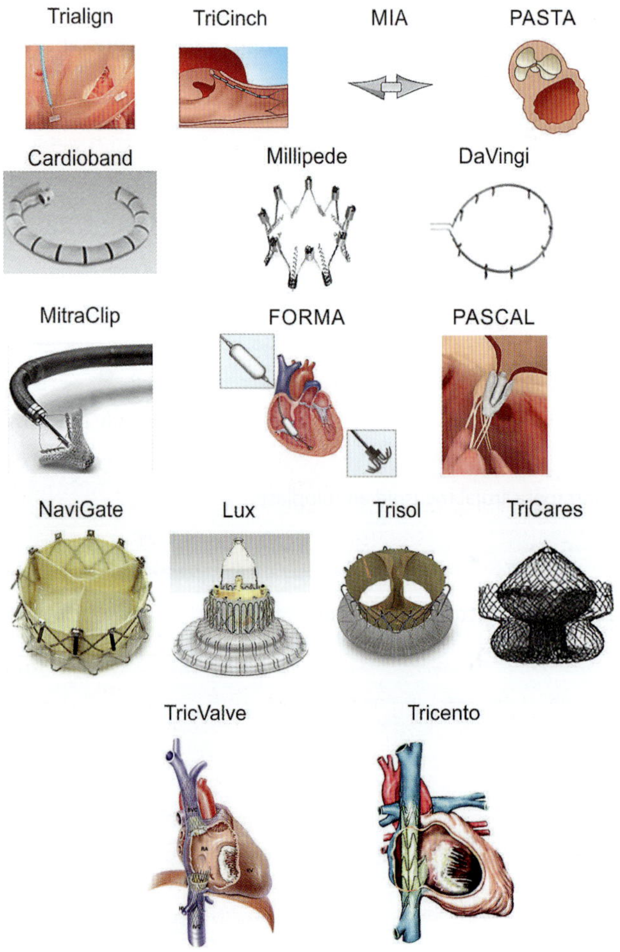

FIG. 3: Transcatheter tricuspid landscape.

Annuloplasty Device

Annuloplasty device aims to reduce annulus diameter and mimic its surgical counterpart. Its advantage is that it preserves leaflet structure. It can be combined with other procedures.

Direct Ring Annuloplasty

- *Cardioband*: This device (as shown in **Figs. 6 and 7**) improves TR via annular size reduction. It consists of a polyester sleeve with radiopaque markers. 12–17 stainless steel anchors are implanted through the sleeve along the annulus. The implant is cinched to reduce the size of annulus. It was previously used for patients with functional MR.

  TRI-REPAIR trial was conducted on 30 patients over a period of 6 months. The device was successfully implanted in all the patients. Complications included three deaths (one device-related due to RV obstruction), cardiac tamponade, pacemaker requirement, VT, stroke, renal failure, and bleeding. The triband trial also showed favorable outcomes at discharge and at 30 days.
- *IRIS Millipede ring*: The millipede ring is a complete semirigid annuloplasty ring made of nitinol. It has eight anchors that fix the device to the TA. It has integrated intracardiac echo. This device is currently under development.[23]

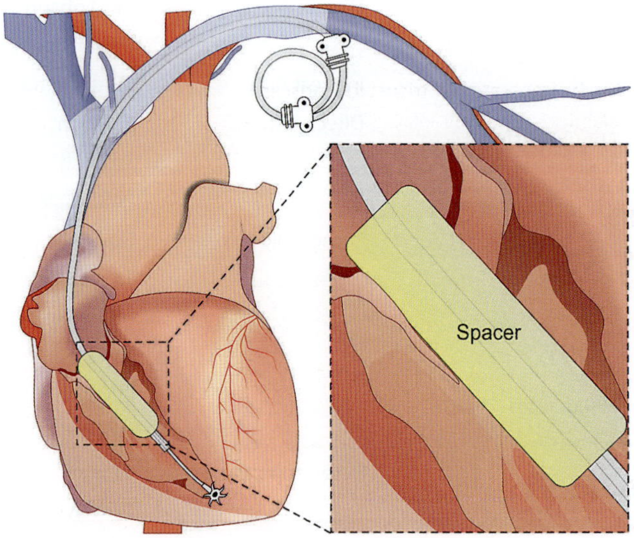

FIG. 4: TR and echo parameters.

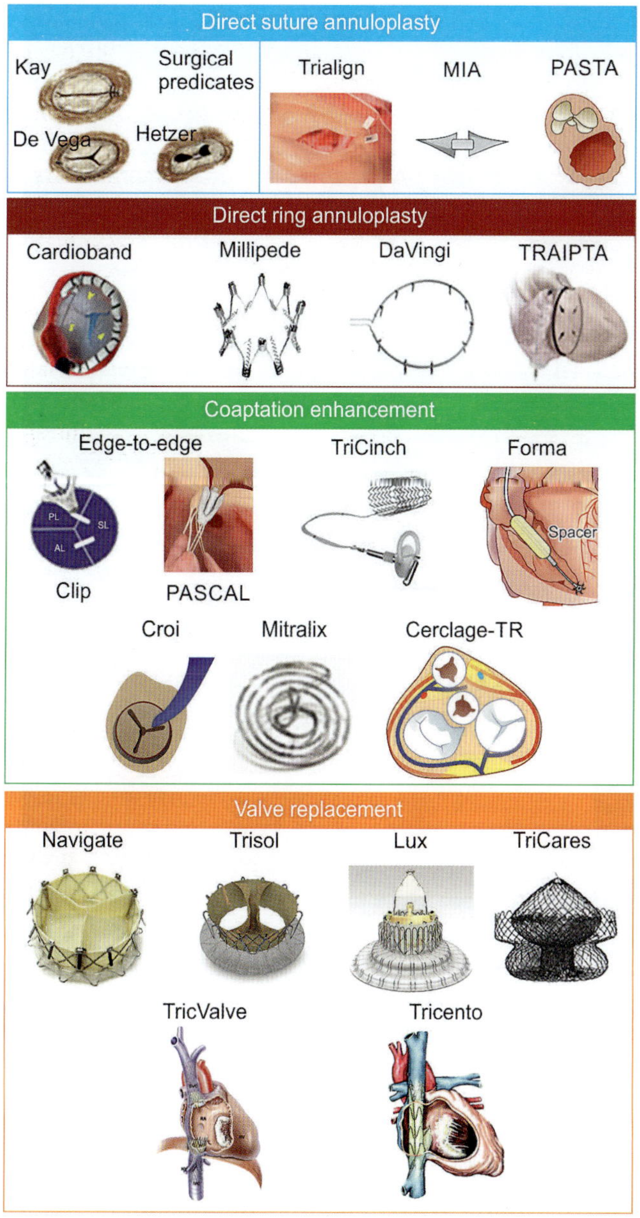

FIG. 5: Transcatheter tricuspid landscape.

(MIA: minimally invasive annuloplasty; PASTA: pledget-assisted suture tricuspid valve annuloplasty; TRAIPTA: transatrial intrapericardial tricuspid annuloplasty)

Indirect Annuloplasty

- Transatrial intrapericardial tricuspid annuloplasty (TRIAPTA): It is a circumferential implant and exerts a compressive force to reduce the TA size[6,24] as shown in **Figure 8**. The pericardium is accessed by puncturing the RA appendage, and nitinol loop of the device is opened inside the pericardium to encircle the heart. The RA appendage defect is closed by a closure device.

Direct Suture Annuloplasty

- *Trialign system*: It mimics the modified Kay surgical technique, that is, obliteration of the posterior leaflet making a tricuspid valve into a bicuspid valve. Pledgets are fixed at the posteroseptal and anteroposterior commissure and cinched resulting in plication of posterior leaflets. RCA angiography is performed to check for complications. The SCOUT trial[26] enrolled 15 patients. One patient required RCA stenting, and three pledget detachments occurred in the remaining patients. Reduction of TR is noted and an increase in LV stroke volume was observed.

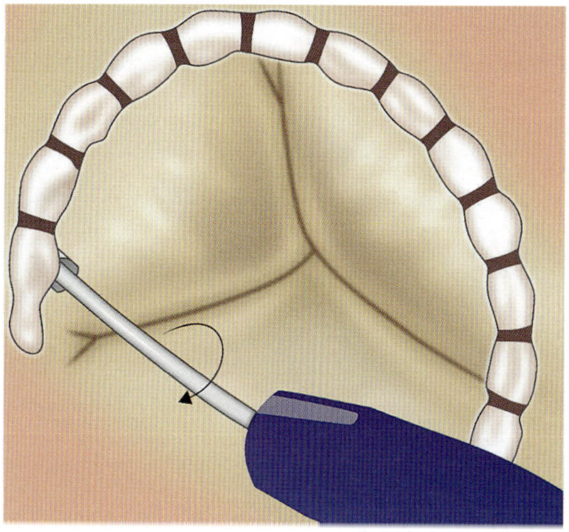

FIG. 6: Cardioband device.

Source: With permission from Arnold et al. (2021).[21]

- *The TriCinch system*: The TriCinch system consists of two components—stainless steel screw that is placed in the anteroposterior portion of the TA and a self-expandable nitinol stent. This device is placed via the transfemoral route. RCA angio is needed to rule out RCA damage. The PREVENT[27] study was done in 24 patients and successfully implanted in 18 patients. One TR grade reduction is observed in 94%. Complications such as hemopericardium 2 patients, RCA damage 1 patient, and late annular detachment 5 patients were noted.
- *Minimally invasive annuloplasty-tricuspid (MIA-T)*: It consists of ultra-low-mass polymeric, biocompatible PolyCor anchors that are tensed by thermoplastic MyoLast polymer. It is designed to obliterate the posterior leaflet.
- *PASTA*: This is similar to the Hetzer double orifice suture technique. This was first implanted in an 84-year-old man, with torrential TR and RV dysfunction. The patient was discharged with recurrence of severe TR.[28]
- *DaVingi tricuspid regurgitation system*: This system offers a two-stage procedure to reduce the tricuspid annular size. In the first part, a flexible ring is placed in the annulus featuring a balloon and by firing all the anchors simultaneously, and the adjustment chord is fixed at IJV. The chronic healing secures the implant to the tissue. In the second part, cinching of the annulus is performed using a 16-French adjustment tool.

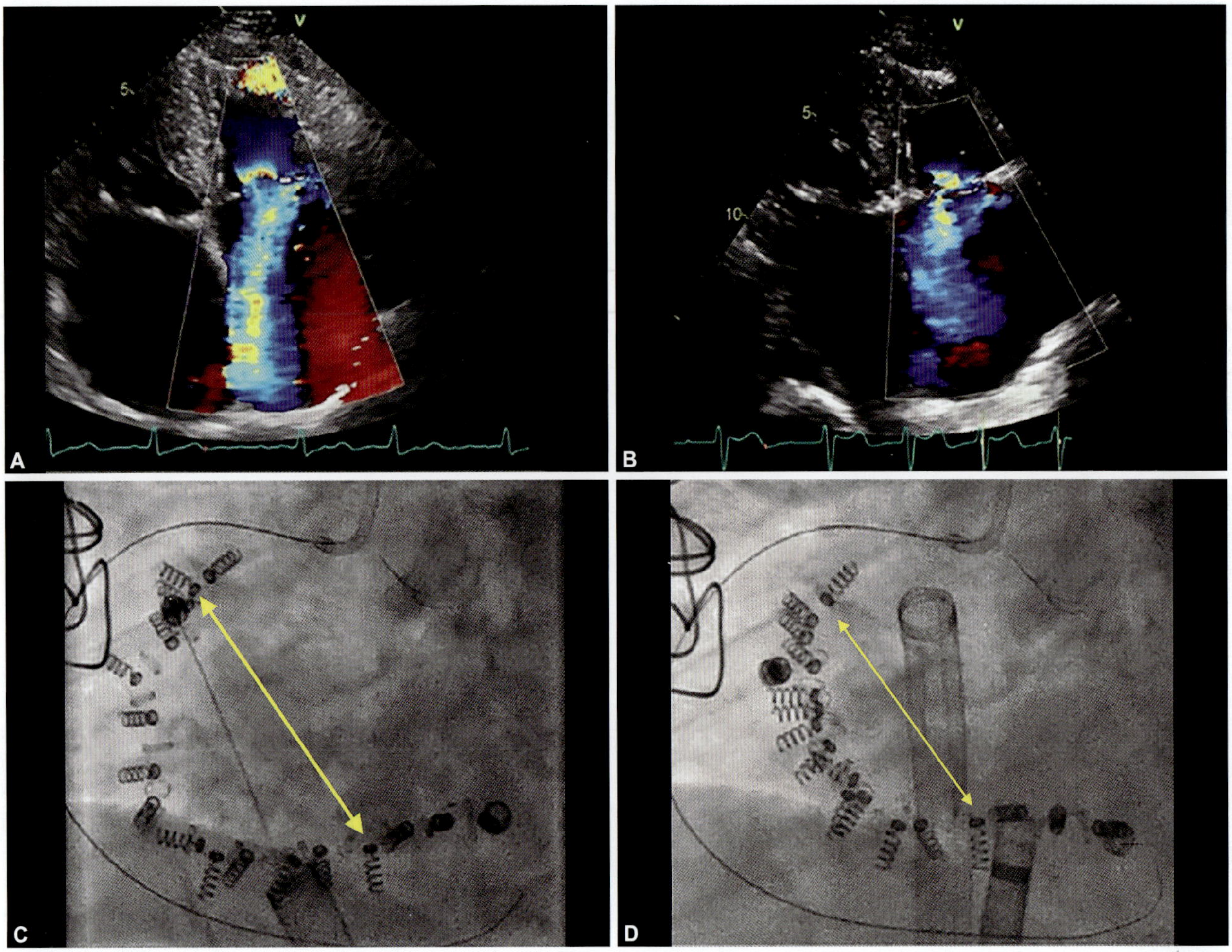

FIGS. 7A TO D: Apical four-chamber view showing severe tricuspid regurgitation at baseline (A) reduced to mild immediately after implantation (B). Left anterior oblique projection demonstrating the direct annuloplasty implanted before (C) and after (D) contraction with resulting decrease in the annular size (shown in yellow).
Source: With permission from Simard and Eleid (2022).[22]

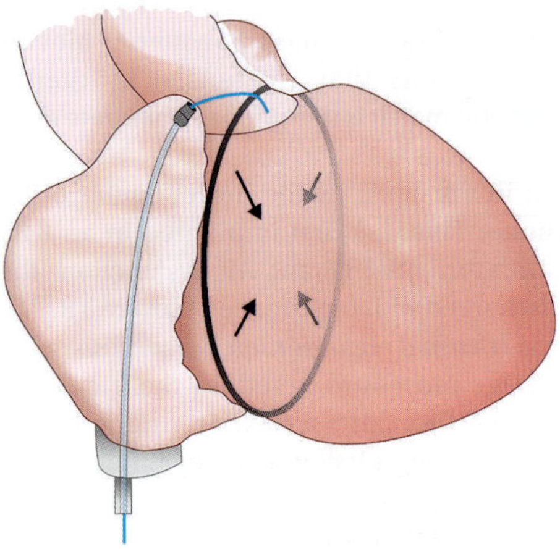

FIG. 8: TRAIPTA.
Source: With permission from Asmarats et al. (2018).[25]

Transcatheter Tricuspid Valve Replacement

There are two types of TTVR—orthotopic and heterotopic. Orthotopic valves are placed in the TA and heterotopic is a prosthetic device placed in SVC or IVC.

Orthotopic valves require favorable anatomy. Large annulus, coaptation gap, device leads, etc., can pose challenges during implantation.

Orthotopic Tricuspid Valve Replacement

- *NaviGate:* It is a self-expanding tricuspid bioprosthesis as shown in **Figures 9A and B**. It is an atrioventricular valved stent with trileaflet design. It is conical in shape and reduces a transvalvular gradient and minimizes right ventricular outflow tract (RVOT) obstruction. It requires a 42-French delivery catheter via transtubular access. Transatrial approach can also be done through minimally invasive thoracotomy.

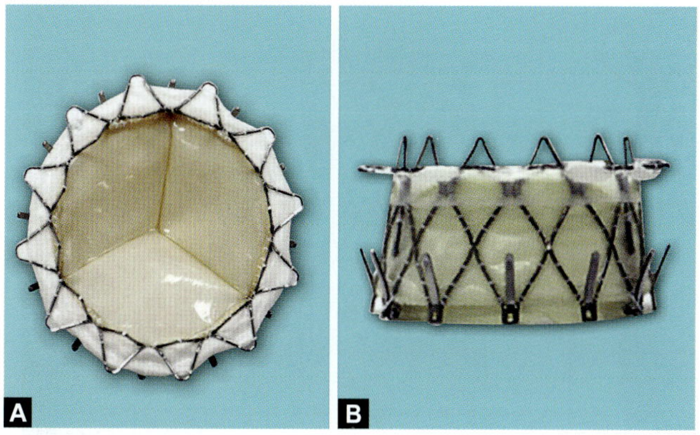

FIGS. 9A AND B: NaviGate inflow and lateral views.
Source: With permission from Asmarats et al. (2018).[25]

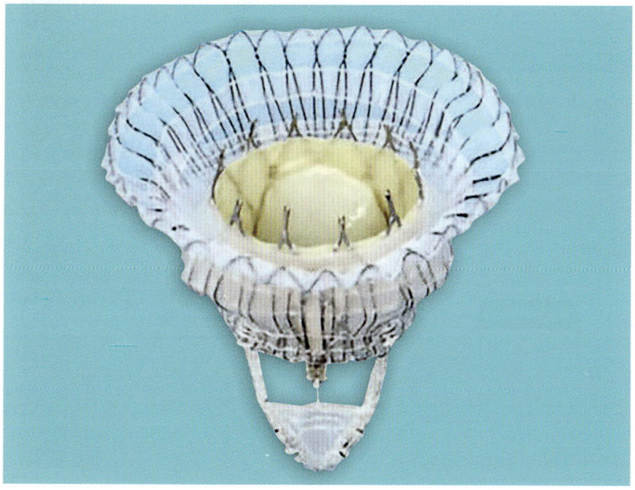

FIG. 10: Atrial view of LUX-Valve.
Source: With permission from Ning et al. (2022).[29]

- *LUX valve:* Valve is delivered using minithoracotomy using a transatrial approach **(Fig. 10)**.
- *TriSol*: TriSol consists of an atrial polyester skirt and a ventricular porcine pericardial skirt. The dome-shaped leaflet of the valve is made of bovine pericardium and creates a bileaflet valve. It is delivered via a 30-French steerable delivery system, and its valve is retrievable and repositionable. The first-in-human case is reported from Israel.
- *EVOQUE system*: It is the largest prosthesis available in trials and is 52 mm. It resembles its mitral counterpart. It consists of a nitinol self-expanding frame, bovine pericardial leaflets, and a fabric skirt to minimize paravalvular leaks. It has a 28-French delivery sheath.[6] The initial experience with 25 patients showed a 92% device success with TR reduction to <1% in 92% of the patients.[30] The TRISCEND trial showed 3.2% all-cause mortality at 6 months in 132 patients. 100% of the patients had mild or less TR post procedure. Improvement in quality of life and NYHA class was also noted.
- *Intrepid*: The Intrepid is composed of a nitinol frame with tri-leaflet bovine pericardium. It uses a 35-French sheath. It was first presented as a compassionate use in three patients.

Heterotopic Valves

In this strategy, the valve is deployed in the SVC or IVC to limit the effects of severe TR on surrounding organs but sparing the right atrium. CAVI uses both self-expandable and balloon-expandable devices. The backflow into the SVC is low compared to the IVC due to the hydrostatic pressure. Hence, CAVI with balloon-expandable valves is performed only in the IVC. CAVI suitability includes the presence of pulsatile caval backflow and adequate vena cava measurements (≤30 mm for balloon expandable and <42 mm for self-expandable valves).

Some of the heterotopic valves are:
- Sapien Valve
- TricValve
- TriCentro

Sapien valve: It is used for severe aortic stenosis patients and is a balloon-expandable valve. It has been implanted either in SVC or in both SVC and IVC after deploying a stent in vena cavae for anchoring. This was an off-label use. TRICAVAL study compared CAVI versus GDMT in patients with severe TR, high surgical risk, and NYHA class > II. Patients with severe LV dysfunction and CKD and IVC landing zone diameter exceeding 31 mm were excluded. Prosthesis was successfully installed in all the patients. The trial was stopped prematurely due to high failure rates.

TricValve: As depicted in **Figure 11**, the TricValve device consists of two pericardial tissue, self-expandable valves on a nitinol stent frame, one for SVC and another for IVC. The IVC valve has an upper segment protruding into the right atrium and the biological valve located above the diaphragm to prevent backflow into hepatic veins. For the SVC valve, the stent frame has a funnel shape with upper and lower segments tapered to facilitate fixation at the cavo-atrial inflow. The proximal stent segment is mounted with a tri-leaflet woven pericardial valve.

TriCentro: The TriCentro CAVI device consists of a bicavally anchored nitinol stent deployed top-down from SVC into IVC. A lateral bicuspid porcine pericardial valve allows implant into the right atrium. The device needs to be custom-made for each patient.

PATIENT SELECTION/DEVICE SELECTION (FLOWCHART 1)

A heart team approach is ideal for patient selection. Isolated severe TR patients who are symptomatic despite

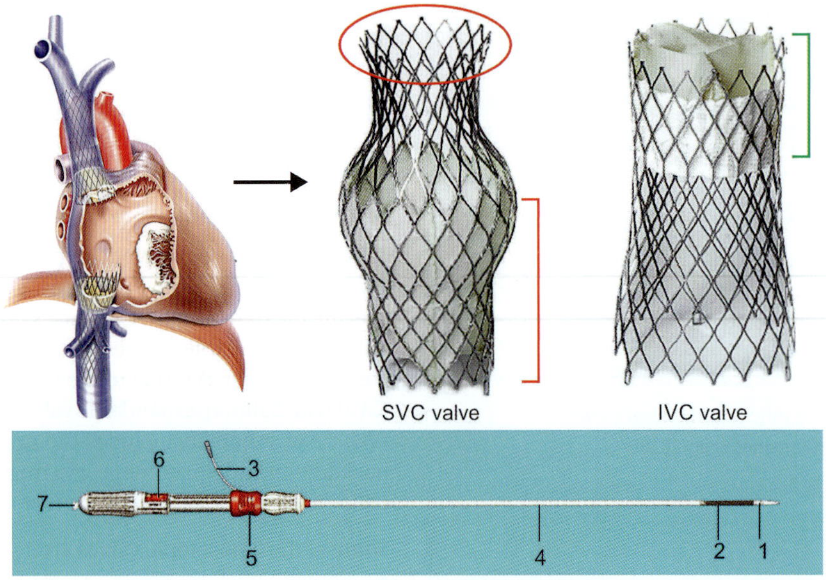

FIG. 11: 1—Catheter tip, 2—capsule, 3—tube flush port, 4—catheter shaft, 5—macro slider, 6—micro knob, and 7—Luer lock connector flush port.

Source: With permission from Wong et al. (2022).[31]

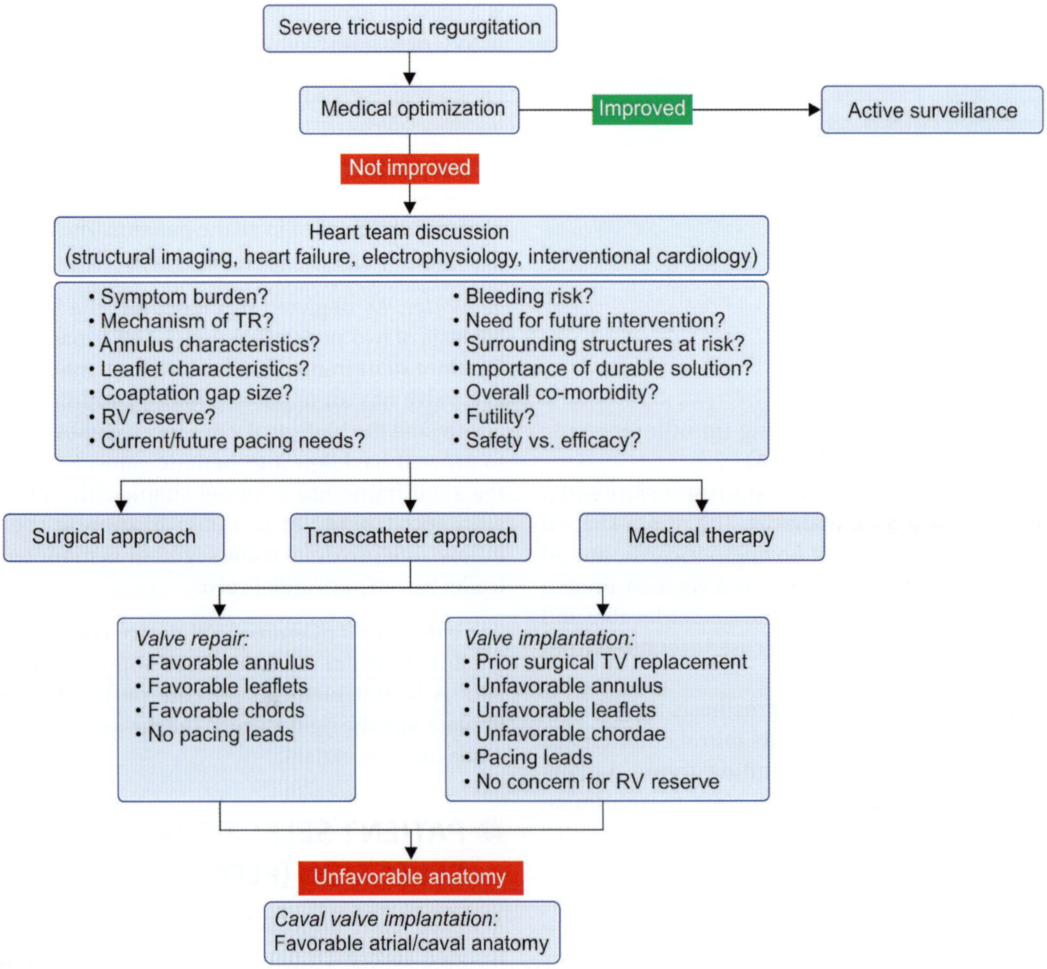

FLOWCHART 1: Patient selection/device selection.

Source: With permission from Seligman et al. (2023).[32]

medical therapy and at high surgical risk are considered. TRI-SCORE helps in decision making where high score patients are unsuitable. Once a patient is deemed suitable for transcatheter procedure, various clinical and anatomical features help in choosing the correct device as shown in the algorithm below.

TRI-SCORE[33]

TRI-SCORE is a simple risk-score model to predict outcomes after isolated tricuspid valve surgery for severe TR at an individual level based on preoperative clinical, biological, and echocardiographic presentation. It has been developed from 466 adult patients who underwent isolated TV surgery on native valve for noncongenital severe TR. Its aim is to guide the clinical decision-making process in routine practice.

Parameters:
- Age ≥ 70 years
- NYHA functional class III or IV
- Right-sided heart failure signs
- Daily dose of furosemide ≥ 125 mg
- eGFR < 30 mL/min
- Elevated total bilirubin
- LVEF < 60%
- Moderate/severe right ventricular dysfunction

TRI-SCORE is a good prognostic score and the higher the score, the poorer the outcome irrespective of the treatment modality.

A summary of factors affecting device choice in the transcatheter treatment of severe TR is given in **Table 4**.

EXAMPLE FROM OUR EXPERIENCE WITH TRIC VALVE

A patient who is a case of CRHD, s/p DVR in 1999 who presented with severe TR, moderate PAH- had AF with CVR and good LV function. She underwent successful TRIC valve implantation as shown in **Figures 12 and 13**.

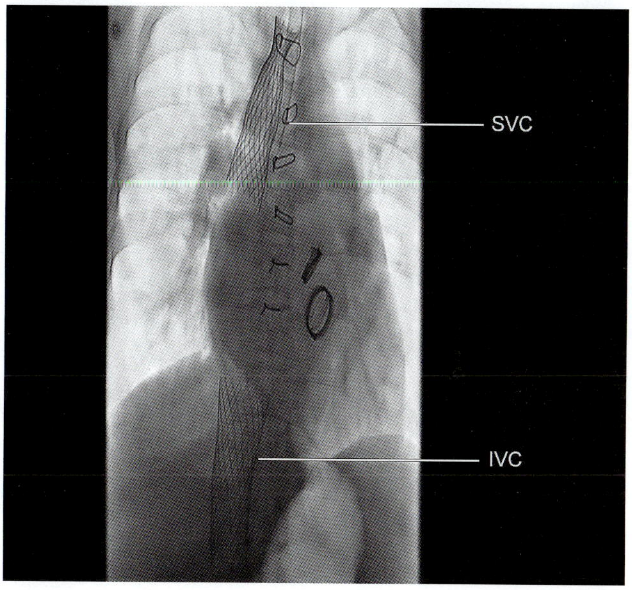

FIG. 12: Fluoroscopic image showing TRIC valve position in SVC and IVC.

TABLE 4: Summary of factors affecting device choice in the treatment of severe TR.

Domain	Valve replacement	Coaptation device	Annular device
Etiology	Suits most etiology patterns where annular dimensions do not exceed the device's own sizing	Pure annular dilation with coaptation defect of ≤10.0 mm without excessive leaflet tethering	Pure annular dilation with coaptation defect of ≤10.0 mm without excessive leaflet tethering
RV dysfunction	Caution in severe RV dysfunction as TR completely abolished—loss of "pop-off" phenomenon	Better suited to patients with RV dysfunction	Better suited to patients with RV dysfunction
Presence of pacemaker lead	Affects implantation but can safely be jailed by some devices	Affects imaging and strategy	Affects imaging
Contraindication to anticoagulation	Avoid in this cohort	Acceptable in this cohort	Acceptable in this cohort
Damage to surrounding structures	Caution in those where coronary damage or heart block would be especially poorly tolerated	Acceptable in this cohort	Acceptable in this cohort
Need for future procedures	Limits options for reintervention but valve-in-valve approach, likely possible	Limit options for reintervention but electrosurgical detachment might be possible	Least restrictive on future procedures
Durability	Untested, concern about risk of deterioration and thrombosis due to bulkiness and low flow	Untested	Untested
Safety versus efficacy	Greater efficacy but more invasive	Often only 1–2 grades TR reduction but less invasive	Often only 1–2 grades TR reduction but less invasive

Source: With permission from Seligman et al. (2023).[32]

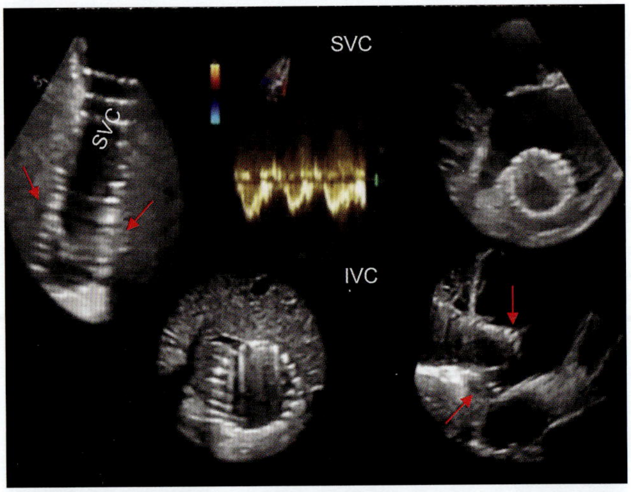

FIG. 13: 2-D echo showing TricValve in SVC and IVC.

CONCLUSION

Patients with severe TR need to be closely followed up as it carries significant mortality. Surgery can be considered in early stages and during other concomitant surgeries. Newer risk score models like TRI-SCORE are available and help in predicting mortality for isolated TR surgery. Heart team approach should be made based on hemodynamics, NYHA class, and various imaging methods to aid in the type of TTVI. TTVI is done in the form of repair (reduce leaflet gap, annuloplasty) or replacement. TEER is the most commonly done procedure with positive results. TricValve is the most common heterotopic valve done in high-risk patients not suitable for other devices.

Recent advances in imaging and treatment options have renewed interest in treating this important condition. Due to high surgical risk, TTVI offers an alternative. Transcatheter therapies have shown reduction in NYHA class and improvement in quality of life. TTVI should be considered early in the course of the disease and patients should be referred to a valve center.

ONLINE REFERENCES

Please scan the QR code provided at the end of the table of contents for References of this chapter.

CHAPTER

177

Transcatheter Mitral Valve Repair for Mitral Regurgitation: Is it Now Choice for Selected Patients

Balbir Singh, Sneha Garg

ABSTRACT

Transcatheter mitral edge-to-edge repair (TEER) is a well-established procedure for managing mitral regurgitation (MR) in high-risk patients. It has proven effective in treating both primary and secondary MR, as documented in surgical and interventional literature. Over time, TEER has become increasingly popular, demonstrating success across various anatomical conditions. Its minimally invasive nature, coupled with a strong safety profile and immediate hemodynamic improvements, suggests potential benefits for high-risk populations often excluded from major clinical trials. These patients, typically considered unsuitable for surgery, are usually managed conservatively, despite growing evidence that reducing MR through TEER could lead to clinical improvement. This includes cases such as postmyocardial infarction MR, patients with hypertrophic obstructive cardiomyopathy, and those experiencing recurrent MR after surgical intervention. This chapter also explores the use of TEER beyond its established indications, assessing outcomes and limitations in a range of patient populations. Further research is needed to evaluate the benefits of TEER in clinical scenarios outside its current indications.

Keywords: Mitral regurgitation, TEER, MitraClip

INTRODUCTION

Mitral regurgitation (MR) is common valvular lesion and leads to poor prognosis both short term and long term. MR leads to symptoms of heart failure (HF), left ventricular (LV) enlargement, and fall in LV ejection fraction (LVEF) over a period of time.

Mitral regurgitation is of two types:

1. *Primary MR*: is caused due to damage to the mitral valve apparatus (leaflets, chordae tendineae, papillary muscles, and/or annulus).
2. *Secondary MR*: The mitral valve apparatus is normal, and MR is attributable to a dilated left ventricle, which causes papillary muscle displacement, leading to annular displacement and consequent MR.

Many patients with MR are at a high surgical risk due to LV dysfunction, age, pulmonary disease, or frailty, hence the need for transcatheter procedures. In the 1990s, Ottavio Alfieri developed the edge-to-edge repair technique, a groundbreaking method for restoring mitral valve function in complex cases. By improving leaflet coaptation, this technique proved effective across various causes of regurgitation and quickly became the most versatile method for mitral valve repair. Its simplicity also paved the way for the development of transcatheter mitral edge-to-edge repair (TEER), which has become the most successful percutaneous approach for treating MR. Edge-to-edge repair has been the procedure after the first in-man study in 2003. After the initial slow development, it got the CE approval in 2008 and FDA approval in 2013 (for primary MR) and 2019 (for secondary MR).[1]

Current guidelines recommend TEER as a safe alternative for patients with severe MR who are either contraindicated for surgery or at high operative risk. Several registries and two randomized trials have assessed the impact of TEER in patients with severe secondary MR (SMR) compared to guideline-directed medical therapy—the MITRA-FR[2] (Multicenter Randomized Study of Percutaneous Mitral Valve Repair MitraClip Device in Patients With Severe Secondary Mitral Regurgitation) and COAPT[3] (Cardiovascular Outcomes Assessment of the MitraClip Percutaneous Therapy for Heart Failure Patients with Functional Mitral Regurgitation) trials. The MITRA-FR study found no improvement in outcomes, while the COAPT trial demonstrated a mortality benefit for TEER. Due to these conflicting results, subsequent guidelines recommend TEER for selected patients with severe SMR who meet the COAPT inclusion criteria. TEER is an appealing option for high-risk populations who do not meet the COAPT criteria, thanks to its minimally invasive nature, strong safety profile, and often immediate hemodynamic improvement. This includes patients needing urgent mitral intervention and patients with complex mitral anatomies, advanced HF, cardiomyopathies, or congenital heart disease (CHD). However, it is important to recognize the diversity within these high-risk groups and understand that the supporting evidence for TEER may vary depending on the specific underlying causes or mechanisms of MR **(Fig. 1)**.

PREPROCEDURAL EVALUATION AND CASE SELECTION

Case selection is extremely important for the success of procedure:

- *Clinical assessment:* Procedure is reserved for Class III–IV patients having symptomatic status despite guideline-directed medical treatment; 6-minute walk is useful for baseline assessment.
- *Transthoracic echocardiography:* It is essential to assess the degree of MR to distinguish between primary- and secondary-cause MR. Several parameters can be used to assess the degree of MR, most important are regurgitant volume and vena contracta. In addition, assessing LV dimensions, LVEF, pulmonary artery pressures, and RV function are important part of entire assessment scheme.
- *Heart team approach:* For primary MR, the high-risk surgical patients should be offered TEER and rest should be offered a surgical MV repair. For secondary MR, selecting COAPT-like patients for TEER **(Box 1)**:
    - Ischemic or nonischemic cardiomyopathy with a LVEF of 20–50%,
    - Moderate-to-severe secondary MR and remained symptomatic (New York Heart Association (NYHA) functional class II, III, or IVa (ambulatory)] despite the use of guideline-directed medical therapy and cardiac resynchronization therapy (if appropriate)

Procedural Steps:

1. *Femoral venous puncture:* It is done with ultrasound guidance with patient in general anesthesia, ventilated,

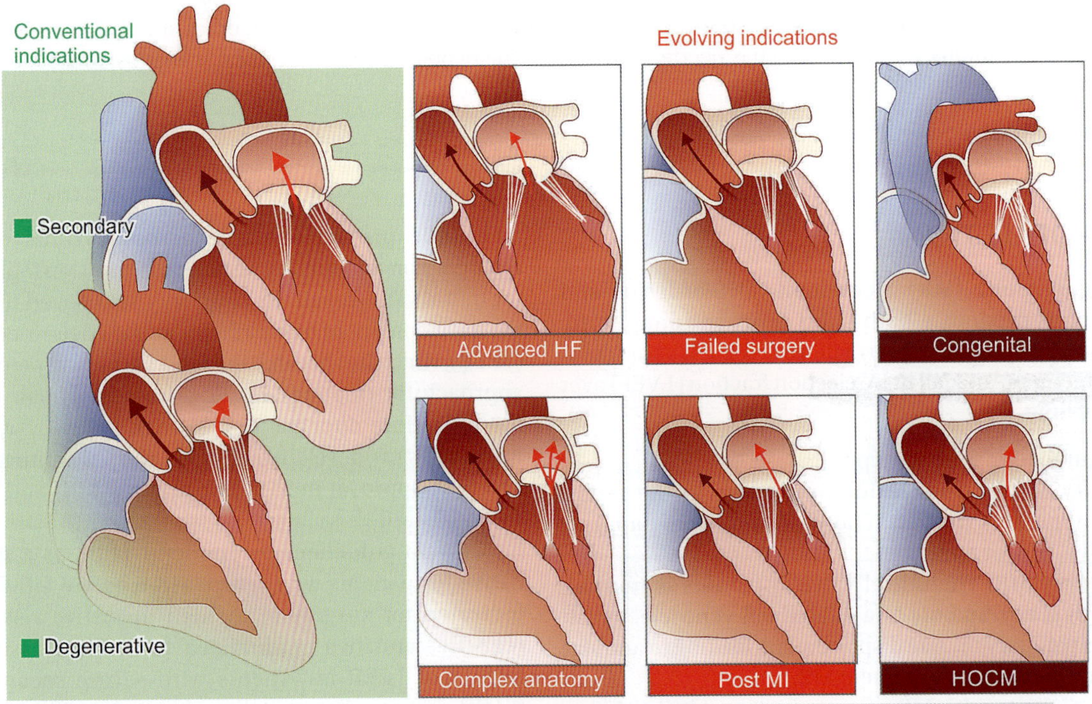

Conventional and evolving indications for TEER, according to the available supportive data, from the most established (advanced HF and complex anatomy, depicted in orange) to the more limited evidence (HOCM and congenital heart disease, represented in dark red).

FIG. 1: Clinical indications for Mitral TEER.[4]

(HF: heart failure; HOCM: hypertrophic obstructive cardiomyopathy; MI: myocardial infarction; TEER: transcatheter mitral edge-to-edge repair)

Source: Shuvy et al. (2024).

BOX 1 The inclusion and exclusion criteria of the COAPT trial.[3]

Major inclusion criteria:
- The primary jet originates from the malcoaptation of A2–P2.

Major exclusion criteria:
- MV orifice area < 4 cm^2
- Severe MV calcification
- Calcification at tips of A2–P2 at the site of grasp
- Cleft mitral leaflets
- Previous MV surgery
- History of rheumatic MV
- Presence of LA thrombus or vegetations
- Leaflet length <8 mm

and TEE probe inserted. After which half dose of heparin is given **(Fig. 2)**.

2. *Transseptal puncture:* It is done with TEE guidance using bicaval and X-plane at the needle position. It is imperative to direct this puncture inferiorly and posteriorly to obtain the best trajectory to enter the mitral valve. **Figure 3** depicts the bicaval view with needle being pulled down to achieve an inferior position.
3. Introducing the steerable guiding catheter over, generally, Amplatz wire or a Safari wire. **Figures 4 and 5** depict the guiding sheath in the LA with the clip being pushed up in the sheath.
4. Medial flexing of the steering handle leads to clip facing towards the mitral valve, this is confirmed on TEE examination **(Fig. 6)**.

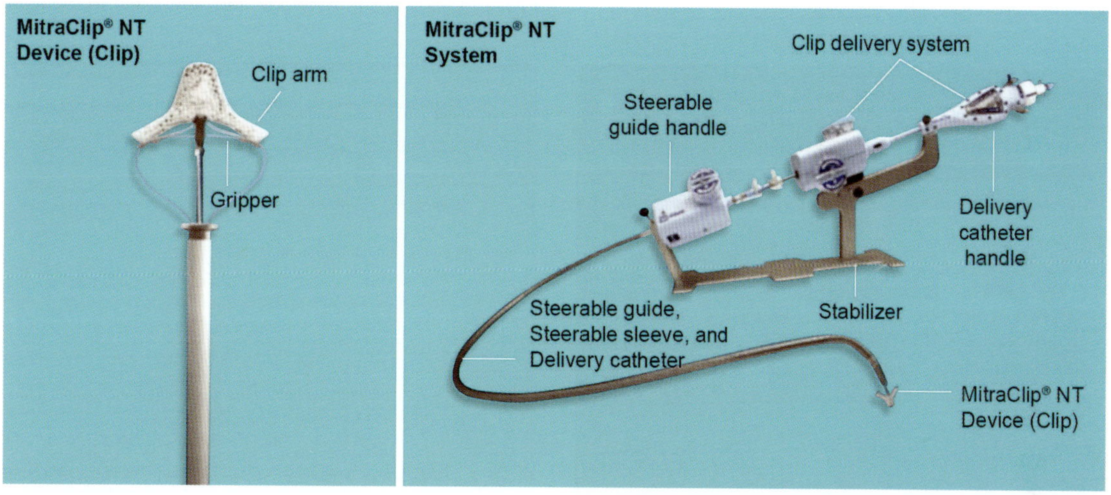

FIG. 2: Mitra Clip comes in NT and XT shapes, the difference is in only the length of the arm, another dimension has been added, which is the width of the clip; extra wide clip is called NTW or XTW. The clip also has gripers that hold on to valve leaflet. Steerable guide handle which is 24F can be steered in anterior and posterior directions. Clip delivery system allows delivery of clip and movements in medial and lateral directions along counterclockwise or clockwise directions. Clip delivery handle has controls for grippers, opening or closing of clip, and final release.

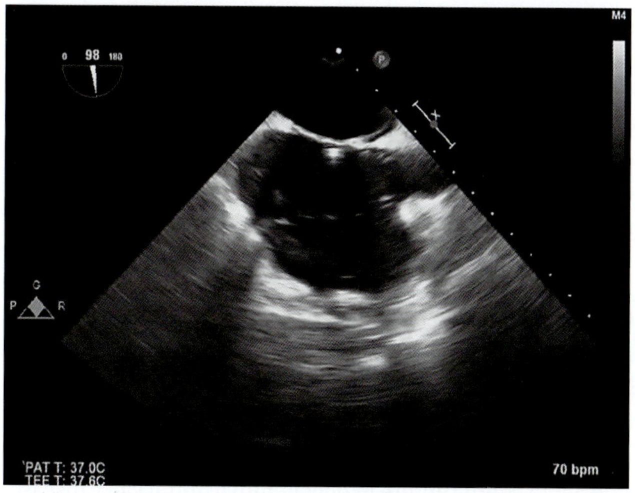

FIG. 3: Bicaval view on TEE for transseptal puncture.

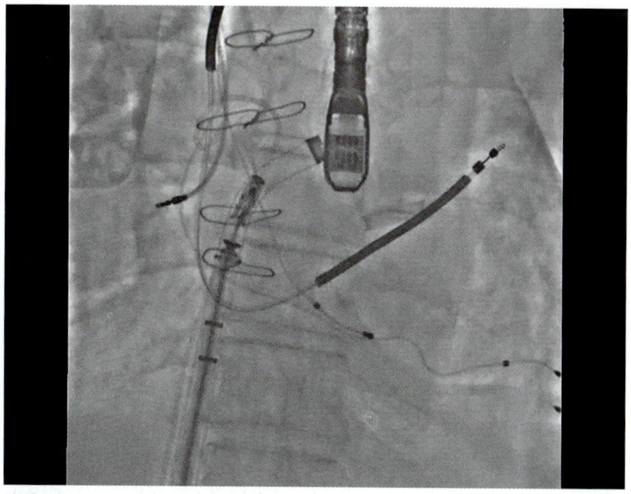

FIG. 4: Steerable guide catheter in LA.

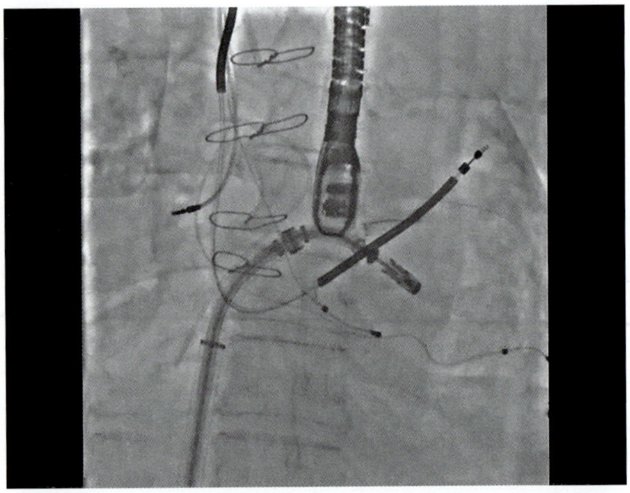

FIG. 5: Clip being pushed in LA.

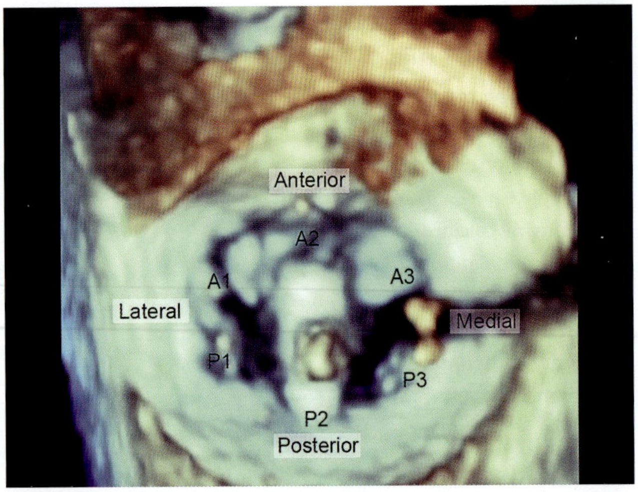

FIG. 7: Clip is positioned to be perpendicular to the leaflets.

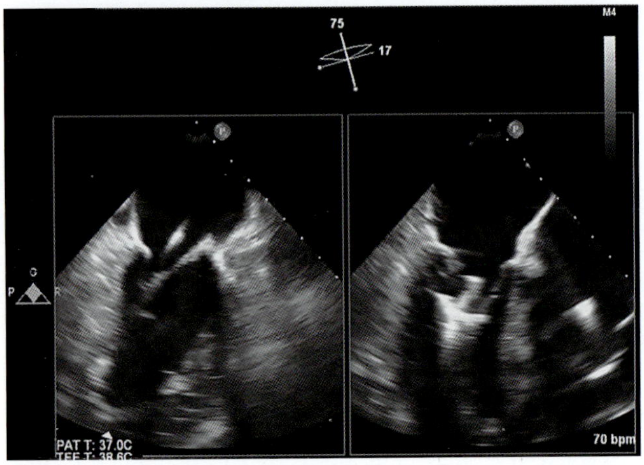

FIG. 6: Clip facing toward the mitral valve.

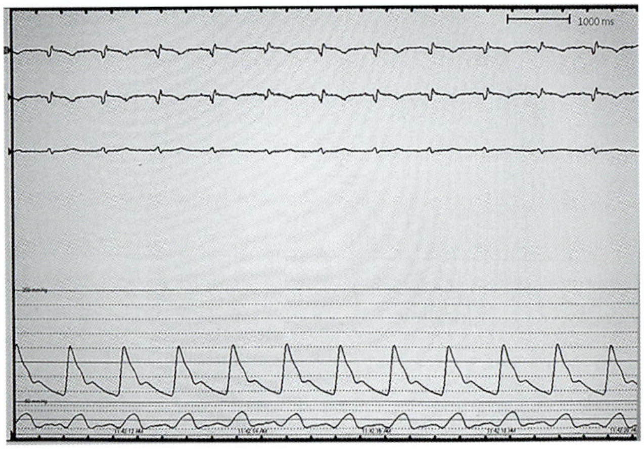

FIG. 8: LA pressure before TEER.

5. Clip arms are then opened to 60° and by rotation movement, the clip is positioned to be perpendicular to the leaflets. This is confirmed by two views—Bicom and LVOT views and rechecked on 3D TEE **(Figs. 6 and 7)**.
6. After a satisfactory position, the grippers are dropped and clip arms are closed, and before the release a thorough MR assessment is done. The clip is released with a safe and elaborate mechanism.
7. LA pressures can be monitored by placing a 4F pigtail catheter in LA at the beginning. **Figures 8 and 9** show LA pressures before and after the procedure, note the fall of v wave and normalization of pressure.

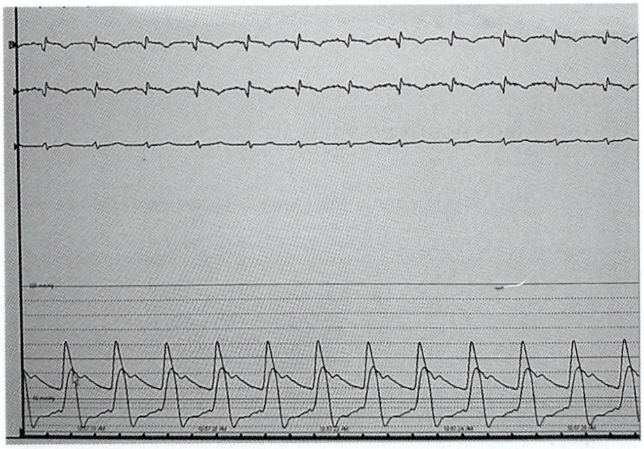

FIG. 9: LA pressure after TEER.

URGENT TRANSCATHETER MITRAL EDGE-TO-EDGE REPAIR FOR ACUTE MITRAL REGURGITATION

Acute mitral regurgitation (AMR) is a serious condition that requires urgent treatment. Common causes include postmyocardial infarction (MI), primary or secondary MR, and acute chord rupture in degenerative mitral valve disease. Patients with HF exacerbated by acute MR are typically at high-risk for surgery and were excluded from previous TEER trials, including COAPT. Medical management aims to stabilize these patients, using treatments like intravenous diuretics, vasodilators, and possibly mechanical support. Surgery is considered for those with persistent symptoms despite optimal medical care, but high-risk patients often face poor outcomes, with a 30-day mortality rate of 22.5% for surgical mitral valve replacement (SMVR), especially after recent MI.[5]

Transcatheter mitral edge-to-edge repair has shown clinical improvement in many AMR patients, including those with severe LV dysfunction and cardiogenic shock, provided they are stabilized before the procedure. The IREMMI study on 471 post-MI patients with SMR found that while surgical and TEER success rates were similar, inhospital and 1-year mortality were lower with TEER, suggesting it may be a better option for high-risk patients.[6] An analysis from the STS/ACC TVT Registry also reported lower 30-day and 1-year mortality rates for successful TEER procedures in patients with cardiogenic shock.[7]

However, TEER is still evolving, and its long-term efficacy and safety are not fully established. The fibrosis that occurs post-TEER can complicate future surgical repair, making this approach more suitable for SMR cases where valve replacement is common. TEER may not be suitable for all AMR patients, and in some cases, surgical repair or replacement may be necessary. Overall, TEER shows promise as a salvage procedure, particularly in critically ill patients with AMR following recent MI and may even serve as a bridge to SMVR.

TRANSCATHETER MITRAL EDGE-TO-EDGE REPAIR IN PATIENTS WITH ADVANCED HEART FAILURE OR SEVERE LEFT VENTRICULAR DYSFUNCTION

Patients with severely reduced LV function and severe MR often face poor outcomes. These patients, similar to those in the MITRA-FR trial, are typically debilitated by symptoms and have limited options for medical therapy due to comorbidities like low blood pressure and kidney dysfunction. The effectiveness of TEER in this group is still unclear, with most data coming from registries.

For example, the TRAMI registry compared 256 patients with severely reduced LV function [ejection fraction (EF) <30%] and found that TEER with the MitraClip device provided significant clinical benefits, which persisted for at least 1 year, similar to patients with better LV function. Another study showed that NYHA Class IV patients treated with MitraClip had marked improvement in functional status and quality of life at 1 year, although their mortality and HF hospitalization rates remained high.[8,9]

The MitraBridge registry, which included 119 patients with severe SMR and advanced HF (median EF: 26%), found that TEER as a bridge to heart transplantation was safe, with two-thirds of patients being free of adverse events after 1 year.[10] However, the MITRA-FR trial did not show a significant reduction in death or HF hospitalizations with TEER, while the COAPT trial demonstrated improved survival and reduced HF hospitalizations with TEER. A subanalysis of COAPT suggested that even patients with severely impaired LV function (EF ≤30%) could benefit from TEER.[11]

A critical concern for patients with low EF undergoing mitral valve interventions is afterload mismatch, where the sudden elimination of MR can lead to acute hemodynamic instability. About 20% of patients may experience a significant drop in EF after TEER, particularly those with low baseline EF, high left atrial pressure, and preexisting right ventricular dysfunction. This condition is typically reversible with time, but close postprocedural monitoring and inotropic support may be necessary.

Treating patients with advanced HF, whether elderly with comorbidities or younger with depressed LV function, requires a careful balance of risks and benefits. While newer mechanical circulatory support technologies show promise, many patients may still require bridging therapies to manage their HF effectively.

TRANSCATHETER MITRAL EDGE-TO-EDGE REPAIR IN SYSTOLIC ANTERIOR MOTION-RELATED MITRAL REGURGITATION AND HYPERTROPHIC CARDIOMYOPATHY

In hypertrophic obstructive cardiomyopathy (HOCM), systolic anterior motion (SAM) of the mitral valve often causes dynamic left ventricular outflow tract (LVOT) obstruction and MR. Standard treatment includes medications, septal reduction therapy, and/or mitral valve surgery. For high-risk patients where septal ablation is not feasible, TEER can be a viable alternative to manage LVOT obstruction and reduce MR by addressing SAM. In a small series of patients, MitraClip successfully reduced intraoperative LVOT gradient, left atrial pressure, and MR grade, improving cardiac output and symptoms, with most reaching NYHA Functional Class I or II. While these results are promising, further studies are needed. TEER should be considered for symptomatic patients with SAM-related MR and LVOT obstruction who cannot undergo alcohol septal ablation or are at high surgical risks.[12]

TRANSCATHETER MITRAL EDGE-TO-EDGE REPAIR AFTER A FAILED SURGICAL INTERVENTION

Patients with recurrent MR after mitral valve surgery are often high-risk candidates for additional surgical intervention, which can be complex and associated with higher mortality, morbidity, and longer hospital stays. Valve replacement is commonly required during redo-surgery due to factors like anatomical complexity and tissue condition. While percutaneous options like valve-in-valve or valve-in-ring procedures are sometimes suitable, they may pose risks such as LVOT obstruction or paravalvular leaks.

Transcatheter mitral edge-to-edge repair presents a promising alternative to redo-surgery, aiming to stabilize the previous repair and avoid valve replacement. Although imaging challenges and residual tissue from previous surgeries can complicate the procedure, TEER has shown success. Data from 57 patients across 11 centers from 2010 to 2016 indicated an 84% success rate in achieving postprocedural MR ≤2, though issues with imaging and mitral stenosis were noted. A more recent study of 104 patients after failed surgery found TEER feasible and safe, with a 90% success rate, suggesting that improved imaging techniques may help overcome technical challenges.[13]

Transcatheter mitral edge-to-edge repair remains a viable option in selected patients at experienced centers, emphasizing the need for careful patient selection in high-volume facilities.

TRANSCATHETER MITRAL EDGE-TO-EDGE REPAIR IN COMPLEX MITRAL VALVE ANATOMY

The EVEREST II trial established anatomical criteria for successful TEER, which include primary regurgitant jets originating from malcoaptation of the A2 and P2 scallops, sufficient leaflet size, and no large flail gaps. As TEER has become more popular, its success has improved even in complex anatomies, thanks to advances like the fourth-generation MitraClip and the PASCAL Ace, as well as 3D transesophageal imaging. This progress has enabled more effective treatment of challenging mitral valve anatomies, such as wide coaptation gaps and large flail gaps.[14]

Recent data show that out of 386 patients treated with TEER, 70 previously deemed unsuitable for the procedure (due to factors like prior valve surgery or anatomical complexity) saw a reduction in MR with no adverse events, and 52% had mild or no symptoms at 1 year. The PASCAL IID registry found a 92.9% implant success rate, with 92.4% of patients achieving MR ≤2+ and 56.1% achieving MR ≤1 at 6 months.[15]

Two ongoing randomized trials are evaluating TEER against surgical repair for severe primary MR. The REPAIR MR trial compares TEER to surgery in older or moderate-surgical-risk patients, aiming to confirm TEER's noninferiority. The PRIMARY trial focuses on patients aged 65 or older with primary degenerative MR. Both trials are expected to significantly impact treatment guidelines and clinical practice.[16]

Transcatheter mitral edge-to-edge repair has limitations in certain anatomies, such as chronic rheumatic disease, severe mitral annular calcification with stenosis, a very small mitral valve area (<3.5 cm^2), and MR due to cleft anatomy.[17] In these cases, transcatheter mitral valve replacement (TMVR) devices, with various anchoring mechanisms and delivery approaches, may be a viable alternative. TMVR offers longer-lasting MR reduction but has a high screening failure rate, with only 10% of screened patients eventually treated. Common exclusions include severe frailty, tricuspid disease, prior aortic valve therapy, and severe annular calcification. Future approaches should combine replacement and repair strategies. The choice between TMVR and TEER depends on anatomical factors, clinical parameters, patient health, and preferences. For elderly patients with complex anatomies, TEER might be preferred despite less MR reduction, while younger patients at high surgical risk may be better suited for TMVR.

TRANSCATHETER MITRAL EDGE-TO-EDGE REPAIR IN CONGENITAL HEART DISEASE

Congenital heart disease often affects younger adults who face higher surgical risks and may have had previous open-heart surgeries. Currently, no percutaneous devices are approved for atrioventricular valve regurgitation (AVVR) in adults with CHD. For symptomatic mitral and tricuspid regurgitation in these patients, TEER could be a viable option, although their complex anatomy and prior surgeries make the procedure challenging.

Patients with congenitally corrected transposition of the great arteries (ccTGA) and systemic right ventricle (SRV) often develop AVVR and SRV dysfunction, impacting their health. TEER in such cases may be complicated by anatomical differences, such as the trileaflet atrioventricular valve in ccTGA or the need to navigate surgical baffles from previous procedures like the Senning or Mustard operations.[18]

Advanced imaging, such as CT, MRI, and 3D printed models can aid in planning and simulation. Procedural techniques may also need adjustments, such as higher positioning for transseptal puncture and modified device steering. TEER has shown promise in CHD patients, but more research is needed to confirm its long-term safety and effectiveness.

POTENTIAL FUTURE INDICATIONS OF TRANSCATHETER MITRAL EDGE-TO-EDGE REPAIR

In current practice, the choice between surgical and percutaneous mitral valve interventions depends on the risks and benefits of surgery, which has traditionally been the standard. TEER, being minimally invasive with a quick recovery, is increasingly considered for earlier stages of mitral valve disease.

For primary MR, intervention is usually guided by symptoms or complications like LV dysfunction or pulmonary hypertension. Early TEER might prevent these complications in asymptomatic patients. The role of TEER in patients with mild ischemic MR soon after MI is unclear, as they are often not ideal candidates for surgery. However, early TEER might mitigate severe MR effects and prevent adverse LV changes, although this needs further research.[19,20]

Additionally, patients with atrial myopathy and atrial fibrillation might benefit from mitral intervention.[21] Studies suggest that MR in these patients reflects atrial myopathy, worsening heart function, and disease severity. The impact of early mitral intervention on atrial myopathy and atrial fibrillation remains unstudied.

CONCLUSION

The edge-to-edge repair technique is highly versatile and effectively addresses various causes of atrioventricular valvular regurgitation. Its safety and adaptability prompt ongoing exploration of its applications beyond current evidence. Consequently, TEER has become a valuable complement to other treatments for patients previously considered inoperable or high-risk. Although case reports and series highlight its effectiveness and safety in these scenarios, its definitive role remains unclear, necessitating further prospective studies. Meanwhile, TEER provides a simple and safe solution for many patients who might otherwise go untreated.

ONLINE REFERENCES

Please scan the QR code provided at the end of the table of contents for References of this chapter.

CHAPTER 178

Transcatheter Pulmonic Valve Therapies: Techniques, Current Roles, and Future Implications

Nirat Beohar, Sanjay Tyagi

ABSTRACT

Patients with congenital heart defects survive well into adulthood as effective therapies have emerged to treat such defects. However, as such patients survive into adulthood, they often require preservation of right ventricular function and management of the right ventricular outflow tract. In the past, surgical pulmonic valve replacement (SPVR) had been the mainstay of treatment for such patients and was considered the standard of care. However, transcatheter pulmonic valve implantation (TPVI), which was first reported in 2000, has made strides, and has emerged as a comparable alternative to SPVR. The present comprehensive chapter provides indications for TPVI, procedural details, and an up-to-date review of the literature regarding outcomes of TPVI. TPVI has been shown to have favorable medium-term outcomes free of reinterventions. Procedural mortality and complications are uncommon. With more experience, the risk of dreaded outcomes like coronary compression has declined and other complications such as conduit rupture are also increasingly managed by transcatheter techniques. The risk of endocarditis still prevails in the TPVI population. While data on head-to-head comparisons with SPVR are still limited, available data suggest equivalence. With improved techniques and technologies, its use is being expanded to increasingly complex anatomy.

Keywords: Pulmonary valve, congenital heart defects, pulmonary atresia, pulmonary valve stenosis, surgical pulmonic valve replacement, transcatheter pulmonic valve implantation

INTRODUCTION

A variety of congenital heart diseases including tetralogy of Fallot (TOF), pulmonary atresia, or stenosis and other conotruncal abnormalities are associated with right ventricular outflow tract (RVOT) obstruction. Surgical repair of such abnormalities, while effective, often results in the development of residual RVOT abnormalities such as pulmonic stenosis (PS) and/or insufficiency of their native outflow tract or right ventricle (RV) to pulmonary artery conduits. Other surgeries such as the Ross operation for aortic valve disease also have sequelae that lead to RV to pulmonary artery conduit dysfunction. Surgical pulmonic valve replacement (SPVR) has been the mainstay for these patients and has been considered the standard of care. Transcatheter pulmonic valve implantation (TPVI) was first reported in 2000 and has emerged as a comparable alternative to SPVR.[1-3] While initially developed for treating regurgitant or stenotic RV to pulmonary artery conduits, the indications for TPVI have been extended to treating dilated RVOTs with patch placement utilizing TPVs. This obviates the need for repeat surgical repairs needed over the patient's lifetime.

APPLICATION OF TRANSCATHETER PULMONIC VALVE IMPLANTATION

Indications for Intervention

The indications for pulmonary valve replacement (PVR), and in particular TPVI, are evolving. There is agreement among clinical societies on the need for PVR in symptomatic patients in the TOF spectrum with moderate to severe PS or pulmonary insufficiency (PI) **(Table 1)**. However, treatment of asymptomatic PI remains controversial. The deleterious effects of progressive RV dilation leading to

TABLE 1: Summary of consensus criteria for pulmonary valve replacement (PVR) in patients with repaired TOF.

2018 American Heart Association/ American College of Cardiology adult CHD guidelines	2020 European Society of Cardiology adult CHD guidelines	2022 Canadian Cardiovascular Society adult CHD guidelines
Moderate or greater PR, plus cardiovascular symptoms not otherwise explained, or ≥2 of the following: • RVEDVi ≥ 160 mL/m² • RVEDV ≥2 × LVEDV • RVESVi ≥ 80 mL/m² • Mild or moderate RV or LV systolic dysfunction • Objectively reduced exercise capacity • Significant RVOTO (RV pressure ≥2/3rd systemic pressure) • Ventricular tachyarrhythmias	Severe PR, plus ≥1 of the following: • Cardiovascular symptoms not otherwise explained • RVEDVi ≥ 160 mL/m² • RVESVi ≥ 80 mL/m² • Moderate or greater TR • Progressive RV systolic dysfunction • Objectively reduced exercise capacity • Significant RVOTO (RV pressure > 80 mm Hg)	Severe PR (regurgitant fraction >25% on CMR or qualitatively severe by echocardiography), plus ≥ 1 of the following: • Cardiovascular symptoms not otherwise explained • RVEDVi ≥ 160 mL/m² • RVESVi ≥ 80 mL/m² • RV systolic dysfunction • Objectively reduced exercise capacity • Significant RVOTO (RV pressure ≥2/3rd systemic pressure) • Sustained ventricular tachyarrhythmias

Source:
- 2018 American Heart Association/American College of Cardiology adult CHD guidelines. Stout KK et al.[3]
- 2020 European Society of Cardiology adult CHD guidelines. Baumgartner H et al.[2]
- 2022 Canadian Cardiovascular Society adult CHD guidelines. Marelli A, Beauchesne L, Colman J, et al. Canadian Cardiovascular Society 2022 Guidelines for Cardiovascular Interventions in Adults with Congenital Heart Disease. Can J Cardiol. 2022;38(7):862-96.

increased mortality are well known. However, it has not been convincingly shown that SPVR improves mortality or the incidence of ventricular arrhythmias.[4-6] Thus, the need to balance the deleterious effects of progressive RV dilation with those of repeated operations and cardiopulmonary bypass need to be weighed together. With the increase in use of TPVI, the repeated surgeries/exposure to cardiopulmonary bypass can be circumvented and with solutions for native RVOT also on horizon, it is likely that more asymptomatic patients may benefit from the procedure. Generally accepted indications for TPVI in asymptomatic patients include: (1) RV indexed end-diastolic volume >160 mL/m^2 or RV indexed end-systolic volume >80 mL/m^2; (2) RV end-diastolic volume >2 times of left ventricular end-diastolic volume; (3) significant RV dysfunction (RV ejection fraction <45%); (4) progressive tricuspid regurgitation in the setting of a dilated RV; and (5) ventricular arrhythmias with a dilated RV.[3]

For patients with native or bioprosthetic pulmonary valve dysfunction, TPVI is preferred.[2,3,7,8] Underlying conditions in which TPVI is performed in selected patients with RVOT/pulmonary valve dysfunction include the following settings: (1) repaired native RVOT—conditions include TOF and pulmonary atresia; (2) conditions such as TOF, pulmonary atresia, or truncus arteriosus that have been previously treated with RV to pulmonary artery conduit that is now dysfunctional can be treated with TPVI; (3) TPVI is recommended for valve-in-valve approach for failed bioprosthetic pulmonary valves;[9] (4) TPVI is an alternative to SPVR for patients with native pulmonary valve stenosis (PS) of regurgitation (PI); (5) for patients with severe PS (Doppler-based peak gradient >64 mm Hg or a mean gradient >35 mm Hg) or moderate PS with associated symptoms, balloon valvotomy is indicated when feasible. Patients with moderate PS who are asymptomatic are closely monitored for development of symptoms or worsening of gradient across the valve[2]; (6) TPVI is an option for patients with PS who have failed balloon-based or surgical valvotomy and have significant residual stenosis or regurgitation.

CHOICE OF PROCEDURE BETWEEN SURGICAL PULMONIC VALVE REPLACEMENT AND TRANSCATHETER PULMONIC VALVE IMPLANTATION

Transcatheter pulmonic valve implantation rather than SPVR is the preferred approach for RVOT dysfunction when feasible unless there are other considerations that are better served with surgery such as concurrent need for coronary artery bypass or tricuspid annuloplasty.

EXCLUSION CRITERIA

Technical and/or safety concerns preclude TPVI in the following conditions[2]:

- Non-balloon dilatable severely stenotic dysplastic pulmonary valve stenosis such as thickened cusps and redundant tissue as seen in Noonan's syndrome
- Native or conduit RVOT size that exceeds the limit of available devices. While there is no lower limit for landing zone size, the RVOT size must be small enough (≤29 mm for balloon-dilatable TPVI) to provide a suitable landing zone for a covered stent. In selected cases, a slightly larger diameter may be successfully treated after presenting to

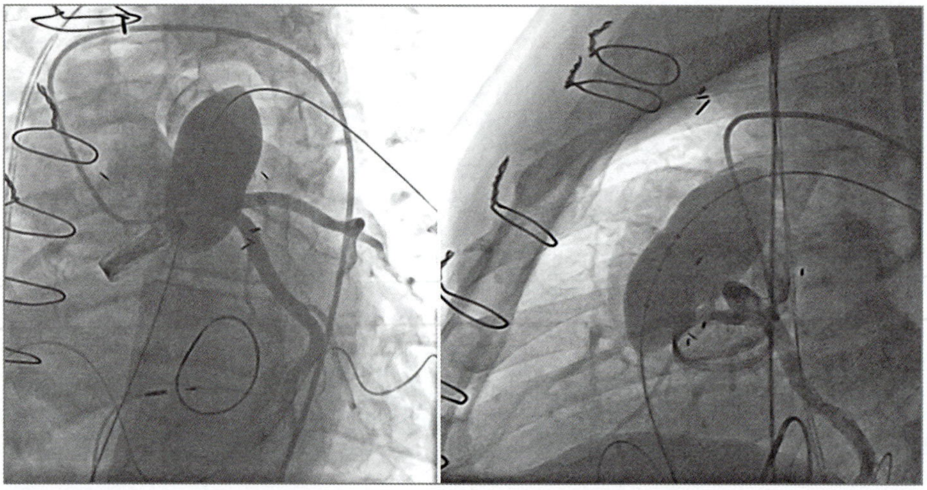

Note:
- Angiogram performed during a balloon test prior to planned TPVI.
- Patency of the left main coronary artery and the left coronary system shown.
- The right coronary artery also remain patent (not shown).

FIG. 1: Balloon testing to evaluate safety of transcatheter pulmonary valve implantation.

a smaller diameter to create a suitable "landing zone" or by overdilating an Edwards SAPIEN valve 29–31 mm. Self-expanding pulmonary valves enable treatment of larger RVOT anatomies.
- Inadequate femoral or jugular venous access caused by: (1) Conditions such as central vein occlusion and (2) small body size (e.g., body weight ≤20 kg)
- Risk of coronary compression by the expanded implant as determined by balloon testing **(Fig. 1)**[10]
- Active systemic infection (such as endocarditis) or high risk of systemic infection (such as intravenous drug abuse)

CHOICE OF TRANSCATHETER PULMONARY VALVES

Transcatheter pulmonary valves (TPV) are available as balloon-expandable or self-expanding valves. The choice of TPV is based on RVOT size.

Two *balloon-expandable* valves are approved by the US FDA and are CE marked. The diameter of the RVOT determines the choice of the Medtronic Melody or the Edwards SAPIEN valves.

The Medtronic Melody valves has a 34-mm cobalt chromium stent scaffold into which a Contegra bovine jugular vein is hand-sewn in. It comes as a 16-mm valve (expandable up to 20 mm) or an 18-mm valve (expandable up to 22 mm).

The Edwards SAPIEN 3 valve has a balloon-expandable stainless steel scaffold with a trileaflet bovine pericardial valve hand-sewn inside while a fabric cuff covering the proximal part of the stent prevents paravalvular leaks. It comes in 23-, 26-, or 29-mm sizes and is approved for RVOT conduit diameters in the 16.5- to 29-mm range or for failed bioprosthetic valves with internal diameter of 16.5–28.5 mm.[11]

Three *self-expanding valves* are US FDA and CE mark approved. Typically, self-expanding valves are used for the largest RVOTs, such as native RVOTs.

The Medtronic Harmony self-expanding TPV **(Fig. 2)** has a nitinol scaffold within which a porcine pericardial valve is mounted within a pericardial tube. It is the preferred option for larger-diameter native RVOTs. It comes in various valve housing sizes (22 mm: inflow 41 mm, outflow 32 mm, length 55 mm; or 25 mm: inflow 54 mm, outflow 43 mm, length 51 mm) to accommodate native outflow tract sizes.[12]

The Edwards SAPIEN 3 Alterra prestent is a two-part system designed for larger-diameter native RVOTs. A self-expanding, 48-mm-long, nitinol stent, covered with polytetrafluoroethylene with a 40-mm inflow and outflow, is deployed first. The central waist of the prestent enables deployment of a 29-mm Edwards SAPIEN 3 valve inside the prestent scaffold.[13]

PROCEDURAL EVALUATION

In order to determine candidacy for replacement of pulmonary valve, the strategy, i.e., TPVI versus SPVR, and to determine the type of TPV, a multidisciplinary approach is preferred. Coronary CT angiography, cardiac MRI, or invasive angiography is often performed as part of this assessment.[2]

IMPLANTATION TECHNIQUE

Transcatheter pulmonic valve implantation is usually performed using general anesthesia. Venous access is generally obtained through the femoral vein and less

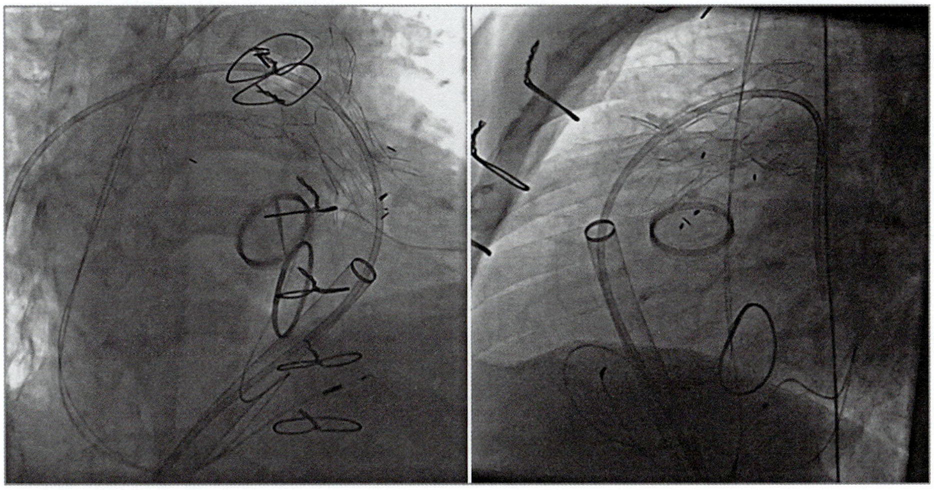

Note:
- 42-year-old male with symptomatic severe prior pulmonic valve/homograft valvular insufficiency.
- History of prior pulmonic valve surgery for congenital pulmonic stenosis following prior balloon valvuloplasty and resultant pulmonary insufficiency.
- Successful transcatheter pulmonic valve implantation with a 25 mm medtronic harmony valve.

FIG. 2: Transcatheter pulmonary valve implantation of Medtronic Harmony valve.

commonly through the jugular venous approach. After a complete hemodynamic and angiographic study, a guidewire is positioned distally into a pulmonary artery.

- *Balloon test* **(Fig. 1)** is performed in the RVOT to exclude the risk of coronary artery compression which is a life-threatening complication of TPVI especially with the balloon-expandable valves. While coronary compression has not been seen with self-expanding TPV, the balloon test is often performed. In case of enlarged native RVOTs, total occlusion of the RVOT during balloon inflation should be ensured. The size of the valve should be 2–4 mm larger than that of the waist seen during balloon inflation. To test for coronary occlusion, a balloon is inflated simultaneously with an aortogram (rather than a selective angiogram) to demonstrate adequate coronary flow.[10] If coronary compromise is found during balloon test, TPVI should not be performed.
- *Conduit preparation and prestenting:* Conduit balloon angioplasty and stenting is required to reduce the RVOT gradient if there is significant conduit stenosis. The role of prestenting varies depending on the type of valve:
    - Prestenting of the conduit with a covered stent (in order to avoid bleeding if there is conduit rupture) before deployment of the Melody valve has been shown to reduce the risk of stent fracture of the TPV.[14] Additional stenting may be required if there is recoil at landing zone. If a noncovered stent is preferred, it is expected to jail one of the branch pulmonary arteries. Stent fracture has not been reported with the SAPIEN valve and therefore it is typically implanted directly.[15] Self-expanding valves such as the Harmony or the Venus P-valves do not require prestenting.
- *The implantation techniques* for the Edwards SAPIEN **(Fig. 3)** and the Melody valves are similar. Both are crimped onto the balloon delivery system. The Melody valve requires a 22-Fr delivery sheath while the SAPIEN valve requires a 14- or 16-Fr sheath for the 23-, 26-, or 29-mm valve. In order to avoid entrapment on the tricuspid valve, it is preferable to use a 65-cm, 16-Fr Gore DrySeal sheath which is advanced across the tricuspid valve into the RVOT and the THV is then directly implanted in the RVOT. The self-expanding valves are advanced over a stiff wire and unsheathed at the deployment site. The Medtronic Harmony valve is typically deployed through a 60-cm, 16-Fr Gore sheath.

PROCEDURAL SUCCESS AND COMPLICATIONS

With growing experience, procedural success has improved, being 96.2% in observational reports.[16] The most dreaded complications for TPVI are conduit rupture and coronary compression.

- *Conduit rupture* is uncommon and estimated to be approximately 4.1%, more so in homografts. It is more common when off-label TPVI is performed in conduits sized <16 mm. Most of these ruptures are limited and can usually be managed with a covered stent implant.[16]
- *Coronary compression* had declined considerably as experience has accrued and procedural planning has improved. The US post-market approval study reported that only 1 out of 100 implants had coronary compression which required conversion to surgery. The anomalous origin of the left coronary arising from the right cusp is a strong predictor of coronary compression.[17,18]

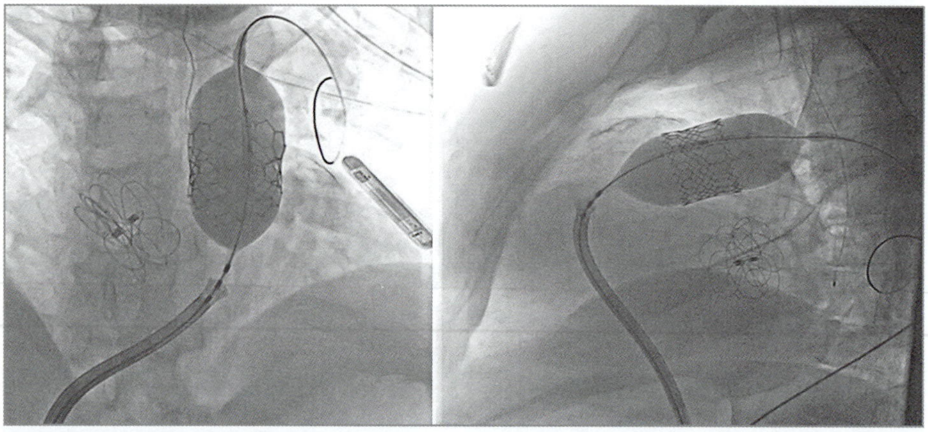

Note:
- A 54-year-old woman with history of tetralogy of Fallot status post left BT shunt followed by a complete repair at 5 years of age.
- Ischemic CVA s/p ASD closure with Gore 37 mm ASD closure device.
- AP and lateral angiogram showing deployment of an Edwards SAPIEN Pulmonic Transcatheter Heart Valve dilated to 29 mm for TPVI.

FIG. 3: Transcatheter pulmonary valve implantation of Edwards SAPIEN valve.

- *Reintervention:* Approximately 20–25% of patients with TOF undergoing TPVI require reintervention within 5–10 years.[19] The reasons for reintervention include stent fracture, device failure with recurrent stenosis, residual stenosis not relieved by the stent, or infection.[20] Presenting may reduce the risk of stent fracture in patients receiving the Melody TPV.
- *Infective endocarditis (IE):* At 1- to 4-year follow-up after TPVI, approximately 1–7% of patients develop IE.[21] Risk factors for IE include younger age, history of endocarditis prior to valve implantation, and higher residual gradient after TPVR. The type of valve does not appear to be an independent risk factor for IE. However, the rate of IE after TPVI may be higher than that seen after RVOT reconstruction with a homograft.[22]

COMPARISON OF TRANSCATHETER PULMONIC VALVE IMPLANTATION WITH SURGICAL PULMONIC VALVE REPLACEMENT

Limited data exist regarding comparison of SPVR with TPVI. Consistent with a smaller study,[23] a recent meta-analysis also did not show any difference in mortality or repeat interventions between TPVI and SPVR. However, there were fewer procedure-related complications, a shorter length of hospitalization, and higher rate of endocarditis with TPVI in other studies.[24]

FUTURE DIRECTIONS

Additional TPVs are being developed to further improve outcomes and provide devices suitable for varying anatomical requirements. Among others, two additional self-expanding valves are being evaluated. *The Venus P-Valve* is composed of a self-expandable nitinol framework with a trileaflet porcine pericardial valve that has received CE mark in Europe in 2023 and is investigational in the United States. This valve is an investigational device in the United States. *The Pulsta TPV* is a trileaflet valve that consists of a double-strand nitinol wire covered with treated porcine pericardium. The valve is approved in South Korea and is awaiting CE mark in Europe. As all the existing valves have been implanted for a short time with limited follow-up, future data are necessary to understand their overall longevity and types of valve failure. In the future, smaller and more flexible delivery systems are likely to be developed.

CONCLUSION

Over the last decade, TPVI has dramatically evolved and has emerged as being a safe and efficacious less invasive therapy to manage many patients with dysfunctional RVOT. Overall, the short-term and midterm results of TPVI demonstrate low and acceptable morbidity and mortality. TPVs will continue to evolve to accommodate a variety of native and surgically altered anatomies.

ONLINE REFERENCES

Please scan the QR code provided at the end of the table of contents for References of this chapter.

CHAPTER

179

Tricuspid Valve Endovascular Interventions

Viveka Kumar, Purneshwar Pandey, Sangeeta Dhir

ABSTRACT

Tricuspid valve (TV) diseases are very common and undertreated diseases with significant mortality and morbidity. Classically, valve replacement or surgical repair were the only option which were also underutilized owing to high mortality. Endovascular TV interventions are newer developing and potential modalities and provide effective therapeutic option for the treatment of significant TV disease. Valvular anatomy of every valve is essential and an essential prerequisite for device planning and explore available options at every cardiac center. Most importantly, appropriate patient selection after clinical examination and imaging with proper timing of the procedure are crucial for the successful procedures.

Keywords: Tricuspid valve diseases, endovascular tricuspid valve intervention

INTRODUCTION

Tricuspid valve (TV) disease especially tricuspid regurgitation (TR) is very common, and its prevalence increases with age.[1] Recent data suggest that the age-adjusted prevalence of TR is approximately 0.55%.[1] Severe TR is associated with poor prognosis independent of the pulmonary artery and right ventricular (RV) systolic pressure and the degree of RV failure.[2] Isolated TR also significantly worsens survival without treatment and in a recent study, 5-year event-free survival was only around 60%.[3] A subanalysis of the COAPT trial in patients with TR and mitral regurgitation (MR) showed that patients with MR and moderate or severe TR had higher NYHA class and BNP levels, as well as more severe MR, highlighting the overall worse clinical outcomes in patients with coexistent TR and MR.[4] In the setting of heart failure with reduced ejection fraction, TR was associated with a more severe heart failure presentation as well as worse survival independently of other baseline markers.[5]

However, it has been seen that several patients with TV disease are refused for cardiac surgery in view of comorbidities and advanced heart failure symptoms. Hence, in the last decade a large number of endovascular therapies for TV have been developed to treat such patients and fulfil the unmet clinical need of treating such patients.

TRICUSPID VALVE ANATOMY

The TV is the largest of the heart valves measuring between 7 and 9 cm^2. It is an easily accessible valve for transcatheter interventions from venous access, so it does not require any arterial access or septal puncture decreasing access related complication in such interventions.[6] However, the TV apparatus has some specific difficulties and challenges for endovascular interventions:

- It has got complex subvalvular apparatus including papillary muscles and multiple chordae tendineae which substantially elevate the risk of entrapment and difficulty in device maneuverability.
- Annulus is an asymmetric and saddle-shaped ellipsoid structure which is dynamic over the cardiac cycle.
- Close proximity of the tricuspid annulus and the conduction system (atrioventricular node and His-Purkinje system) pose a high risk for conduction disturbances, especially in orthotropic replacement.
- Right coronary artery (RCA) reside in the atrioventricular groove, lying in close proximity to the tricuspid annulus, which increases the risk for RCA compression in annuloplasty and replacement cases.
- There is very less space between the inferior vena cava (IVC) opening into the right atrium (RA) and the tricuspid

annulus making the appropriate coaxial positioning of the intended systems more difficult, as they need more sharp bends within a relatively small cavity.

PATHOPHYSIOLOGY

There are three types of TR: *Primary, secondary, and cardiac electric implantable device-related (CEID)* each with different etiology.[7] Primary TR is due to a congenital or acquired defect in the TV structure. The most common congenital pathology affecting TV is *Ebstein's anomaly*. Other causes of primary TR include damage from infection (rheumatic heart disease), carcinoid, or trauma.

Secondary TR is due to situations which increase volume or pressure on the right side of the heart or change the morphology and anatomy of the right-sided cardiac chambers including pulmonary hypertension, left sided heart failure, or right atrial enlargement with annular dilation.

Finally, CEID-induced TR is a result of RV pacing or can be due to direct interaction between the device and the tricuspid valvular apparatus interfering with its normal function.

PATIENT SELECTION AND PREPROCEDURAL WORKUP

The assessment of TV function and associated pathological conditions typically involve meticulous medical history taking, physical examination, and diagnostic tests. Multimodality imaging is necessary for proper planning and execution of device-based therapy of TV. Transthoracic echocardiography (TTE) is the initial cardiac imaging examination to be performed to assess RV size, function, valvular morphology, severity of TR, pulmonary artery, and pulmonary valve, and to rule out any significant left-sided disease. Transesophageal echocardiography (TEE) is the most important investigation for procedural planning, especially a transcatheter procedure **(Table 1)**.

Despite the adequate and good information obtained from TEE, cardiac computed tomography (CCT) is a necessary imaging modality to plan most of the endovascular procedures planned for TV, with the exception of edge-to-edge repair.

FACTORS AFFECTING DEVICE CHOICE IN TRANSCATHETER THERAPY FOR TRICUSPID VALVE DISEASE

Anatomy, leaflet pathology, mechanism of TR, RV function, etc., are important factors in considering device therapy for endovascular interventions. When the predominant mechanism of TR is annular dilation, annular reduction therapy can be considered for such patients, provided the dilation is not too much (massive annulus size, extreme leaflet tethering, and excessively large coaptation gaps of >10.0 mm). Preintervention CCT can help in identifying unfavorable features for annular reduction, such as shallow tricuspid annulus shelf depth, severity of annular calcification, or proximity to the coronaries (RCA).

For planning edge-to-edge repair, coaptation gaps ≥7.5 mm and not originating from either antero- or posteroseptal commissure or severe leaflet tethering are also unfavorable anatomy for edge-to-edge repair. Additional leaflet morphology not amenable for transcatheter edge-to-edge repair include leaflet thickening, restriction, and leaflet

TABLE 1: Basic features of transesophageal echo for tricuspid valve repair.

Preprocedural TEE	Intraprocedural TEE
Severity of tricuspid regurgitation (TR) and stenosis of tricuspid valve	*Annuloplasty repair*: • 3D imaging showing surgical-like atrial view and multiplane 2D views to assess the position of the anchors • Assess depth of annulus from the hinge point of the leaflet • Evaluate distance from the RCA
Quality of the TEE imaging for procedural guidance with the patient in the supine position	
Coexistence of valvular disease other than tricuspid valve	
Annular dimensions and leaflet length	
Morphologic characterization of tricuspid leaflets	*Edge-to-edge repair*: • Biplane sweeping views from the 60° mid esophageal to assess trajectory, position relative to the target jet and leaflet clinching • Deep transgastric view to assess rotation and perpendicularity
Location of regurgitation jet origin and evaluation of coaptation defect(s)	
Rule out right chamber thrombus and lead-related complications.	
Subvalvular apparatus: Calcification, number, and position of chordae tendineae	*Replacement*: • High-support guidewire localization in the tricuspid annulus • System coaxiality and depth • *Final hemodynamic assessment*: Residual TR, tricuspid gradients
Rule out thrombus	

(RCA: right coronary artery; TEE: transesophageal echo; TR: tricuspid regurgitation)

perforation. Valve replacement may be the best treatment option for patients found unsuitable or unfavorable anatomy for annular reduction or leaflet-directed therapy. In patients who are found unsuitable for any of these procedures, Caval therapy remains the only alternative to reduce congestive features. Procedural planning with CCT and CT venography is necessary to demonstrate favorable RA and vena cava anatomy. **Figure 1** shows devices for transcatheter treatment of TV.

Figure 2 shows an ECHO image for a case of TR and **Figure 3** demonstrates the preprocedural CT findings for sizing the TricValve in respective planes.

COAPTATION DEVICES

TriClip

Similar to MitraClip device, TriClip system is an edge-to-edge repair technique which includes two parts: (1) The clip delivery system (CDS), (2) the steerable guide catheter (SGC).[9] The CDS includes an implantable clip with grippers, a delivery catheter, and a steerable sleeve used for manipulating and moving the clip. The SGC includes a dilator. Two methods have been described: The triple orifice technique (or clover) and the bicuspidization technique (or zipping). While in former method the clips are put centrally

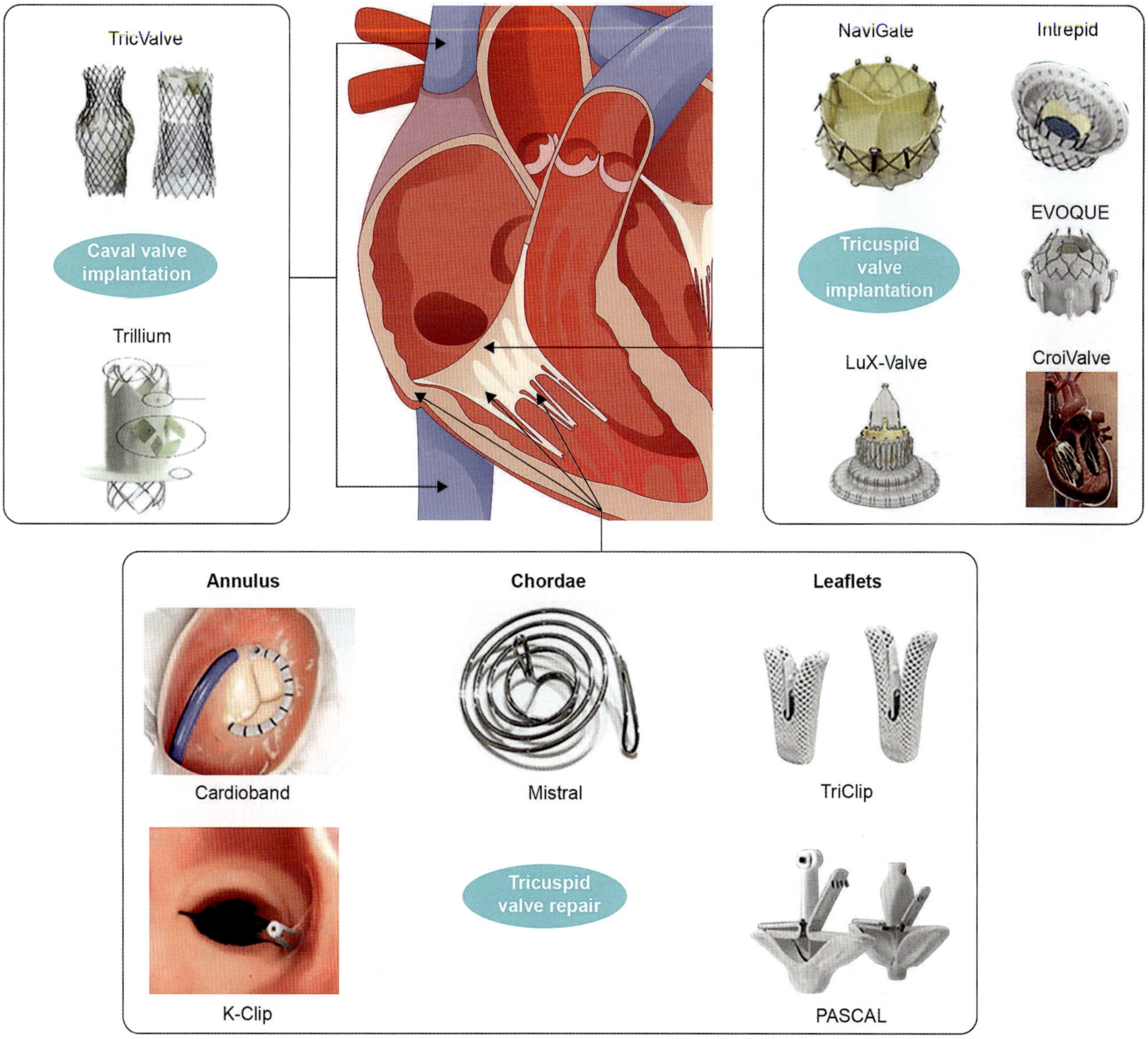

FIG. 1: Devices for transcatheter treatment of tricuspid valve.[8]

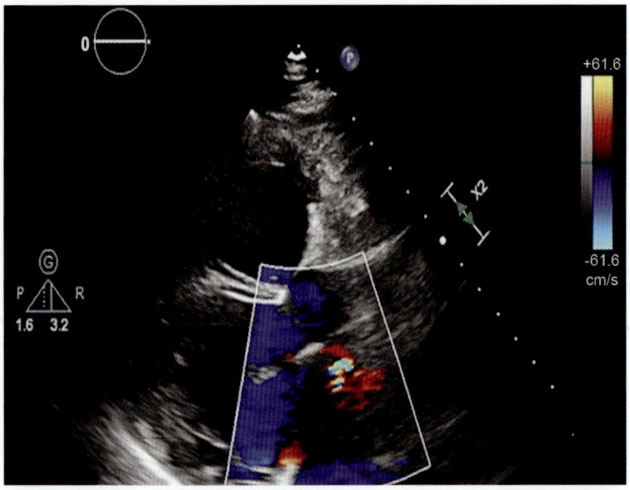

FIG. 2: Preprocedural ECHO showing severe tricuspid regurgitation.

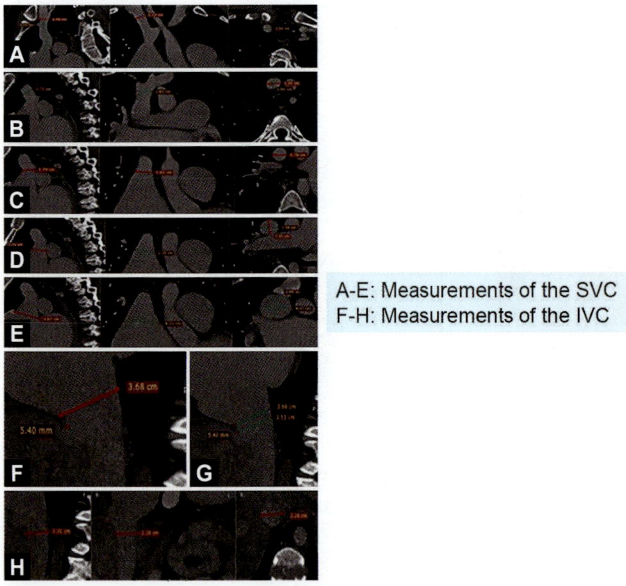

FIGS. 3A TO H: Preoperative computed tomography showing dimensions of superior vena cava (SVC) and inferior vena cava (IVC) for sizing the tricuspid valve in respective planes.

between the septal, anterior, and the posterior tricuspid leaflet, in the latter method the clips are placed between the septal and anterior tricuspid leaflets. The bicuspidization technique has been found to be more feasible and is being frequently done.[10] In the TRILUMINATE trial by Lurz et al.,[11] 85 patients having symptomatic TR receiving a TriClip were evaluated. Greater than 85% of subjects had a sustained decrease in TR of at least 1 grade after 1 year, with around 70% of patients having moderate or less TR, as compared to around 8% at baseline and approximately 60% at 30 days of follow-up. Greater than 50% (22 of 39) of patients with baseline massive or torrential TR achieved decrease-to-moderate or less TR at 1 year, with 90% achieving at least a 1-grade reduction in TR. Patients in NYHA functional class I/II improved from 31% at baseline to >80% at 1 year ($p < 0.0001$) and 6MWT distance was also improved significantly. At the end of 1 year, the hospitalization rate decreased from 1.30 to 0.78 events/patient-year ($p = 0.0030$).

Pascal

The PASCAL system includes a 1 cm central spacer that acts as a filler in the tricuspid orifice with two paddles and clasps. The paddles are broad (25 mm width) and the device can be elongated for safer maneuverings. Similar to other transcatheter edge-to-edge repairs, it needs to cross the valve and grasp the leaflets while pulling the entire system back. All the procedural steps and device positioning is guided by intraprocedural TEE. In a recent study of use of PASCAL in symptomatic TR involving 74 individuals with a follow-up for 1 month and 6 months, a total of 72 patients finally underwent the procedure out of which 97% successfully received the device. At 1 month, 88% of patients had at least 1 TR grade reduction and around 90% had moderate or lower regurgitation. The composite major adverse event rate was only 3.0%. At 6 months follow-up, 88% of patients had sustained reduction in regurgitation with moderate or less TR, while 83% had at least 1 TR grade decrease.[12]

DEVICES FOR ANNULAR REPAIR

Cardioband

The implant includes a contraction wire and polyester fabric wrapping with radiopaque markers attached to an adjustment mechanism. It reduces regurgitation by annular reduction, and it is placed and fixed along the annulus of the valve utilizing the radiopaque anchors as a fluoroscopic reference. After implantation at the anterior and posterior portion of the annulus under fluoroscopy and TEE guidance, it is cinched to decrease the anteroposterior and septolateral diameters. After cinching, coronary angiography should be performed to see RCA occlusion.

In the early feasibility study[13] of 30 patients, procedural success was accomplished in 93% of patients, and without any 1 month mortality. The septolateral diameter of annulus was decreased by 13% successfully and approximately 85% of patients had at least 1 grade in TR reduction with associated improvements in NYHA functional class. The 6-month follow-up results from the study[14] showed a 92% survival rate and a 19% decrease in annular diameters. TR reduction was also sustained with >1 grade reduction in 93% of patients with significant improvements in functional class and quality-of-life metrics.

Trialign

Trialign device (Mitralign, Inc) is a percutaneous annuloplasty method that needs two access sites via the right jugular vein. During the procedure, two polyester pledgets are delivered across the tricuspid annulus in close proximity to the antero- and septoposterior commissure, cinched by a polyester suture to obliterate the posterior leaflet of TV and locked on the atrial side. A radiofrequency guidewire is used to cross the tricuspid annulus from the ventricular side into the atrial chamber at the septoposterior portion of the tricuspid annulus, followed by snaring it through the second access and the first pledget installed. The second device requires similar technique and positioned similarly at the anteroposterior commissure. Finally, a dedicated plication lock delivery catheter is advanced over both pledget sutures to the atrial side of the tricuspid annulus, helping in the plication of the portion of the tricuspid annulus in between the two pledgets.

Results of the Trialign (SCOUT) trial.[15] showed that all 15 patients underwent successful procedure with no adverse event but for an ST elevation myocardial infarction due to plication of the RCA requires stent implantation. Three patients (20%) had single pledget detachment at 1 month echocardiographic follow-up. At least a 1-grade TR decrease was seen for the other successfully treated population (patients without detachment).

DEVICES FOR CHORDAL REPAIR

Mistral

The Mistral device (Mitralix) improves leaflet coaptation by cinching the chordae into a "flower bouquet" shape. The device implantation is performed under TEE guidance utilizing an 8.5F off-the-shelf steerable guide catheter and the 7.5F delivery system. A spiral-shaped wire is deployed in the RA and then delivered into the RV and rotated within the cords until a desired result is achieved. TR severity was reduced from severe-to-moderate with normalization of tricuspid annular plane systolic excursion (TAPSE) and RV fractional area change with significant improvement in NYHA class and KCCQ scores.[16]

Other Devices

The TriCinch system (a stainless-steel corkscrew placed in the anterior annulus with a self-expanding nitinol stent deployed at the IVC) was tried in a series of 24 patients[17] with procedural success rate of 75%. Two (8%) cases of hemopericardium and four (17%) cases of annular detachment, respectively, were of concern. This system is no longer in clinical use.

The Millipede IRIS device is semirigid nitinol ring with multiple independent anchors that function as a full annuloplasty ring. Its development focuses primarily on the mitral position, although a dedicated tricuspid delivery system is in progress.

The pledget-assisted suture tricuspid annuloplasty (PASTA) technique makes a dual-orifice TV via a dual pledgeted polyester suture which is percutaneously attached to the tricuspid annulus. The first-in-human procedure was reported, although the subject presented with annular dehiscence requiring further intervention.[18]

TRANSCATHETER TRICUSPID VALVE REPLACEMENT

Orthotopic Bioprosthesis

NaviGate

The NaviGate system (NaviGate cardiac structures) is a nitinol self-expanding valve with trileaflet (pericardial valve) available in many sizes (36.0, 40.0, 44.0, 48.0, and 52.0 mm), with <10% oversizing to the tricuspid annulus size recommended.[19] In early experience with this device of 30 consecutive patients, 26 had technically successful implantations; four suffered malpositioning, and two required conversion to open surgical procedure. All successfully treated patients experienced good reduction in regurgitation, with 75% experienced ≥2 grade reduction and 76% of patients having mild regurgitation at discharge. In-hospital mortality of high risk patients was 10%, but there were no late device-related events.[20]

LuX-Valve

The LuX-Valve (Ningbo Jenscare Biotechnology Co., Ningbo, China) is a bovine pericardial with three leaflets delivered through a minimally invasive thoracotomy and subsequent transatrial approach using a 32F steerable system. The annulus (50.0, 60.0, and 70.0 mm) and inner valve (26.0 and 28.0 mm) are measured separately. The only experience with this device has been in China with an initial report of 12 patients[21] showing a procedural success rate of 100% with no conversion to open surgery. Only single in-hospital death and all others survived to 1 month, and all but 1 patient experienced less than or equal to mild residual TR.

The second-generation platform, *LuX-Valve Plus*, is implanted via a transjugular approach, with the first-in-human study being reported.[22]

EVOQUE

The EVOQUE valve replacement system for TV (Edwards Life sciences) is comprised of bovine pericardial leaflets with an intra-annular sealing skirt and anchors. It is mounted on a 28F delivery catheter and delivered via transfemoral venous access; its steerable delivery system can be rotated on multiple planes allowing for coaxial deployment of the valve. The valve frame has been specifically designed to conform to the tricuspid annulus, hence respecting the native morphology and achieving optimal retention force.

The feasibility study of the EVOQUE system and its effect on short-term clinical outcomes revealed 92% technical success and without any mortality or conversion to open surgery.[23] 2 year outcomes from a retrospective analysis of 38 patients showed 2-year survival rate of 71% with significant improvements in right cardiac failure symptoms. RV reverse remodeling was maintained at this longer-term follow-up. Adverse events were less, with 11% having major bleeding, 8% requiring pacemaker, and 1 patient requiring surgical TV replacement due to early migration of the device.[24]

HETEROTROPIC CAVAL VALVE IMPLANTATION

Hetertotropic caval valve implantation is the method to put a valved device in superior and inferior venae cavae to decrease the systematic back flow due to TR. It is deployed in patients with presence of caval flow reversal and an appropriate venous anatomy. There are three devices available: device 1 (Sapien) is balloon expandable valve, device 2 (TricValve) and device 3 (Tricento) are self expanding valves. TricValve is the most commonly used device for such indications and consists of two self-expandable valves, one in SVC and other in IVC, while Tricento has one valve implanted in the IVC only. There is currently a limited number of trials regarding these systems.

The TRICUS EURO study[25] enrolled 35 patients getting TricValve implanted, which showed 1 month procedure success of 94% and no periprocedural deaths. At the 6 months follow-up, functional class of the patients were significantly improved, with around 80% of patients in NYHA class I or II. 6 months mortality rate was only 8.5%.

POSTPROCEDURAL ANTITHROMBOTIC THERAPY

Transcatheter TV implants increase the risk of thrombosis due to the low pressure circulation of the right side of the heart. However, optimal antithrombotic therapy following such implants remains controversial.[26] Majority of patients (around 90%) undergoing TV procedures have atrial fibrillation as a comorbid condition and, as such, anticoagulants are reintroduced after the procedure and continued lifelong.[27] Patients with no indication for systemic anticoagulation may benefit from dual antiplatelet therapy of 4 weeks primarily consisting of aspirin and clopidogrel, followed by aspirin daily for life.

CONCLUSION

Tricuspid valve disease is a very common condition associated with increased mortality and morbidity, if left untreated or not treated in time. Surgical repair or replacement were the only therapeutic options available earlier which were mostly deferred in view of high rates of complications. TTVIs have been found to be feasible, effective, and affordable with easy learning curve and associated with excellent outcome and low mortality rates providing good benefits to such patients.

ONLINE REFERENCES

Please scan the QR code provided at the end of the table of contents for References of this chapter.

CHAPTER

180

Valve Thrombosis and Valve Degeneration: How to Detect

John Jose E, Paul V George

ABSTRACT

Prosthetic dysfunction—thrombosis and degeneration can affect mechanical (surgical) or biological prostheses (surgical or transcatheter), and can cause valve obstruction or regurgitation with or without development of valve-related symptoms. In this chapter, we briefly discuss the modes of failure and steps for diagnosing prosthetic valve dysfunction.

Keywords: Valve thrombosis, hypoattenuated leaflet thickening, pannus, structural degeneration, surgical bioprosthesis, transcatheter valve, mechanical valve

INTRODUCTION

Prosthetic heart valves including transcatheter valves have revolutionized the management of valvular heart disease, offering life-saving interventions for patients with severe valve dysfunction. Over the past 50 years, almost 4 million prosthetic heart valves have been implanted[1] and despite their benefits, complications such as thrombosis and degeneration pose significant challenges. This chapter delves into these issues, offering insights into their occurrence and diagnostic approaches.

PROSTHETIC HEART VALVE TYPES

Prosthetic heart valves may be broadly classified as biological (transcatheter or surgical) or mechanical (surgical). Commonly used prosthetic valves are summarized in **Table 1**.

Mechanical Prosthetic Heart Valve Dysfunction

There are four primary processes that might lead to mechanical valve dysfunction—thrombosis, endocarditis, structural, and nonstructural deterioration including fibrotic pannus ingrowth.

Magnitude of the Problem

Despite being more durable than bioprostheses, mechanical prosthetic heart valves are more thrombogenic and require life-long anticoagulation. Mechanical valve thrombosis is a rare but potentially life-threatening complication with an annual rate ranging from 0.1 to 8%, with higher rates for valves in the mitral or tricuspid position compared with the aortic position.[2] Valve thrombosis is the most common cause for mechanical valve dysfunction. Mechanical valve thrombosis can be obstructive or nonobstructive and may or may not be associated with thromboembolic events, which occur at a rate of 2.5–3.7% per year.[3,4] Fibrotic pannus ingrowth is a differential for mechanical valve thrombosis (albeit less common than thrombus) and represents excessive fibroblast and collagen proliferation with infiltration of endothelial and inflammatory cells, occurring as a result of biological reaction to the prosthetic material. Occasionally, pannus may coexist with valve thrombosis. Apart from pannus formation, nonstructural dysfunction may also be caused by patient-prosthetic mismatch, paravalvular leak, valve dehiscence, inappropriate position, and valve migration. Mechanical mitral valve dysfunction may rarely be caused by residual chordae tendineae stuck in the prosthetic sewing ring, extremely long residual papillary muscles in left ventricle or calcified tissues under the prosthesis hampering leaflet mobility.

Structural deterioration of mechanical valves is very rare but has been noted with older valves such as Björk-Shiley and Starr Edwards (ball fracture and fabric wear and tear). Strut or disk fractures, leaflet escape (missing disk), separation of sewing cuff from housing, and occluder dysfunction (due to lipid adsorption) are rare with newer mechanical valves.

TABLE 1: Prosthetic valve types.

Biological	Mechanical
Stented: • Porcine bioprosthesis: ○ Hancock and Hancock II ○ Mosaic ○ Carpentier–Edwards standard and supra-annular ○ Biocor ○ Epic • Pericardial bioprosthesis ○ Carpentier–Edwards perimount ○ Carpentier–Edwards Magna ○ Mitroflow synergy ○ Biocor pericardia ○ Trifecta ○ Sorin Pericarbon More ○ Meril Dafodil and Dafodil Neo ○ Meril Flomero	*Bileaflet*: • St Jude Medical: Standard, HP, Masters, and Regent Carbomedics: Standard, reduced cuff, Optiform, Orbis, and supra-annular (TopHat) • Edwards Tekna • Sorin Bicarbon • Edwards Mira • ATS • On-X • Medtronic advantage • Meril Miltonia
Stentless: • Porcine bioprosthesis: ○ Medtronic Freestyle ○ Edwards Prima Plus ○ St Jude Medical Toronto ○ Shelhigh super stentless aortic porcine valve ○ AorTech Aspire ○ St Jude Biocor ○ Labcor ○ St Jude Quattro stentless mitral • Pericardial bioprosthesis: ○ Freedom Solo ○ Sorin Pericarbon Freedom ○ Medtronic ATS 3F (Equine)	*Tilting disk* • Björk–Shiley Monostrut • Sorin Monoleaflet Allcarbon • Medtronic-Hall • Omnicarbon • Ultracor
Aortic homograft	*Caged ball*: • Starr–Edwards • Smeloff–Cutter
Pulmonary autograft (Ross procedure)	
Suture less: • Perceval S (Sorin) • Edwards Intuity (Edwards Lifesciences) • 3F Enable (ATSMedical) • Trilogy (Arbor Surgical Technologies)	
Transcatheter: • Myval • Octacor • Sapien 3 • Evolut Pro • ACURATE neo2 • Navitor • Hydra • Vienna	

Prosthetic valve endocarditis occurs at a rate of 1–6% and may be complicated by abscess formation, thrombosis, valve dehiscence, paravalvular leak, abscess, pseudoaneurysm (more common with aortic valves), and development of fistulous communication between cardiac chambers.[5,6] Most cases of mechanical valve infection occur during the initial 3 months postvalve replacement.

DIAGNOSIS OF MECHANICAL PROSTHETIC VALVE DYSFUNCTION

Clinical Findings

Prosthetic valve malfunction can result in stenosis or regurgitation; however, symptoms might range from none at all (incidental finding during routine imaging) to acute decompensated heart failure, cardiogenic shock, or even sudden cardiac arrest. Differentiating the most commonly encountered causes for mechanical valve dysfunction—thrombus and pannus are essential from a therapeutic point of view **(Table 2)**. Likelihood of thrombosis is high if there is a history of poor anticoagulant drug adherence, brief interruption, or documented subtherapeutic anticoagulation and embolic manifestations. Fever is present in about 70% of patients with prosthetic valve endocarditis.[5] Timing of presentation after valve surgery can provide clues to the etiology of prosthetic valve dysfunction. Early presentation is usually due to infection or technical factors related to surgery (patient-prosthesis mismatch, valve dehiscence, and paravalvular leaks).

A significant mechanical prosthetic valve obstruction caused by thrombosis, vegetation, or pannus development is typically indicated by a decrease in intensity or even lack of opening or closing sounds on auscultation. While physiologic flow murmur may be commonly appreciated (lower effective orifice area compared to native valves), significant para-or transvalvular regurgitation need not be always audible.

Imaging

Transthoracic echocardiography remains the main initial diagnostic tool for identifying prosthetic valve dysfunction. Visualization of thrombus, vegetations, and pannus may be limited by acoustic shadowing, and transesophageal echocardiography may be required for a more accurate assessment of the pathology.

TABLE 2: Differential diagnosis of thrombus and pannus.

	Thrombus	Pannus
Timing	• Occurs at any time (if late, usually associated with pannus) • Sudden symptom onset or subclinical	• Minimum 1 year from surgery (usually >5 years from surgery) • Progressive onset of symptoms or subclinical
Relation with anticoagulation/ subtherapeutic INR	More commonly associated	Poor association
Location	• More frequent mitral valve • Supra/subvalvular	• More frequent mitral valve • Subvalvular
Morphology	• Larger mass than pannus • Detected at TEE • Irregular mass attached to valves/hinge point • Centrifugal growth • Valve restriction • More commonly located on the atrial side for mitral prostheses and on the aortic side for aortic prostheses	• Small mass • Undetected at TEE • (Semi)circular mass involving the suture line • Centripetal growth • Valve restriction may be absent • More commonly located on the ventricular side for both mitral and aortic prostheses
Echo-density ultrasound video intensity ratio (video intensity of the mass to that of the prosthetic valve)	<0.4	>0.7
Impact on gradient	Mitral > aortic	Aortic > mitral
Impact on valve orifice	Mitral > aortic	Aortic > mitral
Impact on disc mobility	Yes	May be
MDCT attenuation value	<145 HU	>145–200 HU

(HU: hounsfield units; INR: international normalized ratio; MDCT: multidetector computed tomography; TEE: transesophageal echocardiography)

Following are the parameters that need to be assessed on echocardiography for evaluating prosthetic valve dysfunction:

- *Two dimensional echocardiography and color flow imaging:* Opening and closing of occluders (mobility), abnormal densities on the various components of the prosthesis or adjacent to prosthesis, sewing ring and disk integrity and prosthesis stability. Zoom imaging is needed for optimal visualization. Occluder or leaflet or excursion may be better appreciated on M-mode echocardiography. Independent or rocking motion indicates valve dehiscence for valves in the aortic position, while normal increased mobility may be encountered in the mitral position due to annular motion, atrial or annular reconstruction, or location of the sewing ring within the left atrium. Presence of paravalvular leak along with increased mobility suggests valve dehiscence in mitral position. Usually, mechanical valves have small regurgitant jets (physiological)—multiple jets located just inside the sewing ring, homogeneous in color and aliasing confined mostly to the base. Small hemodynamically insignificant paravalvular leaks may be observed immediately postsurgery. Pathological regurgitation can be either transvalvular (impaired closure motion of the valve discs by vegetations, pannus, or thrombus) or paravalvular (surgical technical factors, suture failure, annular disruption, prosthesis dehiscence, or endocarditis).
- *Doppler echocardiography:* Peak and mean gradients, Doppler velocity index (DVI), acceleration time (for aortic prosthesis), pressure half time (mitral), and calculated indexed effective orifice area. The prosthetic valve effective orifice area is calculated using the continuity equation; effective orifice area = stroke volume/prosthetic valve velocity-time integral (VTI).

In patients with elevated transvalvular gradients, high-flow states such as fever, anemia, hyperthyroidism, and atrioventricular shunts need to be excluded.

The Doppler parameters that suggest significant obstruction are as follows[6]:

- *For aortic valve:*[6]
  - Symmetric rounded Doppler jet
  - Peak velocity > 4 m/s
  - Mean gradient > 35 mm Hg
  - Doppler-velocity index (DVI) < 0.25
  - Effective orifice area < 0.8 cm^2 or indexed values < 0.65 cm^2/m^2
  - Acceleration time > 100 ms
  - Acceleration time/ejection time ratio > 0.37
- *For mitral valve:*[6]
  - Peak velocity > 2.5 m/s
  - Mean gradient > 10 mm Hg
  - Prosthetic mitral valve to left-ventricular outflow tract VTI ratio > 2.5
  - Effective orifice area < 1 cm^2
  - Pressure half time > 200 ms
- *For tricuspid valve:*[6]
  - Peak velocity > 1.7 m/s
  - Mean gradient > 6 mm Hg
  - Pressure half time > 230 ms
- *For pulmonary valves*:
  - Peak velocity > 3.2 m/s for bioprosthesis and >2.5 m/s for homograft
  - Mean gradient > 20 mm Hg for bioprosthesis and >15 mm Hg for homograft

Prosthesis-patient Mismatch

Patient-prosthetic mismatch occurs when the effective orifice area of the prosthetic valve is too small for the patient's resting blood flow requirements.

Patient prosthesis mismatch in aortic position is diagnosed if effective orifice area is <0.85 cm^2/m^2 if BMI < 30 kg/m^2 and <0.70 cm^2/m^2 if BMI > 30 kg/m^2.

For mitral position, patient prosthesis mismatch is diagnosed if effective orifice area is <1.2 cm^2/m^2 if BMI < 30 kg/m^2 and <1.0 cm^2/m^2 if BMI > 30 kg/m^2.

The echocardiography parameters that suggest significant regurgitation are as follows.[6] Severe prosthetic aortic regurgitation is identified on echocardiography by vena contracta width and area of >6 mm and 3 mm^2, respectively, circumferential extent of paravalvular leak > 30%, residual volume > 60, and regurgitant fraction > 50.[6]

Severe prosthetic mitral regurgitation is recognized on echocardiography by a large dense central jet (usually >8 cm^2 or >50% of left atrial area) with early peaking triangular jet contour, systolic blunting of pulmonary flow, vena contracta >7 mm, residual volume > 60, regurgitant fraction > 50, and effective regurgitant orifice area > 0.40 cm^2.[6]

Cardiac Computed Tomography

- Leaflet mobility, opening/closing angles, and mass characterization
- Detect thrombus/pannus

Cinefluoroscopy

Leaflet Mobility ± Opening/Closing Angles

The opening and closing angles (angle between disks in the fully open and closed positions) of bileaflet mechanical valves can be measured in orthogonal views and compared to those reported by the manufacturer **(Figs. 1A to H)**.

Cinefluoroscopy should be carried out in following projections—(1) the posteroanterior and lateral; (2) the "in profile" projection for calculation of opening and closing angles (radiographic beam parallel to both the valve ring plane and the tilting axis of disks) and; (3) the "en face" projection for mitral prostheses (radiographic beam parallel

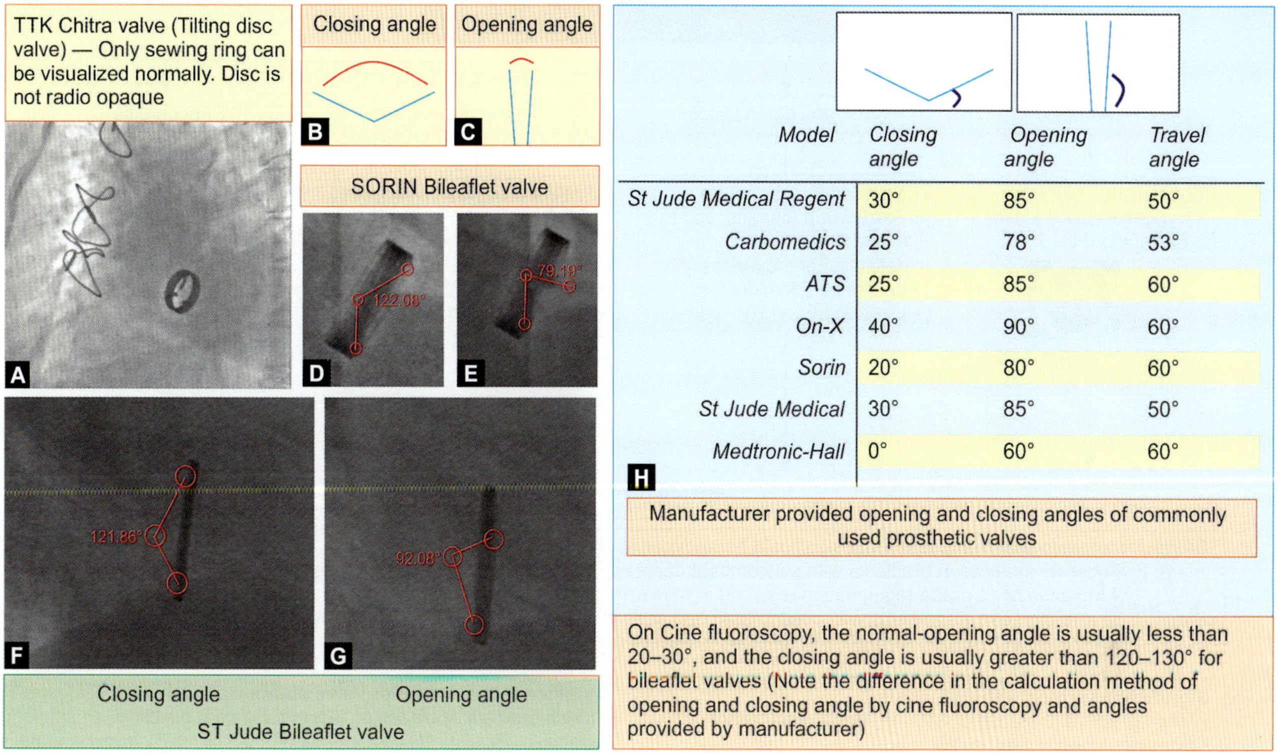

Model	Closing angle	Opening angle	Travel angle
St Jude Medical Regent	30°	85°	50°
Carbomedics	25°	78°	53°
ATS	25°	85°	60°
On-X	40°	90°	60°
Sorin	20°	80°	60°
St Jude Medical	30°	85°	50°
Medtronic-Hall	0°	60°	60°

FIGS. 1A TO H: Cine fluoroscopy for diagnosing mechanical valve dysfunction. (A) Cine fluoroscopy of TTK Chitra valve; (B and C) Measurement of closing and opening angles on fluoroscopy; (D and E) SORIN valve with reduced leaflet excursion; (F and G) St Jude valve with reduced leaflet excursion; (H) Manufacturer provided opening and closing angles of commonly used valves.

to the valve outflow tract) **(Figs. 1A to H)**. Abnormal tilting of the ring base may indicate valve dehiscence.

Bioprosthetic Valve Dysfunction

Both surgical and transcatheter bioprosthetic heart valves are at risk of dysfunction owing to their bioprosthetic nature. In 2021, the Valve Academic Research Consortium-3 provided an updated common standardized definition for characterizing transcatheter and surgical bioprosthetic valve dysfunction.[7] The four main processes of bioprosthetic valve dysfunction that eventually lead to hemodynamic deterioration (stages 1–3) and valve failure (stages 1–3) are identical to those for mechanical valves—thrombosis, endocarditis, nonstructural valve dysfunction, and structural valve degeneration **(Flowchart 1)**. Bioprosthetic valve thrombosis can be further classified as subclinical or clinical. Subclinical leaflet thrombosis is characterized by hypoattenuated leaflet thickening (HALT) and reduced leaflet motion (RLM) detected by multidetector computed tomography (MDCT).[8] HALT is a meniscal-shaped lesion situated on the aortic side of the leaflet and mostly easily visible during diastolic phase. The hypoattenuation affecting motion (HAM) is defined by the cooccurrence of HALT and RLM. A four-tiered scale is used to grade the severity of both HALT and RLM. Recent evidence from noninvasive imaging suggests occurrence of HALT in both porcine and pericardial surgical and transcatheter valves.

A recent meta-analysis of randomized clinical trials and observational studies showed a greater incidence of left sided bioprosthetic valve infective endocarditis than mechanical valves.[9] Early prosthetic valve endocarditis rarely affects the leaflets; it typically affects the paraprosthetic tissue which is a nidus for infection (sewing rings, annuluses, and sutures that have not endothelialized), and leads to valve dehiscence, abscess formation, paravalvular leaks, and fistula formation. Late bioprosthetic valve infections originate in the leaflet cusps and may involve the sewing ring or paravalvular region.

Mechanisms for structural and nonstructural degeneration are mentioned in **Flowchart 1**. Pannus ingrowth and structural valve degeneration might result in stenosis or regurgitation, which can trigger early valve failure. Bovine pericardial valve is more likely to develop stenosis, whereas porcine valves are likely to present with regurgitation.

In the recently published 10 year outcome of NOTION (Nordic Aortic Valve Intervention) trial, severe structural degeneration occurred less frequently in patients receiving transcatheter valve (1.5% vs. 10.0% HR 0.2; 95% CI 0.04–0.7;

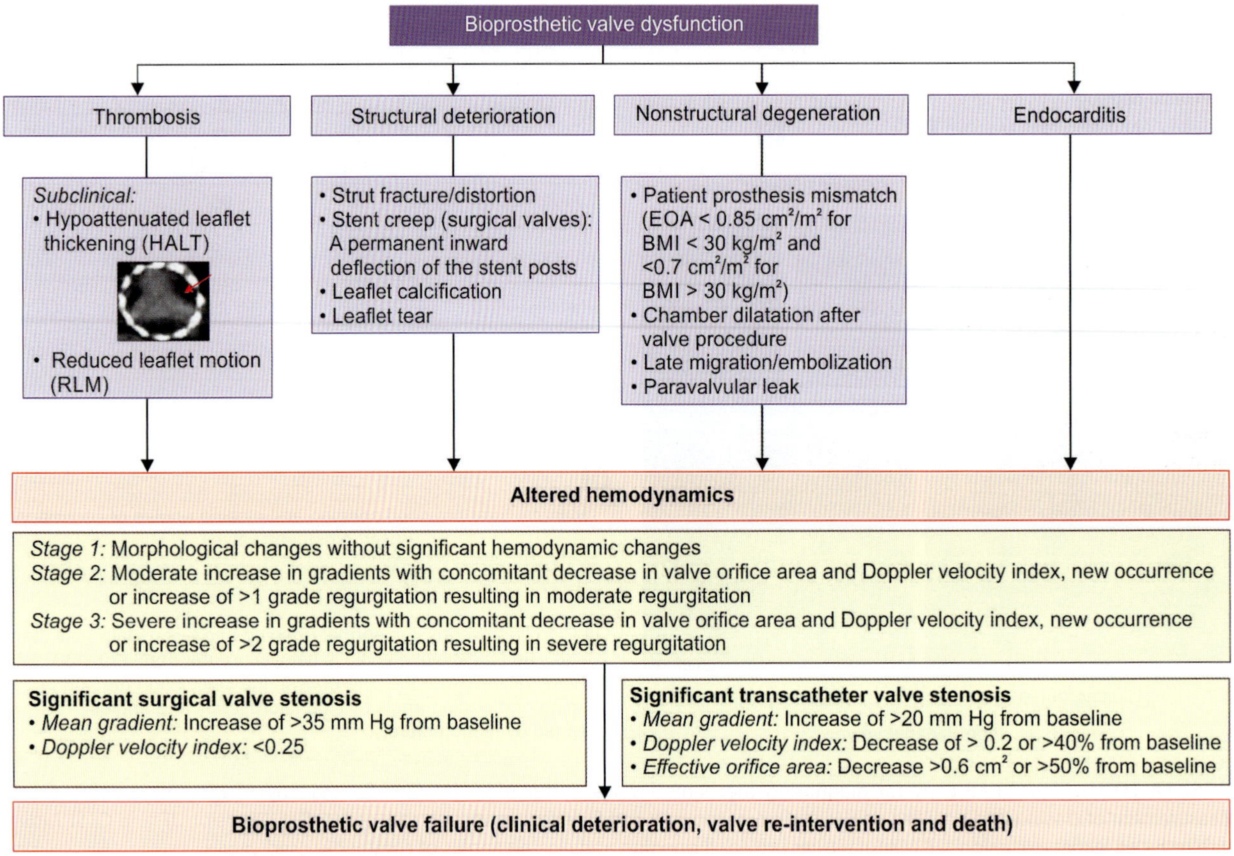

FLOWCHART 1: Bioprosthetic valve dysfunction.

$p = 0.02$) at 10 years. The cumulative incidence for severe nonstructural valve degeneration was 20.5% and 43.0% ($p < 0.001$) after transcatheter aortic valve implantation and surgical valve replacement, respectively while there was no significant difference in the endocarditis rates between the two groups.[10] The rates of structural valve degeneration and valve failure using recent standardized definitions in a low-risk population randomly assigned to receive transcatheter or surgical aortic valve replacement were assessed. While the rates of valve failure in both valve types were comparable over 6 years (6.7% for surgical vs. 7.5%), the rate of structural valve degeneration was substantially greater for surgical valves (24.0% vs. 2.8%). The rates of subclinical thrombosis of transcatheter and surgical bioprosthetic valves are presented in **Table 3**.[11-18]

DIAGNOSIS OF BIOPROSTHETIC VALVE DYSFUNCTION

Clinical manifestations of bioprosthetic valve dysfunction may vary from asymptomatic status to new symptoms, thromboembolic phenomenon, and heart failure with worsening of the left ventricular size and function, pulmonary hypertension, valve re-intervention, and/or death. Echocardiography is the main tool for assessing prosthetic valve function. Routine postprocedure follow-up assessments for transcatheter valve patients are performed predischarge, at 1 month, 1 year, and yearly thereafter. European Society of Cardiology guideline recommends yearly echocardiography for all bioprostheses while the American guidelines recommend yearly assessment only for transcatheter patients while surgical valve patients are given echocardiographic consideration at 5 years or if any symptom change.[19-21] In our clinical practice, surgical bioprosthetic valve recipients get echocardiography evaluations at 1-year intervals. Transthoracic echocardiography can identify the morphological changes of degenerated bioprosthetic valves and the hemodynamic consequences (stenosis or regurgitation) of structural and nonstructural valve degeneration. Transesophageal echocardiography offers greater precision compared to transthoracic echocardiography in detecting leaflet thickening, thrombosis, vegetations, abscess, paravalvular regurgitation, leaflet calcification, and tearing. In case of signs or symptoms of bioprosthetic valve dysfunction or clinical suspicion of endocarditis, a transthoracic echocardiography should be promptly performed. The echocardiographic evaluation should include anatomical

TABLE 3: Hypoattenuated leaflet thickening (HALT) after surgical bioprosthesis and transcatheter aortic valve implantation.

Author, year	Patients (*n*)	Type of valve	Study design	Summary of findings
Makkar et al.[11]	55 patients	Portico	• Substudy of the multicenter randomized controlled Portico IDE trial • CT analysis at 30 days	*CT-defined HALT at 30 days*: • 40% (22 of 55 analyzable CT's) • Portico: 43% (16/37) • SAPIEN XT 43% (6/14) • CoreValve 0% (0/4)
Hansson et al.[12]	405 patients	SAPIEN XT/3	• Single center, single-arm observational study • CT analysis at 1- and 3-month post-TAVI	*CT-defined valve thrombosis*: 7% of patients
Chakravarty et al.[13]	• 890 patients • 752 TAVR • 138 SAVR	• SAPIEN/3/XT • CoreValve/ Evolut • Lotus • Portico • Direct flow • Centera • Acurate • Multiple SAVR valves	• Combined results of the RESOLVE and SAVORY registries • CT analysis at ~3 months (but timing not prespecified)	*CT-defined HALT at 3 months*: • 12% of patients • HALT more common in TAVR than SAVR (13% vs. 4%, $p < 0.001$)
Khan et al.[14]	• 193 patients • 170 SAPIEN • 23 Evolut R/Pro	SAPIEN 3 Evolut R/Pro	• Subanalysis of the Low Risk Trial: Multicenter prospective trial with historical cohort as a comparator • 4DCT scan at 30 days	*CT-defined HALT at 30 days*: • SAPIEN 3: 16% (27/170) • Evolut R/Pro: 0% (0/23)
Blanke et al.[15]	*30-day outcomes*: • 318 patients • 179 TAVI • 139 SAVR *1-year outcomes*: • 268 patients • 152 TAVI • 116 SAVR	Evolut	• Pre-specified substudy of Evolut low-risk randomized controlled trial • Scheduled CT analysis at 3- and 12-month post-TAVI	• *CT-defined HALT at 30 days*: TAVI: 17.3%, SAVR 16.5%, $p = 0.86$ • *CT-defined HALT at 1 year*: TAVI: 30.9%, SAVR: 28.4%, $p = 0.66$
De Backer et al.[16]	• 231 patients • 115 patients Rivaroxaban • 116 patients on dual antiplatelet	• SAPIEN 3/XT • Evolut R/PRO • Accurate Neo • Portico • Lotus	• Prespecified substudy of the GALILEO • Randomized controlled trial. 4DCT at 3-month post implantation	• *CT-defined leaflet thickening at 3 months*: 2.1% rivaroxaban group versus 10.9% DAPT group (between group difference −8.8 percentage points, 95% CI −16.5 to −1.9, $p = 0.01$) • *CT-defined HALT at 3 months*: 12.4% Rivaroxaban group vs 32.4% DAPT group (between group difference −20.0 percentage points 95% CI −30.9 to −8.5)
Kim et al.[17]	204 patients	Acurate Neo2	• Multicenter single-arm observational study • Scheduled 4D-CT analysis at 30 days	*CT-defined HALT at 30 days*: 24.5% (50/204)
Brunner et al.[18]	50 patients	Acurate Neo/ Neo2	Scheduled CT analysis at 6 months	*CT-defined HALT at 6 months*:16% of patients

(CI: confidence interval; CT: computed tomography; HALT: hypoattenuated leaflet thickening; LVOT: left ventricular outflow tract; RR: relative risk; SAVR: surgical aortic valve replacement; TAVI: transcatheter aortic valve implantation) assessment of the prosthesis, color Doppler assessment of stenosis and regurgitation (intravalvar or periprosthetic), and hemodynamic evaluation using flow-dependent and independent parameters (mean transvalvular pressure gradient and calculation of effective orifice area). The 2D images should be compared with the baseline postprocedure images. The main echocardiographic characteristics of structural valve deterioration are thickening (>2 mm) and reduced mobility of hyperechogenic leaflets, calcifications of the leaflets and sewing ring (surgical bioprosthesis) and torn or flail leaflet. Significant structural deterioration is identified by an (1) increase in mean gradient > 20 mm Hg resulting in a mean gradient ≥30 mm Hg with concomitant decrease in effective orifice area ≥ 0.6 cm^2 or ≥50% and/or decrease in DVI ≥ 0.2 orm ≥ 40% compared with the baseline (1–3 months) postprocedural assessment. (2) New occurrence or increase of at least two grades of intraprosthetic leak resulting in moderate or greater to severe aortic regurgitation.[21,22] Pannus is characterized by a hyperechoic fixed layer in the vicinity of the leaflet base and ring and coupled with normal or RLM. Typically, thrombus is less echoic (iso or hypoechogenic mass) and adheres to the surface of the leaflets which appear hypomobile and thickened. Egbe and colleagues[23] suggested a combination of clinical and echocardiographic criteria to diagnose prosthetic valve thrombosis (76% sensitivity, 93% specificity, 85% positive predictive value, and 89% negative predictive value). The diagnostic criteria included a >50% increase in mean echo-Doppler gradient from baseline within 5 years, paroxysmal atrial fibrillation, subtherapeutic international normalized ratio, increased cusp thickness, and abnormal cusp mobility. 3-dimensional transesophageal echocardiography can precisely identify the location of a paravalvular leak and useful for percutaneous leak closure.

CT scan provides superior spatial resolution and may be an alternative diagnostic tool in patients with suboptimal acoustic window and in situations where transesophageal echocardiography is not possible. While CT cannot distinguish between fibrotic valve thickening and thrombus, it can be useful in distinguishing between these two processes from pannus, which occurs circumferentially below the valve level and usually spares the leaflets. Cardiac magnetic imaging is relatively safe for imaging at both 1.5-T and 3.0-T for several valve types, but has a limited role in the evaluation of bioprosthetic valve dysfunction. It has a poorer temporal resolution than echocardiography, which can limit its capacity to detect tiny lesions, like vegetation,

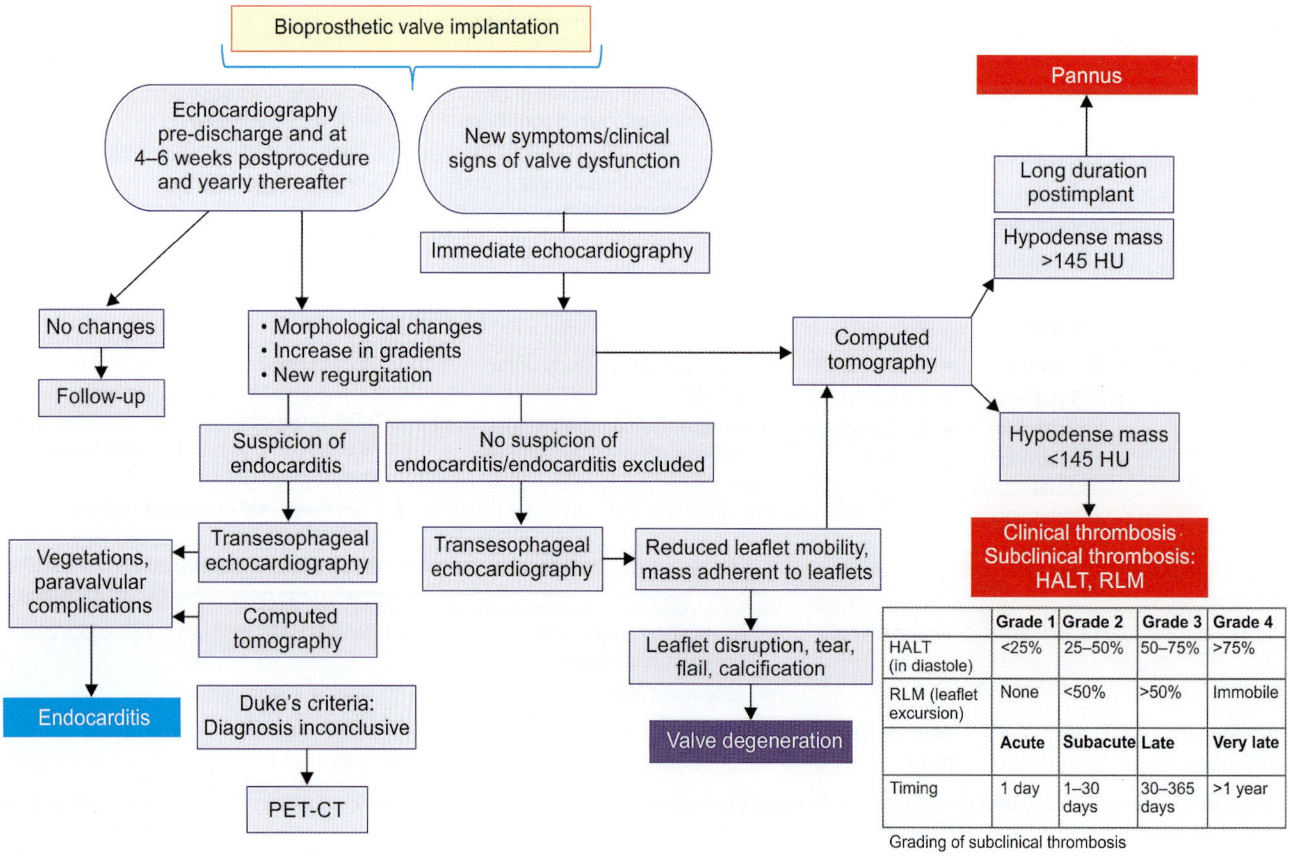

	Grade 1	Grade 2	Grade 3	Grade 4
HALT (in diastole)	<25%	25–50%	50–75%	>75%
RLM (leaflet excursion)	None	<50%	>50%	Immobile
	Acute	**Subacute**	**Late**	**Very late**
Timing	1 day	1–30 days	30–365 days	>1 year

FLOWCHART 2: Diagnostic algorithm for bioprosthetic valve dysfunction.
(CT: computed tomography; HALT: hypoattenuated leaflet thickening; RLM: reduced leaflet motion)

although having great spatial resolution. Nevertheless, MRI-calculated effective orifice area has been shown to correlate with effective orifice area determined by echocardiography even for dysfunctional valves. MRI can also be useful in the quantification of regurgitant volume and fraction in regurgitant valves. Very large thrombus can also be identified by cardiac MRI utilizing postcontrast first pass (nonenhancing mass) and LGE (hypointense border and a brighter center zone). Thrombus may appear completely dark in LGE sequences with long inversion time. For individuals with suspected prosthetic valve endocarditis with inconclusive echocardiogram and blood culture results, nuclear imaging with ^{18}F-fluorodeoxyglucose positron emission tomography/CT can identify active infection.

Finally, an algorithm is provided for the diagnosis of bioprosthetic valve dysfunction **(Flowchart 2)**.

CONCLUSION

In summary, mechanical and bioprosthetic valve dysfunction can be caused by thrombosis, endocarditis, structural degeneration, and nonstructural degeneration. They can impact the lifespan of the prosthetic valve and present with overlapping clinical manifestations. Multimodality imaging with echocardiography, cinefluoroscopy, and CT are needed to diagnose mechanisms of prosthetic valve dysfunction. For bioprosthetic valves, CT complements echocardiography for identifying clinical and subclinical thrombosis.

ONLINE REFERENCES

Please scan the QR code provided at the end of the table of contents for References of this chapter.

CHAPTER 181

Tips and Tricks of Transseptal Puncture in Different Structural Heart Interventions

A Sreenivas Kumar, Ramakrishna J

ABSTRACT

Advancements in left-sided structural heart interventions have increased the need for transseptal puncture, a crucial technique for mitral valve interventions. Since its introduction in the 1950s, it has evolved into a safer and more effective procedure, with a focus on indications, techniques, complications, and site-specific punctures.

Keywords: Transseptal puncture, techniques, complications

INTRODUCTION

Over the last decade, advancements in left-sided structural heart interventions have driven an increased need for transseptal puncture (TSP). TSP is an essential interventional technique, particularly for accessing the left atrium and performing various structural heart disease interventions involving mitral valve. Since its introduction in the late 1950s, TSP has evolved significantly, becoming safer and more effective procedure due to advancements in technology and a deeper understanding of cardiac anatomy with better utilization of imaging modalities. This chapter delves into the application of TSP in the management of various structural heart diseases, exploring its indications, techniques, complications, innovations, and site-specific punctures.

HISTORICAL BACKGROUND

The TSP was developed by Ross, Braunwald, and Morrow at National Heart Institute in the 1950s to allow left heart catheterization[1] for assessment of left-sided valvular heart disease. Later minor modification of the needles and sheaths led to safe and effective procedure with minimal complications. The use of TSP for diagnostic purpose has decreased significantly with advances and knowledge of echocardiography.[2] With recent advances in structural heart interventions which require site-specific TSPs to allow navigation of large size devices across IAS[3] easily. Initially, the procedure was associated with significant risks, but over the years, improvements in equipment and techniques have reduced these risks, making TSP a cornerstone in the treatment of structural heart diseases.

INDICATIONS FOR TRANSSEPTAL PUNCTURE[3]

Transseptal puncture is indicated in a range of structural heart disease interventions, including **(Figs. 1A to H)**:

- *Mitral valve interventions*:
  - Mitral balloon valvuloplasty [percutaneous balloon mitral valvotomy (PBMV)]
  - Mitral valve repair
  - Mitral valve replacement [transcatheter mitral valve repair (TMVR)]
  - Closure of mitral paravalvular leaks
- *Left atrial appendage closure*:
  - *Electrophysiological procedures*: Catheter ablation for atrial fibrillation/left-sided accessory pathway ablation
  - *Percutaneous left ventricular assist device (LVAD) placement*: Hemodynamic support in high-risk patients
- Antegrade treatment of aortic valve disease—not in use nowadays
- Balloon atrial septostomy for severe pulmonary hypertension

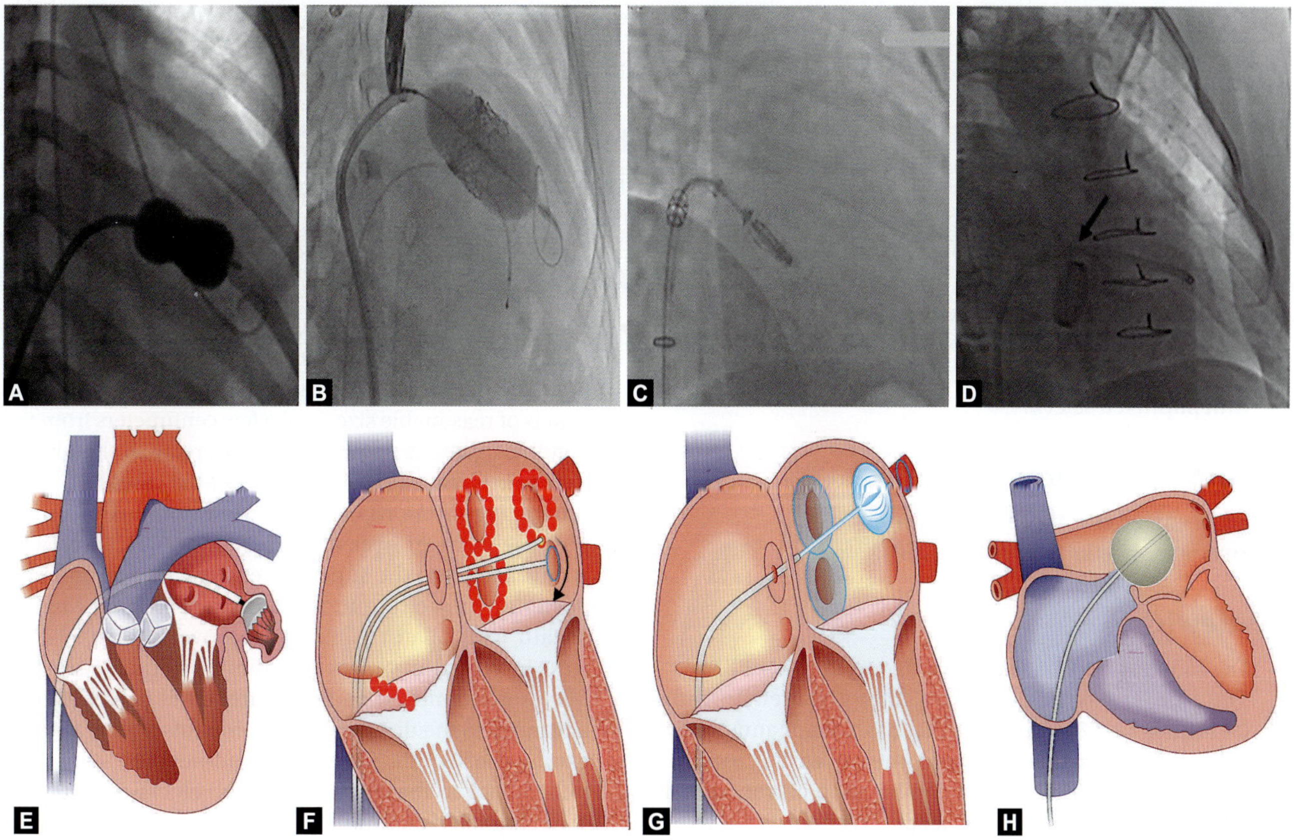

FIGS. 1A TO H: Various indications for transseptal puncture. (A) Percutaneous balloon mitral valvotomy; (B) Transcatheter mitral valve replacement in degenerated previous bioprosthetic surgical valve; (C) Mitra clip for severe MR; (D) Mitral PVL closure; (E) LAA closure; (F and G) RF and cryoablation of atrial fibrillation; (H) Balloon atrial septostomy.

CONTRAINDICATIONS FOR TRANSSEPTAL PUNCTURE[4]

Absolute: Septal thrombus, mobile LA cavity thrombus, or tumor

Relative:[4]

- Distorted anatomy
- Hugely dilated LA and RA
- Enlarged aortic root
- Interrupted IVC
- Bleeding disorders
- Post ASD patch closure or device closure

TECHNIQUES OF TRANSSEPTAL PUNCTURE

Preprocedural Planning

Successful TSP begins with thorough preprocedural planning. Imaging modalities such as preprocedural chest X-ray, echocardiography, transesophageal echocardiography (TEE), intracardiac echocardiography (ICE), and cardiac computed tomography (CT) are invaluable in assessing atrial septal anatomy and identifying potential difficult anatomies. Crossing the IAS through fossa ovalis under fluoroscopy will be sufficient for simple procedure like measuring LA pressure.[3] But for complex structural interventions, the utilization of multimodality imaging makes superior anatomic approach to TSP than fluoroscopy-based procedure, enabling safe and efficacious TSP in increasingly complex anatomies. Preprocedural TEE is performed to rule out LA thrombus and thrombus attached to interatrial septum, which also allow us to study the characteristics of IAS including length, thickness, and presence of PFO or ASD.[5]

Left atrium is the most posterior structure of the heart and in patients with mitral valve diseases like mitral stenosis or regurgitation there could be large LA enlargement. A transseptal sheath and needle assembly pointing toward the spinous process of the left spinal border will invariably encounter the left atrium. Posteriorly directed TSP needle will avoid trauma to the aorta and avoid perforation in the vast majority (exceptions exist) of patients undergoing TSP for structural heart interventions.[6]

EQUIPMENT

Transseptal Needle

The Brockenbrough stainless steel needle (Medtronic) is the most commonly used needle for mechanical puncture of the fossa ovalis **(Fig. 2)**.

- *The BRK needles* (St. Jude Medical) are similar in design to the Brockenbrough needle but are available in multiple lengths and curves.
- *The NRG RF transseptal needle* (Baylis) uses radiofrequency (RF) energy and allows the operator to cross the IAS in a controlled manner without using excessive force with improved safety.[6,7]

Sheath and Dilator

- Fixed curved sheaths (e.g., Mullins)
- Steerable sheaths (e.g., Agilis)

Guidewires

- The stainless steel LA wire is used commonly for PBMV.
- *The SafeSept wire* is a 120-cm nitinol guidewire with 0.014-inch or 0.035 diameter that has a sharp and floppy "J tip". The sharp tip of safe sept wire can easily cross the fossa ovalis when used with combination of transseptal dilator and sheath without needle. Without the dilator and sheath, the tip of the guidewire assumes a "J" shape, thereby reducing the complications during TSP.[8]
- *Confida* 0.035-inch wire (Medtronic) and the *Safari* 0.035-inch wire (Boston Scientific) can also be used for stable LA guidewire position.

Imaging Tools

TEE, ICE, and fluoroscopy are the tools for real-time guidance.[9]

Procedural Steps

- *Vascular access*: Typically, the right femoral vein for index procedure and femoral or radial artery access for pressure monitoring are used during TSP. The femoral vein is of reasonable size until a few centimeters from the inguinal ligament and it does not bifurcate so slightly low puncture is reasonable in majority of the cases.[6]
- *Advancing to the right atrium*: The Judkins or multipurpose catheter over a 0.032-inch or 0.035-inch wire is advanced into the superior vena cava in the anterior-posterior projection under fluoroscopy. Then Mullins sheath with dilator is exchanged over the 0.035-inch wire in superior vena cava; the 0.035-inch wire and dilator are removed and the transseptal needle is then advanced to the distal end of the Mullins sheath without exiting the sheath. The sheath and needle assembly is pulled back to the right atrium with clockwise rotation. Two characteristic "jumps" of the dilator tip are usually described: One as the tip passes under the SVC-RA junction, and one as the tip passes under the muscular

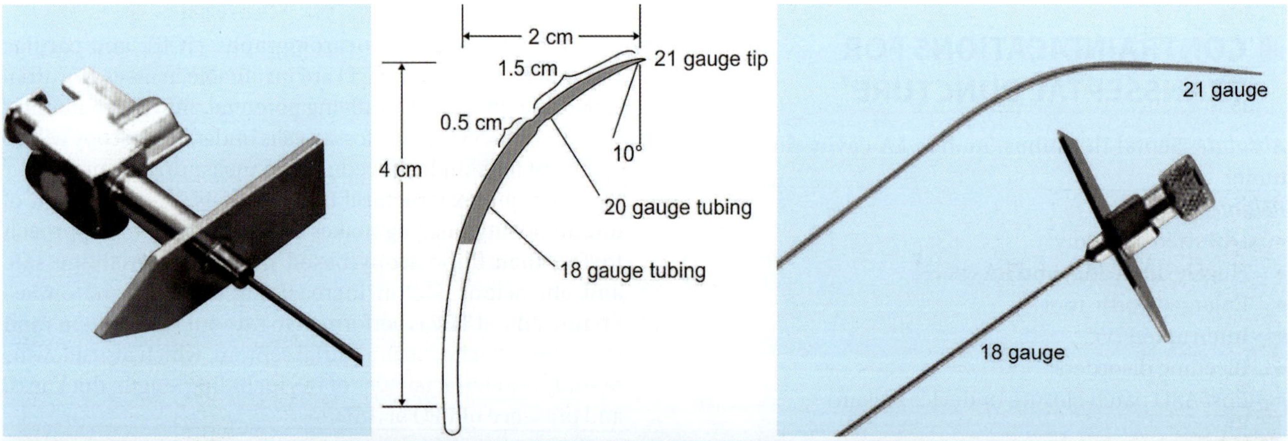

Brockenbrough needle (Medtronic Inc.)		
Shaft size	**Tip size**	**Length**
	Adult	
18 gauge	21 gauge	71 cm
	Pediatric	
19 gauge	22 gauge	56 cm

FIG. 2: Brockenbrough needle.

septum in to the fossa. A pigtail catheter is placed in the noncoronary sinus as an anatomical marker of the aortic root.[9]

- *Imaging guidance for localization of the puncture site*: Traditionally, the fluoroscopy has been the main imaging modality for localization of the fossa ovalis with multiple angiographic projections.[10] Various fluoroscopic projections like lateral view, AP, left anterior oblique (LAO), and right anterior oblique (RAO) views were used to confirm the position below the aortic root. Once the TS sheath is just below the pigtail catheter in the RAO view or AP view, the angle is changed to LAO, and in LAO view the sheath and needle assembly is pointing in between the spine column and pigtail catheter in aortic root.[11] After wedging, the septal puncture needle tip against the IAS—the septal "staining" technique—can be used by injecting 1–2 mL of diluted contrast through the septal puncture needle tip before entering the LA **(Fig. 5B)**.[3] In difficult cases, right atrial angiography with delayed filling LA angiography can help visualize the interatrial septum. Though many operators are comfortable with fluoroscopy-guided septal puncture, use of ultrasound-guided imaging like TEE and ICE allows direct visualization of IAS and provides reassurance that the site-specific location of the puncture and is optimal with increased safety and success. TSP in difficult cases, such as in patients with thickened septum, aneurysmal septum, patients with abnormally rotated hearts, and those with thickened or fibrotic IAS due to patch repair, the TEE guidance allows precise location of TSP with real-time guidance for operator. In more complex anatomies, 3D TEE provides a more precise location of the TSP needle position in relation to adjacent vital cardiac structures. TEE-guided septal puncture allow us to ensure coaxial alignment of devices and catheters, and to ensure adequate space to maneuver within the left atrium for various structural heart procedures.[11]
- *Positioning at the fossa ovalis*: The position is confirmed using fluoroscopy and TEE. The fundamental maneuvers to achieve needle positioning against interatrial septum, including clockwise rotation for posterior and counterclockwise rotation for anterior rotation.[11]
- *Needle advancement and puncture*: The needle is carefully advanced to puncture the interatrial septum with contrast injection or visualization of tenting of interatrial septum in TEE in biplane view away from aorta visualizing its anteroposterior orientation **(Figs. 3A and B)**.[11]
- *Left atrial access*: Once the left atrium is accessed, we can confirm it by detecting the LA pressure tracings, aspirating oxygenated blood, or with contrast injection.[3] The Mullins sheath or Agilis sheath is advanced over the broken borough needle and then LA wire or other stiff wire is placed in LA.

Radiofrequency Ablation of IAS

Electrocauterization of IAS with the existing apparatus can be performed using a standard surgical cautery by very briefly touching the proximal part of the transseptal needle. RF ablation using the NRG Baylis needle or Versa Cross combined system (Baylis Medical) is used in some laboratories and can be helpful in difficult cases.[12] The RF catheter is substituted for Brockenbrough needle that is introduced into the dilator/sheath assembly (TorFlex™ Transseptal Guiding Sheath; Baylis Medical). This catheter can perforate the atrial septum by delivering 5 W energy for 2–5 seconds after 1–4 pulses. This RF ablation technique will be more useful in scarred, calcified, thick fibrous or patched atrial septa, where excess force could result in perforation of the LA free wall due to overshoot phenomenon or unsuccessful puncture.[12]

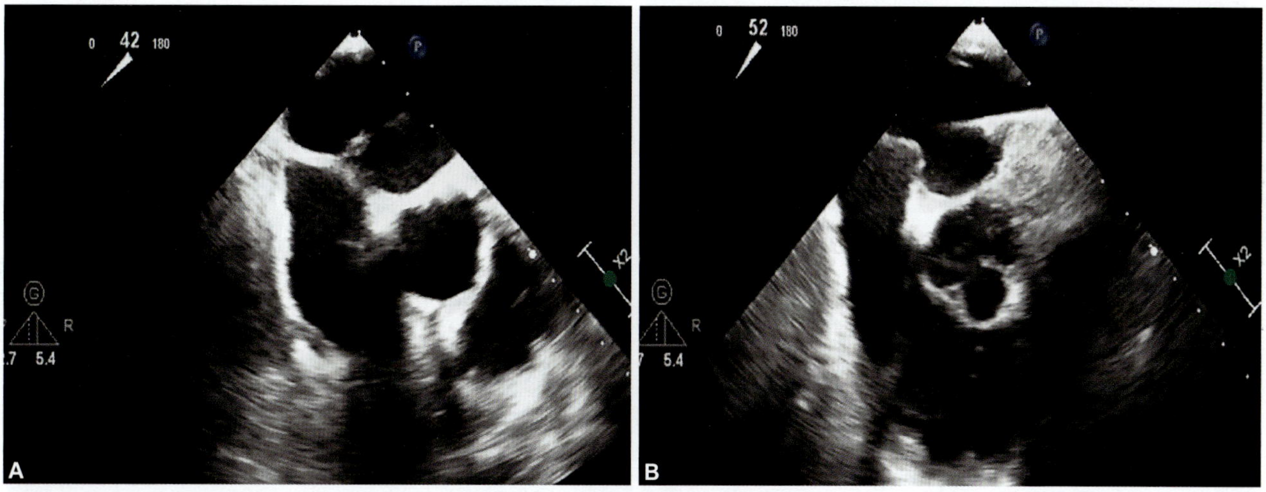

FIGS. 3A AND B: TEE image showing tenting of IAS away from aorta in short-axis view.

APPLICATIONS IN STRUCTURAL HEART INTERVENTIONS

Mitral Valve Interventions

Percutaneous Balloon Mitral Valvotomy

Percutaneous balloon mitral valvotomy is primarily indicated for symptomatic severe mitral stenosis with suitable pliable valve. TSP is essential for crossing the interatrial septum to position the balloon across the stenosed mitral valve. The Inoue balloon technique, widely used in PBMV, relies heavily on accurate TSP **(Fig. 4)**.

For PBMV, a mid-posterior puncture is usually adequate and provides a favorable working height in the left atrium and a coaxial plane with the mitral valve, which is usually associated with enlarged left atrium.[13,14]

Mitral Valve Repair and Replacement

Transcatheter mitral valve repair (e.g., MitraClip or TEER) and replacement procedures (e.g., TMVR) require site-specific TSP with proper guide catheter placement to deliver large bore devices to the middle of the diseased mitral valve. Biplane TEE is essential to provide simultaneous visualization of the orthogonal short-axis view, which allows visualization of the anterior-posterior axis of the atrial septum along with bicaval view. TEE-guided 4-chamber (0–20) view or reverse 4-chamber (160–180) view can be used to measure the anterior-posterior distance from the mitral valve (or annulus) to the TSP site for various mitral procedures.[6] In the case of MitraClip procedures, TEE operator should measure the height of the puncture (the distance between the tenting and the mitral annulus) in four chamber view. A height of at least 4 cm is required in patients with degenerative mitral regurgitation, whereas in functional mitral regurgitation a 3–4 cm distance is acceptable for device manipulation in LA.[15]

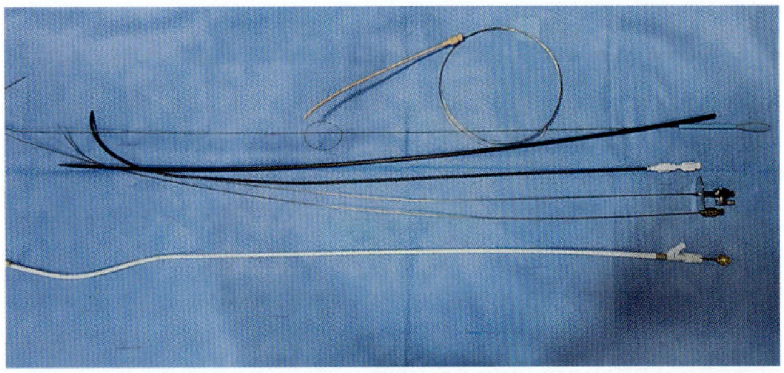

FIG. 4: PBMV with Inoue balloon, transseptal needle, Mullins sheath, septal dilator, and LA wire.

The location of TSP like posterior and slightly superior TSP for central MR jet and a posterior and slightly lower puncture site for lateral MR jet is appropriate for catheter movement in left atrium. Higher TSP heights are needed for more medial jets, while lower transseptal sites are more appropriate when lateral jets for paravalvular leak device closure.[6] The location of TSP affects procedural success and outcomes, which allows the room for device orientation toward the mitral valve **(Figs. 5A to F)**.[11]

Left Atrial Appendage Occlusion

The appropriate location of TSP enables the coaxial navigation and deployment of the occlusion device into the left atrial appendage, necessitating precise puncture. As long axis of LAA is anteriorly oriented, so a more posterior TSP will provide the more favorable sheath orientation with LAA long axis. A TSP that is too anterior or too superior can make it difficult to align the sheath and device delivery with the long axis of the LAA, especially in patients with retroverted LAAs. The ideal height of TSP also depends on particular device like for the Watchman device and the Amplatzer Cardiac Plug; midseptal to slightly inferior TSP is ideal and for the LARIAT device, a more superior location has been suggested.[3,4]

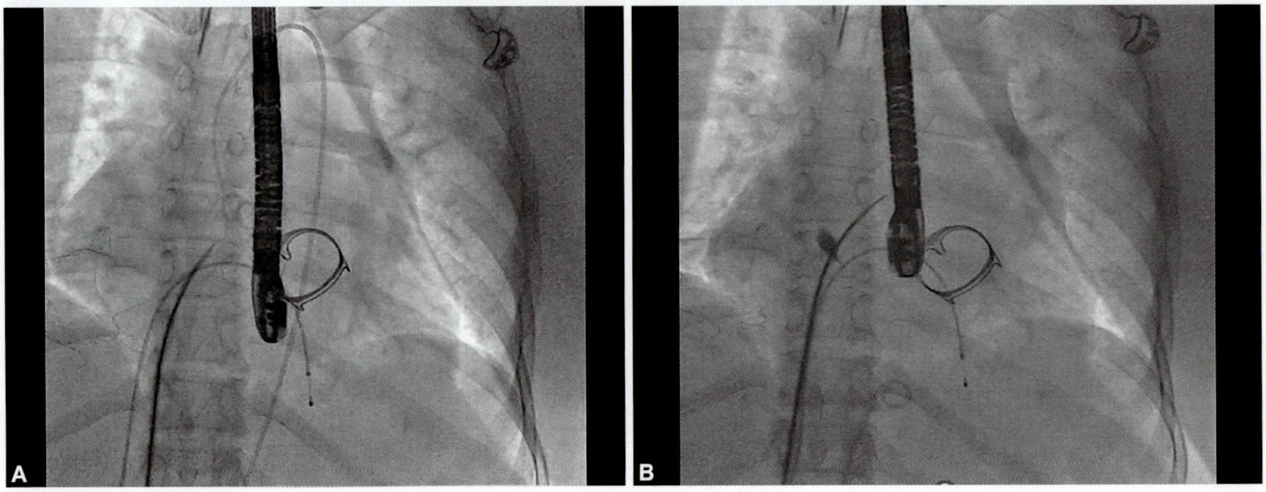

FIGS. 5A TO F: *Continued*

Continued

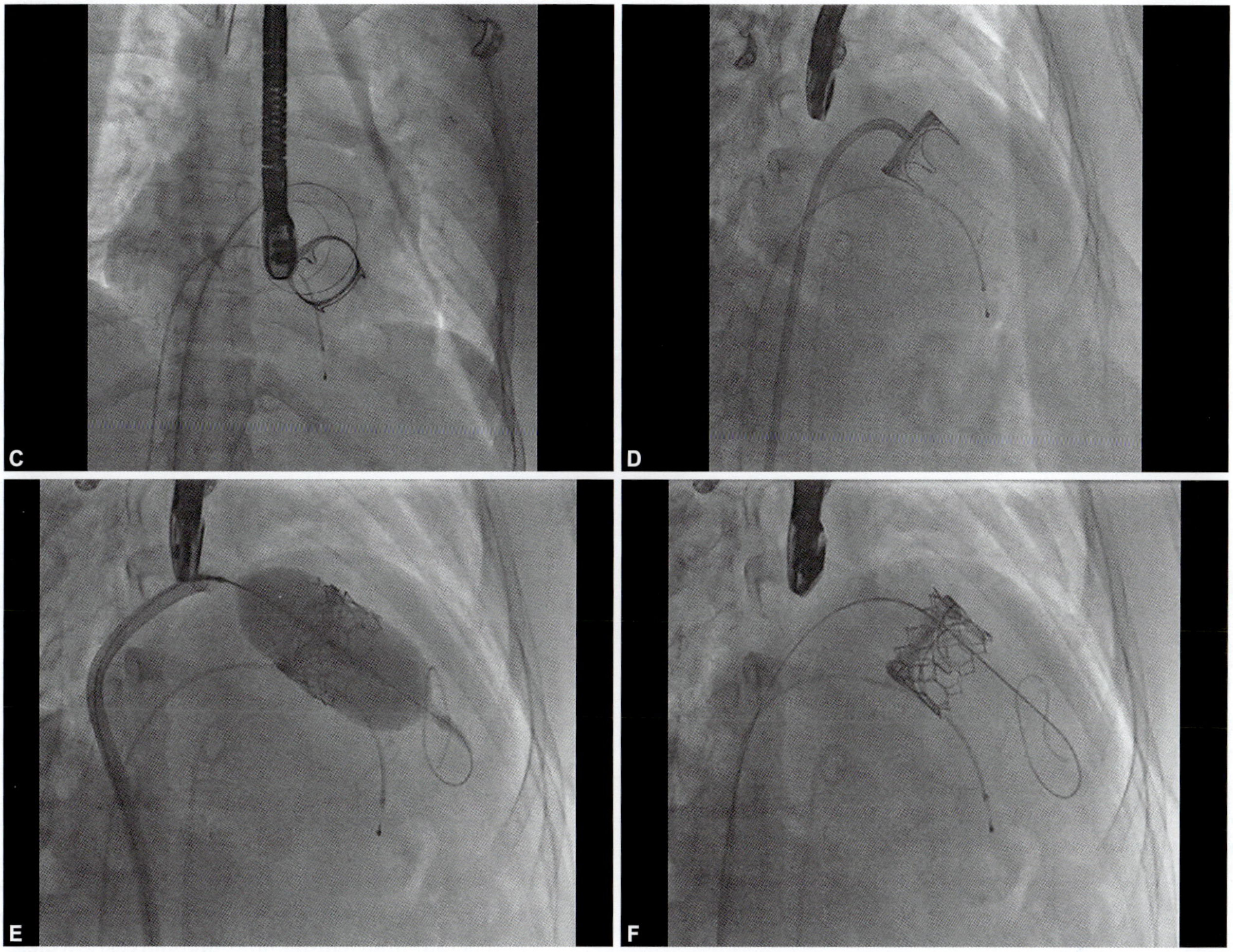

FIGS. 5A TO F: (A) TSP under TEE and fluoroscopy (AP view) with pigtail catheter in NCC; (B) Septal staining with diluted contrast just before TSP needle entry to LA; (C) Placing LA wire; (D) Tip deflectable Agilis sheath with mitral valve crossing; (E and F) TMVR with valve in degenerated tissue mitral valve. Transcatheter mitral valve implantation for degenerated tissue valve.

Electrophysiological Procedures

Accessing the left atrium with TSP is essential for pulmonary vein isolation and other ablation strategies in AF rhythm control. Ablation of left-sided accessory pathways for the treatment of other supraventricular tachycardias also requires TSP. A more anterior crossing of the IAS provides the most favorable approach for accessing all PVs, which are most posterior structures in LA with the Cryoballoon, particularly the right inferior PV.[16]

Percutaneous Left Ventricular Assist Device Placement

In high-risk patients requiring hemodynamic support, percutaneous LVADs (e.g., TandemHeart) are deployed via TSP. Mid-Fossa ovalis access for central transseptal catheter positioning allows more room in the left atrium and reduces the likelihood of device malfunction because of cannula–LA wall contact.[3,4,6]

Challenging Anatomies for Transseptal Puncture

- The extreme venous tortuosity can make the procedure difficult and may need large bore, long sheaths to enter RA. The other difficulties for venous access include venous obstructions, presence of IVC filters, and interrupted IVC. The other accesses like left femoral vein or right internal jugular vein and direct right atrial access provide good alternative venous sites in select cases.
- Chest wall abnormalities such as scoliosis and kyphoscoliosis will change the fluoroscopic orientation to the operator. In these cases TEE-guided septal puncture is safe and associated with less complications.
- Grossly dilated left or right atrium, abnormally rotated heart due to prior surgery, and dilated ascending aorta pose significant challenges during TSP. These intrinsic challenges can be successfully overcome by real-time imaging guidance with TEE or ICE and by using a large-

curved transseptal needle or by manually adding a secondary bend to the transseptal needle.

- *Difficulty at septal puncture site*: Some patients with thickened or hypertrophied IAS, fibrosis of IAS due to prior procedure or surgery will pose significant challenges during puncture. The use of a large-curved transseptal needle (e.g., BRK-1), advancement of transseptal needle stylet or sharp-tipped wires (the back of a 0.014-inch exchange angioplasty wire) through the needle to facilitate needle crossing, and using an RF transseptal needle can overcome some of these challenges. IAS aneurysm is another challenging subset leading more complications such as LA perforation due reduced distance between tented IAS and LA opposite wall. The different types of IAS aneurysms and the slight modifications of the septal puncture with different needle directions so as to enable stable uncomplicated puncture were described before.[17] Application of electrocautery or RF energy can be useful in these cases.

INNOVATIONS AND FUTURE DIRECTIONS

Imaging Advances

Recent advancements in imaging techniques have enhanced the safety and efficacy of TSP. Real-time 3D TEE and ICE provide detailed visualization of the interatrial septum, facilitating precise puncture and device deployment. A novel imaging software (EchoNavigator; Philips Healthcare, Best, the Netherlands) allows the integration between fluoroscopic and TEE images: It acquires patient-specific imaging data from both fluoroscopic projections and bi-/tri-dimensional TEE volumetric data sets and finally overlaps them. By integrating both imaging modalities, the limitations of each imaging modality can be counterbalanced leading to better visualization of cardiac valves and septum, resulting in more safe and effective procedures.

Robotic Assistance

Robotic systems are being developed to assist in TSP, aiming to improve precision and reduce operator fatigue. These systems leverage advanced imaging and robotic control to enhance procedural outcomes.

Novel Sheath Designs

Innovations in sheath design, such as steerable sheaths, provide greater control and flexibility during TSP. These designs enable better navigation through complex anatomical structures and improve access to target sites.

COMPLICATIONS AND MANAGEMENT

- *Cardiac tamponade*: Mostly due to overshoot with TSP needle, leading to LA-free wall perforation. It is managed with pericardiocentesis.
- *Atrial perforation*: It requires immediate attention and possible surgical repair.
- *Aortic puncture*: This complication can occur with inadequate experience in septal puncture and the correct method described is not followed for the TSP. In case of suspected aortic puncture or when the puncture site is in doubt, the dilator and sheath should not be advanced nor the needle to be pulled out in panic, but small contrast puff injection and checking the pressure tracings through needle will sort out the problem and aid in safe puncture. Only small needle puncture in wrong site without advancement of dilator or sheath mostly will not lead to effusion or tamponade if detected before we fully heparinize the patient. So we recommend full heparinization of the patient once we make sure of the correct puncture and entry into LA from proper site after checking with contrast injections and LA entry confirmation by proper pressure tracings.
- *Systemic embolization*: It is prevented by meticulous technique and anticoagulation management.
- *Air embolism*: It is totally preventable complication, and sometimes could lead to catastrophe, especially when the air traverses from LA to aorta and coronaries.
- *Iatrogenic ASD*: It may need device closure in some cases with large defects.
- *ST-segment elevation*: Sometimes we observe inferior segment ST elevation and is accompanied by vagal signs (hypotension, bradycardia, and diaphoresis), which is mostly due to the Bezold–Jarisch-like reflex. It is probably caused by the high density of parasympathetic fibers in the septum, leading to cholinergic vasospasm. If ST elevation persists, air or thrombus embolism might be the cause and should be treated accordingly.

CONCLUSION

With expanding indications of minimally invasive transcatheter solutions for structural heart diseases, the TSP has become a fundamental skill in interventional cardiology. TSP provides an easy access to the left atrium and enabling a variety of interventional procedures on left heart. The ongoing evolution of imaging modalities, device designs, and robotic assistance will further enhance the safety and effectiveness of TSP, solidifying its role in the future of cardiovascular interventions.

ONLINE REFERENCES

Please scan the QR code provided at the end of the table of contents for References of this chapter.

CHAPTER

182

Acute Emergencies in Cardiac Valves

Smit Shrivastava

ABSTRACT

The rheumatic valvular heart diseases (VHDs) are on a decline; yet with effective treatment and increased longevity, the degenerative VHDs are on a rise. Therefore, cardiac emergencies arising out of valve pathologies are not uncommon. However, the recommendations for managing such emergencies desire a need for standardization and update. The first step is to have a low threshold for suspecting VHD as a cause for emergency clinical presentation in patients with known and unknown VHD, and then to proceed to confirmation of the suspicion and assessment of the severity of VHD for appropriate treatment. The final step should include assessment of the natural and unnatural courses of the disease.

Keywords: Valvular heart disease, heart valves, heart valve prosthesis, emergency medicine

INTRODUCTION

The valvular heart disease (VHD) in developing countries has a bimodal incidence with rheumatic valve disease presenting from the third to the fourth decade and degenerative valve diseases presenting after the sixth decade of life. The VHD affects about 2.5% of the general population.[1] Most of the untreated VHD end up with heart failure and death. The natural course is often castrated by infective endocarditis, acute decompensated heart failure, arrhythmias, and thrombotic events. Any and all of these can present with a valve-associated cardiac emergency. Acute valvular emergencies comprise approximately 8% of coronary care unit admissions.[2] The cardiac symptoms are no different than any other cardiac disease and, therefore, often require a high degree of suspicion. The early recognition of valvular emergency can prompt rapid evaluation followed by surgical or percutaneous interventions that presage the best prognosis.

SUSPICION AND PROMPT RECOGNITION OF ACUTE VALVE EMERGENCY

It is vital to recognize the signs and symptoms of a presenting valve emergency from the history and clinical scenario to be able to direct further evaluation by cardiac imaging **(Box 1 and Table 1)**. The common valvular emergencies are the following:

- Acute aortic regurgitation (AR)
- Acute mitral regurgitation (MR)
- Critical aortic stenosis presenting with cardiogenic shock (CS) or pulmonary edema
- Critical mitral stenosis presenting with pulmonary edema and CS
- *General complications*:
    - Heart failure
    - Atrial fibrillation (AF)
    - Valvular thrombosis
    - Rheumatic fever
    - Infective endocarditis
    - Implantation complications

BOX 1 Symptoms of valve emergency.

- Dyspnea
- Orthopnea
- Paroxysmal nocturnal dyspnea
- Edema
- Chest pain
- Syncope
- Palpitation
- Embolic stroke

TABLE 1: Signs of valve emergency.

General examination	Sign	Suspected valve pathology
Dermatological	Subcutaneous nodules	Acute rheumatic fever
	Erythema marginatum	Acute rheumatic fever
	Osler nodules	Infective endocarditis
	Janeway lesions	Infective endocarditis
	Petechiae nails/skin	Infective endocarditis
Fingers	Capillary pulsation with light compression of the nail (Quincke)	Aortic regurgitation
	Nail clubbing	Congenital heart diseases, infective endocarditis
	Nail bed splinter lesions	Infective endocarditis
Head	Rosy–purple malar cheeks	Mitral stenosis
	de Musset's head—bobbing head	Aortic regurgitation
	Müller's pulsation of the uvula	Aortic regurgitation
Eye	Landolfi's pulsation of pupils	Aortic regurgitation
	White-centered retinal hemorrhage (Roth spots)	Infective endocarditis
Neck	Lancisi's giant systolic pulsations with prominent V waves	Tricuspid regurgitation
	Corrigan's dancing carotids	Aortic regurgitation
Abdomen	Gerhardt's pulsation of the spleen	Aortic regurgitation
	Rosenbach's pulsation of the liver	Aortic regurgitation
Pulse	Corrigan's bounding pulse (Watson's water hammer)	Aortic regurgitation
	Parvus et tardus	Aortic stenosis
Murmur	Apical holosystolic	Mitral regurgitation
	Systolic crescendo–decrescendo at the right upper sternal border	
	Diastolic rumble at the apex, often with an opening snap	
	Diastolic decrescendo usually heard at the third left intercostal space	
	Holosystolic, increasing during inspiration at the left lower sternal border	
	Short mid-diastolic rumble heard loudest at the apex in the absence of an opening snap associated with holosystolic murmur	

ACUTE VALVE INCOMPETENCE

Almost all acute VHDs involve MR or AR. There are cardinal differences in the pathophysiologic mechanisms implicated in acute versus chronic valve regurgitation. The fundamental difference is that the chronic regurgitation is well remodeled and compensated for high-volume and low-pressure hemodynamics while acute valve regurgitation is primarily high-pressure and high-volume hemodynamics. The pressure elevation in acute mitral and aortic valvular regurgitation is witnessed by sudden rise in left ventricular end-diastolic volumes (LVEDV), leading to rapid elevations in left ventricular end-diastolic pressure (LVEDP), left atrial (LA) pressure, and pulmonary venous pressures with resultant pulmonary congestion. The sudden flood of large regurgitant volume results in small augmentation in total stroke volume by the Frank–Starling mechanism, but more in decreased forward flow by a low effective cardiac output and compensatory tachycardia.

THE COMPLEMENTARY TEST AND IMAGING FOR SUSPECTED VALVE EMERGENCY

Once the signs and symptoms raise a suspicion for an acute valve emergency, the next step is to confirm the diagnosis and severity to plan proper treatment. The acute valve emergencies occur often because of sudden catastrophic anatomical valve alterations and the suspicion can be confirmed by a series of tests including electrocardiogram chest radiography, POCUS, and echocardiography. The computer tomography and magnetic resonance imaging (MRI) are often not required in acute emergency situations.

THE TREATMENT OF VALVE-ASSOCIATED EMERGENCY AND PLANNING THE FUTURE COURSE

The treatment of valve-associated emergency either surgical, medical, or interventional is particular to the valve pathology and its emergent symptomatology. However, the general principles include treating complicating arrhythmias like AF, heart failure, and complications of infective endocarditis and thrombosis **(Table 2)**.

THE ACUTE VALVE EMERGENCIES

Acute Aortic Regurgitation

Carpentier classification for AR based on cause is as follows.[3]

- Type I (normal leaflet excursion, i.e., annular dilation or leaflet perforation)
- Type II (cusp prolapse or flail)
- Type III (cusp restriction)

Causes of Acute Aortic Regurgitation

- Endocarditis—leaflet destruction or aortic root abscess
- Aortic dissection (type A)
- Ruptured congenitally fenestrated cusp
- Blunt chest trauma/deceleration injury
- Prosthetic valve dysfunction
- *Iatrogenic*: Complication of procedures such as aortic balloon valvotomy or transcatheter aortic valve implantation (TAVI)

Hemodynamics of Acute Aortic Regurgitation

In case of acute AR, the acute severely elevated LVEDP may prematurely close the mitral valve and cause a diastolic MR that further impairs effective cardiac output and results in elevated pulmonary venous pressures. The ensuing compensatory tachycardia is often inadequate to preserve forward stroke volume. The tachycardia can be counterproductive in a type A aortic dissection or concomitant ischemia, diminishing the cardiac output further **(Table 3)**.[3]

Clinical Presentation

The severe acute AR presents with hemodynamic instability and dyspnea, syncope, or altered mentation. The pulmonary congestion is acute onset and severe needing ventilatory support. The clinical signs are drowned and often not useful for clenching the diagnosis. A systolic ejection murmur due to increased stroke volume and an S3 due to ventricular dilatation may be audible. In the lateral decubitus position, a mid-diastolic rumble (Austin Flint murmur) may be appreciated using the bell of the stethoscope at the cardiac apex. Patients often have a widened pulse pressure. In contrast to the chronic AR, the pulse pressure in acute severe AR will be either normal or decreased due to the rapid equalization of the aortic and left ventricular (LV) pressures.[4] The rapid increase in LV diastolic pressure can cause premature mitral valve closure and LV volume overload leading to soft first and third heart sounds. The low-pitched early diastolic murmur is not a reliable marker of severity as minimal gradient from rapid equalization of pressures between the LV and the aorta.

ECG

ECG findings in patients include sinus tachycardia and are generally nonspecific. Ischemic changes or ST elevation may be seen from aortic dissection involving the coronary arteries.

Chest Radiology

Chest X-ray may show acute pulmonary edema without cardiac enlargement.

Computed Tomography

Computed tomography (CT) with contrast is needed to assess the aorta, and transesophageal echocardiography is needed to assess valvular function.

TABLE 2: Suggested treatment principles for acute valve emergencies.[5]

Treatment	AR	MR	AS	LVOTO	MS
Preload reduction		Diuresis	Diuresis	Infusion	Diuresis
Afterload reduction	Vasodilator	Diuresis	Cautious	Harm	Harm
Heart rate	High	Vasodilator	Normal/low	Low	Low
Inotropy	Useful	Normal/high	Useful if EF low	Harm	Harm
Preferred vasopressor	Epinephrine	Useful	Norepinephrine	Vasopressin/phenylephrine	Vasopressin/phenylephrine
Supportive agent	Isoproterenol	Norepinephrine	–	Beta blocker	Esmolol/amiodarone/digoxin
Positive pressure ventilation	Variable	–	Useful	Harm	Harm
IABP	Harm	Useful	Useful	Harm	Harm
ECMO	Harm	Caution	Useful	Useful	Useful
Intervention	TAVR	MitraClip	BAV/TAVI		BMV/TMVR

TABLE 3: Acute and chronic aortic regurgitation.

	Aortic regurgitation	
	Acute	**Chronic**
Hemodynamics	Heart rate increased	Not much increased
Cardiac output	Decreased	Near normal
Pulse pressure	Not much increased	Increased
Left ventricular end-diastolic pressure	Markedly increased	Normal
Left ventricular size	Not increased	Large dilatation
Aortic systolic pressure	Not increased	Increased
Aortic diastolic pressure	Not decreased	Marked decrease
LV compliance	Not increased	Increased
LV ejection velocity	Not increased	Increased
Effective stroke volume	Not increased	Increased

TABLE 4: Echocardiography in aortic regurgitation.

Severity	A vena contracta (narrowest neck of the AR jet) width of greater than 6 mm
	More than 65% of the LVOT width occupied by the color jet
	Holodiastolic flow reversal within the abdominal aorta (indicating flow back through the aortic valve during diastole)[10]
Doppler	A dense continuous wave signal with steep diastolic slope of AR velocity indicating rapid equalization of pressures
M mode	Premature closure of the mitral valve, suggested with a very short mitral valve deceleration time (<150 ms) may indirectly indicate the severity of the AR jet
Other	LV dysfunction and valvular vegetations, LV/LA size, LV systolic function, LV hypertrophy, aortic dissection, pericardial effusion
TEE	Presence of aortic dissection
2D	*Leaflet morphology*: Leaflet thickening, calcifications, vegetation *Leaflet motion*: Valve coaptation defect, flail leaflets

Echocardiography

Echocardiography is the diagnostic modality of choice in severe AR **(Table 4)**.

Treatment

Acute AR with hemodynamic collapse is a surgical emergency. Stabilization of the patient should be focused on afterload reduction and supporting the volume-overloaded ventricle in preparation for surgery. Intravenous vasodilators or inotropic agents depending on the hemodynamic support are required.[6] Beta blockers are the first line in treatment of patients with acute aortic dissection but they are detrimental to tachycardia essential for survival in acute AR.[6] Mechanical circulatory support (MCS), including intra-aortic balloon counterpulsation, venoarterial extracorporeal membranous oxygenation, or percutaneous ventricular assist devices such as the Impella (Abiomed, Danvers, MA), is contraindicated.[7]

Acute Decompensation in Severe Aortic Stenosis

Aortic stenosis is increasing especially in the elderly population with about 1–2% in patients aged 65 years or less and 29% in patients aged 65 years or more. It remains a life-threatening disease, despite gradually worsening symptoms like dyspnea, angina, dizziness, or even syncope at exertion. However, the presenting symptoms for AS may be severely decompensated heart failure or even CS.

Pathophysiology

Left ventricular obstruction increases LV systolic pressure and LV ejection time (LVET), decreases aortic pressure, and increased LV end-diastolic pressure. The increased LV mass leads to LV dysfunction and failure by increased myocardial oxygen consumption increasing with increased LV systolic pressure, LV mass, and LVET, while myocardial perfusion time decreases with increased LVET.[7]

Triggers

The decompensation can be triggered by an intercurrent illness, such as acute myocardial infarction, arrhythmia like AF, systemic infection, hypovolemia, and uncontrolled hypertension.

Echocardiography

The AV VTI automatically calculates the mean gradient; however, the pressure gradient is a flow-dependent measure and inaccurate in reduced LVEF, MR, mitral stenosis, RV dysfunction, and tricuspid regurgitation.

ECG

In severe AS, ECG may show LVH with a strain pattern and possible triggers like myocardial infarction or AF.

Cardiac Computed Tomography

It is used when noninvasive tests are inconclusive or as preimplant TAVI protocol.

Cardiac Magnetic Resonance Imaging

It can assess LV mass, function, and volume when it cannot be obtained readily in echocardiography.

Treatment/Management

- Patients with critical AS have a *fixed cardiac output* and *cannot* meaningfully increase cardiac output to meet the physiologic demands of critical illness.
- *The cornerstones of resuscitation include*:
  - Avoiding systemic hypotension
  - Maintaining sinus rhythm
  - Avoiding excessive tachycardia
  - The goal of medical therapy and MCS is stabilization prior to definitive correction of the lesion **(Table 2)**.[5]
- Surgical and percutaneous interventions for VHDs
- Treat reversible triggers.
- Medical therapy does not significantly affect disease progression in aortic stenosis.[3]
- Aortic valve replacement (AVR) is superior to medical therapy in severe symptomatic aortic stenosis, as proven in observational studies and randomized controlled trials.[8]

Acute Mitral Regurgitation

Causes of Acute Mitral Regurgitation

- Chordal rupture
- Endocarditis
- Papillary muscle rupture
- Functional papillary dysfunction due to ischemia
- Acute rheumatic fever with carditis
- Functional MR in acute cardiomyopathy
- Prosthetic valve dysfunction

The three primary mechanisms are: (1) rupture of the chordae tendineae, (2) rupture of the papillary muscles, and (3) MR in the setting of dynamic LV outflow tract obstruction and functional LV dilatation.

Pathophysiology

In acute MR, the LA has not had time to adapt to the abrupt increase in volume of regurgitant blood, causing a marked increase in LA pressure and pulmonary edema. Owing to the high regurgitant volume, SV and cardiac output may decrease precipitously, leading to global hypoperfusion.

Clinical Presentation

Severe acute MR usually presents as cardiovascular collapse, including signs of poor tissue perfusion and CS, as well as lung auscultation indicating pulmonary edema. With increased right-sided filling pressures, large "v" waves can be seen in the jugular venous pulsation. A systolic murmur is often heard, but owing to a markedly diminished pressure gradient between the LA and the LV, the murmur is often low pitched and ends well before S2. A large proportion of patients may have no murmur on auscultation, or "silent MR." The low intensity of the murmur may also be due to low systemic blood pressures in patients with hemodynamic collapse, further decreasing the LV–LA gradient.

ECG

Findings are usually nonspecific, unless diagnostic of ischemia as the causative etiology.

Chest Radiography

X-ray reveals the presence of pulmonary edema.

Echocardiography

- Absent or mild leaflet thickening, calcification in secondary MR
- Tethering *or* tenting of mitral leaflets caused by papillary muscle displacement, regional, global or local LV remodeling, and mitral annular dilation
- *Annular enlargement*: It can happen secondary to mitral valve prolapse (MVP).
- Systolic anterior motion (SAM) of the mitral valve

Treatment

Acute severe MR with low blood pressure (cold and wet):

- Oxygenation
- BiPAP
- Intubation
- Protect MAP
- Dysrhythmias

Acute severe MR with normal blood pressure (warm and wet):

- Oxygenation
- Reduce preload and afterload.
- Dysrhythmias
- Interventional cardiology for possible intra-aortic balloon pump and MitraClip
- *Cardiothoracic surgery*:
  - Patients with acute MR due to endocarditis require broad-spectrum *antibiotic* treatment.
  - Operative intervention may be required as well.

Acute Decompensation of Chronic MR

- Other than the above principles of management, consider treating *triggers* for the acute decompensation of chronic MR including:
  - New-onset *arrhythmia* such as AF, decompensated comorbidities like pulmonary hypertension, volume overload, or deteriorating myocardial systolic performance in AMI

Acute Valve Emergency in Mitral Stenosis

As the disease evolves, chronic elevation of the LAP eventually leads to pulmonary hypertension, tricuspid and pulmonary valve incompetence, and secondary right heart failure and/or LA dilatation resulting in loss of atrial kick in AF.

Overall, the 10-year survival rate in untreated patients is 50–60%. The acute valve emergency can be due to congestive cardiopulmonary failure (60–70%), systemic embolism

(20–30%), pulmonary embolism (about 10%), and infection (1–5%).[4]

Triggers

Complications of mitral stenosis may include all of the following:

- Thromboembolism
- AF
- Bacterial endocarditis
- Pulmonary hypertension
- Pulmonary edema
- Complications of balloon valvotomy like stroke, cardiac perforation, and MR
- Complications of mitral valve replacement like paravalvular leak, thromboembolism, infective endocarditis, mechanical dysfunction, and bleeding due to anticoagulants

Presentation

The emergency patient can present as paroxysmal nocturnal dyspnea, frank pulmonary edema, chest pain from right ventricular ischemia or failure and concomitant coronary atherosclerosis, and hemoptysis from pulmonary venous hypertension.

The classic murmur of mitral stenosis may be drowned in pulmonary edema.

Electrocardiography

Ninety percent of patients with significant mitral stenosis and sinus rhythm display electrical evidence of LA enlargement.

Echocardiography

Two-dimensional echocardiography evaluates the morphology of the mitral valve, orifice size, and other valves.

Doppler echocardiography is an accurate noninvasive technique to quantify the hemodynamic severity.

3D echocardiography is superior to 2D echocardiography in the evaluation of mitral valve stenosis in valve area measurements.[9]

Chest Radiography

Left atrial, pulmonary artery, right ventricle, and/or right atrium enlargement and calcification of the mitral valve may be seen.

Treatment

- IV diuretic bolus and infusion
- CPAP
- Rate-limiting drugs—beta blockers and calcium channel blockers
- Emergency PTMC
- Open surgery with MVR or open mitral valvotomy
- Unstable AF with rapid ventricular response—consider synchronized direct current (DC) cardioversion after anticoagulation and transesophageal echocardiography
- Anticoagulation

DIAGNOSIS AND TREATMENT OF VHD-RELATED EMERGENCIES

Heart Failure

Heart failure eventually progresses in chronic valvular heart patients leading to repeated emergency presentations. The findings are typical of the other causes: dyspnea, orthopnea, tachycardia, abnormal apical impulse, low systolic blood pressure, third heart sound, jugular venous distention, and edema. The rapid progression to pulmonary edema and hemodynamic compromise is commonly witnessed.[10] The hemodynamic principles are different from other causes of heart failure and exclusive to each VHD. The pressure-volume (PV) curves are altered in both chronic and acute valve diseases. The understanding of PV curves prohibits increase in inotropism in the presence of low output in mitral stenosis, a substantial reduction in LV volume with diuretic therapy in aortic stenosis, and vasoconstriction in regurgitant lesions. Therefore, specific medications and interventions are required according to each valvulopathy, often different from those used in other HF etiologies.

Atrial Fibrillation

Valvular heart disease may present with arrhythmias, commonly AF. More than 30% of patients with AF have VHD. AF cardioversion in the ED is performed exclusively whether patient instability is due to arrhythmia. In most cases, the safest approach is heart rate control and starting anticoagulation if indicated.

Valvular Thrombosis

Prosthesis thrombosis is characterized by a thrombus formation on the prosthetic structures, with subsequent valve dysfunction with or without thromboembolism. This is more common in the mechanical prostheses, ranging from 0.1 to 5.7%, especially in the early perioperative period, mitral position, and subtherapeutic anticoagulation. Patients may present as asymptomatic with incidentally detected thrombus to embolism, hypotension, syncope, dyspnea, pulmonary congestion, and sudden death.[6] Diagnosis is classically confirmed by transesophageal echocardiogram, but a multidetector CT and radioscopy evaluation may also be useful. Nonobstructive prosthesis thrombosis in stable patients is treated with optimization of oral anticoagulation. Fibrinolysis or surgery is recommended for patients with remaining thrombus after optimal anticoagulation or with thrombus ≥10 mm and/or >0.8 cm^2 associated with emboli.

Hemodynamically unstable patients should promptly be submitted to valve replacement. For patients deemed to be at a prohibitive risk for surgery, fibrinolysis is the main option.

Infective Endocarditis

Infective endocarditis still carries higher than 30% 1-year mortality, despite advanced treatment.[4] The diagnosis is suspected in valve disease in the absence of clear infective foci and with the presence of new heart murmur or fever, suspicion of systemic emboli, and acute/subacute heart failure and generalized symptoms of arthralgia, myalgia, anorexia, weight loss, night sweat, chills, headache, abdominal pain, back pain, dyspnea, and hematuria. The signs of infective endocarditis may ascertain the diagnosis like Roth spots (white-centered retinal hemorrhage), Osler nodules (painful nodes on the tips of fingers or toes), Janeway lesions (painless, nontender, erythematous, or hemorrhagic macular or nodular lesions on the palms or soles), splinter hemorrhage (painless hemorrhages in the distal third of the nail), and petechiae (present in the skin and mucous membranes) **(Box 1 and Table 1)**.

The Duke criteria are a set of diagnostic criteria for IE, but their main limitations are that they are not immediate and the accuracy at admission is around 52–70%. The two pillars for the treatment of IE are antibiotics and surgical treatment.[11]

Valve Emergencies during Implantations

The complications causing emergency during the valve replacement procedure are not limited to arrhythmias, vascular complications, stroke, renal replacement therapy, moderate-to-severe AR, valve embolization, myocardial infarction, and coronary obstruction. The discussion for each is beyond the scope of this chapter.

CONCLUSION

The acute valve emergencies can be a presentation of a new lesion like acute regurgitation or acute deterioration of a preexisting valve lesion. The emergent condition of the patient drowns the early signs and symptoms, and the diagnosis primarily relies on a high index of suspicion. The recent rise in valve-related emergencies dictates evolution of guidelines for early and accurate recognition and treatment. The planning and modification of the natural and unnatural courses remains the final goal of management of acute valve emergencies.

ONLINE REFERENCES

Please scan the QR code provided at the end of the table of contents for References of this chapter.

CHAPTER 183

Atrial Septal Defects Device Closures: Basics and Beyond

Sriram Easwaran, Milind Phadke, Bharat Dalvi

ABSTRACT

Atrial septal defects (ASDs) are the most common congenital heart defects amenable to transcatheter closure. Amongst the various types of ASDs, the most commonly closed defects are the ostium secundum type of ASD (OSASD) while some newer transcatheter therapies are now available for dealing with sinus venosus type of ASD (SVASD). Very few selected cases of coronary sinus types can also be closed using transcatheter techniques, while ostium primum type of ASD (OPASD) is still correctable only by surgery. The common features for all these procedures involving nonsurgical closure include comprehensive clinical evaluation, precise imaging, accurate analysis of the anatomy, appropriate selection of the type and the size of the device followed by perfect, step-by-step execution of the procedure. All the patients also need adequate and systematic postprocedural care to optimize results and avoid complications.

Keywords: Atrial septal defect, transcatheter device closure, congenital heart disease, pulmonary hypertension

INTRODUCTION

Atrial septal defects (ASDs) are a group of defects in the interatrial septum (IAS), which can lead to volume overload of the right ventricle and the pulmonary circulation due to significant left-to-right shunting. Though traditionally surgical closure was offered to these patients, since the mid-1990s, the majority of OSASDs are treated using nitinol-based devices. Since the last 10 years, a large number of SVASDs in adolescents and adults are also being treated in the catheterization laboratory using large and long covered stents to exteriorize the anomalously draining right superior pulmonary vein (RSPV) to drain into the left atrium and simultaneously closing the communication between the left and the right atria.

In this chapter, we will be dealing with the indications, contraindications, patient selection, technical considerations, different clinical scenarios, complications and their management, and follow-up of these patients.

INDICATIONS AND CONTRAINDICATIONS FOR CLOSURE

- Repeated respiratory tract infections requiring antibiotics or a history of pneumonia requiring hospitalization, episodes of wheezing requiring visits to the emergency room for nebulization, failure to thrive, shortness of breath, and easy fatigability are some of the common symptoms indicating closure of the defect.
- In the absence of symptoms, ASD closure should be considered if there is a significant left-to-right shunt as indicated by the volume overload of the right atrium and ventricle on echo or Qp/Qs > 1.5 at cardiac catheterization or history of paradoxical embolism irrespective of the shunt magnitude.
- *ASD with pulmonary arterial hypertension (PAH)*: Closure of such defects requires cardiac catheterization to test for reversibility of pulmonary vascular resistance (PVR); if reversible, one can consider device closure with or without a fenestrated device.[1,2] In cases with a disproportionately high pulmonary artery pressure (PAP), where ASD appears to be an innocent bystander or in those with large ASD having PVR of >8 wood units that is unresponsive to acute pulmonary vasodilators (inhaled nitric oxide, IV sildenafil, or calcium channel blockers), it is prudent to leave such a defect alone and the patient be treated with pulmonary vasodilators. In case of an absence of clinical and hemodynamic response to long-term vasodilatory treatment, the patient may need to be listed for a heart-lung transplant. Similarly, those with

severe pulmonary hypertension having a baseline right-to-left shunt with a resting SaO_2 of <90% on room air should be considered as having Eisenmenger's complex and treated with medical therapy and considered for heart–lung transplant.

- *ASD with acquired left ventricular (LV) diseases*: In patients with congenital or acquired LV diseases like myocarditis and cardiomyopathy or in elderly with restrictive LV physiology or ischemic heart disease with LV dysfunction, a fenestrated device may be considered to prevent pulmonary edema due to unmasking of the LV diastolic dysfunction post closure. In addition, these patients need pharmacological unloading of the left ventricle with diuretics and vasodilators for 4–6 weeks prior to the procedure.

OSTIUM SECUNDUM ATRIAL SEPTAL DEFECTS DEVICE CLOSURE

Patient Selection

- *Defect characteristics*:
  - Size: Defects >40 mm can be challenging to close due to nonavailability of devices >46 mm.
  - Rims: An atrioventricular (AV) rim of <7 mm and all the other rims (excluding the aortic rim) of <4 mm are not ideal for device closure due to high chances of mitral valve injury and device embolization. Deficiency/absence of aortic rim is considered as a risk factor for cardiac erosion, and the same needs to be discussed with the family. Apart from the rim length, rim strength also plays an important role in determining the stability of the device. A "floppy" rim (which cannot be defined objectively) is associated with device migration. One more rim characteristic that is very often overlooked is the rim alignment—malalignment between the septum primum and secundum is prone to device embolization as well as cardiac erosion.
  - Number of defects: Multiple ASDs require careful planning in order to decide the number, size, and type of device to be used and require a tailor-made approach.[3,4]
- *Patient characteristics*:
  - Weight: The size of the patient affects device choice as well as the mode of device delivery. Many small children with large defects need one of the modified approaches of device delivery.
  - Pulmonary hypertension: In the presence of PHT, it is important to assess its severity and reversibility of PAH mentioned under the heading ASD with PAH.
  - Ventricular function and associated cardiac anomalies: The presence of ventricular dysfunction (systolic and/or diastolic) can increase the risk of the procedure mentioned under the heading ASD with acquired LV diseases. Presence of any other congenital or acquired heart defect requiring surgical intervention needs to be precisely diagnosed prior to offering a device closure.

Preprocedural Evaluation

- Detailed history including history of allergy for nickel so as to counsel the patient accordingly
- *Physical examination*: To estimate the approximate shunt magnitude, evidence of ventricular dysfunction, presence, severity and reversibility of PHT, and suggestion of an arrhythmia, especially atrial fibrillation (AF)
- *Imaging*: In children, transthoracic echo is usually adequate to decide preprocedural suitability for device closure. In adults, however, imaging the defect rims may be challenging on transthoracic echocardiography (TTE) and hence preprocedural transesophageal echocardiography (TEE) is recommended **(Figs. 1A to C)**.[5] The following variables need to be clearly defined in echocardiographic imaging:
  - Presence of ASD
  - Site
  - Size
  - Number
  - Rim characteristics: Length, strength, and alignment
  - Direction of the shunt
  - Presence and severity of PHT
  - Sate of ventricular function
  - Presence of other defects requiring transcatheter/surgical intervention
  - Baseline pericardial effusion
- In some cases, cardiac CT or MRI with 3D reconstruction is used for detailed rim evaluation.

Potential issues based on preprocedural assessment:

- *Deficient aortic rims*:
  - Risk: Cardiac erosion[6]
  - Counseling: Inform patients about the risk and the need for careful monitoring
- *Floppy and/or deficient posteroinferior rims or malaligned rims*:
  - Risks: Procedural failures, device embolization, and cardiac erosion
  - Approach: Consider surgical intervention or a thorough understanding of potential complications by the family.
- *Large defects in small children*:
  - Safety: Generally safe and effective in experienced hands and using alternative techniques.[7-11] However, complications may be higher in some cases.[12]
- *Multiple ASDs*:
  - Strategy: Use single or multiple septal occluders or a cribriform device.[3,4,13-17] Balloon interrogation and 3D TEE can aid in closing multiple defects effectively.[18]

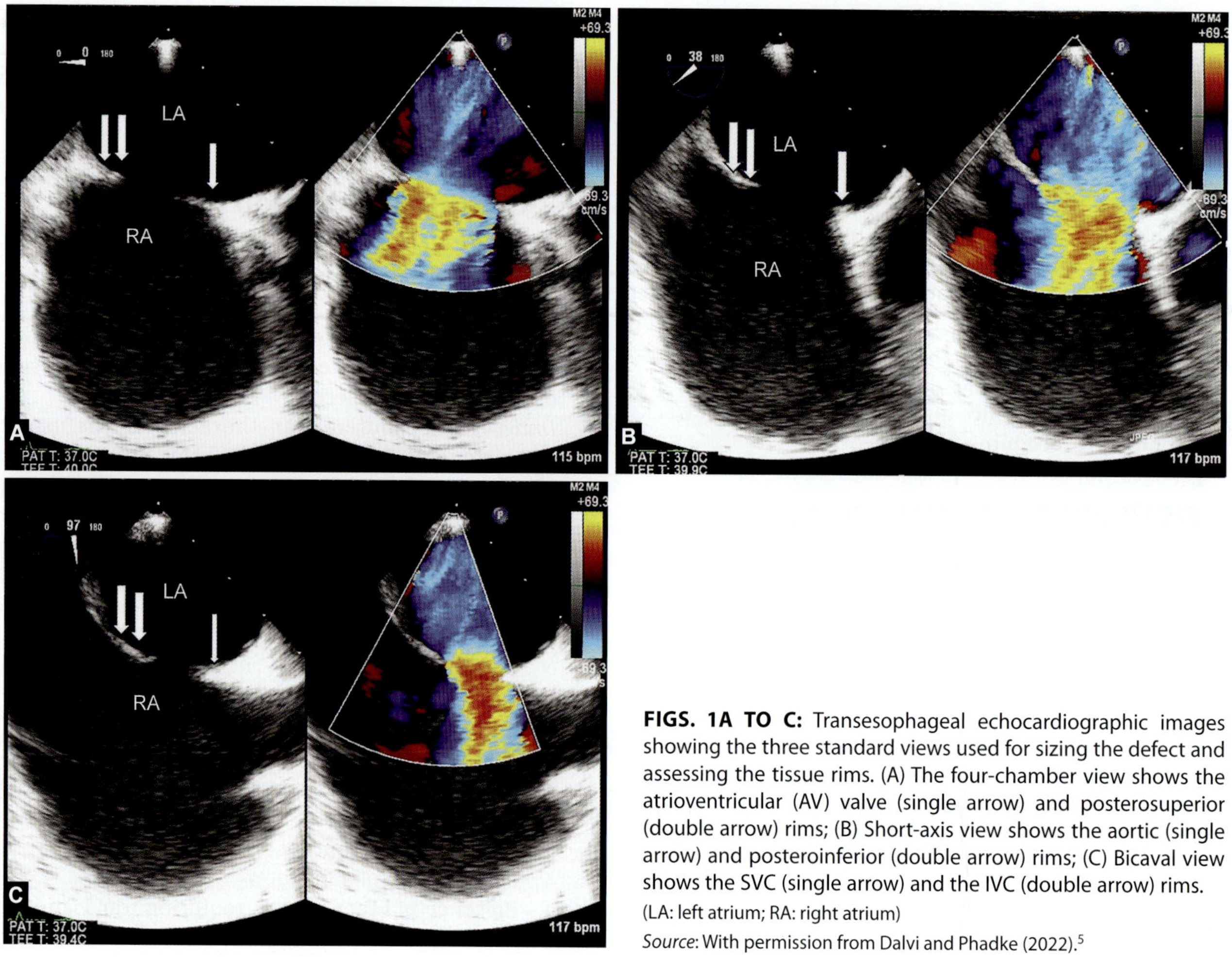

FIGS. 1A TO C: Transesophageal echocardiographic images showing the three standard views used for sizing the defect and assessing the tissue rims. (A) The four-chamber view shows the atrioventricular (AV) valve (single arrow) and posterosuperior (double arrow) rims; (B) Short-axis view shows the aortic (single arrow) and posteroinferior (double arrow) rims; (C) Bicaval view shows the SVC (single arrow) and the IVC (double arrow) rims.
(LA: left atrium; RA: right atrium)
Source: With permission from Dalvi and Phadke (2022).[5]

Intraprocedural Considerations

- *Anesthesia*:
  - Children: General anesthesia is preferred, especially with TEE guidance.
  - Adolescents and adults: Sedation with local anesthesia (LA) is sufficient if TTE or intracardiac echocardiography (ICE) is used for intraprocedural imaging. For TEE imaging, GA is advisable.
- *Imaging*:
  - TTE: It is simple, easily available, inexpensive, and does not require GA but may lack details about the defect as well as the surrounding rims. It is advocated only in those with optimum echo window.
  - TEE: It is preferred for high-resolution imaging of rims and defect size by balloon sizing. Retroflexing the TEE probe can help visualize even some of the difficult areas like the IVC rim.[19]
  - ICE: It is useful for detailed imaging but more expensive and has a steeper learning curve. It negates the use of GA and a single operator can manage imaging as well as the device closure.
- *Access*:
  - Venous access: Single femoral venous access is typical. Additional access may be needed for temporary balloon occlusion to assess change in LV hemodynamics, for balloon sizing, and to assess reversibility of PAH.
  - Arterial access: It is required for ASDs with severe pulmonary hypertension or for small ASDs needing hemodynamic assessment to decide whether to close or not to close. It is also useful to assess coronary anatomy in older patients. In case of IVC interruption, internal jugular vein (IJV)[20] access may be used, with hepatic venous access[21] as an alternative.
- *Heparinization*:
  - Dosage: 100 units/kg IV heparin, with adjustments based on activated clotting time (ACT) > 250 seconds. In resource-limited settings, repeated dosing at 50 units/kg after 1st hour and every 30 minutes thereafter without ACT monitoring may be used.
- *Hemodynamics and angiography*:
  - Baseline variables: Qp, Qs, PVR, and SVR are to be measured in patients with PAH. For severe PAH,

reassess after pulmonary vasodilator challenge using 100% O_2, inhaled NO, or IV sildenafil. Left ventricular end diastolic pressure (LVEDP) monitoring is advisable in patients with suspected restrictive LV physiology.

Choice of Device Size

Sizing: Device size is selected based on the maximum defect diameter in standard TEE imaging planes (four-chamber, short axis of the aorta, bicaval) plus 2–4 mm.[22] Alternatively, balloon sizing is used with the stop-flow technique to determine device size.[23]

DEPLOYMENT TECHNIQUES FOR NITINOL-BASED DOUBLE DISC DEVICES

- *Standard technique* ***(Figs. 2 to 4)***:
  - Deploy the left atrial disc outside the left superior pulmonary vein (LSPV), then pull it back together with the sheath unit until it abuts against the IAS, followed by deployment of the waist and the right atrial disc by withdrawing the sheath **(Figs. 3A to F)**. The two common causes of unsuccessful deployment of the device using this routine technique include a malalignment of the LA disc with the plane of the IAS and the inability of the small LA to accommodate a relatively large opened LA disc resulting in its prolapse across the defect into the right atrium **(Figs. 5A to D)**.
- *Alternative techniques*: Under these circumstances, one may need to take a recourse to these alternative techniques of deployment.
  - Changing the mode of delivery: Try deploying from just outside the RSPV or the LA roof instead of just outside the LSPV.
  - Changing the delivery sheath: Use braided, double-curved Hausdorff sheath, tip deflecting FuStar sheath or a beveled Mullin sheath to aid deployment.
  - Supporting the LA disc to prevent it from prolapsing across the defect **(Figs. 6 and 7)**: Use guidewires or a catheter or a long dilator or a circular/cylindrical sizing balloon.[24,25]

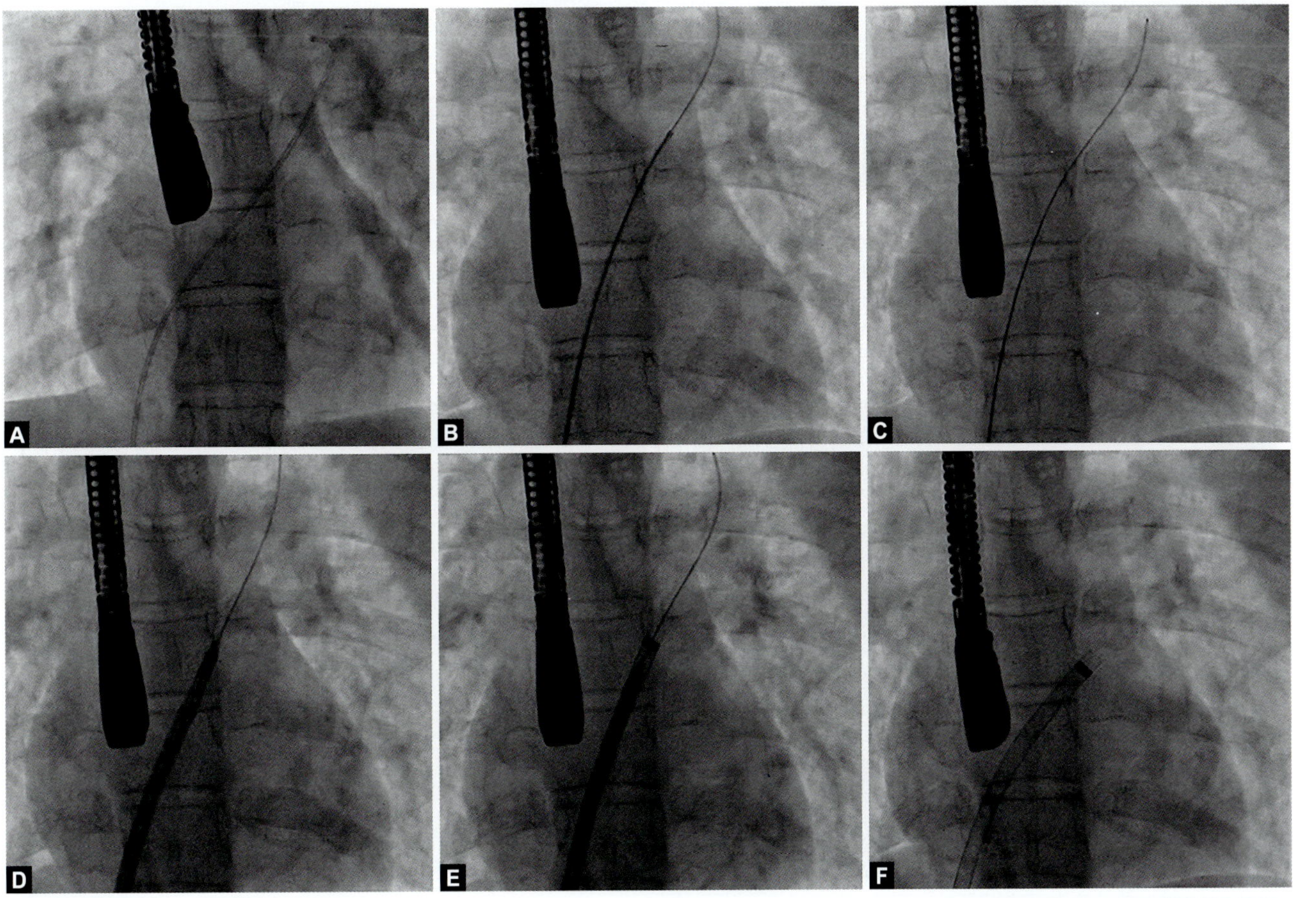

FIGS. 2A TO F: (A) Judkins right (JR) catheter is parked in the left superior pulmonary vein (LSPV). (B) 0.035" Teflon-coated guidewire is exchanged for JR in the LSPV. (C) The wire is seen parked in the LSPV. (D) The delivery sheath with its dilator is then advanced into the LSPV. (E and F) The guidewire and dilator are then removed leaving behind the sheath.

Source: With permission from Dalvi and Phadke (2022).[5]

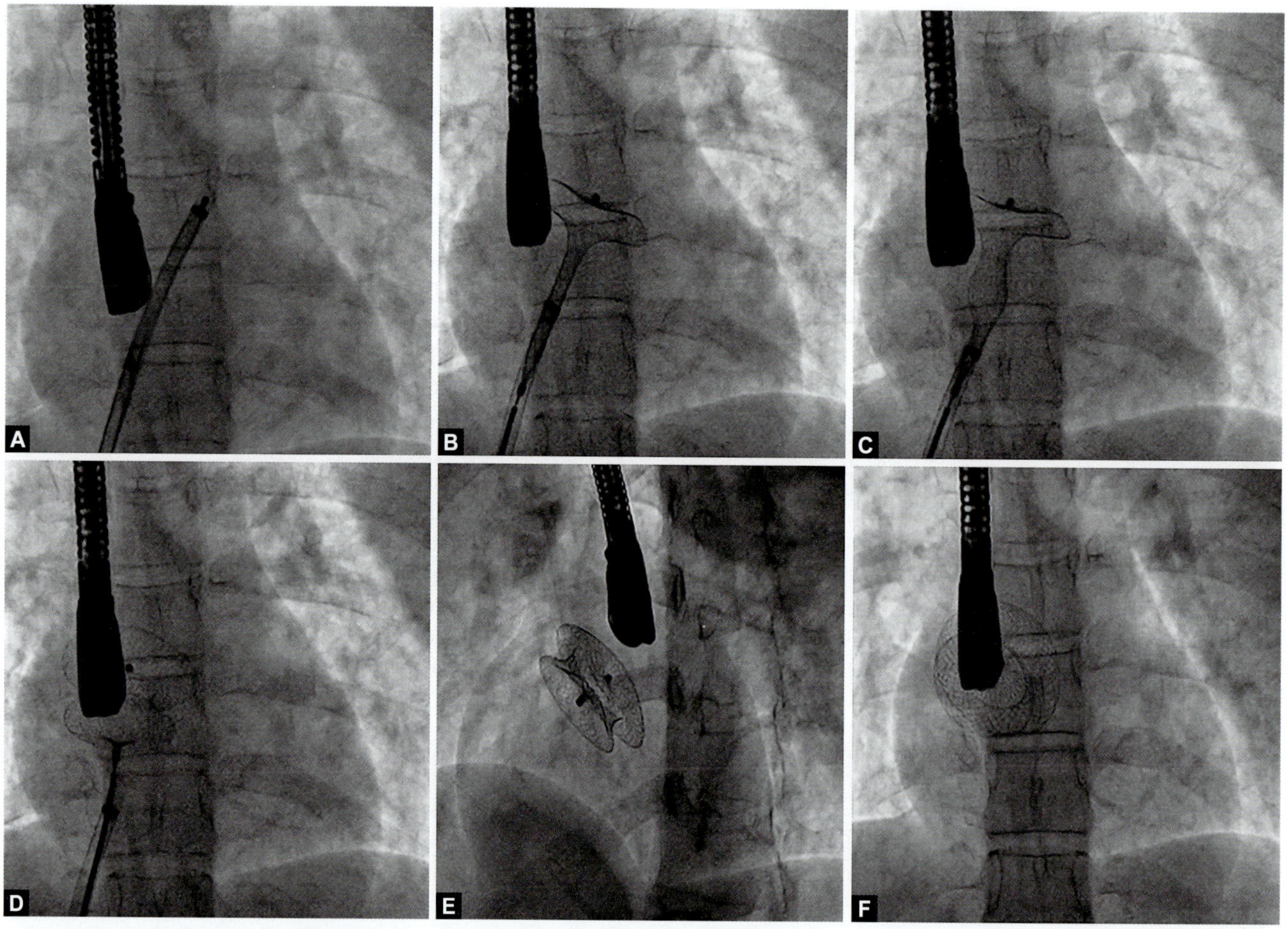

FIGS. 3A TO F: Series of fluoroscopic images showing the device delivery of ASD device. (A) The device is seen at the tip of the delivery sheath; (B) The left atrial (LA) disc is delivered; (C) The waist is delivered after bringing back the LA disc to abut against the interatrial septum; (D) Thereafter the right atrial disc is delivered; (E) The device is released in the left anterior oblique with a cranial angulation view after confirming its position on transesophageal echocardiography; (F) The device is seen after release in the posteroanterior view.

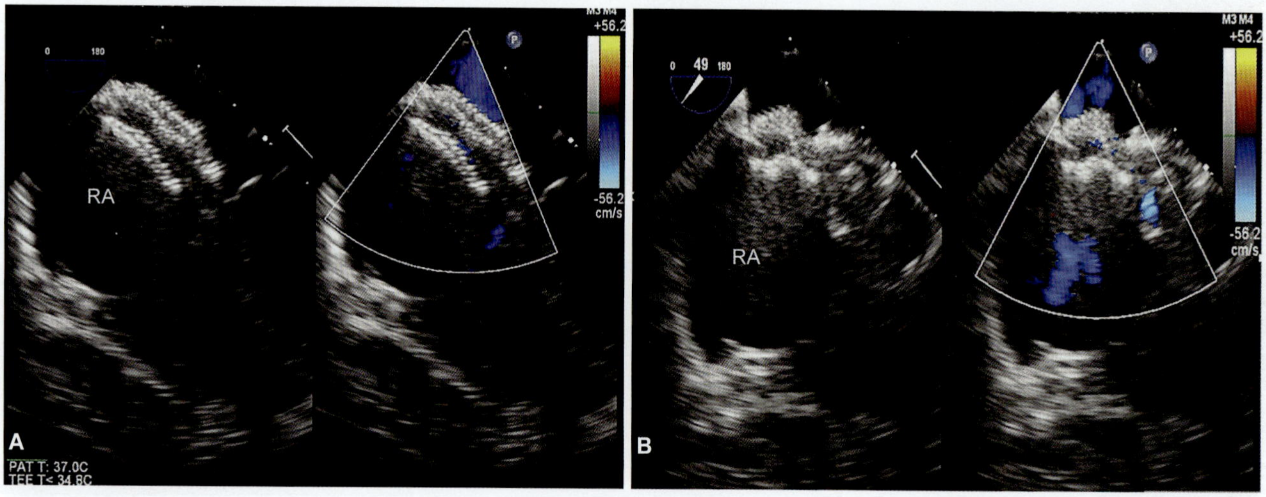

FIGS. 4A TO C: *Continued*

Continued

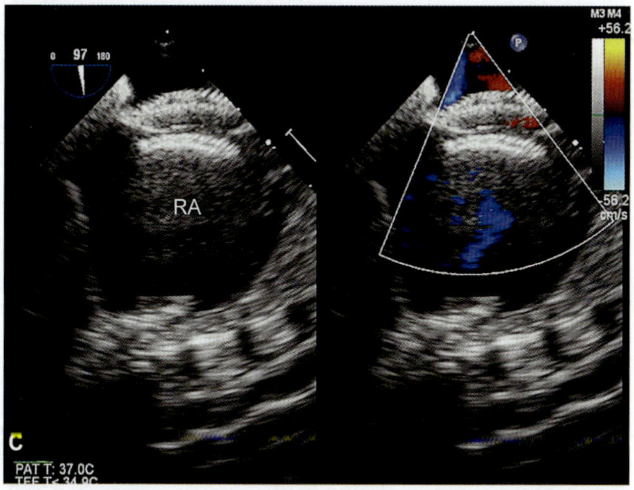

FIGS. 4A TO C: Transesophageal echocardiographic (TEE) images after release, (A) in the four-chamber, (B) short axis, and (C) bicaval views. The device is seen parallel to the plane of the interatrial septum with all the rims adequately caught between the two discs.

(LA: left atrium; LV: left ventricle; RA: right atrium; RV: right ventricle)

Source: With permission from Dalvi and Phadke (2022).[5]

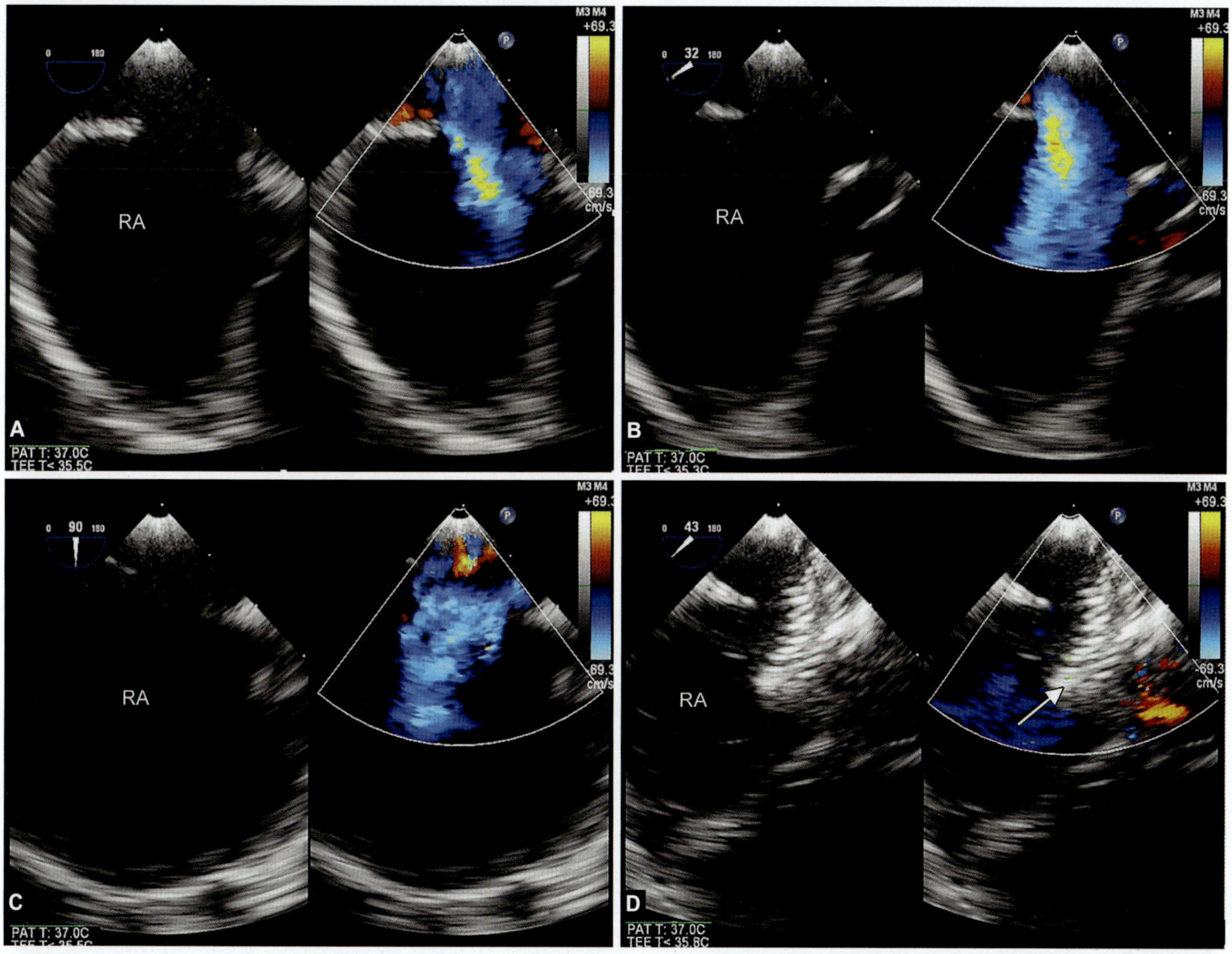

FIGS. 5A TO D: (A) Four-chamber view; (B) Short-axis view; (C) Bicaval view of a large atrial septal defect; (D) Malalignment of the opened-up left atrial disc with the plane of the interatrial septum in the short-axis view of the aorta resulting in the herniation of the left atrial disc (arrow) across the defect.

(LA: left atrium; RA: right atrium)

Source: With permission from Dalvi and Phadke (2022).[5]

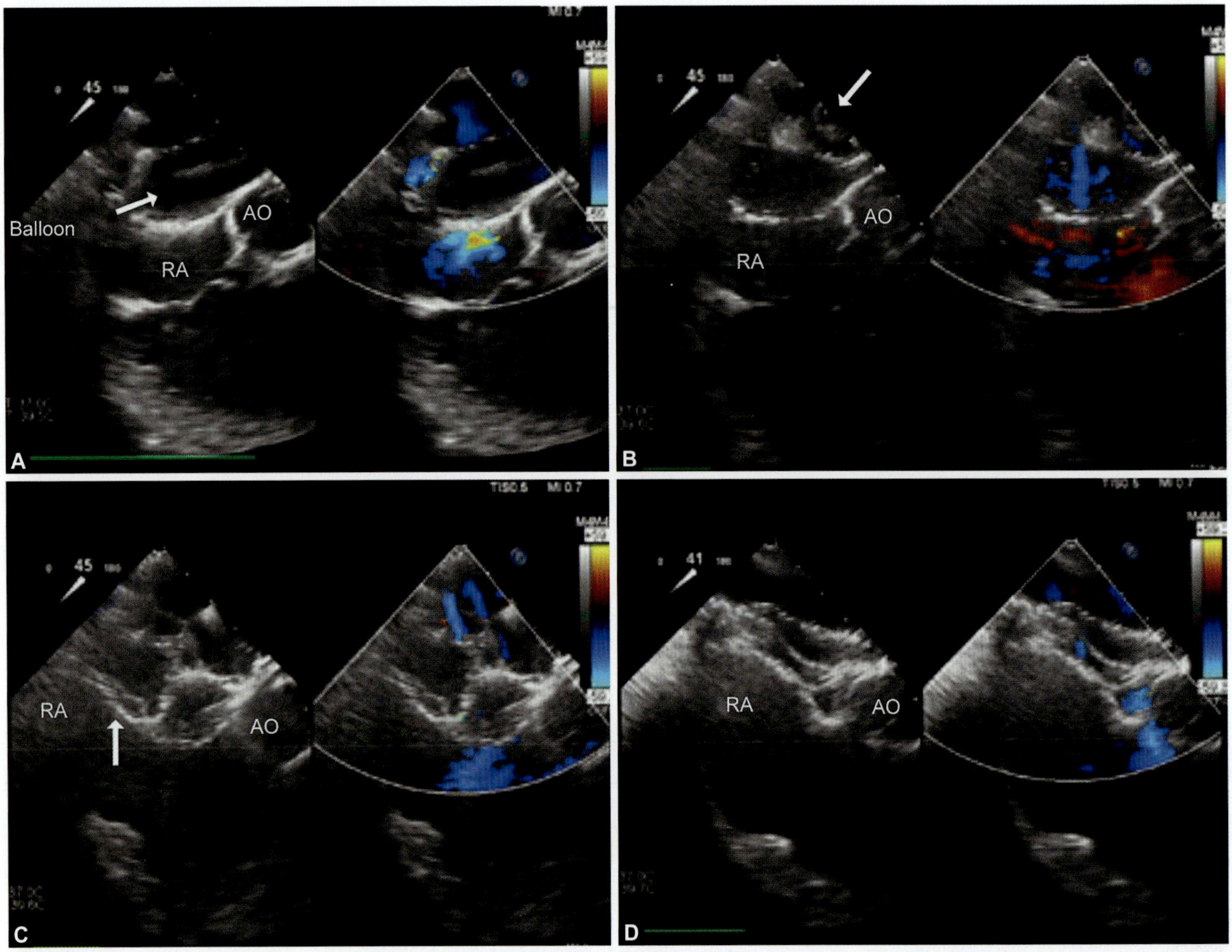

FIGS. 6A TO D: Transesophageal echocardiographic (TEE) images of the balloon-assisted technique using a cylindrical Amplatzer balloon. (A) The balloon is passed over the wire parked in the left superior pulmonary vein (LSPV) and inflated across the defect; (B) The left atrial disc (arrow) has been deployed and positioned against the inflated balloon; (C) The waist and the right atrial disc (arrow) are then deployed with the balloon partially deflated; (D) The device is well formed after complete deflation of the balloon.

(AO: aorta; RA: right atrium)

Source: With permission from Dalvi and Phadke (2022).[5]

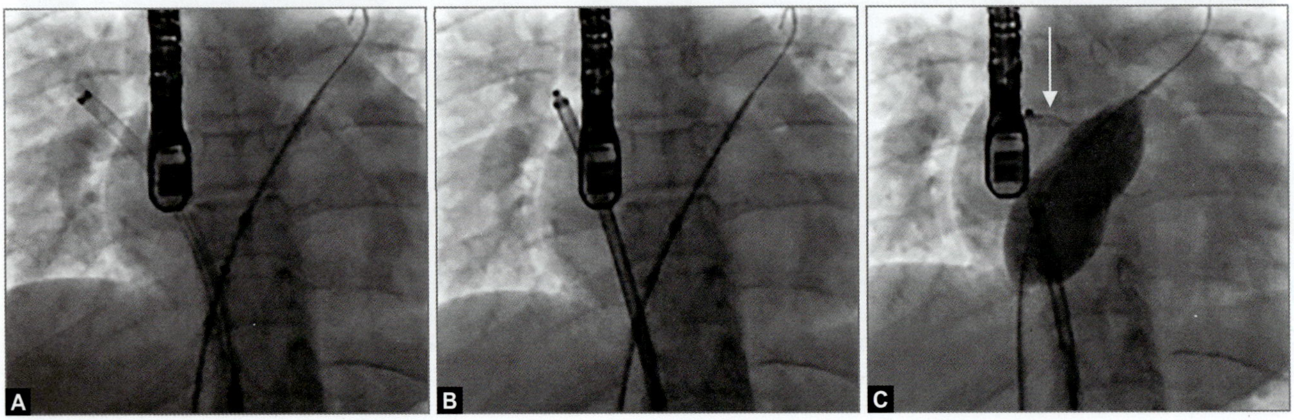

FIGS. 7A TO I: *Continued*

Continued

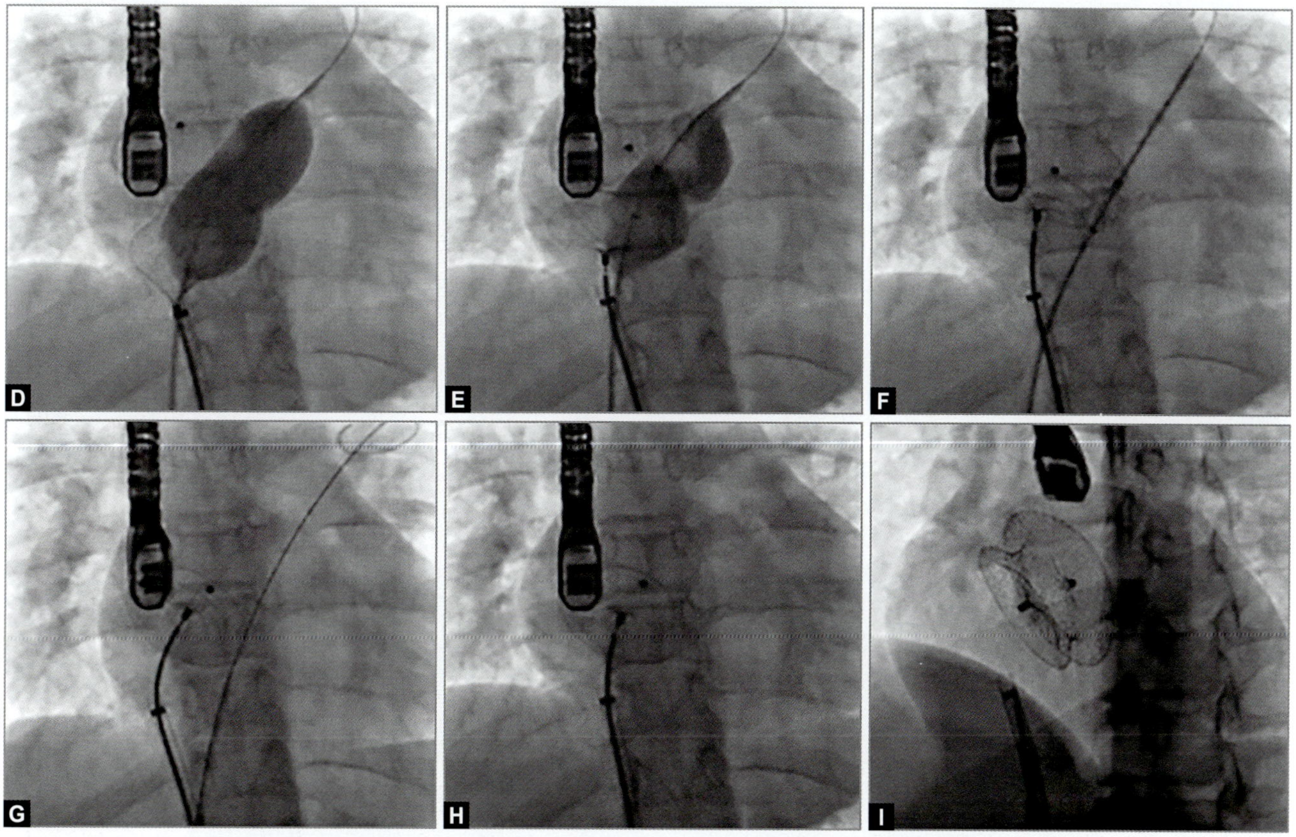

FIGS. 7A TO I: Fluoroscopic images of the balloon-assisted technique using a cylindrical Amplatzer balloon. (A) Delivery sheath positioned in the right superior pulmonary vein and the deflated balloon is seen over the wire parked in the left superior pulmonary vein (LSPV); (B) Slenderized device at the tip of the delivery sheath; (C) Balloon inflated across the defect, with the deployed left atrial disc (arrow) sitting against the inflated balloon; (D) Waist and the right atrial (RA) disc deployed with the balloon still inflated; (E and F) Deflation of the balloon, with the device flattening out; (G) Deflated balloon pulled back into the right atrium; (H) Device position after removal of the guidewire; (I) Postrelease position of the device in left anterior oblique cranial projection.

Source: With permission from Dalvi and Phadke (2022).[5]

- Left atrial disc engagement–disengagement techniques (LADEDT)[26]
- Engage the LA disc in a pulmonary vein **(Figs. 8A to E)** or left atrial appendage (LAA) **(Figs. 9A to E)** followed by release of the waist and RA disc. In case the left atrial disc does not disengage spontaneously, one may have to use one of maneuvers (pull or push) to actively disengage the LA disc.[27-29]

SPECIAL SUBSETS

Multiple Atrial Septal Defects

Closing multiple ASDs is complex due to varying morphologies. Traditionally, defects within 7 mm apart used one device; others required two.[3,30] New techniques using balloon interrogation allow single-device closure for 75% of cases. Large aneurysms or multiple fenestrations might need specialized occluders or combinations, with unimportant defects often left untreated.

Atrial Septal Defects with Pulmonary Arterial Hypertension

ASD with PAH is a subset which comprises a wide spectrum of patients of varying age and weight with different defect sizes and variable severity of PAH. Those with severe and irreversible PAH are better treated medically with pulmonary vasodilators, as complete defect closure is counterproductive; the natural history following the closure is less favorable as compared to the Eisenmenger's syndrome.[31] Those with small defect size but moderate or severe PAH, disproportionate to the size, are likely to have pulmonary vasculopathy with ASD being an innocent bystander. In this subset, too, it is better to leave the ASD open and treat the patient with pulmonary vasodilators. In

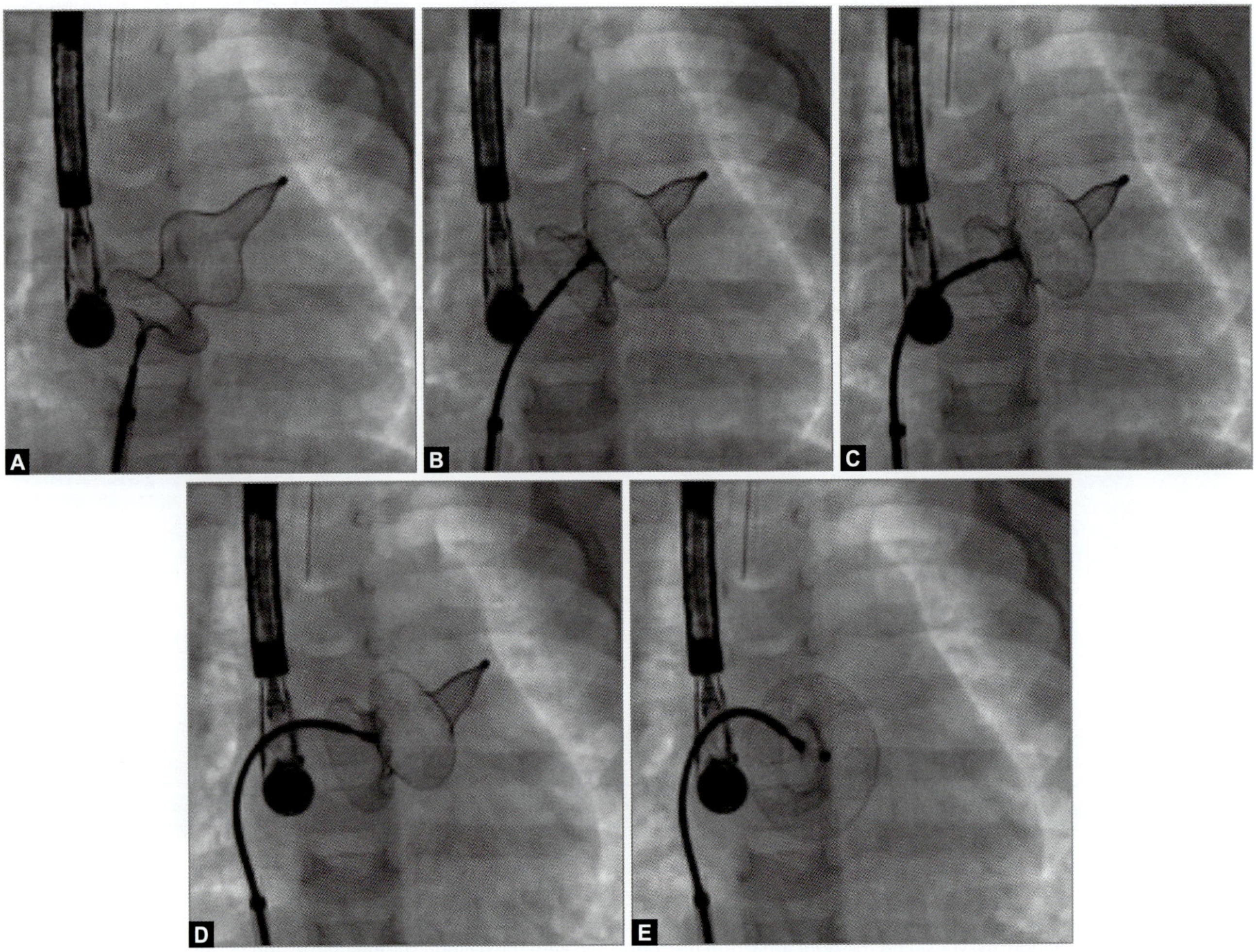

FIGS. 8A TO E: Fluoroscopic images showing the left atrial disc engagement–disengagement technique being performed from the left superior pulmonary vein (LSPV) with active disengagement of the left atrial (LA) disc. (A) The LA disc is engaged in the LSPV followed by the delivery of the waist and the right atrial disc. The LA disc did not disengage spontaneously. (B) The loading cable is pushed gently. (C) The cable is pushed further. (D) Note the redundancy of the cable resulting in the distal part of the cable looking downwards. (E) One of the components of the force acting in the downward direction successfully disengages the LA disc without traumatizing the LSPV resulting in appropriate device position.

Source: With permission from Dalvi and Phadke (2022).[5]

those with large defect and moderate to severe PAH, it is advisable to use a multidimensional approach to decide on the reversibility of the PAH.[32] This approach takes into consideration clinical, radiological, electrocardiographic, and echocardiographic parameters **(Figs. 10A to D)** to decide the pretest probability and then correlates it with the hemodynamic data (Qp, Qs, Qp/Qs, PVR, SVR, PVR/SVR) obtained in the catheterization laboratory to decide on the PAH reversibility **(Figs. 11A and B)**.[2,33-35] When in doubt about the reversibility, despite all efforts, it is better to leave the defect as is or close it with a fenestrated device **(Figs. 12A and B)** to avoid occurrence of idiopathic pulmonary arterial hypertension (iPAH) such as syndrome following complete closure. Most of the patients in severe reversible PAH subset improve significantly in terms of their effort tolerance and feeling of well-being with significant reduction (without normalization) of the PAP but require long term pulmonary vasodilators.[36]

Atrial Septal Defects Closure in Elderly

The group comprising individuals >50 years of age often present late due to the paucity of symptoms during the first five decades of life. No age is considered as a barrier for closing the defect if it is hemodynamically significant because such closure is shown to enhance O_2 delivery, reduce RV dimensions and improve functional status. Issues which need special attention while considering device closure in the elderly include:

- Presence of coexisting coronary artery disease (CAD)
- Reduced LV compliance due to ageing
- Risk of atrial arrhythmias

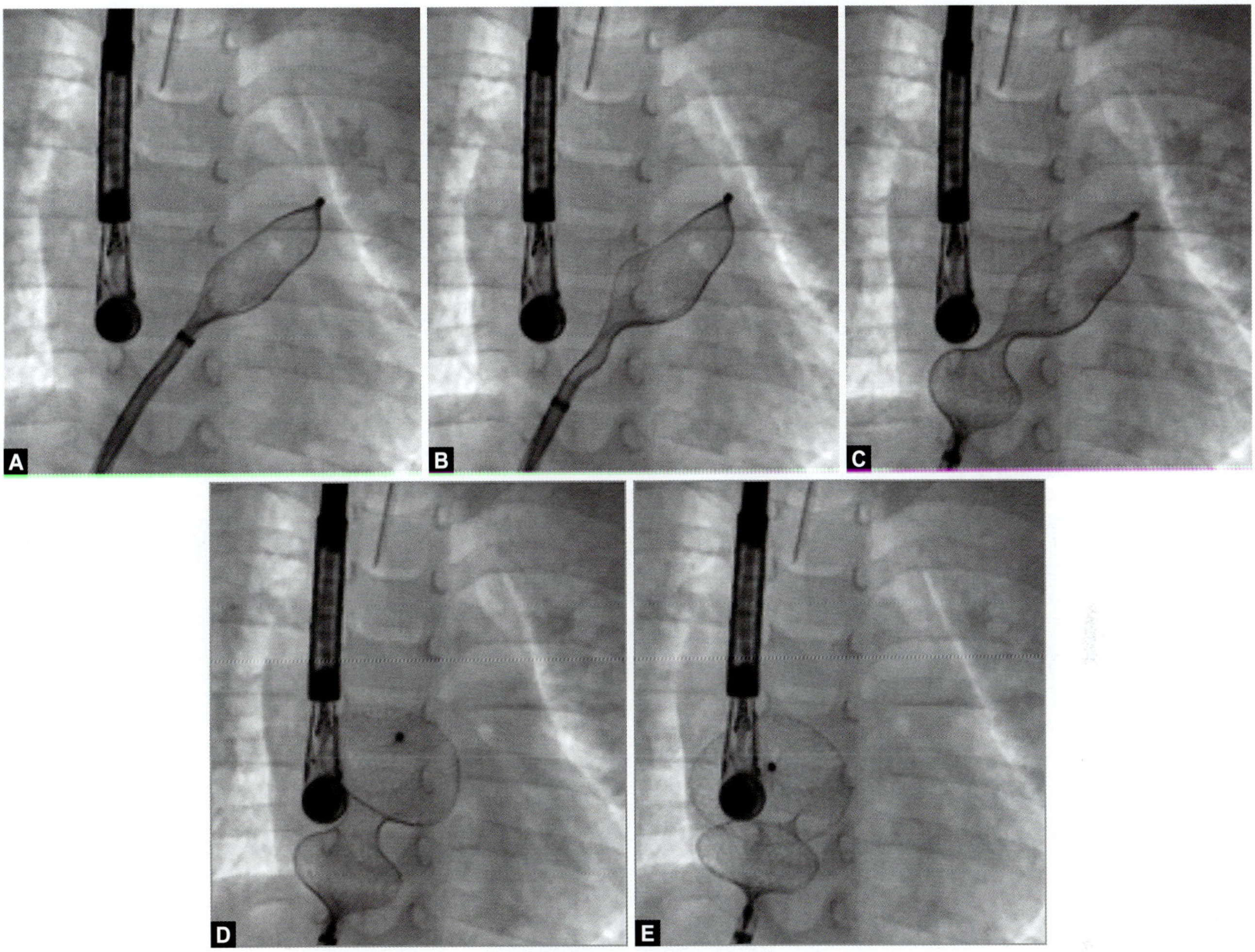

FIGS. 9A TO E: Fluoroscopic images in posteroanterior projection showing the left atrial disc engagement–disengagement technique being performed from the left superior pulmonary vein (LSPV). (A) The left atrial (LA) disc is engaged in the LSPV. (B) The waist is released. (C) The right atrial disc is delivered. (D) Spontaneous disengagement of the LA disc followed by (E) appropriate placement of the device.
Source: With permission from Dalvi and Phadke (2022).[5]

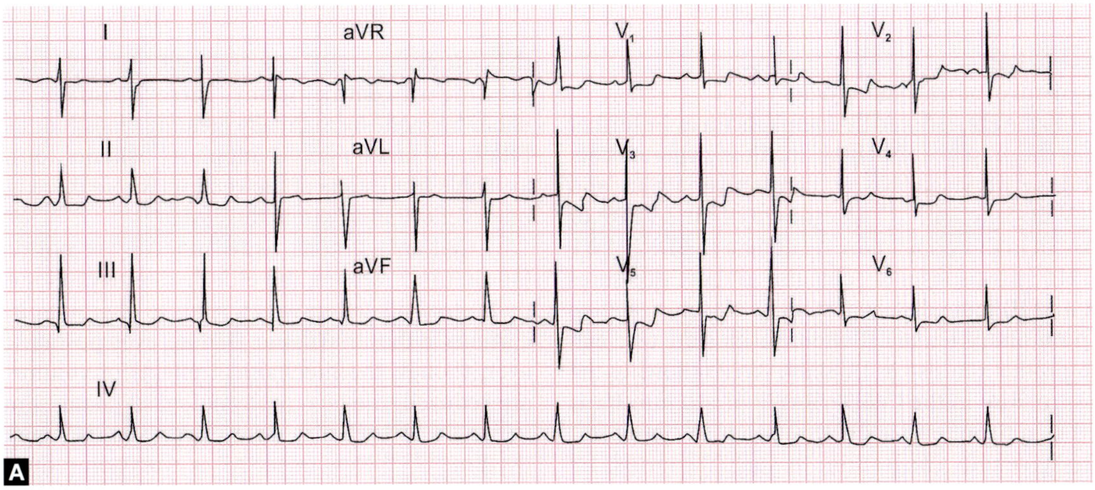

FIGS. 10A TO D: *Continued*

Continued

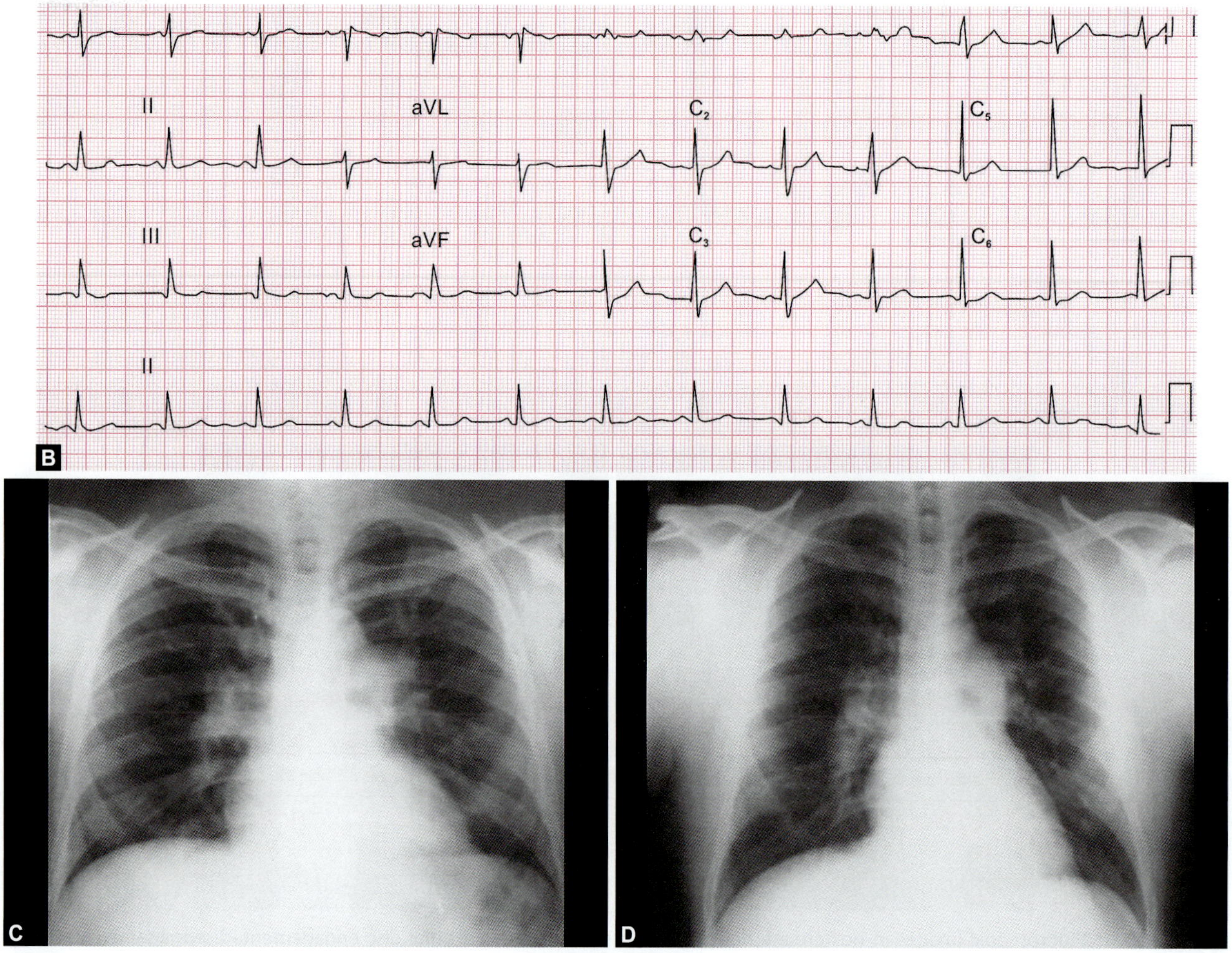

FIGS. 10A TO D: (A and C) Baseline and (B and D) 2-year follow-up ECG and chest X-ray after device closure. The follow-up ECG shows normalization of the QRS axis and significant regression of right ventricular hypertrophy (RVH) with disappearance of the right ventricular (RV) strain pattern. Similarly, follow-up chest X-ray shows mild decrease in heart size with reduction in pulmonary plethora.
Source: With permission from Dalvi and Phadke (2022).[5]

- Presence of PAH
- Management of other comorbidities

Apart from the age, reduced LV compliance may be further enhanced by the presence of diabetes mellitus, hypertension, chronic kidney disease, obesity, cardiomyopathies and ischemic LV dysfunction.[37-41] Assessment of the LVEDP or PAWP is useful in this population. A baseline LVEDP/PAWP if >15 mm Hg[42] predisposes to acute rise in these pressures **(Figs. 12A and B)** immediately postdevice closure resulting in acute pulmonary edema. Balloon occlusion test can be used to predict the rise in LVEDP/PAWP following the device closure. Rise in the LVEDP/PAWP of >10 mm Hg is considered significant and is likely to produce symptoms of pulmonary venous congestion. In such scenarios, LV preconditioning with diuretics and vasodilators prior to the device closure of the ASD is mandatory **(Figs. 13A and B)**.[43] Alternatively, one can use a fenestrated ASD device where the fenestration acts as a "pop off" for any increase in LA pressure with device closure. These fenestrated devices can either be made by manually creating fenestrations with a 12 FR dilator and 6 mm valvuloplasty balloon[44] or are readily available from some of the vendors where there is a factory-made fenestration within the device.[45,46]

Atrial arrhythmias, especially AF, are not uncommon (40–50%)[47-50] among the elderly due to the long-standing right atrial dilatation which leads to alteration in the ionic currents in the atrial tissue. Of note, even postdevice closure, even though the mechanical effects of volume overload are reduced, the electrophysiological changes persist and hence the arrhythmias rarely revert spontaneously to sinus rhythm.[47,51,52] New onset AF is worrisome due to risk of rhythm induced LV dysfunction, which may complicate the scenario. Management includes anticoagulation with vitamin K antagonists or newer OACs as indicated; rhythm

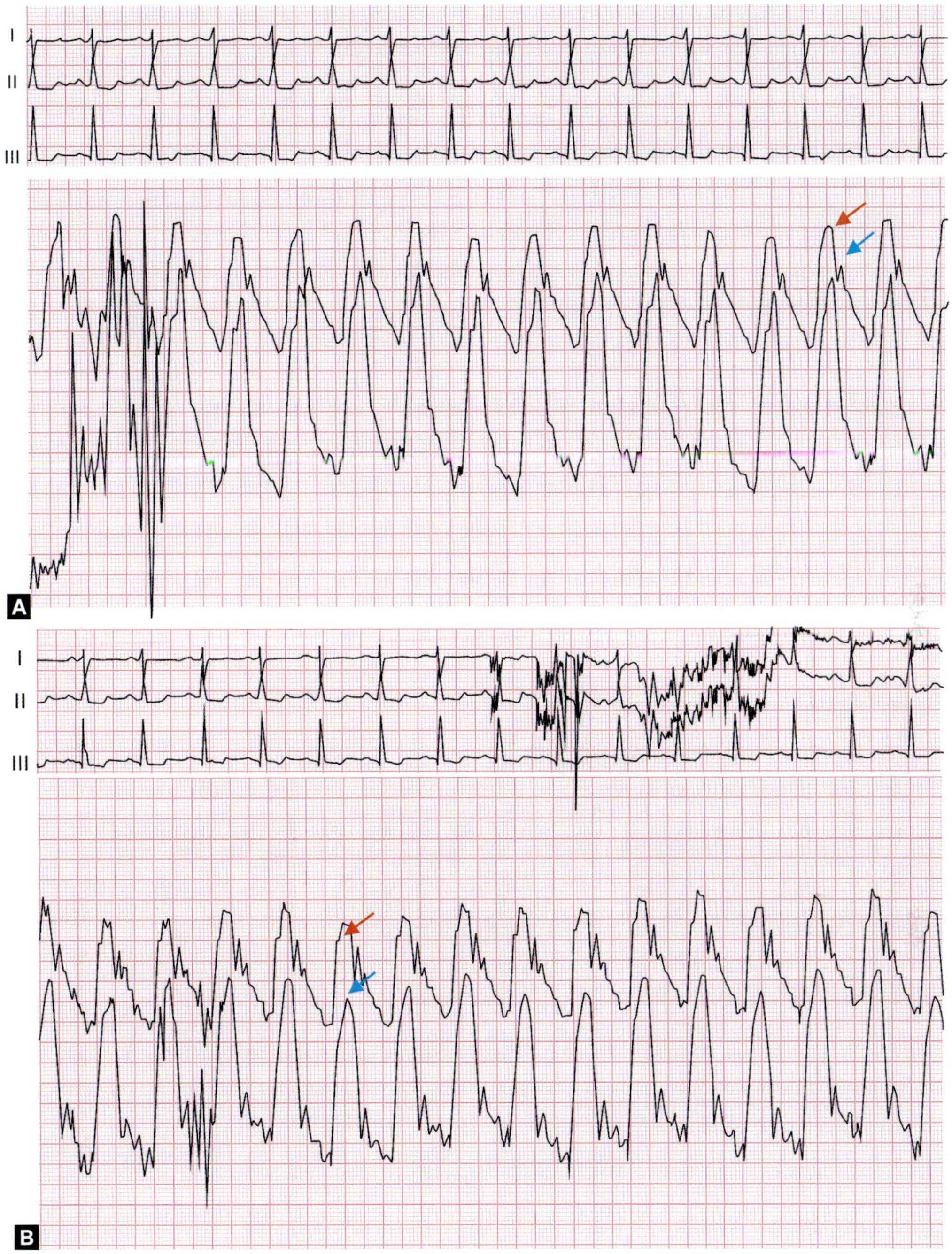

FIGS. 11A AND B: Aortic and pulmonary arterial (PA) pressure tracings in a patient with atrial septal defect and severe pulmonary arterial hypertension. (A) Baseline tracings. (B) After 100% oxygen and IV sildenafil. There was a fall in the PA diastolic and mean pressures after IV sildenafil and 100% oxygen administration. The ASD was subsequently closed based on clinical, radiological, echocardiographic, and hemodynamic criteria (red arrow—Aorta; blue arrow—PA).

Source: With permission from Dalvi and Phadke (2022).[5]

control via pharmacological or ablation therapy is aimed to be achieved. Ablation is always better done prior to device closure of defect to easily access the pulmonary veins; however, in unavoidable circumstances, a smaller transseptal puncture might be needed above or below the device to access the LA postclosure. In patients with contraindication to anticoagulation, LAA closure might be warranted.

Management of CAD is tricky in these patients. Male patients >45 years and female patients >50 years of age need to undergo a coronary angiography prior to the procedure. A heart team approach is used and individualized therapeutic approach is chosen. However, in acute coronary syndromes, coronary treatment takes precedence over ASD.

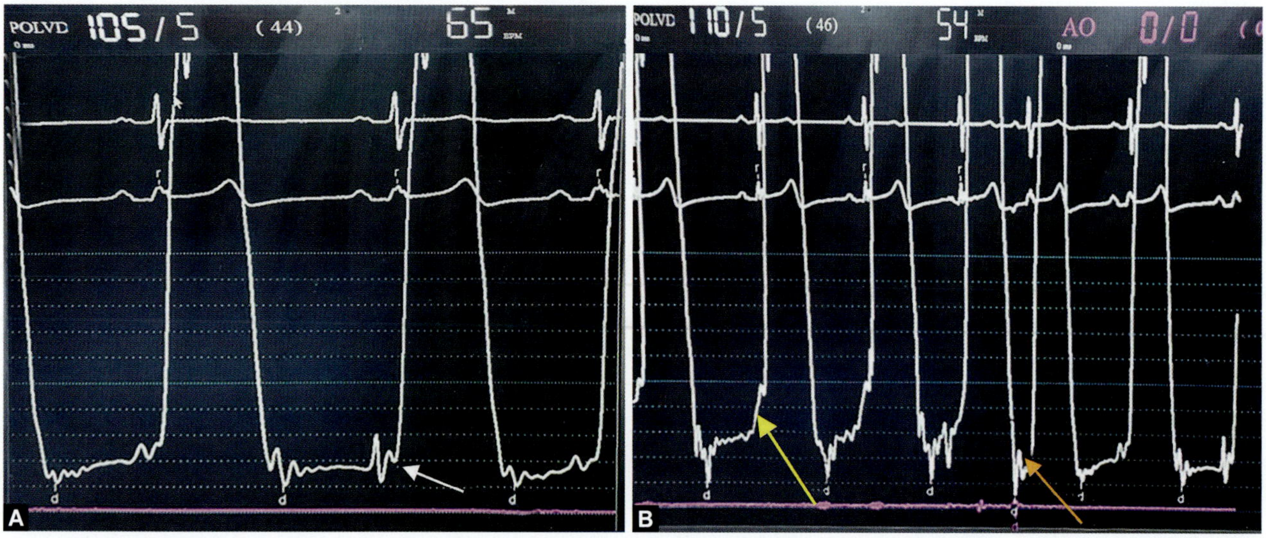

FIGS. 12A AND B: Intraprocedural hemodynamics in elderly ASD device closure before LV preconditioning; LVEDP before (A) and after device deployment without releasing it (B); abrupt rise >10 mm Hg is noted after device deployment (yellow arrow) compared to baseline (white arrow), which returns to the same level after device retrieval (orange arrow).

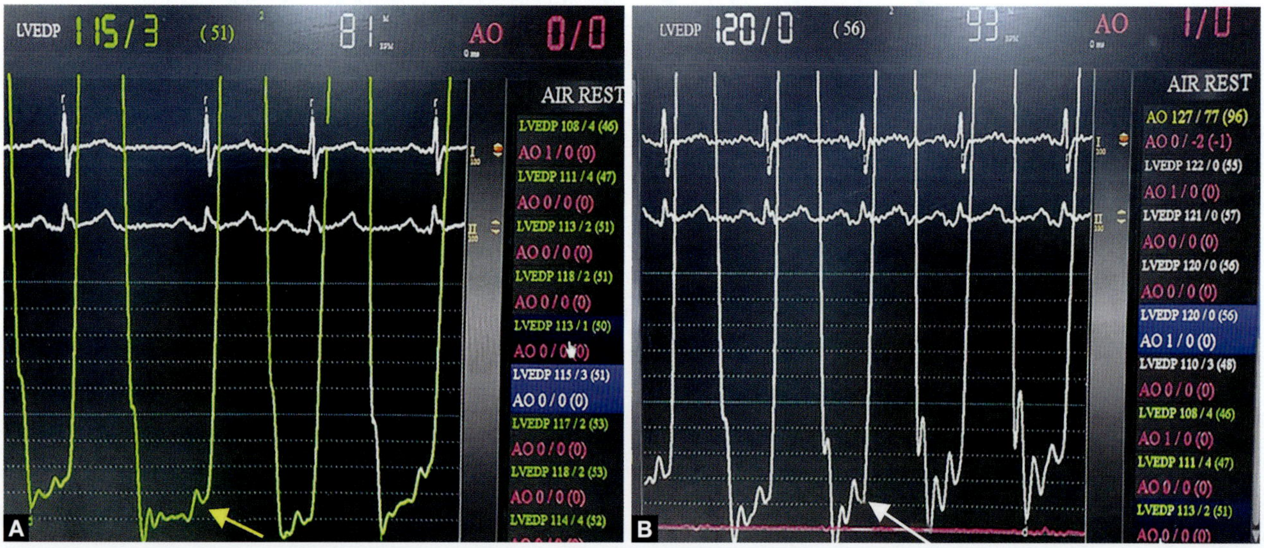

FIGS. 13A AND B: Left ventricular end diastolic pressure (LVEDP) of the same patient in **Figure 12** after LV preconditioning for 4 weeks before (A) and after device deployment (B) showing very little or no variability in LVEDP after device closure; device was subsequently deployed due to <10 mm Hg variability in LVEDP.

ACUTE COMPLICATIONS OF ATRIAL SEPTAL DEFECTS DEVICE CLOSURE

- *Procedural failure*:
  - Incidence: Rare, about 1–2% in high-volume centers. More common in small children, in those with large defects and those having rim abnormalities
  - Management: Proper patient selection and multiple deployment techniques minimize risk.
- *Device embolization*:
  - Predisposing factors: Large defects, deficient or floppy rims, device undersizing, improper placement, accidental unscrewing
  - Timing: Can occur during extubation when patient coughs or retches, or within the hours postdeployment
  - Management: Retrieval in the catheterization lab by snaring and using a larger device if embolization was thought to be due to undersizing. In some cases,

embolized device may require surgical removal with closure of the defect.

- *Arrhythmias*:
  - Types: Atrial tachycardia/flutter/fibrillation. AV conduction disturbances such as first-degree, second-degree, or complete heart block
  - Tachyarrhythmias: Due to catheter manipulation within the atria, especially around free wall of the right atrium (RA) and the pulmonary venous system. More common in the elderly population >50 years and are usually self-limiting. Some may terminate by generating atrial or ventricular premature beats, while some may need pharmacological (IV amiodarone/metoprolol) or electrical cardioversion (preferred in significant hemodynamic compromise due to rapid ventricular rate).
  - Atrioventricular conduction disturbances **(Figs. 14A and B)**: The incremental risk factors include small patient size, use of relatively (with respect to heart size) large devices and inferiorly placed defects.[53,54] Intravenous atropine or isoprenaline may help in improving conduction, sometimes it may be worth giving intravenous steroid therapy to reduce the acute edema in the region of the AV node. If these

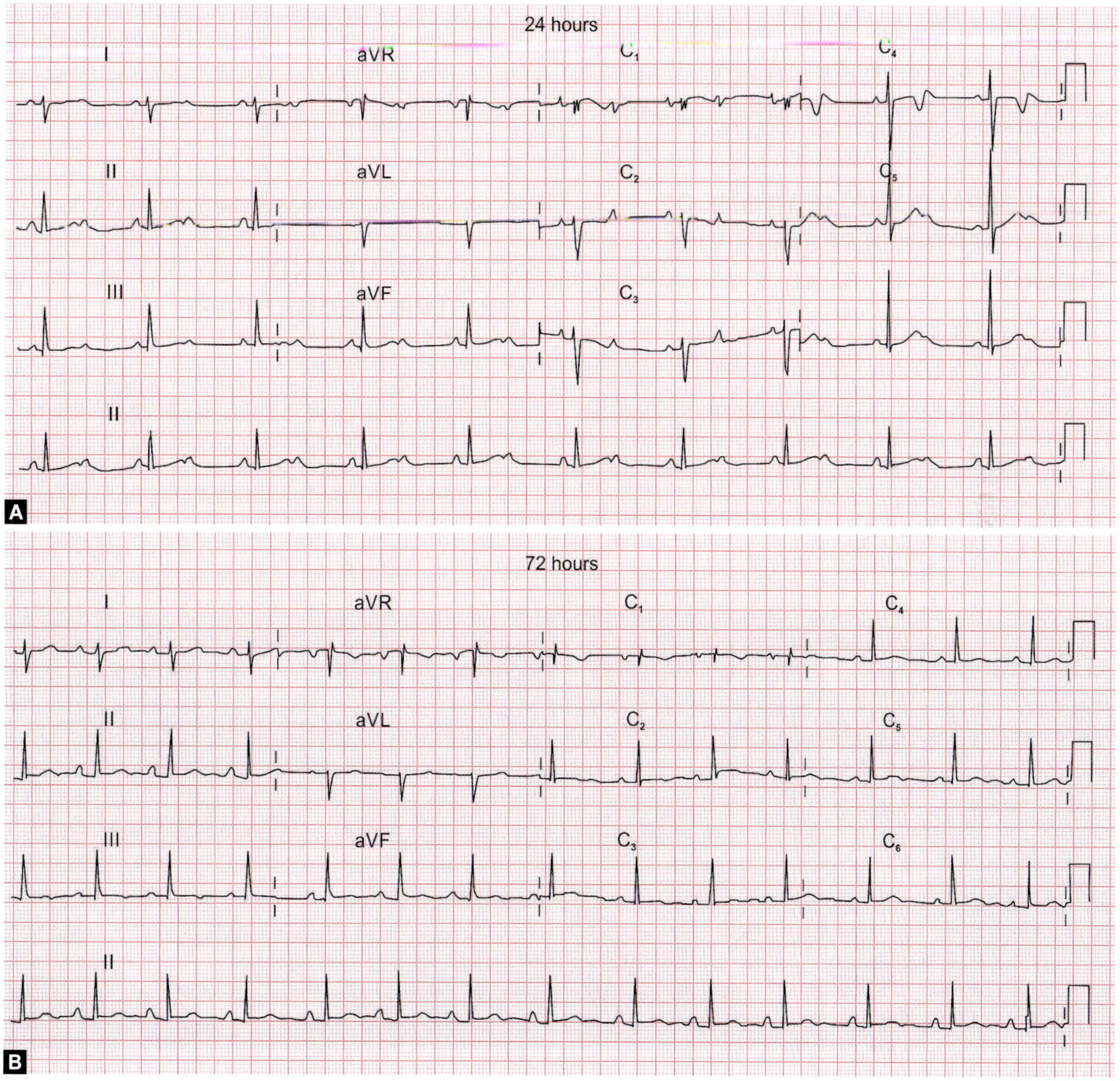

FIGS. 14A AND B: ECGs of a patient following atrial septal defect device closure. (A) ECG at 24 hours postprocedure showing a 2:1 AV block. (B) ECG at 72 hours following a trial of NSAIDs and steroids, showing normalization of AV conduction.

Source: With permission from Dalvi and Phadke (2022).[5]

interventions do not work, and the high degree AV persists, device retrieval may be necessary. If the AV conduction reverts to normal, one can attempt closure with a smaller device after priming the patient with anti-inflammatory drugs or he/she can be referred for surgical closure. If high grade AV blocks (especially complete AV block) persist beyond 48–72 hours, surgical removal and defect closure should be considered as waiting longer may increase the chances of needing permanent pacemaker implantation.

- *Injury to pulmonary veins and AV valves*:
  - Risk factors: Large devices, smaller patients, multiple recaptures and redeployments can result in injuring these structures and hence gentle manipulation advised. The mitral valve may be damaged due to its proximity to the deployed LA disc.
  - Management: Surgical intervention if severe; conservative management with follow-up if mild

LONG-TERM COMPLICATIONS OF ATRIAL SEPTAL DEFECTS DEVICE CLOSURE

- *Delayed embolization*:
  - Timing: Uncommon, within days or weeks, possibly due to trauma[55]
  - Management: Removal in the catheterization lab if freely moving; surgical removal if the device is partially anchored with significant residual shunt.
- *Late-onset arrhythmias*:
  - Types: Most often they include atrial ectopics, atrial tachycardia, or atrial flutter/fibrillation.
  - Management: Do not require treatment if they are self-limiting. If persistent, they require pharmacological treatment with amiodarone or beta blockers or electrophysiological mapping and ablation if resistant to antiarrhythmic medications. Medications for rate/rhythm control and anticoagulants to prevent systemic thromboembolism are the mainstay of pharmacological treatment.
- *Cardiac erosion*:
  - Incidence: Very rare (0.01–0.03%)[56]
  - Risk factors: Absence of aortic rim, device oversizing, deficiencies of the other rims, anterior and superior defects. The most common site is the roof of the right or left atrium.[57]
  - Presentation: Chest pain, breathlessness, syncope, or new continuous murmur (aorto-atrial fistula),[57] rarely sudden death (due to cardiac tamponade) **(Figs. 15A and B)**
  - Management: Surgical removal of the device, repair of the atrial wall, and ASD closure. Preprocedural counseling about cardiac erosion and the symptoms to watch out for needs to be meticulously done.

FOLLOW-UP AND POSTPROCEDURE CARE

- *Initial postprocedure*:
  - Hospital stay: Patient stays overnight in the hospital and is discharged the next morning after confirming normal AV conduction and normal rhythm on ECG and normal device position confirmed by imaging.
  - Medications: Oral aspirin (5 mg/kg, up to 150 mg/day) for 6 months, infective endocarditis prophylaxis, and restrictions on MRI and contact sports for 6 months

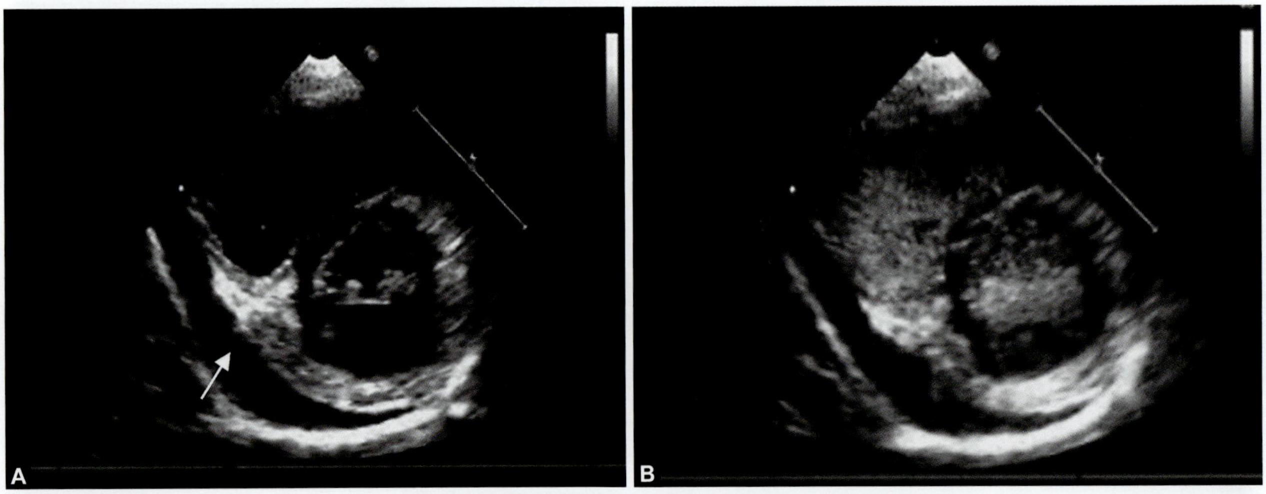

FIGS. 15A AND B: Transthoracic echocardiographic images in a patient following atrial septal defect device closure showing (A) a moderate sized pericardial effusion (arrow). (B) Image of contrast echo showing opacification of the cardiac chambers only, with no evidence of the contrast leaking into the pericardial cavity, ruling out erosion or perforation.

(LV: left ventricle; RV: right ventricle)

Source: With permission from Dalvi and Phadke (2022).[5]

- *Follow-up visits*:
  - Timing: At 1 month, 3 months, and annually for 5 years
  - Investigations: Clinical evaluation, ECG, and echocardiogram. Additional tests if complications arise

Transcatheter Closure of Sinus Venosus Atrial Septal Defect

Has gained recognition over the past decade as a viable alternative to surgical correction, especially in adults, though some cases in children have been reported. The procedure typically involves the use of a covered stent to close the interatrial communication and reroute the RSPV to the left atrium. Preprocedural assessment includes imaging and balloon interrogation to evaluate the feasibility and exclude cases with large defects or residual shunts.[58-62]

The procedure, performed under general anesthesia, requires careful access via bilateral femoral veins, the right jugular vein, and femoral artery. Balloon interrogation ensures there is no RSPV obstruction or residual shunt before deploying the covered stent, which is stabilized using a veno-venous circuit. Postprocedure, patients are monitored with ECG, TTE, and Holter, and prescribed aspirin for 1 year. Complications can include residual shunts, stent embolization, and late atrial arrhythmias, with management options ranging from balloon dilation to pacemaker implantation. The procedure has demonstrated success, particularly in patients where surgical risks are high.

CONCLUSION

The management of ASDs has evolved with advanced closure techniques, improving patient outcomes. Percutaneous closure is preferred for its minimally invasive nature, though surgical options remain vital for complex cases. Individualized care, long-term follow-up, and ongoing research are key to enhancing quality of life and patient survival.

ONLINE REFERENCES

Please scan the QR code provided at the end of the table of contents for References of this chapter.

CHAPTER

184

Ruptured Sinus of Valsalva Device Closure: Current Status

Mohsin Raj Mantoo, Sivasubramanian Ramakrishnan

ABSTRACT

Ruptured sinus of Valsalva (RSOV) aneurysm usually leads to biventricular failure and, if untreated, carries a poor prognosis. Conventional surgical repair of RSOV is considered the gold standard. In selected cases, transcatheter device closure offers an attractive therapeutic option. No strict guidelines exist for selecting appropriate patients for RSOV device closure. This chapter reviews the clinical presentation of RSOV aneurysms, indications, and contraindications for device closure, different techniques of device closure, and the data on outcomes of RSOV device closure.

Keywords: Ruptured sinus of Valsalva (RSOV) aneurysm, transcatheter, device closure, catheterization

INTRODUCTION

Ruptured sinus of Valsalva (RSOV) aneurysm refers to a structural defect of the aortic root characterized by an outpouching of one of the aortic sinuses (part of aortic root between aortic annulus and sinotubular junction) that ruptures into an adjacent cardiac chamber. The sinus of Valsalva aneurysm (SOVA) may be congenital or acquired. Most patients with RSOV present with clinical features of biventricular failure, and if untreated, most patients succumb within a year of diagnosis.[1] Treatment of RSOV has traditionally been open surgical repair. The transcatheter device closure of RSOV has emerged as a suitable alternative in the past few decades.

ETIOLOGY

Ruptured sinus of Valsalva can occur as a result of congenital weakening of the aortic sinus wall or due to a multitude of acquired etiologies. The most accepted theory for the congenital variant is from Edwards and Burchell, which states that a lack of fusion between the aortic media and annulus fibrosus of the aortic valve causes the weakening of the aortic root.[2] Embryologic basis for the same is postulated to be an incomplete fusion of aortopulmonary and interventricular septum, which together form the right and noncoronary sinus. Less commonly, RSOV occurs as a result of acquired causes, including infective endocarditis (IE) (most common acquired etiology), other infections (syphilis and tuberculosis), trauma (accidental or iatrogenic), atherosclerosis, cystic medial degeneration, connective tissue diseases, vasculitic disorders (Behçet's and Takayasu), or prior surgery for congenital heart disease or aortic valve.[3]

EPIDEMIOLOGY

The exact prevalence of SOVA is unclear, with differing estimates from autopsy, surgical, and imaging series—around 0.09% of the general population and around 0.1–3.5% of all congenital heart defects.[4] Around 50% of SOVA rupture, necessitating a repair rather than watchful waiting especially in progressive or symptomatic lesions.[5] RSOV is more common in males and the Asian population [just like supracristal ventricular septal defects (VSDs)].

Ruptured sinus of Valsalva most commonly arises from the right coronary sinus (around 70–75%), followed by the non-coronary sinus (around 20–25%), and rarely the left sinus. The most common receiving chamber is the right ventricle [the most common site being the right ventricular outflow tract (RVOT)], followed by the right atrium (RA).[6,7] Additional lesions associated with RSOV include aortic regurgitation (AR) (around 40%), VSD (around 30%), bicuspid aortic valve (BAV) (around 10%), coarctation of the aorta, atrial septal defect, etc.[6] The most common age at rupture is generally adolescence and young adulthood.

Multiple classification systems have been proposed for RSOV based on imaging. Sakakibara classification is based on the drainage site of RSOV (RVOT just below the pulmonary valve or RV cavity or adjacent to the tricuspid leaflet or RA). In contrast, an angiographic classification is based on RSOV morphology (window-like, aneurysm-like, or tubular).[8,9] Careful attention to the abovementioned is needed for appropriate patient selection for transcatheter closure and appropriate device selection, as shall be discussed subsequently.

PRESENTATION

The clinical presentation of RSOV ranges from incidental detection on clinical examination (murmur) or echocardiography to acute presentations such as pulmonary edema and cardiogenic shock. Most patients are symptomatic, with dyspnea and palpitations being the most typical symptoms, followed by chest pain and fatigability.[6,10] Uncommon presentations include atrioventricular block (as a result of rupture of SOVA into interventricular septum), acute coronary syndrome (as a result of coronary compression or thromboembolism), AR, pericardial tamponade, and RVOT obstruction. Physical examination findings include biventricular failure (orthopnea, pulmonary rales, jugular venous distention, and peripheral edema) due to a sudden large left to right shunt. The murmur of RSOV is continuous, with "sawing" quality heard best at the right and left sternal edge, depending on the rupture site. Associated VSD intensifies the systolic component of murmur, while AR intensifies the diastolic component.

Transthoracic two-dimensional echocardiography (TTE) is the usual imaging modality to confirm the diagnosis. It is characterized by a classic "windsock" appearance of the RSOV protruding from the aortic sinus into the draining chamber. Besides the characteristics of RSOV (site of origin and drainage as well as the size of the defect), TTE enables the diagnosis of associated lesions such as AR, VSD, or BAV and the estimation of left ventricular (LV) volumes, function, and pulmonary hypertension. It is important to note that an associated VSD may escape detection on TTE if the wall of the RSOV or aortic valve cusp occludes it. Other imaging modalities such as transesophageal echocardiography (TEE), 3D echocardiography (3DE), multidetector computed tomography (CT), and cardiac magnetic resonance imaging (MRI) offer superior resolution. They are used in selected cases, especially for procedural planning.[11-14]

OUTCOMES OF RUPTURED SINUS OF VALSALVA SURGICAL REPAIR

Conventional open surgical repair options include aneurysm resection and direct suture approximation of aortic defect, as well as the use of pericardial or prosthetic patches. A large series (n = 100) from China reports 10-year and 15-year actuarial survival rates of 94% and 90%, respectively. Concomitant aortic valve surgery was required in 22 patients in this series.[15] An older series from Mayo Clinic (n = 86) reported a poorer outcome, with a 10-year actuarial survival rate of 63%. Perioperative mortality was 7% in this series, and 84% of patients underwent other cardiac procedures at the time of RSOV repair (aortic valve surgery in 32 patients and VSD closure in 27 patients).[6] Newer series, including one from North India, report improved results.[16,17] A minimally invasive surgical approach has also been described via a parasternal mini-incision and RA puncture followed by the use of a delivery system/sheath to deploy devices such as VSD or patent ductus arteriosus (PDA) occluders.[18]

RUPTURED SINUS OF VALSALVA DEVICE CLOSURE

Cullen et al. reported the first case of transcatheter RSOV device closure in 1994 in a 34-year-old man with right coronary sinus to RVOT communication using a 12 mm Rashkind umbrella device delivered retrograde over a sheath advanced from the aortic root to the RV.[19] Since then, several modifications have been introduced in the closure technique and the devices used for percutaneous closure.

Indications

All patients with RSOV need closure, either via device or through surgery. While there are no strict guidelines for patient selection for percutaneous device closure, the operator must choose the most appropriate patient carefully. The following may be considered as more suitable candidates for device closure:[10,20]

- Body weight > 10 kg
- Defect size < 10 mm
- No or mild AR
- Adequate rims (at least 7 mm from aortic annulus and 5 mm from RCA ostium)
- No other anomaly that requires surgery. Other cardiac defects should be amenable to percutaneous closure.

Contraindications

The following may be considered as contraindications to percutaneous device closure (most are relative):

- More complicated defects such as tunnel-like RSOV or having multiple rupture sites
- More than mild AR
- Associated subarterial VSD (a small perimembranous VSD may not be a contraindication)
- Active IE
- Other anomalies that require surgical intervention.

Note: RSOV device closure has been reported even in the presence of small-outlet VSD or perimembranous VSD, with some reports of concomitant VSD device closure of perimembranous defects.[21] Similarly, device closure has been successful even in patients with multiple rupture sites.[22] There are reports of RSOV device closure even in the presence of mechanical aortic valves.[23] Successful percutaneous closure has been performed even in infants or those with giant aneurysms.[24,25] Hence, the above list of patient selection and contraindications is not absolute.

Cardiac Catheterization

While a routine invasive cardiac catheterization is not necessary for establishing a diagnosis of RSOV, it is generally performed at the time of intervention. Critical information obtained from cardiac catheterization includes pulmonary artery pressure, ventricular filling pressures, amount of left-to-right shunt (Qp: Qs), confirmation of the number, size, and site of the defect (on aortic root angiogram), and presence of associated VSD (on LV angiogram). Usual initial projections for aortic root angiogram include right anterior oblique (RAO) and left anterior oblique (LAO) with slight cranial angulation.

Imaging

Intraprocedural TEE guidance is preferred by most operators. 3D-echocardiography adds to procedural accuracy by demonstrating the exact size and shape of the defect and visualization of guidewire passing through the defect. Baseline AR, as well as any worsening during device deployment, needs to be carefully assessed. Post-deployment, any residual peridevice leak and any impingement of nearby structures such as RVOT or tricuspid valve needs attention. In cases where the defects are clearly delineated and sized on preprocedure TEE, TTE may be enough for procedural guidance (this approach enables the operator to avoid general anesthesia).

Antegrade Closure Technique

This is the most commonly used percutaneous RSOV device closure technique. It involves creation of an arteriovenous loop from the femoral access site and advancing the delivery sheath and device from the venous side. Procedural steps are briefly summarized further **(Figs. 1A to H)**:

- Preprocedural antibiotics, as per institutional policy (cefazolin is the agent of choice), are given intravenous 30–60 minutes before the start of the procedure.
- Femoral artery (FA) and vein access using the conventional Seldinger technique.

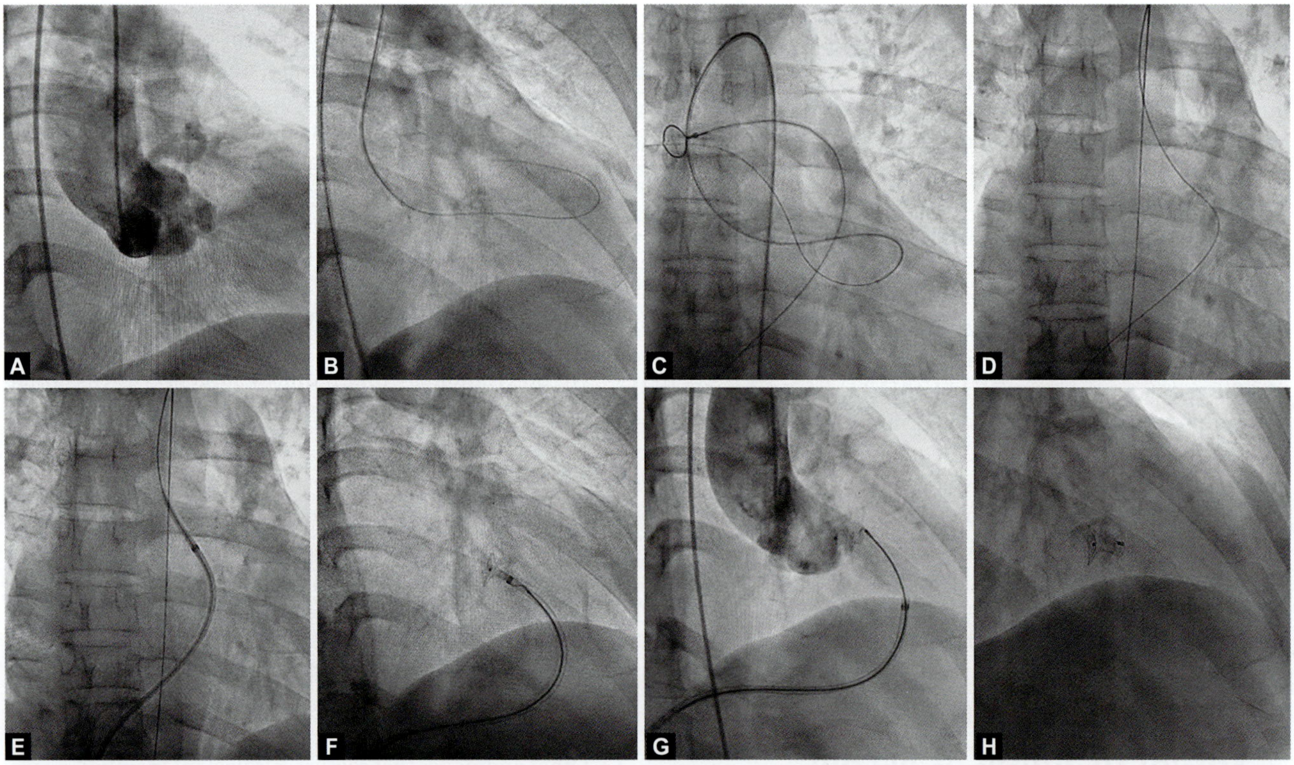

FIGS. 1A TO H: (A) Aortic root angiogram in right anterior oblique view using a 6Fr pigtail catheter demonstrating a sinus of Valsalva aneurysm ruptured into right ventricular outflow tract. (B) Using a Judkins right (JR) catheter introduced from the femoral artery to the aortic root, the RSOV defect is crossed with a 0.035" straight-tip Terumo wire. (C) An exchange length of 0.035" Terumo wire parked in the right pulmonary artery being snared out using a gooseneck snare introduced from the ipsilateral femoral venous side. (D) Arteriovenous loop between ipsilateral femoral artery and vein. (E) Mullin's sheath (Cook Inc. Bloomington, IN) being introduced from the venous end of the arteriovenous loop. (F) An Amplatzer duct occluder (ADOI) is used for defect closure. The disc is released on the aortic side while pulling the delivery sheath. (G) ADOI deployed across the ruptured sinus of Valsalva; repeat aortic root angiogram using a pigtail catheter showing no residual leak. (H) The final device position is after release from the delivery cable.

- Heparinize (100 units/kg unfractionated heparin). Check activated clotting time (ACT) during the procedure to ensure optimum anticoagulation.
- *Aortic root angiogram*: Using a 5–6Fr pigtail catheter in the RAO and LAO projections. This delineates the origin, number, size, shape, and rupture site of RSOV. More than mild baseline AR is generally considered a contraindication to device closure. Selective coronary angiography is performed in patients over 40 years of age or with coronary artery disease risk factors.
- *Crossing the defect*: Using a right Judkins (JR) or multipurpose (MPA2) catheter introduced from the FA to the aortic root, the RSOV defect is usually crossed with a 0.035" straight-tip Terumo wire over which the catheter is advanced. Successful crossing through the defect may be checked on TEE.
- *Establishing an arteriovenous loop*: An exchange length guidewire is next passed through the catheter (JR or MPA2) and parked in the superior vena cava (if the RSOV opens into RA) or pulmonary artery (if RSOV opens into RV/RVOT). This guidewire is snared out using a gooseneck snare introduced from the ipsilateral femoral venous sheath. This creates an arteriovenous loop between the FA and vein over which the delivery sheath is railroaded. It is essential to avoid too much tension/pulling from the venous side, which may injure the structures traversed by the guidewire.
- *Selection of an appropriate device and delivery sheath*: The most commonly used devices are the PDA occluder and Amplatzer duct occluder (ADOI, St Jude Medical Inc. MN) as they are most suitable to the morphology of RSOV (windsock appearance with a wider aortic end). Duct occluders are mainly deployed using a Mullins sheath (Cook Inc. Bloomington, IN) introduced from the venous end of the arteriovenous loop. The device size selected is at least 2 mm more than the smallest diameter of RSOV.
- *Deploying the device*: First, the aortic rim is deployed and the entire assembly is gently pulled (a tug is felt once the disc is against the aortic opening of RSOV), followed by the release of the whole device or disc on the venous side. An aortic root angiogram is taken to confirm the position of the device and any residual shunts. A selective coronary angiogram is generally not needed, as the aortic rupture site is usually away from the coronary ostium.
- *Release of device*: After confirming the desired position of the device and the absence of residual shunt or any significant AR or impingement of adjacent structures, the device is slowly released from the delivery cable.

Retrograde Closure Technique

In this case, bilateral FA access is needed. After obtaining an aortic root angiogram, the defect is crossed (just like the antegrade method) using a JR or multipurpose (MPA2) catheter and a straight-tip Terumo wire. Next, a 0.035" or 0.038" Amplatz exchange length guidewire is advanced across the defect and parked distally (no snaring done in the method). The introducer sheath is advanced over this wire across the defect retrograde from the aortic end. The occluder device (modified duct occluder or muscular VSD occluder) is then advanced through this sheath. The latter is slowly withdrawn to deploy the distal disc in the chamber where RSOV ruptures. The sheath is again slowly withdrawn to deploy the disc on the aortic end. A repeat aortogram (using a pigtail catheter through contralateral FA access) and TTE/TEE are used to confirm the correct device position and any residual shunts or AR, after which the device is released.

While operators most commonly utilize the antegrade technique, it involves longer fluoroscopy time and a steeper learning curve in arteriovenous loop formation. The duct occluders, which are best suited for the morphology of windsock, can generally be deployed only through the venous end (given their single retention disc, which is placed on the high-pressure arterial side). The retrograde technique, on the other hand, avoids the need for AV loop formation at the cost of one extra FA access. Devices that are bulky with retention discs on both sides (like muscular VSD occluders) are better delivered retrograde.

Devices for Percutaneous Closure

No device has been specifically designed for percutaneous RSOV closure. In a systematic review of 407 RSOV device closure cases, the PDA occluder was the most common device used (42%), followed by ADOI (21%), other duct occluders (10%), and VSD occluder (9%). Other devices less commonly used include small-waist double-disc occluder, muscular VSD occluder, Amplatzer septal occluder, Amplatzer vascular plug, patent foramen ovale occluder, and Gianturco coils.[10] The first device used by Cullen et al. in 1994 was a 12 mm Rashkind umbrella.[19] The first use of ADO was reported around 2002–2003 by Fedson et al. and Trehan et al.[26,27] Rittger et al. described the use of Amplatzer vascular plug II (AVP II) and proposed its suitability over ADO in RSOV with tortuous anatomy.[28] Bioptome-assisted delivery of 0.052" Gianturco coil to close the windsock of RSOV has also been reported.[29] Recently, other devices such as the Konar multifunctional device and Cocoon duct occluder have been successfully used to close RSOV defects.[30,31]

Outcomes of Ruptured Sinus of Valsalva Device Closure

Multiple case series from different parts of the world report the short- and intermediate-term outcomes of RSOV device closure. Liu et al. report experience on 25 cases of RSOV from China, with five patients having concomitant VSD. They enrolled patients considered very high-risk for surgery (mean EuroSCORE II was 25%), defects measuring <12 mm, and any other associated defect being amenable to percutaneous closure. Percutaneous closure was successful in 23 (92%) cases. Trivial residual shunts and mild new-onset AR occurred in three and five patients, respectively, which disappeared in most patients on follow-up. Two patients required surgery for device retrieval due to severe hemolysis caused by residual shunt.[32] Such spontaneous resolution of trivial device-related AR is also described in another series by Yang and colleagues.[20] Most patients with successful device closure become NYHA functional class I on follow-up.[33]

Several notable series on RSOV have been published in India. Arora et al. described their experience of RSOV device closure in eight patients as early as 2004. They used the arteriovenous loop and antegrade closure technique to deploy devices, including the Rashkind umbrella and Amplatzer occluders. One patient required surgical intervention due to severe hemolysis post-device closure, one patient died on follow-up, and the six remained asymptomatic.[34] In a series by Mahimarangaiah et al., percutaneous closure was attempted in 25 RSOV patients. The operators used an antegrade or retrograde approach to deploy devices (duct occluder in most cases and muscular VSD occluder in four). Device closure was successful in 21 (84%) cases, with one patient having device embolization, one with device-related severe AR, and two with a significant residual shunt.[35] A concomitant restrictive VSD (especially supracristal VSD) often creates a dilemma and has conventionally been considered a contraindication to device closure. A study from India describes a 92% success rate (12 out of 13 attempted cases) of device closure in patients with concomitant restrictive VSD, eight of which had an outlet VSD. One patient with perimembranous VSD underwent device closure of that defect too. Therefore, the success of the RSOV device closure was not affected by the presence of VSD, which could theoretically lead to a lack of support for the device by the VSD beneath the aortic sinus.[21]

A recent systematic review by Ayati et al. described the outcomes of 407 patients who underwent RSOV device closure. Most patients (90%) were symptomatic, with the majority being in NYHA II and III. The most common site of origin of RSOV was the right coronary sinus (62%), followed by the noncoronary sinus (37%). RA (52%) and RV (46%) were the most common draining sites. The defect size ranged from 3 to 17 mm at the aortic site. The overall procedural success rate was 95.6%. The most common devices used were PDA occluders (42%) followed by ADO (21%). There was a significant residual shunt in 61 (15%) patients, which resolved in most cases (all except six patients) on follow-up. A new-onset or worsening AR was reported in 22 (5.4%) cases, although it was moderate-to-severe in only seven (1.7%) cases. Recurrent RSOV, significant hemolysis, and device embolization were reported in six (1.5%), five (1.2%), and four (1%) patients, respectively. Only two patients died after intervention in this analysis.[10]

Complications of Ruptured Sinus of Valsalva Device Closure

In the systematic review cited earlier, residual shunts and AR were the most common complications. Other less commonly reported complications include hemolysis, device embolization, atrioventricular blocks, RVOT obstruction, thrombosis, LV dysfunction, IE, myocardial ischemia, and femoral access site complications.[36-39]

Postprocedure Antiplatelet Therapy

Most of the series cited earlier have used a single antiplatelet, aspirin 3–5 mg/kg for 6 months postprocedure. One series reported the use of dual antiplatelet therapy starting a day before the procedure and continuing for 6 months postprocedure.[35]

COMPARISON OF RUPTURED SINUS OF VALSALVA DEVICE CLOSURE AND OPEN SURGICAL REPAIR

There are no randomized studies comparing these two modalities of treatment of RSOV. Good quality prospective studies are also scarce. A large comparison study included 34 studies of percutaneous closure and 16 studies of surgical closure of RSOV, enrolling 877 patients (741 in the surgical group and 136 in the percutaneous group).[40] The authors concluded that a direct comparison of outcomes between the two modalities was impossible due to selection bias. Patients with more complicated diseases such as severe AR, tortuous or tunnel-like windsock, extensive and multiple defects, active IE, and associated significant septal defects underwent surgery. In the surgical group, early and late mortality rates were 1.5% and 3.2%, respectively. In the percutaneous group, only one death was reported with limited long-term data.

A recent systematic review of 10 studies (all retrospective data) included 330 patients, 207 in surgical and 123 in percutaneous groups, respectively. The two groups had no significant difference with respect to concerning in-hospital mortality, residual shunts, or postprocedure AR. However, percutaneous group had a significant reduction in length of hospital stay.[41]

Hence, it may be concluded that percutaneous RSOV closure is safe and efficacious but requires careful patient selection and heart team discussion.

CONCLUSION

The RSOV aneurysm needs repair in all cases. Conventional surgical repair is safe and has good long-term survival data. Percutaneous device closure is reported to have high success rates (above 90%) with minimal periprocedural mortality (<1%). Residual shunts, new or worsening AR, and hemolysis sometimes complicate device closure; the former two mostly resolve spontaneously. Long-term outcomes data on device closure is lacking.

ONLINE REFERENCES

Please scan the QR code provided at the end of the table of contents for References of this chapter.

CHAPTER

185

Left Atrial Appendage Closure

Lakshmi Durga Kumaraguruparan, Nagendra Boopathy Senguttuvan

ABSTRACT

Atrial fibrillation is the CHA_2DS_2-VASc most common arrhythmia encountered in elderly populations globally. Assessment of ischemic stroke risk using CHA_2DS_2-VASc score and bleeding risk using HAS-BLED is the paramount step in managing such patients. The LAA is the most common site for thrombus formation in patients with atrial fibrillation. Anticoagulation is the single most important step that reduces the risk of stroke and systemic embolism. The alternative to the same is left atrial appendage occlusion (LAAO) devices. The safety of the deployment of LAAO has been shown in multiple randomized trials and registries. However, the therapy is still highly underutilized in Indian scenarios. The LAAO is still uncommonly used in India predominantly due to cost constraints and absence of superiority of such a therapy over medical therapy in all-comers with atrial fibrillation. A strong data is still required to convince cardiologists to use it in all-comers with atrial fibrillation. Involvement of patients in the process of the "shared decision-making" is an essential tool to convey all the myths and facts about LAAO to them. Till then, it is reasonable to consider the same in patients with atrial fibrillation with high bleeding risk or patients with contraindications to anticoagulation.

Keywords: Left atrial appendage closure (LAAC), left atrial appendage occlusion (LAAO), WATCHMAN device, atrial fibrillation (AF), nonvalvular atrial fibrillation

INTRODUCTION

Left atrial appendage (LAA) is a hollow cylindrical structure situated in the left atrium (LA) and has various morphologies. It is of prime importance in its contribution to thromboembolism and CVA in patients with atrial fibrillation (AF). It is observed that there is an increase in risk of ischemic stroke by 4–5 folds in patients with AF, with doubled risk for all-cause mortality and cognitive dysfunction.[1,2]

LEFT ATRIAL APPENDAGE ANATOMY

Left atrial appendage is a finger-like blind tubular structure from the left atrium with variable lobes and morphologies. Embryologically, it is derived from primordial left atrium, which in turn is formed primarily from adsorption of the primordial pulmonary veins.[3]

Left atrial appendage has three anatomic regions—ostium, neck that serves as the landing zone for devices, and body that has the lobes. Volume of LAA ranges from 0.7 to 9.2 mL, and length varies widely ranging between 16 and 51 mm.[4]

Left atrial appendage is located in the AV groove anteriorly, extending anterosuperiorly mostly, and lies in proximity to left border of RV outflow tract, left circumflex artery, great cardiac vein, left phrenic nerve, and the left pulmonary veins **(Fig. 1)**.

Internally, the ostium is separated from the pulmonary veins by left lateral ridge.[3] The inner surface has both smooth endocardial part and the trabecular part formed by pectinate muscles.[15] The pectinate muscle bundles in the LAA may spuriously resemble thrombus or intra-atrial masses in echo.

The LAA tip can lie in various positions:

- Over the pulmonary artery and the left anterior descending coronary artery
- Pointing posteriorly
- Angled medially facing posterior part of the aorta

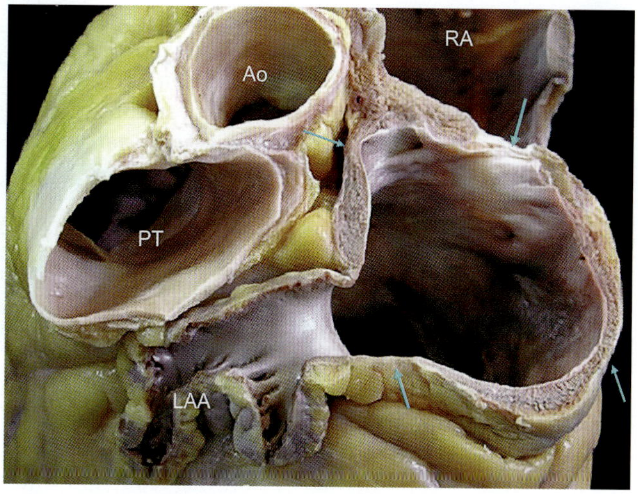

FIG. 1: Short axis section across the left atrial chamber.
(Ao: aorta; LAA: left atrial appendage; PT: pulmonary trunk; RA: right atrium)
Source: Sánchez-Quintana D, López-Mínguez JR, Macías Y, et al. Left atrial anatomy relevant to catheter ablation. Cardiol Res Pract. 2014;2014:289720.

Classification of LAA based on morphology of the body of LAA is as follows **(Figs. 2A to L)**:[5]

- Chicken wing-type LAA has a proximal or mid-prominent bend in the dominant lobe and it is the most common type.
- Cactus-type LAA has a dominant lobe with secondary lobules arising from it both upward and downward.
- *Cauliflower type:* With limited length and distal diameter widening
- *Windsock type:* One dominant lobe

LEFT ATRIAL APPENDAGE FUNCTION: THROMBUS RISK

In sinus rhythm, normal contraction of the LA appendage with normal blood flow reduces thrombus risk.[17] However, when there is reduced contraction and stasis as in AF, manifested by decrease in Doppler velocity in LAA and LA dilatation and fibrosis after remodeling, there appears an

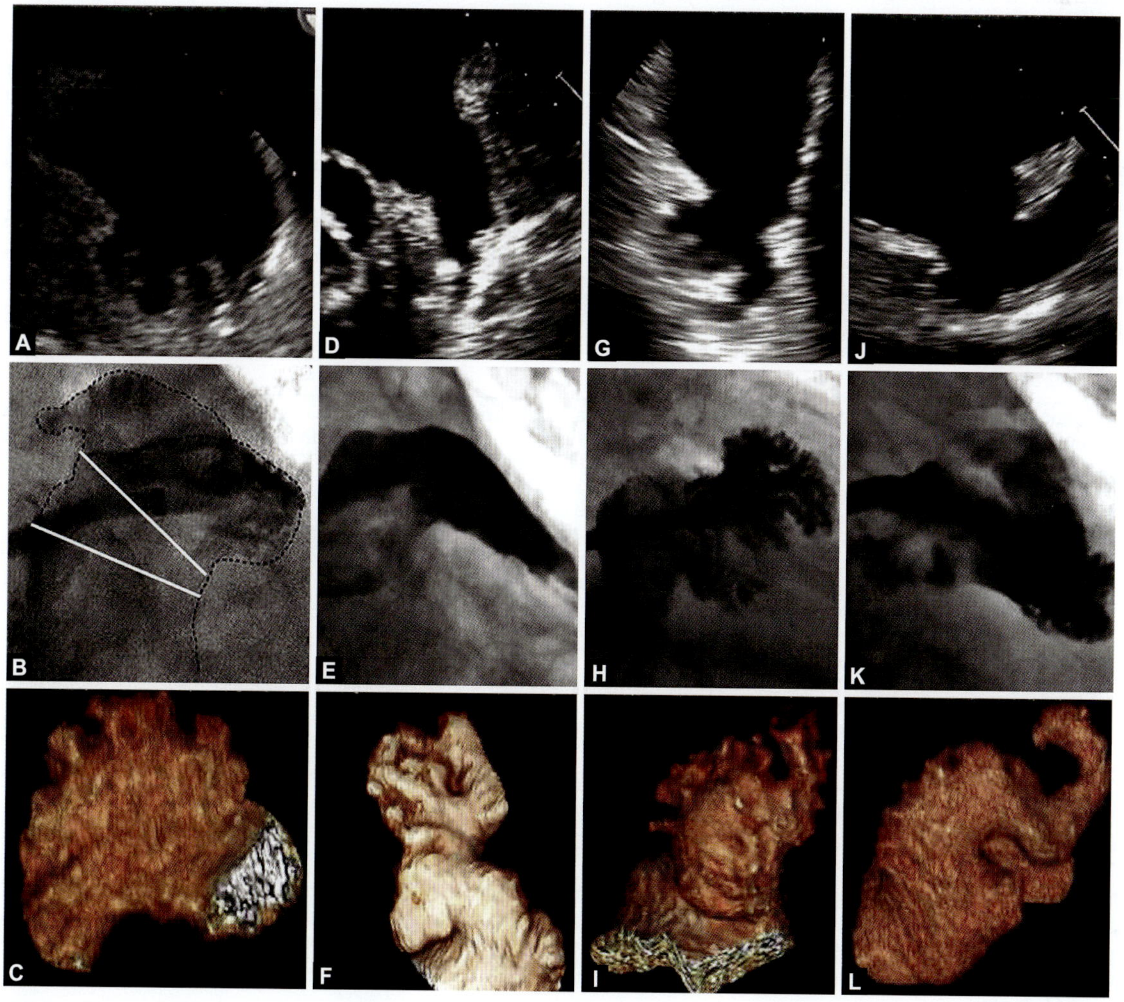

FIGS. 2A TO L: The four different LAA morphologies as shown by TEE (top row), cine angiography (middle row), and 3D computed tomography (bottom row). (A to C) Cauliflower; (D to F) windsock; (G to I) cactus; and (J to L) chicken wing.

increase in risk of thrombosis. Also, with advancing age, LAA contractility decreases with rise in AF incidence, thus risking LAA thrombus formation. In addition, the effect of AF on the neurohormonal properties of LAA such as release of atrial natriuretic peptide and modulation of intravascular volumes is poorly understood and may contribute to other mechanisms of thrombus formation.[16] The CHA_2DS_2-VASc score that is used for risk stratification for CVA in AF patients, does not include LAA contractility.

APPROACHES TO PREVENT LEFT ATRIAL APPENDAGE-RELATED THROMBI IN ATRIAL FIBRILLATION

Approach to stroke prevention in a patient with atrial fibrillation is given in **Flowchart 1**.

Elimination of the underlying arrhythmia and restoring sinus rhythm is the key. However, rhythm control may not be achievable in chronic AF. Oral anticoagulation is the key for stroke prevention, especially direct oral anticoagulants (DOACs) compared to warfarin, due to lower bleeding risk.[13] In addition, transcatheter LAA closure/surgical LAA closure can be done.

CHALLENGES IN TREATING ATRIAL FIBRILLATION WITH ORAL ANTICOAGULANTS

Traditionally, the cornerstone for decreasing the stroke risk in a patient with AF has been anticoagulation, which brings its own set of risks to the table. Especially in the older population and patients with high bleeding risk, many a times physicians end up in a situation where oral anticoagulants (OACs) are not started or have to be discontinued in spite of the stroke risks due to the comorbidities. Hence, risk stratification for thromboembolic events and bleeding is important before starting OACs.

Some of the common risk factors for increased risk of ischemic stroke in AF patients include history of stroke or transient ischemic attack (TIA), mitral stenosis, hypertension, diabetes, age >70 years, and heart failure. CHA_2DS_2-VASc score is the most recommended for calculating stroke risk.[6]

Warfarin and NOACS are the cornerstone of therapy. Assuming 51 ischemic strokes/1,000 patient-years, adjusted standard dose of warfarin prevented 28 strokes at expense of 11 fatal bleeds and aspirin prevented 16 strokes at expense of 6 fatal bleeds.[7] Warfarin has 60–70% risk reduction when compared with no treatment and 30–40% risk reduction versus aspirin.[8]

RATIONALE FOR LEFT ATRIAL APPENDAGE CLOSURE

In patients with nonvalvular AF, in whom conventional therapy with anticoagulation is high risk, left atrial appendage occlusion (LAAO) is a possible safe alternative to OAC.

Left atrial appendage is found to be the source of >90% of thrombi seen during transesophageal echocardiography (TEE).[9] LAA thrombus and decreased LAA peak flow velocity have been observed to be independent predictors of risk of thromboembolism and stroke[10,11] among nonvalvular AF patients. Hence, exclusion of LAA either by surgery or transcatheter device closure is paramount for CVA risk

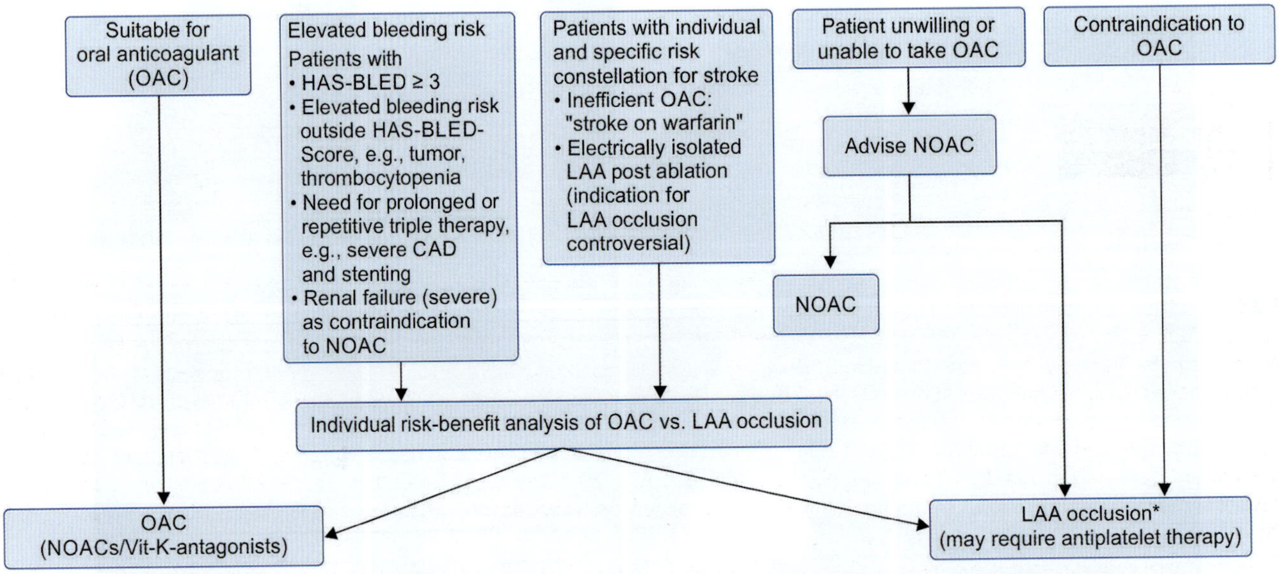

* In case of strict contraindication to antiplatelet therapy, patient may not be eligible for LAA occluder implantation but for epicardial LAA occlusion or thoracoscopic LAA clipping.

FLOWCHART 1: Approach to stroke prevention in a patient with atrial fibrillation.

reduction in patients with atrial fibrillation. In LAAOS III trial, for patients on anticoagulation, surgical LAAO during cardiac surgery had added benefit in regard to stroke risk reduction.[12]

HISTORY OF LEFT ATRIAL APPENDAGE OCCLUSION

The first device for transcatheter LAAO was percutaneous left atrial appendage transcatheter occlusion (PLAATO), which was designed by Dr Michael Lesh and was implanted by him and Dr Horst Sievert on 30 August 2001. This device had difficult implantation technique and some drawbacks and was withdrawn from market.[14] Since then, various transcatheter devices for LAA closure have been designed, studied, and Food and Drug Administration (FDA) approved for usage.

LEFT ATRIAL APPENDAGE CLOSURE DEVICES

Among transcatheter endocardial devices **(Figs. 3A to E)**, FDA approval for CVA prevention has been obtained for the WATCHMAN FLX (Boston Scientific) and Amulet (Abbott) devices for stroke prevention without OAC for the long run.

The principles behind LAAC devices are:

- *Plug:* The device obstructs the neck of the LAA, seals the lobe, then endocardialization of the device lobe occurs (WATCHMAN, WaveCrest), thereby excluding the LAA.[18]

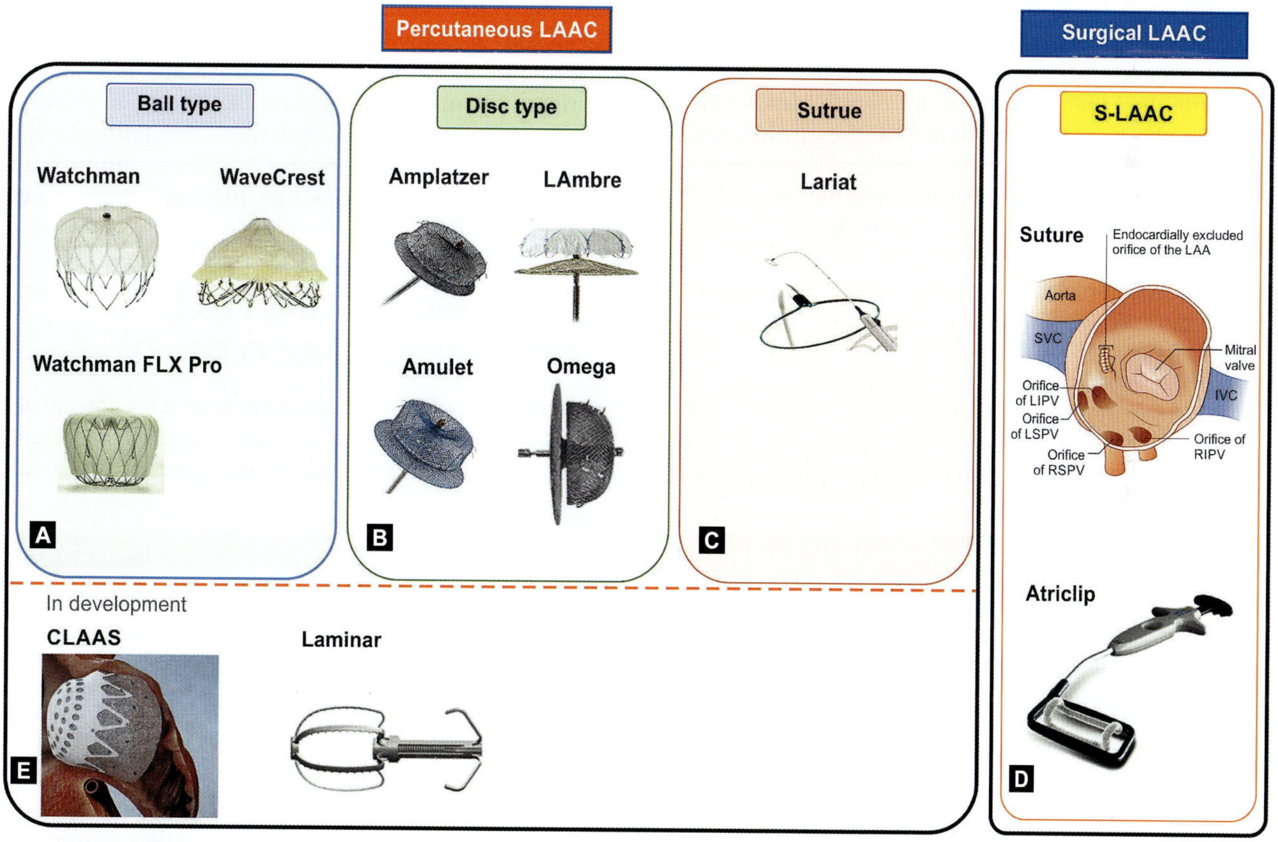

FIGS. 3A TO E: Percutaneous left atrial appendage closure devices and methods for surgical left atrial appendage closure. (A) Ball-type device (plug): Endovascular delivery of a lobe or umbrella and closure by obstructing the neck of the left atrial appendage (WATCHMAN, WAveCrest). (B) Disc-type device (pacifier): Endovascular device of a lobe or umbrella (anchoring/obstructing the neck of the left atrial appendage) with an additional disc attached (sealing of the left atrial appendage ostium; Amplatzer Amulet, LAmbre). Left atrial appendage closure is dependent on sealing and endothelialization of the corpus/umbrella and/or disc (pacifier principle). (C) Ligation: Endocardial and epicardial snaring and percutaneous suture ligation of the left atrial appendage (Lariat). (D) Surgical left atrial appendage closure: Amputation by suture or Atriclip is depicted. (E) Future devices: Aims of future developments are better conformability (foam-based devices such as CLAAS), reducing the footprint of foreign material (left atrial appendage obliteration, i.e., Laminar device), and causing less thrombogenicity by antithrombotic covering.

(IVC: inferior vena cava; LIPV: left inferior pulmonary vein; LSPV: left superior pulmonary vein; RIPV: right inferior pulmonary vein; RSPV: right superior pulmonary vein; S-LAAC: surgical left atrial appendage closure; SVC: superior vena cava)

Source: Landmesser U, Skurk C, Tzikas A, et al. Left atrial appendage closure for stroke prevention in atrial fibrillation: Current status and perspectives. Eur Heart J. 2024;45(32):2914-32.

- *Pacifier principle:* Examples include ACP, Amulet, LAmbre where there is an umbrella with an additional disc to seal the LAA ostium from the LA side.[18]
- *Ligation:* LARIAT device is used for snaring and completely ligating the neck of the LAA by an epicardial/endocardial approach.[18]

Device choice is based mostly on operator's experience and preference, excepting some anatomies that require specific devices.

EVIDENCE TO SUPPORT LEFT ATRIAL APPENDAGE CLOSURE

- *PROTECT AF* tested the efficacy and safety of the WATCHMAN device for LAAO in patients with nonvalvular AF.[19]
  - The trial demonstrated that the WATCHMAN device was noninferior to warfarin in prevention of stroke, systemic embolism, and cardiovascular death. This trial laid the groundwork for considering LAAC as an alternative to long-term OAC therapy in patients with AF.[19]
- *PREVAIL trial*: Participants were randomized to receive either the WATCHMAN device or continue with warfarin therapy in this RCT.[20] 5-year results indicated that when evaluating ischemic stroke or systemic embolism beyond 1 week postprocedure, LAAC did demonstrate noninferiority to warfarin.
- *PRAGUE-17 trial:*
  - It compared LAAO with DOACs in patients with AF.
  - LAAO was noninferior to DOACs in preventing stroke, systemic embolism, and bleeding events. It provided important evidence supporting the use of LAAO in patients at high risk of bleeding who may not be ideal candidates for long-term anticoagulation.
- *Patient-level meta-analysis (PROTECT AF and PREVAIL combined)*:
  - Analysis outcomes: LAAC was compared with warfarin:
    - All-cause stroke: Equivalent rates of all-cause stroke compared to warfarin.
    - Hemorrhagic stroke: LAAC showed significant decrease in hemorrhagic stroke and disabling/fatal stroke.
    - Ischemic stroke: No significant differences were observed in rates of ischemic stroke between the two.

In conclusion, based on the evidence from all these trials, the WATCHMAN device for LAAC provides stroke prevention in nonvalvular AF and is non-inferior to warfarin. In addition, LAA closure helps in reducing the risk of hemorrhagic stroke likely due to reduced need for long-term anticoagulation. The findings from PRAGUE-17 further support LAAC as a noninferior alternative to newer DOACs in high-risk populations **(Tables 1 and 2)**.

SELECTING PATIENTS FOR LEFT ATRIAL APPENDAGE CLOSURE

Transcatheter LAAC is specifically indicated for nonvalvular AF patients at high risk of thromboembolism who are not fit for long-term OAC and with minimum 1-year life expectancy.

TABLE 1: LAAC randomized controlled trial showing noninferiority.

Trial	Design	*n*	Key findings
PROTECT AF	Noninferiority WATCHMAN versus warfarin	Device ($n = 463$), control ($n = 244$)	• The primary efficacy endpoint (stroke, SE, and CV/unexplained death) event rate was 3.0 per 100 patient-years (95% CrI 1.9–4.5) in the device group and 4.9 per 100 patient-years (2.8–7.1) in the control group (RR 0.62; 95% CrI 0.35–1.25). • Primary safety events were more frequent in the intervention group (7.4 per 100 patient-years, 95% CrI 5.5–9.7 vs. 4.4 per 100 patient-years, 95% CrI 2.5–6.7; RR 1.69, 1.01–3.19)
PREVAIL	Noninferiority WATCHMAN vs warfarin	Device ($n = 269$), control ($n = 138$)	• First coprimary efficacy endpoint (stroke, SE, and CV/unexplained death) event rate at 18 months was 0.064 in the device group versus 0.063 in the control group (RR 1.07; 95% CrI 0.57–1.89])[a] • Second coprimary efficacy endpoint (stroke or SE >7 days after randomization) was 0.025 versus 0.020 (risk difference 0.005; 95% CrI 0.019–0.027) • Adverse events lower than PROTECT AF (4.2% vs. 8.7%; $p = 0.004$)
PRAGUE-17	Noninferiority LAAC device versus DOAC	Device ($n = 201$), control ($n =201$)	• The annualized rate of the primary composite outcome (stroke, TIA, SE, CV death, major or nonmajor clinically relevant bleeding, or procedure/device-related complications) was 10.99% with LAAO and 13.42% with DOACs ($p = 0.44$ and $p = 0.004$ for non-inferiority) • Major LAAO-related complications occurred in 9 (4.5%) patients

(CrI: credible interval; DOAC: direct oral anticoagulant; LAAO: left atrial appendage occlusion; RR: rate ratio; SE: systemic embolization; sHR: subdistribution hazard ratio; TIA: transient ischemic attack)

TABLE 2: Latest trials in LAA closure.

Study name	Device/Intervention	Population	Key outcomes	Published date	Status
OPTION trial	WATCHMAN device, WATCHMAN FLX	Patients undergoing AF ablation	Comparable safety and efficacy; FLX device shows reduced device-related complications	August 2024	Ongoing
Amulet IDE trial	Amplatzer Amulet versus WATCHMAN	Patients at risk of stroke	Amulet showed higher early complications but better appendage sealing; similar long-term stroke prevention	July 2024	Completed
LAAO registry	Various LAAO devices	Multicenter, varied risk AF patients	Preprocedural imaging reduces device-related complications, improving procedural safety	March 2024	Ongoing

TABLE 3: 2019 AHA/ACC/HRS focused update of the 2014 AHA/ACC/HRS guideline for the management of patients with atrial fibrillation.

Recommendations	Class of recommendation	Level of evidence
After surgical occlusion or exclusion of the LAA, it is recommended to continue anticoagulation in at-risk patients with AF for stroke prevention	I	B
LAA occlusion may be considered for stroke prevention in patients with AF and contraindications for long-term anticoagulant treatment (e.g., those with a previous life-threatening bleed without reversible cause)	IIb	B
Surgical occlusion or exclusion of the LAA may be considered for stroke prevention in patients with AF undergoing cardiac surgery	IIb	B
Surgical occlusion or exclusion of the LAA may be considered for stroke prevention in patients undergoing thoracoscopic AF surgery	IIb	B

TABLE 4: 2020 European Society of Cardiology Guidelines for the management of atrial fibrillation.

Recommendations	Class of recommendation	Level of evidence
LAA occlusion may be considered for stroke prevention in patients with AF and contraindications for long-term anticoagulant treatment (e.g., intracranial bleeding without a reversible cause).	IIb	B
Surgical occlusion or exclusion of the LAA may be considered for stroke prevention in patients with AF undergoing cardiac surgery.	IIb	C

Physician–patient discussion is crucial for shared decision-making **(Tables 3 and 4)**.

According to the AHA and ESC guidelines, LAAC is recommended for stroke prevention in patients with a high risk of thromboembolism (CHA_2DS_2-VASc score ≥ 2) who also have contraindications to OACs due to a history of significant bleeding, such as intracranial or life-threatening hemorrhage. Additionally, LAAC is suggested for patients with a high bleeding risk associated with long-term OAC use, including: (i) those with a HAS-BLED score ≥3, (ii) those who require extended triple therapy (anticoagulant and dual antiplatelet therapy) following stent placement for severe coronary artery disease, and (iii) patients with creatinine clearance of 15–30 mL/min.

IMAGING

Preprocedural Imaging

For preprocedural planning, TEE or cardiac CT is essential. During the preprocedural evaluation with TEE, it is important to record and analyze the measurements, look for presence of LAA thrombus, check technical considerations like a lipomatous or aneurysmal septum, and LAA size/morphology to anticipate possible technical difficulties. LAA is imaged in two-dimensional (2D) images at 0, 45, 90, and 135 degrees, when there is maximal LAA filling (LV systole) to measure the landing zone width. Depth is measured between 2 points—midpoint of the landing zone and LAA body. Alternatively, three-dimensional (3D) TEE imaging can be done with double-oblique multiplanar views and it yields more accurate measurements for sizing.

Role of Cardiac CT in terms of pre-procedural planning is superlative to TEE with regards to spatial resolution. Ideally, 0.5 to 1.5 mm slices are required to look for LAA thrombus. Landing zone in LAA is measured using 3D multiplanar reformatted LAA images at the level of the LCX artery in the mid-to-late systolic phase.

There can be a discrepancy in device sizing between cardiac CT measurements and TEE. CT measurements are usually 2–3 mm larger than TEE measurements, as patients are usually fasting for TEE. In patients with challenging anatomies, it is beneficial to use software simulations to see how various device sizes would fit in individual patient anatomy.

Intraprocedural Imaging

Intraprocedural imaging is necessary to check for LAA thrombus, and pericardial effusion; it is also necessary for transseptal puncture guidance, guidance for device implantation, device stability, peridevice leaks (PDL), and the residual iatrogenic ASD assessment.

Transesophageal echocardiography is preferred over ICE as ICE requires the probe to be in LA, which may complicate the procedure. Placement of ICE probe in RA does not give adequate imaging resolution.

STEPS IN LEFT ATRIAL APPENDAGE CLOSURE

The steps in LAA closure are as follows:

1. Transcatheter LAAO is generally done under TEE and fluoroscopic guidance. Antibiotic prophylaxis is given prior to procedure.
2. *Venous access:* For access, using ultrasound guidance and micropuncture technique are beneficial and recommended. Access is via a femoral vein. Right femoral vein is preferred over left in case of trans-septal puncture, as sheath manipulation will be difficult through left femoral vein. Closure of the access site can be done with figure-of-eight sutures or by manual compression. Both are equally effective and can be chosen as per operator preference. If hemostasis is not achieved, protamine administration can be considered.
3. *Anticoagulation:* The choice of anticoagulant during procedure is unfractionated heparin (UFH). The activated clotting time (ACT) needs to be maintained in the range of 250–300 seconds.
4. *Trans-septal puncture:* For TSP, the ideal site is usually inferior and posterior, so that the access sheath will be coaxial to LAA. The exact site can be adjusted based on the LAA's position as seen on TEE or preprocedural cardiac CT. Typically, the LAA is anteriorly directed, so a posterior puncture is the norm. For an LAA directed superiorly, an inferior puncture is chosen, and for a mid-to-inferior LAA, a slightly less inferior puncture is made.[18]
5. Delivery sheath selection is based on the device selected.
6. *Advancing the delivery sheath into the LAA*:
   - *Introduction of delivery sheath*:
     - The delivery sheath can be introduced into the LA using either of the following methods:
       - Anchoring a stiff support wire in pulmonary vein
       - Usage of a "pigtail" type wire positioned in the LA.
   - *Troubleshooting*:
     - If there is difficulty advancing the sheath into the LA:
       - Predilation of atrial septum with 14F: Inoue dilator
       - Atrial septostomy: With a balloon of 5 mm or larger
   - *Preparation in LA*: After advancing the sheath into the LA, carefully deair and flush it with saline to ensure it is free of air.
   - *Advancement into the LAA*: Over a 5F or 6F straight pigtail catheter that has been positioned deep in the LAA, advance the delivery sheath into the LAA.
7. *LA pressure measurement:* Measurement the left atrial pressure is done to confirm delivery sheath placement and to ensure adequate pressure for preventing device undersizing. A mean LA pressure of 12 mm Hg helps in precise LAA measurements and to select the proper device sizing.
8. *Deployment of LAAC device:* The deployment procedure varies depending on the specific LAAC device used. Care should be taken to ensure that proper device sizing, anchoring, and positioning within the LAA are achieved. Additionally, check for the absence of significant peridevice leaks (PDLs).

DEVICES AVAILABLE IN INDIA

Details of Devices available in India are given in **Table 5**.

COMPLICATIONS

The common immediate complications include pericardial effusion and device embolization and late complications include device-related thrombus and PDL **(Table 6)**.

Managing Complications

Pericardial effusion and tamponade: It can be caused by LAA perforation or can be TSP-related and can result in tamponade, necessitating emergency pericardiocentesis, then surgical repair. Factors that contribute to the decrease in occurrence of this complication include experienced

TABLE 5: Common LAA closure devices and their characteristics.

Device name	Watchman	Amulet	LAmbre
Produced by	Boston Scientific	Abbott	Lifetech
Approved	FDA, CE	FDA, CE	CE
Design	Self-expanding nitinol frame covered by a 160 µm polyester membrane on its atrial-facing side; 18 fixation barbs in FLX versus 10 in the original WATCHMAN around the mid-perimeter secure the occluder to the wall of the left atrial appendage, unlike earlier generations, WATCHMAN FLX device has enfolded distal tines, dual-row anchors, more numerous struts, and reduced exposed metal	Pre-loaded, double-seal structure; distal lobe which sits inside the appendage, and proximal disk that closes the ostium are connected by a waist. It has hooks that are attached to the distal body enabling the occluder to engage the wall of the left atrial appendage	Self-expanding dual membrane design (hook-embedded umbrella and fabric cover) connected by a short, central waist
Shapes and sizes	The device is available in diameters ranging from 20–35 mm	The proximal disks are 4 mm larger for lobe sizes 16–22 mm and 6 mm larger for lobe sizes 24–30 mm; Amulet also available in 31 and 34 mm sizes	Two designs. The standard design is for a cover that is 4–6 mm larger than the umbrella, and the special design is for a cover that is 12–14 mm larger. These designs are intended to accommodate LAA morphologies that are single-lobed or multilobed 16–36 mm for the umbrella and 22–40 mm for the cover
Sheath	12 F	12–14 F	8–10 F
Technique	Unsheathing the device after placement inside the LAA	Unsheathing the device after placement inside the LAA	• The delivery sheath is placed at the ostial LAA • To deploy the umbrella, the delivery cable is pushed forward • Unsheathing releases the cover over the LAA ostium

TABLE 6: Periprocedural and postprocedural complications.

Periprocedural complications	**Postprocedural complications**
Death (<0.2%)	Late pericardial effusion and tamponade (~1%)
Stroke (<0.2%): • *Ischemic*: Air or thromboembolism • Hemorrhagic	Peridevice leak: • *>5 mm on TEE*: l–3% • *>3 mm on TEE*: 10–25%
Systemic embolism (rare)	Device-related thrombus (3–5%)
Pericardial tamponade (~1%)	Late device migration/embolization (infrequent)
Device embolization (~0.2%)	Device erosion (rare)
Vascular complications: Retroperitoneal bleed, arteriovenous fistula, and pseudoaneurysm	Iatrogenic atrial septal defects (rare to require intervention)
Other: • Major bleeding, renal failure, respiratory failure, sepsis, and MI • Endotracheal/esophageal damage and interfering surrounding structures • Device/contrast allergy and pericarditis	

operator, meticulous assessment planning before the procedure, image-guided TEE or ICE during the procedure, and usage of less stiff guidewires. More importantly, consistently using a pigtail catheter for LAA entry, prevents damage to the thin-walled LAA, as the larger sheaths can be advanced safely. Timely recognition of effusion and tamponade and subsequent pericardiocentesis is needed.

Periprocedural stroke: Careful preprocedure screening is critical to exclude LAA thrombus, and proper flushing is essential to prevent air embolism. During the procedure, intravenous UFH is used to maintain ACT within the range of 250–300 seconds, minimizing the risk of thrombus formation. If a thrombus is detected, give additional doses of heparin. A timely decision regarding procedure discontinuation should be made, after confirming if the thrombus has resolved. Resolution of thrombus needs to be checked. After which, a timely decision regarding procedure discontinuation should be made.

Device embolization: Although rare, proper device sizing is crucial to prevent embolization. If a device becomes dislodged, it can end up in aorta, LA, or LV. The retrieval method largely depends on the location of the embolized device. Surgery is preferred when the device has migrated to the left ventricle, especially if it gets tangled in the mitral valve apparatus or causes hemodynamic compromise. Percutaneous retrieval is possible for embolization into the descending aorta or LA, necessitating the operators to be skilled in the usage of large sheaths and snares.

Device-related thrombosis (DRT): DRT occurs in approximately 3–5% of LAAC procedures (SCAI)[1] and is more frequent in patients with a history of CVA, large LAA size, permanent atrial fibrillation (AF), or prior history of thrombus in LA. If DRT is detected in postprocedure imaging, OAC should be continued. Follow-up imaging every 45–90 days is recommended to monitor for resolution, with the goal of eventually discontinuing anticoagulation.

PDLs: These are observed in 11–57% of percutaneous LAAO procedures, depending on the device and imaging method used. Analysis from the PROTECT AF trial indicated no significant difference in adverse event rates between leaks smaller than 1 mm, leaks between 1 and 3 mm, and those larger than 3 mm; however, larger leaks were not assessed with the WATCHMAN device. The management of PDLs remains unclear due to limited data and the lack of established guidelines. PDLs <5 mm are generally considered significant, and in these cases, the continuation of OAC is currently recommended.

FOLLOW-UP IMAGING

Usually, follow-up imaging after LAAC device implantation is recommended as follows:

- Immediate postprocedure imaging with TEE or ICE to detect pericardial effusion should be done.
- Before discharge from hospital, check for device embolization and appearance of pericardial effusion.
- At 45 days follow-up postprocedure, TEE or TTE is done to check device sealing and PDLs.

ANTITHROMBOTIC THERAPY AFTER LEFT ATRIAL APPENDAGE CLOSURE

If anticoagulation is contraindicated, DAPT is recommended for 6 months followed by single antiplatelet therapy. If anticoagulation is not contraindicated, a 6-week of anticoagulation will help prevent device-related stroke in the initial period till it gets re-endothelized.

CONCLUSION

Atrial fibrillation is the most common arrhythmia encountered in elderly populations globally. Assessment of ischemic stroke risk using CHA_2DS_2-VASc score and bleeding risk using HAS-BLED is the paramount step in managing such patients. The LAA is the most common site for thrombus formation in patients with AF. LAA is the most common site of thrombus origination. LAAO is still uncommonly used in India predominantly due to cost constraints and absence of superiority of such a therapy over medical therapy in all-comers with AF. A strong data is still required to convince cardiologists to use it in all-comers with AF. Till then, it is reasonable to consider the same in patients of AF with high bleeding risk or patients with contraindications to anticoagulations.

ONLINE REFERENCES

Please scan the QR code provided at the end of the table of contents for References of this chapter.

SECTION 16

Mechanical Circulatory Support

Section Outline

CHAPTER

186

Recent Advances in Cardiogenic Shock

Dev B Pahlajani, Kayan Siodia

ABSTRACT

Despite increasing use of coronary artery revascularization, acute myocardial infarction (AMI) continues to be the most common cause of cardiogenic shock (CS) and accounts for more than two-thirds of the cases of CS. Invariably, the clinical condition is the result of left or right heart or biventricular failure. Recently, it has also been understood that irreversible extensive myocardial damage could be a systemic response due to complement activation and release of inflammatory cytokines. Role of expression of inducible nitrite oxide synthase and inappropriate vasodilation that plays an important role in the clinical situation of CS is being widely recognized. The incidence of CS might have fallen due to prompt treatment of AMI with primary angioplasty in acute myocardial infarction or fibrinolysis with rapid transportation to the PAMI-capable centers. Yet all over the world, excluding the Western world, the treatment eludes large number of victims of AMI. Initial treatment is to stabilize the patient's hemodynamics and maintain oxygenation with inotropes and well-monitored fluid administration to protect kidneys and vital organs. Whenever feasible and indicated, percutaneous coronary intervention (PCI) is the gold standard and life-saving treatment and should be performed without delay. In those who do not improve on this conventional treatment currently, there are several mechanical circulatory systems (MCS) available. Until about few years back, intra-aortic balloon pump (IABP) was considered the main tool for management of CS. Recent studies have failed to show its impact on morbidity and mortality and is no more indicated except maybe while performing PCI. Various other support systems like Impella with flow rates of 2.5–5.5 liters, extracorporeal membrane oxygenator (ECMO), and TandemHeart have been used at some of the well-equipped cardiovascular centers. However, the impact on the mortality and morbidity and long-term benefit data is yet to be established.

Keywords: Cardiogenic shock, Impella, IABP, acute MI

INTRODUCTION

Cardiogenic shock (CS) is a state of circulatory failure resulting in low cardiac output, hypotension, and reduced organ and tissue perfusion leading to fluid and biochemical derangement. While the most common cause of CS is acute myocardial infarction (AMI), which accounts for 70–80% of cases, it could also result from chronic heart disease due to left, right, or biventricular failure. It is reported that 5–8% cases of AMI develop CS. Despite advances in treatment, mainly early revascularization, the overall mortality in patients presenting with AMI complicated by CS remains very high (≅50%), especially in the first 48 hours.[1] *Though inhospital mortality has decreased from 45 to 34%, the mortality in patients 75 years or above is 55%* The clinical situation arises due to irreversible extensive myocardial or vital-organ damage. However, systemic inflammatory response, complement activation, release of inflammatory cytokines, expression of inducible nitric oxide (NO) synthase (iNOS), and inappropriate vasodilation may play an important role not only in the genesis of shock but also in outcome after shock.

Thus, CS is a state of critical end-organ hypoperfusion primarily due to cardiac dysfunction, as described by the European Society of Cardiology (ESC) and the American Heart Association (AHA).[1,2]

INCIDENCE AND MORTALITY

Cardiogenic shock complicates approximately 5–10% of acute coronary syndromes (ACS) and is considered a powerful determinant of mortality. The SHOCK trial registry reported that the most common cause of CS during AMI is left ventricular (LV) failure (78.5%), followed by severe mitral regurgitation (6.9%), ventricular septal rupture (3.9%), right ventricular failure (2.8%), and cardiac tamponade (1.4%)

Even with widespread availability of PAMI and SHOCK centers in the developed world, impact on mortality and morbidity has been insignificant. In the Indian context, the prognosis would be grave due to paucity of such centers, trained medical and paramedical staff, financial constraints, nonavailability or delay in time to revascularization in large majority of patients with AMI.

SCORING SYSTEM

There are various scoring systems that help to categorize patients with CS to ascertain prognosis and guide patient therapy.

Sleeper score[3] obtained from the SHOCK trial cohort provides one of two scores that are different on the basis of the availability of invasive data from pulmonary artery catheterization **(Table 1)**. The score uses eight variables for patients when invasive monitoring is not available [age, shock on admission, clinical evidence of end-organ-hypoperfusion, anoxic brain damage, systolic blood pressure, prior coronary artery bypass grafting (CABG), noninferior myocardial infarction (MI), and creatinine ≥1.9 mg/dL] or five variables for patients when right heart catheterization data are accessible [age, end-organ hypoperfusion, anoxic brain damage, LV ejection fraction (EF) <28%, and stroke work].

The CardShock includes only clinical and laboratory data: Age, confusion at presentation, previous cardiac revascularization, ACS etiology, LV systolic dysfunction, blood lactate, and estimated glomerular filtration rate (eGFR) **(Table 2)**.

The most recent IABP-SHOCK II risk score[4,5] demonstrated strong correlation with short-term prognosis and includes six variables proven to be independent predictors of 30-day mortality: Age, prior stroke, thrombolysis in myocardial infarction (TIMI) flow grade <after PCI, and admission levels of glucose, creatinine, and arterial blood lactate **(Table 3)**.

The different risk profiles showed to be associated with a stepwise increase in short-term mortality rates: Low, i.e., 20–30%, intermediate, i.e., 40–60%, and high, i.e., 70–90%, respectively.

BOS, MA2 score[6] considers blood urea >25 mg/dL, minimum oxygen saturation 88%, minimum systolic blood

TABLE 1: Sleeper score.

Sleeper (2010)	
Scoring system without invasive hemodynamics	**Scoring system for invasive hemodynamic cohort**
Age	Age
Shock on admission	—
End-organ hypoperfusion	End-organ hypoperfusion
Anoxic brain damage	Anoxic brain damage
—	Stroke work
Systolic blood pressure	—
Prior CABG	—
Non-inferior MI	—
Creatinine ≥1.9 mg/dL	—
—	LVEF <28%

(LVEF; left ventricle ejection fraction; MI: myocardial infarction)

TABLE 2: CardShock (2015).

Variable	Points
Age >75 years	1
Confusion at presentation	1
Previous MI or CABG	1
ACS etiology	1
LVEF <40%	1
Blood lactate	0 point if <2 mmol/L 1 point if 2–4 mmol/L 2 points if >4 mmol/L
$eGFR_{CKD-EPI}$	0 point if >60 mL/min/1.73 m^2 1 point if 30–60 min/mL/1.73 m^2 2 points if <30 mL/min/1.73 m^2
Maximum	9

(ACS: acute coronary syndrome; CABG: coronary artery bypass grafting; CKD-EPI: chronic kidney disease Epidemiology Collaboration Formula; eGFR: estimated glomerular filtration rate; LVEF: left ventricle ejection fraction; MI, myocardial infarction)

Source: Harjola VP, Lassus J, Sionis A, et al. Clinical picture and risk prediction of short-term mortality in cardiogenic shock. Eur J Heart Fail. 2015;17(5):501-9. Erratum in: Eur J Heart Fail. 2015;17(9):984.

TABLE 3: IABP-SHOCK II (2017) risk score.

Variable	Points
Age >73 years	1
History of stroke	2
Glucose at admission >10.6 mmol/L (191 mg/dL)	1
Creatinine at admission >132.6 μmol/L (1.5 mg/dL)	1
Arterial lactate >5 mmol/L	2
TIMI flow grade <3 after PCI	2
Maximum	9
Risk category	
Category	**Points**
Low	0–2
Intermediate	3–4
High	5–9

(PCI: percutaneous coronary intervention; TIMI: thrombolysis in myocardial intervention)

Source: Pöss J, Köster J, Fuernau G, et al. Risk stratification for patients in cardiogenic shock after acute myocardial infarction. J Am Coll Cardiol. 2020; 69(15):1913-20.

pressure 80 mm Hg, mechanical ventilation, and maximum anion gap >14 mm/L, and age >60 years during first 24 hours of ICU stay. Those with score of 6 had highest mortality of around 70%, whereas it was lowest in patients with score of 0.

PATHOPHYSIOLOGY

The complex pathophysiology of CS after AMI has been elucidated over the past two decades. A severe depression of myocardial contractility is responsible for LV systolic dysfunction leading to reduced cardiac output, hypotension, and resulting coronary hypoperfusion. Impaired right ventricular (RV) systolic function and deranged vasculature functionality may also contribute toward establishment and/or worsening of CS.

The observed LVEF in the SHOCK trial was ≃30%, the value commonly noted in many of the trials evaluating heart failure and post-MI therapies. Not only systolic impairment but also diastolic dysfunction and associated restrictive filling patterns are common findings in patients presenting with CS. Similarly, isolated RV dysfunction can also result in CS, albeit in a very small number of patients (~5%), whereas in the majority of patients, it coexists with LV dysfunction.

Thus, vicious cycles are sequentially triggered: (1) Coronary ischemia further decreases myocardial contractility, and (2) the compensatory pathway to systemic hypoperfusion includes vasoconstriction and augmented serum arterial lactate levels, LV afterload, and cardiac oxygen consumption, contributing to myocardial dysfunction **(Flowchart 1)**.

The initial compensatory vasoconstriction is partly counteracted by the pathological vasodilation induced by capillary leakage and microcirculation impairment that is provoked by systemic inflammation. The composite of systolic and diastolic dysfunction increases the LV end-diastolic pressure and predisposes to pulmonary edema.

A NEWER PARADIGM OF INFLAMMATION[7]

Patients with large MIs often have elevated body temperature, white blood cell count, complement, interleukins, C-reactive protein, and other inflammatory markers. NO, synthesized at low levels by endothelial and myocardial cell endothelial nitric oxide synthase (eNOS), is a cardioprotective molecule. In contrast, many cell types express iNOS at pathological levels after trauma or exposure to inflammatory mediators (i.e., bacterial lipopolysaccharide, tumor necrosis factor-alpha, and interleukin-1). Such expression may lead to toxic levels of NO and the cytotoxic NO-derived species, peroxynitrite, formed by reaction with superoxide. In experimental models, high iNOS and NO levels are seen after MI and subsequent reperfusion. Release of cytokines by the heart after MI has been documented in patients. These levels markedly increase after primary PCI in AMI patients but not in control patients. This suggests that in patients post-MI, activation of inflammatory cytokines leads to high levels of iNOS, NO, and peroxynitrite, all of which have multiple deleterious effects.

Effects of high levels of no and no-derived species:
- Direct inhibition of myocardial contractility
- Suppression of mitochondrial respiration in nonischemic myocardium
- Effects on glucose metabolism
- Proinflammatory effects

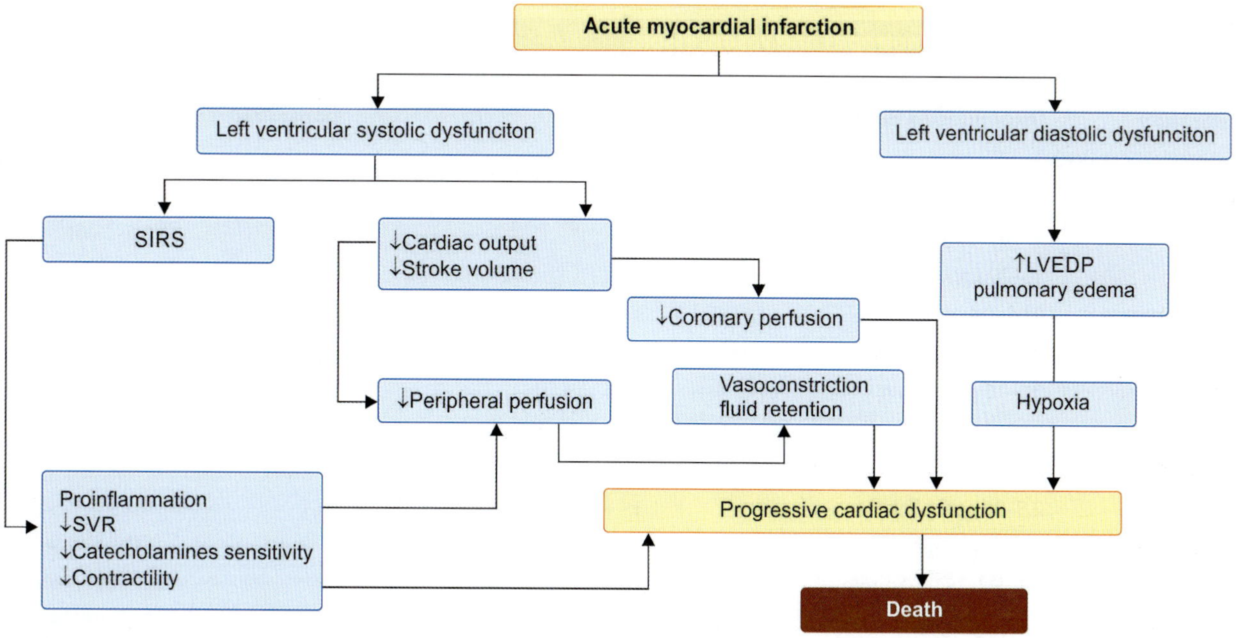

FLOWCHART 1: Acute myocardial infarction.

- Reduced catecholamines responsivity
- Induction of systemic vasodilation

POTENTIAL PRESENTATIONS

The potential presentations are given in **Figure 1**.

General Approach

Initial therapeutic intervention in patients with AMI complicated by CS (AMI-CS) is to achieve coronary reperfusion, at the earliest possible. Hemodynamic instability should be managed by ensuring adequate oxygenation and ventilation, preserving euvolemic state, and restoring adequate cardiac output and tissue perfusion. Such supportive therapy will include:

- Prevention of hypoxia
- Supplemental oxygen for saturation <94%
- However, avoid giving supplemental oxygen to nonhypoxic patients as oxygen can increase coronary resistance.

Inotropes and Vasopressors

Doses and effects of inotropes and vasopressors are given in **Table 4**.

- Improve cardiac output and tissue perfusion
- Increase myocardial contractility and systemic vascular resistance
- Amongst the commonly used vasopressors, norepinephrine alone or in combination with dobutamine has favorable hemodynamic effects and are preferred form of pharmacological treatment.
- Epinephrine use could be associated with tachycardia and lactic acidosis and has prothrombotic effects.
- Vasopressin is the second line inotrope to be used.
- Levosimendan, a calcium-sensitizing agent, increases contractility, causes vasodilation, and decreases afterload.

However, long-term outcomes have failed to show favorable outcomes.

Peripheral circulation		Volume status: Wet	Volume status: Dry
	Cold	Classic cardiogenic shock (↓CI; ↑SVRI; ↑PCWP)	Euvolemic cardiogenic shock (↓CI; ↑SVRI; ↔PCWP)
	Warm	Vasodilatory cardiogenic shock or Mixed shock (↓CI; ↑/↔SVRI; ↑PCWP)	Vasodilatory shock (Not cardiogenic shock) (↑CI; ↓SVRI; ↓PCWP)

FIG. 1: Potential hemodynamics during presentation of cardiogenic shock.

TABLE 4: Doses and effects of inotropes and vasopressors.

Medication	Usual infusion dose	Receptor binding: α1	β1	β2	Dopamine	Hemodynamic effects
Vasopressor/inotropes						
Dopamine	0.5–2 μg/kg/min	–	+	–	+++	↑CO
	5–10 μg/kg/min	+	+++	+	++	↑↑CO, ↑SVR
	10–20 μg/kg/min	+++	++	–	++	↑↑SVR, ↑CO
Norepinephrine	0.05–0.4 μg/kg/min	++++	++	+	–	↑↑SVR, ↑CO
Epinephrine	0.01–0.5 μg/kg/min	++++	++++	+++	–	↑↑CO, ↑↑SVR
Phenylephrine	0.1–10 μg/kg/min	+++	–	–	–	↑↑SVR
Vasopressin	0.02–0.04 U/min	Stimulates V_1 receptors in vascular smooth muscle				↑↑SVR, ↔PVR
Inodilators						
Dobutamine	2.5–20 μg/kg/min	+	++++	++	–	↑↑CO, ↓SVR, ↓PVR
Isoproterenol	2.0–20 μg/min	–	++++	+++	–	↑↑CO, ↓SVR, ↓PVR
Milrinone	0.125–0.75 μg/kg/min	PD-3 inhibitor				↑CO, ↓SVR, ↓PVR
Enoximone	2–10 μg/kg/min	PD-3 inhibitor				↑CO, ↓SVR, ↓PVR
Levosimendan	0.05–0.2 μg/kg/min	Myofilament Ca^{2+} sensitizer and PD-3 inhibitor				↑CO, ↓SVR, ↓PVR

REPERFUSION THERAPY

Reperfusion should be seriously considered for all patients with CS if seen within window period **(Flowchart 2 and Fig. 2)**.[4,5]

- For patients within 12 hours of symptom onset and with persistent ST-segment elevation or new or presumed new left bundle branch block, early mechanical or pharmacological reperfusion should be performed as early as possible.
- The reperfusion therapy should be considered if there is clinical and/or electrocardiographic evidence of ongoing ischemia between 12 and 24 hours. Primary PCI is preferred in these patients.
- Routine PCI of a totally occluded artery >24 hours after symptom onset in stable patients without signs and symptoms of ischemia is not recommended.
- Primary PCI should be performed in patients with STEMI and ischemic symptoms of <12 hours duration who have contraindications to thrombolytic therapy, irrespective of the time delay from first medical contact (FMC).
- Primary PCI should be performed in patients with STEMI presenting with cardiogenic shock and hemodynamic and electrical instability irrespective of time delay from symptom onset.
- Thrombolytic therapy is recommended within 12 hours of symptom onset in patients without contraindications if primary PCI cannot be performed by an experienced team within 120 minutes of FMC (preferably within 90 minutes).
- Fibrin-specific agents have some advantages over streptokinase but are more expensive and not widely available. Whereas streptokinase is cheap, easily available, and is the most frequently used thrombolytic agent in India. However, the final decision of choice of thrombolytic agent is at the discretion of the treating physician and the patient.

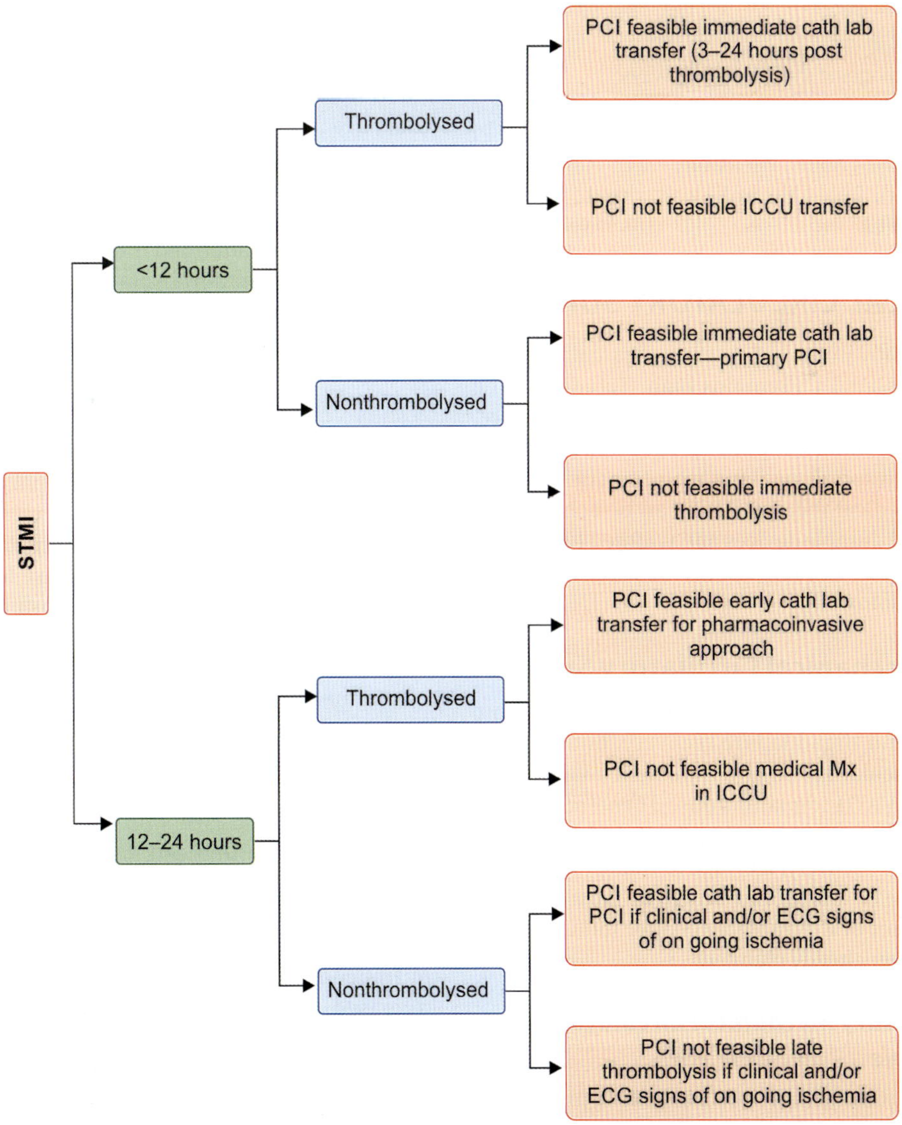

FLOWCHART 2: ST-elevation myocardial infarction (STEMI) and timeline.

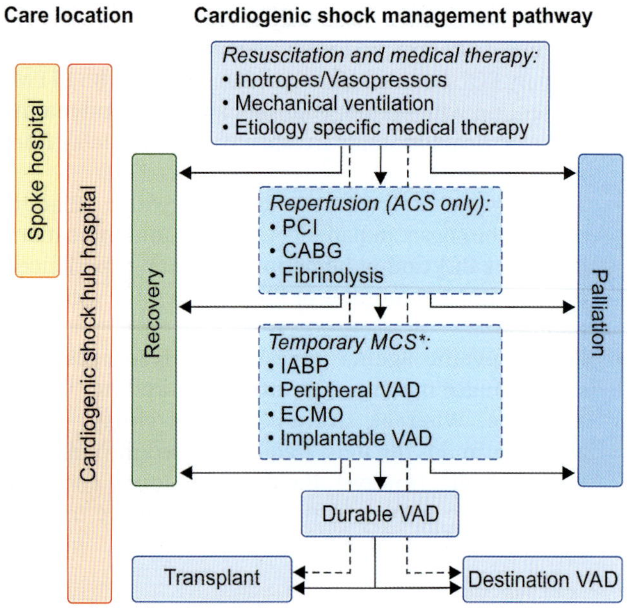

*Mechanical circulatory support.

FIG. 2: Potential cardiogenic shock-care pathways.

- All thrombolysed patients should be considered for PI therapy within 3–24 hours, if feasible.
- All patients with failed thrombolysis should undergo prompt rescue PCI.

MECHANICAL CIRCULATORY SUPPORT

Despite being recently improved by early revascularization, mortality of AMI-related CS remains high. To address the organs hypoperfusion and consequent multiorgan failure, the mechanical circulatory support (MCS) appears to be a hopeful approach for all patients who remain unstable despite optimal medical therapy. MCS can be achieved by both temporary and durable devices and is aimed to improve cardiac output and/or reduce the use of catecholamines reducing their cardiotoxicity.[5]

Temporary Mechanical Circulatory Support

The temporary devices are intended for hemodynamic stabilization and end-organ failure recovery, but they can also facilitate revascularization and durable left ventricular assisted device (LVAD) implantations. These temporary supports are indeed identified as "bridge" solutions and might represent a bridge to recovery, a bridge to transplantation, a bridge to decisions, or a bridge to-bridge in those patients in whom the implant of a durable MCS after initial cardiac stabilization has been already planned.

Different Temporary Mechanical Circulatory Support Available

Figure 3 highlights the different MCS available at present.

An IABP: A balloon in the descending aorta is inflated with helium during diastole (counterpulsation) and actively deflated in systole. The inflated balloon helps direct blood flow to the coronary arteries during diastole (black arrows) and into the aorta during systole.

Despite decades of familiarity with the IABP, only in recent years has conclusive evidence established a lack of benefit in AMI-CS.

The IABP-SHOCK II trial randomized 600 patients with AMI-CS to early revascularization with or without IABP.[6,7]

No difference in primary endpoint of 30-day mortality was noted.

Hence, they are used only for the mechanical complications group.

Currently ESC has a class IIIB recommendation for routine use of an IABP for patients with CS after AMI, although it might still be considered in patients with severe MR and VSD.

Active LV temporary MCS: The TandemHeart is a percutaneous ventricular assist device (VAD) consisting of an extracorporeal centrifugal continuous flow pump that drains blood from the left atrium and pumps it into the femoral artery at a flow rate of up to 4 L/min **(Flowchart 3)**.

The TandemHeart increases cardiac output and mean arterial pressure and decreases cardiac filling pressure by venting the left atrium. This effect might be partly offset by the increased LV afterload due to retrograde blood flow up the aorta toward the aortic root. TandemHeart was associated with improvement in hemodynamic and metabolic outcomes compared with an IABP in two small randomized trials. However, survival was not improved[8] and more complications were seen in patients fitted with the TandemHeart.

Impella: Impella CP, 2.5, 5.0, and 5.5 are catheter-based, continuous axial flow pumps with propellers at the tips of the catheters, which are positioned in a retrograde way across the aortic valve **(Flowchart 3)**. Impella pumps actively deliver blood to the aorta and decrease left ventricular size, pressure, wall tension, and oxygen consumption. The Impella 2.5 and Impella CP are inserted percutaneously through the femoral artery and provide low- (1.5–2.5 L/min; Impella 2.5) to-intermediate (2–4 L/min; Impella CP) blood flows. The larger Impella 5.0 and 5.5 require surgical insertion through the axillary or subclavian artery and can provide blood flow rates up to 5.0 L/min. The use of this device could reduce the left ventricular scar size, improve cardiac function, reduce apoptosis, and improve cardioprotective signaling.

Two small randomized trials evaluated Impella devices against the IABP in CS caused by an acute MI. The ISAR-SHOCK trial[8] randomly assigned 25 patients with CS to either an Impella LP2.5 or an IABP. Cardiac index was slightly increased after 30 minutes of support with the Impella LP2.5. This finding was not seen at later time points. After 24 hours, no significant differences were seen in urine output, vasopressor requirement, or duration of mechanical

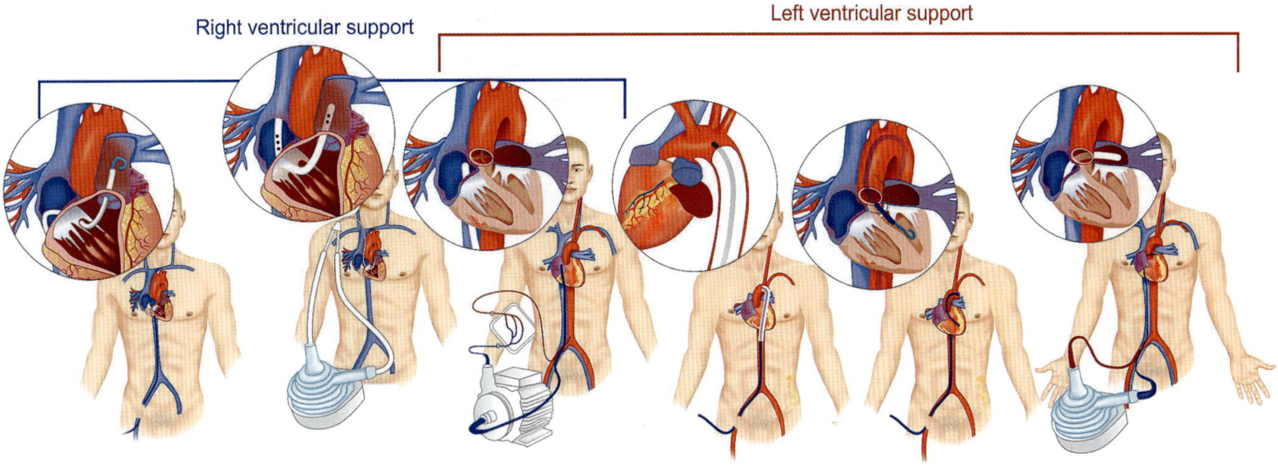

	Impella RP	TandemHeart RA-PA	VA-ECMO	IABP	Impella (2.5, CP, 5.0, 5.5)	TandemHeart LA-FA
Flow	Max 4.0 L/min	Max 4.1 L/min	Max 7.0 L/min	0.5 L/min	2.5–5.5 L/min	Max 4.0 L/min
Pump speed	33,000 rpm	Max 7,500 rpm	Max 5,000 rpm	NA	Max 51,000 rpm	Max 75,000 rpm
Mechanism	Axial flow continuous pump (RA-to-PA)	Centrifugal flow continuous pump (RA-to-PA)	Centrifugal flow continuous pump (RA-to-AO)	Balloon inflation-deflation (AO)	Axial flow continuous pump (LV-to-AO)	Centrifugal flow continuous pump (LV-to-AO)
Cannula size	22F venous	29F venous	14–19F arterial 17–21F venous	7–8F arterial	13–21F arterial	12–19F arterial 21F venous
Insertion/ placement	Femoral vein	Internal jugular vein	Femoral vein Femoral artery	Femoral artery Axillary artery	Femoral artery Axillary artery	Femoral artery Femoral vein
LV unloading	–	–	–	+	+ to +++	++
RV unloading	+	+	++	–	–	–
Cardiac power	–	–	↑↑	↑	↑↑	↑↑
Afterload	–	–	↑↑	↓	↓↓	↑
Coronary perfusion	–	–	–	↑	↑	–
Considerations	• Recover right: 73% survival-to-30 days in RVF post LVAD, AMI post cardiotomy • May 2019-FDA post-approval study: 33% survival-to-30 days	• IJ access may facilitate early ambulation	• BiV+ oxygenation support for CS following: – AMI, ADHF or cardiac arrest – Cardiotomy – Myocarditis – Allograft rejection	• Requires stable cardiac rhythm and native heart function • May consider in select cases of post-AMI mechanical complications	• June 2008–FDA 510(k) approval for HR-PCI • April 2016: Expanded indication for CS • Contraindicated with mechanical aortic valve, LV thrombus	• Requires transseptal access • Oxygenator may be added to the circuit

FIG. 3: Brief overview of available MCS.

ventilation. Overall 30-day mortality was similar in both groups.

In a recent study, Javaid et al.[9] compared outcomes in AMI-CS undergoing PCI. They compared outcomes in patients who received Impella without vasopressors, IABP without vasopressors, and vasopressors without MCS. Among 17,762 patients, Impella use when compared with IABP was associated with significantly higher bleeding (31% vs. 31.6%) without any mortality benefit (34% vs. 26%). Further, Impella use had worse outcomes when compared to CS with vasopressor and without MCS (33.9% vs. 22.7%).

In a meta-analysis of 6,484 patients with AMI CS that compared outcomes with Impella versus IABP, Jeet Upadhyay et al.[10] reported higher incidence of inhospital mortality as well major bleeding with impella compared to IABP.

While incidence of complications with Impella is higher in patients with AMI with CS, AJ Lansky et al.[11] reported favorable outcomes in patients who underwent nonemergent high-risk PCI with Impella as compared to IABP. In 2,156 patients who were treated with Impella or IABP, use of Impella was associated with improved survival and less MI and CS.

Thus, further studies are required to recommend widespread use of Impella, particularly considering the cost constraints.

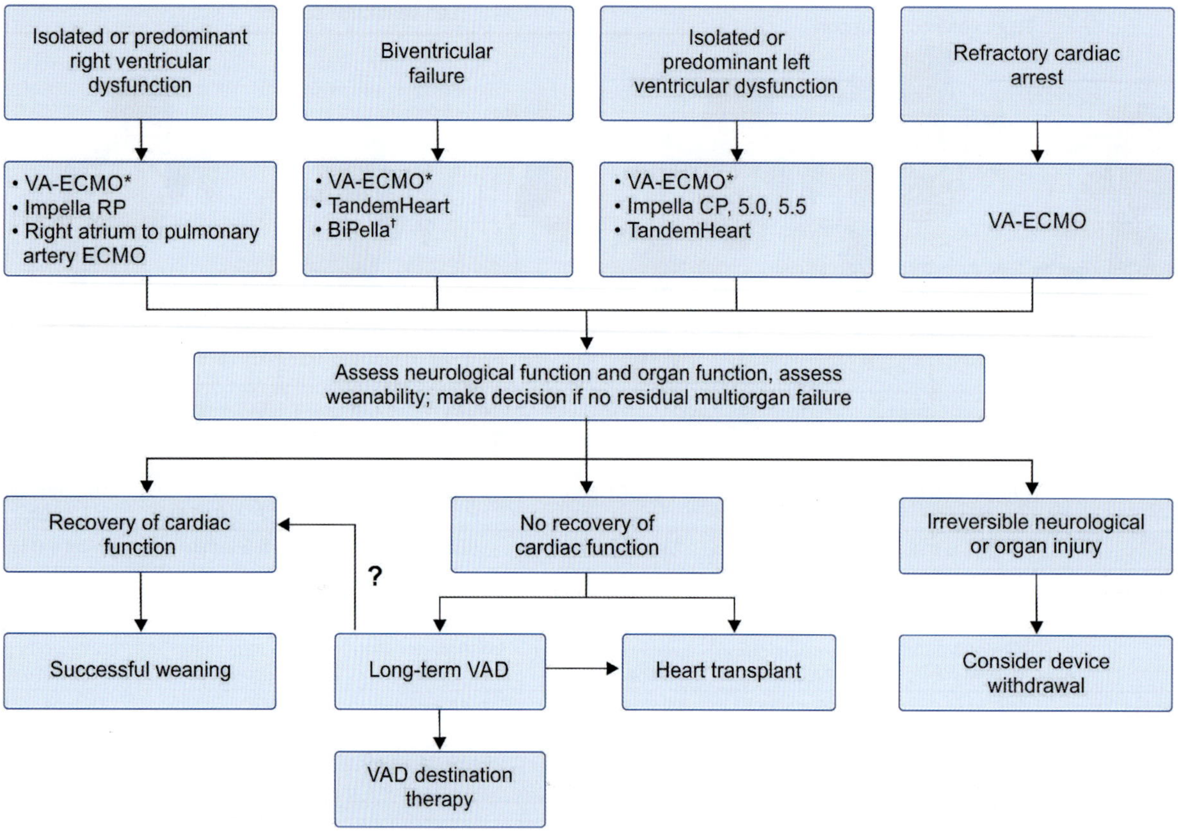

*VA-ECMO is the first line of MCS used.

+BiPella is still not a proven modality.

?Recovery of cardiac function post VAD has limited data.

FLOWCHART 3: Use of temporary MCS protocol.

EXTRACORPOREAL MEMBRANE OXYGENATION

Extracorporeal membrane oxygenation (ECMO) performs partial circulatory and respiratory life support. Multiple types of ECMO are available which include but are not limited to venoarterial (VA), AA, venovenous (VV), etc. Appropriately selected patients with isolated respiratory failure despite MV and no significant cardiac dysfunction are often treated with ECMO. Venoarterial ECMO, on the other hand, is used to support both the cardiovascular and respiratory systems and is frequently used in CS. Data from International Extracorporeal Life Support Organization (ELSO) that included 8,619 patients concluded that delayed initiation of ECMO beyond 24 hours from admission was associated with higher inhospital mortality emphasizing the importance of prompt ECMO initiation. In another study by Petr Ostadal et al.,[12] there was no difference in the 30-days incidence of resuscitate cardiac arrest, all-cause mortality, and desirous adverse events between immediate VA-ECMO and no-immediate VA-ECMO.[13,14]

Relative contraindications to ECMO include:

- Advanced age (>75 years)
- Life expectancy <1 year
- Severe peripheral vascular disease
- Advanced liver disease
- Contraindications to systemic anticoagulation
- Neurological injury

Potential complications of veno-arterial ECMO include:

- Distal limb ischemia
- Thromboembolism
- Stroke
- Bleeding
- Hemolysis
- Infection
- Aortic valve insufficiency

A common issue related to peripheral insertion is the resulting increase in LV afterload, which may lead to inadequate unloading of the LV. In these cases, combining VA ECMO with IABP, Impella support, atrial septostomy, or other venting maneuvers may help to achieve more complete LV unloading. Recently, in an observational study of 15,980 patients with CS, IIhwan et al.[15] reported that LVU with Impella, particularly 2.5/CP did not show improved survival at 40 days when compared with IABP. Impella was associated with increased adverse outcomes **(Fig. 4)**.

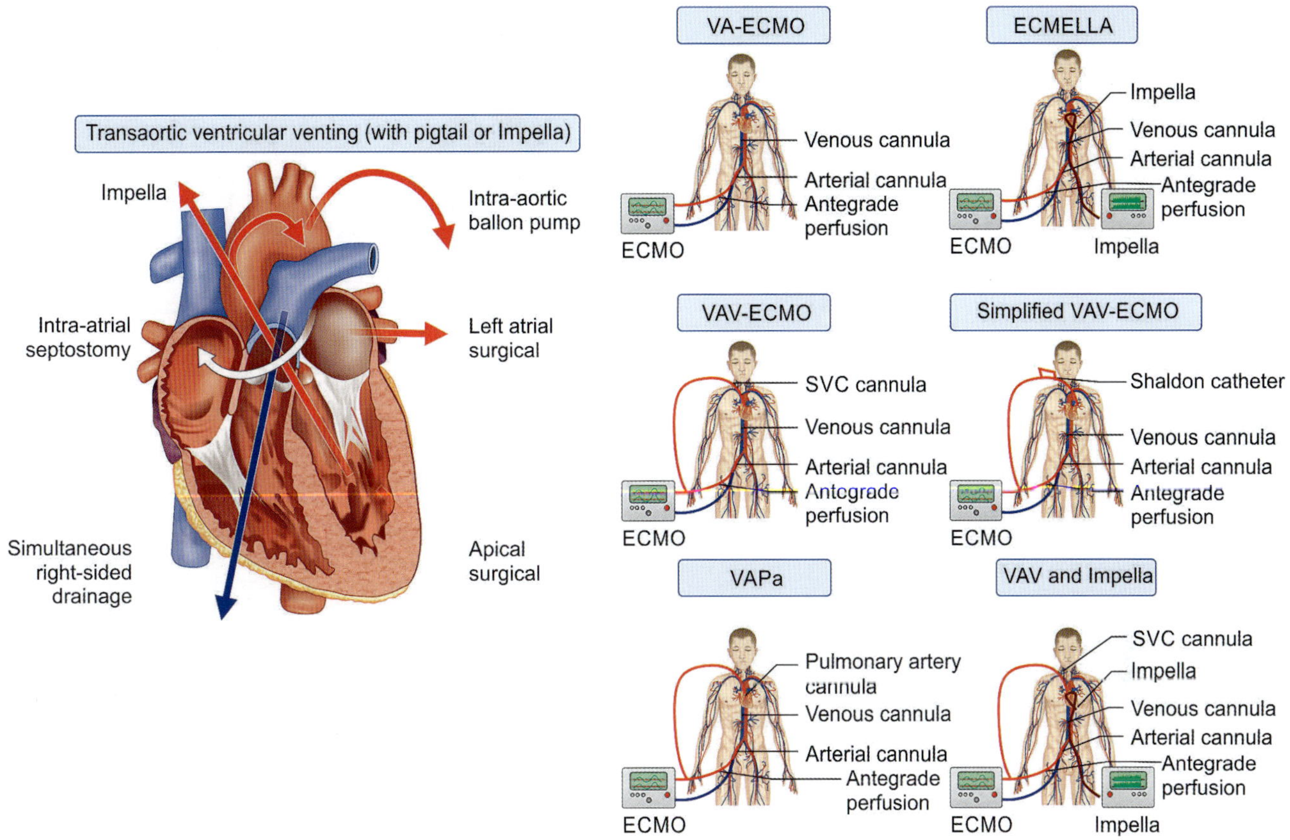

FIG. 4: Potential approaches to unload ventricle.

VENTRICULAR ASSIST DEVICES

Ventricular assist devices can be used either in univentricular or biventricular configuration. Central cannulation needs medial sternotomy. Central motor can give up to 10 L/min. Inflow cannula can be placed in the LA or the apex and outflow sutured into the aorta. Although approved only for short-term use, there are reports of it being used as a bridge to transplant.

Finally, as previously mentioned, percutaneous MCS devices can be useful tools for managing refractory shock. The newly introduced HeartMate percutaneous heart pump features a novel design with a collapsible elastomeric impeller and nitinol cannula, which gives this device a low profile but high flow rate. Once placed in a retrograde fashion across the aortic valve, the cannula can expand to 24F and support a continuous mean blood flow of >4 L/min. Although current data for this device are limited, ongoing trials should help to clarify its role in the treatment of CS **(Fig. 5)**.

CONCLUSION

Cardiogenic shock is a serious complication in patients with AMI. It could also result from severe left, right, or biventricular dysfunction and could be a terminal event of chronic heart disease. It is multifactorial with varied clinical and hemodynamically diverse presentations. Various scoring systems have been devised from several recent trials of CS, particularly those due to AMI. Current pathophysiological studies have also indicated contributory role of inflammation since various inflammatory markers have been identified. These could determine the ultimate prognosis and their significance is yet to recognized. While initial treatment is to stabilize the patient, maintain appropriate fluids and electrolyte balance, preserve vital organ function, and inotropes like sympathomimetic agents, timely restoration of blood flow by PCI or fibrinolytic is the sheet anchor of treatment. Various MCS have been advocated to improve outcomes. IABP has been found to be of no therapeutic value in CS. Impella and ECMO offer short-term inhospital benefits but long-term, i.e., 30-day data in most of the studies has been shown to have insignificant impact on outcomes. Moreover, bleeding and access-site complication rates are quite significant with currently available MCS. Further data on use of LVAD is awaited.

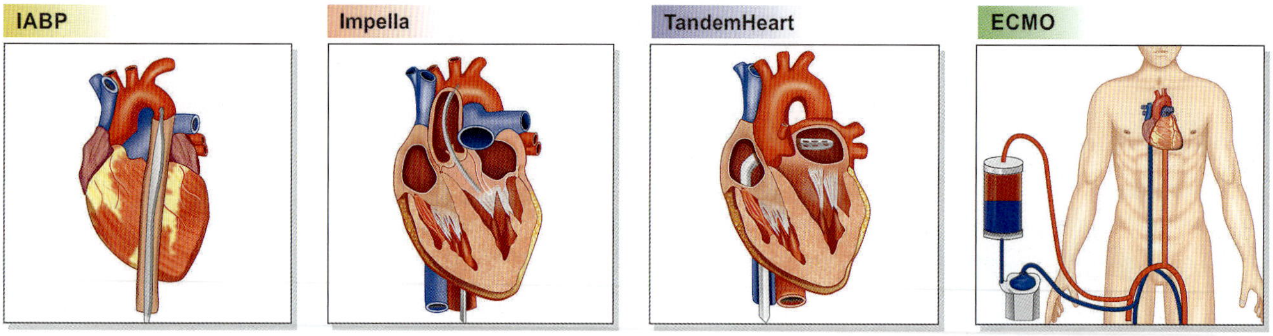

Device-specific complications

IABP:
- Spinal cord ischemia

Impella:
- Frequent hemolysis*
- Valvular lesions

TandemHeart:
- Air embolism
- Cardiac perforation
- Tamponade
- Residual atrial septal defect
- Massive right atrium to aorta shunt

ECMO:
- Air embolism
- Increased left ventricular afterload
- Left ventricular dilation
- Left ventricular blood stasis
- Pulmonary edema
- Differential oxygenation
- Circuit clots
- Disseminated intravascular or intraoxygenator coagulation
- Oxygenator failure
- Altered drug pharmacokinetics

Common complications

Device insertion site:
- Infection
- Bleeding
- Vessel perforation
- Retroperitoneal hematoma

Limb ischemia:
- Compartment syndrome
- Fasciotomy
- Amputation

Neurological:
- CNS hemorrhage
- CNS infarction
- Brain death
- Seizures

Acute kidney injury:
- Hemolysis-induced
- Other causes

Haematological:
- Hemolysis
- Acquired von Willebrand disease
- Thrombocytopenia
- Heparin-induced thrombocytopenia
- Venous thromboembolism
- Gastrointestinal or pulmonary bleeding
- Bacteremia or sepsis

*Hemolysis seen in more than 10% individuals but is not life threatening.

FIG. 5: Potential complications with temporary MCS use.

ONLINE REFERENCES

Please scan the QR code provided at the end of the table of contents for References of this chapter.

CHAPTER 187

Management of Right Ventricular Shock

Anil Sharma, Akash Shah, Anushree Kumbhalkar

ABSTRACT

Right ventricular (RV)-predominant heart failure (HF) causing shock is routinely underdiagnosed. RV shock is associated with significant morbidity and mortality irrespective of the etiology. RV shock requires timely diagnosis guided by echocardiographic and hemodynamic data and immediate resuscitative efforts targeting the etiology. The need for MCS is determined by the degree of target organ perfusion and response to pharmacological therapies. This review elaborates on the pathophysiology, clinical features, hemodynamic monitoring, medical and interventional management, and mechanical circulatory support (MCS) for RV shock.

Keywords: Right ventricular-predominant cardiogenic shock, mechanical circulation devices, management of RV shock

INTRODUCTION

Historically the term "Choc," French for "push" was published in 1743 by physician LeDran who believed that symptoms arose from fear.[1] Shock is an inadequate perfusion of the body's cells with oxygenated blood. It is classified into four types: Hypovolemic, distributive, obstructive, and cardiogenic.

Cardiogenic shock (CS) is a life-threatening syndrome defined as clinical and biological evidence of systemic tissue hypoperfusion secondary to inadequate cardiac output despite adequate circulatory volume and ventricular filling pressure.

DIAGNOSTIC CRITERIA FOR CARDIOGENIC SHOCK

The clinical definition of CS includes hypotension [systolic blood pressure (SBP) < 90 mm Hg] despite adequate filling pressures, and signs of organ hypoperfusion.

Cardiogenic shock is an acute hemodynamic state of hypoperfusion caused by decreased cardiac output (CO), which results in multiend-organ damage. SHOCK trial defined cardiogenic shock as follows:[2]

- *Hypotension*: An SBP < 90 mm Hg for at least 30 minutes or the requirement of supportive measures to maintain the SBP at 90 mm Hg
- Cardiac index (CI) < 1.8 L/min/m^2 without hemodynamic support or <2.2 L/min/m^2 with support
- Pulmonary capillary wedge pressure (PCWP) ≥ 15 mm Hg

CLASSIFICATION OF CARDIOGENIC SHOCK

The SCAI classification **(Fig. 1)** defines the severity based on biochemical findings, clinical examination, and hemodynamic parameters. Patients are classified into one of five stages, ranging between A and E, with stage E being the most severe.[3]

Cardiogenic shock from left ventricular (LV) failure is a common presentation. In contrast, right ventricular (RV)-predominant heart failure (HF) causing shock is less well recognized.

HOW RV ANATOMY AND PHYSIOLOGY ARE DIFFERENT FROM LV?

Right Ventricle Anatomy and Physiology

Right ventricle is triangular in side-section and crescent-like in cross-section. It is made up of superficial and deeper longitudinal fibers. The RV has a thin free wall (2–3 mm) wrapped around the more muscularized LV medial wall. The superficial fibers are continuous with the subepicardial fibers of the LV. The shortening of deep longitudinal fibers contributes to the majority of the RV output. Traction by LV contraction contributes about 20–40% of RV output.

Right ventricle contracts against low-pressure, high-compliance pulmonary circulation. Output is facilitated by dilatating the outflow tract and expanding the proximal pulmonary artery (PA). Hence, RV stroke volume continues to move into the proximal PA even during diastole. The more compliant RV is better suited to accommodate an increase in right-sided venous return but tolerates acute increases in afterload poorly. As RV afterload increases, the RV dilates limiting its contractility. The inflow region of the RV contracts about 25–50 ms before the outflow region.[2]

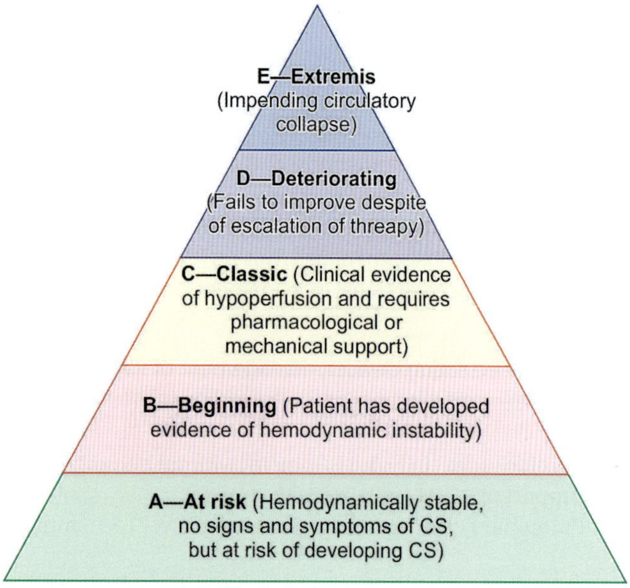

FIG. 1: SCAI SHOCK classification.

(CS: cardiogenic shock; SCAI: Society of Cardiovascular Angiography and Interventions)

Despite increased CO during heavy exertion, pulmonary arterial pressure (PAP) increases minimally and pulmonary vascular resistance (PVR) falls. This is based on the ability to recruit partially collapsed vessels and the lower vasomotor tone in the proximal pulmonary vessels. RV function is influenced by venous return, PAP, myocardial contractility, and pericardial compliance.[2]

RV Function and Pressure-volume Loop

Generating RV output requires one-sixth the energy expenditure of the LV. This difference is exemplified by the trapezoid shape of the RV pressure-volume (PV) loop, which lacks isovolumic phases of contraction and relaxation and has a lower peak systolic pressure.[3] The RV has a tremendous capacity to hypertrophy and dilate due to chronic pulmonary hypertension (PH) leading to tricuspid annular dilatation and tricuspid regurgitation (TR) as well as RV ischemia.[2] However, in an acute setting, the RV response is much more blunted. Hence, RV shock is a hemodynamic problem caused by the sudden change in preload, afterload, and/or impaired ventricular contractility **(Figs. 2A to D)**.[2,4]

Acute dilatation of the RV, e.g., in RVMI or pulmonary embolism, increases RV end-diastolic pressure (EDP) over LVEDP. An acute rise of PAP results in rapid RV dilatation and dysfunction manifesting as hypotension and shock. A chronic increase in PAP dilates RV using Starling's law to preserve CO. Eventually, the RV fails, becomes more spherical, TR worsens causing more right heart failure and a vicious cycle starts leading to systemic congestion and hypoperfusion.[5]

In acute RV dysfunction, RV dilation and worsening TR increase venous congestion and reduce LV preload. The septum shifts toward the LV during diastole, creating a flattened septum and a "D" shaped LV cavity which impedes LV filling and compromises LV function. This cascade of events can result in multiorgan dysfunction, shock, and death.

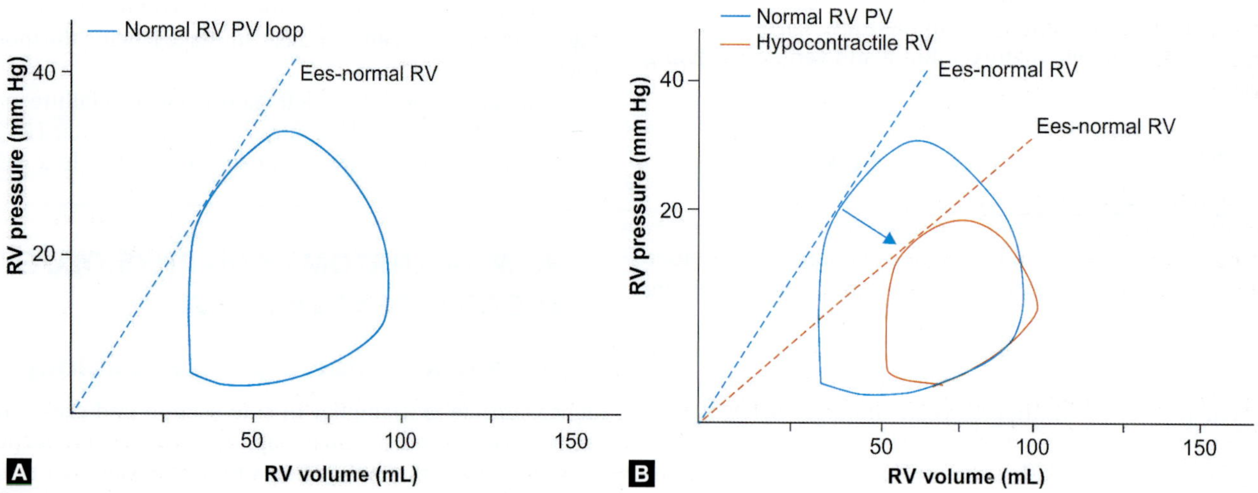

FIGS. 2A TO D: *Continued*

Continued

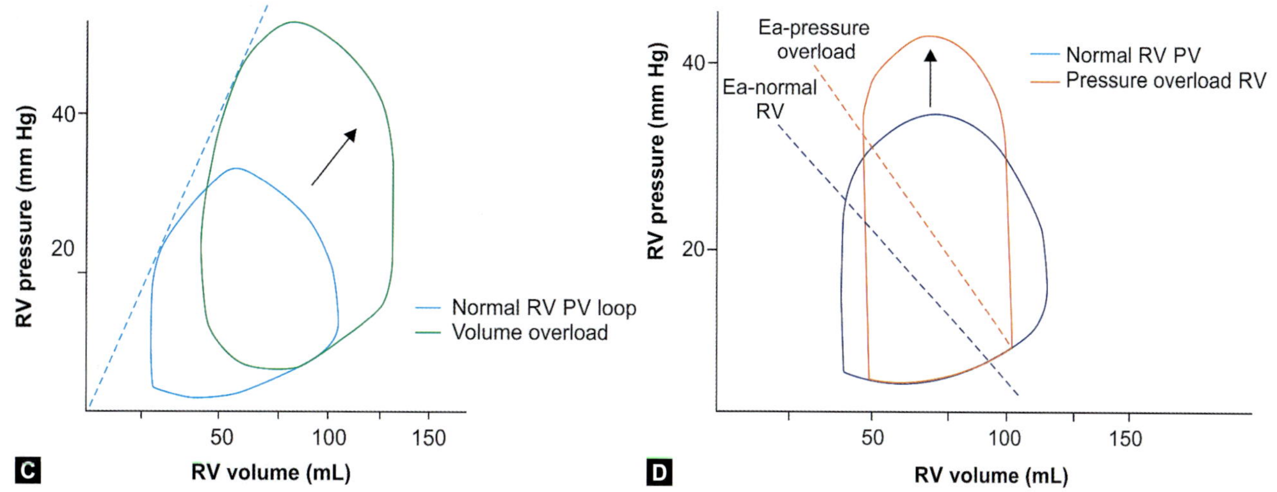

FIGS. 2A TO D: Changes in the pressure–volume relationship that occur with RVD precipitated by normal (A), pure contractile dysfunction (B), volume overload (C), and pressure overload (D).

(Ea: arterial elastance; Ees: end systolic elastance; PV: pressure volume loop; RV: right ventricle)

Defining Right Ventricular Shock and Right Ventricular Failure

Multiple invasive hemodynamic variables are considered along with the clinical history, physical examination, and echocardiographic indices.[6]

Right ventricular dysfunction (RVD) is suggested by:

- Central venous pressure (CVP) > 12 mm Hg
- CVP: PCWP ratio > 0.8
- Pulmonary artery pulsatility index (PAPi) <1
- RV stroke index (RVSI) < 300 g/m^2/beat

Causes of Right Ventricular Failure and Shock (Table 1)

Right ventricular failure accounted for 2.2% of HF admissions in the CHARITEM registry. They are divided into three categories: Secondary to RV hypercontractility, RV volume overload, and RV pressure overload.[7]

Diagnosis of Right Ventricular Shock

Meticulous clinical history and simple investigations can determine the diagnosis. However, the diagnosis of less common causes like PAH, chronic thromboembolic PH (CTEPH), or constrictive pericarditis can be challenging.

Clinical Features

Symptoms are secondary to hypoperfusion and systemic congestion like exertional dyspnea, fatigue, giddiness, ankle swelling, and right upper abdominal discomfort or pain. Relevant history should be enquired.

TABLE 1: Causes of predominant RV cardiogenic shock.

	Decreased contractility	RV volume overload	RV pressure overload
Acute	Sepsis		Acidosis
	LVAD support		Hypoxia
	RVMI	Excessive transfusion	Acute PE
	Myocarditis		ARDS
	Postoperative injury/ischemia (postcardiotomy)		Positive pressure ventilation
Chronic	RV cardiomyopathy	LH disease	
	ARVC	Single ventricle	
	Ebstein's anomaly		Pericardial disease
		PR	PAH
		TGA	CTEPH
		TR	PS
			Left-sided valvular heart disease
			Restrictive cardiomyopathy

(ARDS: acute respiratory distress syndrome; ARVC: arrhythmogenic right ventricle cardiomyopathy; CTEPH: chronic thromboembolism pulmonary hypertension; LH: left heart; LVAD: left ventricular assist device; PAH: pulmonary arterial hypertension; PE: pulmonary embolism; PR: pulmonary regurgitation; PS: pulmonary stenosis; RV: right ventricle; RVMI: right ventricular myocardial infarction; TGA: transposition of great arteries; TR: tricuspid regurgitation)

Shock is characterized by hypotension, signs of systemic congestion, and clear lungs.[8]

Noninvasive Investigations

Electrocardiography in patients with PH shows right axis deviation, dominant R in V_1, dominant S in V_5 or V_6, and P pulmonale. An elevated ST in V3R and V4R denotes RVMI.

Echocardiography provides evidence of RVF, including RV size, depressed RV ejection fraction, eccentricity index, flattening of septum, tricuspid annular plane systolic excursion (TAPSE), RV S' pulmonary artery systolic pressure (PASP), pulmonary artery acceleration time (PAT), size and distensibility of inferior vena cava (IVC) and pericardial disease.[8]

Contrast echocardiography is useful to detect intracardiac shunts.

Magnetic resonance imaging (MRI)/CT has the advantage of volume, size, and etiological diagnosis; however, their use in the setting of acute RV shock is limited.

Biochemical Markers

Markers for end-organ damage reflect poor prognosis and may improve with diuretics. There are no specific biomarkers for RV failure. However, raised BNP, troponins, and lactate reflect stress and severity.[8]

TABLE 2: Invasive hemodynamic parameters to assess RV function.

Cardiac filling pressures	mRAP/PCWP	>0.63 (RVF after LVAD) >0.86 (RVF in acute MI)
PAPi	(PASP-PADP)/mRAP	<1.85 (RVF after LVAD) <1.0 (RVF in acute MI)
PVR	mPAP-PCWP/CO	>3.6 (RVF after LVAD)
Transpulmonary gradient	mPAP-PCWP	Indeterminant
Diastolic pulmonary gradient	PADP-PCWP	Indeterminant
RV SW	(mPAP-RAP) × SV × 0.136	<15 (RVF after LVAD) <10 (RVF after acute MI)
RV SWI	(mPAP-RAP) × SV index	<0.3–0.6 (RVF after LVAD)
PA compliance	SV/(PASP-PADP)	<2.5 (RVF in chronic heart failure)

(CO: cardiac output; LVAD: left ventricle assist device; MI: myocardial infarction; mPAP: mean pulmonary artery pressure; mRAP: mean right atrial pressure; PA: pulmonary artery; PADP: pulmonary artery diastolic pressure; PAPi: pulmonary artery pulsatile index; PASP: pulmonary artery systolic pressure; PCWP: pulmonary capillary wedge pressure; PVR: pulmonary vascular resistance; RV SW: right ventricle stroke work; RV SWI: right ventricle stroke work index; RVF: right ventricle failure; SV: stroke volume)

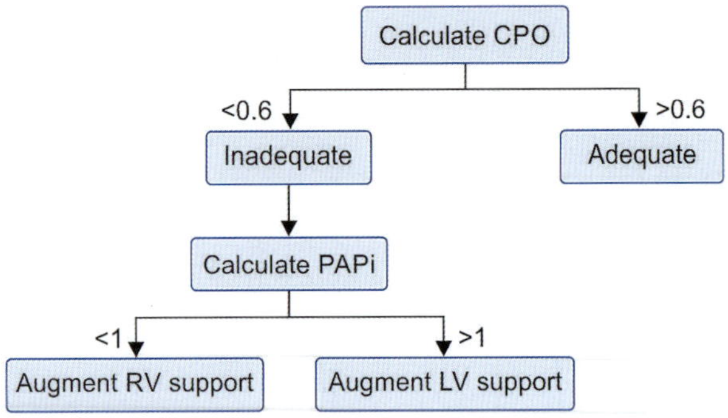

FLOWCHART 1: Ensuring adequate support.

(CPO: cardiac power output; LV: left ventricle; PAPi: pulmonary artery pulsatile index; RV: right ventricle)

Invasive Hemodynamic Assessment

Right heart catheterization (RHC) with a PA catheter remains the cornerstone in the management and formulating strategy for RV shock **(Table 2 and Flowchart 1)**.[9]

Diagnostic Algorithm

A useful algorithm **(Flowchart 2)** comprises the presence of PH and primary myocardial or pericardial disease. If a meticulous history, chest X-ray and an ECG raise suspicion of PH, the next step is to perform transthoracic echocardiography to look for biventricular function and PASP. If PH is present without LV dysfunction, we should exclude lung diseases like OAD, ILD, or OSA. A ventilation-perfusion scan is the next step for CTEPH exclusion. A positive V/Q scan necessitates CT pulmonary angiography for confirmation, while a negative scan increases the probability of type 1 PAH. RHC and connective tissue disease screening may be required in selected cases.

MANAGEMENT OF RIGHT VENTRICULAR-PREDOMINANT HEART FAILURE AND SHOCK

Principles of Management

The triage of patients presenting with RVF and shock aims to assess clinical severity and focus on rapid identification and management of the etiology. Early recognition is essential, as undertreated RV shock can potentiate hemodynamic collapse and end-organ damage.

Initial Management of Right Ventricular Failure

Medical Therapy

General Measures

Medical therapy for acute RVF is based on fundamental principles to optimize preload, afterload, and contractility.

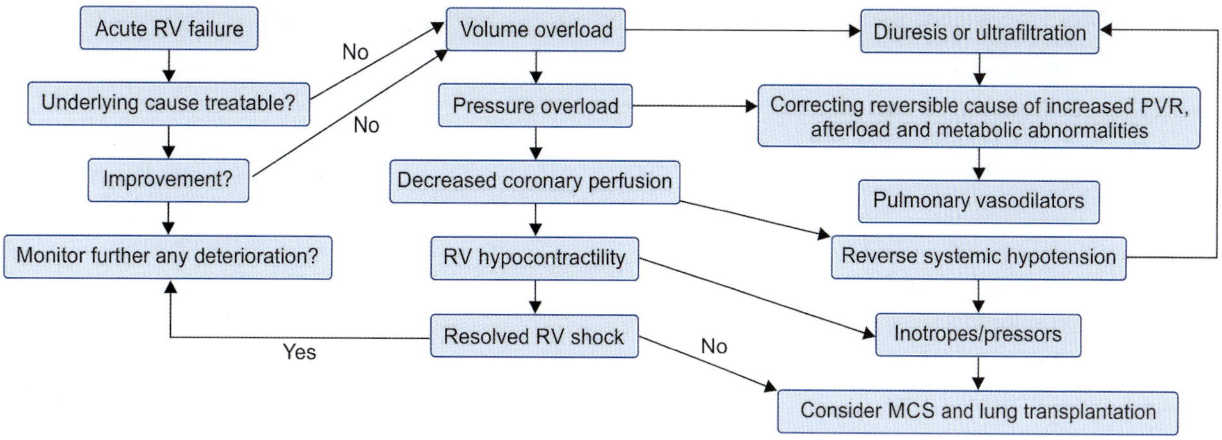

FLOWCHART 2: Proposed algorithm for management of acute right ventricle (RV) failure.

Volume Optimization and Preload Management

Acute RV shock is preload dependent. Hence, reducing venous pressures is key for improving cardiac output and reducing systemic congestion while avoiding systemic hypotension **(Figs. 2A to D)**.

In patients with RVF, renal venous pressure is often elevated. Hence either bolus or continuous infusion of loop diuretics is required to maintain a decongestive effect.[10] Monitoring urine output is crucial to identify patients with an inadequate diuretic response. Escalation of the same or ultrafiltration is needed if decongestion is insufficient. However, no trial has demonstrated the superiority of ultrafiltration in reducing mortality over diuretics.

Afterload Reduction

Pulmonary vasodilator therapies: The use of pulmonary vasodilator therapies can relieve RV afterload in patients with PH and acute RVF. Intravenous epoprostenol has long-term benefits, including improved survival and functional capacity. However, in cases of RV shock, it may cause hypotension and worsen oxygenation. Short-acting inhaled nitrous oxide is recommended in this setting.[10]

Thrombolytic therapy for acute high-risk or intermediate high-risk pulmonary embolism restores pulmonary blood flow and reduces RV afterload.

Revascularization

In the setting of RVMI causing RV shock, myocardial reperfusion is crucial for the rapid restoration of RV function. In the SHOCK registry, these patients had a similar mortality as compared to LV-predominant shock. Restoration of TIMI III flow in the right coronary circulation leads to dramatic recovery of RV CO and improved survival.[10] Temporary pacing can treat vagal-mediated bradycardia or heart block. If these measures fail, MCS may be necessary.

Pressors and Inotropic Agents

Vasopressors and inotropes are the keys in treating RV shock.[10] They restore coronary perfusion pressure and increase CO and renal perfusion. Combined inotropic and vasopressor properties are ideal for hypotension. Alpha-1 agonists like dopamine, norepinephrine, and epinephrine have dose-dependent vasopressor effects that can augment contractility. Dobutamine, levosimendan, and phosphodiesterase III inhibitors (milrinone) are also recommended, because they affect ventricular-arterial coupling by combining RV inotropy and pulmonary vasodilation. However, caution is recommended in acute RVMI due to increased oxygen demand and arrhythmogenicity.[10]

Vasopressin can restore systemic hemodynamics without affecting PVR and causing tachyarrhythmias while supporting renal perfusion. In small studies, digoxin was associated with acute increases in CO when administered to patients with PH and RVD **(Table 3)**.

Mechanical Ventilation

Mechanical ventilation can negatively impact RV preload and afterload but appropriate use of PEEP and other parameters can minimize these effects.

Interatrial Shunt

Initial human studies of iatrogenic interatrial shunt creation demonstrated high mortality due to refractory hypoxia.[11] Robust trial data is lacking and the use of such devices remains controversial.

Mechanical Circulatory Support

A multidisciplinary shock team should be incorporated while approaching patients with cardiogenic shock. Such patients should be identified early in the course of the disease to avoid irreversible end-organ damage. The approach should include timing, hemodynamic parameters, underlying etiology, technical feasibility, and exit strategies while choosing such patients. The MCS helps to rapidly stabilize patients with RV shock by bypassing the RV and is able to (1) LV cardiac output augmentation and thereby increasing end-organ perfusion, and (2) decongesting the end organ by decreasing RV preload **(Flowchart 1)**.

TABLE 3: Various inotropes and vasopressors and their effects.

Types	Effects					Dosage
	Mechanism	Contractility	Heart rate	SVR	Venous tone	
Dobutamine	β1 β2	↑↑	↑↑	↓		2–20 μg/kg/min (maximum 40 μg/kg/min)
Milrinone	PDE-3 inhibitor	↑↑	↑	↓↓	↓	50 μg/kg loading F/B 0.375–0.75 μg/kg/min
Epinephrine	α1α2 β1β2	↑	↑↑	↑	↑	0.05–0.2 μg/kg/min
Norepinephrine	α1α2 β1β2	↑	↑	↑↑	↑↑	2–4 μg/kg/min
Phenylephrine	α1			↑↑		0.4–10 μg/kg/min
Dopamine	α1 β1 Dopa	↑	↑	↑		5–15 μg/kg/min
Vasopressin	V1			↑		0.03 units/min

(α: alpha receptors; β: beta receptors; Dopa: dopamine receptors)

OVERVIEW OF RECENT RIGHT-SIDED MECHANICAL CIRCULATORY SUPPORT (TABLE 4 AND FLOWCHART 3)

Percutaneously Deployed Mechanical Circulatory Support

Right Atrium to Pulmonary Artery

Impella RP

Impella RP (right peripheral; Abiomed Inc., Danvers, MA) is a percutaneous, single access, microaxial flow catheter. An 11F catheter on which a 22F pump is mounted which bypasses the failing RV and pumps blood directly in PA (outflow) from right atrium (RA) (inflow). The device is inserted in the peripheral vein (usually the right femoral vein) via a 23F peel-away sheath and advanced under fluoroscopic guidance and ultimately deployed onto PA. It delivers 4–5 L/min of blood into PA at 33,000 RPM. It cannot be used to support concomitant respiratory failure as lacks oxygenator support.[4] In the RECOVER RIGHT trial (2015), Impella RP support was studied in 30 patients with medically refractory RV failure where it showed reduction in RAP (19.2 ± 0.7 to 12.6 ± 1 mm Hg; $p < 0.0001$), improvement in cardiac index (1.82 ± 0.04 to 3.3 ± 0.23 L/min/m^2; $p < 0.001$), and 73% of patients survived to 30 days or hospital discharge.[12]

The beneficial effects of Impella RP are attributed to a reduction in RA pressure, an increase in PA pressures, and an increase in LV preload. Optimal use has been reported in RV CS secondary to acute MI, massive PE, postcardiotomy syndrome, following LVAD implantation, and in primary graft dysfunction after orthotopic heart transplantation, among others. The disadvantages include a challenge to navigate the device, which is prone to migration, bleeding, and hemolysis; the obligate need for femoral access which limits mobilization; and the risk of thromboembolic episodes. A novel Impella RP device is under development for ease of access which can negate this limitation.[4]

TandemHeart RVAD and ProtekDuo RVAD

TandemHeart (21F cannula) and ProtekDuo (29 or 31 Fr dual-lumen cannula) MCS are centrifugal extracorporeal pump to simultaneously displace blood from the RA to PA. This device delivers 4–5 L/min blood into the PA. However, due to the need for a dual access site in TandemHeart (typically right femoral vein and right internal Jugular vein or bilateral femoral vein), ProtekDuo device was developed which had the major advantage of eliminating the obligate femoral venous access allowing the patient to be mobilized early. Also, this device can be used in combination with an oxygenator in cases of persistent hypoxemia and hypoxic respiratory failure. Several case series have illustrated the efficacy of the ProtekDuo Cannula. The hemodynamic profile of TandemHeart-RVAD/ProtekDuo is similar to that of Impella RP.[4]

PERKAT RV (PERkutane KATheterpumptechnologie Right Ventricle)

The PERKAT RV is the first pulsatile, right-sided MCS device inserted percutaneously into the femoral vein via an 18F catheter and advanced under fluoroscopic guidance unto the PA (outflow), bypassing the RV. The PERKAT RV system relies on a standard intra-aortic balloon pump (IABP) connected to an external IABP console. The balloon is encapsulated within a 2.2-m self-expanding nitinol stent cage and is electrocardiogram-gated, inflating during diastole and deflating during systole. Inflation of the balloon during diastole causes blood to displace from IVC and distal veins into the PA. It can generate nearly 4 L/min of flow. Advantage is due to its smaller bore access compared to other percutaneous right-sided MCS devices, and also its pulsatile support to the failing RV while avoiding complications that have been reported with continuous flow devices. The PERKAT RV is yet to be approved and currently undergoing clinical human trials hence data supporting its efficacy is lacking.[13]

TABLE 4: Types of current mechanical circulatory support.

Device type	Mechanism	Access site and size	Advantages	Disadvantages	Remarks
Impella RP	Percutaneous use. RA to PA	Right femoral vein, 23F	Single access, ease of deployment	Risk of thrombosis, limits ambulation with femoral access	Optimal in RV infarct, and in presence of thrombus in RA or IVC
ProtekDuo RVAD	Percutaneous implantation, RA to PA	Right IJV, 29F–31F	Single site access, ambulation, addition of oxygenator	Larger bore size, need quick weaning, may cause SVC syndrome	Optimal after LVAD implantation
TandemHeart	Percutaneous use, RA to PA	B/L femoral or right femoral + right IJV access, 21F and 15–19F	Allows addition of oxygenator, durable for longer period	Dual access site, immobilization, may cause thrombosis	C/I in IJV, severe TV/PV stenosis
PERKAT RV	Percutaneous use, IVC to PA	Femoral vein, 18F	Single access and smaller bore	Limited mobility	Not yet approved
Peripheral VA ECMO	Percutaneous use, RA to Ao	Femoral or IJV for venous access (21–25F) and femoral artery for arterial access (17–21F)	Ease of cannulation as can be done at bedside, durable for 1–2 weeks.	Augments LV afterload, risk of limb ischemia and thromboembolic episodes	High-risk pulmonary embolism or decompensated PHTN
CentriMag RVAD	Surgical implantation into RA or RV to PA		Allows addition of oxygenator, durable for longer period, low chances of hemolysis	Surgical implantation, risk of thrombosis	Optimal when used in combination with LVAD
Heartmate 3	Surgical implantation, RV to PA		Patient can be discharged with a device in situ	Surgical implantation	In combination with LVAD for dischargeable patients

(IJV: internal jugular vein; RP: right peripheral; IVC: inferior vena cava; LVAD: left ventricular assist device; PA: pulmonary artery; PERKAT RV: PERkutane KATheterpumptechnologie Right ventricle; PV: pulmonary valve; RA: right atrium; RV: right ventricle; RVAD: right ventricular assist device; SVC: superior vena cava; TV: tricuspid valve)

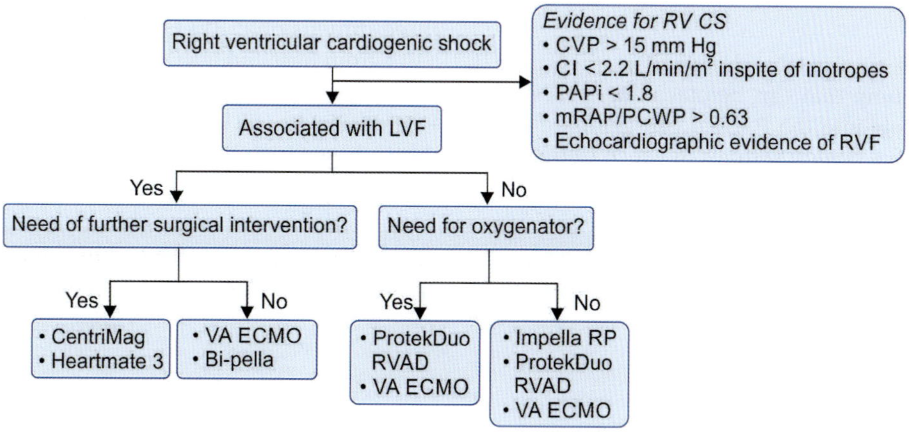

FLOWCHART 3: Approach to mechanical circulatory support in RV CS.

(CI: cardiac index; CS: cardiogenic shock; CVP: central venous pressure; mRAP: mean right atrial pressure; PAPi: pulmonary artery pulsatile index; PCWP: pulmonary capillary wedge pressure; RV: right ventricle; RVAD: right ventricular assist device; RVF: right ventricular failure; VA-ECMO: veno-arterial extracorporeal membrane oxygenation)

Intra-aortic Balloon Pump

The use of an intra-aortic balloon pump (IABP) is known to improve cardiac hemodynamics by increasing coronary artery perfusion and reducing LV afterload. Its role in RV cardiogenic shock is not as well characterized however in a trial with CS secondary to acute MI with RVI, survival was 81%, attributed to increased coronary perfusion capacity before and after revascularization.[14]

RA to Ao

Veno-arterial Extracorporeal Membrane Oxygenation

Veno-arterial extracorporeal membrane oxygenation (VA-ECMO) is by far the most widely used MCS for cardiogenic shock. It simultaneously provides extracorporeal gas exchange and circulatory support in the setting of left, right, or biventricular failure. The circuit consists of a venous inflow (femoral vein or IJV) cannula, centrifugal flow pump, oxygenator, heat exchanger, and outflow arterial (femoral artery) cannula.[13]

Typically, VA-ECMO provides 3–5 L/min of blood flow via the central venous vein and pumps into the peripheral arterial circulation thereby decreasing the RV preload but at the same time increasing preload and LA pressure and over-distending LV and augmenting LV afterload and worsening pulmonary edema. It has been increasingly used in specific cases of fulminant myocarditis, allograft failure after cardiac transplantation, acute RV failure due to PE, RV failure during LVAD support, and severely decompensated heart failure. Hence in contrast VA ECMO establishes a parallel circulation as opposed to being an actual ventricular assist device. Because of this, the risk of device thrombosis increases when used for RV support after LVAD implantation. Therefore, many clinicians will initiate a "venting" strategy to prevent the complications of LV pressure overload.[13]

Other potential complications of peripheral VA ECMO include lower extremity ischemia, and major bleeding which has been shown to occur in 12–25% of patients.

Surgically Deployed MCS

CentriMag RVAD

The CentriMag is a surgically deployed extracorporeal centrifugal-flow pump that can be placed into RA or RV (inflow) and outflow into the PA and can generate up to 10 L/min of flow. The clinical settings in which CentriMag-RVAD has most commonly been used are postcardiotomy cardiogenic shock, primary graft dysfunction after orthotopic heart transplantation, and RV failure post-LVAD implantation. The major advantage is that it can be used for a longer duration up to 30 days like in a meta-analysis of 999 patients supported with the CentriMag found that it was used as a ventricular assist device in 72% of cases where at 30 days, survival in per-cardiotomy cardiogenic shock was 66%, 61%, 54% and 41% in precardiotomy cardiogenic shock, post-LVAD placement, post-transplant allograft failure, and postcardiotomy cardiogenic shock, respectively.[13]

Heartmate 3

Heartmate 3 is another surgically deployed MCS similar to CentriMag, which can be placed into RA/RV and outflow into the PA. The advantage of this device is that the patient can be discharged with the device in situ and thus can be used as a strategy to bridge to transplant or bridge to recovery[12] **(Table 5)**.

Management and Weaning Strategy of the Device

Prior to the selection of the device, the goal should be adequately defined as to whether to use it as a bridge to transplant or a bridge to recovery. Hence frequent monitoring and reassessment for readiness to wean the device is crucial. This includes adequate anticoagulation, frequent hemodynamic, biochemical (hemolysis and end-organ damage), and echocardiographic monitoring, reasonable goals include CVP < 14 mm Hg, PCWP < 18 mm Hg, and cardiac index (CI) >2.2 L/min/m^2. Most echocardiographic predictors like three-dimensional RVEF of >24.6% or improvement in *S*′ >10% from baseline have both been associated with higher weaning success. With that said, sufficient data and protocols for weaning are still lacking in many studies and need further device-based trials to formulate an algorithm.

TABLE 5: Consequences of mechanical circulatory support on hemodynamics.

Device	Inflow	Outflow	RV preload	RV afterload	mPAP	LVEDP or PCWP	LV afterload	MAP	RV CO
Impella RP	RA	PA	↓	↓	↑	↑	↔	↑	↑
ProtekDuo RVAD	RA	PA	↓	↓	↑	↑	↔	↑	↑
Tandemheart	RA	PA	↓	↓	↑	↑	↔	↑	↑
VA ECMO	FV	FA	↓	↓	↓	↑↑	↑↑	↓	↓↔
IABP			↑	↓	↑	↓	↓	↑	↓↔
CentriMag	RA/RV	PA	↓	↓	↑	↑	↔	↑	↑
Heartmate 3	RA/RV	PA	↓	↑	↑	↑	↔	↑	↑

(FA: femoral artery; FV: femoral vein; Impella RP: Impella right peripheral; LV: left ventricle; LVEDP: left ventricular end diastolic pressure; MAP: mean arterial pressure; mPAP: mean pulmonary artery pressure; PA: pulmonary artery; PCWP: pulmonary capillary wedge pressure; RA: right atrium; RV CO: right ventricle cardiac output; RV: right ventricle; VA ECMO: veno-arterial extracorporeal membrane oxygenation)

Finally, routine critical care management should not be ignored during the period of MCS. This includes lung-protective ventilation, minimization of sedation and paralytics, and stress ulcer prophylaxis. In addition, aggressive physical therapy should be initiated whenever possible.

CONCLUSION

Right ventricular shock is associated with significant morbidity and mortality irrespective of the etiology. It requires timely diagnosis guided by echocardiographic and hemodynamic data and immediate resuscitative efforts targeting the etiology. Initial management should focus on targeting the etiology. Efforts should be directed toward optimizing RV preload and afterload. Inhaled short-acting pulmonary vasodilators can be used. Vasopressors and inotropes should be considered to improve RV function. The need for MCS is determined by the degree of target organ perfusion and response to pharmacological therapies. MCS is the bridge to surgical interventions, like pulmonary endarterectomy or transplantation.

ONLINE REFERENCES

Please scan the QR code provided at the end of the table of contents for References of this chapter.

CHAPTER

188

Mechanical Circulatory Support in Severe Heart Failure

Ashmit Bhardwaj, Mukesh Goel

ABSTRACT

Heart failure, a chronic and progressive condition, can progress to advanced stages, where conventional medical therapy fails. When this happens, a heart transplant becomes necessary. However, given the scarcity of donor hearts combined with how quickly a patient with advanced heart failure deteriorates, preserving a patient's life becomes challenging.

To bridge the gap between diagnosis of heart transplantation and keeping the patient alive until a donor is found, ventricular assist devices (VADs) are used, namely, the HeartMate 3 and the Berlin Heart; these are highly successful in adult and pediatric patients, respectively.

This chapter will explore the efficacy, complications, and advancements of these VADs in treating patients with advanced heart failure.

Keywords: Mechanical circulatory support (MCS), ventricular assist device (VAD), HeartMate 3, EXCOR Berlin Heart

INTRODUCTION

Heart failure is recognized as a chronic and progressive condition that results from structural or functional cardiac disorders that are marked by the heart's inability to pump blood to the body's systemic requirement.

Advanced heart failure denotes a stage where the condition becomes refractory to medical therapy, and the patient's symptoms worsen rapidly. This stage is marked by the failure of conventional medical therapy, necessitating more curative interventions, such as heart transplantation.[1]

Heart transplants wait-lists are very long. Donor hearts are naturally scarce resources, with some sources reporting the average wait-time being 36 months for a recipient to obtain a heart in India.[2]

With a rapidly deteriorating heart and prolonged wait-list times for cardiac transplantation, ventricular assist devices (VADs) are utilized to "bridge" a patient to a heart transplant.

The rationale behind using these devices is to ensure the survival of the patient's vital organs, by taking on the role of one or both ventricles of the failing heart, until a suitable donor is found.

Some patients with refractory heart failure are not suitable candidates for heart transplants. VAD can be the final solution, i.e., "destination therapy" for these patients.

The Interagency Registry for Mechanical Assisted Circulatory Support (INTERMACS) is used to assist clinicians with informed decision-making. The INTERMACS is a database that helps clinicians track and analyze the outcomes of patients who have been implanted with mechanical circulatory support devices, including VADS.

The INTERMACS can improve the quality of care for patients who are diagnosed with advanced heart failure, by guiding physicians with evidence-based insights.

The INTERMACS uses a standardization system of "profiles", which range from profiles 1–7, with "1" indicating a patient who is critically ill, and "7" being a patient who has advanced heart failure but is stable on medical therapy.

Patients who are receiving VADs are enrolled in the INTERMACS registry, which categorizes the patient based on the severity of their heart failure to guide device implantation. Regular reports are generated to provide insights into the performance of the device and the patient's outcomes, allowing clinicians to benchmark their patients' examples against national averages, to improve and identify the best practices.[3]

When a patient is enrolled in the registry, various outcomes include their quality of life, functional status, and VAD performance.

This registry also provides crucial information to device manufacturers and regulatory agencies, supporting the continuous improvement of VAD technology.

Heart failure can occur in both pediatric and adult patients. The HeartMate 3 device is considered the most effective among the adult patient population. For pediatric patients, the Berlin heart device is used.

This chapter seeks to provide a review of these two VADs: The Berlin Heart and HeartMate 3. This chapter will describe how the devices work, how they compare to other VADs, and possible adverse events.

BERLIN HEART

The Berlin Heart provides mechanical circulatory support, aimed at pediatric patients with severe heart failure.[4]

The Berlin Heart's underlying engineering involves it having a simple air-driven pump, which takes over the work of one or both sides of the child's heart. Therefore, the Berlin Heart is known as a biventricular assist device (BiVAD), capable of taking over the role of either one or both the ventricles of the heart, enabling perfusion of vital organs in the body, until a suitable donor is available.[5]

This BiVAD system includes an external pump, which takes over the role of the left ventricle, by circulating blood through the body. These pumps are connected to cannulas and carefully sewn onto the patient's heart through surgery. This device can be powered pneumatically or via an electric motor and is controlled by a console, which carefully regulates the pump's speed and pressure. Through this device, blood is drawn from the heart into a pump, and it is then sent back into the circulatory system **(Figs. 1A and B).**

Currently, the Berlin Heart EXCOR is the only VAD specifically designed for pediatric patients, as it is the most well-suited for a pediatric patient's heart size and physiological needs.

A prospective, multicenter, single-arm study evaluated the safety of the Berlin Heart EXCOR, comparing it to a historical control population supported by "ECMO" as a bridge to heart transplantation.[6]

The study revealed that the subjects in the "all-implant group" were supported for a median of 47 days (range 0–504) and were successfully weaned or bridged to transplant in 73% of the subjects.

Further, the rate of adverse events, including ischemic/hemorrhagic events decreased over the years and was only 15.6% in the overall group **(Fig. 2)**.

Although the Berlin Heart functions as a bridge to heart transplant, due to its nonbiological inner surfaces through which blood passes, neurological events (largely strokes) are common, with a cohort study noticing an incidence rate of 29% experiencing at least one neurological event.[7] Other possible side effects and complications to Berlin Heart use include major bleeding in 44% as per one study.[7]

Complications also include infection, which frequently occurs in patients who have been implanted with the Berlin Heart. The incidence of infection varies from study to study, where infection rates in previous VAD studies vary from 18 to 59%.[8-10]

HEARTMATE 3

Similar to the Berlin Heart, the HeartMate 3 device is indicated for older children and adult patients with advanced heart failure, who risk dying without any intervention. The HeartMate 3 was introduced as the latest advancement in left ventricular assist devices (LVADs) after it received approval from the FDA after extensive clinical trials demonstrated the device's reliability, efficacy, and safety.[11]

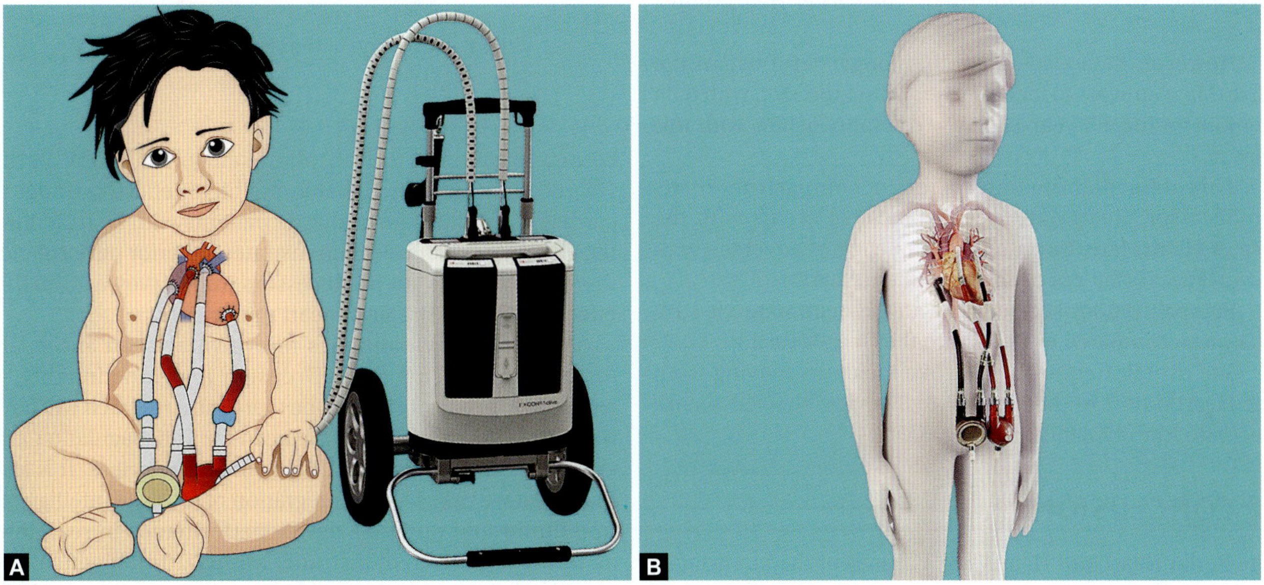

FIGS. 1A AND B: Berlin Heart EXCOR product overview.
Courtesy: Berlin Heart GmBH, Berlin, Germany.

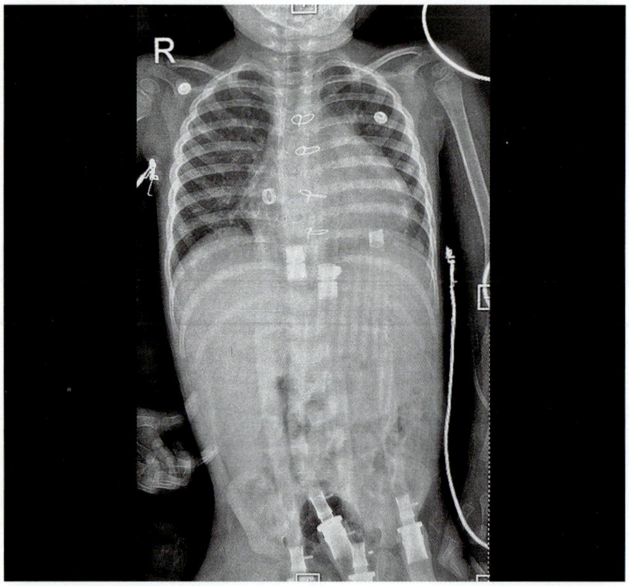

FIG. 2: Anonymized patient with the Berlin Heart device (implanted at Indraprastha Apollo Hospital, New Delhi).

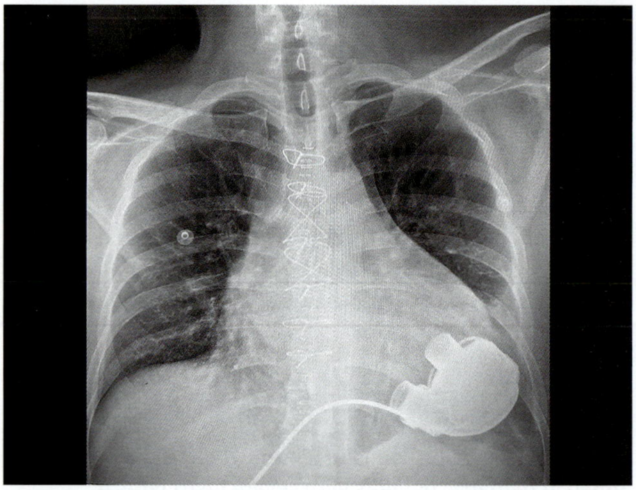

FIG. 3: Anonymized patient with the HeartMate 3 device (implanted at Indraprastha Apollo Hospital, New Delhi).

The engineering of the HeartMate 3 device uses a centrifugal flow mechanism, with a magnetically levitated rotor. This design effectively allows for a frictionless environment, reducing damage to blood components.[12] Its design also allows for it to mimic the natural pulse, reducing the risk of clot formation and improving hemocompatibility. The full Maglev flow technology employed in the HeartMate 3 helps minimize complications and hemocompatibility-related adverse events **(Figs. 3 and 4)**.[13]

Long-term data on the HeartMate 3 device also demonstrates that the patients who have been implanted with the device show an overall survival of 83% at 2 years, as opposed to 69% with the use of the earlier HeartMate 2 device.[14,15]

However, data also shows that longer-term use of the HeartMate appears to increase the risk of mortality, with data demonstrating a 5-year-all-cause mortality of 38% with this device.[16]

This data demonstrates that in comparison to its predecessor, HeartMate 2, whilst adverse events with the use of HeartMate 3 occur, the frequency of adverse event occurrences is far less common with the HeartMate 3.

Pump thrombosis incidence with the HeartMate 3 is 1.1% at 2 years, compared to 10.1% with the HeartMate 2.[17]

The overall frequency of stroke incidents moving from the HeartMate 2 to the Heartmate 3 device, showed a stark decrease from 19.2 to 10.1% **(Fig. 5)**.[18]

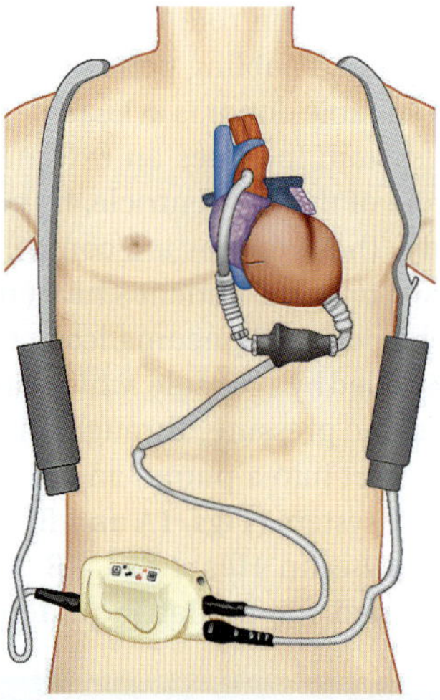

FIG. 4: Illustration of the HeartMate 3 device.

CONCLUSION

The Berlin Heart and HeartMate 3 represent the forefront of mechanical circulatory support, having successfully bridged countless patients to transplant safely. While the Berlin Heart continues to be a reliable and highly effective bridge to cardiac transplants for pediatric patients with heart failure, the HeartMate 3 device demonstrates superior performance in comparison to its predecessors and serves as a highly effective tool as a bridge to heart transplants.

As technology continues to evolve, we can anticipate further refinements in VAD design and functionality. A reasonable prediction would be that future research will have a strong focus on reducing the need for anticoagulation and enhancing the hemocompatibility of these devices. It is also likely that we may see the integration of artificial intelligence to monitor and optimize device performance in real time, as new research demonstrates artificial intelligence and machine learning to predict adverse events.

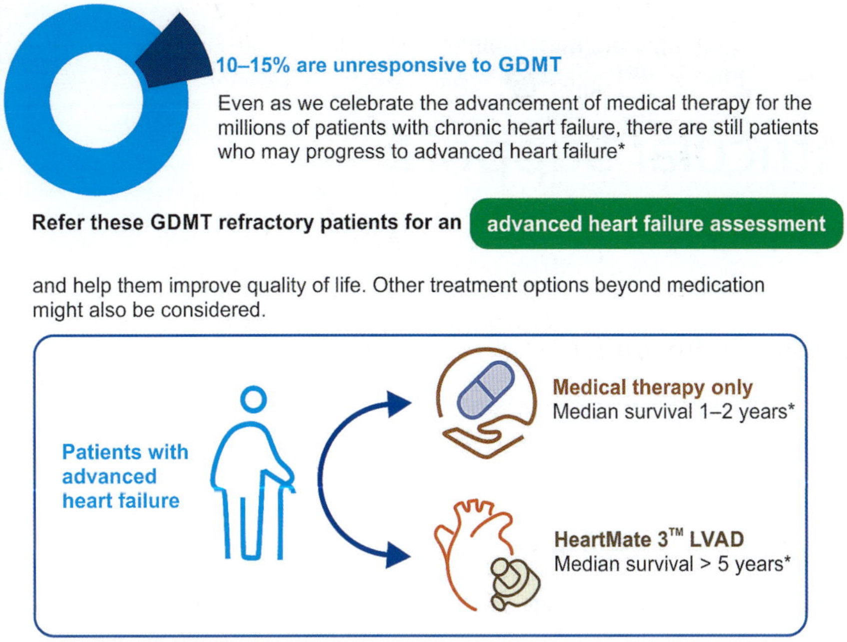

*Median survival with HM3 versus medical therapy.

FIG. 5: Some patients are still unresponsive to GDMT.

ONLINE REFERENCES

Please scan the QR code provided at the end of the table of contents for References of this chapter.

CHAPTER

189

Right Ventricular Support: When and How

Pawan Sharma, Himanshu Jindal

ABSTRACT

The right ventricle (RV) of the heart is anatomically and functionally distinct from the left ventricle (LV). Right ventricular failure (RVF) is often underestimated but significantly impacts long-term morbidity and mortality rates. It affects 3–9% of acute heart failure cases, with in-hospital mortality ranging from 5 to 17%. Following LV assist device implantation, RVF prevalence can vary widely, affecting between 9 and 40% of cases. Conditions causing RV dysfunction include congenital heart disease, myocardial infarction, pulmonary embolism, pulmonary hypertension, and cor pulmonale. Early detection of RV dysfunction is crucial for effective management. Diagnostic strategies encompass a comprehensive understanding of pathophysiological mechanisms and the identification of biomarkers indicative of RV stress and injury. Management strategies for RV dysfunction include mechanical, surgical, and interventional approaches (RV support). This chapter focuses on dysfunction and indication of RV support along with several management strategies.

Keywords: Right ventricle, RV dysfunction, mechanical, biomarkers, RV support

INTRODUCTION

The right ventricle (RV) of the heart possesses distinctive anatomy and physiology that are pivotal in regulating hemodynamics and various cardiovascular functions.[1] Its crucial role extends across a spectrum of medical conditions.[2] The function, regulation, and structure of RV differ significantly from those of the left ventricle (LV).[3] It generates a lower pressure compared to the LV, ensuring efficient blood flow through the pulmonary circulation. Its function is crucial in maintaining a balanced circulation between the heart and the lungs.[1]

Right ventricular failure (RVF) is uncommon post-routine cardiac surgery but remains a substantial contributor to perioperative and long-term morbidity and mortality due to its significant impact on patient outcomes. In perioperative settings, it is more difficult to diagnose and more challenging to treat.[4] The RVF is frequently overlooked but affects 3-9% of acute heart failure cases with in-hospital mortality rates ranging from 5 to 17%. Post-LVAD implantation, RVF prevalence varies significantly, affecting 9-40% of cases.[5] The various causes of RV dysfunction are also responsible to induce prevalence. The birth prevalence of congenital heart disease (CHD) was found to be 17.8/1,000 live births.[6] The right ventricular myocardial infarction (RVMI) is often silent and clinical evidence can only be seen in 20% of patients.[7] The prevalence rate of RV infarction in patients with acute inferior wall MI varies between 26.5 and 39%,[8] while cor pulmonale represents 5-10% of all heart disease cases, contributes to 20-30% of admissions for HF, and is found in 9.2% of cardiac autopsies.[9]

Their dysfunction is often overlooked by LV dysfunction, despite rising prevalence of heart failure-related disorders. Therefore, RV support is crucial. This chapter explores the critical issue of RVF, a condition linked with increased mortality and morbidity. It underscores early diagnostic methodologies to efficiently manage this complex clinical scenario. Furthermore, it emphasizes on management strategies, including pharmacological treatments, mechanical support modalities, and advanced surgical techniques as a RV support.

CLINICAL INSIGHTS AND PATHOPHYSIOLOGICAL PERSPECTIVES OF RIGHT VENTRICULAR DYSFUNCTION

Right Ventricular Failure

The RVF typically arises from LV failure, volume overload, or pressure overload.[10] It can manifest as both acute and chronic. Acute events like pulmonary embolism rapidly lead to RVF due to maladaptive responses. Conversely, chronic conditions such as congenital heart defects allow the RV to develop adaptive mechanisms over time before eventual decompensation.[11] Several acute and chronic RVF causes are presented in **Box 1**.

Right Ventricular Failure in Congenital Heart Disease

The CHD is the most significant condition worldwide, affecting millions of newborns.[6] The RV and its outflow tract develop specifically from the second heart field.[12] During fetal development, RV is underdeveloped and does not connect with pulmonary circulation, enduring high afterload. It acts as a systemic ventricle due to high pulmonary vascular resistance and low systemic vascular resistance within placental circulation.[13] In CHD with a systemic RV, structural adaptations mimic the LV to support systemic circulation efficiently, characterized by elevated NT-pro-B-type natriuretic peptide (NT-proBNP) and troponin T levels, abnormal NYHA class, reduced exercise tolerance, and hypotension.[12]

BOX 1 **Causes of acute and chronic RVF.**

Acute RVF:
- Pulmonary embolism
- RV infarction
- Sepsis
- Acute lung injury
- Acute respiratory distress syndrome
- Transfusion-related acute lung injury
- Acute chest syndrome
- Pulmonary hypertensive crisis

Chronic RVF:
- Tricuspid valve regurgitation
- Pulmonic valve regurgitation
- Congenital heart disease
- Anomalous pulmonary venous return

Source: Adapted from Sayer and Semigran.[11]

Right Ventricular Myocardial Infarction

This condition has a high rate of in-hospital mortality attributed to hemodynamic compromise, cardiogenic shock, and electrical complications.[14] The RVI mostly occurs due to dysfunction of the left circumflex artery in left dominant coronary circulation.[7] The RV myocardium is thin and requires less oxygen than LV. Occlusions occurring proximal to the RV marginal artery are associated with larger infarction sizes, leading to an increased risk of cardiogenic shock and cardiac death. Acute thrombotic occlusion, catheter-induced dissection, thromboembolism from AF, spontaneous dissection, etc., are several causes of RVMI.[14] The signs and symptoms of RVMI are presented in **Table 1**.

Right Ventricle in Pulmonary Embolism

After MI and stroke, PE is the most common cause of CV death. Among patients with PE, approximately 45% experience compromised RV function.[15] PE is characterized by acute obstruction of the pulmonary artery by a thrombus, leading to impaired RV filling and reduced output,[16] which increases RV afterload. When thrombus obstruction affects >50–75% of the pulmonary circulation and pulmonary artery pressure (PAP) exceeds 40 mm Hg, it exacerbates RV afterload, potentially reducing coronary artery perfusion and increasing intramyocardial pressure, which can lead to RV ischemia. Symptoms of PE generally include worsening shortness of breath, dyspnea on exertion, fatigue, and sometimes hemoptysis.[15]

Right Ventricular Pulmonary Hypertention

The RV dysfunction commonly signifies PH, defined as a mean PAP ≥ 25 mm Hg at rest.[17] In RV function regulation, preload, afterload, and contractility play a vital role. Elevated

TABLE 1: Signs and symptoms of RVMI.

Common signs	Signs indicating impending hemodynamic instability	Signs of RVMI along with inferoposterior MI
Chest pain	Kussmaul's sign (increase in jugular venous pressure during inspiration)	Lower level of consciousness
Diaphoresis	Pulsus paradoxus (rapid decrease in systolic blood pressure during inspiration)	Hypotension (low blood pressure)
Nausea and vomiting	Tricuspid regurgitation murmur (heard on auscultation)	Elevated jugular venous pressure

RV afterload primarily induces RV wall stress during ejection. In RVPH, intricate interaction involving neuroendocrine and paracrine signaling is exacerbated by elevated afterload, resulting in myocardial ischemia, inflammation, fibrosis, and myocyte loss.[18] Prolonged elevation of pulmonary arterial pressure results in RV hypertrophy, eventual RVF, and death. Chronic pressure overload typically initiates RV hypertrophy, resulting in a change in the thickness of myocardium.[19] Typical signs of PH include dyspnea, fatigue, and syncope. Physical examination findings may show a parasternal lift, jugular venous distention, and a tricuspid regurgitant murmur.[10]

Cor Pulmonale

Cor pulmonale results from increased resistance in the pulmonary circulation due to conditions like chronic obstructive pulmonary disease or pulmonary hypertension, causing strain and enlargement of RV as it pumps against higher pressure in the lungs.[9,20] It arises from elevated right-sided filling pressures caused by PH associated with lung diseases. Elevated pulmonary vascular resistance refers to increased resistance to blood flow in the pulmonary circulation. This increased resistance causes higher pressure in the pulmonary arteries, which subsequently increases workload on RV of the heart, which further causes enlargement.[20] Symptoms include cough with expectoration, peripheral edema, distension of the abdomen, and hemoptysis. Common signs are tachypnea, tachycardia, cyanosis, barrel-shaped chest, crepitation, rhonchi, ascites, and obliteration of cardiac/liver dullness.[9]

DIAGNOSIS OF RIGHT VENTRICULAR DYSFUNCTION

Electrocardiography

Electrocardiography (ECG) serves as the initial diagnostic tool in the evaluation of patients suspected to have right heart (RH) issues. The AF is a common finding in these cases.[21] In patients with acute PE, RV dysfunction can manifest with specific ECG findings, including T-wave inversions in leads V_1–V_3, an S1Q3T3 pattern, and occasionally a right bundle branch block. The T-wave inversions in leads V_1–V_3 demonstrate the highest sensitivity and diagnostic accuracy for early detection of RV dysfunction associated with acute PE. Additionally, RVMI can be diagnosed using right precordial leads, where it typically presents as ST elevation in leads V3R and/or V4R. These ECG changes are pivotal in the prompt identification and management of RV dysfunction and MI involving the RV.[21] A QRS width of 140 ms demonstrates good sensitivity for diagnosing RV dilatation (>80%) and dysfunction (>95%). QRS duration prolongation ≥ 4 ms/year in TOF patients is associated with higher risks of sustained ventricular tachycardia and sudden cardiac death **(Box 2)**.[12]

BOX 2 Assessment of RV function through several devices and parameters.

ECG

- RV hypertrophy:
  - $RV_1 \geq 7$ mm
  - $SV_1 < 2$ mm
  - R/S ratio ≤ 1 in V_5–V_6
  - qR pattern in V_1
  - $RV_1 + SV_5/V_6 > 10.5$ mm
  - $RV_1 > RV_6$

Echo

- RV systolic function:
  - TAPSE < 17 mm
  - FAC < 35%
  - RVS′ < 10 cm/sec
  - RIMP (TDI) > 0.54
- RV diastolic function:
  - Tricuspid E/A, E/E′
- Global RV function:
  - MPI, FAC, 2D/3D strain
  - 3D volume, EF
- Regional RV function:
  - TAPSE, TDIS′
- RV–PA coupling:
  - TAPSE-PASP, RVFWL
  - PASP
- Other:
  - RVEF < 45%
  - RVGLS < –20%
  - RVLS apical, mid, basal

CMR

- Structure:
  - RV mass index
  - RVEDV index
  - RVESV index
  - Fibrosis assessment
  - RV SV and Svi
  - 4D flow
  - RV strain imaging
  - LGE

Hemodynamic parameters:

- PASP
- PADP
- PA pulse pressure
- CVP
- PAPi

(CVP: central venous pressure; EF: ejection fraction; FAC: fractional area change; LGE: late gadolinium enhancement; MPI: myocardial performance index; PA: pulmonary artery; PADP: pulmonary artery diastolic pressure; PAPi: pulmonary artery pulsatility index; PASP: pulmonary artery systolic pressure; RIMP: right ventricular index of myocardial performance; RV: right ventricular; RVEDV: right ventricular end-diastolic volume index; RVEF: right ventricular ejection fraction; RVESV: right ventricular end-systolic volume; RVFWL: right ventricular free wall longitudinal; RVGLS: right ventricular global longitudinal strain; RVLS: right ventricular longitudinal strain; RVS′: right ventricular stroke volume; SV: stroke volume; Svi: stroke volume index; TAPSE: tricuspid annular plane systolic excursion; TDIS′: right ventricular systolic wave on tissue Doppler imaging)

Echocardiography

Echocardiography (echo) is pivotal in imaging diagnostics for its accessibility, noninvasiveness, and cost-effectiveness. One of its significant advantages is its capability to be performed at the patient's bedside, making it particularly useful in critically ill patients. In intensive care settings, both point-of-care cardiac ultrasound and transesophageal echo are commonly employed for the assessment of RH function. These modalities provide detailed and real-time information crucial for managing critically ill patients with suspected RH issues.[21]

Cardiac Magnetic Resonance

Cardiac magnetic resonance (CMR) imaging is considered a golden standard in the assessment of RV morphology, mass, volumes, and systolic function. In CHD, CMR is invaluable for high-quality 3D anatomical reconstruction and is essential for volumetric measurements, assessing myocardial fibrosis, evaluating great vessels, and analyzing flow-related parameters in the PA. Generally, CMR is used for the visualization of PA, aorta, and systemic and pulmonary veins. On CMR, signs of RV dysfunction include a large RV volume, reduced right ventricular ejection fraction (<45%), and reduced LV volume.[12] The CMR is applicable in assessing the RV despite its variable geometric configuration, but its use may be limited by cost and availability in certain countries and centers **(Box 2)**.[21]

Biomarkers

Biomarkers play a crucial role in the identification and monitoring of RVF progression. They are classified into two types: Inflammatory and stress biomarkers.[21] Elevated troponin levels signify RVMI, while elevated plasma natriuretic peptides such as N-terminal proBNP indicate RVF.[22] The BNP levels are high in atrial and ventricular septal defects, linked to shunt severity and PH. In tetralogy of Fallot, BNP relates to RV dilation, pulmonary regurgitation severity, and exercise ability. It also correlates with tricuspid regurgitation severity and predicts HF, transplantation need, and mortality in systemic RV.[12] High-sensitivity troponins (hsTns) are utilized to forecast adverse outcomes and RV dysfunction in acute PE and precapillary PH. In CHD, increased levels of blood hsTns are associated with RV dysfunction.[12] In PH and ischemic cardiomyopathy, cartilage intermediate layer protein 1 (CILP1) serves as a novel biomarker indicating cardiac dysfunction.[21] The CILP1 concentrations were higher in PH patients with maladaptive RV remodeling.[22] Inflammatory biomarkers such as suppressor of tumorgenicity 2 (ST2) and soluble ST2 reflect RV remodeling, hypertrophy, and fibrosis, while galectin-3 correlates with RV function in isolated PH.[12,21] Elevated levels of microRNA-21 are generally associated with a high

TABLE 2: Specific biomarkers for diagnosis of RV dysfunctions.

RV dysfunction-related conditions	Biomarker	Release characteristics
RV ischemia	Troponin I, Troponin T	Troponin released into systemic circulation; released from RV ischemia-induced myocardial injury
Acute PE	Troponin	Released into the systemic circulation in response to RV myocardial ischemia in acute PE
	BNP or NT-proBNP	Released as a result of increased myocardial wall stress in the setting of RV dysfunction due to PE
PH	BNP, NT-proBNP	–
Acute PE	hFABP, GDF-15, copeptin	–
		–
		–

(GDF: growth differentiation factor; hFABP: heart-type fatty acid–binding protein; NT-proBNP: N-terminal pro-B-type natriuretic peptide; PE: pulmonary hypertension; RV: right ventricle)

Source: Pradhan et al.[23]

occurrence of myocardial fibrosis and worsening RV function in TOF.[12] Thus, diagnosis plays a crucial role in identifying conditions and formulating effective management strategies **(Table 2)**.

MEDICAL MANAGEMENT STRATEGIES FOR RIGHT VENTRICULAR SUPPORT

The HF Association and the Working Group on Pulmonary Circulation and Right Ventricular Function of the European Society of Cardiology (ESC) have recently released comprehensive guidelines for managing acute RVF. These guidelines emphasize the importance of assessing severity, understanding the underlying causes, and promptly identifying anatomical and physiological specifics to initiate appropriate treatment.[1] An overview of acute RVF management strategies is depicted in **Flowchart 1**. Medical management of acute RVF involves addressing reversible causes like acute coronary syndrome or PE. Initial interventions include coronary revascularization or thrombolytic therapy, followed by medical treatments aimed at optimizing RV function and reducing pulmonary vascular resistance. It involves optimizing fluid volume, administering inotropic therapy, and providing vasopressor support.

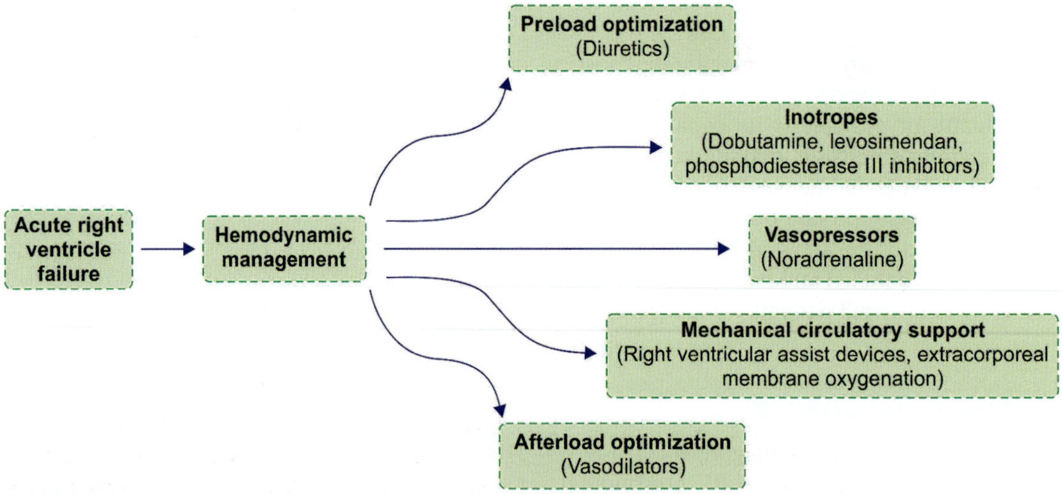

FLOWCHART 1: Overview on the management of acute RVF.

TABLE 3: RV support strategies and indications.[1,25]

Strategies	Specific treatment/drugs	Indication/use
Volume optimization	Diuretics	Managing volume overload in the RV
Restoration of perfusion pressure	Vasopressors—noradrenaline	To restore arterial blood pressure
Improvement of myocardial contractility	RV inotropy—dobutamine, levosimendan, phosphodiesterase III inhibitors	To improve contractility and cardiac output
Mechanical circulatory support devices	Extracorporeal membrane oxygenation (ECMO) or life support (ECLS)	Can provide short-term mechanical support, cost-effective, and easy insertion
	Paracorporeal right ventricular assist devices (RVADs)	Can be used for 4 weeks and can be combined with oxygenators
	Percutaneous catheter-mounted microaxial pumps	Can be used in high-risk percutaneous coronary intervention

Volume optimization is done in case of overload where diuresis is indicated. In case of hemodynamic instability, vasopressors are recommended. Norepinephrine is preferred for systemic hypotension and organ perfusion. Inotropes like dobutamine, levosimendan, and milrinone enhance cardiac function; dobutamine is optimal for RVF but can decrease systemic pressure, necessitating vasopressor use if needed.[10,24] The strategies and drug indications are depicted in **Table 3**.

Management Strategies for Right Ventricular Dysfunctions

A PE is the major cause of RVF which causes mortality. In August 2019, the ESC and the European Respiratory Society issued updated guidelines for diagnosing and managing PE.[1] According to ESC guidelines (2019), treatment for acute PE involves several strategies aimed at preventing early mortality and restoring pulmonary perfusion. Oral anticoagulants like dabigatran or edoxaban are commonly used in order to avoid further clot formation and manage long-term anticoagulation. For patients at a high risk of PE, initial treatment often includes parenteral anticoagulants such as intravenous unfractionated heparin, subcutaneous low-molecular-weight heparin (enoxaparin, tinzaparin, dalteparin), or subcutaneous fondaparinux. These agents have been rigorously studied for safety and efficacy in clinical trials. Thrombolytic therapy is another option, preferred for its ability to rapidly restore pulmonary perfusion compared to anticoagulants alone. When anticoagulant therapy is contraindicated, venous filters may be implanted to prevent further embolism.[26]

The PH results in high mortality and morbidity and the main consequence of PH is RVF which can further affect many organs.[25] In a patient with PAH presenting with signs of acute decompensated RVF, careful assessment for impaired venous return is crucial, distinguishing between pressure and volume overload in RVF.[27] Several pharmacological options for PH in acute RVF are presented in **Flowchart 2**.

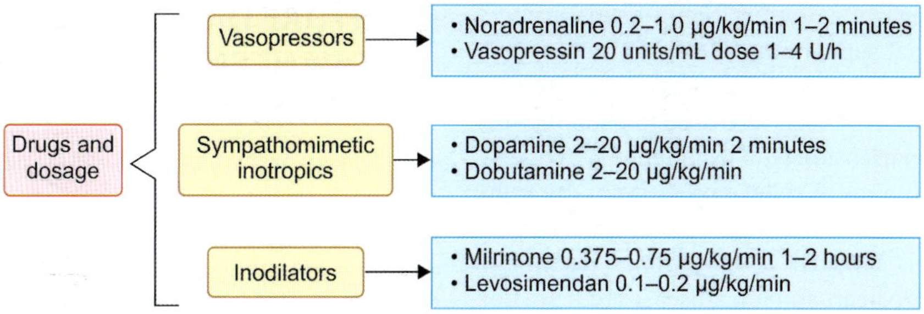

FLOWCHART 2: Recommended drugs and dosage for PH patients with a risk of RV failure.[27]

The occurrence of acute RV infarction alongside acute MI is significantly influenced by age.[25] Initial management includes preload optimization followed by the usage of inotropes like dobutamine and milrinone to improve contractility. Several devices for mechanical circulatory support (MCS) are commonly used.[28] Studies have confirmed that digitalis has a modest beneficial effect on the failing RV in patients with chronic cor pulmonale.[20] Moreover, the RV in cases of pressure overload, particularly in young patients, is often highly dependent on preload. Therefore, loop diuretics usage approached cautiously.[12]

SURGICAL AND INTERVENTIONAL THERAPIES

For patients with refractory RVF despite medical therapy, or those with progressive disease despite maximal treatment, surgical or percutaneous interventions are recommended.[29]

Mechanical Circulatory Support for Right Ventricular Failure

Some patients may find relief from persistent RVF through MCS. This approach is expanding with the utilization of both percutaneous and surgical devices designed to assist the RV.[29]

Percutaneously delivered advanced mechanical circulatory support (AMCS) devices for RVF (RV-AMCS) represent a modern approach allowing early intervention without surgery. Options include venoarterial extracorporeal membrane oxygenation (VA-ECMO), the TandemHeart® centrifugal-flow pump, and the Impella RP® catheter. These devices can be categorized by their mechanisms: Direct RV bypass (Impella RP®, TandemHeart-RVAD®, ProtekDuo®) and indirect RV bypass (VA-ECMO) **(Table 4)**. Direct bypass devices redirect blood from the right atrium to the pulmonary artery, bypassing the RV directly. In contrast, VA-ECMO reroutes blood from the right atrium to the femoral artery for oxygenation before returning it to the systemic circulation, indirectly bypassing the RV. The choice between direct and indirect RV bypass systems influences hemodynamic effects, especially in scenarios of isolated RVF versus biventricular failure.[24] The Impella RP® involves the insertion of a microaxial flow pump with inflow from the inferior vena cava or right atrium and outflow into the pulmonary trunk, resulting in adequate gas exchange through the lungs.[30] Understanding these distinctions is crucial for selecting the most appropriate device based on the clinical context.

Short-term extracorporeal CF-RVADs offer significant advantages over traditional surgical temporary RV assist devices temporary right ventricular assist device (t-RVAD). Unlike older models that require an open sternotomy or thoracotomy for implantation and removal, CF-RVADs can be inserted and removed without reoperation. This system provides up to 30 days of support with blood flow up to 10 L/min, offering extended and robust assistance to patients with RVF. These advancements significantly reduce the invasiveness and complexity of temporary RVAD therapy. For more durable and long-term support, surgically deployed rotary-flow RVADs, isolated pulsatile RVADs, and biventricular support with pulsatile VADs or total artificial heart replacement are better options during hospitalizations.[1]

Surgical Procedures

The CentriMag™ device (Thoratec Corporation) is the leading choice among surgically implanted centrifugal pumps, capable of producing flows up to 10 L/min. It has shown promising outcomes in effectively weaning patients with HF who need temporary right ventricular support.[31] Pulmonary thromboendarterectomy is the preferred curative treatment for chronic thromboembolic PH, benefiting functional status, exercise tolerance, quality of life (QoL), and survival. It is effective for proximal lesions but unsuitable for those with greatly elevated pulmonary vascular resistance exceeding 1,000–1,200 dyn/cm. Surgical embolectomy or percutaneous embolectomy is a potential intervention for acute RVF in cases of massive PE.[10] The surgical procedure is performed through median sternotomy and extracorporeal circulation, which involves aortic and bicaval cannulation. Both venae cavae are snared to isolate the inflow of the RH. The embolic material is typically removed using forceps and suction, with Fogarty catheters being used rarely.[30] Similarly, balloon atrial septostomy (BAS) is an emergent and essential cardiac interventional procedure used to stabilize neonates with CHD.[32] It is also used in patients with pulmonary arterial hypertension who experience syncope or have refractory RVF. It aims to relieve pressure in the right atrium and RV, thereby increasing cardiac output. Heart-lung transplantation is considered the ultimate treatment option for certain severe heart and lung diseases that are not responsive to other therapies, offering a potential cure and significant improvement in QoL for eligible patients.[10] The summary of surgical t-RVADs is depicted in **Table 5**. Other surgically implanted t-RVADs include Capiox® or Gyro pump, Deltastream, AB5000, Thoratec PVAD, and Rotaflow.[33]

FUTURE DIRECTION AND ADVANCEMENT IN RIGHT VENTRICULAR SUPPORT

Research in the RV is increasingly emphasizing pharmacological and device-centered therapies. Advancement in RVF management emphasizes the need for innovative therapies and early detection using molecular imaging and novel biomarkers. PERKAT-RV, also known as NovaPump, is an advanced device designed to provide minimally invasive mechanical support for the RH. It builds upon the pulsatile support technology used in intra-aortic balloon pump therapy, aiming to enhance treatment with a less invasive approach.[29]

TABLE 4: Mechanical circulatory support (MCS) for RV failure.

Mechanical support devices	
Microaxial flow transvalvular right ventricular assist devices (RVAD)	Impella RP® catheter
Extracorporeal centrifugal-flow percutaneous RVAD	TandemHeart® centrifugal-flow pump
	Venoarterial extracorporeal membrane oxygenation (VA-ECMO)
	ProtekDuo®

TABLE 5: Summary of frequently used t-RVADs.

Device	Implantation and configuration	Feature	Advantage	Disadvantage	Contraindication
ProtekDuo®[34-36]	A percutaneously inserted dual-lumen cannula placed via the right IJV, which extends to the main PA with inflow ports in the RA and distal outflow ports in the main PA	Provides flow up to 3.9 L/min for RV support	Early ambulation, reduced dependency on mechanical ventilation, enhanced RV function, decreasing RV transmural filling pressure, patient comfort and mobility	Bleeding, infection, air embolism, and device clotting	With internal jugular vein stenosis or thrombosis, right-sided mechanical valves, severe tricuspid or pulmonic stenosis
Impella RP®[24,33,36]	The device is introduced through a 23F venous peel-away sheath into the PA using a 0.018-inch wire as a monorail system, accessed via one venous site, commonly the RFV; after placement, the 23F sheath is exchanged with a staged 11F to 23F repositioning sheath	Microaxial pump capable of achieving flow rates up to 4.5 L/min	In isolated RV failure, reduce RA pressure, increase mean PA pressure, and increase LV preload	Bleeding and hemolysis	In right-sided mechanical valves, severe tricuspid or pulmonic stenosis, mural thrombus of the RA or inferior vena cava
TandemHeart®[36]	Two 21F cannulas are used: one placed in the RA for inflow, typically via the LFV, and the other in the PA for outflow, typically via the RFV; if anatomical constraints prevent placing the outflow cannula via the femoral vein, a right internal jugular approach can be employed	Capable of delivering up to 4 L/min of blood flow	Allows addition of oxygenator	Limited patient mobility	With right-sided mechanical valves and severe tricuspid or pulmonic stenosis

Continued

Continued

Device	Implantation and configuration	Feature	Advantage	Disadvantage	Contraindication
CentriMag™[33,36,37]	Surgically (sternotomy) via direct cannulation of RA (inflow) and PA (outflow), minimally invasive surgical approach via left-sided mini-thoracotomy to suture the outflow cannula of t-RVAD with PA and t-RVAD inflow via Fem. V, by peripheral cannulation of the Fem. V and direct cannulation of the PA, percutaneously via ProtekDuo,® percutaneously peripheral cannulation of the femoral vein and a percutaneous PA cannula	Extracorporeal centrifugal-flow pump capable of generating up to 10 L/min of flow	Variable configurations enable the addition of an oxygenator as needed	Increased risks of bleeding and infection	To use as a cardiotomy suction device and patients who are unable or unwilling to be treated with heparin or an appropriate alternative anticoagulant
Peripheral VA-ECMO[33]	A drainage cannula (inflow) is typically inserted within RA via a femoral vein approach, and a reinfusion cannula is positioned within the descending aorta, typically in the iliac artery	Used for isolated LV failure, RV failure, biventricular failure, or other causes of cardiopulmonary collapse	Ease of cannulation	LV distension and necessitates secondary arterial access for LV unloading in biventricular failure	Severe peripheral arterial disease, aortic regurgitation, and intolerance to anticoagulation

(F: French; IJV: internal jugular vein; LFV: left femoral vein; PA: pulmonary artery; RA: right atrium; RFV: right femoral vein)

The development of ambulatory RV-AMCS systems aims to enhance patient mobility and QoL. Fully implantable devices represent a step toward reducing infection risks associated with percutaneous drivelines and improving long-term patient management.[24]

High-dose dapagliflozin (DAPA) treatment in PAH-induced right heart failure (RHF) rats improves RV structure/function, attenuates Cx_{43} remodeling, enhances conduction velocity, and reduces arrhythmia susceptibility. Even low-dose DAPA treatment exhibited notable antiarrhythmic effects in pulmonary artery hypertension-induced RHF, underscoring its potential therapeutic utility across different dosages in managing cardiac complications associated with PH-induced RHF. These findings highlight dapagliflozin as a promising candidate for mitigating both structural and functional cardiac impairments in this pathological condition.[38] A recent multicenter study recommends simultaneous implantation of RV-MCS during LVAD placement, linking it to enhanced 1-year survival and a greater likelihood of successful RV support withdrawal compared to delayed insertion postoperatively,[39] thus suggesting a significant step forward in therapeutic strategies for RV conditions.

CONCLUSION

Enhancing RV function not only complements LV care but also plays a pivotal role in comprehensive HF management. By focusing on pharmacological, surgical, and mechanical interventions tailored to RV support, clinicians can address the multiple challenges of HF more effectively. Improved RV function translates not only to enhanced hemodynamics but also to better patient QoL, offering a holistic approach to optimizing outcomes in HF management.

ONLINE REFERENCES

Please scan the QR code provided at the end of the table of contents for References of this chapter.

SECTION 17

Vascular Interventions

Section Outline

CHAPTER

190

Advances in the Management of Chronic Limb Ischemia

Manoj Kumar Agarwala, Rufus Demel X

ABSTRACT

Chronic limb ischemia is the most severe type of peripheral artery disease, with high mortality and morbidity. Revascularization, whether surgical or endovascular, is the treatment option for the majority of patients. Despite advances in revascularization, there are still individuals who do not qualify for revascularization due to insufficient targets or the disease's diffuse nature. Several creative approaches and technologies are in development or in early use, which could give new answers.

Keywords: Peripheral arterial disease, chronic limb ischemia

INTRODUCTION

Peripheral arterial disease (PAD) is one of the most underappreciated and undertreated atherosclerotic vascular illnesses in India. PAD is more prevalent in low- and middle-income countries than in high-income countries. In India, PAD prevalence ranges from 7.6 to 26.7%.[1,2] Medical management and revascularization remain the foundation for treating chronic limb ischemia (CLI). Chronic limb ischemia is becoming more common, necessitating the development of new treatment alternatives that are both effective and long-lasting. This review discusses current advancements in the management of CLI.

ADVANCES IN THE MANAGEMENT OF CHRONIC LIMB ISCHEMIA

- Tools to assess perfusion and evaluate wounds
- *Endovascular techniques for lower extremity reconstruction*:
  - Retrograde pedal access
  - Below-the-knee (BTK) angioplasty
- *New endovascular devices*:
  - Implants for postangioplasty dissections
  - Bare-metal stent in BTK arteries
  - Drug-eluting stent (DES) in BTK arteries
  - Bioabsorbable scaffolds
  - Serrated balloon angioplasty
  - Intravascular lithoplasty (IVL)
- Percutaneous deep venous arterialization
- *Advances in drug delivery*:
  - Drug delivery to the adventitia
  - New delivery systems for sirolimus
- Gene and cell-based therapy

TOOLS TO ASSESS PERFUSION AND EVALUATE WOUNDS

Perfusion plays a crucial role in wound healing as well as enabling the survival of healthy tissue. Up to 20% of CLI patients may not recover after revascularization.[3] Microvascular flow and alterations in tissue perfusion that impact wound healing cannot be evaluated by angiography.

There are two ways to measure intraoperative perfusion—(1) perfusion angiography and (2) laser-assisted fluorescence angiography. Reconstructive plastic surgery already uses laser-assisted fluorescence angiography assessment to monitor tissue flap perfusion. Using this technology, Colvard et al.[4] prospectively analyzed 93 patients both pre- and postrevascularization, showing a significant increase in perfusion after an intervention. With digital subtraction angiography, perfusion angiography measures perfusion based on the time-density curve of contrast volume flow in the foot using postprocessing software. Reproducibility is very poor. Perfusion readings will be considerably distorted by even tiny movements.[5]

External perfusion monitors that are capable of measuring changes in perfusion after an intervention includes laser speckle imaging, hyperspectral imaging, and laser Doppler flowmetry. To see tissue perfusion, laser speckle imaging calculates backscatter from coherent laser light. It is unaffected by calcification, in contrast to ABI.[6] Hyperspectral imaging uses the visible and infrared spectral range to quantify superficial tissue oxygenation by measuring oxyhemoglobin and deoxyhemoglobin, both correlated with ulcer healing.[7]

An early window of opportunity to intervene will be provided by "smart" real-time remote monitoring of perfusion during or after an intervention, allowing for the prompt identification of hemodynamic alterations. An implantable biosensor that integrates with tissue, the Lumee Oxygen Platform (Profusa, Emeryville, CA, USA) continuously monitors subcutaneous oxygen levels. A prospective, single-arm, open-label, and multicenter study OMNIA (oxygen monitoring near ischemic areas) enrolled 35 CLI patients who had endovascular procedures in order to investigate the relationship between revascularization success, conventional measures of gross hemodynamic characterization, and Lumee measurement of tissue perfusion. According to the OMNIA data, individuals who underwent wound healing had notably greater increase in tissue oxygenation during interventions compared to those who did not.

Wireless interfaces and embedded sensors are being developed into "smart" stents. These sensors provide real-time data to a remote detector by utilizing microelectromechanical systems (MEMS) to forecast changes in local pressure distribution brought on by in-stent stenosis or thrombosis.[8]

NEW TECHNIQUES FOR LOWER EXTREMITY RECONSTRUCTION IN CLI

Retrograde Access

Antegrade crossing techniques via transfemoral access can be difficult and lead to technical and clinical failure when treating patients with CLI due to a lengthy or calcified lesion. Subintimal methods are similarly unsuitable in BTK arteries due to lack of reentry devices and difficulties in reentering the true lumen using standard techniques.

After an antegrade effort failed, retrograde access via the popliteal artery was first used. Retrograde pedal access can be carried out with ultrasound guidance or under fluoroscopy. 90% of lesion crossing cases and 94% of successful retrograde access cases were found in a systematic review.[9] Research has also revealed commendable rates of limb salvage—55% at 24 months and 77% at 18 months.[10,11] A review of 554 retrograde tibioperoneal access procedures was conducted by Schmidt et al.,[12] and found 95% of the instances resulted in effective lesion crossing. At 1 year, freedom from target lesion revascularization (TLR) and restenosis for CLTI were 62% and 36%, respectively. In 14.8% of cases, there was a vessel spasm; vascular site problems were uncommon (3.3%), and vessel occlusion was reported in three cases.

BTK Angioplasty

Several clinical researches have shown that the presence of pedal artery disease leads to poor wound healing. As a result, supplemental revascularization for pedal artery disease may speed up wound healing time. The pedal-plantar loop approach has been defined as a method for recanalizing blocked pedal arteries and the plantar arch. Patency after revascularization improves with patent pedal vessels and plantar arch, which is related with faster wound healing. The RENDEZVOUS registry[13] was a multicenter registry that included patients with CLI presenting with infrapopliteal arterial disease who underwent endovascular therapy (EVT) at five experienced cardiovascular centers in Japan. The study concluded that patients who underwent pedal artery angioplasty had a higher rate of wound healing and a shorter time to heal. Pedal angioplasty's long-term patency, however, has not been evaluated and is probably restricted.

NEW DEVICES FOR REVASCULARIZATION IN CLI

Treatment of Postangioplasty Dissection

Balloon angioplasty works by expanding the artery wall, which results in adventitial straining, plaque breakage, and local dissection. Angiographically apparent postangioplasty dissection occurs in up to 56% of instances and is related with poor patency and a 3.5-fold increased risk of TLR. Flow-limiting postangioplasty dissections have historically been treated with a stent placed along the length of the dissection. However, stents can fracture, limit future revascularization options, and cause chronic inflammation, which leads to intimal hyperplasia and in-stent restenosis. There are currently no FDA-approved stents for the BTK arteries. Development has proven difficult due to the high mobility and dynamic character of these arteries, as well as the tiny caliber and significant heterogeneity of different tibial segments. In general, spot repair has had better results than full metal jacket coverage.

The Tack Endovascular System is a first-of-its-kind, minimal-metal dissection repair device designed specifically for the precise treatment of post-PTA peripheral artery dissections to promote healing, improve outcomes, and save limbs. It is a short-segment, self-expanding nitinol scaffold designed for focal repair of postangioplasty dissections, with an 81% reduced metal burden than conventional stents **(Figs. 1 and 2)**.

The TOBA (Tack Optimized Balloon Angioplasty) trial, which included 130 patients with superficial femoral and popliteal artery disease, showed a 12-month patency rate

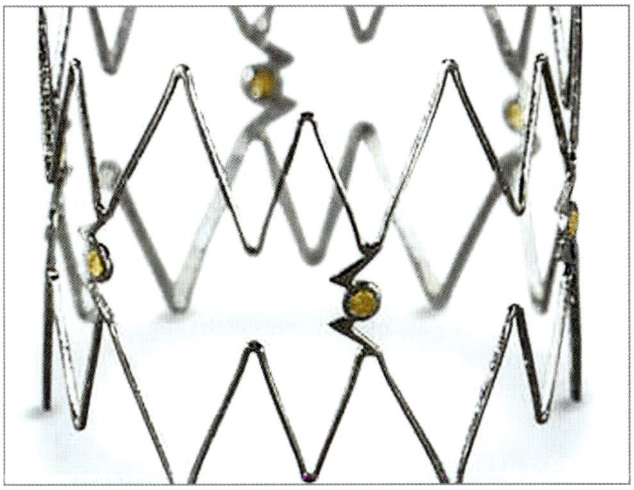

FIG. 1: Tack endovascular system.

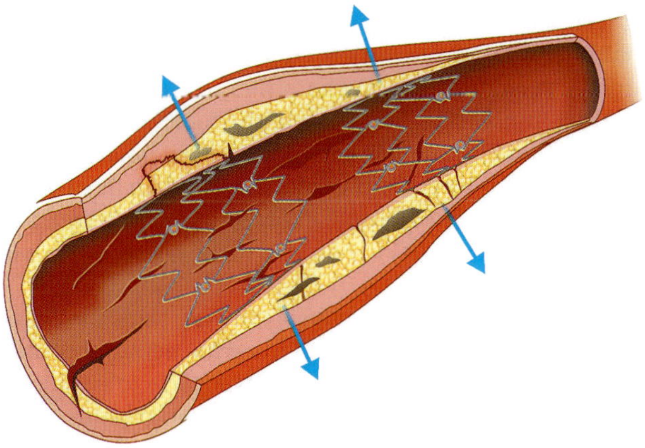

FIG. 2: Tack endovascular system implanted at the site of dissection.

of 76.4% and 89.5% independence from TLR.[14,15] The TOBA III trial[16] evaluated the safety and effectiveness of the Tack Endovascular System in patients with superficial femoral artery (SFA) and/or proximal popliteal artery (PPA) dissection after PTA with a drug-coated balloon (DCB) and found that the Tack Endovascular System was safe and effective at 24 months in patients who required post-PTA dissection repair in the SFA and PPA following DCB angioplasty for claudication and rest pain. In 233 patients with popliteal, tibial, and peroneal artery disease, the Tack Endovascular System was assessed as part of the TOBA II BTK study, With a 92% 6-month absence from clinically-driven TLR and an 87% 6-month target lesion patency, there was 100% technical success.[17]

Bare-metal Stent in Below the Knee Arteries

Treatment for BTK vascular disease has mostly consisted of angioplasty and off-label coronary stents for short lesions. The MicroStent peripheral vascular stent system (MicroMedical Solution, Wilmington, MA, USA) is a woven nitinol self-expanding bare-metal stent intended for the BTK arteries that may be deployed using either antegrade or retrograde access. Micro Medical Solutions has provided updates on its European HEAL postmarket registry and the United States STAND investigational device exemption (IDE) randomized controlled trial. The studies are assessing the company's MicroStent technology for the treatment of patients with chronic limb-threatening ischemia (CLTI)/critical limb ischemia, with results expected in early 2025.

Drug-eluting Stent in BTK Arteries

The purpose of the SAVAL trial was to evaluate the safety and efficacy of the SAVAL DES, a specially designed longer and flexible nitinol DES combined with paclitaxel for use in the arteries BTK. Patients with CLTI and infrapopliteal artery lesions with a total lesion length of at least 140 mm, stenosis of at least 70%, and Rutherford category 4–5 were enrolled in the prospective, multicenter, and randomized SAVAL trial and were divided 2:1 between treatment with the SAVAL DES, which is an expandable paclitaxel stent, or percutaneous transluminal angioplasty (PTA) using an uncoated balloon. When compared to PTA, this trial did not provide any advantages in terms of efficacy or safety using nitinol DES in infrapopliteal artery lesions up to 140 mm in length.

Bioabsorbable Scaffolds

Endovascular intervention's durability and success are severely hampered by the distinct pattern of infrapopliteal illness. The lower extremity vascular bed has relatively low flow with high resistance outflow. Although femoropopliteal endoluminal therapies have been developed, infrapopliteal occlusive disease still presents a therapeutic challenge. Drug-eluting resorbable scaffolds (DRS), which were first created for use in the coronary circulation, have become a potentially revolutionary treatment for BTK.

The CREDENCE BTK-1 (Clinical Outcomes of Sirolimus-Eluting Bioresorbable Peripheral Scaffold System Following Percutaneous Transluminal Angioplasty of Below-the-Knee Arteries in Patients With Critical Limb Ischemia) study a first-in-man, prospective, multicenter, and open-label study, was carried out at 12 different clinical centers throughout India. The study concluded that the Sirolimus-Eluting Bioresorbable Peripheral Scaffold System has favorable safety and performance in the treatment of CLI with no target lesion revascularization and scaffold thrombosis up to a 12-month follow-up following percutaneous transluminal angioplasty of below-the-knee arteries.[18]

TLR goal of the LIFE-BTK trial[19] is to assess the safety and effectiveness of a novel everolimus-eluting resorbable scaffold (Esprit BTK, Abbott Vascular) for the treatment of infrapopliteal artery disease in patients with CLI. It is a single-blind, randomized, controlled trial. The use of an everolimus-eluting resorbable scaffold was superior to angioplasty in 173 patients with CLTI caused by infrapopliteal artery disease in terms of freedom from amputation above the ankle of the target limb, occlusion of the target vessel, clinically driven revascularization of the target lesion, and binary restenosis of the target lesion at 1 year. The use of the scaffold was noninferior to angioplasty with regard to the primary safety end criterion (freedom from significant adverse limb events at 6 months and perioperative death).

There is a lot of attraction to a scaffolding system that prevents neointimal hyperplasia and leaves nothing behind. There are still unanswered concerns regarding the best antiproliferative medication, resorption kinetics, and material. Future research and clinical application of BTK DRS depend heavily on familiarity with the mechanical characteristics of the implanted device, the deployment protocol, and particular imaging modalities.

Scoring and Serrated Balloon Angioplasty

In order to aid in artery preparation during dilatation, the Serranator PTA Serration Balloon Catheter (Cagent Vascular, Wayne, PA, USA) is a balloon with four inserted exterior serrated metal strips designed to create linear interrupted scoring patterns. Microserration balloon angioplasty minimizes vascular damage while yielding a regulated, predictable lumen gain outcome. 25 patients with femoropopliteal lesions, were prospectively included in the PRELUDE (PRospective Study for the TrEatment of Atherosclerotic Lesions in the Superficial Femoral and/or Popliteal Arteries Using the Serranator Device) study[20] and found 1- and 6-month patency rates of 100% and 64%, respectively. The PRELUDE BTK study was conducted to assess the safety and efficacy of the Serranator PTA serration balloon catheter in patients with infrapopliteal peripheral artery disease, which demonstrated excellent lumen gain with minimal evidence of arterial injury and a low 6-month CD-TLR.[21]

Intravascular Lithoplasty

Angioplasty in calcified lesions is associated with limited patency and a high rate of bailout stenting. Calcification also hinders medications from being transferred to the artery wall during DCB angioplasty, which increases the likelihood of poor outcomes. IVL is a revolutionary technique for treating vascular calcification that employs acoustic shock waves. The Shockwave Medical Peripheral Lithoplasty System (Shockwave Medical, Fremont, CA, USA) uses pulsatile mechanical force to disrupt calcium while reducing artery stress, allowing for low pressure balloon angioplasty. The device has two types of catheters, the Shockwave M for the treatment of iliac and femoropopliteal lesions, and the Shockwave S for BTK lesions.

The Disrupt PAD I and Disrupt PAD II trials used IVL in 95 patients with femoropopliteal lesions with moderate-to-severe calcifications. Investigators observed low rates of bailout stenting and acceptable patency in this difficult group of patients.[22,23] The Disrupt PAD III RCT enrolled 306 patients with moderately-to-severely calcified femoropopliteal arteries treated with IVL (n = 153) or PTA (n = 153) prior to DCB treatment or stenting and found superior 1-year primary patency.[24] The Disrupt BTK trial demonstrated the safety of IVL in tibial artery disease with moderate-to-severe calcification in 20 patients with one posttreatment dissection and no evidence of embolization.[25] The Disrupt PAD BTK II Study is ongoing in a larger population.

PERCUTANEOUS DEEP VENOUS ARTERIALIZATION

Revascularization remains the primary mode of treatment for CLI. However, a considerable number of patients are unable to undergo revascularization due to a lack of eligible targets. In circumstances where there is no other option for providing arterial perfusion to the foot's capillary bed, venous arterialization has emerged as a potential solution. It was first introduced by Hastead and Vaughan in 1912 and has since been refined several times. The goal is to create an arteriovenous fistula (AVF) proximal to the diseased segment of the tibial arteries.

Transcatheter arterialization of the deep veins was found to be feasible and safe in patients with persistent limb-threatening ischemia who were unresponsive to traditional surgical or endovascular revascularization treatments by PROMISE I trial.[26] The PROMISE II trial[27] is a prospective, single-group, multicenter study that will assess the efficacy of transcatheter arterialization of the deep veins in patients with nonhealing ulcers and no surgical or endovascular revascularization therapy alternatives. The composite primary endpoint was 6-month amputation-free survival (defined as the absence of above-ankle amputation or death from any cause). A total of 105 patients were enrolled, and 66.1% of them survived without amputation after 6 months. This study showed that transcatheter arterialization of deep veins was safe and effective in individuals with persistent limb-threatening ischemia and no conventional surgical or endovascular revascularization therapy choices.

The meta-analysis revealed a technical success rate of 96.2% (95% CI 91.5–98.4), an overall survival rate of 82.8%, and a limb salvage rate of 77.2% throughout the follow-up. Amputation-free survival rates at 30 days, 6 months, and 1 year were 87.8%, 68.7%, and 65.6%, respectively. The arterialization of the deep veins resulted in a complete wound healing rate of 53.4%. The pooled reintervention rate reached 46.7%.[28] For individuals who do not have access to routine CLTI treatment, transcatheter arterialization of the deep veins appears to be a viable alternative. However, due to the small number of research, the strength of the evidence is limited.

NOVEL DELIVERY SYSTEMS FOR DCBs

Trials using sirolimus and everolimus in the lower extremities found no advantage over bare-metal stents. DCBs have transformed the treatment of peripheral artery disease. Despite their clinical usefulness, rates of restenosis, and bailout stenting remain high, particularly in more complicated lesions.

A novel over-the-wire angioplasty balloon catheter, the Chocolate Touch paclitaxel-coated PTA balloon catheter (TriReme Medical) divides the inflated balloon into sections that expand independently, producing a "pillow effect." The dilation component is mounted on a nitinol structure. This differential dilatation technique may reduce the risk of dissections and shield the vessel from harm. The Chocolate Touch Study is a prospective, multicenter, randomized trial that compared Lutonix paclitaxel DCB with the second-generation Chocolate Touch DCB. It found that, at 12 months, Chocolate Touch DCB was safer, more effective than Lutonix DCB for treating femoropopliteal disease, and noninferior in terms of primary patency.[29]

The Selution sirolimus-coated balloon (MedAlliance, Switzerland) employs a novel drug delivery technology that includes microreservoirs of biodegradable polymer intermixed with sirolimus, allowing for regulated and sustained release of sirolimus into the target tissue. Furthermore, it reduces wash off during balloon insertion and enhances target drug distribution during angioplasty, delivering roughly eight times more medication than existing DCBs. The SELUTION4BTK trial is a prospective, multicenter, single-blind, randomized, controlled experiment that found sirolimus-eluting technology can reduce distal embolization, improve wound healing, and increase amputation-free survival.[30]

GENE AND CELL-BASED THERAPY

Therapy for CLI is still restricted by further disease development and eventual limb ischemia, despite advancements in medicine and technology. Even now, not all patients can achieve long-term success with interventional and surgical revascularization, and many CLI patients may not be able to receive this treatment technically. Patients for whom revascularization is not an option now have new hope thanks to gene and cell therapy.

In refractory situations, the therapeutic application of viruses or proteins (angiogenic gene and protein therapies), as well as stem and progenitor cells (cell-based therapies), has emerged as viable approaches for targeting CLI. Despite promising preclinical and early-phase clinical investigations, further studies failed to establish the efficacy of gene and cell-based treatments, albeit their safety profile remains favorable. While the underlying causes of the failure of randomized large-scale studies have been extensively disputed, the implementation of alternative therapy is not recommended by current guidelines. While the medical demands of patients with CLI remain unmet, innovative treatment methods show significant promise in the clinic.[31]

CONCLUSION

The recent advances gives us a newer preview of the future management and treatment of CLI.

ONLINE REFERENCES

Please scan the QR code provided at the end of the table of contents for References of this chapter.

CHAPTER

191

Advances in Management of Acute Limb Ischemia

NN Khanna, Saurabh Bhardwaj

ABSTRACT

Acute limb ischemia (ALI) is a sudden decrease in blood supply threatening limb viability. Caused by embolism, atherosclerotic disease, hypercoaguable states, thrombophilia, occlusion, vasospasm, dissection, aneurysmal occlusion, compartment syndrome, adventitial cystic disease, foreign body embolization, iatrogenic, and trauma, it requires immediate attention.

Keywords: ALI, threat, causes

INTRODUCTION

Acute limb ischemia (ALI) is defined as a sudden decrease in the blood supply that threatens the viability of the limb. It is a condition that requires immediate attention to salvage the limb with prompt diagnosis and revascularization of the affected extremity, within 14 days.[1]

It is caused by multiple factors of which the most common is embolism, most commonly from the heart. Other important causes are atherosclerotic disease, hypercoaguable states (especially postCOVID), thrombophilia, occlusion of a previous bypass graft, vasospasm (Raynaud's phenomenon), dissection, aneurysmal occlusion, compartment syndrome, adventitial cystic disease, foreign body embolization in intravenous drug abusers, iatrogenic, and trauma **(Box 1)**.[2]

Embolization from a cardiac source passes easily through the large arteries and lodges peripherally, usually at an arterial bifurcation, where vessels naturally narrow. Emboli can occlude any artery, but in the legs, the common femoral and popliteal arteries are commonly obstructed. In the upper extremity, the brachial artery bifurcation and the brachial artery at the takeoff of the profunda brachialis artery are frequent locations for emboli.[3]

Another precipitating factor is arrhythmia like an underlying atrial fibrillation. Rarely embolism is caused by bacterial endocarditis, cardiac tumor, or paradoxically from the PFO.[4]

CLINICAL PRESENTATION (BOX 2)

As sensory and motor function is lost progressively from the distal to proximal part of the limb, a simple test of viability to assess the intactness of motor function is dorsiflexion of the big toe to resistance.[3]

Rutherford's classification[6] is used for clinical assessment and management. Assessment determines whether the limb is viable or irreversibly damaged. The distinction between

BOX 1 **Causes of acute limb ischemia.**

Causes:
- Embolism
- Atherosclerotic disease
- Hypercoaguable states (especially postCOVID)
- Thrombophilia
- Occlusion of previous bypass graft
- Vasospasm (Raynaud's phenomenon)
- Dissection
- Compartment syndrome
- Aneurysmal occlusion
- Foreign body embolization (IV drug abusers, iatrogenic)
- Embolization caused by bacterial endocarditis, cardiac tumor, or paradoxically from PFO
- Trauma

grade IIa and IIb, and between grade IIb and III, can sometimes be challenging. Prompt diagnosis and revascularization by means of catheter-based thrombolysis and/or thrombus-aspiration or by open surgery reduces the risk of limb loss and death. Primary amputation is recommended in patients with irreversible (Class III) ischemia **(Table 1)**.

IMAGING MODALITIES

Investigations are valuable in confirming the clinical diagnosis and planning the appropriate treatment for patients with acute ischemia.

Depending upon the emergency/urgency of the clinical scenario, a number of methods can be used to definitively determine the site and nature of the arterial occlusion.

Based on current evidence, duplex ultrasound (DUS), computed tomographic angiography (CTA), digital subtraction angiography (DSA), and contrast enhanced-magnetic resonance angiography (CE-MRA) can all be considered for imaging in patients with ALI, and may be used on the basis of local expertise, availability, and clinician preference.

BOX 2 Classic symptoms of 6 Ps.

Classic symptoms of 6 Ps:[5]

- *Pain*
- *Pallor*
- *Pulseless*
- *Poikilothermia (a cold limb)*
- *Paresthesia, and*
- *Paralysis*

The DUS is the preferred initial choice of investigation because it permits rapid bedside assessment.[7] CTA is the most commonly used imaging modality used and should be performed for treatment planning.[8] New-generation CT scanners acquire images at very high speed and are available in most emergency department. Barring concerns about contrast-induced nephropathy, CT angiography has thus become the investigation of choice for urgent investigation of acute arterial ischemia. The role of CE-MRA is limited, mainly because of limited availability and log examination time.[9]

MANAGEMENT

Once the diagnosis of acute ischemia has been established and its severity should be determined. Management constitutes the following:

- Anticoagulation
- Endovascular procedures
- Surgery
- Ancillary measures include analgesia, intravenous hydration, supplementary oxygen, and lowering the foot end of the bed (anti-Trendelenburg position).

The acuity of symptom onset and clinical manifestation of limb ischemia guides treatment strategies.[10]

Rutherford class I ischemia is a viable limb which is not immediately threatened, a window of time does exist to allow for completion of diagnostic studies, optimization of medical therapy, and appropriate risk stratification. If revascularization is opted, endovascular-first approach should be preferred.

Rutherford class II ischemia represents threatened limbs, mandating timely revascularization for limb salvage. This

TABLE 1: Rutherford's classification.[6]

Rutherford class	Prognosis	Sensory exam	Motor exam	Arterial Doppler	Venous Doppler	Skin exam	Initial therapy	Definitive therapy
Class I: Viable, not threatened	Not immediately threatened	Normal	Normal	Audible	Audible	Normal capillary return	Anticoagulation	Imaging and urgent revascularization
Class IIa: Marginally threatened	Salvageable with prompt therapy	Minimal loss	Normal	Often inaudible	Audible	Decreased capillary return	Anticoagulation	Imaging and emergency revascularization
Class IIb: Immediately threatened	Salvageable If treated immediately	Mild sensory loss and rest pain	Mild-to-moderately abnormal	Usually inaudible	Audible	Pallor	Anticoagulation	± Imaging and emergency revascularization
Class III: Irreversible	Irreversible tissue and nerve damage	Profound loss	Paralysis and rigor	Inaudible	Inaudible	No capillary return	Anticoagulation	Amputation

Source: Rutherford RB, Baker JD, Ernst C, et al. Recommended standards for reports dealing with lower extremity ischemia: revised version. J Vasc Surg. 1997;26:517-38.

class is subdivided into marginally (IIa) and immediately (IIb) threatened limbs based on severity of ischemic neurologic deficits.

In the marginally threatened limb (IIa), a less severe ischemic insult allows for greater consideration of an endovascular-first approach and emergent availability of vascular surgeons for failed endovascular intervention should all be considered in decision making.

With progression in extent of the sensory and the motor neurologic deficits, ALI is classified as immediately threatened (IIb) and requires emergent revascularization.

At this level of ischemia, the salvage of neurologically intact viable tissue is time-sensitive, favoring traditional open revascularization. An endovascular approach with more rapid means of revascularization, including aspiration or pharmacomechanical thrombectomy devices, may be considered.

In the most severe class of ALI (Rutherford class III), primary limb amputation should be elected as definitive therapy. The profound extent or duration of limb ischemia results in irreversible damage to nerve sensory and motor function, with limb paralysis.[10]

Initial management includes analgesia and intravenous (IV) heparin. Heparin anticoagulation has no direct thrombolytic effect; it is used to stabilize clot formation and prevent further secondary thrombosis. Anticoagulation for stable class I ischemia, followed several weeks later by intervention (usually endovascular) if collaterals do not become established, is safe and effective. Anticoagulation has been shown to improve results after embolectomy.

Endovascular Strategies

The primary goal of any endovascular intervention for ALI is rapid clearance of clot burden for restoration of normal limb perfusion **(Box 3)**.[11]

Catheter-directed Thrombolysis

Catheter-directed thrombolysis (CDT) remains a highly utilized therapy for management of viable (class I) and marginally threatened (class IIa) ALI. The procedure can be used for acute embolism or thrombosis of native arterial atherosclerotic lesions, autogenous vein and prosthetic bypass grafts, as well as intraluminal stents.[12] Thrombolysis is catheter-directed to minimize systemic effects, though contraindications do exist for use in patients at heightened risk of hemorrhagic complications. Clinical judgment and operator experience must guide the use of thrombolytic agents to maximize benefits against the risks, and minimize potential hemorrhagic complications. The technical aspects for arterial access, diagnostic imaging, and crossing occlusive lesions are similar for all endovascular therapies.

Usually a retrograde contralateral femoral approach is preferred for initial access as it allows placement of diagnostic catheters in patent vessels proximal to the thrombus.[8]

Antegrade approach is acceptable, and at times anatomically required, though care must be taken to minimize entrance and disruption of thrombus while obtaining access.[13]

Once a decision is made for endovascular therapy the patient is anticoagulated and a delivery sheath (usual size—45 or 55 cm 6-F) is placed over the aortic bifurcation. Delivery sheaths increase support for recanalization, and provide a more stable platform for indwelling lytic catheters. An angled wire of 0.035 inch is used to cross an acute occlusion. Judkins Right catheter is used upfront to facilitate wire advancement. The ease with which a guide wire passes through a thromboembolic occlusion ("guide wire traversal test") does correlate with technical success of CDT. A multitude of wires are available to help navigate tortuous stenoses. Coronary 0.014 inch wires are also used, but hydrophilic 0.018 inch wires provide greater support than 0.014 inch wires. After crossing the occlusion, aspiration of blood from the catheter suggests post-thrombus position, and a distal angiogram is performed to confirm true lumen and distal patency[14] (Refer to **Figs. 1 and 2**).

It is preferred to place a 5-F multipurpose catheter with multiple side holes for delivery of thrombolytic agents. The recommended thrombolytic agents are tissue plasminogen activator (TPA)—alteplase, tenecteplase, or urokinase. Usually 1–2 mg/hour of TPA or 2,000–4,000 unit/min of urokinase is given.

Monitoring can be done by measuring fibrinogen levels. Heparin infusion at a fixed rate of 500 units/h is instilled through the delivery sheath side port to prevent thrombosis.[8]

The results of the STILE trials helped frame our understanding of the increased benefit of thrombolysis for patients with acute ischemia of <2 weeks' duration, and the superior long-term freedom from recurrent ischemia and major amputation with surgical revascularization.[15,16]

BOX 3 Endovascular therapies.

Endovascular therapies may include any one the following:
- Catheter-directed thrombolysis (CDT)
- Pharmacomechanical thrombectomy (PMT), or
- Mechanical thrombectomy (MT)

Pharmacomechanical Thrombectomy

Pharmacomechanical thrombectomy (PMT) combines thrombolytic therapy with mechanical clot extraction, with the advantages of decreasing total lytic dose and duration of thrombolysis.[17] Procedural technique follows the same sequence as noted for CDT with ultrasound-guided arterial access, selective catheterization, and sheath placement, and diagnostic angiogram prior to endovascular therapy. The

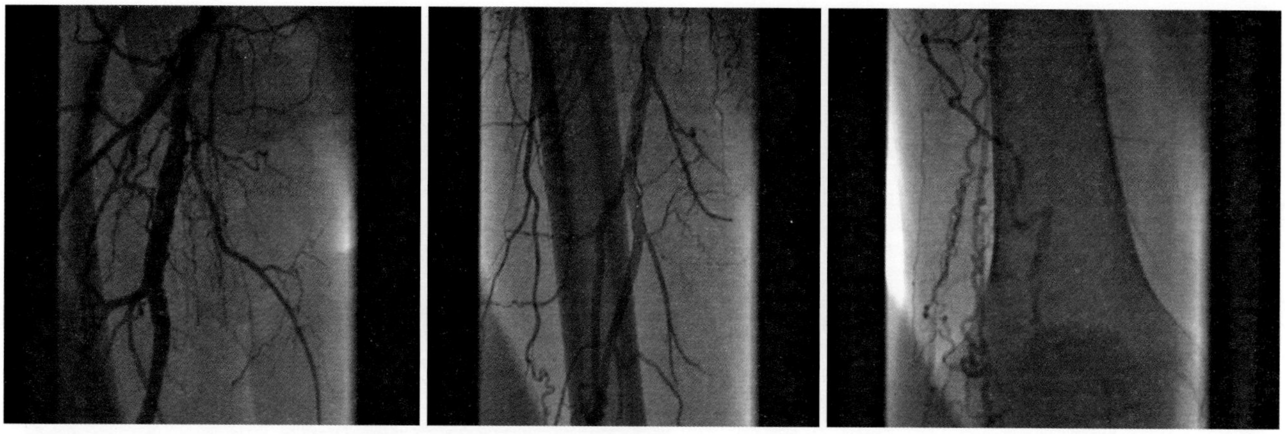

FIG. 1: Cine picture depicting complete occlusion of right superficial femoral artery (SFA).

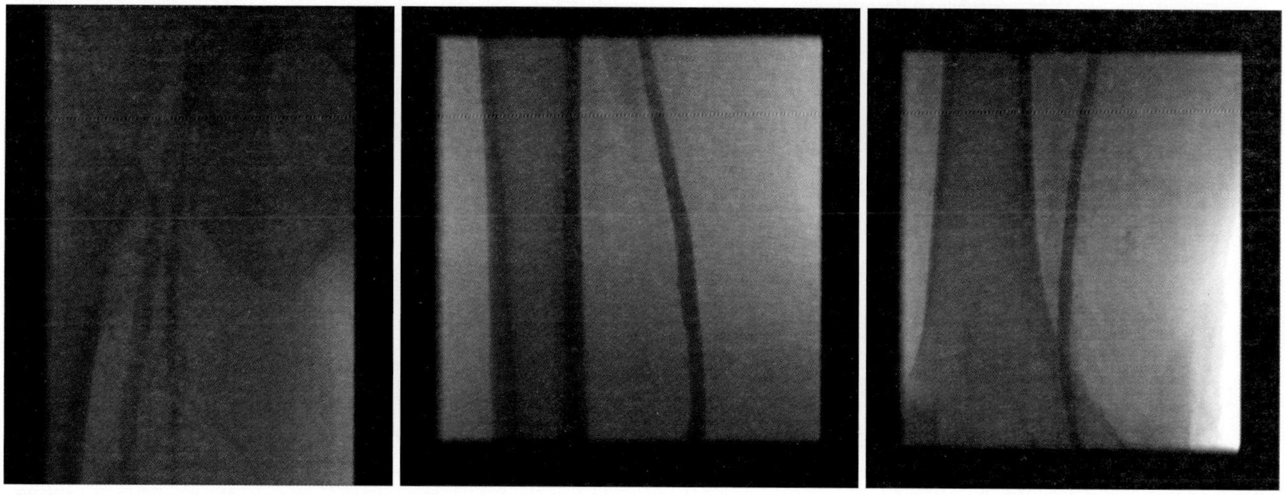

FIG. 2: Cine picture depicting opening of occluded artery.

Angiojet Rheolytic Thrombectomy System (Boston Scientific, Marlborough, MA) combines mechanical thrombectomy via high-velocity saline injection (creating venturi effect) with pulsatile delivery of thrombolytic agent[18] **(Fig. 3)**.

A wide range of catheter treatment lengths and diameters are available to complement arterial and venous obstructions. A control system console monitors the system and energizes a pump, which delivers high-velocity saline toward the catheter tip. The pressurized saline jets create an incredibly low-pressure zone at the distal catheter facilitating thrombus disruption, aspiration, and extraction. Clot extraction is enhanced with use of a "power-pulse spray" (P-PS) mode. Common protocols use 10 mg of rtPA in 50 mL of saline, with the system pump delivering 0.6 mL of lytic solution per pedal pump/pulse. A single antegrade and retrograde pass in P-PS mode is recommended advancing the catheter slowly at 0.5–1.0 mm increments, with the console monitoring maximum run times. The concentrated pulsed lytic agent dwells for 15–20 minutes prior to returning the AngioJet system to thrombectomy mode for clot extraction with a single antegrade and retrograde pass, followed by angiography. The PEARL Registry[19] (PEripheral use of Angiojet Rheolytic thrombectomy with a variety of catheter lengths) reported the contemporary use of the AngioJet system **(Fig. 3)** in management of ALI, with a focus on defining patient and anatomic factors associated with procedural success.

An alternative PMT device is the EKOS catheter[20] (EkoSonic Endovascular System, Boston Scientific, Marlborough, Massachusetts) **(Fig. 4)**. The catheter is a 5.4-F multi-lumen catheter with channels for lysis delivery, a central lumen for the ultrasonic core wire, and an adjacent central coolant lumen. Catheter working lengths come in 106 cm and 135 cm options, with treatment zones ranging

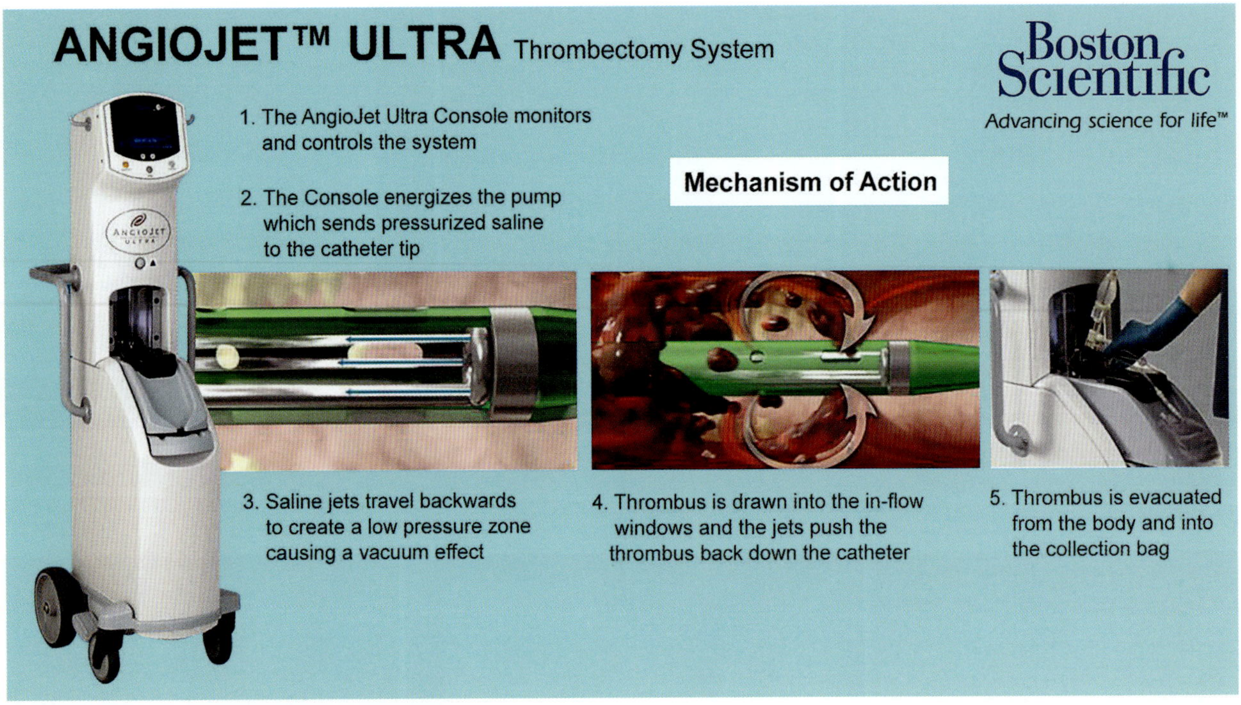

FIG. 3: Cartoon showing thrombectomy system.

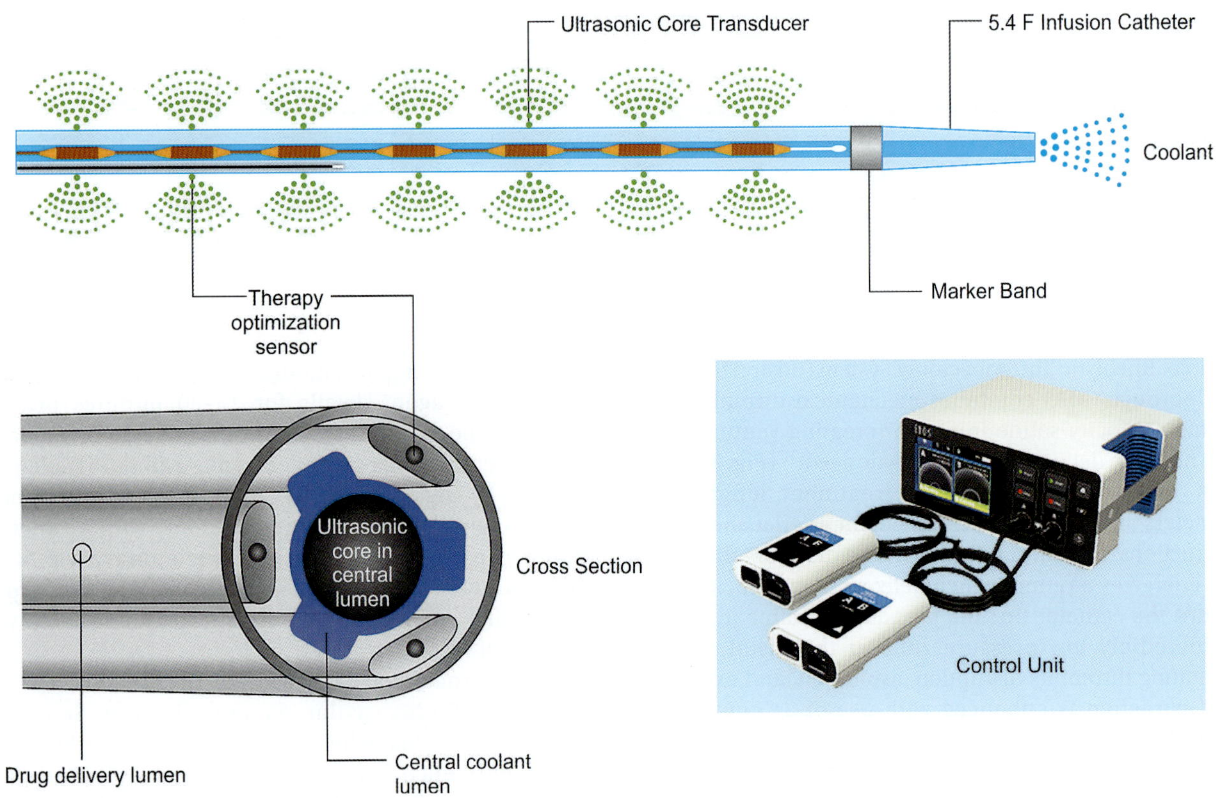

FIG. 4: EKOS catheter (EkoSonic Endovascular system).

6–50 cm. The ultrasonic core wire transducer elements are spaced 1 cm apart, with the ultrasound energy delivered simultaneously with infusions of lytic agent and coolant. Catheter temperature is monitored by the control unit, which can adjust ultrasound power to prevent overheating. The ultrasound waves propel lytic agent deeper into the thrombus and expose a greater surface area for thrombolysis. Studies have reported increased exposure of thrombus to rtPA with use of ultrasound, decreased procedure time and volume of lytic agent while increasing technical success. The DUET trial,[21] reported the results of a Dutch randomized trial comparing outcomes of ultrasound-accelerated thrombolysis (UST) against standard catheter directed thrombolysis (ST) for ALI **(Fig. 4)**.

Mechanical Thrombectomy

Mechanical thrombectomy uses aspiration, mechanical/rotational, or hydrodynamic forces to fragment and clear thrombus without infusion of a thrombolytic agent. A variety of devices exist with defined indications for use in arterial, venous, or dialysis graft occlusions.[22] Aspiration mechanical thrombectomy (AMT) catheters have gained popularity recently for the ability to remove fresh thrombus and emboli from peripheral arterial and venous vessels across a wide range of diameters.

The Indigo Aspiration Catheters (CAT, Penumbra, Inc, Alameda, CA) and Pronto catheter (Teleflex, NC) come in a range of catheter diameters and lengths to accommodate all arterial sizes.[23] Arterial access and sheath positioning are performed as with other endovascular devices. The aspiration catheters engage the angiographically localized thrombus. Robust data is limited on the technical success of AMT for ALI. The Mayo Clinic has recently reported a retrospective experience with use of Indigo aspiration catheters (Penumbra, Inc) in management of limb ischemia.[24]

Mechanical and rotational thrombectomy devices rely on fragmentation and simultaneous aspiration of thrombus to restore arterial flow. Several on-market devices are available, though none are used with great frequency in management of ALI.[25] Various mechanical thrombectomy catheters are enlisted in **Table 2**.

TABLE 2: Types of mechanical thrombectomy catheters.

Company	Device
Argon Medical Devices, Inc.	Cleaner 15, Cleaner XT
Boston Scientific Corporation	• AngioJet AVX thrombectomy catheter • AngioJet Solent (Dista, proxi, omni) thrombectomy catheter
Codman Neuro (Johnson & Johnson)	Revive PV peripheral vascular thrombectomy device
Inari Medical	Clot retriever, flow retriever system
Medtronic	Solitaire platinum
Penumbra Inc.	• *Indigo system catheters*: CAT8, CATD, CAT6, CAT5, CAT3, and CAT RX • *Indigo system separators*: SEP8, SEPD, SEP6, SEP5, SEP3, and SEPC4

POSTPROCEDURE COMPLICATIONS

The management of ALI is associated with significant systemic end-organ insults related to ischemia-reperfusion injury. With restored perfusion to tissue beds, rhabdomyolysis with myoglobinuria, as well as extremity compartment syndrome, must be monitored for.[26,27]

Lab evaluation should include baseline and surveillance creatine phosphokinase (CPK) levels, electrolyte abnormalities and acid-base status, as well as urinalysis for hemoglobinuria or myoglobinuria if oliguria or discolored urine is noted.[28,29]

In compartment syndrome, increased capillary permeability at the time of ischemic reperfusion causes localized edema and increased intramuscular compartment (compartmental) pressure, which leads to circulatory disturbance and neuromuscular dysfunction.[2,30] The lower limbs comprise four muscular compartments, and when the pressure within each compartment exceeds 30 mm Hg, irreversible nerve and muscle necrosis occurs, and in some instances, lower limb amputation is necessary even if revascularization is successful.[8]

If leg swelling is observed after revascularization, the pressure within each compartment is measured (via needle insertion), and if the pressure exceeds 30 mm Hg, then relaxation incision (fasciotomy) should be positively considered.[30]

CONCLUSION

The expansion and refinement of catheter-based interventions for ALI has allowed for a more patient-centric approach to limb salvage regardless of ischemic class. Recently published meta-analyses have confirmed comparable rates of limb salvage for catheter-based and surgical revascularization. The results of these large reviews suggest clinical equipoise in mortality and limb-salvage outcomes. Endovascular-first approach is probably a practical and useful approach in selected patients of ALI **(Flowchart 1)**.

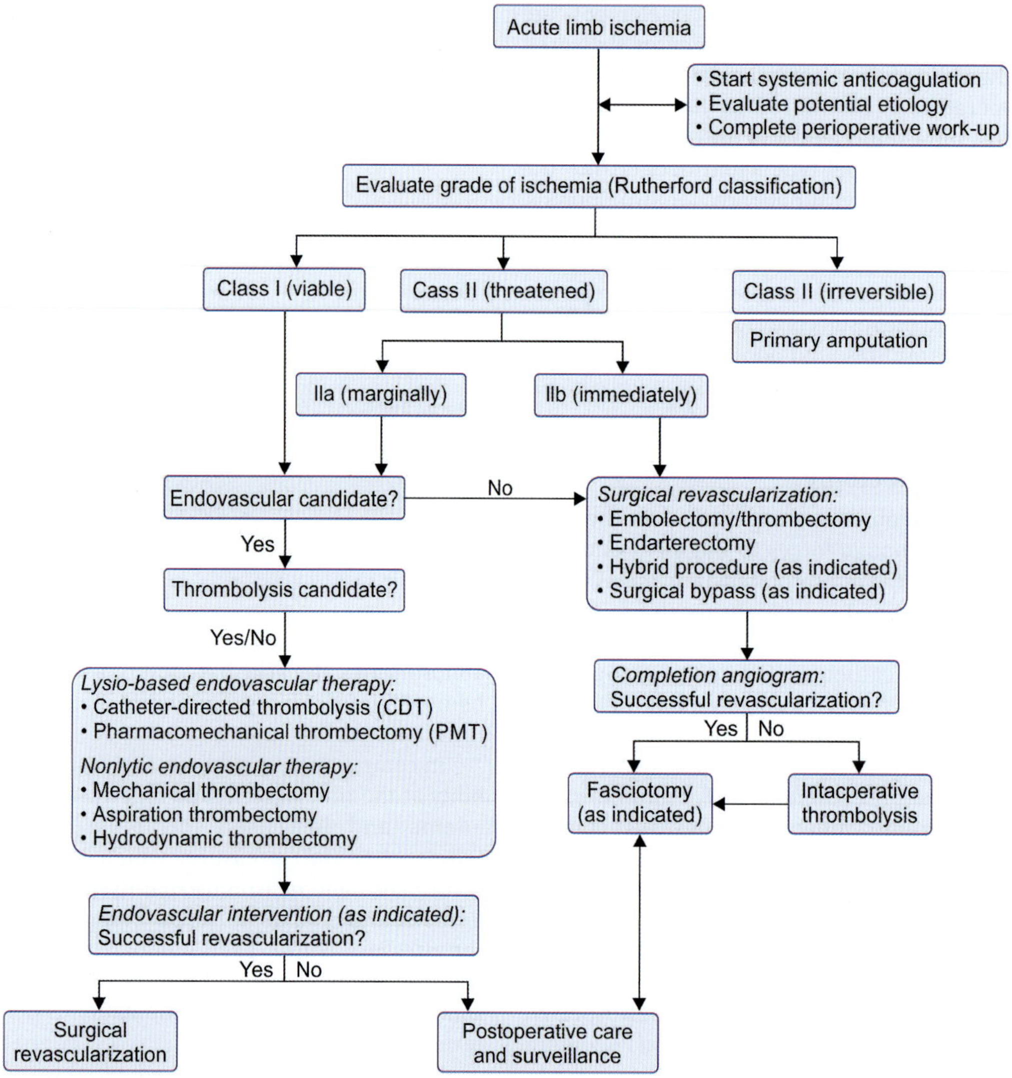

FLOWCHART 1: Algorithm approach to acute limb ischemia.

ONLINE REFERENCES

Please scan the QR code provided at the end of the table of contents for References of this chapter.

CHAPTER

192

Advances in the Management of Endovascular Treatment of Aortic Dissection

Sanjay Mehrotra

ABSTRACT

Aortic dissection is a devastating disease with high mortality and morbidity. Imaging is crucial for management. Most type B aortic dissections (TBADs) progress to aneurysms, increasing adverse events and mortality. Early thoracic endovascular aortic repair prevents aneurysm formation. Young patients may require reintervention, including further endovascular or surgical repair.

Keywords: Aortic dissection, disease, crucial, repair

INTRODUCTION

Aortic dissection is the most common catastrophe of aortic diseases that is two to three times more common than rupture of the abdominal aorta. A classic aortic dissection involves the formation of a dissection flap that divides the aorta into true and false lumens **(Figs. 1A to D)**.

CLASSIFICATION OF AORTIC DISSECTION

The standard classifications of aortic dissection that have been used traditionally and are widely accepted and recognized have been the Stanford classification and DeBakey classification.

Data from the International Registry suggested that acute aortic dissection is the most common emergency that involves the aorta and is associated with high mortality and morbidity more so in patients who have connective tissue disorders such as Marfan syndrome.[1]

Stanford classification is simple and is described to be of two types: Type A aortic dissection, when the dissection entry point is located proximal to the left subclavian artery, and type B, when the entry tear is located distal to the left subclavian artery.

On the other hand, in DeBakey classification, the aortic dissection was described as three types, which are as follows **(Fig. 2)**:

1. *DeBakey type I* includes dissection tear starting in the ascending aorta and involving the whole aorta, both ascending and descending.
2. *DeBakey type II* includes dissection confined to the proximal aorta.
3. *DeBakey type III* is further subdivided into two types: Type IIIa, which is confined to postsubclavian thoracic aorta only, and type IIIb, which involves both thoracic and abdominal aorta going up to the iliac arteries **(see Fig. 2)**.[2]

In the year 2020, the Society of Vascular Surgery and the Society of Thoracic Surgery reported a new classification, which may be a more descriptive anatomical classification incorporating the location of the tear in the classification where the aorta, in addition to the type based on Stanford (type A and type B), also divided the aorta into 12 zones locating the entry tear and extension, which was described as proximal and distal **(see Fig. 3)**.

A more descriptive classification includes type A and type B differentiation and extent location with numbers written along which expands the understanding **(Fig. 4)**.

Aortic dissection can also be described according to the clinical presentation, which may be as risk stratification

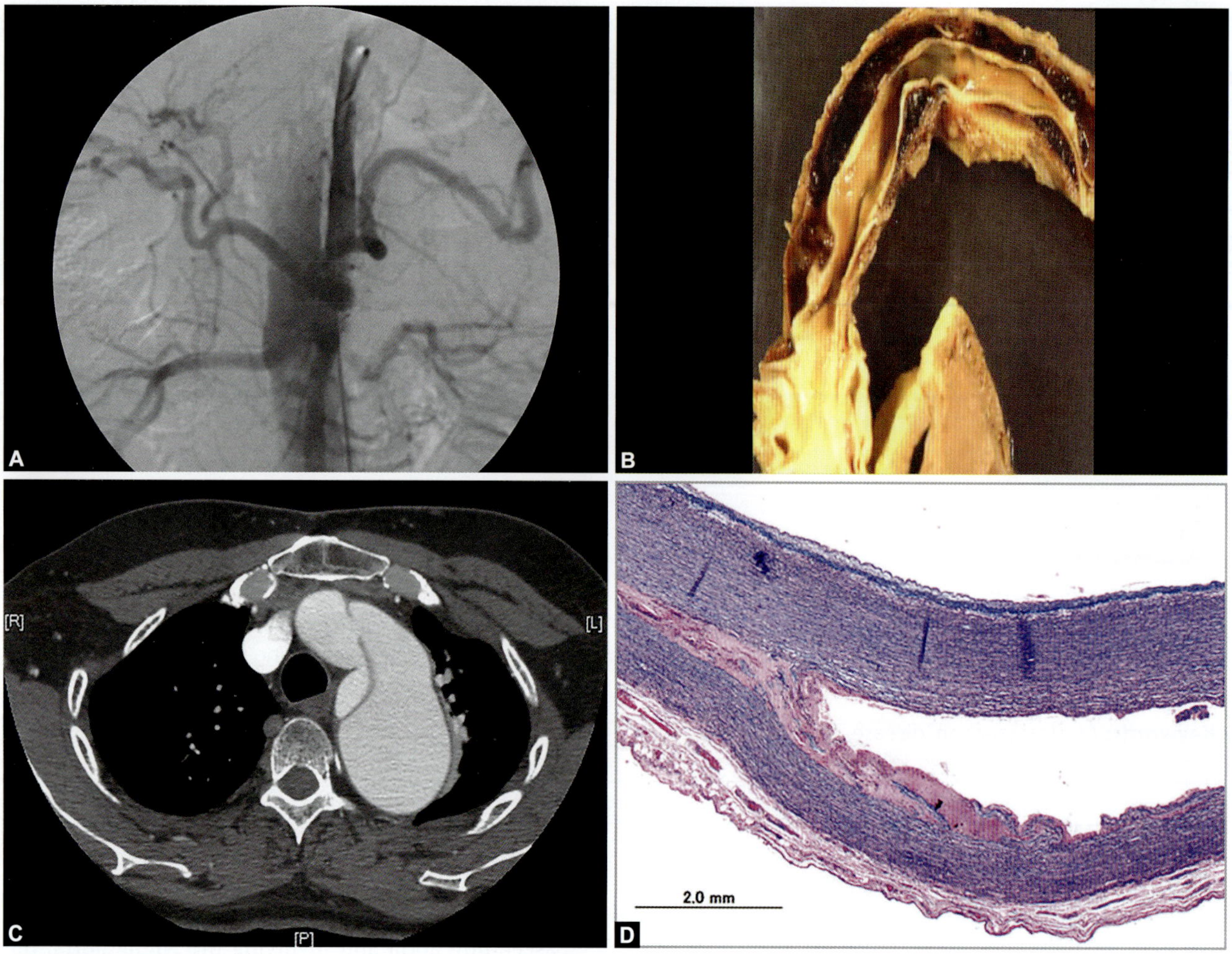

FIGS. 1A TO D: Aortic dissection with intimal flap showing entry tear, with false and true lumen.

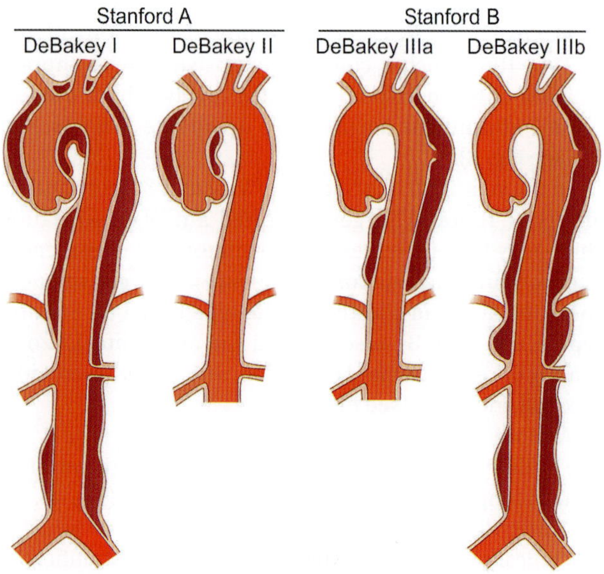

FIG. 2: Classification of dissection of aorta.

of the clinical status or chronicity of aortic dissection. Dissections are hyperacute within 24 hours of the index event, acute from 1 to 14 days, subacute from 15 to 90 days, and chronic if it is >90 days.[2] Uncomplicated dissection has no complications like rupture and no malperfusion and no high-risk features. Complicated dissection is a dissection, which presents with rupture and perfusion.

High-risk dissection would cause refractory pain and hypertension. There may be pleural effusion with blood. The aortic diameter is >40 mm with radiographic malperfusion. Entry tear located on the lesser curvature is also considered to be high risk and those patients where the false lumen (TL) diameter is >22 mm.

Acute type A dissection mortality is higher in the initial period and needs surgical treatment but is stable in the later period.

International Registry of Acute Aortic Dissection Database[3]

- In-hospital mortality with surgical treatment was 27% and 56% with medical treatment.

Examples

Type A_9:
- Entry tear identified in zone 0 (A)
- Distal extent in zone 9

Type $B_{4,10}$:
- Entry tear is identified > zone 0 (B)
- Proximal extent in zone 4
- Distal extent in zone 10

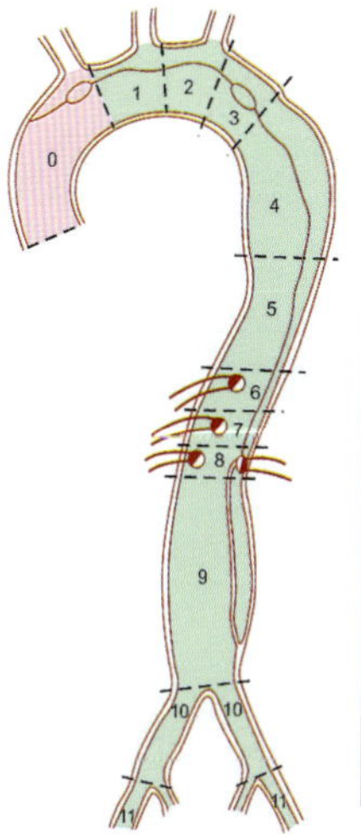

Type	Proximal extent	Distal extent
A_D	0	0
	1	1
Entry tear: **Zone 0**	2	2
	3	3
	4	4
B_{PD}	5	5
	6	6
Entry tear: **≥Zone 1**	7	7
	8	8
I_D	9	9
Unidentified entry tear involving **Zone 0**	10	10
	11	11
	12	12

FIG. 3: Anatomic reporting of aortic dissection is based on the location of the entry tear (A or B) and proximal and distal extent.
Source: With permission from Lombardi et al. (2020).[2]

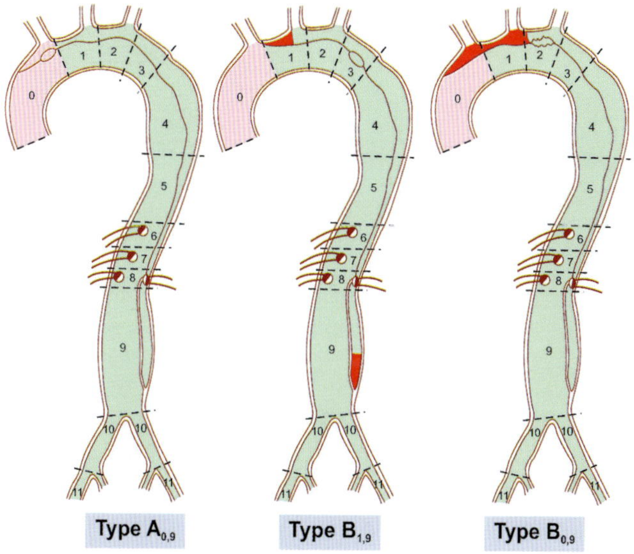

FIG. 4: Descriptive classification including entry tear and extent description.

- There is no role of conservative medical treatment in acute type A aortic dissection. The primary aim is to not treat the whole aortic dissection but come out with a live patient.
- Acute type B dissection mortality is relatively low in the initial period.
- Uncomplicated type B dissectionsurvival is 89% at 1 month, 84% at 1 year, and 80% at 5 years.[4] Type B aortic dissection (TBAD)can also be uncomplicated and complicated.
- Uncomplicated dissection is well tolerated and the initial treatment is medical.

WHAT ARE THE GOALS OF THERAPY FOR TYPE B AORTIC DISSECTION?

The main aim of treatment is to reduce wall stress and FL depressurization.

This is achieved by control of heart rate and blood pressure, which reduces the d_p/d_t, thus reducing the tension on the wall of the aorta to reduce the risk of rupture.

The target heart rate is <70 beats/min, and the target blood pressure is to keep systolic blood pressure <120 mm Hg.

Medicines which are used to achieve this are:
- Beta-blockers
- Alpha and beta-blockers (labetalol)
- Sodium nitroprusside + beta-blockers
- Adequate analgesia

COMPLICATED TYPE B AORTIC DISSECTION

There may be malperfusion of aortic branches and the blood pressure may be refractory to treatment or there may be CT evidence of impending FL rupture preceded by an increase in the size of periaortic hematoma or pleural effusion.
- Thoracic endovascular aortic repair (TEVAR) for the treatment of TBAD has changed the management of aortic dissection.
- TEVAR is associated with a lower risk of mortality and morbidity.

A meticulous understanding of the anatomy using the imaging modalities is the key to a successful procedure and avoidance of complications.
- TEVAR is the first-line treatment for TBAD. It helps to seal the proximal entry tear which favors remodeling of the aorta.
- Indications are now expanding for uncomplicated dissections.

False lumen thrombosis (FLT), true lumen (TL) expansion, and FL regression are the initial aims of treatment with endovascular aneurysm repair (EVAR). Below is a simple case description for anatomical delineation of the entry and subsequent closure of the entry tear in a stable TBAD. The aim is to locate the entry tear, measure the size of the aorta above the entry tear which will be the proximal landing zone of the endovascular stent graft, and subsequently length assessment of the graft after the location of the landing site of the lower end of the graft **(Figs. 5A to C)**.

After planning the procedure and the location is understood, the endovascular stent graft procedure is

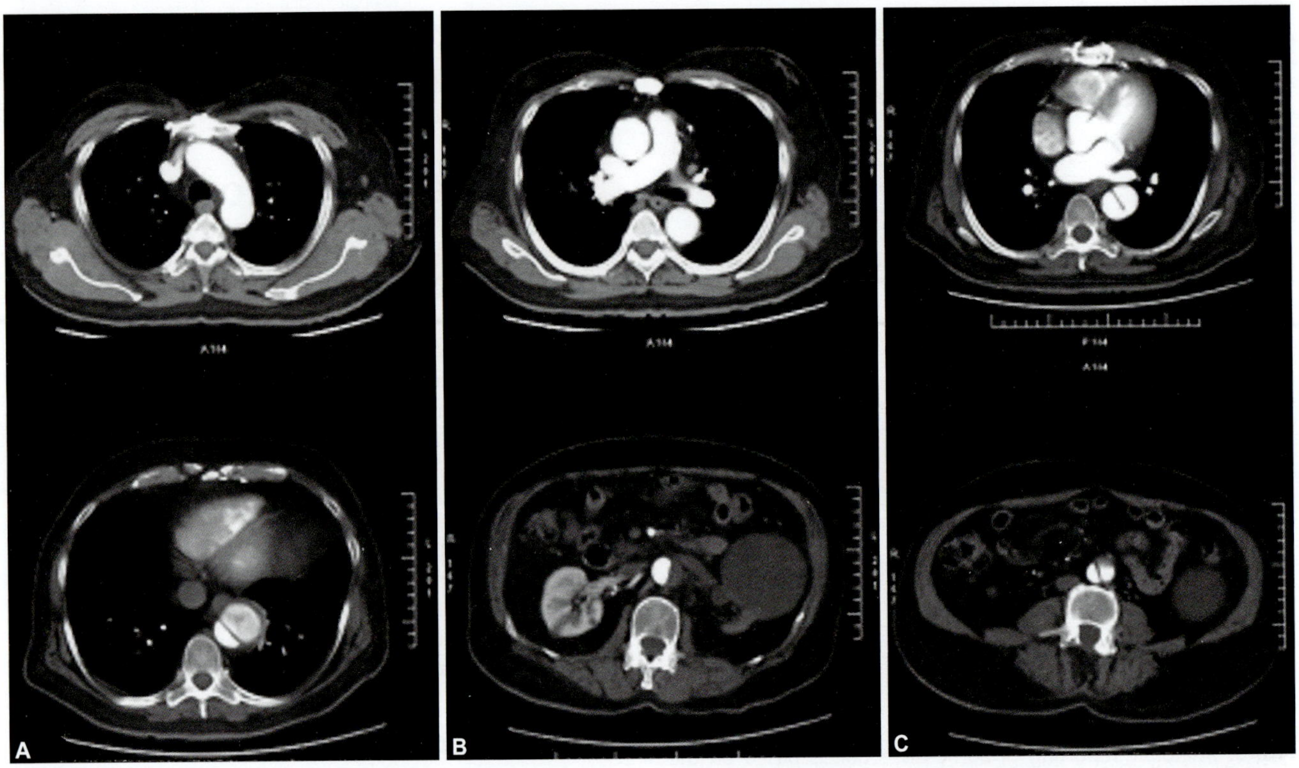

FIGS. 5A TO C: Contrast CT slices showing the type B aortic dissection with entry tear and true and false lumen.

performed using a transfemoral approach, which was done, using a percutaneous approach using the preclosure device—Proglide (Abbott Inc).

Some patients may require a surgical exposure of the common femoral artery which is used as an access. The endovascular stent graft is inserted and deployed at the previously planned location as depicted in **Figure 6**.

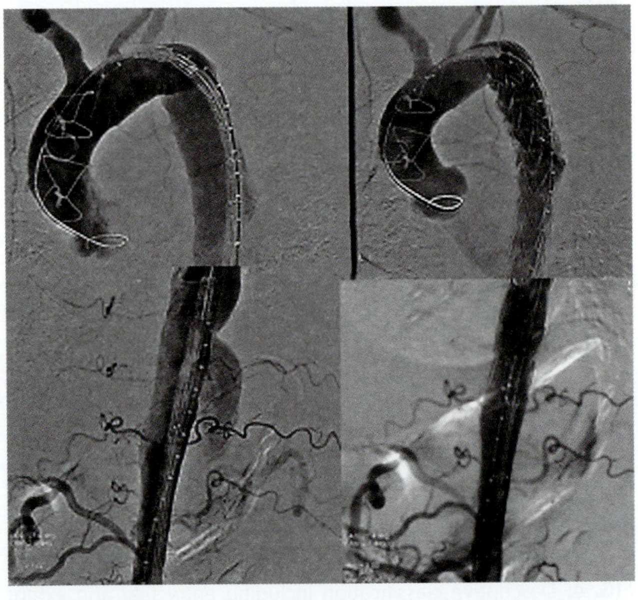

FIG. 6: Positioning of the stent graft using endovascular repair.

CASE EXAMPLE FOR EVALUATION AND TREATMENT PLAN OF A PATIENT WITH AORTIC DISSECTION

A 32-year-old man developed sudden chest pain followed by severe pain in his right lower limb. His clinical examination confirmed significantly elevated blood pressure, and the right lower limb was cold and painful. A contrast CT performed showed a type A dissection, along with occlusion of the right iliac artery causing right lower limb ischemia. This patient presented to another hospital with cold right lower limb and pain, which was evaluated at another hospital, and a CT was performed which confirmed type A aortic dissection **(Figs. 7A and B)**.

This patient required fenestration of the intimal flap as there was no flow into the TL, followed by stenting of the right iliac artery to improve flow into the right lower limb. As this patient was primarily a type A dissection, after initial stabilization with improvement the patient was sent for surgical treatment.

Thoracic endovascular aortic repair is associated with a lower risk of mortality and morbidity but follow-up patients may present with:

- Endoleak
- Stent graft migration
- Retrograde aortic dissection
- Distal dissection and aneurysm formation

These events require reinterventions in such patients.

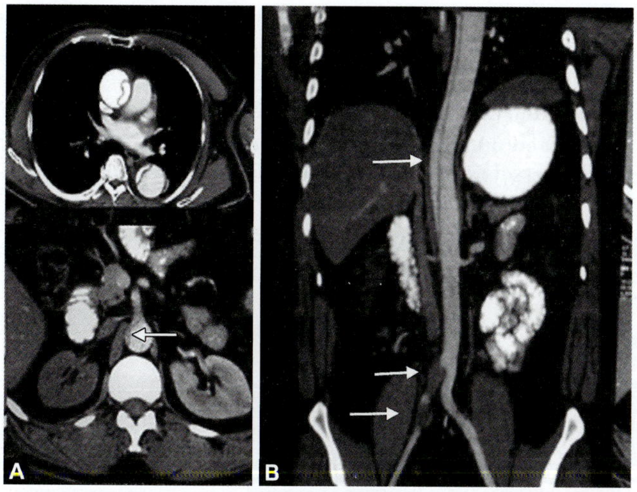

FIGS. 7A AND B: Type A aortic dissection with compromised true lumen and ischemic right lower limb.

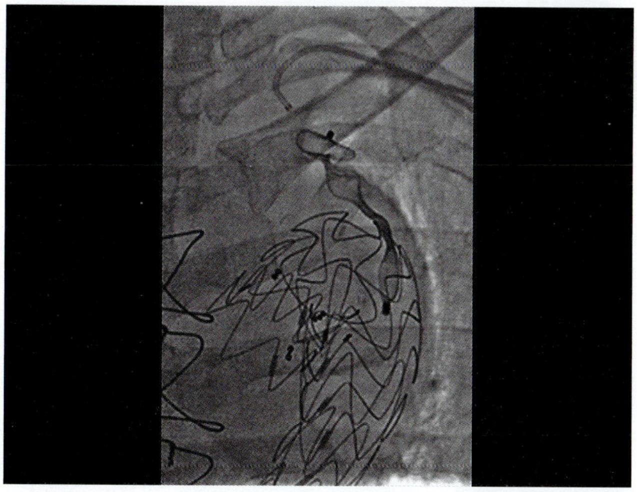

FIG. 8: Reintervention in a patient with type 2 endoleak requiring a vascular plug.

Reintervention is defined as second intervention for the management of complications **(Fig. 8)**.

POTENTIAL RISK FACTORS FOR REINTERVENTIONS

What are the risk factors for reinterventions?
- Age, male gender, follow-up period
- Technical success of the prior aortic intervention
- Marfan syndrome, connective tissue disorder, and other comorbidities

Endoleak is the most common cause of reintervention while other causes may include:
- FL perfusion
- Continued aortic dilatation
- Extension of the dissection

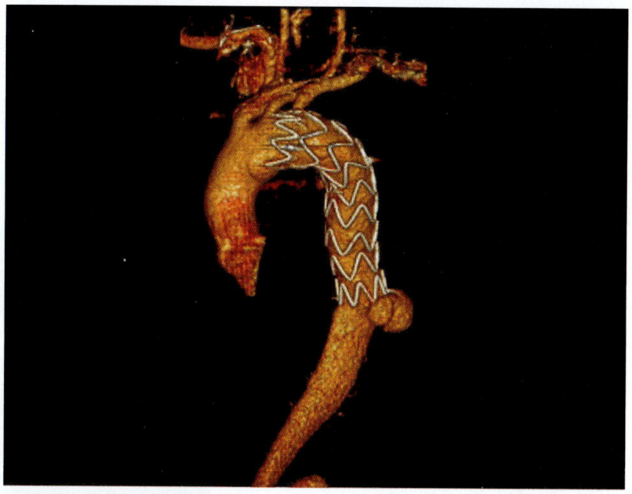

FIG. 9: Stent graft causing distal edge injury leading to the formation of a new saccular aneurysm.

Another cause of reintervention is retrograde thoracic aortic dissection (RTAD), which though uncommon is a devastating complication in type B dissection—the most common cause for which is excessive oversizing of stent graft, especially in a recent dissection.

False lumen perfusion causes aortic growth/dilatation. Complete thrombosis is good but partial thrombosis may lead to further growth. Also, the distal intimal flap tear extends the dissection **(Fig. 9)**.

There may be various causes of endoleaks:
- Inadequate landing zone
- Usage of scallops, chimney, and fenestration
- Anatomy of the vascular segment
- Stent graft design which may be prone to degeneration

In a meta-analysis of 27 studies with 2,403 patients, pooled evidence of interventions 33.7 months after endovascular repair, endoleak was 33.2%, FL perfusion and dilatation were 19.8% and new dissection was 6.9%.[4]

TREATMENT OPTIONS FOR POSTDISSECTION THORACIC AORTIC ANEURYSM

For patients who develop further aneurysm formation and require treatment, the following options can be considered:
- Open surgical repair—which although carries more risk, especially in older Individuals, is more definitive in nature.
- FL can be treated with some other endovascular methods.
- A complex endovascular repair can be offered.
- Further aneurysm formation can be prevented by doing a more complete treatment of patients on their first intervention so that further complications are prevented.

FALSE LUMEN TREATMENT

False lumen treatment is technically a less complex procedure in those patients who develop thoracic aortic aneurysm (TAA) and can be of use in limiting the coverage of the aorta by a stent.

This can be achieved by FL embolization which can be obtained by various methods. Some of them are described in **Figure 10**.

Further treatment of post-EVAR development of TAA can also be done by extension of the graft and fenestration for the vessels and lastly, as described earlier, open surgical

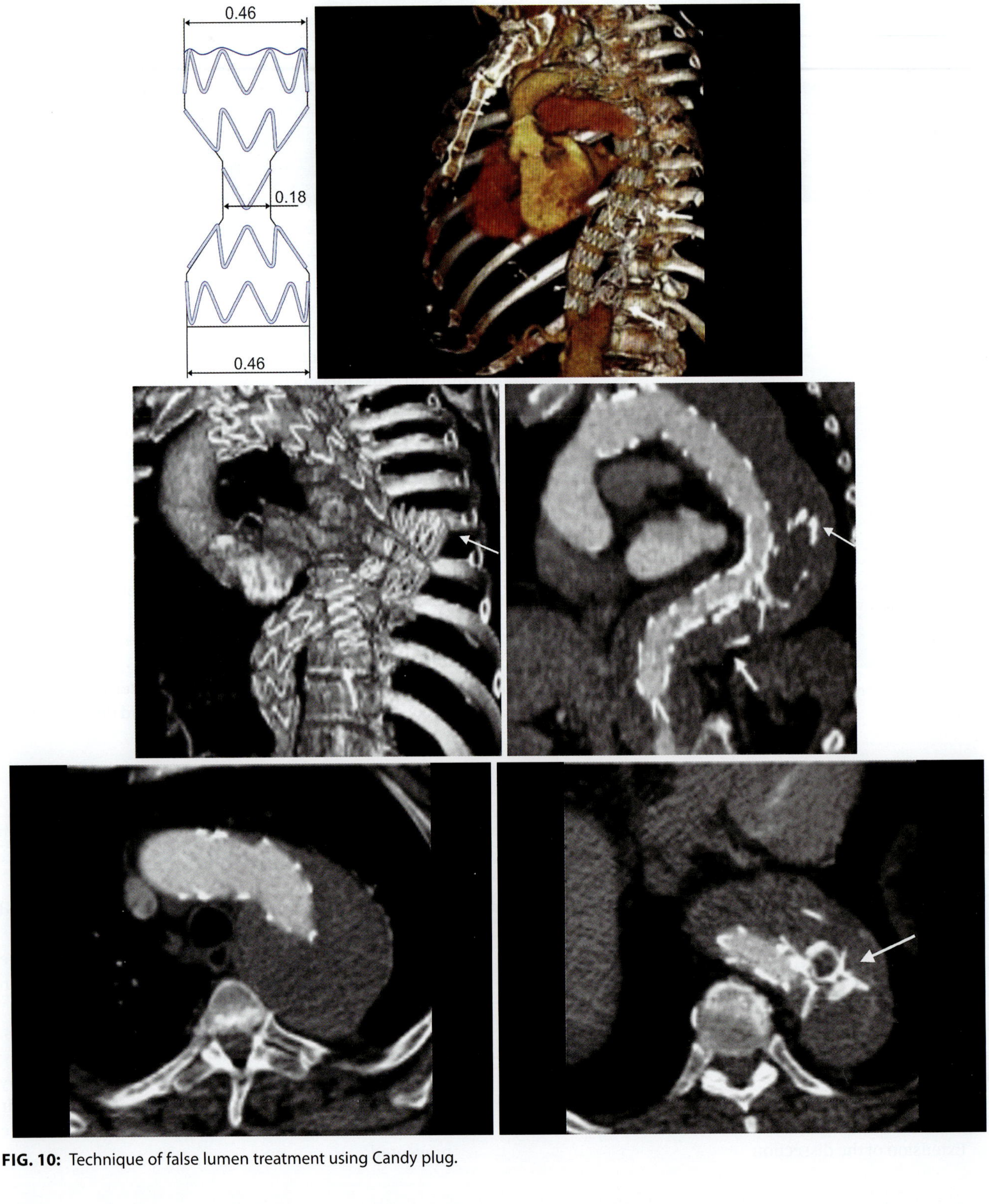

FIG. 10: Technique of false lumen treatment using Candy plug.

repair can be offered with good long-term results when performed by an experienced surgical team in an experienced center resulting in long-term symptom and complication-free clinical status.

CONCLUSION

Dissection of aorta is a devastating disease with high mortality and morbidity.

Understanding the disease using imaging is the most important step in its management. Most TBADs that are medically managed progress to aneurysms, increasing the evidence of adverse events and mortality.

Early TEVAR results in favorable aortic remodeling, which prevents aneurysm formation. To avoid aortic complications in uncomplicated acute TBAD, early TEVAR may be selectively considered. Those patients who are young and are treated with endovascular repair may require reintervention which may be further endovascular repair or surgical repair which may encompass removal of the stent graft, or it can be used as well for surgical repair after repair of the aneurysm.

ONLINE REFERENCES

Please scan the QR code provided at the end of the table of contents for References of this chapter.

CHAPTER 193

Atherosclerotic Carotid Disease: Revascularization—When, Why, and How

Bhavuk Jaiswal, Ashish Jai Kishan, Atul Mathur

ABSTRACT

Stroke is one of the major causes of death and disability globally. Atherosclerotic carotid disease accounts for a significant burden in the elderly to cause stroke and hypoperfusion. Revascularization for carotid artery stenosis can be challenging, and the therapeutic option of carotid endarterectomy (CEA) or carotid artery stenting (CAS) should be selected based on timing, presenting symptoms, ongoing or worsening neurological symptoms, concomitant heart disease, and other comorbidities. In this review of atherosclerotic carotid disease, we discuss about atherosclerotic carotid disease with a focus on when, why, and how to pursue revascularization strategies.

Keywords: Atherosclerosis, carotid artery, carotid artery stenting, carotid artery endarterectomy

INTRODUCTION

Atherosclerotic carotid artery disease (>50% stenosis) accounts for 3–4% of the general population.[1] Stroke is one of the leading causes of disability and death, with up to 15–20% linked to significant carotid artery disease.[2] Patients with atherosclerotic carotid disease are at a higher risk of recurrent stroke. Stroke prevention and treatment strategies include carotid revascularization strategies along with medical therapy. Carotid endarterectomy (CEA) has been the gold standard treatment of choice for a long time; however, newer advancements have improved revascularization strategies with carotid artery stenting (CAS) with outcomes similar to the surgical technique.

CAROTID REVASCULARIZATION STRATEGY

When?

The European Society for Vascular Surgery (ESVS) 2023 Clinical Practice Guidelines on the Management of Atherosclerotic Carotid and Vertebral Artery Disease recommends carotid artery revascularization in patients:[3]

- Symptomatic patients with carotid stenosis of >50%
- Asymptomatic patients with carotid stenosis of >70%

Symptoms of carotid artery disease are defined as recent history of TIA or ischemic stroke of <6 months' duration and of an ipsilateral vascular supply. Other symptoms of carotid territory can be higher cortical dysfunction such as aphasia, apraxia, dysgraphia, visuospatial and visual field defects, hemianopia, amaurosis fugax or transient monocular blindness, blurring, chronic ocular ischemia syndrome, weakness, paresthesia of face/arm/leg, and upper or lower limb clumsiness. "Limb-shaking TIAs" (hemodynamic events in patients with severe carotid stenosis and exhausted cerebral vascular reserve) can also occur. "Nonhemispheric" symptoms such as isolated episodes of syncope (blackout, drop attack), presyncope (faintness), isolated dizziness, isolated double vision (diplopia), tinnitus, and isolated vertigo can be attributed to carotid artery disease and absence of any other etiologies. Patients can also present with posterior circulation symptoms and syndromes but with a significant carotid artery disease due to carotid emboli if a persistent fetal PCA origin from the ICA via the posterior communicating artery exists, which requires an intracranial MRA/CT imaging. Routine investigation for carotid artery disease is not recommended, but in cases of high clinical suspicion and clinical phenotypes [coronary artery disease (CAD), hypertension, history of smoking, dyslipidemia, left ventricular dysfunction, increasing age, prior history of TIA/stroke > 6 months, PAD, diabetes mellitus, familial hypercholesterolemia], it is warranted.[4] First line for diagnosis is color Doppler ultrasound with a sensitivity and specificity of 89% and 84%, respectively, for carotid stenosis of >50%.[5] Noncontrast- or contrast-enhanced MRA and CTA can simultaneously image the aortic arch, supra-aortic trunks, carotid bifurcation, distal ICA, and intracranial course along with location, extent, burden, and calcification of atherosclerotic plaque which is important for a revascularization procedure if being planned. A combination of two imaging modalities (DUS + CTA or DUS + MRA) improves accuracy and is routine practice in many centers.

Timing of Revascularization

Asymptomatic

Patients with asymptomatic carotid stenosis can initially be managed with both CEA and CAS if the predicted 30 days postoperative stroke/death risk is <3% or with "best medical therapy" (BMT) with the latter being the first choice.[3] BMT along with monitoring with semiannual or annual follow-ups with DUS surveillance and other investigations (lipid profile, blood pressure monitoring, neuroimaging, ECG, glycosylated Hb) can delay or halt revascularization and its risks. However, patients with silent infarction on CT/MRI, increase of >20% stenosis progression, baseline of >60% stenosis, large plaque area or large juxtaluminal black area (JBA) on computerized ultrasound plaque analysis (defined as an area of pixels with a grayscale value < 25 adjacent to the lumen without a visible echogenic cap after image normalization), plaque echolucency, interplaque hemorrhage on MRI, impaired cerebral vascular reserve, or at least one spontaneous microemboli signal during 1 hour of transcranial Doppler monitoring are considered higher risk for stroke and are advised for a CEA/CAS over BMT.[6-12]

Symptomatic

Patients with symptomatic carotid stenosis should be managed with a revascularization strategy when predicted 30 days postoperative stroke/death risk is <6%.[3] Patients with an acute history of TIA/stroke (<24 hours) should be initially managed medically with antiplatelet regimens and anticoagulants as recommended. The incidence of recurrent stroke in previous natural history studies after a TIA ranges from 5 to 8% at 48 hours, 4 to 17% at 72 hours, 8 to 22% at 7 days, and 11% - to 25% at 14 days which is higher than those reported in revascularization studies and newer randomized controlled trials (RCTs) due to changes in medical therapy in the modern era, patient selection of lower risk of stroke and early revascularizations.[13] New data suggest that early carotid revascularization within 6–14 days is beneficial to prevent recurrent stroke/TIA.[3] However, in selected patients with smaller infarcts, crescendo TIAs and stroke in evolution revascularization can be performed early with urgent CEA within 24 hours provided the risk is <8%. Delayed (>14 days) revascularization in symptomatic carotid stenosis increases the risk of recurrent stroke up to 2% at 120 days.[3]

The size of the infarct is an independent predictor of postoperative ICH and encephalopathy. In patients with a disabling stroke (modified Rankin Score of >3), having an area of infarction exceeding one-third of MCA territory and those in altered sensorium should be deferred from the revascularization strategy till neurological improvement.

About 10–20% of patients with acute stroke managed with antithrombolytic therapy have significant carotid stenosis and early carotid revascularization strategies in this subset of patients have higher peri- and postprocedural complications such as neck hematoma and stroke. Perioperative stroke/death was 13% when the revascularization strategy was performed after 3 days of thrombolysis and 10.6% after 4 days. The risk was predicted to decrease within the currently accepted risk of <6% threshold after 6 days had elapsed, suggesting that revascularization should be deferred until 6 days after post-thrombolysis.[14]

Why?

Asymptomatic

In patients with asymptomatic carotid stenosis, the decision to pursue revascularization has been contentious, as it parallels a primary prevention strategy. The benefits of such an approach must clearly outweigh the potential risks of future stroke, given the associated perioperative risks of stroke and death compared to medical therapy alone. Previous trials have not demonstrated a clear advantage of CEA or CAS in asymptomatic patients. SPACE 2 trial (2022), which included 513 patients, found that neither CEA plus BMT nor CAS plus BMT showed superiority over BMT alone in reducing the risk of any stroke or death within 30 days or ipsilateral stroke during a 5-year follow-up. However, this trial's conclusions were limited by the small number of patients in each treatment arm.[15] The ongoing CREST-2 trial (Commitment to Rigorous Assessment of Carotid Stenting for Primary Prevention of Stroke) holds promise for contributing valuable data to this discussion.[16] A meta-analysis comparing CEA, CAS, and BMT in asymptomatic patients with significant carotid stenosis found that CEA was associated with a lower early risk of stroke compared to CAS, with no significant differences in other early or late outcomes. Moreover, CEA appeared to offer an advantage over BMT in preventing long-term ipsilateral stroke, although the short-term outcomes were less favorable after CEA.[17] Therefore, it is recommended that revascularization be considered for patients with a life expectancy exceeding 5 years, to ensure that the long-term benefits of the procedure outweigh the short-term and perioperative risks.

Symptomatic

A meta-analysis of 5-year risks of any stroke, including perioperative stroke or death, from European Carotid

Surgery Trial (ECST), North American Symptomatic Carotid Endarterectomy Trial (NASCET), and Symptomatic Veterans Affairs Carotid Study (SVACS) RCTs showed an absolute risk reduction of 7.8% at 5 years in patients with carotid stenosis of 50–69% and 15.6% at 5 years in patients with stenosis severity of >70%. Excluding perioperative risks, a meta-analysis conducted by CSTC of four RCTs reported that the 5-year rates of ipsilateral stroke were 3.1% following CEA compared to 3.2% after CAS [hazard ratio (HR) 1.06; 95% confidence interval (CI) 0.73–1.54]. This corresponds to an average annual ipsilateral stroke rate of 0.62% for CEA and 0.64% for CAS. At 9 years, the ipsilateral stroke rates were 3.9% for CEA and 4.5% for CAS, translating to an average annual ipsilateral stroke rate of 0.43% after CEA and 0.5% after CAS.[18] These findings suggest that CAS is as durable as CEA once the perioperative period has passed, similar to findings in asymptomatic carotid stenosis. Health-related quality of life was assessed in the CREST study in which 365 patients who underwent CAS reported a better quality of life during the postoperative period after 1 year, particularly in terms of physical limitations and pain ($p = 0.010$). Using disease-specific scales, CAS patients experienced fewer issues with driving, eating, swallowing, neck pain, and headaches but reported greater difficulty with walking and leg pain ($p < 0.050$).[19] However, these differences had disappeared as 1-year postprocedure elapsed. Additionally, perioperative stroke was associated with poorer 1-year quality of life across all SF-36 domains, while periprocedural myocardial infarction (MI) and cranial nerve injury (CNI) did not have the same impact.

How?

Open Surgical Techniques

Carotid Endarterectomy

Surgical CEA has been the mainstay treatment for over three decades prior to CAS and is commonly opted as the first choice in both asymptomatic and symptomatic carotid stenosis at many centers. The standard approach is a longitudinal anterior sternomastoid incision, but a transverse skin crease incision has a better cosmesis and a lower CNI rate but a difficult insertion of a shunt with transverse incisions. A modified approach involves DUS marking of the bifurcation and a smaller longitudinal incision, which is extended if required. This reduces incision length and also offers good cosmesis. CEA is associated with a higher risk of postprocedural MI, longer hospital stay, and concerns in patients with cardiopulmonary disease, hemodynamic instability, risk of neck hematoma, CNI, and hyperperfusion syndrome.

Carotid Bypass

Carotid bypass may be indicated in the treatment of patch infection, carotid stent explantation, restenosis, or technical problems during CEA (arterial wall thinning, damage to arterial wall). Other indications include extensive atherosclerotic disease, ICA fibrosis secondary to radiotherapy, or revascularization after en bloc removal of a neck tumor.

Carotid Stenting

Carotid artery stenting is routinely done via the transfemoral route; however, transradial or transbrachial routes are well described but can be challenging. Technique and hardware for CAS have advanced over the years with newer generation stents, specialized protection devices, and wires which help CAS achieve better outcomes comparable to CEA. Technical success in CAS firstly depends on CCA access using a long introducer sheath or guiding catheters. Baseline anatomy of the aortic arch, supra-aortic branches, and the access site is essential for planning CAS. CCA catheterization can be performed using different techniques: (1) Direct approach requires a guiding catheter (6–8F) advanced over a standard hydrophilic guidewire (0.035″/180 cm, angled tip) into the aortic arch and then advanced up to 2–3 cm below carotid bifurcation; (2) telescopic approach needs a diagnostic catheter (5F) which is first advanced over a standard hydrophilic guidewire (0.035″/180 cm, angled tip) placed into ECA where the guidewire can safely be exchanged with a stiff wire (e.g., Amplatzer Super Stiff wire, Supracore stiff wire) over which a guiding catheter can be exchanged with a long introducer sheath (6–7F/90 cm) with its inner dilator advanced up to 2–3 cm below carotid bifurcation; and (3) in the telescopic approach with coaxial technique, a 4–5 F diagnostic catheter (>110 cm in length) is preloaded into a long introducer (6–7 F/90 cm) or a guiding catheter (6–8 F/90–100 cm). The entire coaxial system is advanced into the aortic arch and then into the CCA using a hydrophilic guidewire (0.035″/260 cm, angled tip). The choice of the technique depends on the patient's anatomical configuration and the practitioner's experience. Following catheterization of CCA lesion is crossed with a 0.014″ wire or specialized wire with a preloaded EPD (Emboshield NAV) over which CAS is performed. Various carotid stents are available with a closed-cell nitinol design (Xact-Abbott vascular, Nex Stent-Endotex) or open-cell nitinol design (RxAcculink-Guidant, ExponentRx-Medtronic, Vivexx-Bard, Precise-Cordis) which are self-tapering with a proximal–distal diameter size difference (10/8, 9/7, 8/6 mm). To reduce the risk of plaque protrusion, three types of dual-layered stents have been developed. These are CGuard (Inspire-MD), Roadsaver (Microvention), and Scaffolds (W.L. Gore and Associates). In a large multicenter registry involving 725 patients treated consecutively with the CGuard stent, the 1-year stroke and death rate was 1.9%. In an RCT involving 100 patients who underwent CAS, a head-to-head comparison was conducted between the CGuard dual-layered covered stent and the Acculink single-layer open-cell stent. The group with the covered stent experienced significantly fewer periprocedural and 30-day embolic events, with a 78% reduction in periprocedural new lesion volume, as documented using diffusion-weighted magnetic resonance imaging. The Roadsaver stent was evaluated in the CLEAR-ROAD (Physician-initiated Carotid Trial Investigating the Efficacy of Endovascular Treatment of Carotid Arterial Disease With the Multi-layer Roadsaver Stent) study, which enrolled 100 patients and documented a 30-day major adverse event rate of 2.1%.[19] The 30-day stroke rate in the SCAFFOLD (Carotid Stent Clinical Study for the Treatment of Carotid Artery Stenosis in Patients at Increased Risk for Adverse Events from Carotid Endarterectomy) study was found to be 2.9%.[20]

Embolic Protection Devices

Embolic protection devices (EPD) decrease the risk of perioperative stroke and make CAS more feasible and safer. An EPD should be selected based on anatomical consideration and plaque characteristics and morphology. Distal protection with balloon occlusion was the first method to be used by occluding the blood flow across ICA and once the lesion is treated, the catheter is advanced to the balloon with proximal aspiration of blood across the balloon and then deflated. However, new distal protection filter wire systems help in maintaining flow throughout the procedure and retrieval of emboli and devices is done together upon completion of the procedure. Several types of distal filters are now available in the market with varying rigidity of metallic structure, pore size, basket length, and stiffness of wire (Accuent-Abbott vascular, Angioguard-Cordis, Emboshield NAV6-Abbott Vascular, SpiderFX-Medtronic).

Transcarotid Revascularization

Transcarotid revascularization (TCAR) is a hybrid procedure in which a surgical cut down at the level of the carotid is done following which a small sheath is passed at the level of bifurcation which is connected to either a femoral vein or an ipsilateral jugular vein via a filter device, thus reversing flow from the internal carotids into the low pressure venous system. During this reversal of flow, thromboemboli plaques can be collected into the specialized filter system.

Best Medical Therapy

Medical therapy has evolved over the years and is the first line of management in asymptomatic carotid stenosis and is necessary for both asymptomatic and symptomatic carotid stenosis. BMT includes good glycemic control, ideal blood pressure targets, lipid levels, optimal antiplatelet therapy and NOACs, diet and lifestyle modifications, smoking cessation, use of newer drugs such as PCSK 9 inhibitors, ezetimibe, bempedoic acid for dyslipidemia, SGLT-2 inhibitors for glycemic control, optimized antihypertensive and DUS surveillances and neuroimaging. Medical therapy helps in delay and cessation of plaque progression and any adverse events and should be targeted in all patients.

CONCLUSION

Atherosclerotic carotid disease has a significant contribution to disabling/death-related strokes, and revascularization in significant asymptomatic or symptomatic carotid stenosis with either CEA or CAS outweighs the risk associated. No major difference exists in long-term outcomes between CEA and CAS. While CEA is associated with a lower risk of short-term stroke but a small risk of perioperative MI, CNI, and neck hematoma, CAS is more suitable in patients with preexisting cardiopulmonary disease such as CAD, heart failure, and prior history of previous surgery and neck radiation but at a risk of small emboli stroke post procedure. Optimizing the BMT for all patients is necessary.

ONLINE REFERENCES

Please scan the QR code provided at the end of the table of contents for References of this chapter.

CHAPTER

194

Interventional Approach to Central Venous Occlusion

BC Srinivas, Disha Shetty, Vijay Kumar, Babu Reddy, CM Nagesh

ABSTRACT

Central venous obstruction (CVO) is a common complication of central venous catheterization, complicating dialysis and leading to access failure in hemodialysis-dependent chronic kidney disease (HDCKD) patients. CVO causes venous hypertension, edema, ulceration, and tissue loss. Long-term repetitive use of catheters is the main cause, with up to 40% incidence. Endovascular therapy, less invasive and safer, is currently the first-line treatment. Routine evaluation of central veins is crucial before creating arteriovenous fistulas.

Keywords: CVO, HDCKD

INTRODUCTION

Central venous obstruction (stenosis or occlusion; CVO) commonly occurs as a complication of central venous catheterization, it complicates dialysis and is the cause of access failure in hemodialysis-dependent chronic kidney disease (HDCKD) patients. CVO causes venous hypertension producing edema, ulceration, and tissue loss **(Figs. 1 and 2A and B)**. Long-term repetitive use of central venous catheters is the main cause of CVO with reported incidence of up to 40%.[1,2] The surgical reconstruction of the central vein had high patency rates of 80–90% at 1 year,[2] but it is associated with significantly high rate of perioperative mortality and morbidity due to the intrathoracic location of deep veins and difficult to execute. Endovascular therapy being less invasive, safer with experienced interventional team has good success rate and is currently the first-line treatment.

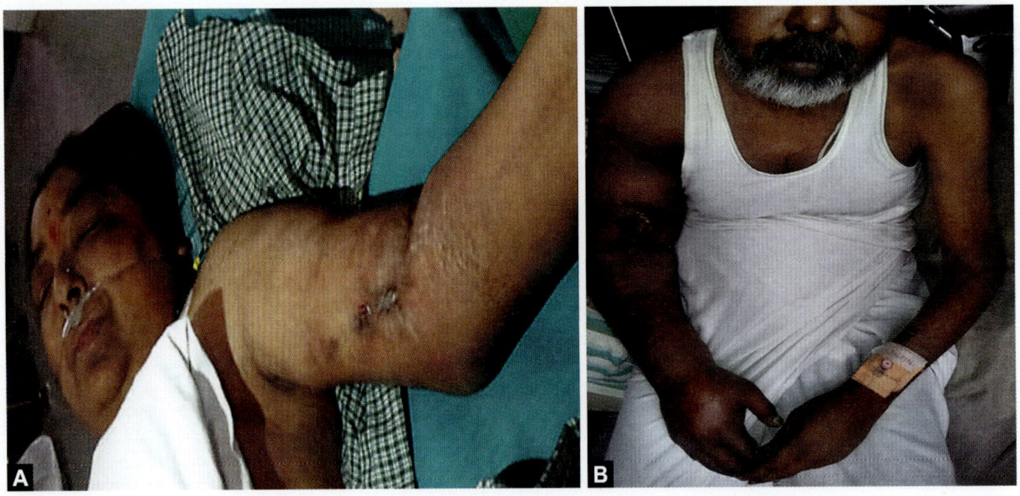

FIGS. 1A AND B: Patient with SVC syndrome with facial, neck and left upper limb edema.

ETIOLOGY

Mechanisms of CVO are predominantly vein wall thickening, endoluminal thrombofibrotic obstruction, and extrinsic compression.[3] There is a strong association of CVO with previous placement of central venous catheters.[4] The incidence of CVO is significantly higher in patients with a history of subclavian catheterization (42–50%) as compared to 10% with internal jugular vein use.[5,6] Risk factors for developing CVO include the number and duration of central vein catheters, left-sided catheterization, and catheter-related infections. Peripherally inserted central catheters (PICC), central venous port catheters, pacemaker, and defibrillator wires also cause CVO. The suggested mechanisms for the development of CVO include central venous catheter-induced trauma to the venous endothelium, secondary inflammatory damage within the vessel wall at the time of insertion, and high blood flow leading to abnormal shear stress, turbulence, and platelet aggregation.[5] The inflammatory state of CKD and underlying risk factors also contribute to the development of central venous occlusion.

CLINICAL MANIFESTATION

The CVO patients usually remain asymptomatic before the creation of the arteriovenous fistula because the collaterals can compensate the normal venous flow.[7] After the fistula formation they fail to compensate the increased flow and the patients develop the signs/symptoms of venous obstruction including incapacitating arm edema, ulceration, tissue loss, varicosity, and pain **(Figs. 1 and 2A and B)**. Symptoms of CVO depend on the location of obstruction. Innominate and subclavian vein occlusion presents with ipsilateral limb edema **(Figs. 2A and B)**. Patients with bilateral innominate vein obstruction and or SVC obstruction present with superior vena caval syndrome with upper limb edema, facial puffiness, neck engorgement, and chest wall edema **(Figs. 1A and B)**. CVO causes dysfunction of the ipsilateral access, increases the risk of thrombosis of the access, increases the risk of infection, and shortens the life of the hemodialysis access. In extreme cases, patient can have cellulitis, gangrene and ultimately amputation of the limb adding to severe disability **(Fig. 2C)**. The decreased flow rate in the fistula will make dialysis difficult.

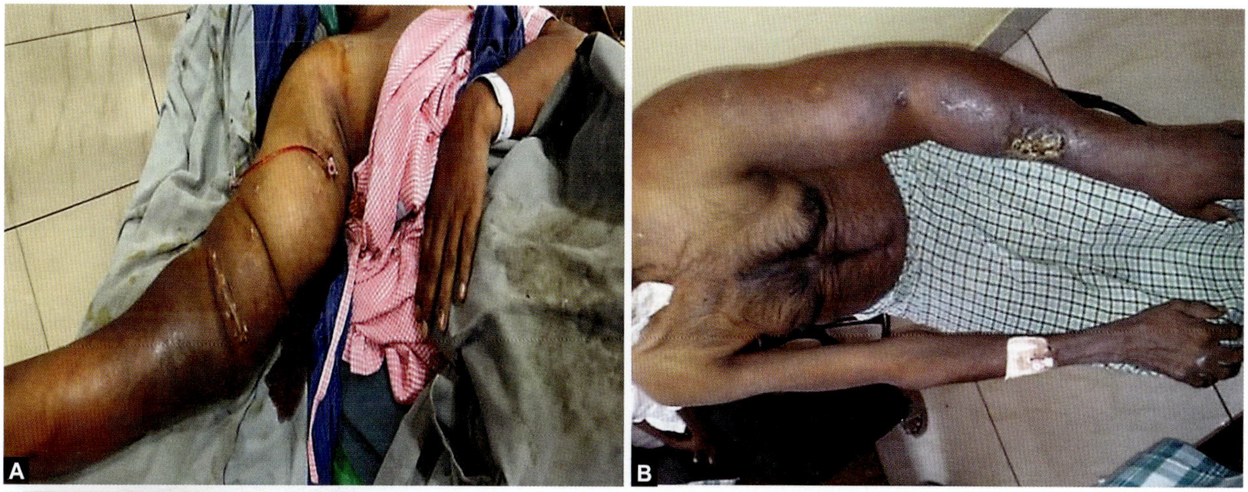

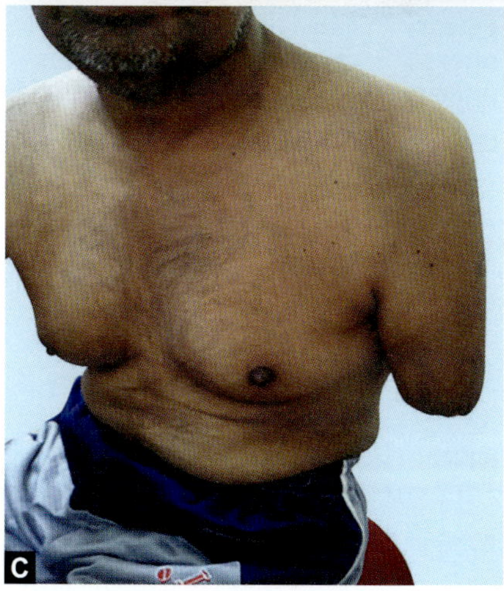

FIGS. 2A TO C: (A) Limb edema and features of venous hypertension; (B) Ulceration and tissue loss; (C) Amputation of left arm due to gangrene.

DIAGNOSIS

Combination of clinical features, history of previous catheters use, and imaging help in diagnosing CVO. Duplex ultrasound, Doppler shows an absence of normal respiratory variation in the central vein diameters, absence or decreased flow in central veins and polyphasic atrial waves in patients with CVO. Digital subtraction central venography is the gold standard for the diagnosis of CVO. Magnetic resonant angiography remains alternative to conventional angiography in selective cases for diagnosing CVO.

ENDOVASCULAR INTERVENTION

Endovascular intervention was first reported by Glanz et al. in 1984.[6] Percutaneous transluminal angioplasty (PTA) with or without stent implantation is currently the first-line management to treat CVO. It is less invasive, safe, and effective in maintaining the patency of central veins, vascular access for dialysis. It relieves the symptoms and signs of venous hypertension. PTA has demonstrated a variable technical success rate ranging from 70 to 90%.[1] The procedure failure is mainly related to inability to cross the long segment of total occlusion. Short-segment obstruction and focal restenosis are managed with balloon angioplasty alone **(Figs. 3A to D)**. Recoiling of the vessel is commonly seen after the balloon angioplasty and the restenosis rate are high. Primary stent implantation has got the advantage of immediate successful and complete expansion of the occluded segment with good flow **(Figs. 4A to H)**. Restenosis remains the Achilles heel of both balloon angioplasty and stent implantation. They need to be followed up meticulously and treated with repeat balloon angioplasty of the restenosis to facilitate hemodialysis and relieve venous hypertension. The primary patency rates at 3 months, 6 months, and 12 months in various studies were ranging between 65 and 95%, 54 and 90%, and 33 and 70%, respectively. The assisted patency rate with repeat balloon angioplasty of restenosis varies between 85 and 100%. Clinically, the limb edema resolves over one week in majority of the patients and facilitates the use of fistula for dialysis. The restenosis occurs due to intimal hyperplasia, fibrothrombosis, or progression of remote lesion. The stent shortening and stent movement are rare causes of restenosis.[8] The possibility of stent shortening increases with increasing nominal diameter and with use of stainless steel stent in comparison to nitinol. The number of reinterventions required for maintaining the high patency rates is dependent on experience of the operator, morphology of the lesion, optimal predilatation, liberal use of postdilatation, hardwires, and the stents.

OUR EXPERIENCE

We have performed endovascular intervention in 355 cases of central vein occlusions from January 2011 to March 2024. Technical success was achieved in about 94% of the patients during the index procedure and balloon angioplasty alone achieved satisfactory result in 24% of patents. In 76% of our patients having suboptimal angioplasty result are long occlusive lesions, we used self-expanding stents. Primary patency rate in our experience is 85%, 70%, and 60% at 3 months, 6 months, and 1 year, respectively **(Table 1)**.

TIPS AND TRICKS FOR INTERVENTIONAL APPROACH IN CENTRAL VENOUS OCCLUSION

Several key points noted below guide the procedure improve, procedural success and patency rates.

TABLE 1: CVO cases treated from 2011 to 2024.

Study	Total patients	Repeat procedures	Technical success	3 months patency rates primary	3 months patency rates assistant	6 months patency rates primary	6 months patency rates assistant	1 year patency rates primary	12 years patency rates assistant
Hagge et al. 1999	50	73 with 19 additional stents	NA	92%	NA	84%	97%	56%	97%
Hogel et al. 2004	15	NA	NA	815	NA	74%	NA	67%	NA
Christi duo et al. 2006	22	17 stents in 13	95.4%	85.3%	95.4%	65.3%	79%	45.6%	74%
Bakken et al. 2007	26	17 stents in 10 of 13 repeat procedures	96%	65%	72%	54%	55%	45%	46%
Ozyer et al. 2009	43	80 repeat procedures	NA	85%	98%	68%	91%	33%	67%
Our experience	355	195	91.2%	85%	100%	70%	95%	60%	89%

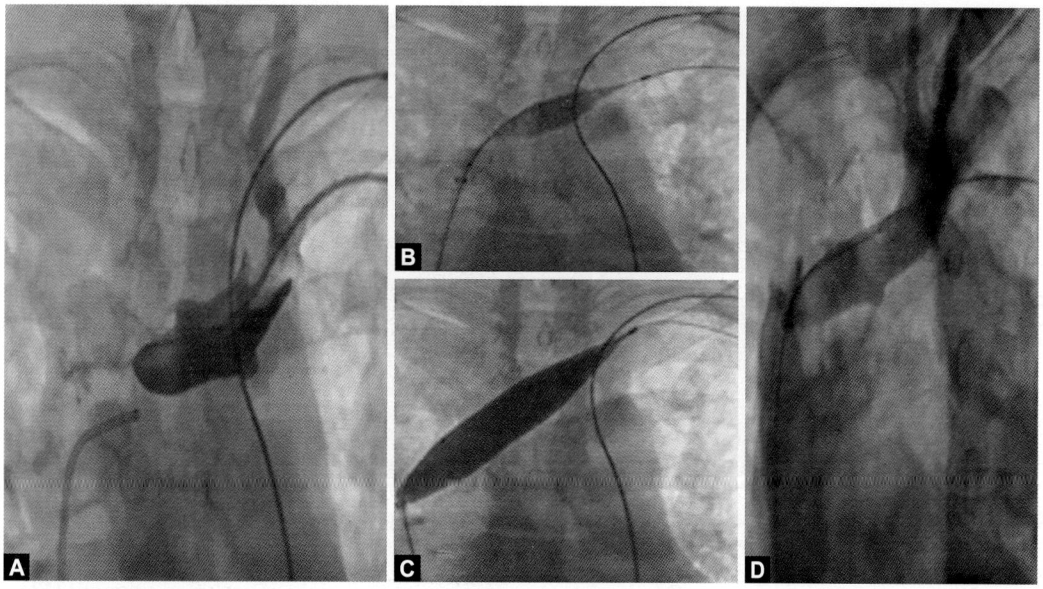

FIGS. 3A TO D: (A) Severe stenosis of left innominate vein; (B and C) Balloon angioplasty with 14 × 40 mm Atlas balloon; and (D) Adequately dilated left innominate vein with good flow and no residual lesion.

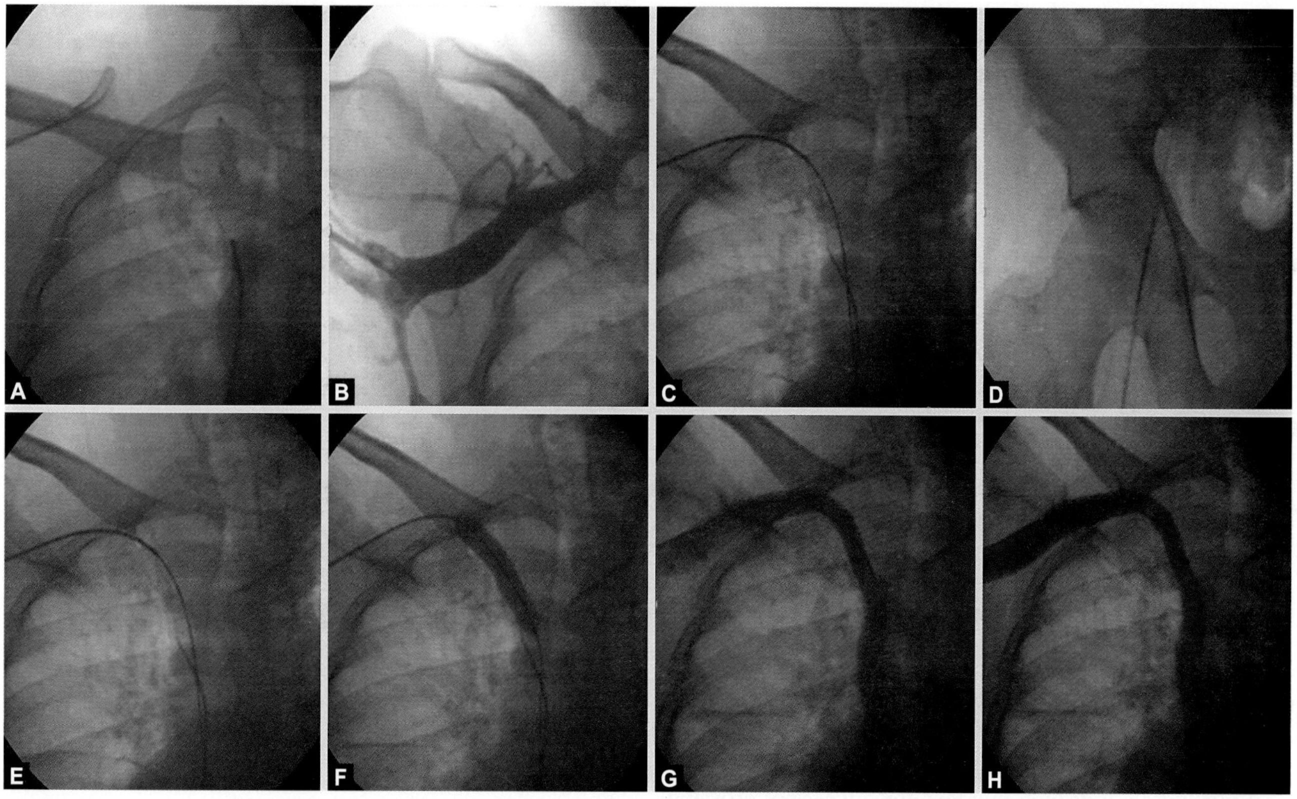

FIGS. 4A TO H: (A) Total occlusion of entire right innominate vein from ostium; (B) Occlusion extending till distal subclavian vein; (C) Lesion crossed with short cook catheter, straight tip 0.035" Terumo GW; (D) Terumo GW exteriorized by snaring from right femoral vein; (E) Venovenous loop established; (F) Lesion predilated with 10 × 40 mm balloon; (G and H) Postballoon expandable stent 10 × 39 mm implantation well open Innominate vein with good flow.

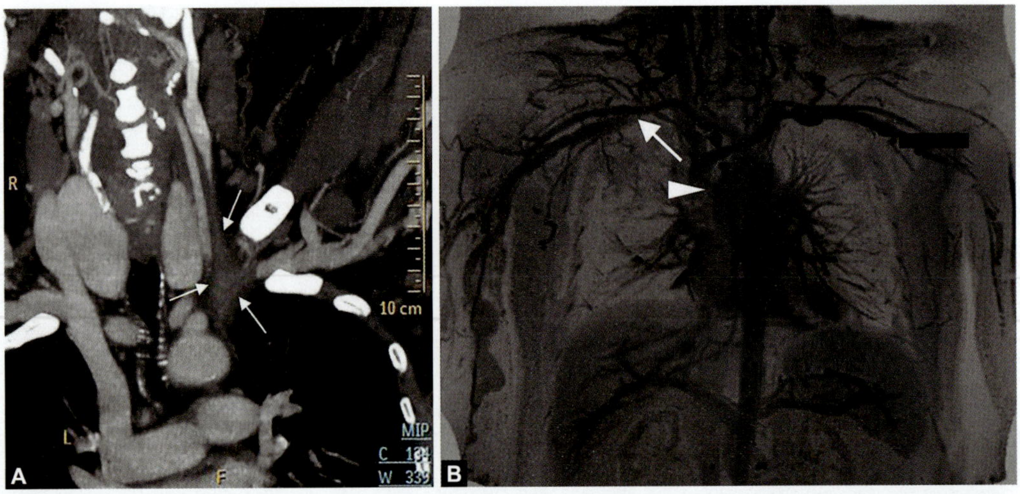

FIGS. 5A AND B: (A) Left innominate, subclavian and IJV stenosis; (B) Right innominate vein and subclavian stenosis.

Role of Imaging in Preprocedure Planning

To completely elucidate the lesion anatomy using appropriate imaging techniques such as CT venography **(Figs. 5A and B)**, magnetic resonance venography, or conventional venogram is essential and key to success in CVO intervention. It helps in planning the procedure such as the venous access, strategy to cross the occlusion (blunt or sharp recanalization), the size of balloon, and stent required. Long occlusions will be difficult to cross and recanalize. Knowing morphology of the occluded segment helps in planning access and intervention.

Preprocedure Ultrasound

Preprocedure ultrasound of the upper extremity is done to select the access vein for interventional approach and facilitate venous access.

Choice of Vascular Access

Being coaxial in the occluded central vein and being nearer to occlusion using ante grade puncture of brachial, cephalic, axillary vein, subclavian vein, and external or internal jugular vein facilitate in engaging and crossing the lesion, which is the most important step for successful intervention **(Figs. 3A to D)**. The antegrade puncture can be performed successfully using fluoroscopic guidance during levophase of brachial artery angiogram or ultrasound Doppler guidance. The engorged veins are palpable with a bruit and help in access. The knowledge and the use of both the antegrade and retrograde approach increase the success of crossing and recanalization in long occlusion **(Figs. 4A to H)**.

Diagnostic Venography

Diagnostic venogram is done to map the venous occlusion. Doing angiogram close to the occluded segment antegradely and retrogradely reveals length of occlusion, exact anatomical features of the origin of occluded segment **(Figs. 3, 4, 6 to 8)**. A tapered end at the beginning of occlusion helps in engaging the catheter to cross the lesion with the guidewire as there is better support **(Fig. 7A)**. Lesion with blunt end is difficult to engage and cross, and may need sharp recanalization as last resort.

Crossing the Lesion

From the upper or lower limb approach 0.035" Terumo guidewire (straight tip or angulated) through an 6F (JR/Multipurpose) catheter is routinely used to navigate through the occlusion. In case of chronic tough fibrotic lesions, 8F/9F COOK long sheath may be used for better stability and support while attempting to cross the lesion**(Figs. 8D and E)**. There are two ways of crossing the lesion, blunt **(Figs. 4C and D and 6C and D)** and sharp recanalization methods **(Fig. 8H)**. For simple lesions 0.035" Terumo hydrophilic wire with slow drilling can be used to cross lesions, which is called blunt recanalization. In long occlusion while maneuvering the guidewire if the tip gets stuck in the occlusion and loops, the loop with the catheter backup, when advanced knuckles the occluded site and traverses through the lesion and facilitates crossing the occlusion **(Figs. 6C and 8D)**. In case of resistant tough lesion when routine GW with back up catheter fails to engage the lesion, sharp recanalization can be used to engage and cross the lesion.

Sharp Recanalization

We have done sharp recanalization in chronic CVO with hard end of GW hard end of GW (0.035 terumo GW hard end of Teflon GW). If the above methods fails, Brokenborough needle can be used as last resort **(Fig. 8H)**. Hard end of Teflon-coated guidewire can be shaped, as it retains that memory, unlike hard end of Terumo GW which cannot be shaped. When occluded segment of vein is straight hard end of Terumo can be utilized to pierce through the

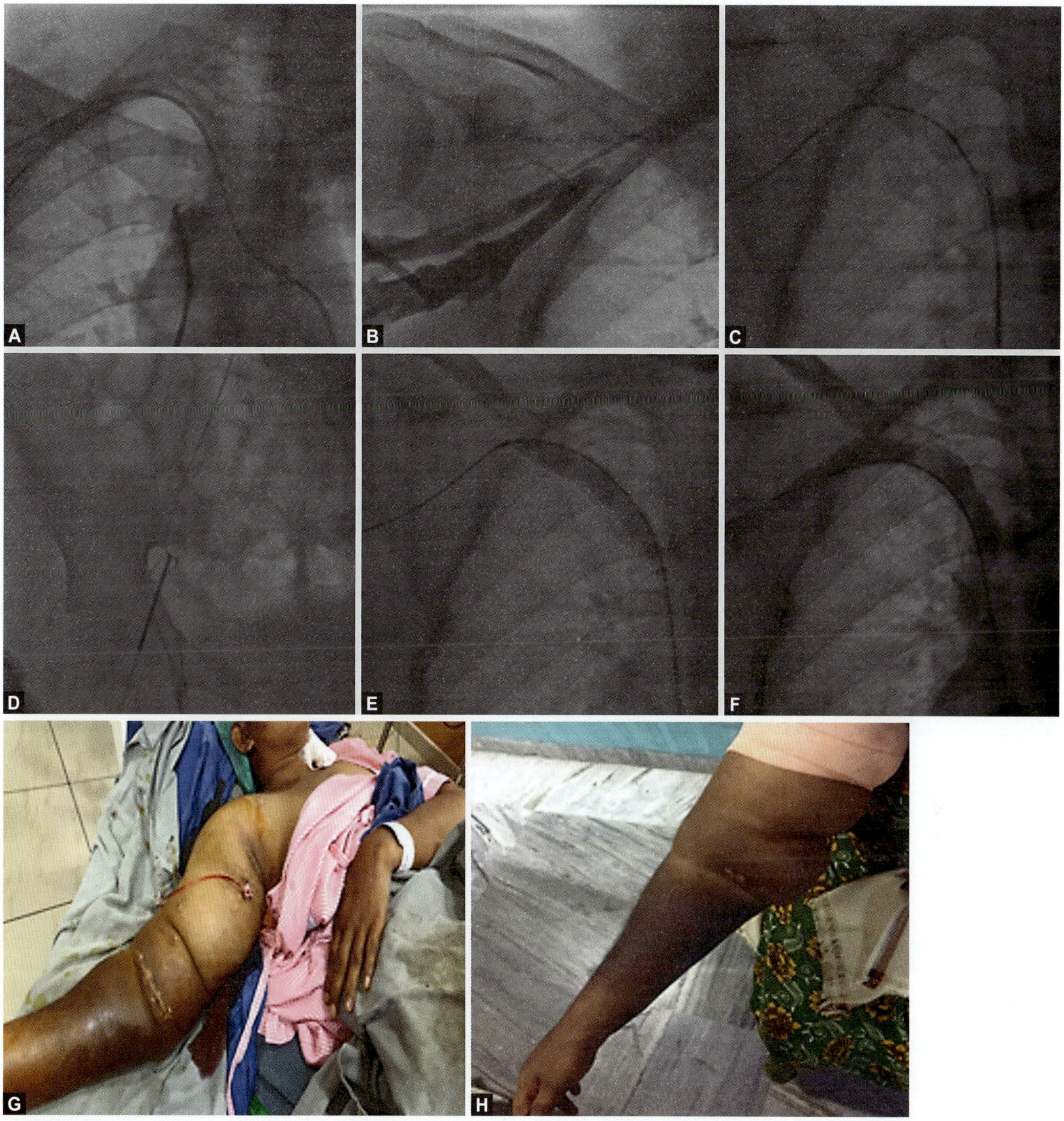

FIGS. 6A TO F: (A) Right innomiate vein, subclavian vein, distal axillary vein—long segment occlusion; (B) Crossing with Terumo guidewire/multipurpose catheter assembly; (C) Guidewire got stuck in the lesion and looped, loop when advanced knuckled to cross the occlusion; (D) Guidewire exteriorized by snaring and formed a venovenous loop; (E) Lesion predilated with 12 × 40 mm Atlas balloon; (F) 12 × 80 mm self-expanding Nitinol stent deployed with good result; (G) Preprocedure severe chronic edema of right upper limb; (H) Significant reduction in the limb edema postprocedure.

occlusion. If the occluded segment is curved with an angle, appropriately shaped hard end of Teflon-coated GW can be used to cross the lesion. Half-way into the occlusion, GW hard end is changed to softer end, and reattempted to cross the rest of lesion with soft end of GW. Brokenborough needle can be shaped according to occluded vein anatomy and needle advancement can be facilitated with small diluted contrast injection within the occlusion. Once sharp recanalization facilitates crossing, we exchange wire for a 360 cm exchange length GW.

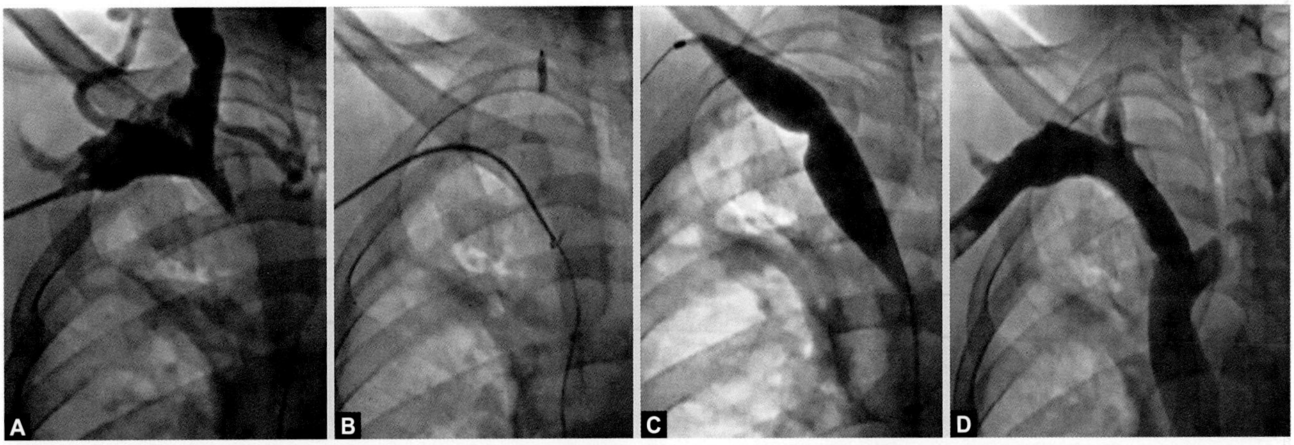

FIGS. 7A TO D: (A) Right innominate vein occlusion with tapered end from above; (B) Engaged with multipurpose catheter and crossed with Terumo guidewire; (C) Predilated with Atlas 14 × 40 mm balloon; and (D) Final result—post 14 × 40 mm self-expanding stent.

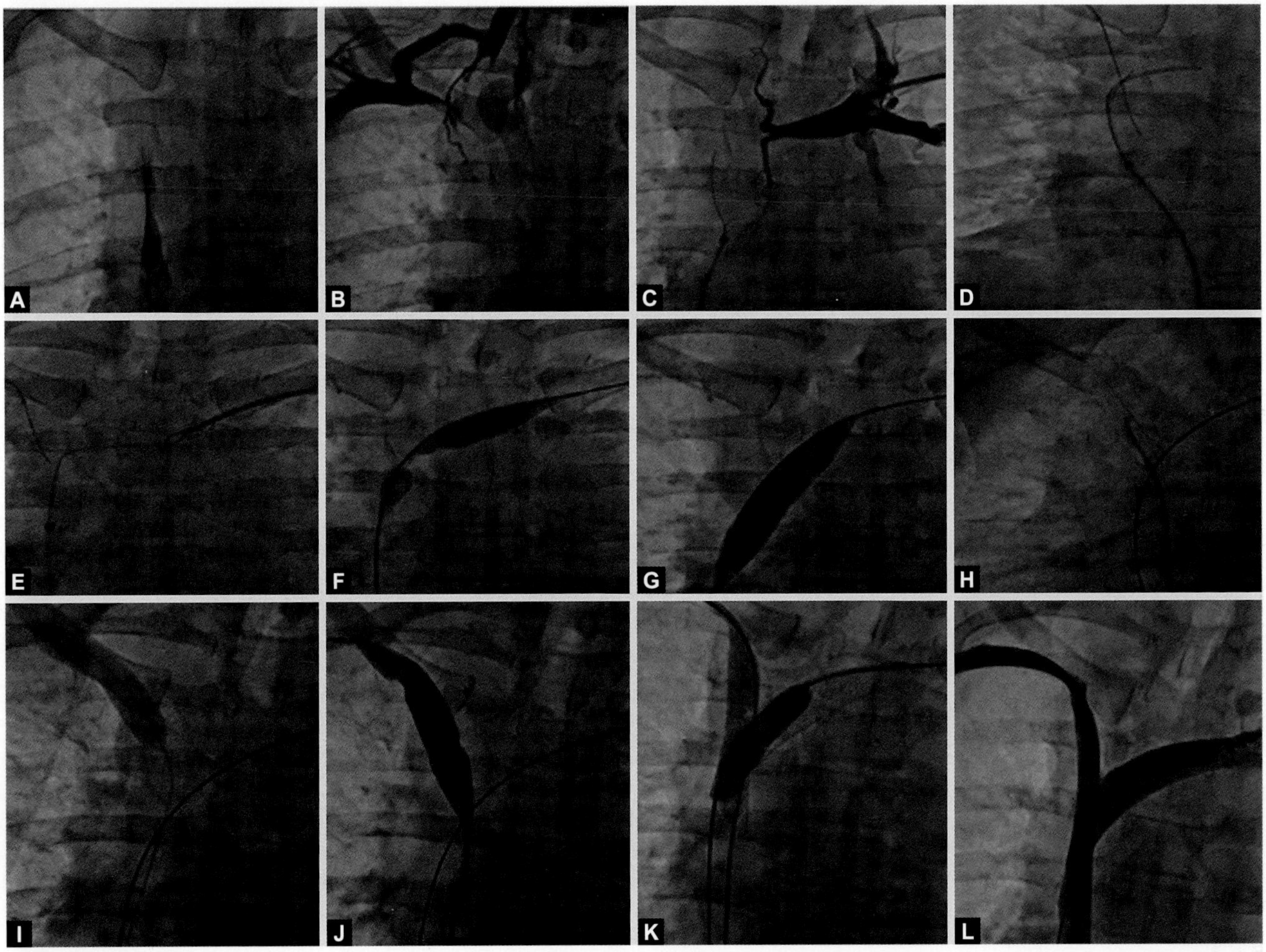

FIGS. 8A TO L: (A) Completely occluded right innominate vein; (B) Occluded right subclavian vein; (C) Occluded left innominate vein; (D) SVC and left innominate vein occlusion crossed with Terumo guidewire through backup long sheath; (E) Guidewire looped and knuckled through the occlusion. Wire exteriorized by snaring from left subclavian vein; (F and G) Predilated with 14 × 40 mm Atlas balloon; (H) Right innominate vein occlusion crossed with Brockenbrough needle; (I) Predilation with 10 × 40 mm ATLAS balloon; (J) Predilation with 14 × 40 mm ATLAS balloon; (K) 18 × 80 mm wall stent (from right subclavian to SVC); and (L) 22 × 60 mm wall stent (from left innominate vein to SVC) is deployed. Adequately opened innominate veins and SVC with good flow.

Venovenous Loop

In long occlusion, as we approach antegradely from upper limb vein (axillary, basilic, and subclavian) and retrogradely from femoral vein, once we cross the lesion, GW is exteriorized with snare from either end or venovenous loop is created. Veno venous loop between upper limb vein and femoral vein gives stability and facilitates to push or pull balloon across chronically occlusive lesions which otherwise would be difficult **(Figs. 4D, 6D, and 8E)**.

Predilation

The lesions are gradually adequately predilated 8 × 40 or 9 × 40 mm balloon initially and then 12 × 40 mm ATLAS noncomplaint balloon (BARD) **(Figs. 3C and D, 6E, 7C, 8G, and 8J)**.

Stent in CVO

Stent deployment is recommended in chronic long venous occlusion and in cases of recoil following balloon angioplasty as the stents provide effective mechanical support **(Figs. 6F, 7D, 8K and L, and 9A to F)**.[7] The choice of stent is also important. Central veins are tortuous and have larger diameter making the self-expandable stents more suitable in CVO. Self-expandable stents are preferred in axillary and peripheral brachiocephalic segments because of significant external compression by expiratory phase of respiration. Though ballon expandable stents can be used for SVC and central brachiocephalic veins, it is preferable to use self-expanding stent. Dedicated venous stents are available for management of CVO [sinus venous (Optimed), zilver vena (Cook), Venovo (Bard), and Vici (Boston)]. Covered stents, drug-eluting stents, and drug-eluting balloon may help in reducing restenosis and are being evaluated in studies.

COMPLICATIONS

Complications such as venous perforation or rupture are extremely rare **(Figs. 10A to M)**. It can lead to hemorrhage into pleural and pericardial space. It can be managed with prolonged balloon dilatation with or without stenting. In case of cardiac tamponade, urgent pericardiocentesis and autologous blood transfusion are performed as a bail out **(Figs. 10J to M)**. Rarely pneumothorax can occur. Inadvertent

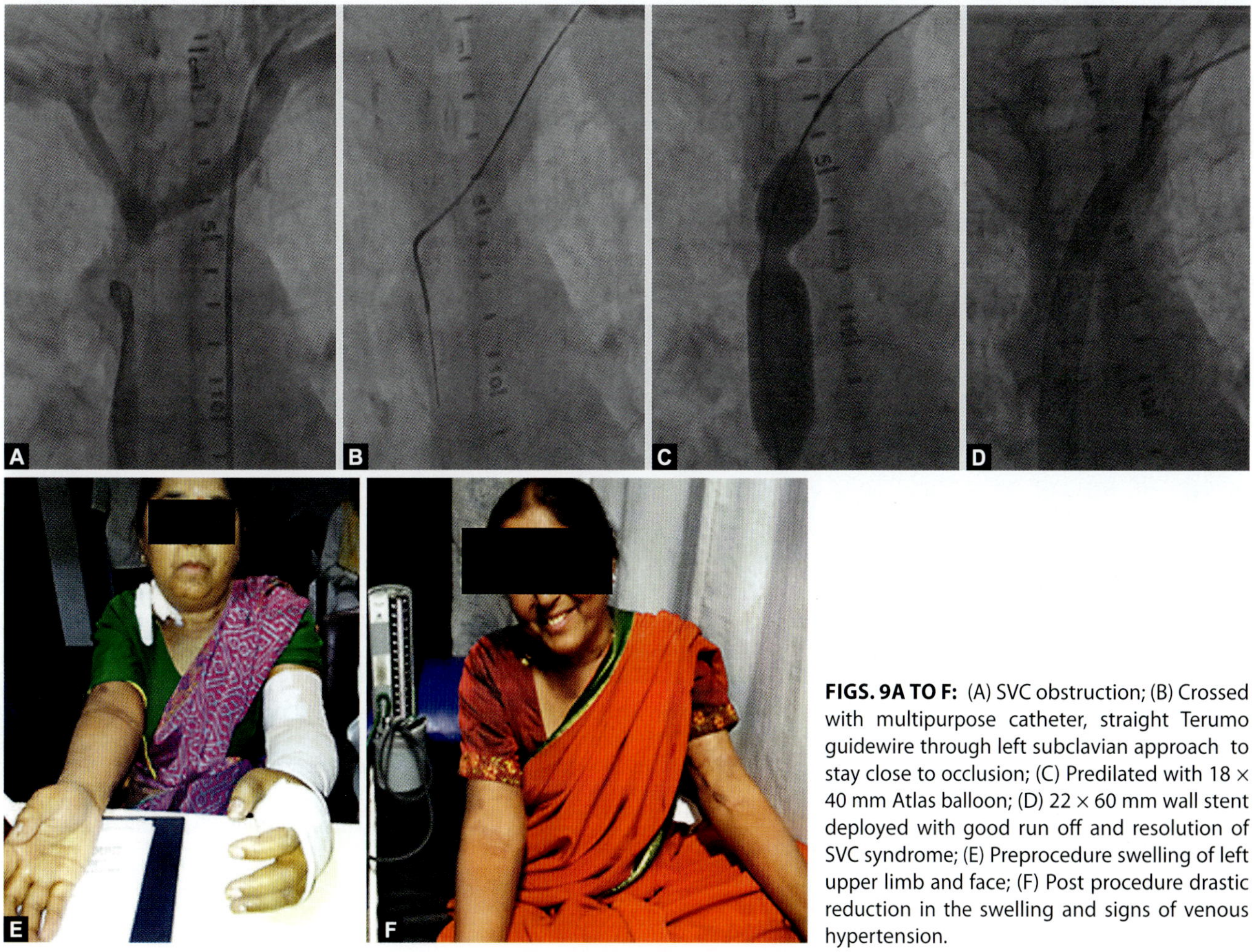

FIGS. 9A TO F: (A) SVC obstruction; (B) Crossed with multipurpose catheter, straight Terumo guidewire through left subclavian approach to stay close to occlusion; (C) Predilated with 18 × 40 mm Atlas balloon; (D) 22 × 60 mm wall stent deployed with good run off and resolution of SVC syndrome; (E) Preprocedure swelling of left upper limb and face; (F) Post procedure drastic reduction in the swelling and signs of venous hypertension.

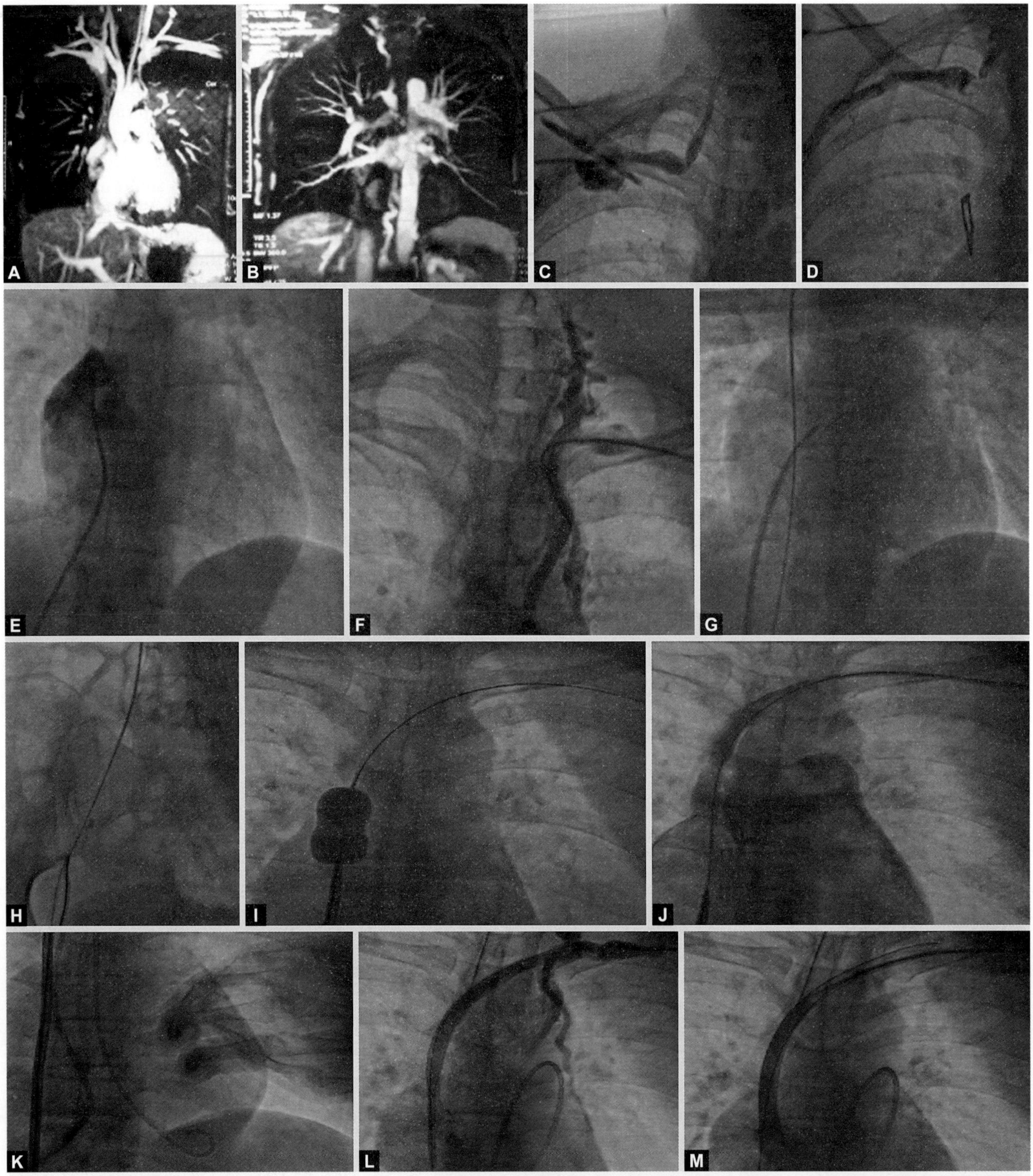

FIGS. 10A TO M: (A and B) CT venogram showing SVC occlusion with significant collaterals; (C and D) Contrast injection by subclavian venous and right internal jugular vein showed occlusion of SVC; (E) Contrast injection by multipurpose catheter at right atrium with SVC obstruction showed proximal extent of obstruction; (F) Trying to cross via left subclavian venous approach; (G and H) Terumo wire crossed by loop method from left subclavian vein and snared through right femoral vein using goose neck snare; (I) Predilatation using 22 mm Accura balloon; (J) SVC rupture leading to large pericardial effusion; (K) Pigtail in situ, with simultaneous aspiration and autotransfusion done; and (L and M) 8 × 60 mm wall stent deployed and perforation sealed.

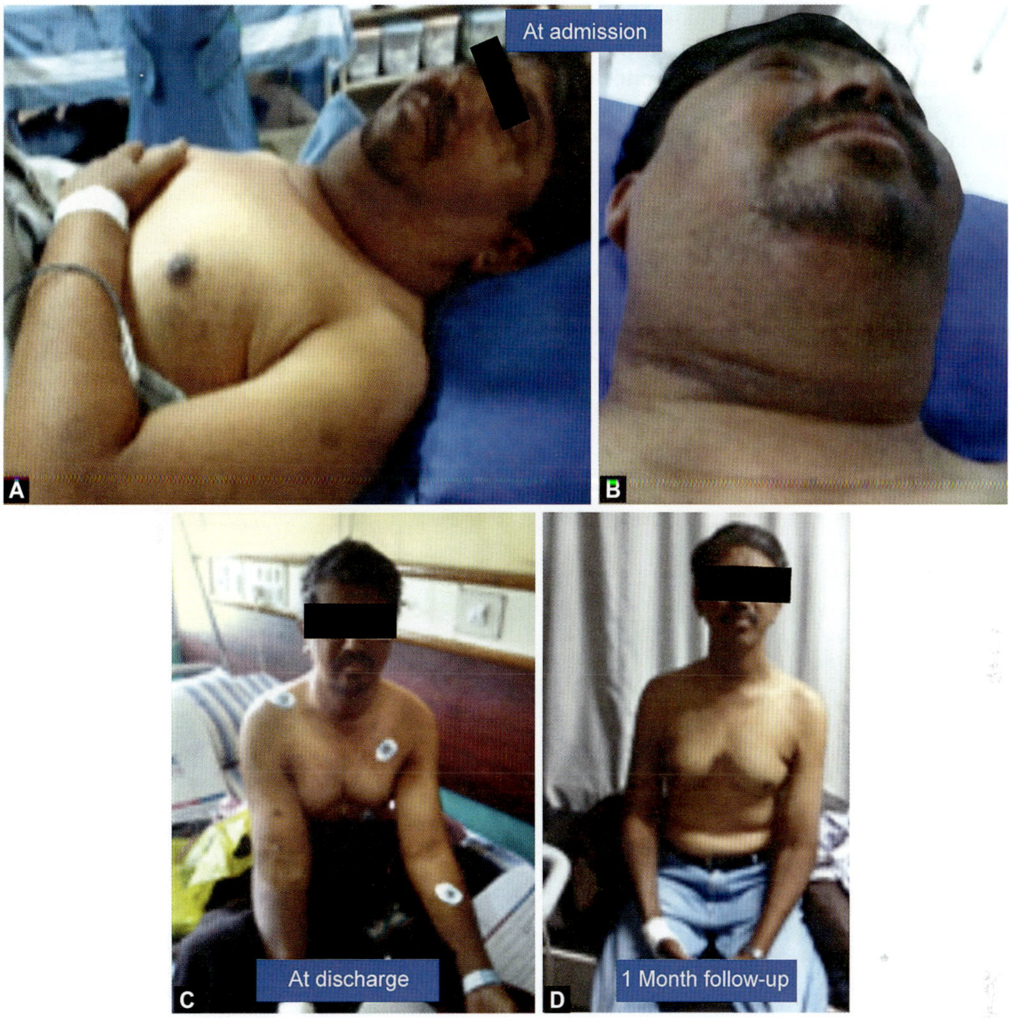

FIGS. 11A TO D: Case of SVC syndrome with gross edema due to bilateral innominate vein occlusion. Used to sleep in semirecumbent posture as he was unable to lie down flat. Post-CVO recanalization needed daily dialysis with extrafluid removal in each setting to relieve the gross volume retention. Edema resolved rapidly and completely.

arterial puncture can also occur with sharp recanalization techniques and RF wire.

Pharmacotherapy

DAPT for 1 month and single antiplatelet for life long is recommended.

POSTPROCEDURE

Once CVO is relieved with intervention, fluid shifts from third space to central circulatory system, which can cause flash pulmonary edema as many of them have comorbidities with systolic or diastolic LV dysfunction. They have to be dialyzed with extrafluid removal after intervention. Some of them with gross edema need dialysis more frequently than usual to remove the accumulated extravolume **(Figs. 11A to D)**.

CONCLUSION

Central venous occlusion is an important cause of dialysis failure in CKD patients on maintenance hemodialysis and contributes to morbidity. There is strong association of prolonged and repeated central venous catheterization with the CVO. Routine evaluation of central veins using either Doppler or venography studies should be done before creating the arteriovenous fistula. In CVO, the endovascular interventions are safe and effective for achieving and maintaining the patency of central veins, fistula access and alleviating the symptoms of venous hypertension. In view of higher restenosis following balloon angioplasty or stent implantation, meticulous follow-up and repeat intervention to maintain patency are mandatory. Long-term outcomes are determined by associated comorbidities.

ONLINE REFERENCES

Please scan the QR code provided at the end of the table of contents for References of this chapter.

SECTION

18

Rhythm and Conduction Abnormalities

Section Outline

CHAPTER

195

Top Ten Papers in Arrhythmia Treatment: 2023–2024

Sanjeev Asotra, Rajesh Sharma, Sachin Maggo

ABSTRACT

Cardiac arrhythmias remain a common cause of death and disability. Atrial fibrillation remains an ever-increasing global pandemic with a complex pathophysiology that contributes to significant patient morbidity and mortality. Ever-increasing understanding and focused research in primary prevention, early detection, risk prediction, drugs, and ablation therapy are trying to fill voids in the gaps in knowledge. Arrhythmogenic right ventricular cardiomyopathy (ARVC) is a progressive fatal disorder characterized by lethal arrhythmias and sudden cardiac death (SCD). Current approaches are the use of antiarrhythmic drugs and the use of AICD. There is a critical need to identify the targets of underlying drivers of the pathogenesis of ARVC. The gene therapy though tried in the murine model holds promise for prevention, but the challenge will remain to translate this proof-of-concept study into clinical application.

Keywords: AF, NOAC, ARVC

INTRODUCTION

The year 2023–2024 witnessed some major landmark trials in atrial fibrillation (AF), primarily focusing on primary prevention with paradigm shifts in screening tools and treatment of subclinical AF. There is a ray of hope for gene therapy in patients with progressive disease like arrhythmogenic right ventricular dysplasia, which carries high morbidity and mortality.

SCREENING AND DETECTION OF HIGH-RISK ATRIAL FIBRILLATION

As with other swiftly expanding lifestyle diseases, the need for assessment of lifestyle-related risk factors for the development of AF cannot be underestimated. The HARMS2-AF score is a novel lifestyle risk score that may help identify individuals at risk of AF in the general community and assist in population screening **(Table 1)**. The score developed using UK Biobank and Framingham heart study population cohorts performed comparably with the CHARGE-AF risk score and outperformed the Framingham-AF and ARIC risk scores in predicting incident AF in patients with no prior history of AF. A summed score of 5–9 or >9 is associated with an increased risk of incident AF with hazard ratios of 13 and 39, respectively.[1] The tool assists in rapid decision-making either in public health, in emergency wards, or even at the bedside and allows the identification of people at risk of incident AF and perhaps initiates early intervention. It may also reduce the number of screens needed to find one AF case, and thereby improve the cost-effectiveness of screening.

TABLE 1: HARMS2-AF score.

Parameter	Score
Hypertension	4
Age: 60–64 years ≥ 65 years	1 2
BMI > 30 kg/m^2	1
Male gender	2
Sleep apnea	2
Smoking	1
Alcohol 7–14 standard drinks/week ≥15 drinks/week	1 2

Atrial fibrillation, apart from causing hemodynamic compromise, can also lead to other disabling consequences like ischemic stroke, making it prudent to screen the elderly population for early detection and anticoagulation. The same was demonstrated in STROKESTOP trial, a multicenter RCT conducted in Sweden. 7,165 elderly patients were subjected to twice daily ECG for 14 days. If AF was detected, they were initiated on anticoagulation. With a median follow-up of 6.9 years, they demonstrated a significant reduction in the primary endpoint (ischemic or hemorrhagic stroke and systemic embolism) of 31.9% versus 33% in the control group with a hazard ratio of 0.96. This health economic study implies that population-based AF screening for individuals of age 75/76 years is cost-effective at a probability of 99.7% and a cost-saving probability of 92.7%. The major limitation of STROKESTOP trial was that the participation rate in this population-based screening study was low.[2]

Another study that deserves mention here is the LOOP trial including 6,004 patients with a mean age of 74.7 years,[3] which demonstrated that in individuals with stroke risk factors, implantable loop recorder screening resulted in three times increase in AF detection and anticoagulation. However, the benefit did not translate into stroke risk reduction. Nevertheless, subgroup analysis did show screening for AF is most effective in those with N-terminal pro-B-type natriuretic peptide (NT-proBNP) >15 pmol/L with fewer thromboembolic complications (amongst others stroke) and cardiovascular death. The number needed to screen to avoid one stroke/SE after 6 years was 31 for participants with NT-proBNP > 28 pmol/L and 21 for participants with NT-proBNP >76 pmol/L. The study had limitations as the study population was mainly comprised of the elderly population. This was not a prespecified analysis of the LOOP study and there was a lack of echocardiographic data and there was lack of echocardiographic data in the study.

Overall, the last decade has seen a paradigm shift in our approach toward preventing AF. The focused screening (based on lifestyle factors, age, and advanced hemodynamics) has helped us to cater to high-risk populations systematically, thereby making it both more efficient as well as cost-effective.

ORAL ANTICOAGULATION IN SUBCLINICAL ATRIAL FIBRILLATION

Non-vitamin K oral antagonists (NOACs) have gradually become the preferred oral anticoagulant drug to prevent thromboembolic complications in patients with AF. The role of NOACs was studied in patients with subclinical AF as defined by atrial high-rate events, recorded by an implanted electronic device, lasting at least 6 minutes in NOAH-AFNET 6 and ARTESiA trials. The composite of cardiovascular death, stroke, or systemic embolism was not reduced by edoxaban compared to the placebo group in NOAH-AFNET 6, despite 54% of patients being on aspirin in this trial, with annual event rates of 3.2% versus 4.0%. The major bleeding occurred significantly more often, 2.1% versus 1.0% per year. There was no difference in ischemic stroke rates, i.e., 0.9% versus 1.1% per year. The trial was terminated early at the median follow-up of 21 months based on safety concerns. Though the results of both trials are consistent with each other in the form of the same stroke risk, the primary endpoint of ischemic stroke and systemic embolism occurred significantly less often compared to aspirin in ARTESiA (0.7% vs. 1.24% per year). ARTESiA trial had higher patient numbers and longer follow-up, thus better statistical power than NOAH-AFNET 6 trial.[4,5]

Both trials had major issues and had to be stopped prematurely, NOAH-AFNET 6 for futility and unsafety of NOAC therapy, and ARTESiA for slower recruitment. Pooled data of both trials together showed that ischemic stroke rates are low in subclinical AF and treatment on NOACs could result in delayed and restricted stroke preventive benefits at the cost of early onset bleeding risk. The clinical implication supports the use of NOAC in patients with device-detected AF through a shared decision-making process considering treatment benefits, event rates, strokes or bleeding, and patient's values and preferences.

TREATMENT OF ATRIAL FIBRILLATION: INSIGHTS INTO NEW MANAGEMENT STRATEGIES

With technical advancement and greater confidence in ablation strategies, there is rising advocacy for early definitive treatment for AF. This has been validated by promising results of several studies in the last few years. Be it studies on early AF ablation, pulsed-field ablation, or AF catheter ablation in end-stage heart failure (HF), all have opened new avenues giving interventional cardiologists food for thought.

As the boom of electrophysiology (EP) reaches its teenage, it was assumed that EP interventions would answer all the unmet challenges in the field of arrhythmias, AF being the most prominent. This led to a strong enthusiasm for early catheter ablation for AF. However, Kalman study enrolled 100 patients with AF who were randomized in a 1:1 ratio for early ablation within 1 month and delayed AF ablation after initial antiarrhythmic drugs therapy followed by AF ablation at 1 year. The results included the primary endpoint of freedom from recurrent AF (56.3% vs. 58.6%) and secondary endpoints of median AF burden [0% (IQR 3.2) vs. 0% (IQR 5)], and the use of antiarrhythmic drug therapy (33% vs. 37%) 12 months after AF ablation did not show any difference.[6] The study did have limitations such as fewer patients with relatively few comorbidities; still, the study did bring out that initial drug therapy and delayed ablation a feasible approach. This is especially relevant for a country like India with limited resources, and thus may release the pressure on healthcare systems to perform instantaneous ablations. The critics attribute the results to a low rate of AF progression in patients qualifying for ablation, low comorbidity burden, and effects of antiarrhythmic drugs. Also, the study does not answer many questions including its application for patients with severe symptoms or tachycardia-induced HF, patients with higher comorbidity burden, or whether the timing of ablation affects the rate of major adverse cardiovascular and cerebrovascular events differentially. Nevertheless, it does lay down foundation for further research.

Another imperative trial, the ADVENT trial, conducted in 607 drug-refractory paroxysmal AF patients compared pulsed field ablation (PFA) with thermal ablation. The results concluded that PFA was noninferior to thermal ablation in terms of freedom from initial procedural failure, arrhythmia recurrence, antiarrhythmic drug use, cardioversion, or repeat ablation (73.3% vs. 71.3%).[7] With statistically insignificant device- and procedure-related adverse events (2.1% vs. 1.5%) and shorter and less variable procedure times, the study supported the noninferiority of PFA. Though PFA's shorter and more predictable operation times are alluring, its role in ablation still needs further studies. Importantly, PFA requires general anesthesia or deep sedation, and notwithstanding a high initial procedural success, long-term rhythm control is not better than with conventional approaches. Adverse effects include silent cerebral lesions, coronary artery spasms, and phrenic nerve injury, the impact of these is yet to be studied.

One of the major challenges confronted by each physician in cardiac ICUs is the management of patients with symptomatic AF and end-stage HF. The CASTLE HTx trial was a single-center, open-labeled trial including 194 patients with symptomatic AF and end-stage HF. The trial compared the combination of catheter ablation and guideline-directed medical therapy versus medical therapy alone. Patients were initially evaluated for left ventricular assist device (LVAD) or heart transplantation and then were given catheter ablation while awaiting HF intervention. The study concluded that a combination of catheter ablation and guideline-directed medical therapy at 18 months is associated with a reduction in primary outcomes, a composite of all-cause mortality, LVAD implantation, or the need for urgent heart transplantation compared to medical therapy alone (8% vs. 30% primary endpoint event). This effect was driven primarily by a reduction in all-cause mortality and LVAD implantation.[8] The study had a highly selected patient population and open-label design and higher rates of crossover from the ablation group attenuated the primary outcomes. Still, the Castle HTx study supports that catheter ablation is an important and promising add-on HF therapy and possibly slows the progression and clinical course in end-stage HF patients.

ATRIAL FIBRILLATION RECURRENCE: DO WE NEED TO REDEFINE THE TERM?

A working definition for recurrences of AF in clinical trials is taken as an event lasting at least 30 seconds. This definition is similar to that for sustained ventricular arrhythmias, permitting comparison of outcomes between intervention studies. The CIRCA-DOSE study was designed to evaluate cryoballoon versus irrigated catheter ablation and the effectiveness of pulmonary vein isolation by contact force guided RF ablation and second generation cryoablation using double and standard exposure duration. The study demonstrated the efficacy of PVI for the patients of paroxysmal AF, there was no difference between contact-based RF ablation and cryoballoon ablation on reoccurrence and complications. The sub-analysis of CIRCA dose study has challenged the very definition, questioning the basis of such a low cut-off duration to define AF recurrences after rhythm intervention since it does not reflect the pathophysiology of clinical AF very well or clinical outcomes. The gold standard definition of an AF episode of >30 seconds lacked clinical relevance concerning healthcare utilization and quality of life outcomes. There is a relationship between AF duration and AF burden on healthcare utilization along with quality of life. Healthcare utilization is represented by emergency department consultation, cardiovascular hospitalization, cardioversion, and repeat ablation. The study demonstrated that the cutoff for the duration of AF with a meaningful impact on healthcare utilization to be 1 hour, paralleled by an AF burden cutoff of 0.1%. Above those thresholds, risks of emergency department consultation, cardiovascular hospitalization, cardioversion, and repeat ablation rose significantly, and disease-specific quality of life indices became impaired.[9] This study looks at the definition from a practical point of view, thereby advocating a paramount shift towards redefining AF recurrences after intervention as lasting more than 1 hour. Such a definition will abolish the need for costly and infeasible continuous monitoring. These shall be replaced by more practical options, such as repeated 12-lead ECG, Holter, or even more patient-friendly intermittent telemonitoring. Also, the efficacy data of the interventions done would be more representative taking into account the clinical effects of arrhythmia recurrence rather than the arrhythmia per se.

ACUTE REDUCTION IN RAPID VENTRICULAR RATE IN PATIENTS OF SYMPTOMATIC ATRIAL FIBRILLATION

Fast ventricular rate in AF can precipitate HF and is associated with worsening symptoms including palpitations, breathlessness, chest pain, and anxiety requiring medical therapy in the form of intravenous beta blockers, IV calcium channel blockers (CCB), or electric cardioversion. There is a need for a self-administered medication that can rapidly reduce the heart rate. Etripamil is a fast-acting CCB that is rapidly absorbed by nasal mucosa and the drug achieves maximum concentration within 7 minutes. ReVera is a multicenter, randomized, double-blind, placebo-controlled study that evaluated the efficacy and safety of etripamil nasal spray 70 mg in patients presenting to emergency with AF with rapid ventricular rate. Etripamil, a fast-acting CCB, administered intranasally was able to achieve heart rate reduction in 60 minutes and ventricular rate reduction persisted up to 150 minutes. A greater proportion of patients achieved ventricular rate reduction to <100 bpm compared to placebo. There was a significant improvement in satisfaction with symptom relief and treatment effectiveness with etripamil compared to placebo. Serious adverse effects of etripamil were rare. An intranasal spray of etripamil may have a future in self-administration by patients outside the healthcare setting.[10]

REPLACEMENT OF DYSFUNCTIONAL GENES COULD PROLONG SURVIVAL IN ARRHYTHMOGENIC RIGHT VENTRICULAR CARDIOMYOPATHY

Arrhythmogenic right ventricular cardiomyopathy is a progressive incurable genetic heart disease predominantly involving the right ventricle manifesting by early electrical cardiac defects progressing to the structural phase in which there is a fibrofatty replacement of myocardium. Electrical dysfunction is a key hallmark of ARVC causing ventricular arrhythmias and a major contributor to sudden cardiac death (SCD) in patients. ARVC involves 1 out of 2,000-5000 people. Human genetic studies have shown that half the patients with ARVC carry genetic mutations involving desmoplakin (*DSP*), desmoglein (*DSG2*), desmocollin (*DSC2*), plakoglobin (*JUP*), and plakophilin2 (*PKP2*). The *PKP2* mutations make up for the majority of mutations leading to haploinsufficiency causing a reduction in myocardial PKP2 protein levels. The altered PKP2 RNA levels act as a critical trigger of ARVC pathogenesis. Bradford et al. demonstrated in the murine model that in vivo-based AAV-PKP2 strategies were sufficient to restore PKP2 in the myocardium to prevent not only the striking cardiac desmosomal dissolution but also the gap junction deficits, thus preventing electrical and structural cardiac deficits in ARVC. It represents an effective future therapy for preventing and stabilizing ARVC disease progression.[11] The future challenge remains in the translation of proof-of-concept study into clinical application.

CONCLUSION

It was an exceptional year of research for arrhythmia trials. AF research remained in focus looking for answers in screening, detection, reoccurrences, role of NOAC, treatment, and current understanding of catheter ablation. Some trials have shown encouraging results and may change the present-day guidelines.

ONLINE REFERENCES

Please scan the QR code provided at the end of the table of contents for References of this chapter.

CHAPTER

196

Electrocardiogram Approach to Narrow QRS Complex Tachycardia

Sundaram Chandrashekhar, Yash Lokhandwala

ABSTRACT

Supraventricular tachycardia (SVT) can be either AV node-dependent [atrioventricular nodal reentrant tachycardia (AVNRT) and atrioventricular reentrant tachycardia (AVRT)] or AV node-independent [atrial tachycardia (AT), atrial flutter (AFL), and atrial fibrillation (AF)]. This chapter covers the fundamental ECG approach to distinguishing between various forms of narrow QRS tachycardia.

Keywords: SVT, AVNRT, AVRT, AT, AFL, AF

INTRODUCTION

Narrow QRS complex tachycardia (NCT) is any cardiac rhythm above 100 beats per minute (bpm) with a QRS duration of <120 ms. The ventricles get activated through the His–Purkinje system, hence the narrow QRS complex. The majority of NCT seen in the emergency room are supraventricular tachycardias (SVT) or those arising above the branching of the bundle of His (HB). Patients often present with persistent palpitations, chest discomfort, lightheadedness, breathing difficulty, or rarely syncope due to associated hypotension in the presence of other comorbidities or due to frailty.[1] A diagnosis of NCT can be made with a 12-lead ECG (considered the gold standard), ambulatory Holter monitoring, telemetry, an implantable loop recorder, and using smartwatch or smartphone devices.[2] This chapter focuses on the systematic approach to differentiating different types of NCT based on clues from ECG **(Box 1)**.

BOX 1 Differential diagnosis of narrow QRS (≤120 ms) tachycardia.

- *Regular*
  - Physiologic sinus tachycardia
  - Inappropriate sinus tachycardia
  - Sinus nodal reentrant tachycardia
  - Focal AT
  - Atrial flutter with fixed AV conduction
  - AV nodal reentrant tachycardia
  - Junctional ectopic tachycardia
  - Orthodromic AV reentrant tachycardia
  - Idiopathic VT (especially upper septal VT)
- *Irregular*
  - Atrial fibrillation
  - Focal atrial tachycardia or atrial flutter with varying AV conduction
  - Multifocal atrial tachycardia

CLASSIFICATION

Based on the consistency of R–R interval during NCT:

- *Regular NCT*: Variability of R–R interval < 20 ms
- *Irregular NCT*: Variability of R–R interval > 20 ms

Based on the ventricular–atrial (VA) relationship during NCT (refers to the number of P waves for every QRS complex):

- *1:1 AV conduction*: Can be either AV node-dependent or nondependent
- *Atrial rate > ventricular rate*: Non-AV node (AVN) dependent

Based on the RP interval, when there is 1:1 VA conduction (refers to timing of the P wave in relation to the R–R interval):[3]

- *Short RP tachycardia*: The P wave following the preceding R wave falls within half of the R–R interval.
- *Intermediate RP tachycardia*: The P wave falls midway between the QRS complexes.
- *Long RP tachycardia*: The P wave following the preceding R wave falls after half of the R–R interval.

MODE OF INITIATION AND TERMINATION OF TACHYCARDIA

- *Typical AVNRT*: A premature atrial complex (PAC) is followed by sudden prolongation of PR interval, which initiates the tachycardia, suggestive of antegrade conduction through the slow pathway.
- *Atrial tachycardia (AT)*: Initiated by an ectopic atrial beat; however, it is not dependent on PR prolongation.
- *Atypical AVNRT*: Frequently triggered by premature ventricular complex
- *AVRT*: Triggered by premature atrial or ventricular complex
- Termination of NCT in a QRS can be AVNRT/AVRT/AT, whereas termination in a P wave rules out AT **(Fig. 1)**.

BUNDLE BRANCH BLOCK DURING SUPRAVENTRICULAR TACHYCARDIA

The presence of SVT with and without bundle branch block (BBB) helps in localizing the pathway in AVRT.

Ipsilateral BBB (RBBB in a right-sided AP; LBBB in a left-sided AP): Due to ipsilateral BBB, the impulse from the atrium travels through the contralateral bundle followed by transeptal conduction to reach the AP, which results in prolongation of ventriculoatrial (VA) interval.[4] A rise in the VA interval frequently leads to a corresponding decrease in the AH interval, which helps to reduce a rise in cycle length (CL) **(Fig. 2)**. Contralateral BBB (RBBB in a left-sided AP; LBBB in a right-sided AP) has no effect on the VA interval.

P-WAVE MORPHOLOGY

- *Similar to sinus P wave*: Appropriate or inappropriate sinus nodal tachycardia, sinus nodal reentrant tachycardia, or focal AT arising close to the sinus node
- *Different from sinus P wave with PR interval equal to or longer than the PR in sinus rhythm*: Focal AT and atypical AVNRT
- *Retrograde P wave*: The presence of pseudo r′ in V_1 and pseudo S wave in the inferior leads favors typical AVNRT **(Figs. 3A and B)**. Specificity is 91–100%, while sensitivity is 58 and 14%, respectively.[5,6]

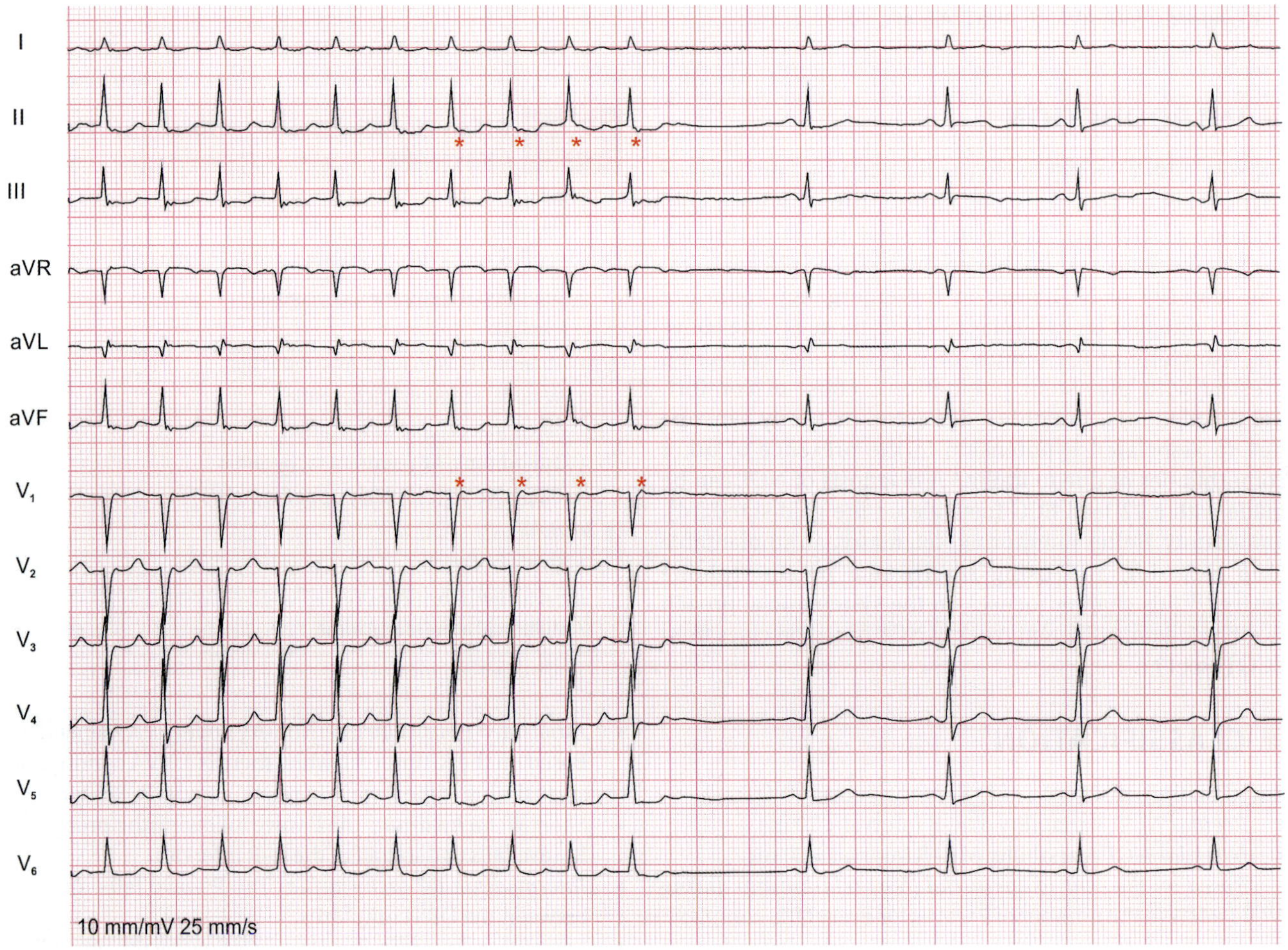

FIG. 1: Termination of tachycardia: ECG strip of a patient with typical AVNRT showing termination in a P wave (*), which rules out atrial tachycardia.

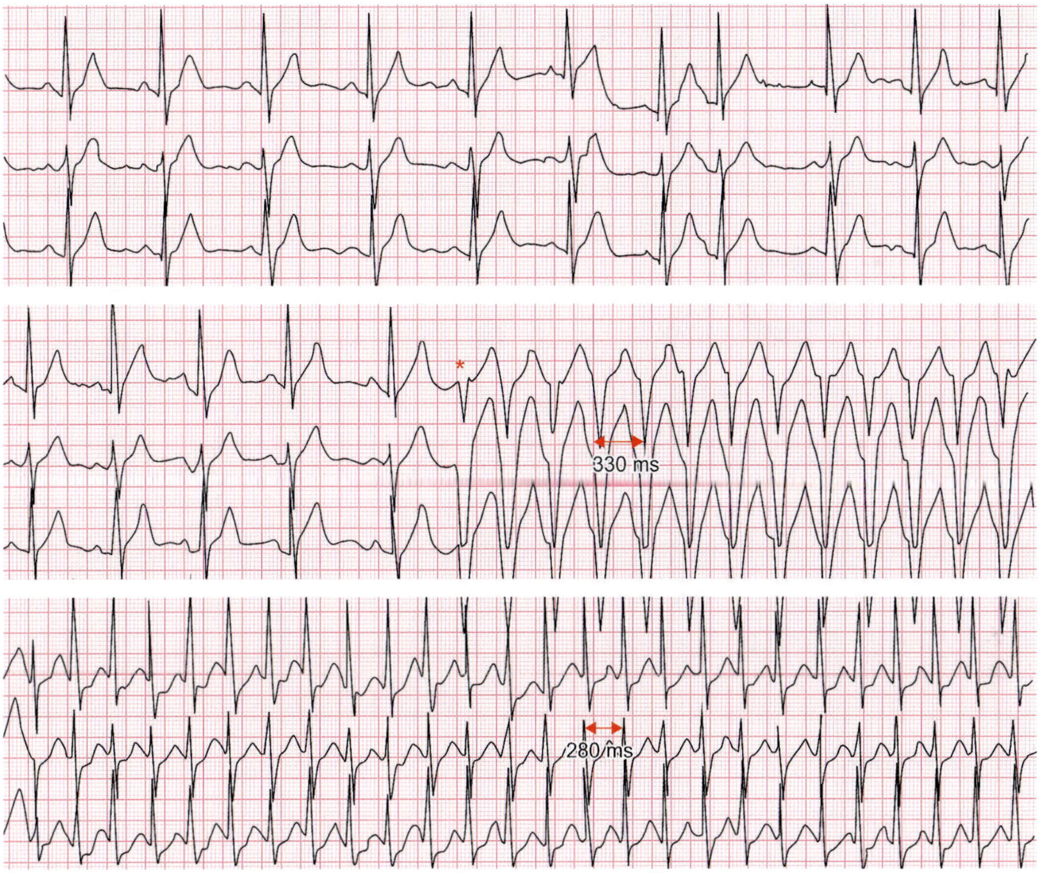

FIG. 2: Holter strip of orthodromic AVRT, with and without LBBB in a concealed left lateral AP: PVC (*) initiates regular tachycardia with initial LBBB. The LBBB complexes exhibit greater R–R intervals compared to the narrow QRS tachycardia.

ATRIOVENTRICULAR BLOCK DURING NARROW QRS COMPLEX TACHYCARDIA

The presence of AV block during an NCT is seen with AT and, in certain cases, AVNRT, but rules out AVRT as atria and ventricles are part of the reentrant circuit.

VAGAL MANEUVERS AND ADENOSINE IN NARROW QRS COMPLEX TACHYCARDIA

- *Sudden termination*: AVNRT, AVRT **(Fig. 4)**, and sinus node reentry
- *Gradual slowing, then reacceleration of rate*: Sinus tachycardia, automatic AT, and nonparoxysmal junctional tachycardia (JT)
- *No change in rate*: Inadequate dose and high septal VT
- *Persistent AT with high-grade AV block*: Atrial flutter and macro (micro) reentrant AT

ATRIOVENTRICULAR NODAL REENTRANT TACHYCARDIA

Atrioventricular nodal reentrant tachycardia is the most common form of SVT seen in clinical practice.[7,8] It can be seen at any age. It is a type of micro-reentrant tachycardia involving two functional pathways referred to as a slow pathway and a fast pathway, which form a microcircuit that is confined to the AV node and perinodal tissue.[9]

Typical Atrioventricular Nodal Reentrant Tachycardia

A slow–fast AVNRT is generally referred to as typical AVNRT. The antegrade limb of the circuit has slow conduction properties, while the retrograde limb has fast conduction properties, hence the name. Due to rapid conduction via retrograde limb, the ventricular and subsequent atrial activation occur almost simultaneously ("A on V"). On surface ECG, this is manifested as short RP tachycardia with P waves either buried in the QRS or occurring immediately

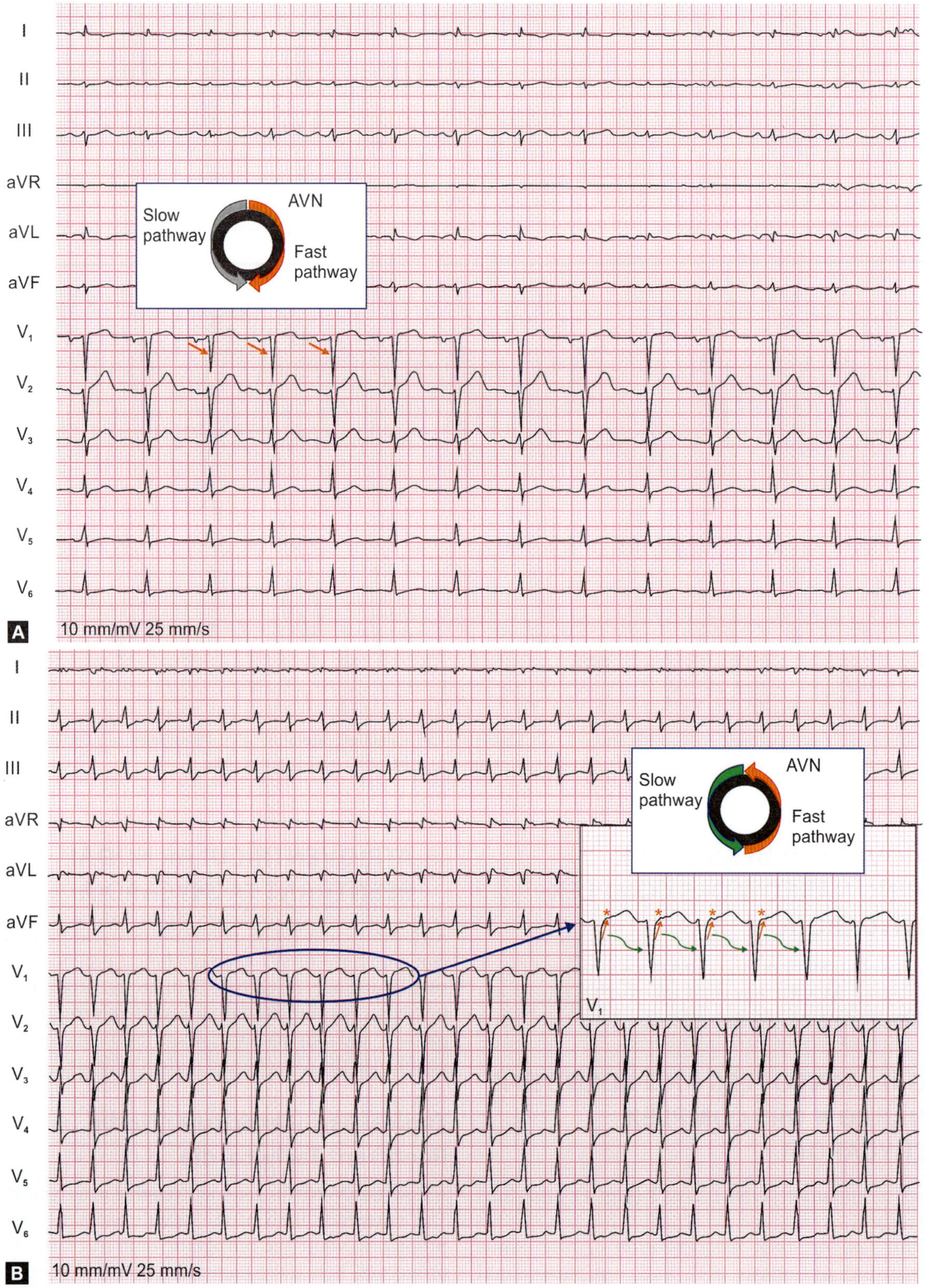

FIGS. 3A AND B: Typical AVNRT. (A) ECG during sinus rhythm. Antegrade conduction through the normal "fast" pathway. (B) ECG during tachycardia. There is a block in conduction through the fast pathway and the impulse goes antegrade through the slow pathway; retrograde conduction through the fast pathway back to the atrium results in pseudo r′ wave (*) in V_1.

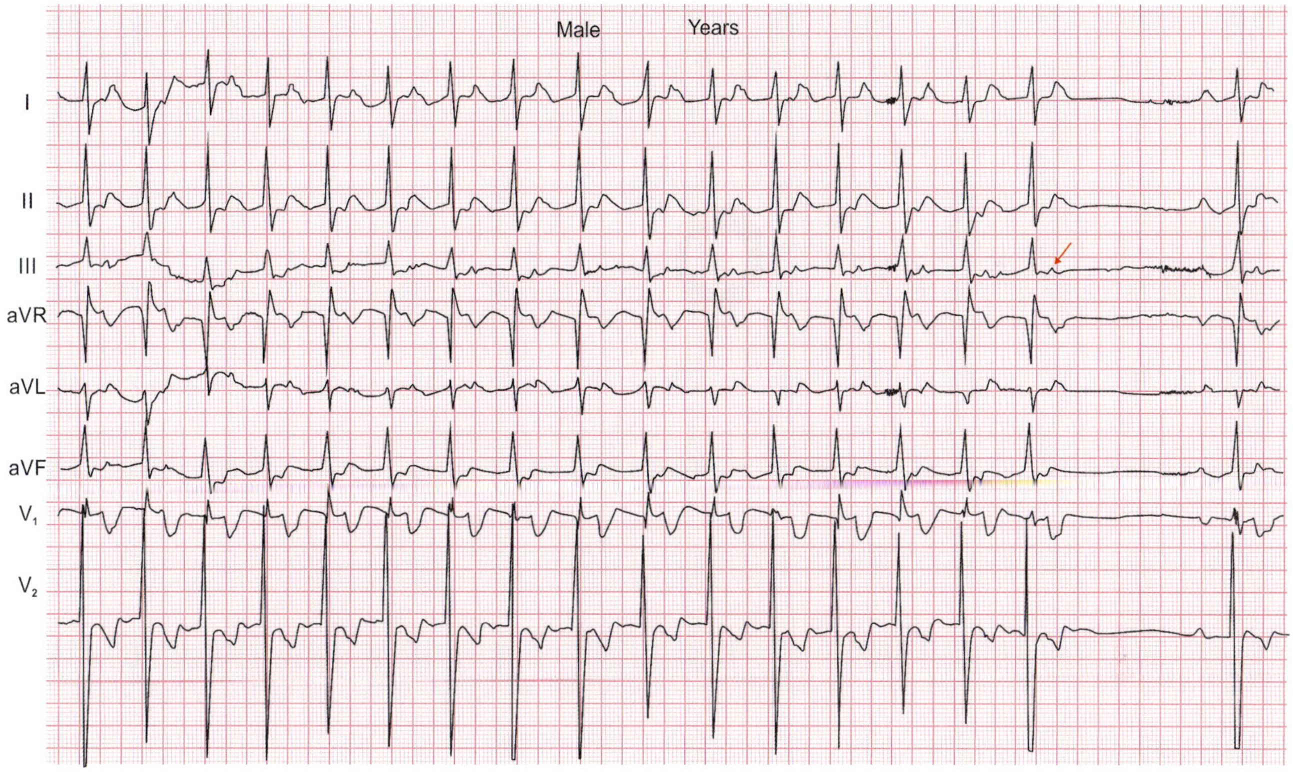

FIG. 4: Response to adenosine: ECG of a 6-year-old boy with orthodromic AVRT, which terminates after a P wave (arrow) after administration of 6 mg IV adenosine.

after the QRS. The P waves that fall at the end of the QRS are seen as pseudo S waves in the inferior leads and pseudo R waves in V_1 during tachycardia, which are not seen in sinus rhythm.

In sinus rhythm, conduction usually happens via the fast pathway of the AV node. Dual AV nodal conduction can sometimes be seen as changing PR intervals on the surface ECG with no change in heart rate. Holter monitoring may show PACs and atrial echo beats (antegrade conduction occurs through the slow pathway, and the impulse returns via the fast pathway to depolarize the atria resulting in P wave and subsequently fails to conduct antegrade due to refractoriness) between episodes. Initiation of narrow complex tachycardia may be seen with a PAC followed by a sudden prolongation of PR interval,[10] which denotes the block in the antegrade fast pathway and shift of conduction through the slow pathway.

Atypical Atrioventricular Nodal Reentrant Tachycardia

This is an uncommon form of AVNRT, which is often classified as "fast-slow," "slow-slow," or "slow-intermediate" types. The prevalence of atypical AVNRT is 5–10% of all AVNRT.[11] AH > 200 ms denotes an antegrade slow pathway, and HA > 70 ms denotes a retrograde slow pathway. As a result of the slow conducting retrograde limb, the P wave falls outside the preceding QRS complex, resulting in an intermediate RP **(Fig. 5)** or a long RP tachycardia. Atypical AVNRT is more likely to be initiated and terminated by a PVC.

ATRIOVENTRICULAR REENTRANT TACHYCARDIA

Atrioventricular reentrant tachycardia is the second most common SVT, occurring in approximately 30% of all reentrant SVT.[7] There is an associated bypass tract that connects the atrium directly to the ventricle. An atrial impulse can conduct to the ventricle through the AV node and return to the atria via the bypass tract or conduct to the ventricle through the bypass tract and return to the atria through the AV node. AVRT is commonly seen in young adults with no structural heart disease. Multiple bypass tracts can sometimes be seen in patients with Ebstein anomaly.[12] Less common bypass tracts with a septal location include atrionodal, atriofascicular, nodofascicular, and nodoventricular.

Atrioventricular reentrant tachycardia may be seen with narrow or wide QRS complexes:

- *AVRT with narrow QRS complexes (orthodromic AVRT)*: This type comprises 90–95% of AVRT.[12] A narrow QRS complex is seen when the antegrade conduction is through the AV node and retrograde conduction is through the bypass tract.

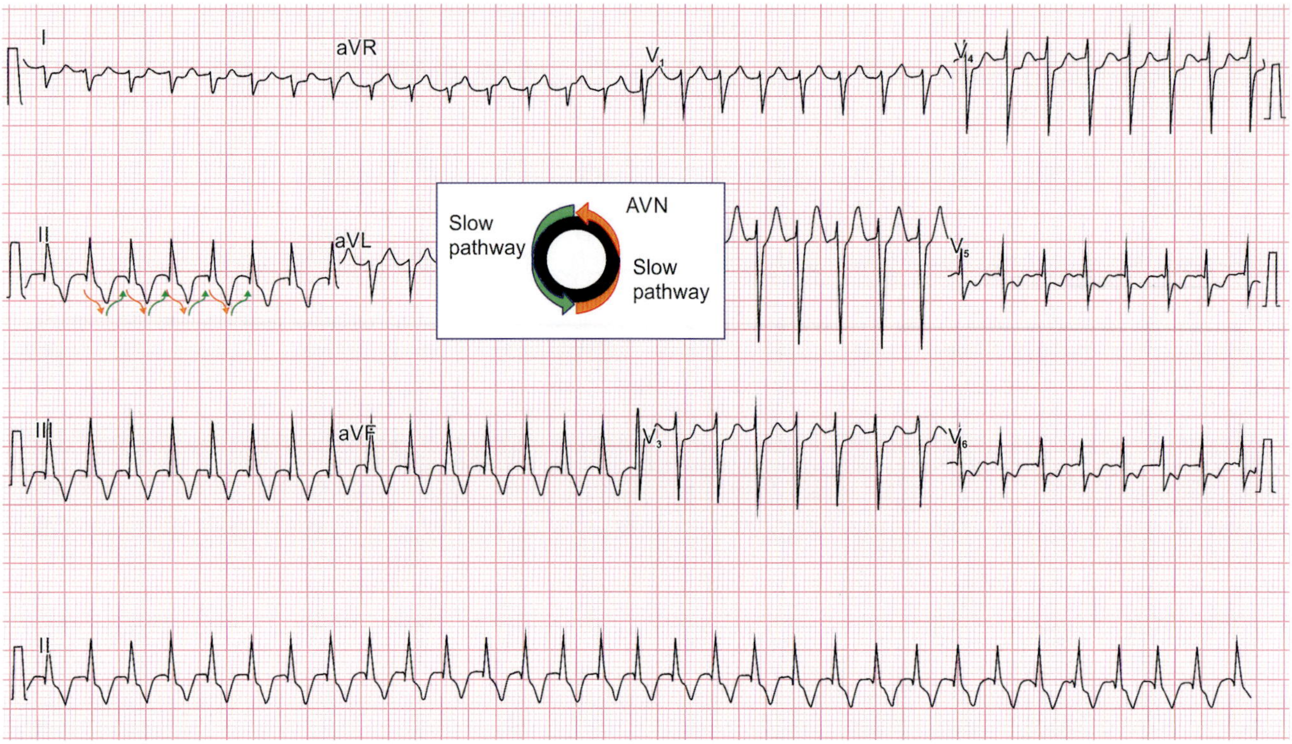

FIG. 5: Atypical AVNRT. ECG of a patient during intermediate RP tachycardia with retrograde P waves in leads II and III.

- *AVRT with preexcited QRS complexes (antidromic AVRT)*: A wide QRS complex is seen when the antegrade conduction is through the bypass tract and retrograde conduction is through the AV node.[12,13]

Orthodromic AVRT is a type of macro-reentry where the circuit involves the atria, AV node, bundle of His, bundle branches and fascicles, ventricles, and bypass tract before returning to the atria.[14,15] The bypass tract may be right- or left-sided; conduction may be unidirectional or bidirectional and generally has rapid and nondecremental conduction unlike the AV node.

The bypass tract (accessory pathway) can be of two types:

1. *Manifest bypass tract (preexcitation)*: During sinus rhythm, the impulse conducts through both the AV node and the bypass tract, thus producing a short PR interval and a widened, fused QRS complex with a delta wave **(Fig. 6A)**. Localization of the bypass tract can be made on surface ECG with the preexcitation using certain algorithms.[16,17]
2. *Concealed bypass tract*: Absence of preexcitation on ECG (narrow QRS) in a patient with a bypass tract. This may be due to the following: Weak antegrade conduction through the bypass tract, retrograde-only conducting bypass tract, or distant location of bypass tract from sinoatrial and AV nodes.

Mechanism of orthodromic reentrant tachycardia (ORT): A premature impulse from either atria or ventricles can initiate AVRT with narrow QRS complexes. The perfectly timed PAC (AV node has fully recovered and bypass tract is still refractory) enters the AV node and activates the ventricles antegradely, resulting in a narrow QRS complex. The impulse returns back to the atrium rapidly via the bypass tract, activating the atrium, then reenters the AV node, and the circuit starts all over again, resulting in short RP tachycardia **(Fig. 6B)**. A PVC finds the His bundle refractory and conducts retrograde to atria via the bypass tract.

Here, ventricle and atrium are activated in series (ventricular activation followed by atrial activation through the bypass tract); hence, the RP interval is >90 ms.[18] Whereas in AVNRT, there is parallel activation of the ventricle and atrium (A on V), and hence the RP interval is <90 ms. Permanent junctional reciprocating tachycardia (PJRT) is an example of a slowly conducting decremental pathway, where the slow retrograde conduction results in a long RP tachycardia **(Fig. 7)**.[19] AV block during NCT rules out AVRT as atria and ventricles are essential components of the circuit. Development of BBB during NCT with subsequent delay in R–P interval and slowing of the tachycardia CL (R–R interval) points toward ORT and localizes the bypass tract to the side of the functional block.

ATRIAL TACHYCARDIA

Atrial tachycardia is a type of NCT that arises from a particular site from either of the atrium. The most common mechanism of focal AT is abnormal automaticity from an ectopic source, other mechanisms being triggered activity or

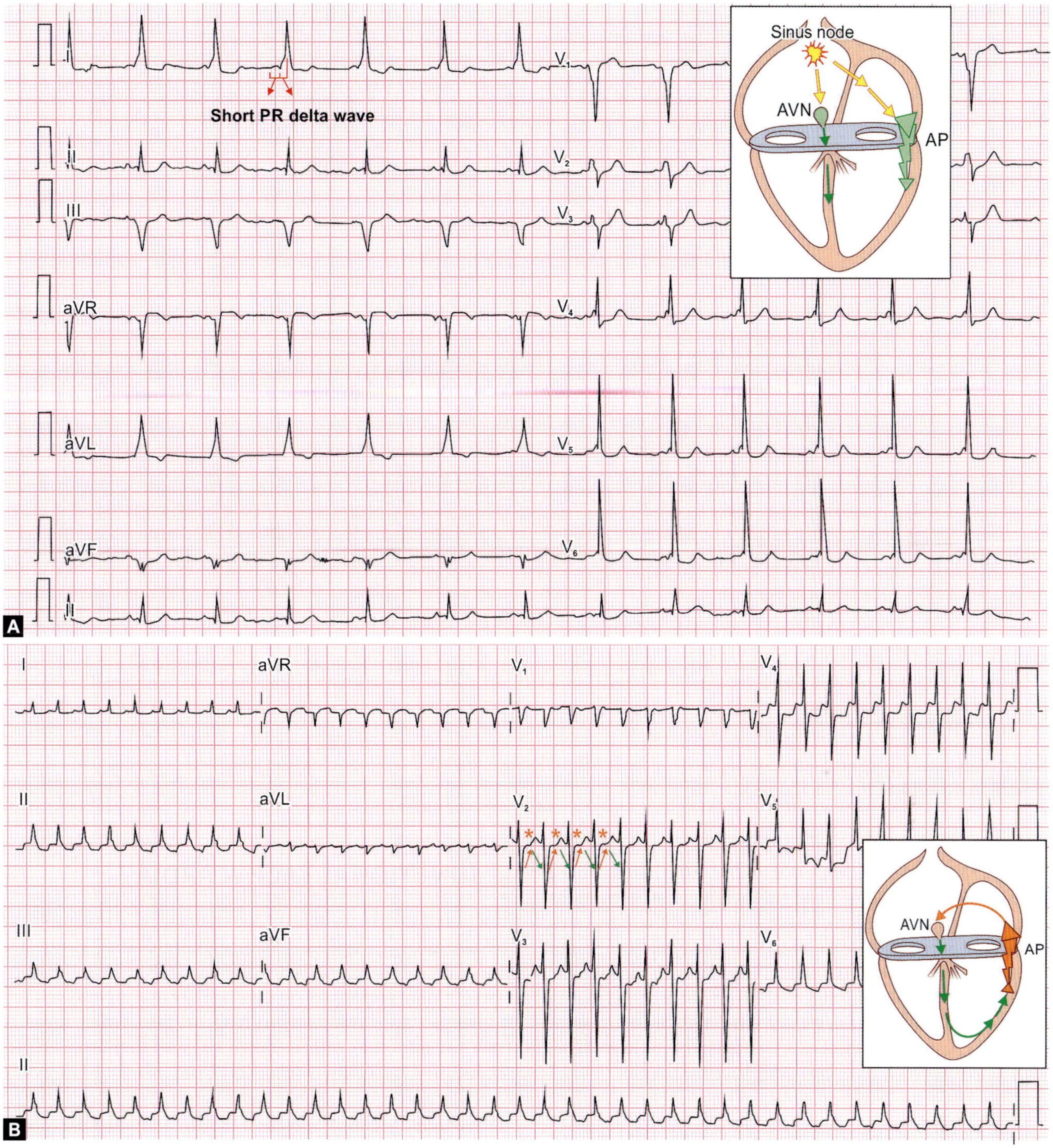

FIGS. 6A AND B: Wolff–Parkinson–White syndrome, orthodromic AVRT. (A) ECG during sinus rhythm with preexcitation; short PR interval and a delta wave are seen. (B) ECG during orthodromic AVRT in the same patient; antegrade conduction through the AV node and retrograde conduction through the accessory pathway, resulting in retrograde P waves (*) and a short RP tachycardia.

micro-reentry.[20] AT may manifest in young individuals who possess a structurally normal heart as well as in those who have structural heart disease characterized by an affected atrium.[21] The atrial rate varies from 100 to 250 bpm with A > V in ECG as ectopic atrial firing continues independent of the AV node or ventricular activation.[21] AT can be 1:1 or variable **(Fig. 8)**, depending on the vagal tone and AV nodal conduction. Localization is based on the comparison of P-wave morphology during tachycardia and sinus rhythm.[22] The tachycardia terminates with a QRS in contrast to other

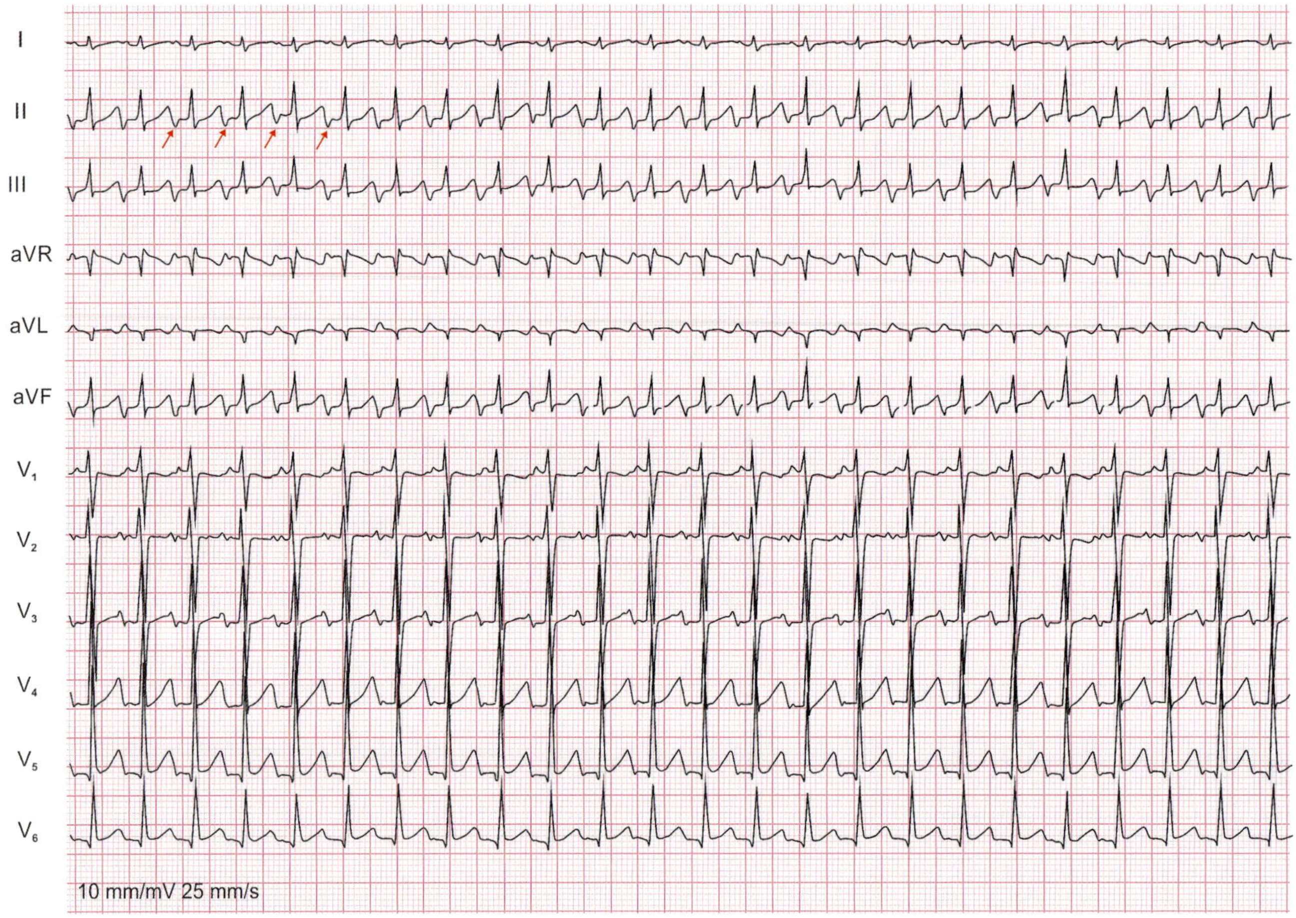

FIG. 7: Permanent junctional reciprocating tachycardia (PJRT): ECG showing PJRT in a 3-year-old child; long RP tachycardia with inverted P waves in leads II and III.

SVT (AVNRT/AVRT), which usually terminates with a retrograde P wave. Sites of origin include crista terminalis, ostium of coronary sinus, tricuspid annulus, pulmonary veins, and mitral annulus.[23] Holter monitoring may show initiation of tachycardia with a PAC, with similar P-wave morphology to tachycardia. Warm-up and cool-down phenomena may be seen. Adenosine may terminate AT resulting from triggered activity or perinodal reentrant AT, while it results in AV block with marching P waves due to other mechanisms.

MULTIFOCAL ATRIAL TACHYCARDIA

Multifocal atrial tachycardia is a rare type of NCT seen usually in children or in patients with preexisting pulmonary disease. It is characterized on ECG by the presence of consecutive three or more different P-wave morphologies with an isoelectric baseline between P waves, rate > 100 bpm, and irregular PR/RR intervals.

JUNCTIONAL TACHYCARDIA

Junctional tachycardia is a type of focal NCT arising from the site of AV junction, which may be due to abnormal automaticity or triggered activity. It is usually seen in children, where it may present as congenital JT or postoperative JT.[24] It gives an appearance of AVNRT on ECG when there is 1:1 VA conduction with negative P waves in inferior leads. Sometimes, JT is seen in adults after prior ablation for AVNRT. Here, AV dissociation is often noted during NCT with marching sinus P waves on ECG. Differential diagnoses for VA dissociation during NCT include AVNRT with blocked retrograde conduction, concealed nodofascicular/nodoventricular tachycardia, and upper septal VT. Clues from surface ECG include initiation of JT with junctional beats and no PR prolongation as seen in AVNRT. Warm-up and cool-down phenomena may be seen. Termination with adenosine suggests focal JT with triggered activity.[21,25]

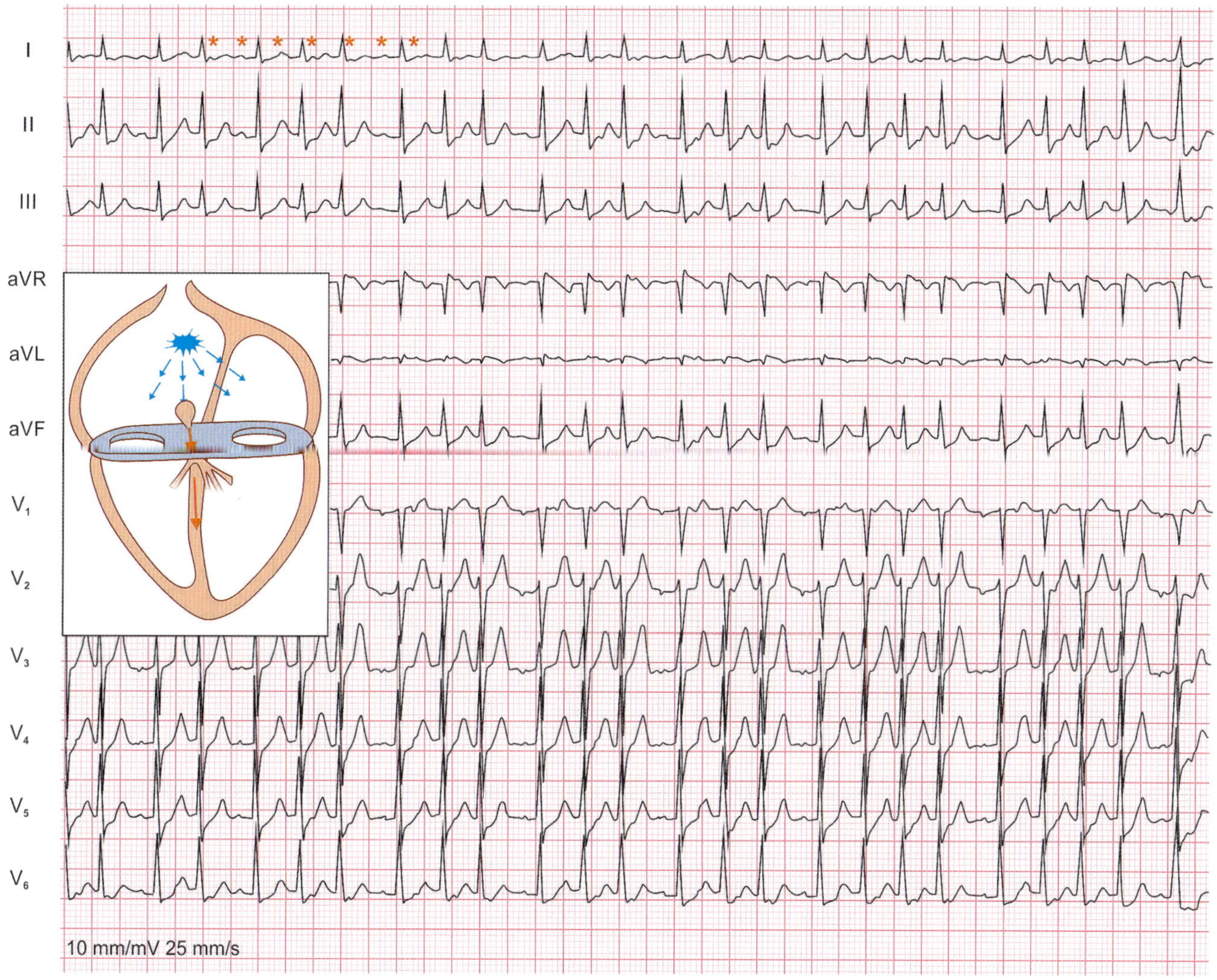

FIG. 8: Focal atrial tachycardia. ECG showing ectopic atrial tachycardia [ectopic P waves are marked as (*) with variable atrioventricular nodal conduction].

ATRIAL FLUTTER

Atrial flutter is a supraventricular arrhythmia with an atrial rate between 250 and 350 bpm. It is due to macro-reentry within the atria. The origin can be from either the right or the left atrium. It can arise as a result of previous surgery, structural heart disease, or ablation.[26] Based on ECG, atrial flutter can be classified as either typical or atypical.

Typical Atrial Flutter

This is the most common form of atrial flutter, seen in 90% of such patients.[22] It is also called cavotricuspid isthmus (CTI)-dependent flutter, where the critical isthmus is between tricuspid annulus and IVC. The trajectory of the impulse is typically in a counterclockwise pattern around the tricuspid annulus, which gives rise to negative flutter waves in the inferior leads (II, III, aVF) and positive flutter waves in V_1 **(Fig. 9)**. The negative flutter waves are in a sawtooth pattern. The typical CTI-dependent flutter can also be in a clockwise fashion.

Atypical Atrial Flutter

This is a non-CTI-dependent atrial flutter. It involves the part of the atrium affected by previous surgery (atriotomy scar, atrial septal defect repair, Mustard/Senning procedure, Fontan surgery, etc.),[27] de novo atrial scar, or due to prior catheter ablation for AF (involving mitral annulus, roof of left atrium, or around the pulmonary veins).[28]

The most common AV conduction in atrial flutter is 2:1, where every other atrial impulse is followed by a QRS complex. An NCT with a ventricular rate of 120–150 bpm should raise the suspicion of AFL with 2:1 conduction. The AV conduction can also be variable in the same patient.

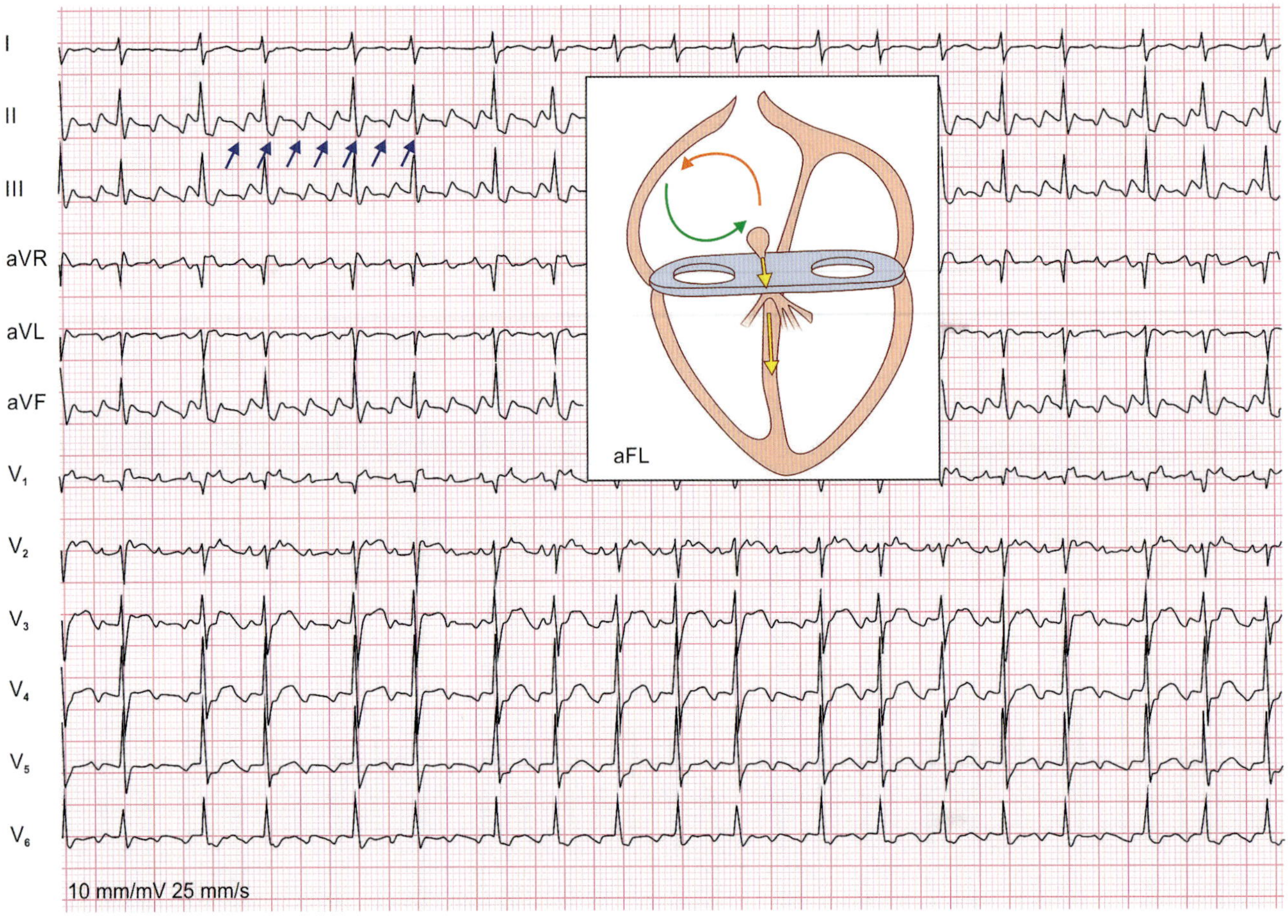

FIG. 9: Typical atrial flutter (cavotricuspid isthmus-dependent, counterclockwise): ECG showing typical atrial flutter with variable AV nodal conduction. Flutter waves (arrows) are negative in inferior leads and positive in V_1.

Differentiating AFL from SVT: Vagal maneuvers like carotid sinus massage can help differentiate AFL from other regular NCT.

- *Atrial flutter*: Carotid sinus massage or administration of AV nodal blockers will slow AV nodal conduction, which slows ventricular rate and brings out flutter waves, but will not convert it to sinus rhythm.
- *Regular NCT (AVNRT/AVRT)*: Here, the tachycardia may revert to sinus rhythm with carotid stimulation.

Differentiating AFL from AT: AFL with 2:1 AV conduction may be mistaken for AT with 2:1 AV block.

- *Atrial rate*: In AFL with 2:1 conduction, the atrial rate is roughly 250–350 bpm. In AT with 2:1 AV conduction, the atrial rate is roughly 150–250 bpm.
- *Morphology of the P wave*: In AFL, the flutter waves are typically inverted in the inferior leads, with a wavy and undulating baseline between QRS complexes. In AT, the P waves are typically upright in the inferior leads, with a flat baseline between P waves.

CONCLUSION

Good quality ECG recordings are needed to discriminate amongst the several underlying mechanisms of narrow QRS tachycardia. A systematic approach, starting with regularity or irregularity, helps narrow down the differential diagnoses. While comparison with the sinus rhythm ECG, if available, if very helpful to identify the P wave during tachycardia, these may still not be identifiable. Response to vagal maneuvers and to IV verapamil/diltiazem also help clinch the diagnosis.

ONLINE REFERENCES

Please scan the QR code provided at the end of the table of contents for References of this chapter.

CHAPTER 197

Recent Advances in the Management of Ventricular Tachycardia

Vinayaga Pandian, Ravikishore Amancharla

ABSTRACT

Ventricular tachyarrhythmias (VTs) are the most common cause of sudden cardiac death. The treatment of VTs has undergone a drastic change over the last few decades. The role of antiarrhythmic drugs in preventing the recurrence of VTs is well established, but its side effects limit their use in the long term. Flecainide and quinidine have remerged as potent new drugs for the treatment of VT. Catheter ablation is a class I indication of drug-resistant VTs. With the availability of 3D mapping technology, different catheters, and newer mapping methods such as Ripple mapping, ILAM, etc., precise substrate identification is possible, thereby improving the efficacy of ablative therapy.

Keywords: Ventricular tachycardia, Ripple mapping, catheter ablation, pulse field ablation, stereotaxic radiotherapy

INTRODUCTION

Ventricular tachycardia (VTs) are life-threatening and are the most common cause of sudden cardiac death (SCD), especially in structural heart disease (SHD). Intracardiac defibrillator (ICD) is a Class I indication for therapy of recurrent VTs. Antiarrhythmic drug (AAD) therapy along with ICDs has been able to reduce the number of inappropriate ICD shocks, but the side effects of prolonged use of AADs are a major limitation. However, ICDs are unable to prevent the occurrence of VT episodes and significantly alter the quality of life (QOL) by delivering recurrent therapies.[1] Catheter ablation has been used for more than three decades in the treatment of VTs. It is a class I indication in recurrent sustained VTs with ischemic substrate and failure of AADs. Improved understanding of mechanism of VT with rapid technological advances has led to innovations in this field. Recent advances in the management of VTs can be classified as diagnostic and therapeutic.

DIAGNOSTIC ADVANCES

The main purpose of catheter ablation is to target the isthmus area of reentrant VT circuit or the origin of automaticity in focal VTs. Activation mapping, entrainment mapping, pace mapping, and substrate mapping are the different mapping techniques used in VT ablation.

The currently available mapping systems have a 3D electroanatomical map (EAM), with different color-coded annotations, which record the activation time of different sites in order to identify the localization of the earliest activation.[1]

The CARTO system, NavX system, and Rhythmia platform are the latest available systems for substrate mapping of VTs. These mapping are done during sinus and paced rhythm based on 3D EAM systems which can combine both voltage maps and activation maps, thereby revealing critical re-entry components having slow or delayed activation and defining scar areas.

Ripple mapping is a feature of the CARTO 3 system which shows bipolar electrogram (EGM) amplitude from each point as a white moving bar. It is used to differentiate the border zone slow conduction areas from the ventricular scar.[1] Conducting tissue is seen as areas supporting the ripple activation and electrical scar as areas devoid of ripple activation.

Isochronal late activation map (ILAM) is a mapping technique described by Tung et al. which defines the zones of deceleration (DZ) during sinus rhythm acquisition **(Fig. 1)**. Targeted ablation of these DZs have shown drastic reductions in arrhythmia event relapses.

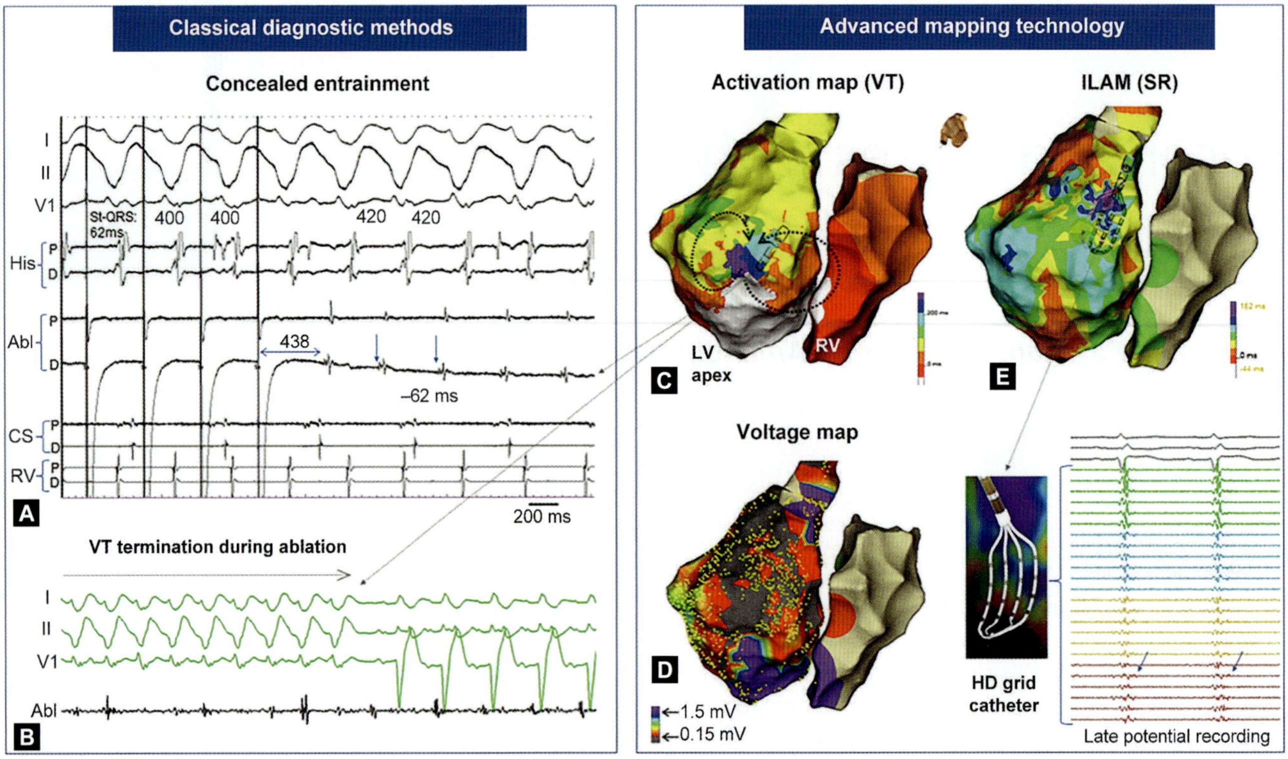

FIGS. 1A TO E: The newer and classical arrhythmia mapping methods.
(ILAM: isochronal late activation map; SR: sinus rhythm; VT: ventricular tachycardia)

THERAPEUTIC ADVANCES

Antiarrhythmic Drug Therapy

Flecainide

Flecainide is a class IC antiarrhythmic drug which blocks the fast sodium current and causes slowing of conduction velocity with prolongation of HV interval and QRS duration and also a ryanodine receptor (RNR) blocker. Primarily used in the maintenance of sinus rhythm in atrial fibrillation, it has now been advocated for treatment of VTs in the absence of ischemic heart disease, LV systolic dysfunction, or SHD based on the results of CAST (Cardiac Arrhythmia Suppression Trial) study.[2]

It is used along with beta-blockers in the treatment of catecholaminergic polymorphic ventricular tachycardia (CPVT), long QT syndrome 3 (LQTS 3), Anderson-Tawil syndrome (LQTS 7), ventricular bigeminism, arrhythmogenic RV cardiomyopathy (ARVC), and PVC-induced tachycardiomyopathy. However, the CAST study did not involve those with revascularized coronary artery disease patients with VAs. Studies in this direction are warranted.

Quinidine

Quinidine is a class IA antiarrhythmic agent which blocks both the rapid inward sodium current and rapidly activating component of delayed rectifier potassium current. It has been advocated for acute use in controlling refractory polymorphic VT in high-risk patients with failed conventional treatment options.[2] With minimal negative inotropic effect, it can be safely used in LV systolic dysfunction presenting with polymorphic VT. The combination of mexiletine with quinidine has synergistic antiarrhythmic effects as opposed to amiodarone quinidine combination which increases the proarrhythmic potential of quinidine. Long-term therapy with quinidine is limited with modest antiarrhythmic effect and gastric intolerance.

Other drugs in the investigational phase for therapy for VTs are azimilide (class III antiarrhythmic action) Botulinum toxin type A and celivarone (noniodinated benzofuran derivative similar to amiodarone).[2]

Device Therapy

Automated external defibrillators (AEDs) and ICDs for the treatment of VTs use shock algorithms to classify ECG tracings as shockable and nonshockable.

With artificial intelligence (AI), machine learning (ML) algorithms are assessed for shock decision classification with improved precision, in the diagnosis of causes of SCD, prediction of successful defibrillation, and rhythm classification without the need to interrupt cardiopulmonary resuscitation.[3]

By applying these ML to ICD-acquired EGMs, ventricular tachycardia events can be predicted seconds before they occur **(Flowchart 1)**. Mid-term and long-term prediction models are in the nascent phase.

Catheter Ablation Therapy

Catheter ablation is a class I recommended acute treatment modality for recurrent drug refractory VTs, electrical storms, and poor tolerance to AADs, especially in patients with CAD, in ESC (2022), ACC/AHA/HRS (2017), and CCS/CHRS (2019) guidelines.[4]

The conventional radiofrequency (RF) ablation uses a unipolar current between the catheter tip and a dispersive patch on the patient skin. An improvisation to this technique is with the use of two ablation catheters in a bipolar method, where one catheter connects to the ground port instead of the dispersive patch.

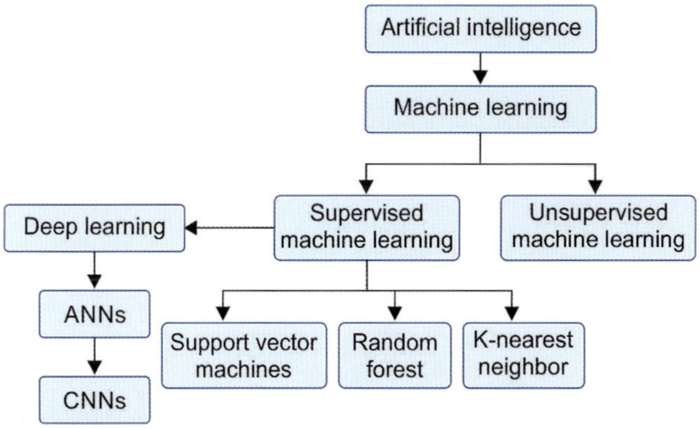

FLOWCHART 1: Use of machine learning to predict VT events.
(ANN: artificial neural network; CNN: convolutional neural network)

Newer Radiofrequency Ablation Catheters

They are contact force sensing catheter with six thermocouples and three microelectrodes (QDOT Micro, Biosense Webster) **(Fig. 2)** and another flexible mesh-shaped irrigation tip with contact force sensing catheter (Tactiflex, Abott) which allows high-resolution mapping of the substrate and optimal temperature ablation.[4]

Pulsed Field Ablation

Pulsed field ablation is a novel ablation method which selectively targets cardiac tissue responsible for the arrhythmia by using ultrashort electrical pulses to induce irreversible electroporation, thereby reducing collateral damage to adjacent normal tissues **(Fig. 2)**.[5]

Ethanol Ablation

Difficult substrates, which are intramural deep in the septum, can be delineated by injecting ethanol into the coronary veins using a double-balloon technique to reduce ethanol dispersion. The results are immediate cell destruction and elimination of clinical VT.[5]

Stereotaxic Radiotherapy

Another newer noninvasive modality of ablation is by using stereotaxic radiotherapy to arrhythmogenic substrate region.[5]

Neuromodulation

Targeting the autonomic nervous system by sympathetic cardiac denervation and modulation of nerve activity has

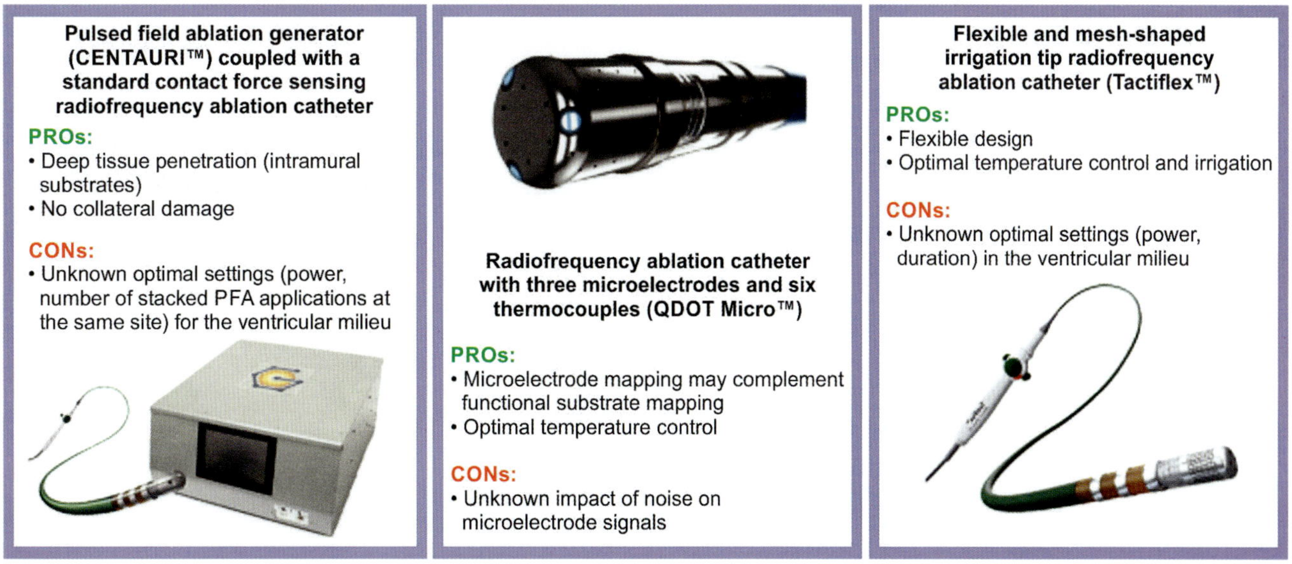

FIG. 2: Technological advancement in catheter ablation in VTs.

shown promise in managing refractory VTs. The following are the methods applied with encouraging results:[1]

- Stellate ganglion modulatory therapy
- Spinal cord stimulation
- Thoracic epidural anesthesia
- Vagal stimulation
- Renal denervation

CONCLUSION

The management of VTs should be on a trifront approach of initial drug therapy for control of the acute episode, use of ICDs, and substrate mapping with catheter ablation to prevent recurrences, reduce the number of ICD shocks, and restrict long-term use of AADs as standard of care.

ONLINE REFERENCES

Please scan the QR code provided at the end of the table of contents for References of this chapter.

CHAPTER

198

Cardiac Channelopathies

Sudipta Mondal, Ajit Kumar Valaparambil

ABSTRACT

Cardiac channelopathies or inherited arrhythmia (IA) syndromes predispose individuals who may appear otherwise healthy to a heightened risk of experiencing sudden cardiac arrest (SCA) and subsequent sudden cardiac death (SCD). Three of the most prevalent IA syndromes stand out: Brugada syndrome (BrS), long QT syndrome (LQTS), and catecholaminergic polymorphic ventricular tachycardia (CPVT). While each syndrome presents unique characteristics, there is also a degree of overlap in their clinical manifestations and the genetic underpinnings that contribute to their development. A critical gap exists in the clinical guidance for these syndromes. Management strategies for channelopathies encompass a multipronged approach, including risk mitigation through lifestyle modifications, medical therapies, interventional procedures, and device implantation. All elements require collaborative decision-making between the healthcare provider and the patient.

Keywords: Cardiac channelopathies, Brugada syndrome, BrS, long QT syndrome, LQTS, catecholaminergic polymorphic ventricular tachycardia, CPVT

INTRODUCTION

The cells and intracellular organelles are covered by membranes comprised of a lipid layer that regulates the movement of water and solutes for biological function. Specific evolved proteins comprise (1) ion channels, (2) transporters, and (3) pumps that take on the function of transporting the ions across it.

- *Ion channels*: Transport ions passively down the electrochemical gradient.
- *Ion pumps*: Transport ions against the electrochemical gradient with ATP energy.
- *Transporters*: Ion moves against the electrochemical gradient by the downhill movement of the other.

Ion channels are pore-forming membrane proteins that mediate ion conduction across these cell membranes.[1] Ion channels are composed of pore-forming alpha subunits and their regulatory beta subunits. The channel complex is thus comprised of pore-forming proteins, pumps, and transporters. The accessory subunits specify the location and presence of ion channels. They modulate and tune their sensitivity to ligands and pharmacological drugs. The ion channels have the property of ion selectivity and gating. The property of the channels to discriminate between ion species to allow them to move through is selectivity. Gating is the transition process of opening and closing.

WHAT ARE CHANNELOPATHIES?

Channelopathies are diseases related to primary ion channel dysfunction due to mutation in genes encoding for ion channels, their subunits, or associated proteins. Channel dysfunction can arise due to functional or structural alterations of the ion channels, pumps, or transporters, and can arise from loss or gain of function. Secondary cardiac channelopathies arise due to altered expression or regulation of ion channels in the context of diseases such as heart failure or drugs.

CHANNELOPATHIES

While there is substantial overlap between ion channel abnormalities and their associated syndromes, these conditions primarily cluster into broad categories. The mutations related to cardiac diseases can be related to those affecting (1) sodium channels, (2) potassium channels, and (3) calcium channels.

Sodium channel-related channelopathies:
- Brugada syndrome (BrS)
- Lev-Lenegre syndrome
- Atrial fibrillation (AF)

Potassium channel-related channelopathies:
- Long QT syndrome (LQTS)
- Short QT syndrome (SQTS)
- AF

Calcium channel-related channelopathies:
- Polymorphic ventricular tachycardia (VT): CPVT
- Timothy syndrome
- Miscellaneous

SODIUM CHANNEL MUTATIONS

The cardiac isoform of the sodium channel is primarily composed of the Nav1.5 α-subunit and is encoded by the *SCN5A* gene.[1] Nav1.5 is a membrane protein containing a 2015 residues variant, with a molecular weight of 227 kDa. The malfunction of cardiac sodium channels has been identified as a causal factor in several primary arrhythmia syndromes. Specifically, genetic mutations affecting sodium channel function are associated with four main disorders: BrS, Lev-Lenegre syndrome (familial progressive conduction disease), LQTS, and familial AF. The above mutations can lead to diverse phenotypes and features increased or reduced channel activity.

Brugada Syndrome

What is Brugada Syndrome?

Brugada syndrome is a clinical syndrome characterized by syncope and a well-defined electrocardiogram (ECG) phenotype. It is also a classic sodium channelopathy-related inherited cardiac arrhythmic syndrome, predisposing individuals to potentially fatal cardiac arrhythmias. Genetic mutations that affect the Na channel happen 25% of the time in BrS, in the *SCN5A* gene that encodes the alpha subunit of the cardiac Na channel. Over 200 *SCN5A* BrS-related mutations have been described. Initially described by Joseph and Pedro Brugada in 1992, the syndrome is characterized by electrocardiographic findings of the right bundle branch block pattern and ST-segment elevation in the right precordial leads (V1–V3).

Genotype–Phenotype

SCN5A gene encodes for the alpha subunit of the sodium channels in the heart. Mutations in the gene lead to reduced expression of Nav1.5-subunit proteins, loss of functional sodium channels, and impaired phase 0 action potential. While mutations resulting in loss of function within the *SCN5A* gene represent the most frequently identified genetic etiology of BrS, a significant portion of cases lack a single identifiable genetic variant. This observation suggests a polygenic inheritance pattern for BrS, wherein the interplay of multiple genes contributes to disease susceptibility.

ECG

Asymptomatic individuals with abnormal ECG are common presentation of BrS. A definitive diagnosis of the condition is established by the presence of spontaneous type 1 ECG changes specifically localized to leads V1 and V2.

Three different ECG patterns have been described in BrS patients: (1) Coved ST elevations >2 mm accompanied by an inverted T wave (type I). (2) Saddle-back-shaped ST elevation >2 mm (type II). (3) Saddle-back-shaped ST elevations <2 mm (type III).

The ESC definition of BrS diagnosis states that patients must display a BrS ECG pattern with ST-segment elevation ≥2 mm in at least one lead (V1–V2) placed in the second, third, or fourth intercostal spaces. The BrS type I ECG pattern may also be induced by fever and exercise tests. In the absence of spontaneous findings, a diagnosis can be considered probable if a type 1 ECG pattern is provoked, either by the presence of a fever or through the administration of a sodium channel blocker challenge.

Diagnosis

The Shanghai scoring system for BrS diagnosis is based on ECG, family history, clinical symptoms, and genetics **(Table 1)**.[2]

Provocative Testing

Provocative tests to unmask type I pattern can be achieved by sodium channel blocker (flecainide, procainamide, mexiletine, and ajmaline) challenge. The dose of flecainide is 2 mg/kg over 10 minutes as an infusion. Since the IV preparation is not available in the country, an oral dose of flecainide can be given: 400 mg stat and ECG taken every 10 minutes for 30 minutes and every 30 minutes for 6 hours.[3] The sodium channel blockers increase the conduction delay or increase the area with conduction delay to result in type I BrS ECG.

Electrophysiological Study

Electrophysiology studies are generally not routinely recommended for BrS diagnosis due to their limited ability to predict VT. Nevertheless, in select cases, these studies may be considered as a diagnostic option, to risk stratify patients for inducible VT. The meta-analysis data on VT inducibility and predictability does not favor its routine use.

TABLE 1: Shanghai scoring for diagnosis of BrS.

Criteria	Points
ECG (12-lead/ambulatory)*:	
• Spontaneous type I Brugada pattern	3.5
• Fever-induced type I Brugada pattern	3
• Type II or III Brugada pattern that converts to type I on provocative testing	2
Clinical history:†	
• Unexplained cardiac arrest or VT/VF	3
• Nocturnal agonal respiration	2
• Suspected arrhythmogenic syncope	2
• Syncope with unclear etiology	1
• Atrial flutter/fibrillation in patients of <30 years without alternative etiology	0.5
Family history:	
• First- or second-degree relative with definite BrS	2
• Suspicious SCD (fever, nocturnal, and Brugada-aggravating drugs) in first or second-degree relative	1
• Unexplained SCD <45 years of age in first- or second-degree relative with negative autopsy	0.5
Genetic testing:	
• Probable pathogenic mutation	0.5

*One item from this category must apply.

†Only award points once for the highest score within this category. Score (requires at least 1 electrocardiographic finding): >3.5 points: Probable and/or definite Brugada syndrome (BrS); 2–3 points: Possible BrS: <2 points: Nondiagnostic.

Treatment

Management strategies for BrS encompass lifestyle modifications, pharmacological interventions, and, in select cases, interventional procedures. Patients presenting with a spontaneous type I ECG pattern and a documented history of cardiac arrest or arrhythmic syncope are considered to be at the highest risk for future events.

Implantable cardioverter-defibrillator (ICD) is recommended in patients with BrS who are survivors of aborted sudden cardiac death (SCD) and documented spontaneous VT/ventricular fibrillation (VF).[4-7] It can also be considered in type 1 Brugada ECG and an arrhythmic syncope. In asymptomatic BrS with inducible VF, it may be considered in specific selected cases.

Pharmacological interventions play a crucial role in managing electrical storms, serving as both an adjunct to ICD therapy and a preventive measure for asymptomatic patients at high risk for developing life-threatening arrhythmic events.

In BrS, the arrhythmogenic substrate arises from an outward shift in the balance of currents during phase 1 of the epicardial action potential. The primary objective of drug therapy in this context is to achieve an inward shift in this current balance. This can be accomplished through two main mechanisms:

1. *Enhancing inward calcium current*: This can be achieved by using beta-adrenergic agents or phosphodiesterase III inhibitors.
2. *Suppressing outward currents*: Agents such as quinidine, which target the transient outward current (Ito), fall under this category.

Quinidine is suggested as an antiarrhythmic treatment in patients with BrS, but its efficacy in preventing life-threatening arrhythmic events in this population is unproven. A prospective multicenter randomized (HQ vs. placebo) double-blind study (QUIDAM) suggested that although HQ appears to be effective in preventing life-threatening VA, it could not be an alternative for an ICD implant.[8] However, Quinidine prevented VF induction in 88% when evaluated for VF inducibility. Because of gastrointestinal side effects, a dose of 600 mg is recommended for long-term use.

The potential utility of focal endocardial/epicardial radiofrequency ablation of sites generating monomorphic extrasystoles is being explored. There are well-defined EP substrates characterized by abnormal fragmented, prolonged, low-frequency ventricular electrograms. Few recent studies have shown that ablation of such substrates in RVOT epicardial sites normalized the ECG and resulted in noninducibility of VT/VF.

Lev-Lenegre Syndrome

The disease was reported in 1995 on chromosome 19q13.2-13.3. The mutation was localized to *SCN5A* in 1999. The mutation results in reduced velocity of impulse conduction, a consequence of the mutation in *SCN5A* and reduction of Na current. It leads to progressive disease and fibrotic involvement of the conduction system. It progresses to cardiac arrhythmias and asystole.

POTASSIUM CHANNEL DISEASE

Repolarization is based on the actions of the outward delayed potassium-mediated currents: I_{Ks} (slow), I_{Kr} (rapid), and IK1. The pore-forming alpha subunit of I_{Ks} is called KCNQ1 (or Kv7.1), of I_{Kr} HERG (or Kv11.1), and for IK1 Kir2.1.[1] Prolongation of action potential duration can be the result of either a reduction in the repolarizing current or an increase in the depolarizing current.

The potassium channels that are involved in the channel dysfunctions are:

- Slowly activating delayed cardiac rectifier K^+ channel: I_{Ks}
- Voltage-gated inward rectifying K^+ channel: I_{Kr}

The affected alpha subunits of these two potassium channels are KvLQT1 and KCNH2. The manifest diseases due to mutations in the genes that encode the K channels are LQTS, SQTS, and AF.

Long QT Syndrome

What is Long QT Syndrome?

Long QT syndrome is a potassium-related cardiac channelopathy caused by abnormalities of repolarization of K^+ channels. The mutations reported are loss-of-function of the K^+ channels. Six different K-channel genes are affected in 50%. The inheritance pattern follows autosomal dominant or recessive modes. Type I LQTS which is the most common LQTS is caused by mutation in KCNQ1 which encodes the alpha subunit of the slowly activating delayed rectifier cardiac K^+ channel: I_{Ks}. Type II LQTS is caused by a mutation in *KCNH2* that encodes for the alpha subunit of the voltage-gated inwardly rectifying K channel that mediates the rapidly activating component of I_{Kr}. This accounts for 50% of type II LQTS.

Congenital LQTS is characterized by a prolongation of the cardiac repolarization phase as measured on an ECG. The Schwartz score is a clinical scoring system employed to stratify patients into risk categories for LQTS **(Table 2)**.[9] This score is derived from a combination of historical features and ECG findings, and it categorizes patients into three groups: unlikely (≤1.5 points), possible (2–3 points), or probable (≥3.5 points) LQTS.

Geno Phenotype

Genetic testing is recommended for patients categorized as possible LQTS, following pretest genetic counseling.

TABLE 2: LQTS diagnostic criteria (updated in 2015).

Electrocardiographic findings	Points
QTc interval:	
• ≥480 ms	3
• 460–479 ms	2
• 450–459 ms (men)	1
QTc ≥ 480 ms during 2nd–4th minute of recovery from an exercise stress test	1
Documented Torsade de pointes (TdP)	2
T-wave alternans	1
Notched T wave in three leads	1
Resting heart rate below second percentile forage	0.5
Clinical history	
Syncope:	
• With stress	2
• Without stress	1
Congenital deafness	0.5
Family history	
Relatives with clinically definitive LQTS	1
Unexplained sudden cardiac death in immediate relative <30 years of age	0.5

Total score indicates the probability of LQTS: 1 point (low), 2–3 points (intermediate), and ≥3.5 points (high).

This recommendation is based on the observation that approximately 80% of individuals with genetically confirmed LQTS harbor mutations within specific genes.[10] At present, LQTS is pathogenetically linked to mutations in around 16 different genes, all of which prolong the QT interval by decreasing potassium current (loss-of-function) or increasing sodium or calcium current (gain-of-function). 75% of patients possess a pathogenic mutation in one of the three major LQTS-causing genes (*KCNQ1*, 35%; *KCNH2*, 30%; and *SCN5A*, 10%). Patients with LQT1 more frequently experience cardiac syncope triggered by adrenergic stimuli (e.g., physical exertion or emotional stress). The development of cardiac events in LQT2 patients is associated with emotional stress and sudden exposure to auditory stimuli, such as noise from telephones, alarm clocks, and crying babies. In LQT3, about 65% of cardiac syncope occurs during sleep or rest (bradycardia-triggered arrhythmias). A causative role of sinus bradycardia is strongly associated with *SCN5A* mutations. Slow heart rate-induced excessive action potential duration predisposes individuals with LQT3 to fatal arrhythmias, typically at rest or during sleep without emotional arousal.

ECG

The typical ECG features of LQTS are prolonged QT interval, abnormal T wave, often accompanied by T wave alternation (TWA), and Torsades de Pointes. (TdP), a serious, mostly self-limiting type of VT that can produce syncope, can degenerate into VF, and cause SCD. T wave morphology may help differentiate LQTS 1 to 3. Typically, a broad T wave is observed in LQT1, a biphasic T wave in LQT2, and a late-appearing T wave in LQT3, which has a narrow and tall shape and appears at the very end of the QT interval.[11] The implementation of a standardized approach to QT interval measurement can enhance the reliability and accuracy of detection for prolonged QT intervals. In clinical practice, heart rate correction of the QT interval is most commonly performed using Bazett's formula.

The definitive diagnosis of LQTS is based on (1) presence of LQTS score >3.5, (2) pathogenic mutation in proven LQTS genes, and (3) QTc > 500 ms in repeated ECG. LQTS can also be diagnosed in the presence of QTc 480-499ms in repeated ECG, with unexplained syncope. A 24-hour Holter monitor is not a routine recommendation; however, it may be done on a case-to-case basis.

Provocative Testing

The percentage of patients exhibiting a normal QTc interval was notably higher in LQTS1 (36%), followed by LQTS2 (19%), with the lowest percentage observed in LQTS3 (10%). Provocative drug testing with epinephrine, in LQTS can be a valuable diagnostic tool for patients who have not undergone genetic testing but exhibit suspected LQTS features, as well as for those with confirmed LQTS1 or LQTS2 diagnoses but a normal resting ECG.

Treatment

The pharmacological management of LQTS centers on two key strategies: Meticulous avoidance of medications known to prolong the QT interval and the initiation of beta-blocker therapy **(Fig. 1)**.[11] The implementation of these interventions in combination has been demonstrated to significantly reduce the risk of both syncopal and SCD events. Beta-blocker therapy is a cornerstone intervention for LQTS, demonstrating exceptional efficacy in reducing the risk of cardiac events. Mexiletine may be considered a therapeutic option for patients with LQTS type II or type III.

Left cardiac sympathetic denervation is recommended when beta-blockers are not effective or not tolerated. ICD implantation is recommended in LQTS patients who have survived cardiac arrest.

Short QT Syndrome

Short QT syndrome is characterized by a short QT interval <330 ms and symmetric tall-peaked T waves. It manifests with syncope at rest or on exertion. Ventricular arrhythmias like PVCs, polymorphic VTs, and SCD are important features. Sinus bradycardia and AF are also seen. A family history of SCD is usually evident, with an autosomal dominant pattern of inheritance.

Genetics

Short QT syndrome is characterized by mutations in three K^+ channels, related to enhanced function with shortened repolarization and reduced QT interval.

- *Type I SQTS*: Mutation in *KCNH2* gene with enhanced I_{Kr} function and shortened ventricular AP.
- *Type II SQTS*: Mutation in *KCNQ1:* Leads to enhanced function and shortened AP. Can be present in neonates.
- *Type III SQTS*: Mutation in *KCNJ2:* Leads to acceleration of phase 3 of AP. Characteristic sharp T wave.

CALCIUM CHANNEL DISEASE

Calcium ions are noted in phase 2 of the action potential and also increase the sarcoplasmic output of calcium. Ca channel activation governs (1) membrane potential changes (voltage-gated), (2) ligand binding (ligand gated), and (3) Ca depletion (Ca release activated).

Voltage-gated calcium channel alpha subunit Cav1.2 is encoded by *CACNAIC,* a membrane protein with a similar pattern to the alpha subunit of the sodium channel.

Ryanodine receptor2 is encoded by *RyR2,* an ion channel that permits the outflow of Ca ions from the sarcoplasmic reticulum (SR) when the cell membrane is depolarized. Mutated RyR2 channels leak Ca ions resulting in leaky ryanodine receptors, triggering arrhythmias.

Calcium channel dysfunction can result in three different arrhythmic syndromes:

1. Polymorphic VT: CPVT
2. Timothy syndrome
3. BrS variation with short QT

Catecholaminergic Polymorphic Ventricular Tachycardia

What is Catecholaminergic Polymorphic Ventricular Tachycardia?

Catecholaminergic polymorphic ventricular tachycardia (CPVT) is essentially a Ca^{2+} ion channelopathy. Calcium ions mediate phase 2 of the action potential. They also increase the Ca output from the SR, which is a storage for Ca ions. The RyR2 and the Calsequestrin 2, encoded by RyR2 and CASQ2, respectively are located at the SR. CPVT is distinguished by the presence of rapid, polymorphic, and bidirectional VT arising in response to abrupt adrenergic stimulation **(Figs. 2A and B)**. It is classified as one of the least prevalent inherited arrhythmia (IA) syndromes. CPVT

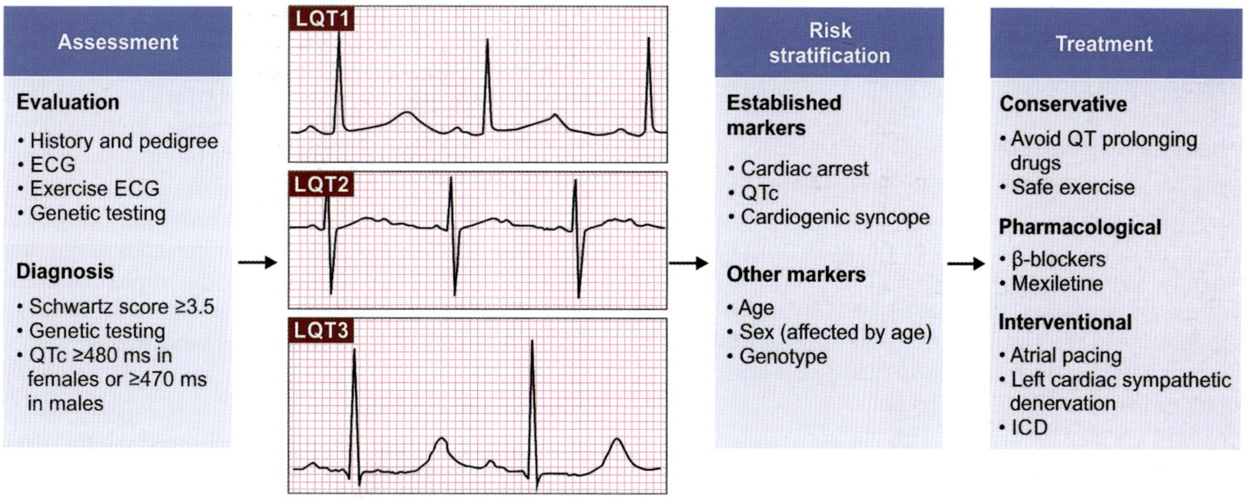

FIG. 1: Clinical approach to congenital long QT syndrome.
Source: Adapted from Krahn et al.[11]

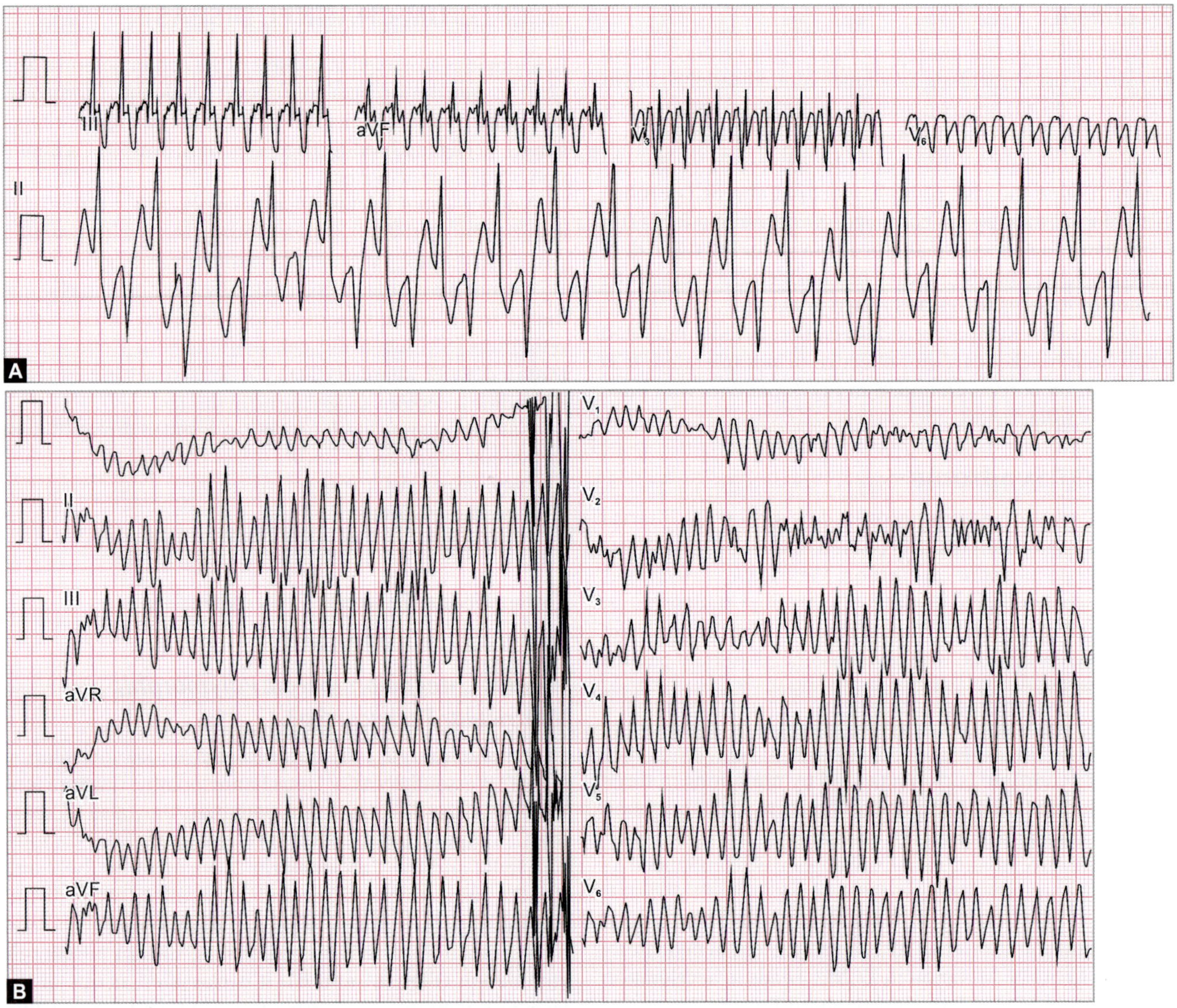

FIGS. 2A AND B: (A) Exercise-induced bidirectional VT in CPVT; (B) Exercise-induced polymorphic VT in CPVT.

arises from a fundamental abnormality in calcium (Ca^{2+}) handling within the SR.

Genotype–Phenotype

Notably, pathogenic variants in RyR2 are identified in up to 60% of patients diagnosed with CPVT.[12] CPVT is noteworthy for the frequent occurrence of de novo mutations in probands. Two primary forms of CPVT have been identified. The first, an autosomal dominant type (CPVT1), is caused by mutations in the cardiac *RyR2* gene. The second, a less prevalent autosomal recessive form (CPVT2), is attributed to mutations in the cardiac *CASQ2* gene.

ECG

In the majority of cases, the resting ECG fails to reveal any pathological findings. Consequently, establishing a diagnosis of CPVT necessitates a comprehensive clinical history and the implementation of provocative testing protocols.

Presentation

The initial presentation of symptoms typically occurs during childhood or young adulthood. However, these symptoms may be subtle and lack specificity, often manifesting as presyncope or palpitations. Furthermore, the triggering adrenergic stimuli can be diverse, ranging from physical exertion to amusement park rides or episodes of emotional distress. Timely diagnosis allows for the implementation of highly effective interventions that can significantly mitigate the risk of sudden cardiac arrest (SCA) and SCD.

Provocative Testing

Exercise stress testing serves as the cornerstone for diagnosing CPVT by replicating the effects of adrenergic stimulation within a controlled clinical environment. However, the sensitivity of conventional Bruce protocols, which involve progressively increasing exercise intensity, is demonstrably low.[10] The diagnosis of CPVT is confirmed when an infusion of epinephrine triggers either nonsustained or sustained polymorphic VT with more than 10 PVCs per minute or new T-wave alternans. When compared with exercise testing, the epinephrine test demonstrated low overall sensitivity (28%) and high specificity (98%).

Treatment

The cornerstone of CPVT management revolves around two key principles: Trigger avoidance and risk stratification. When possible, patients are counseled on identifying and minimizing potential adrenergic triggers.

Following confirmed diagnosis, nonselective beta-blockers, such as nadolol or propranolol, represent the first-line pharmacological intervention.[10] These medications aim to reduce sympathetic activity, thereby mitigating the risk of arrhythmia. Flecainide, a sodium channel blocker, can be employed as an effective adjunct therapy in select patients.

Left cardiac sympathectomy, a surgical procedure that disrupts sympathetic innervation of the heart, has also demonstrated efficacy in CPVT management. However, due to its invasive nature, it is typically reserved for individuals who fail to achieve adequate control with medications. Unlike other IA conditions, ICD placement in CPVT patients is more limited.

CONCLUSION

A meticulous and multifaceted evaluation strategy is paramount for achieving diagnostic accuracy and guiding precise therapeutic interventions in patients and families with suspected IA syndrome. Iatrogenic consequences can be devastating in cases of missed diagnoses, while over-diagnosis also presents a significant concern. The diagnostic odyssey, encompassing both phenotypic and genotypic evaluation, may necessitate a significant investment of time and resources. In such complex scenarios, multidisciplinary consultations with experts are the cornerstone elements in optimizing patient care and providing comprehensive support for families.

ONLINE REFERENCES

Please scan the QR code provided at the end of the table of contents for References of this chapter.

The Role of Radiofrequency Ablation in Management of Ventricular Tachycardia in Ischemic Cardiomyopathy: Two Decades of Advances

CHAPTER

199

Abhishek Goyal, Naved Aslam, Gurpreet S Wander

ABSTRACT

Ventricular tachycardia (VT) in ischemic cardiomyopathy (ICM) is associated with substantial morbidity and mortality. Traditional management approaches include optimization of therapy for heart failure, escalation of antiarrhythmic therapy (AAD) and ICD implantation. AAD is often ineffective and carries significant side effects. Catheter ablation is a very potent tool in managing recurrent VT occurring despite ICD and AAD. In last two decades, various trials have established the role of catheter ablation as a therapy which reduces VT recurrence, ICD shocks, and possibly mortality. Timing of ablation and role of prophylactic ablation at the time of ICD implantation remain debatable. Current chapter discusses all these issues in details based on recent literature.

Keywords: Recurrent ventricular tachycardia, ischemic cardiomyopathy, catheter ablation

INTRODUCTION

Ventricular tachycardia (VT) is associated with significant morbidity and mortality in patients with ischemic cardiomyopathy (ICM). ICM-related myocardial scarring results in creation of reentrant circuits, creating a substrate for VT. Effective management of VT in ICM patients requires a comprehensive understanding of the various available therapeutic strategies.

Conventional management approaches, including antiarrhythmic drugs (AADs) and implantable cardioverter-defibrillators (ICDs), have limitations and are often associated with recurrent VT episodes.[1-4] Radiofrequency ablation (RFA) has emerged as a pivotal therapeutic intervention by directly modifying the arrhythmogenic substrate.[5] It has been shown to reduce VT recurrence, ICD shocks, and composite primary outcomes in various clinical trials. However, RFA has not been demonstrated to improve cardiovascular mortality.

ROLE OF ANTIARRHYTHMIC DRUGS AND ICDS IN CURRENT ERA

Antiarrhythmic Drugs versus Catheter Ablation

In patients with ICM and sustained VT or VF, AADs may be used to reduce recurrent symptomatic arrhythmias among patients with ICD implantation. Among various available AADs, beta-blockers have been shown consistently to reduce mortality and sudden death in various trials.[1,2] and β-blockers can reduce arrhythmia recurrences by various mechanisms. Class III AADs (e.g., sotalol and amiodarone) have been shown to reduce arrhythmia recurrences but not all cause mortality. In a meta-analysis, amiodarone has been shown to decrease the risk of sudden cardiac death and cardiovascular death but effect on all-cause mortality did not reach statistical significance.[3] Most importantly, it is inferior to an ICD in long-term management of these patients.[4] Amongst ICD patients, amiodarone reduces the incidence of ICD therapies when compared to placebo. Also, combination of amiodarone plus β-blocker compared to β-blockers or sotalol alone was more effective in reducing ICD shock. However, amiodarone use is associated with significant side effects as well as low patient compliance with discontinuation rates ranging between 18 and 32%.

In the era of ablation therapy, data suggest that catheter ablation is preferred strategy over AAD escalation. The VANISH trial compared catheter ablation with escalated AAD treatment in ICM patients presenting with recurrent VT despite first-line AAD therapy.[5] Escalated AAD treatment included the initiation of amiodarone if another AAD (e.g., sotalol) had been used previously, a dosage increase dose is <300 mg/day (58% of patients) or addition of mexiletine if the maximum dose was already used (9% of patients). As compared to AAD escalation, catheter ablation decreased the composite primary outcome of death, electrical storm, or appropriate ICD shock.[5] In this trial, mexiletine did not offer any additional benefit in the relatively small number of patients already on amiodarone.[6] Result of this trial indicates that ablation is more effective that escalation of AAD therapy in recurrent VT. This is helpful in patients who develop the side effects of amiodarone or have relevant contraindications.

In another prospective, multicenter, randomized trial (SURVIVE VT) which included patients with ICM and appropriated ICD shock, complete endocardial substrate-based catheter ablation was compared to antiarrhythmic therapy (amiodarone + β-blockers, amiodarone alone, or sotalol ± β-blockers).[7] Ablation led to fewer occurrences of the combined endpoint of cardiovascular death, appropriate ICD shocks, hospitalizations for heart failure, and severe complications from treatment when compared to AADs. This further supports the role of catheter ablation in recurrent ICD shocks. Additionally, VT storm, slow and incessant VT were less in ablation group. Similar to the results of VANISH trial, AAD was associated with significant side effects leading to discontinuation of AAD.

However, further trials are underway such as VANISH-2 and AFTER-VT trial which will clarify these issues further.

Implantable Cardioverter-defibrillator versus Catheter Ablation

The ICDs are crucial for prevention of SCD and are recommended for both primary and secondary prevention in ICM. As compared to AAD, mortality is significantly reduced by ICD implantation. With the current understanding of disease substrate in ICM and emergence of ablation therapy, role of ICD needs to be redefined. Moreover, ICD therapy has certain shortcomings and disadvantages. Both appropriate and inappropriate ICD interventions are associated with worsening of congestive heart failure and may enhance mortality too. ICD shocks are painful which have a significant psychological impact. Anxiety is a very strong predictor of increased 1 year mortality. To address these issues and improve quality of life, ICD shock number needs to be minimized by optimal ICD programming. There are number of studies which show that catheter ablation has a significant role in reducing number of shocks and improving outcomes which is discussed in subsequent sections.

APPROACHES TO CATHETER ABLATION

Patient selection for early catheter ablation requires careful risk stratification to identify those most likely to benefit. Risk factors for recurrent VT and ICD shocks include the extent of myocardial scar, left ventricular ejection fraction (LVEF), and the presence of comorbidities such as heart failure and diabetes. Advanced imaging techniques, such as cardiac MRI with late gadolinium enhancement, can provide detailed information on scar morphology and extent, aiding in patient selection.

Patients with a history of myocardial infarction, significant myocardial scarring, and reduced LVEF are prime candidates for early ablation. Those with frequent VT episodes or electrical storm despite medical therapy may also benefit from early intervention. Additionally, patients with intolerance to AADs due to side effects or contraindications may be considered for early ablation.

The last two decades have witnessed significant advancements in catheter ablation which have made the procedure simpler and safer. More and more number of patients undergo these procedures now which has improved clinical outcomes significantly. However, these patients are sicker, have presence of advanced heart failure, poor ejection fraction, and associated comorbidities such as CKD, COPD which confers high risk of periprocedural and postprocedural complications. Prior risk stratification is of paramount importance to ward off adverse periprocedural outcomes such as worsening of heart failure and possibly, mortality. 2019 HRS/EHRA/APHRS/LAHRS expert consensus statement on catheter ablation of ventricular arrhythmias recommend the use of The PAAINESD risk score. This score includes [chronic obstructive pulmonary disease (five points), age > 60 years (three points), general anesthesia (four points), ICM (six points), New York Heart Association class III or IV (six points), ejection fraction < 25% (three points), VT storm (five points), diabetes mellitus (three points)] and is useful for risk stratification.[8] Also this is very well-validated tool in various studies. It is evident from various published studies suggests that a PAAINESD score ≥ 15–17 (depending on whether the variable "general anesthesia" is included in the risk score calculation or not) identifies patients with SHD and VT at particularly high risk of adverse periprocedural outcomes.

Catheter ablation targets the arrhythmogenic substrate within scar tissue, disrupting reentrant circuits that sustain VT. By creating lesions that interrupt these circuits, ablation can prevent the initiation and propagation of VT. There are various approaches which primarily include activation mapping, entrainment mapping and substrate modification by 3D mapping systems, allowing display of the position and relative timing on the electroanatomical mapping (EAM) system.

Activation mapping **(Table 1 and Fig. 1)** involves recording the electrical activation sequence during ongoing VT which is possible in only hemodynamically stable VT.

Entrainment mapping is performed by pacing at various sites within the heart to determine the relationship between paced and VT cycle lengths. This method helps to identify critical components of the reentrant circuit.

Substrate mapping is typically performed during sinus rhythm, identifying areas of abnormal electrograms (late potentials and fractionated signals) within the scar tissue. These regions are potential targets for ablation, especially when VT is not inducible or is hemodynamically unstable. Activation and entrainment mapping use is limited by noninducibility, self-terminating tachycardia, or hemodynamic instability. These limitations can be overcome by substrate mapping, focusing on characterization of the scar and border zones which represent arrhythmogenic substrate of reentry. Substrate mapping can be done during

TABLE 1: A patient with ICM presenting with recurrent VT despites optimal AAD who received 25 ICD (appropriate) shocks over 8 months.

Arrhythmia episode list								
Arrhythmia episode list: 27-Aug-2020 10:23:51 to 12-Aug-2023 16:18:40 only specified episodes shown below								
Type	**ATP seq**	**Shocks**	**Success ID#**		**Date**	**Time (hh:mm)**	**Duration hh:mm:ss**	**Avg bpm V**
Last programmer session 12-Aug-2023								
VT	2	15J	Yes	368	09-Aug-2023	13:30	:39	154
VT	2	15J	Yes	364	09-Aug-2023	02:55	:37	154
VT	2	15J	Yes	357	07-Aug-2023	23:32	:24	171
VT	2	15J	Yes	356	07-Aug-2023	18:31	:25	171
VT	2	20J	Yes	355	07-Aug-2023	12:27	:26	158
VT	2	20J	Yes	347	05-Aug-2023	12:29	:51	162
VT	2	20J	Yes	316	01-Aug-2023	11:13	:01:06	162
VT	2	20J	Yes	308	27-Jul-2023	07:07	:26	167
VT	2	20J	Yes	307	27-Jul-2023	06:18	:01:04	162
VT	2	20J	Yes	291	24-May-2023	18:29	:24	171
VT	2	20J	Yes	290	22-May-2023	04:17	:25	171
VT	2	20J	Yes	289	11-May-2023	18:38	:01:12	162
VT	2	20J	Yes	277	08-May-2023	12:14	:27	162
VT	2	20J	Yes	271	08-May-2023	07:36	:50	162
VT	2	20 J, 35 J	Yes	266	20-Apr-2023	00:18	:41	167
VT	2	20J	Yes	264	14-Apr-2023	13:13	:25	167
VT	2	20J	Yes	263	14-Apr-2023	02:43	:25	167
VT	2	20J	Yes	262	12-Apr-2023	19:51	:25	171
VT	2	20J	Yes	258	17-Mar-2023	02:01	:26	167
VT	3	20J	Yes	255	13-Mar-2023	03:59	:39	162
VT	3	20J	Yes	244	27-Jan-2023	07:14	.45	167
VT	3	3	Yes	242	27-Jan-2023	06:10	:01:37	162
y^	3	20J	Yes	240	27-Jan-2023	06:07	:02:12	162
VT	3	20J	Yes	216	26-Jan-2023	08:01	:33	167
VT	3	20J	Yes	215	25-Jan-2023	06:53	:01:38	162

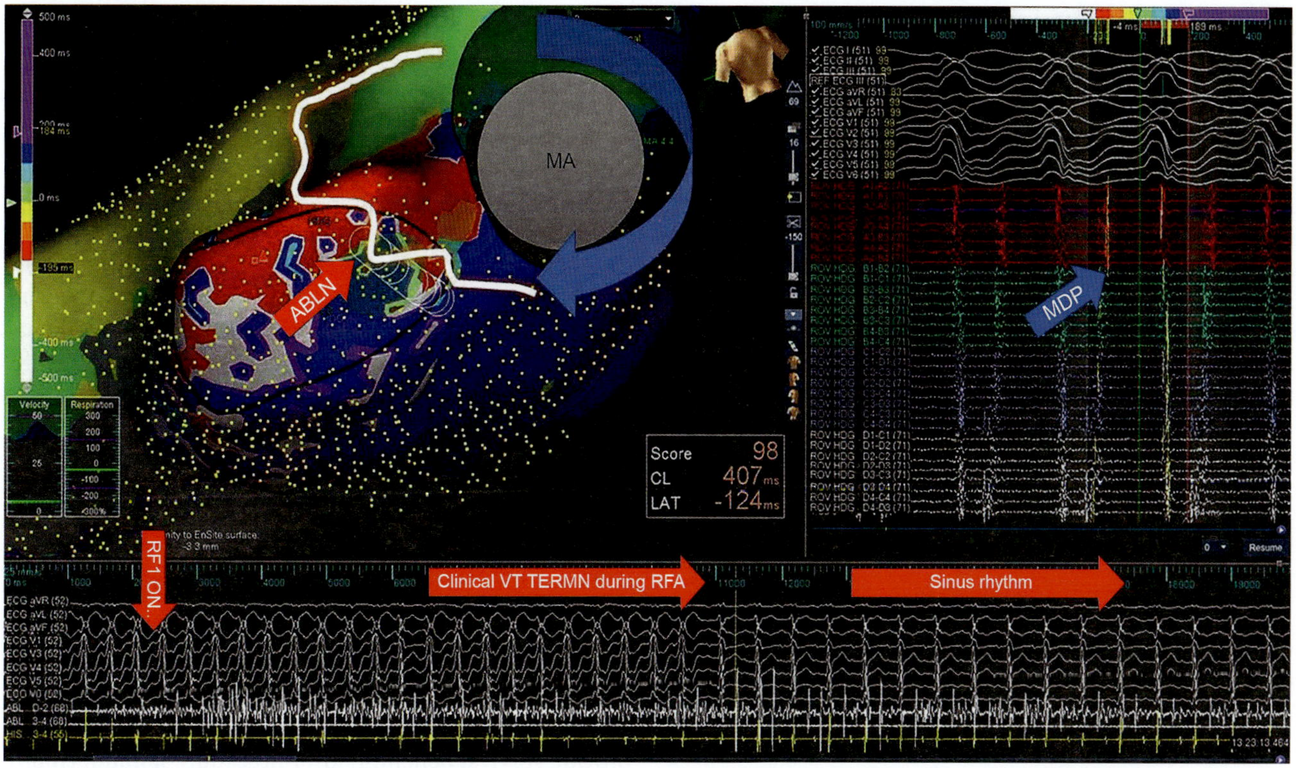

FIG. 1: Since VT of patient was hemodynamically stable, EAM was constructed with EnSite Precision during tachycardia. Reentrant map showed tachycardia reentry around mitral annulus (MA) and areas of slow conduction which represent conduction through scar and border zones which harbor the reentrant channels. Mid-diastolic potentials (MDP) representative of critical isthmus of tachycardia are seen in adjacent intracardiac electrogram trace. First burn in this region terminated the tachycardia which could not be induced again. Subsequently, multiple burns were given in the scar area for ablation of residual channels as a part of substrate modification.

sinus or paced rhythm and does not require tachycardia for mapping.

Preprocedural cardiac imaging to evaluate arrhythmogenic substrate and cardiac function is considered essential in the vast majority of cases. Cardiac imaging not only characterizes underlying substrate in detail, it helps in risk stratification of patients with VT also. Cardiac magnetic resonance imaging is regarded as the gold standard and its use has been shown to increase arrhythmia free survival after ablation. there are several limitations to CMR imaging such as device (pacemaker, ICD)-related artifacts, Frequent ventricular ectopy, etc., patient's clinical condition should be stable enough as this scan requires 45 minutes and breath holding for 10 seconds.

Interestingly, cardiac CT offers higher spatial resolution besides overcoming the shortcomings of MRI. CMR resolution is limited to a voxel size of 1.4 mm^3, whereas CT provides higher voxel resolution of <0.4 mm^3. Additionally, cardiac CT takes only seconds, making it a safer modality as compared to MRI in a sicker patient.

Integration of CT with EAM is another useful tool in VT ablation. Several studies have shown the utility of CT-defined scar and EAM-defined scar integration strategy. The agreement between two modalities is typically good in patients with ICM which is very helpful in ablation. Cardiac MRI is also useful, but the correlation of EAM-defined and CMR-defined scar is not always accurate, with few studies demonstrating a mismatch between these two modalities.

In the last decade, rapid and precise mapping has been possible with high-density mapping, which acquires thousands of mapping points within only a few minutes. High-density mapping systems, such as the CARTO and EnSite platforms, provide detailed maps of the electrical activity within the heart. These systems enhance the precision of substrate identification, allowing for more targeted and effective ablation. Robotic navigation systems and stereotactic radio ablation are emerging techniques that offer greater precision and reduced procedural times. These technologies are in early stages of development but show potential for transforming VT ablation.

The acute success rate of RFA, defined as the elimination of inducible VT at the end of the procedure, is high, typically ranging from 70 to 90%. Factors influencing success include the extent of myocardial scarring and the complexity of the VT substrate. Long-term outcomes studies have demonstrated sustained freedom from VT in a substantial proportion of patients, leading to improved quality of life and reduced hospitalization rates.

INDICATIONS OF CATHETER ABLATION

Patients with recurrent VT episodes despite optimal AAD therapy are prime candidates for RFA. Additionally, in patients experiencing hemodynamically unstable VT, ablation can provide immediate stabilization by eliminating the VT source. Electrical storm, characterized by multiple VT episodes within a short period, poses a high risk for morbidity and mortality. RFA can be lifesaving in these scenarios by interrupting the cycle of recurrent arrhythmias.

The ICDs are effective in terminating VT but do not prevent recurrent episodes. The SURVIVE-VT trial clearly showed that RFA serves as an adjunct to ICD therapy, reducing the frequency of VT and minimizing the psychological and physical impact of repeated ICD shock.

TIMING OF CATHETER ABLATION

The appropriate timing of VT ablation and group of patients that will receive the maximum benefit remains a burning issue. Recently published "The PAUSE-SCD trial" included a total of 121 patients which were randomly assigned (1:1) to ablation plus an ICD versus conventional medical therapy plus an ICD.[9] ICM was present in 35% of enrolled patients. Early catheter ablation performed at the time of ICD implantation resulted in significant reduction in the composite primary outcome of VT recurrence, cardiovascular hospitalization, or death. This was driven by a reduction in ICD therapies in ablation group. At a follow-up of 31 months, the primary outcome occurred in 49.3% of the ablation group and 65.5% in the control group [HR 0.58 (95% CI 0.35–0.96); $p = 0.04$]. There was a significant reduction in VT recurrence in the ablation arm [HR 0.51 (95% CI 0.29–0.90); $p = 0.02$]. A statistically significant reduction in both ICD shocks (10.0% vs. 24.6%; $p = 0.03$] and antitachycardia pacing (16.2% vs. 32.8%; $p = 0.04$) was observed in ablation group compared with control. There were no significant differences in overall mortality [8.9% vs. 8.8%; HR 1.40 (95% CI 0.38–5.22); $p = 0.62$] or in rates of cardiovascular hospitalization [32.0% vs. 33.7%; HR 0.82 (95% CI 0.43–1.56); $p = 0.55$]. 8.3% patients developed ablation-related complications. These results are similar to previously published randomized control trials namely, SMASH-VT, V-TACH, and SMS trial. In a recent meta-analysis that included these three trials, prophylactic catheter ablation was found to significantly reduce the incidence of ICD therapies, including ICD shocks and electrical storms, compared to treatment with ICD alone.[10]

Another strategy of deferring ablation till first episode of VT after ICD implantation seems reasonable according to the findings of recently published PARTITA trial.[11] Of 517 patients, 47.6% suffered from VT episodes during a median follow-up of 2.4 years. Only 10% of these patients received an ICD shock, because most episodes resolved either spontaneously or terminated with antitachycardia pacing. The low frequency of ICD shocks indicates that it is often reasonable to wait for VT to reoccur before starting AAD therapy or considering catheter ablation, especially for patients after their initial VT episode. Subsequently, 47 patients were randomized ablation ($n = 23$) and standard therapy (control group, $n = 24$). The trial was discontinued after the first interim analysis because of strikingly positive endpoints in ablation group. The primary endpoint occurred in one patient in the ablation group versus 10 patients in the standard therapy group [HR 0.11 (95% CI 0.01–0.85); $p = 0.034$]. Additionally, there were no deaths in the ablation group, while the standard therapy group had eight deaths. However, these findings should be carefully extrapolated to clinical practice as number of patients in ablation arm were very small.

Therefore, the timing of catheter ablation does not appear to influence prognosis, as early ablation does not reduce mortality compared to deferred ablation.

Indirect evidence seems to suggest that ablation might provide survival benefit. End-of-procedure noninducibility of VT has been shown to improve all-cause mortality. A retrospective study including 2,061 patients with structural heart disease (53% ischemic) found that ablation improves transplant-free survival by decreasing arrhythmia recurrence.[12] Till date, no trial had sufficient power to demonstrate reduction in mortality with ablation alone.

COMPLICATIONS ASSOCIATED WITH ABLATION

Despite a lower incidence of complications in elective ablations performed at experienced centers, up to 10% of patients may still experience procedure-related issues. These complications include cardiac tamponade, pericardial effusion, and third-degree atrioventricular conduction block, each occurring in 1–4% of cases. Notably, all randomized controlled trials (RCTs) have reported 0% periprocedural mortality. However, early postprocedural mortality is observed in about 5% of cases and is often attributed to poor patient condition and associated comorbidities such as chronic kidney disease, and postprocedural VT recurrence. Incomplete substrate ablation is also another important predictor of overall mortality.

CONCLUSION

Recently published data clearly support the role of VT ablation in ICM patients with recurrent VT despite AAD therapy and ICD implantation. Role of prophylactic ablation remains doubtful and needs to be tested with larger RCTs. Survival benefit with ablation has not been documented though composite endpoints comprising of mortality have shown superior outcomes. Till date, no trial was adequately powered to study the impact of ablation on mortality. Further trials are underway which will include novel mapping and ablation techniques to further improve catheter ablation in this most needy and difficult patient subset to reduce mortality as well as reduce complications with ablation.

ONLINE REFERENCES

Please scan the QR code provided at the end of the table of contents for References of this chapter.

CHAPTER

200

Difficult-to-treat Atrial Fibrillation: Management Options

Ajay M Naik, Aarya A Naik, Aditi A Naik

ABSTRACT

Atrial fibrillation (AF) is the most common arrhythmia, and its prevalence increases with advancing age. AF is associated with an increased risk of thromboembolism resulting in stroke and systemic embolism. Evaluation of the need for anticoagulation and its adjustment as per clinical circumstances is an integral part of AF management.

Atrial fibrillation and associated irregularity of ventricular contraction worsen hemodynamics in the presence of an underlying structural heart disease, such as valvular heart disease or heart failure. Adequate ventricular rate control in AF is necessary to alleviate a patient's symptoms and is primarily achieved with drugs. Restoration of sinus rhythm helps restore hemodynamics; this may need pharmacologic or electrical cardioversion, maintenance of antiarrhythmic drugs, and AF ablation when necessary.

The management plan of AF needs to be revisited and remapped with the passage of time and new clinical events. There may be situations requiring switching from rate control to rhythm maintenance and vice versa as per changing circumstances. Anticoagulation agents may need to be changed or the dosage may need to be adjusted. There may be situations calling for the discontinuation of drugs and the adoption of intervention strategies. All these require discussing the nature of the disease, various treatment options, and shared decision-making with the patient over the long term.

Keywords: Atrial fibrillation, rate control, rhythm control, AF ablation, cardioversion, anticoagulation, pacemaker implantation

INTRODUCTION

Prevalence of atrial fibrillation (AF) increases with advancing age. Modern medicine has increased human longevity; hence, AF is a frequent comorbidity in clinical practice. Whereas in the past, AF associated with rheumatic heart disease (RHD) was a common presentation in the Indian subcontinent, nowadays nonrheumatic AF has also become common.

Evaluation of the risk of stroke and the need for anticoagulation for stroke and systemic embolism prevention should be the initial step in the management of any patient with AF.[1,2] Concurrently, there ought to be efforts for appropriate ventricular rate control during AF to relieve symptoms. Rhythm restoration and maintenance should be the ideal goal. There may be circumstances where AF is difficult to manage despite concerted efforts toward the same **(Box 1)**.

BOX 1 Comprehensive management of AF.

<table>
<tr><td colspan="4">Pillars for AF management</td></tr>
<tr><td colspan="4">Access to all aspects of care for all</td></tr>
<tr><td colspan="2">• Stroke risk
• Assess and treat</td><td>• Optimize
• All modifiable risk factors</td><td>• Symptom management
• AF burden
• Rhythm and rate control</td></tr>
<tr><td colspan="4">Shared decision-making</td></tr>
<tr><td colspan="4">Treat risk factors and enact behavioral changes</td></tr>
<tr><td>Heart failure</td><td>Exercise</td><td>Arterial hypertension</td><td>Diabetes</td></tr>
<tr><td>Tobacco</td><td>Obesity</td><td>Ethanol</td><td>Sleep</td></tr>
</table>

Source: Adapted from 2023 ACC/AHA/ACCP/HRS guideline recommendations for comprehensive management of AF.

DIFFICULT-TO-TREAT ATRIAL FIBRILLATION

- Atrial fibrillation may be particularly difficult to treat in certain clinical scenarios. Some of these are enumerated below and discussed in further detail. In each of these, the primary discussion will be regarding arrhythmia management; options for stroke prevention are discussed only if it is pertinent to a particular disease scenario or treatment option. Paroxysmal AF in young adults
- Paroxysmal AF with frequent breakthrough episodes
- Persistent AF with uncontrolled symptoms
- AF with heart failure (HF)
- AF in valvular heart disease
- AF in hypertrophic cardiomyopathy (HCM)
- AF in athletes
- AF in patients with associated conditions, such as obesity, obstructive sleep apnea (OSA), chronic obstructive pulmonary disease (COPD)
- AF associated with congenital heart disease (CHD) and in the pediatric age group
- AF after previous AF ablations
- AF patient with recurrent transient ischemic attacks (TIAs)/strokes/systemic embolism

The above scenarios would represent some common scenarios that perplex the clinician; the list is *comprehensive but not exhaustive.*

Paroxysmal Atrial Fibrillation in Young Adults

- AF is a rare arrhythmia in a young adult with a normal heart. Hence, the first episode of AF in the young adult should prompt the quest for a precipitating cause. A complete history taking is required to elicit information about febrile illness, use of decongestant medications, bronchodilators, and binge alcohol drinking. Physical examination, ECG in sinus rhythm, and echocardiogram would be necessary to rule out congenital structural heart disease.
- A first episode of AF in a young patient could be treated conservatively by addressing the circumstances with a clearly identified precipitant (such as fever or possible culprit drugs).
- It is not unusual for an underlying paroxysmal supraventricular tachycardia (PSVT) such as accessory pathway (AP) mediated atrioventricular reentrant tachycardia (AVRT) to degenerate to AF in young patients due to high sympathetic or catecholaminergic state. The sinus rhythm ECG may show pre-excitation in some cases. This should prompt an electrophysiology study (EPS) and radiofrequency ablation (RFA), which may be curative and prevent AF occurrence in the future **(Table 1)**.
- A normal sinus rhythm ECG does not rule out PSVT degenerating to AF, as the primary mechanism may be an orthodromic AVRT due to a concealed AP or due to rapid atrioventricular nodal reentrant tachycardia (AVNRT) degenerating to AF. Hence, recurrent AF episodes in young adults should prompt an EPS–RFA procedure.
- If all precipitating circumstances are addressed, a first episode of AF in the young can be managed with a "pill in the pocket/purse" approach with a class IC agent such as flecainide or propafenone.[1,2] It is prudent to use a fast-acting beta blocker such as metoprolol tartrate prior to using an IC agent.

Recurrent episodes of paroxysmal AF would necessitate the use of class IC agents with a beta blocker on a regular basis. In case of breakthrough episodes, escalation to class III antiarrhythmic drugs (AAD) such as amiodarone has been the usual practice. In the current era, rather than using

TABLE 1: Recommendations for AF catheter ablation.

Class of recommendation	Level of evidence	Recommendations
I	A	In patients with symptomatic AF in whom AADs have been ineffective, contraindicated, not tolerated, or not preferred, and continued rhythm control is desired, catheter ablation is useful to improve symptoms
I	A	In selected patients (generally younger with few comorbidities) with symptomatic paroxysmal AF in whom rhythm control is desired, catheter ablation is useful as first-line therapy to improve symptoms and reduce progression to persistent AF
I	A	In patients with symptomatic or clinically significant AFL, catheter ablation is useful for improving symptoms
IIa	B-NR	In patients who are undergoing ablation for AF, ablation of additional clinically significant supraventricular arrhythmias can be useful to reduce the likelihood of future arrhythmia
IIa	B-R	In patients (other than younger with few comorbidities) with symptomatic paroxysmal or persistent AF who are being managed with a rhythm-control strategy, catheter ablation as first-line therapy can be useful to improve symptoms

Source: Adapted from 2023 ACC/AHA/ACCP/HRS guideline recommendations for AF catheter ablation.

class III agents with their attendant adverse effects, it would be better to discuss the pros and cons of AF ablation in these patients. Due to improved success rates and reduction in risks associated with AF ablation following the adoption of new technologies and therapies, this has become a class I recommendation in the recent 2023 ACC/AHA/ACCP/HRS guidelines for AF management **(Table 1)**.[1]

Paroxysmal Atrial Fibrillation with Frequent Breakthrough Episodes

In both older and younger patients, paroxysmal AF is generally primarily managed with a combination of class IC and beta-blocker agents. Frequent breakthrough episodes may result in the progression of the mechanism to persistent AF.

In order to halt this relentless progression, one conservative option is the introduction of a class III agent. However, this strategy may not prevent breakthrough episodes completely and entails the risk of adverse effects. It is necessary to intervene with AF ablation at the appropriate time in these patients to prevent the inexorable progression of the disease **(Table 1)**.[1]

Persistent Atrial Fibrillation with Uncontrolled Symptoms

Patients may progress from repeated paroxysmal AF or present in persistent AF of unknown duration. In the majority of patients, symptoms such as palpitations due to fast ventricular rate or exertional fatigue and dyspnea may need to be managed by a combination of AV node blocking agents for rate control, with a class III agent to help rate control or hope for rhythm restoration to sinus rhythm **(Table 2)**.

- Some patients may continue to be symptomatic despite escalated drugs. At this point in time, the onset of tachycardiomyopathy becomes an issue and needs to be actively looked for.
- Patients pretreated with anticoagulation and AAD should be advised DC cardioversion in an attempt for rhythm restoration. Pretreatment with class III AADs (especially amiodarone) improves the probability of successful cardioversion and maintenance of sinus rhythm subsequently.
- Recurrence of AF after cardioversion may be treated by increased AAD dosage and repetition of cardioversion. However, after repeated recurrences and multiple cardioversions, this strategy appears futile. At this stage, AF ablation again appears as an option. In view of lower overall success rates (compared to AF ablation in paroxysmal AF), this has received a class IIA recommendation in the 2023 ACC/AHA/ACCP/HRS guidelines for AF management **(Table 1 and Flowchart 1)**.[1]
- A significant number of elderly patients may develop sinoatrial node (SAN) dysfunction due to advancing cardiac disease or SAN suppression by AADs. These patients may manifest as tachy-brady syndrome, often revealed after cardioversion. These patients are likely to benefit from dual chamber permanent pacemaker (PPM) implantation. Atrial pacing prevents the occurrence of brady-dependent atrial arrhythmia episodes and reduces AF occurrence. Also, administering AADs at higher doses is possible now that the bradycardia risk is obviated by the pacemaker.

Some of these patients may be candidates for atrioventricular node (AVN) ablation after pacemaker implantation if the ventricular rates are still not controlled. Accordingly, pacing in the form of conduction system pacing (CSP) or cardiac resynchronization therapy (CRT) should be considered upfront in patients where the underlying heart disease suggests the likelihood of worsening of left ventricular ejection fraction (LVEF) in the future **(Table 3)**.

TABLE 2: Recommendations for rate versus rhythm control in AF.

	Favors rate control		Variable		Favors rhythm control
Patient factors	Prefers rate control	⟵	Patient choice	⟶	Prefers rhythm control
	"Older"	⟵	Age	⟶	"Younger"
	Longer history of AF	⟵	Antecedent history of AF	⟶	Shorter history of AF
	Fewer symptoms	⟵	Symptom burden	⟶	More symptoms
Physical examination and anatomy	Easily controlled heart rate	⟵	Rate control in AF	⟶	Difficult-to-control heart rate
	Larger LA	⟵	LA size	⟶	Smaller LA
	Less LV dysfunction	⟵	LV function in AF	⟶	More LV dysfunction
	Less AV regurgitation	⟵	AV regurgitation in AF	⟶	More AV regurgitation

Source: Adapted from 2023 ACC/AHA/ACCP/HRS guideline recommendations for rate versus rhythm control in AF.

Atrial Fibrillation with Heart Failure

- AF and HF are the final frontiers in cardiology. Each on its own may be difficult to manage and when they coexist, they worsen the outcomes considerably.
- Rhythm control is the preferred option in HF, as the outcomes are better than in rate control.
- Guideline recommended medical therapy (GDMT) for HF, anticoagulation for stroke prevention, and AADs for rhythm control are the multipronged therapy strategies for this population. Additionally, revascularization and valvular interventions where indicated should be performed.
- Pharmacological rhythm control is difficult due to frequent breakthrough episodes and the risk of proarrhythmias especially common in HF patients.
- As per the 2023 ACC/AHA/ACCP/HRS guidelines, AF ablation is recommended for rhythm control in HF patients **(Flowchart 2)**.
- Advanced HF and resistant AF may need to be treated with AV node ablation and CRT implantation or conduction system pacing (CSP).

Atrial Fibrillation in Valvular Heart Disease

- The Indian subcontinent still has RHD as a common etiology for AF. They form a distinct population of relatively young patients who are at high risk for thromboembolism. There is also a significant number of

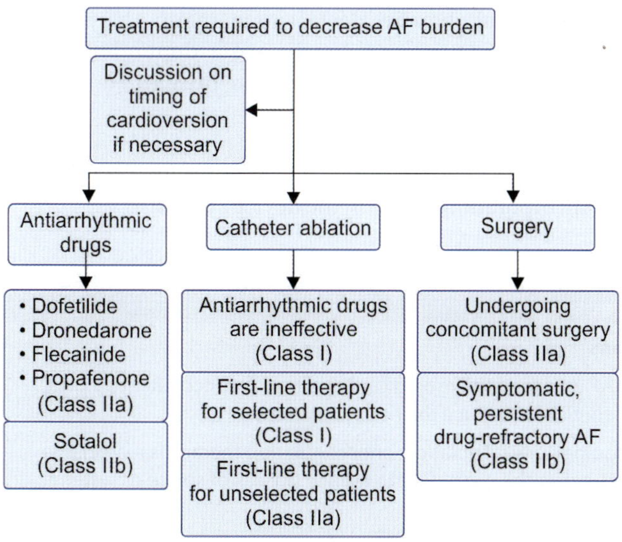

FLOWCHART 1: Treatment choices to reduce the AF burden.

Source: Adapted from 2023 ACC/AHA/ACCP/HRS guideline recommendations for treatment choices to reduce the AF burden.

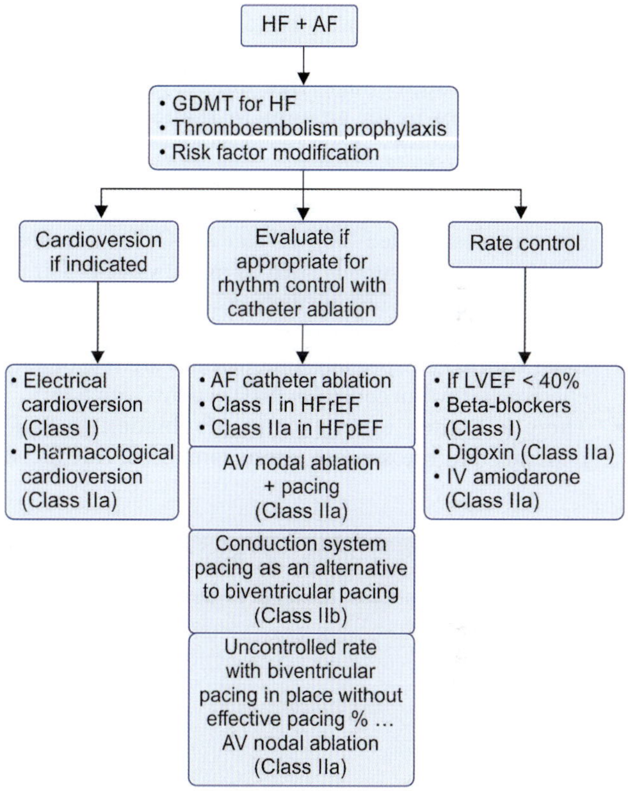

FLOWCHART 2: Management of AF in HF.

Source: Adapted from 2023 ACC/AHA/ACCP/HRS guideline recommendations for management of AF in HF.

TABLE 3: Recommendations for AV node ablation.

Class of recommendation	Level of evidence	Recommendations
I	C-LD	In patients with AF and a persistently rapid ventricular response who undergo AVNA, initial pacemaker lower rate programming should be 80–90 beats/min to reduce the risk of sudden death
IIa	B-R	In patients with AF and uncontrolled rapid ventricular response refractory to rate-control medications (who are not candidates for or in whom rhythm control has been unsuccessful), AVNA can be useful to improve symptoms and QOL
I	B-NR	In patients with AF who are planning to undergo AVNA, implantation of a pacemaker before the ablation (i.e., before or same day of ablation) is recommended to ensure adequacy of the pacing leads before performing ablation
IIb	C-LD	In patients with AF with normal EF undergoing AVNA, conduction system pacing of the His bundle or left bundle area may be reasonable

Source: Adapted from 2023 ACC/AHA/ACCP/HRS guideline recommendations for AV node ablation.

RHD patients who have undergone interventions (such as balloon mitral valvotomy) or surgery (mitral and/or aortic valve replacement) in the course of the disease.

- RHD with AF should be given vitamin K antagonists (warfarin, acenocoumarol) as anticoagulation for stroke prevention. Direct oral anticoagulants (DOACs) (such as dabigatran, apixaban, and rivaroxaban) are not an option for patients with AF and RHD, especially those with stenotic mitral disease.
- If the patients are candidates for surgical valvular interventions, simultaneous RF or electrocautery maze procedure concurrent with the valvular surgery may be a good option **(Table 4)**.
- Left atrial appendage ligation/resection at the same surgery in an attempt to reduce the risk of thromboembolism may also be considered **(Table 5)**.
- Nonrheumatic AF with valvular disease (e.g., coronary artery disease, LV dysfunction with mitral regurgitation) was previously called "nonvalvular AF" (NVAF). If these patients undergo surgery such as mitral valve repair or replacement with bioprosthetic valve, DOACs can be given safely for stroke prevention.
- Class III AADs (especially amiodarone) are reasonably effective in rhythm control in RHD patients with AF.[3,4]
- There is limited experience in AF ablation in RHD patients, and the success rate is tempered. Advanced RHD patients with AF and HF may finally be candidates for AV node ablation and CRT/CSP.[4] This is also applicable for patients who are unsuitable for or have already undergone valvular interventions.

Atrial Fibrillation in Hypertrophic Cardiomyopathy

- Patients with HCM have significant LV wall stiffness. AF in HCM patients critically affects ventricular filling and cardiac output. The onset of AF results in rapid clinical deterioration. These patients are also at high risk for thromboembolism.
- DOACs should be initiated in patients with HCM with the onset of AF to reduce the stroke risk.
- Rhythm control is vital in HCM patients. These are often the patients who benefit the most from AF ablation.
- Patients who are candidates for automatic implantable cardioverter defibrillators (AICD) should preferably be given dual-chamber devices to maintain AV synchrony and prevention of bradycardia-dependent atrial arrhythmias as AADs are often prescribed to these patients.
- Progression of HCM to the dilated phase, LV dysfunction, and HF may need to be treated with CRT-ICD or incorporation of CSP in the device system.

TABLE 4: Recommendations for AF patients undergoing cardiac surgery.

Class of recommendation	Level of evidence	Recommendations
IIa	B-R	For patients with AF who are undergoing cardiac surgery, concomitant surgical ablation can be beneficial to reduce the risk of recurrent AF
IIa	B-NR	In patients undergoing surgical ablation, anticoagulation therapy is reasonable for at least 3 months after the procedure to reduce the risk of stroke or systemic embolism
IIb	B-R	For patients with symptomatic, persistent AF refractory to antiarrhythmic drug therapy, a hybrid epicardial and endocardial ablation might be reasonable to reduce the risk of recurrent atrial arrhythmia

Source: Adapted from 2023 ACC/AHA/ACCP/HRS guideline recommendations for AF patients undergoing cardiac surgery.

TABLE 5: Recommendations for AF patients undergoing cardiac surgery with LAA exclusion/excision.

Class of recommendation	Level of evidence	Recommendations
I	A	In patients with AF undergoing cardiac surgery with a CHA_2DS_2-VASc score ≥ 2 or equivalent stroke risk, surgical LAA exclusion, in addition to continued anticoagulation, is indicated to reduce the risk of stroke and systemic embolism
I	A	In patients with AF undergoing cardiac surgery and LAA exclusion, a surgical technique resulting in the absence of flow across the suture line and a stump of <1 cm as determined by intraoperative transesophageal echocardiography should be used
IIb	A	In patients with AF undergoing cardiac surgery with CHA_2DS_2-VASc score ≥ 2 or equivalent stroke risk, the benefit of surgical LAA exclusion in the absence of continued anticoagulation to reduce the risk of stroke and systemic embolism is uncertain

Source: Adapted from 2023 ACC/AHA/ACCP/HRS guideline recommendations for AF patients undergoing cardiac surgery with LAA exclusion/excision.

Atrial Fibrillation in Athletes

- Endurance/high-performance athletes are a special population. They often have structural changes in relatively dilated cardiac chambers (especially LV and LA dilatation).
- Extreme fitness and hypervagotonia result in resting sinus bradycardia and blunted chronotropy compared to average individuals. AF may complicate this scenario and become rather difficult to manage.
- These individuals cannot be given beta blockers due to resting bradycardia and negative effect on their athletic performance. AADs can at the most be used in a "pill in the pocket/purse" approach. Maintenance therapy with AADs is not possible due to interference with their training and performance schedules. The efficacy of AADs in this population is also not well studied.
- AF ablation becomes the sole remaining therapy in highly affected individuals. This needs to be performed in a high-volume center that has skilled performers with good success rates and a high benefit–risk ratio.

Atrial Fibrillation in Patients with Associated Conditions Such as Obesity, Obstructive Sleep Apnea, Chronic Obstructive Pulmonary Disease

- This is a diverse population with complicated comorbidities that have unique problems that need to be managed individually.
- OSA is a major culprit of AF occurrence and also for recurrence of AF after AF ablation.[1,2]
- Continuous positive airway pressure (CPAP) helps relieve OSA and may also have a positive effect on AF occurrence.
- Obesity coexisting with hypertension and diabetes mellitus also worsens AF-related morbidity. Obesity often coexists with OSA, and weight reduction also helps in relieving OSA **(Table 6)**.
- COPD patients are usually treated with beta stimulants, resulting in an increased incidence of AF. To control ventricular rate, nondihydropyridine calcium channel blockers (CCB) such as verapamil and diltiazem are the main options in these patients, as beta blockers may worsen bronchoconstriction. Amiodarone may be contraindicated if the lung disease is significant. These patients are particularly difficult to manage and maintain.

Atrial Fibrillation Associated with Congenital Heart Disease and in Pediatric Age Group

- Patients with CHD and grown-up congenital heart (GUCH) disease are again a different and unique group. Patients who have undergone surgical correction such as Fontan repair are also prone to atrial arrhythmias later in life. AF causes significant symptoms and adversely affects the hemodynamics in these patients.
- The mainstay of treatment in these patients is beta blockers, lanoxin, and class IC and III AADs as per individual problems.
- AF or intra-atrial reentrant tachycardias (IART) are often seen in postoperative patients. If resistant to drugs, ablation therapy is the only recourse for these patients. This needs to be done in highly specialized centers with highly skilled operators.
- Despite being young, these patients may require anticoagulation therapy due to the hemodynamics and slow flow in some of the postsurgical anatomical chambers.
- Cardiac implantable electronic devices (CIED), commonly pacemakers, may be needed if SAN or AVN dysfunction complicates the situation.

Atrial Fibrillation after Previous Atrial Fibrillation Ablations

- AF recurrence after AF ablation is a bane of progressive disease; it brings both psychological and financial stress to the patient. Patients may undergo multiple AF ablation procedures over the years by multiple different operators at multiple different centers. This is currently true for many patients in the West.
- In India, even the high-volume centers would probably perform a maximum of two or three ablation procedures for a patient over the years. With successive procedures, both the financial and procedural outcomes may become less attractive.
- Newer technologies (e.g., cryoablation, pulsed field ablation, PFA) promise a safer, quicker procedure with predictable outcomes. These may be good options for some patients.
- Elderly patients with severe, recurrent symptoms despite AF ablation procedure may be considered for

TABLE 6: Recommendations for weight loss in individuals who are overweight or obese.

Class of recommendation	Level of evidence	Recommendations
I	B-R	In patients with AF who are overweight or obese [with body mass index (BMI) > 27 kg/m^2], weight loss is recommended, with an ideal target of at least 10% weight loss to reduce AF symptoms, burden, recurrence, and progression to persistent AF

Source: Adapted from 2023 ACC/AHA/ACCP/HRS guideline recommendations for weight loss in individuals who are overweight or obese.

the rate control option. If even this is difficult due to ineffectiveness or adverse effects of drugs, these patients may be candidates for AV node ablation and CSP/CRT.

Atrial Fibrillation Patient with Recurrent Transient Ischemic Attacks/Strokes

- VKAs are effective and DOACs are both effective and safe for AF-associated thromboembolism reduction. However, some patients may get TIAs/stroke/systemic embolism despite appropriate anticoagulation therapy. There is an attendant risk of bleeding complications, especially in the elderly and those with comorbidities [such as chronic kidney disease (CKD)]. Left atrial appendage occlusion (LAAO) is an emerging alternative and a viable option in such patients.
- In RHD, the thromboembolism may be from the LAA in only half the cases; in the rest, it may be occurring from a thrombus harbored in the dilated LA. Consequently, LAAO would not be effective in these patients. Surgery, when indicated with LAA ligation, atrial size reduction, RF maze, and well-monitored VKA anticoagulation, would be needed in these patients.

CONCLUSION

Atrial fibrillation can have myriad presentations due to diverse clinical backgrounds. It increases the risk of stroke and systemic embolism that can have devastating effects with major morbidity and mortality implications. Anticoagulation reduces this risk considerably and should be managed with regular and periodic supervision. Rate and rhythm control alternatives should be discussed with the patient. Advances in each of these fields are emerging rapidly and frequently; hence, these discussions need to be conducted periodically. Management of AF requires shared decision-making with the patient. In the occasional case, it is difficult to achieve a satisfactory outcome despite all efforts.

ONLINE REFERENCES

Please scan the QR code provided at the end of the table of contents for References of this chapter.

CHAPTER

201

Atrial Fibrillation in India: The Burden and the Way Forward

Vivek Chaturvedi

ABSTRACT

Atrial fibrillation (AF) is the most common arrhythmia worldwide including India and is associated with major morbidity and mortality.[1] While there is a rapidly rising burden of nonvalvular AF (NVAF) in India, there also exists a large pool of individuals with AF due to rheumatic heart disease (RHD), a situation which is unlike developed nations. Accordingly, it is imperative that policies and recommendations, for treatment and prevention of AF and its complications, be guided by locally relevant and context specific data. In this article, we attempt to outline the contemporary burden of AF and its complications in India, using available evidence, and possible actions for its comprehensive management.

Keywords: Atrial fibrillation, rheumatic heart disease, risk factors, epidemiological transition, oral anticoagulation, stroke, heart failure, prevention

INTRODUCTION

As far as cardiovascular diseases are concerned, India faces a double whammy due to the differing stages of epidemiological transition that we are in, simultaneously, owing to geographic, socio-economic, and demographic heterogeneity. This is exemplified by the epidemiology of AF in India.

Earlier data regarding the epidemiology of atrial fibrillation (AF) in India was sparse and pointed toward a majority being of rheumatic in origin and in a much younger population.[2] While there have been no studies till now to look at incidence of AF, some community-based data in recent times have documented contemporary point prevalence of AF in India. These studies, mostly done in southern and western India, summarized in **Table 1**, indicate a prevalence of 0.2–1.6% for AF in Indian adults. The actual figure may be higher given that most of these studies were rural-based and urban areas typically have higher burden of degenerative diseases. Another reason for finding low prevalence may be use of single time versus repeated screening given that many patients have paroxysmal episodes. SMART India study[3] found that with single screening prevalence was 1.1% versus 1.6% with repeated screening. The prevalence of AF above age of 50 years in Gujarat was 5.1%, which is consistent with the global prevalence in developed nations.[4] Another indicator for the rising burden of AF is the rising burden of stroke in India, as AF is a major cause for stroke.

TABLE 1: Prevalence of atrial fibrillation in India.

	Year	Setting	Number	Prevalence %
PINNACLE India Registry[5]	2014	Clinic records	630 adults	0.4
Nagpur pilot study[6]	2016	Urban Nagpur city community	4,077 adults	0.2
Soni et al.[4]	2016	Rural Gujarat community	354 adults > 50 years	5.1
Smart India study[3]	2019	Rural Gujarat community	2,100 adults	1.6
AP-AF study[7]	2022	Rural Andhra Pradesh community	4,281 adults	0.3

CLINICAL PROFILE OF ATRIAL FIBRILLATION IN INDIA

As mentioned, rheumatic heart disease (RHD) is a major cause of AF in especially patients with mitral valve disease. Negi et al[8] found that 24% of their patients with RHD had AF. However, with increasing longevity and adverse metabolic profile, degenerative AF is also rising rapidly in India. **Table 2** summarizes the proportion of AF patients with RHD as the etiology in different studies.

As can be seen, the proportion of AF due to RHD varies from 20 to 40% of all patients. Such difference likely reflects regional differences in RHD prevalence and epidemiological transition toward atherosclerotic and vascular disease. For example, burden of mortality due to cardiovascular diseases in Kerala already exceeds that in western nations.[12]

TABLE 2: Proportion of atrial fibrillation due to rheumatic heart disease (RHD) in India.

Study	Setting	Proportion of AF due to RHD
RELY-AF registry[9]	n = 2,536, emergency department visits	31.5%
Kerala–AF registry[10]	n = 3,421, state wide registry	21.4%
IHRS AF[11]	n = 1,537, India wide	47.6%
REALISE AF[8]	n = 301, India wide	40.7%*

*Percentage with valvular heart disease, RHD not mentioned.

CLINICAL FEATURES OF ATRIAL FIBRILLATION IN INDIA

The epidemiology of AF in India shows a convergence toward that is found in western countries with decline of RHD as a major cause for AF. Importantly the risk factors for AF, several of which are also major cardiovascular risk factors, are developing at a much younger age as compared to developed nations, which is a matter of concern. **Table 3** summarizes the prevalence of major clinical features seen in large registries reported in India and compares to to a large global registry. The average age is younger than developed nations, but the metabolic risk factors such as diabetes and hypertension are highly prevalent and vascular diseases such as CAD and stroke are also common. In a study from North India among patients with persistent nonvalvular AF (NVAF), 46% had obstructive CAD while only 30% had normal coronaries.[13] Alcohol use and obstructive sleep apnea are probably under-reported in India. The increased burden of permanent AF is probably due to rheumatic causes as well as the fact that rhythm control strategy is

TABLE 3: Clinical features among individuals with atrial fibrillation.

Parameter	RELY-AF registry[9]	GARFIELD-AF registry[14]	IHRS-AF registry[11]	Kerala-AF registry[10]	GARFIELD-AF worldwide[14]
Mean age years	57.9	65.8	54.7	65	69.7
Mean BMI kg/m^2		24.3		24.2	27.8
% Women	50.3	40.1	51.5	51	44
Alcohol use %		16.4			44.5
HT %	41.6	68.5	31.4	53.8	76.3
Diabetes %	20.2	36.2	16.1	34.5	22.2
Dyslipidemia %		13.6	8.5	42.2	41.6
CAD %		28.1	9.3	34.8	21.6
Heart failure %	17.7	15.5	18.7	26.5	20
Stroke/TIA	7.4	9.1	9.2	14.9	11.4
Chronic kidney disease %		5.2	4.6	10.3	10.3
Mean CHA_2DS_2-VASc score	1.1#	2.9	47% > 3#	2.9	3.2
HAS-BLED score		1.5	30.7% > 3	1.7	1.4
Permanent AF %	46.6	8.5*	45.6	46.2	12.8*
Obstructive sleep apnea	0.8		2.0		
Use of oral anticoagulants	23.5	46	73.9	44.3	
Use of antiplatelets	38.6	40	38.9	36.6	

*GARFIELD-AF had additional classification of AF as new onset/unclassified which was the majority condition.

#$CHADS_2$ score.

still sparingly used in India. The differences seen in various registries likely reflect varied healthcare settings and regional disparities but the epidemiological changes being witnessed suggest that the entire India is transiting toward the demographic profile of Kerala which in turn resembles that of developed nations. Thus, it appears that we are set to see dramatic rise in incidence of degenerative AF in the near future. Use of oral anticoagulants has been rising in India; however, an alarming trend is that use of antiplatelets (which should be discouraged as a choice of anticoagulant in AF) is very high and has stayed at that level over time as was shown in the GARFIELD AF registry[14] and the KERALA-AF study.[10] GARFIELD-AF also found that oral anticoagulant use increased appropriately with increasing thromboembolic risk (by CHADSVASc score), but use of oral antiplatelets remained constant despite higher risk. While a majority of studies from India show that vitamin K antagonists were the predominant form of anticoagulant use, this is likely to be different today given the sharply decreasing prevalence of RHD associated AF and availability of off-patent cheaper direct oral anticoagulants (DOACs). Of concern is that many patients with RHD and MVD with AF still do not receive anticoagulation leading to unacceptably high risk of thromboembolism. Even among those with AF who receive VKA anticoagulation, time in therapeutic range (TTR) was only 33% in RELY-AF India and GARFIELD-AF India data which is much less as compared to a global average of approximately 50%.

OUTCOMES OF ATRIAL FIBRILLATION IN INDIA

Atrial fibrillation is associated with increased all-cause and cardiovascular mortality, stroke, heart failure, hospitalization, and thromboembolism. Among patients with RHD, onset of AF leads to worsening of disease status, deterioration of hemodynamics (especially relevant for mitral stenosis) and increased risk of stroke and thromboembolism multifold.[15] In the study by Negi et al.,[16] the prevalence of heart failure (25.7% vs.12.6%) $p < 0.001$, systemic thromboembolism (8.6% vs. 5.8%) $p < 0.02$ and mortality were significantly higher among patients with AF and RHD as compared to those who did not have AF. As RHD is quite common in women of child bearing age in India, an interesting study from South India[17] compared the outcomes of pregnant women with or without concomitant AF. Among 1,393 pregnant women with RHD, 71 (5%) had coexistent AF. Composite adverse outcome (maternal death, heart failure, or thromboembolic events) and pregnancy outcomes were compared. It found that composite adverse outcome was significantly higher in those with AF as compared to without (77.5% vs. 17%). There were 9.9% maternal deaths in those with AF as compared to 0.7% in controls. There was also a trend toward higher rates of miscarriage, small-for-gestational-age babies, and cesarean rates.

Similar observations have also been made for NVAF which tends to cluster with other metabolic and cardiovascular morbidities in India. **Table 4** summarizes the outcomes observed in patents with AF during follow-up among large registries of India.

As can be seen, Indian registries uniformly show higher all-cause and cardiovascular death as compared to developed nations, while the stroke and major bleeding risks are low (probably due to lower mean age of Indian participants). The higher cardiovascular death is intriguing and implies higher cardiovascular disease burden in these patients. Even if patients with RHD, who are more prone to AF related complications, are excluded, the KERALA-AF registry showed the all-cause mortality and hospitalization at 1 year to be 16.5% and 20.65%, respectively.[18] Of note, among this population of NVAF, almost 40% had CAD, 40% had CKD, and almost a quarter had heart failure. This is also much higher than the complication rate in GARFIELD-AF India,[14] which also had NVAF population. While the embolic complications AF are rightly emphasized, it is worthwhile mentioning that the biggest cause of death and hospitalization in AF are heart failure, myocardial infarction, and sudden death.

These findings are corroborated by global projections. A recent publication utilizing data from Global Burden of Disease Study[19] has highlighted that India has one of the highest death and disability adjusted life years (DALYs) lost attributable to AF/atrial flutter (AFL) with 855,145 DALYs lost and 27,888 deaths in 2021. This is comparable to China and the USA which have a high AF burden.

TABLE 4: Outcomes among patients with atrial fibrillation in large Indian registries.

Parameter	GARFIELD-AF registry[14]	IHRS-AF registry[11]	Kerala-AF registry[10]	GARFIELD-AF worldwide[14]
All cause death %	7.7	6.5	12.9	4.3
Cardiovascular death %	3.4	4.4	10.5	1.6
All cause hospitalization %		8	16.9	
Stroke/TIA/Systemic embolism %	0.85	1.03		1.34
Acute coronary syndrome %	0.38			0.77
Major bleeding	0.31	0.85		0.84

TREATMENT TRENDS FOR ATRIAL FIBRILLATION

In the RELY-AF registry reported in 2014,[9] which had almost 2,500 patients reporting to emergency services across India, rhythm control medications were used in 10% and was almost exclusively amiodarone. Rate control drugs were used in the majority. Of note, several physicians in India continue to use amiodarone also as a rate controlling agent (i.e., amiodarone is not discontinued despite not converting AF to sinus rhythm because it has AV nodal blocking properties also). Similar data were also reported from IHRS AF registry,[11] conducted in 2011, where a majority of patients were on rate controlling agents, of which digoxin was the most common. In the more contemporary KERALA-AF registry[10] also similar patterns were seen with almost three quarter of patients receiving only rate control agents, but β-blockers were the most common medication used. **Table 5** summarizes the rate and rhythm control medications used in various studies.

The KERALA-AF study also looked at the clinical outcomes stratified by the treatment strategy of rate or rhythm control.[20] As mentioned in the previous text, majority of patients were on rate control. The primary outcome studied was a composite of all-cause mortality, arterial thromboembolism, acute coronary syndrome or hospitalization due to heart failure, or arrhythmia at 12 months. The rates of primary outcomes were high at nearly 30% in both groups. Bleeding outcomes were also similar (1.6% rate control and 1.9% rhythm control). These findings are quite different from those of the recently published EAST-AFNET 4 trial[21] which showed superiority of rhythm control strategy when instituted early. Notably, the event rates in this trial, using almost similar primary outcome as KERALA-AF study, were much lower in both rhythm control and rate control arms implying higher level of cardiovascular comorbidity in Kerala participants. Also, it is expected that wider use of radiofrequency ablation primarily for paroxysmal AF will lead to better outcomes for rhythm strategy given the proarrhythmic potential and increased noncardiovascular mortality associated with antiarrhythmic drugs.

TABLE 5: Use of rate and rhythm control medication in atrial fibrillation in India registries.

Parameter	RELY-AF registry[9]	IHRS-AF registry[11]	Kerala-AF registry[10]	RELY-AF worldwide[9]
Rhythm control %	10.2			
Amiodarone %	10.0	17.0	7.4	8.7
Flecainide/ Propafenone %	0.1		0.7	2.8
Sotalol	0.1	1.0	0.1	2.0
Rhythm control %		75.5		
β-blockers	27.7	21.0	30.9	41.8
Calcium channel blockers %	14.3	15.0	–	8.2
Digoxin	37.3	27.0	22.2	23.4

Traditionally, RHD associated AF has not been subjected to rhythm control aggressively in India, but this is changing with generation of evidence by local research. Previously, small studies had shown utility of amiodarone for converting and maintaining sinus rhythm among patients with mitral stenosis.[15] A recent small study found that flecainide was quite effective in maintaining sinus rhythm among patients with RHD and AF who had undergone mitral valve replacement.[22] Another study looked at efficacy of early direct current cardioversion (DCCV) followed by 6-week amiodarone therapy in patients with long standing AF who were undergoing balloon valvotomy.[23] It is found that 87% of patients receiving DCCV were in sinus rhythm as compared to only 5% among those who did not receive DCCV at 7 months follow-up. Both studies also found better clinical and quality of life (QOL) parameters in those who had maintained sinus rhythm. Another small randomized study[24] recruited patients with persistent AF undergoing balloon valvotomy and randomized then to amiodarone assisted DCCV followed by 12 months amiodarone or only DCCV followed by placebo. After 1 year 55% patients in amiodarone group and 17% in placebo group were in sinus rhythm. Another pilot study found ivabradine to be quite useful for rate control in RHD among those with fast ventricular rates despite maximally tolerated rate control agents.[25] The indigenized efforts of surgical ablation of AF during valve surgeries by bipolar cautery devices (replacing costlier cryoprobe) have been quite impressive with maintenance of sinus rhythm in up to two-thirds of individuals in intermediate term.[26]

A recent study from Hyderabad investigated a tailored approach to treatment of persistent AF in patients with RHD with corrected valvular disease.[27] The investigators attempted to restore sinus rhythm in all patients with the help of antiarrhythmic drugs and DCCV. Where these measures failed, patients were offered catheter ablation or atrioventricular junction (AVJ) ablation and subsequent conduction system pacing or cardiac resynchronization therapy (CSP/CRT). The latter strategy was preferred over catheter ablation if the left atrial size on echo was >6 cm, as long-term success of catheter ablation in that subset is very low. A close follow-up was maintained for all. Of the 83 cases recruited, a majority had undergone a surgical or percutaneous procedure for correction of valve disease. Mean age was 56 years, majority were women and the average duration of persistent AF was >5 years. >60% were in NYHA class 3/4, average heart rate was 107/min, and mean

LA size was 4.7 cm. Pharmacological cardioversion alone was successful in 10% patients and additional 50% cardioverted with DCCV. In 32% of patients sinus rhythm could not be achieved at the outset or there was a recurrence of AF within 3 months. Another 25% (n = 20) had an AF recurrence over 9 months. These individuals (n = 52) were offered additional interventions and underwent ablation (n = 1) or pace and ablate strategy (n = 24). Remarkably, 11 of 24 individuals in pace and ablate strategy also reverted to sinus rhythm for a total of >50% of total group in sinus rhythm in long term. Patients who achieved sinus rhythm had lower NYHA class, lower NTProBNP levels, and higher 6-minute walk distance as compared to those who did not. The study also showed that pace and ablate strategy was superior to conventional measures for rate control in terms of clinical outcomes.

Exciting research has also been carried out recently, exploring more safe and effective options for prevention of thromboembolism among patients of AF with RHD. This was necessitated by the problems associated with usage of VKA for AF in RHD (interactions, monitoring, and narrow therapeutic window) leading to low TTR and the fact that embolic events continue to happen despite their use among patients. The INVICTUS trial[28] compared use of rivaroxaban to VKA among patients with AF and predominantly rheumatic MS. In this large trial, 17% of 4,531 participants were from South Asia including India. The primary efficacy outcome was a composite of stroke, systemic embolism, myocardial infarction, or death from vascular (cardiac or noncardiac) or unknown causes while bleeding outcomes were studied separately. The study unexpectedly found that VKA were superior in preventing the composite outcome while having similar bleeding profile as rivaroxaban. With this, the focus has again shifted to improving the "low-quality anticoagulation" in India by systemic and policy measures.

THE WAY FORWARD

India faces unique challenges while tackling the burgeoning cardiovascular disease epidemic in the nation. On one hand, while there has been a decline in incidence of RHD, the legacy burden of established RHD and its high morbidity and mortality is still present in several parts of the country, with AF a major contributor to it. On the other hand, with rising life expectancy, premature acquisition of metabolic risk factors, alcohol intake, and obesity the burden of degenerative diseases like AF is rapidly rising as well. Longer survival of those fortunate enough to receive timely care for cardiovascular disease but left with residual cardiac damage, is also a contributing factor. While the prevalence of AF is still less than that of developed nations possibly due to age and racial differences, poor detection and treatment rates in India have translated to a very high associated morbidity and mortality. While there have been no studies looking at incidence of AF in India, it is likely that this is rapidly rising unlike developed nations where it is on the decline. The data from the KERALA-AF registry[10] should be a wake-up call for the entire nation. So, what should be done, while going forward, to achieve cost effective prevention and management of AF in India?

Improving Detection Rates

Several methods have been proposed for improving detection rates of AF. While population level screening and using digital healthcare devices for detection are certainly comprehensive, perhaps the easiest and cheapest approach is opportunistic detection of irregular pulse level.[29] This should be done at all health encounters by all healthcare providers and individuals can even be taught self pulse-palpation.

Establishment of Systems for Prospective Data Collection

The KERALA-AF registry is an admirable effort in this direction. Such registries, with prospective data collection, are vital for providing informed evidence about future policy and action. Through subtle cues, they also bring about a change in prescriber treatment patterns. In KERALA-AF study,[10] prescription of warfarin increased from 34% at baseline to 51% at 1 month follow-up. Similarly, use of rhythm control drugs (amiodarone use doubled from 7.4 to 14.8%) and rate control (54–78%) also increased.

Comprehensive Cardiovascular Prevention Strategies

The AF is a degenerative cardiovascular disease. It not only coexists with several metabolic and lifestyle-related cardiovascular conditions, but also shares pathophysiology with them. Evidence for this is very clear from the national studies, where a high prevalence of diabetes, hypertension, CAD, stroke, and heart failure was found in patients of AF. Thus, a comprehensive primary and secondary prevention strategy is the need of the hour.[30] While the risk factors are well known, societal awareness and adoption of preventive strategies is sadly lacking. These strategies include quality and performance measures, and adoption of evidence based measures from public health arena.[31] Upstream interventions such as enhanced opportunistic screening for AF in at-risk individuals and evaluation for clustered cardiovascular and metabolic risk factors, as mentioned earlier, go a long way in better prevention and management of AF.

Improving the Low Quality of Oral Anticoagulation

Development of cardioembolic complications such as stroke and acute limb ischemia is a catastrophic event in AF. This is even more true in India, where a significant proportion of strokes are due to AF in RHD. Such strokes are more severe, occur in a much younger age group, and are more common in socio-economically weaker strata. Oral anticoagulation is cheap and widely available in India but its usage is hampered by poor awareness, compliance, and hindrances in regular monitoring. This has resulted in India having one of the lowest TTR rates globally. This can be changed by systematic institution of public and healthcare provider interventions. The IMPACT-AF study,[32] which had 493 patients from India, was a prospective international cluster randomized controlled trial that tested educational intervention in patients and public coupled to regular monitoring and feedback. OAC use over 1 year increased from 68 to 80% in the intervention arm. Importantly, this led to reduction in stroke rates in the intervention arm (HR 0.48 as compared to controls).

Dedicated Centers for Integrated and Comprehensive Management of Atrial Fibrillation

Treatment of established and persistent/recurrent AF is difficult but possible with a tailored approach as reported recently. Several such centers across India are the need of the hour. Furthermore, for comprehensive management of established AF the paradigm is shifting to multidisciplinary and integrated care given that lifestyle modification and behavioral change are critical to maintenance of sinus rhythm and avoidance of vascular events.[33] Such institutions can be the center of a hub and spoke model and spearhead efforts for comprehensive management of AF.

CONCLUSION

Atrial fibrillation is an important cause of death and disability in India and data show that its burden will rise further in future. While AF due to RHD is on the decline, adverse lifestyle changes, better survival after heart disease and increasing life expectancy have translated into a burgeoning population of nonvalvular AF in India. While there are no prospective incidence data, several registries suggest a high burden of co-morbidity and worse clinical outcomes of AF in the Indian population as compared to developed nations. This can be explained to some extent by low awareness and inadequate treatment of AF. Improving detection rates, reinforcing comprehensive cardiovascular prevention strategies and improving low quality anticoagulation is the need of the hour. Finally, institution of dedicated centers for integrated and comprehensive management of AF is the way forward for prevention of AF related morbidity and mortality.

ONLINE REFERENCES

Please scan the QR code provided at the end of the table of contents for References of this chapter.

CHAPTER

202

Premature Ventricular Contraction Localization

Sanjeev Kathuria, Ankit Bansal, Rahul Nijhawan

ABSTRACT

The manuscript focuses on idiopathic ventricular arrhythmias (VAs) in structurally normal hearts, typically seen in younger patients. These arrhythmias often originate from the right or left ventricular outflow tract and can be effectively managed through catheter ablation (CA). The study reviews various electrocardiogram (ECG) algorithms used to predict the site of origin for these arrhythmias, aiding treatment decisions. Specifically, the document evaluates ECG-based methods for differentiating arrhythmias from the outflow tract and other parts of the heart, enhancing the accuracy of ablation strategies. It emphasizes the importance of precise localization using ECG to optimize clinical outcomes.

Keywords: Idiopathic arrhythmias, ventricular tachycardia, outflow tract, catheter ablation, ECG localization

INTRODUCTION

Idiopathic ventricular arrhythmias (VAs) occur in patients with structurally normal hearts.[1] The spectrum of clinical presentation includes isolated premature ventricular contractions (PVCs), repetitive nonsustained or sustained ventricular tachycardia (VT), and PVC-triggered ventricular fibrillation.[2] The majority originate from the outflow tract of the right ventricle (RV) and left ventricle (LV), but they may arise from anywhere in the heart.[3] It typically presents in young patients—and has a notably increasing incidence[4] It is classically a benign, focal arrhythmia, but patients can be highly symptomatic and refractory to medical therapy.[5] Idiopathic VAs can be effectively treated with catheter ablation.[6] Before CA, it is imperative to have an appreciation of the outflow tract ventricular arrhythmia (OTVA) origin. The surface 12-lead electrocardiogram (ECG) is useful to localize the site of origin of VAs when catheter ablation (CA) is being considered.

The anatomical relationship is complex and is important to understand for localizing the site of origin of PVC. Firstly, the aortic valve has a central location at the base of the heart with relationship to all other heart valves and cardiac chambers. Second, the right ventricular outflow tract is anterior and to the left of the LVOT. Third, the proximal coronary arteries and the distal coronary veins have a close and complex anatomic relationship with the outflow tracts and semilunar valves. This has led to the creation of a number of algorithms to refine the predictive accuracy of ECG localization including the development of new ECG configurations. We review various ECG algorithms to assess their applicability in different types of idiopathic VA.[7]

GENERAL CONSIDERATIONS

Electrocardiogram features for PVC localization include:

- *Bundle branch block pattern*: PVCs with a right bundle branch block (RBBB) pattern originate in the LV, while those with a left bundle branch block (LBBB) may arise in the RV or the interventricular septum.
- *QRS duration*: Septal PVCs have a narrower QRS than PVCs from the free wall of both ventricles.
- *QRS axis (vertical and horizontal dimensions)*: An inferior axis (positive leads II and III) suggests an origin in the outflow tract or the superior aspect of the atrioventricular valves (tricuspid or mitral), while a superior axis (negative leads II and III) is observed in PVCs from the inferior aspect of both ventricles. A right axis (positive lead I) indicates an origin rightward from midline, and a left axis (negative lead I) suggests an origin leftward from the midline.
- *Precordial transition*: In PVCs with a RBBB pattern, the transition becomes later as the site of origin moves from

the apex to the base of the heart. In PVCs with a LBBB pattern, the transition becomes later as the site of origin moves from the septum to the RV free wall.

- Since the Purkinje network is located only in the subendocardium, ventricular activation from the epicardial origin requires more time to reach the Purkinje network, resulting in a delayed onset and duration of the QRS during epicardial PVCs.
- When the ventricular activation propagates from an epicardial origin on the LV free wall or ventricular posterior wall, the total activation vector should go from a lateral toward medial or from an inferior toward superior direction, resulting in a QS pattern in lead I or lead aVF.[8] Therefore, a QS pattern in lead I or aVF suggests an epicardial origin in the LV free wall[8,9] or the ventricular posterior wall, respectively.

All these ECG algorithms are more accurate in patients with structurally normal hearts than without structural heart disease as the ventricular activation propagates away from the PVC origins through healthy ventricular myocardium in a predictable manner.

ENRIQUEZ ET AL'S ANATOMIC APPROACH ALGORITHM (FIG. 1)[1]

Step 1: Localize site in vertical plane, i.e., in uppermost part lies the outflow tract and superior part of atrioventricular valves, mid-cavitary structures in the middle, and inferior LV structures in lowermost part. For this purpose, one has to look for axis in the inferior leads. Inferior-axis VAs (positive QRS complex in leads II and III) arise from basal areas of the heart, including the outflow tracts and the superior aspect of the atrioventricular valves, while superior-axis VAs (negative QRS complex in leads II and III) have their origin at the inferior aspect of both ventricles inferior lead discordance portends to mid-cavitary structures or lateral part of atrioventricular valves.

Step 2: Localize site in the horizontal plane, i.e., whether it lies to the right or left of midline of chest. It does not necessarily means RV or LV structure, especially in outflow tract, where complex anatomy causes significant overlap between right ventricular outflow tract (RVOT) and left ventricular outflow tract (LVOT). For outflow tract sites, look at lead I. Rightward structures, such as the posterior aspect of the RVOT, RCC, para-Hisian region, and superior aspect of the tricuspid valve (TV), are positive in lead I, while leftward structures, such as the anterior aspect of the RVOT, LCC, AMC, anterolateral MV annulus, and LV summit, will produce a negative complex in lead I.

For VAs originating in the inferior part of LV, look at lead V_1 (or bundle branch block pattern). VAs with LBBB appearance may arise from RV structures [inferior aspect of the TV or moderator band (MB)] or the cardiac crux. Conversely, VAs with RBBB pattern arise from LV structures [inferior aspect of the MV, posteromedial papillary muscle (PPM), or left posterior fascicle].

Step 3: So, in steps 1 and 2, we have divided heart into four quadrants, and now we apply a more refined localization relies in other characteristics such as precordial transition, QRS width, or QRS morphology in specific leads.

POSTERIOR ECG LEAD LOCALIZATION APPROACH[10]

F Zhang et al. utilized standard V_5 and V_6 leads as posterior leads V_8 (placed at inferior tip of left scapula) and V_9 (placed just left of the spine at same level), respectively.[10] The anteroposterior relationship between the right and left outflow tract was explored by this method. The V_4/V_8 ratio >3 had 88% sensitivity for diagnosing left-sided outflow PVC. When analyzing cases with borderline V_3 transition, the V_4/V_8 index (i.e.,V_4/V_8 in PVC/V_4/V_8 in sinus) value > 2.28 had 100% specificity and positive predictive value.

SPECIFIC PVC SITE OF ORIGIN AND THEIR ECG CHARACTERISTICS

Outflow Tract PVC

Approximately 70% of idiopathic VAs referred for CA originate in the RVOT and LVOT. Although the RVOT has traditionally been the most common site of origin, accounting for 80% of outflow tract PVCs in early series, the proportion of LVOT PVCs undergoing ablation has progressively increased over time, overcoming those from the RVOT in some recent series.[11] The ECGs of idiopathic

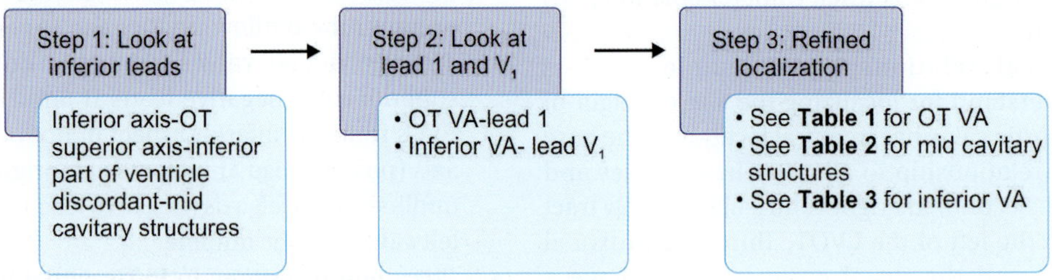

FIG. 1: A stepwise anatomic approach to PVC localization.

TABLE 1: Specific ECG features for PVC localization in outflow tract.

Site	Key morphological features
RVOT	
Free wall	Late transition, inferior notching
PSC (RC)	Taller R wave in lead I, smaller aVL/aVR ratio
PSC (LC)	Negative lead I, taller R-wave amplitude inferiorly
Posteroseptal	Positive lead I, aVR more negative than aVL
Para-Hisian	Narrow LBBB, QS IN V_1, voltage lead II > III
LVOT	
RCAS	Early transition and rS in V_1
LCAS/RCAS	QS notch in V_1 and V_3 transition
LCAS	Multiphasic M or W in V_1
Aortomitral continuity	qR in V_1 with positive precordial concordance
LV summit	V_2 pattern break, negative lead I, more negative aVL > aVR
LV septal	Narrow LBBB, QS ratio lead II and III >1
Anterolateral MA	Late phase notching in the inferior leads

TABLE 2: Specific ECG features for PVC localization in mid-cavitary structures.

Mid-cavitary sites	Key morphological features
RV structures	Negative lead 3 with positive lead 2
Lateral tricuspid valve	Rs V_1, V_4–V_5 transition
Moderator band	QS or Rs V_1, V_5–V_6 transition
Para-Hisian	QS in V_1, V_2–V_3 transition, narrow QRS
LV structures	Negative lead 2 with positive lead 3
Lateral mitral valve	R/S V_6 > 1, R
Anterior papillary muscle	R/S in V_6 < 1

TABLE 3: Specific ECG features for PVC localization in inferior ventricular structures.

Inferior ventricular sites	Key morphological features
RV structures	LBBB
Tricuspid valve septum	Early transition ≤ V_3
Crux	Early transition, QS in inferior leads, pseudo delta wave
Tricuspid valve free wall	Late transition
Moderator band	Late transition
LV structures	RBBB
Inferior mitral valve	R/S V_6>1, R or Rsr′ in V_1
Posterior papillary muscle	R/S in V_6 < 1, R, RSr′ or Qr in V_1
Left posterior fascicle	rsR′ in V_1, narrow QRS

outflow tract PVCs are characterized by positive R waves in all inferior leads and deep S waves in both leads aVR and aVL (almost a QS pattern). An RBBB QRS morphology clearly suggests a VA origin on the left side. However, when PVCs present an LBBB QRS morphology, it is often difficult to differentiate RVOT PVCs from LVOT PVCs. Because anatomically, the LVOT is located posterior to the RVOT, LVOT PVCs exhibit taller and wider R waves in leads V_1 and V_2 than RVOT PVCs. Therefore, the precordial transition is helpful for differentiating RVOT PVCs from LVOT PVCs. When the precordial transition is at lead V_4 or later, the PVCs are very likely to originate from the RVOT, and when the precordial transition is at lead V_2 or earlier, the PVCs are very likely to originate from the LVOT. However, when the precordial transition is in lead V_3, it is most difficult to differentiate RVOT PVCs from LVOT PVCs.[12]

RVOT and Pulmonary Artery

The RVOT is divided into rightward (referred to as free wall), anterior, leftward, and posterior (referred to as septal) parts.[7] Electrocardiographically, PVCs from the RVOT are characterized by an LBBB pattern with transition at V_3 or later: V_3 or V_4 for posterior (septal) sites and V^4 or V_5 for anterior (free wall) sites. PVCs from the RVOT free wall also have a wider QRS duration and more often exhibit notching in the inferior leads. PVCs from the pulmonary artery are characterized by larger R-wave amplitude on inferior leads and greater aVL/aVR ratio due to the more leftward location of the pulmonary artery.[1,7,13]

Figure 2 shows an ECG of RVOT PVC in a 59-year-old male, driver by occupation who presented to us with chest pain and palpitations. His 24-hour holter showed PVC burden of 30%. He was taken up for electrophysiology study and radiofrequency ablation and was successfully ablated in RVOT free wall.

LV Ostium

The LV ostium includes the aortic sinuses of Valsalva, the subaortic LV endocardium, mitral annulus, and LV summit. With exception of PVCs from the right coronary cusp (RCC), right-left commissure, and the septal aspect of the LV summit, most LV ostial PVCs are characterized by an RBBB pattern with positive precordial concordance, with some distinct ECG features pointing to certain particular structures.[1,13] For example, a multiphasic QRS complex in V_1 can be seen in PVCs from the left coronary cusp (LCC), a qR pattern in V_1 is characteristic of the AMC and PVCs from the anterolateral mitral annulus usually have a monomorphic R-wave in V_1 **(Table 4)**.[13]

This is an ECG of an elderly diabetic male with CKD stage 4 and mild LV dysfunction had come to us with intermittent palpitation. His 24-hour holter study revealed high PVC burden. His PVC was ablated from left coronary aortic sinus in LVOT **(Figs. 3 and 4)**.

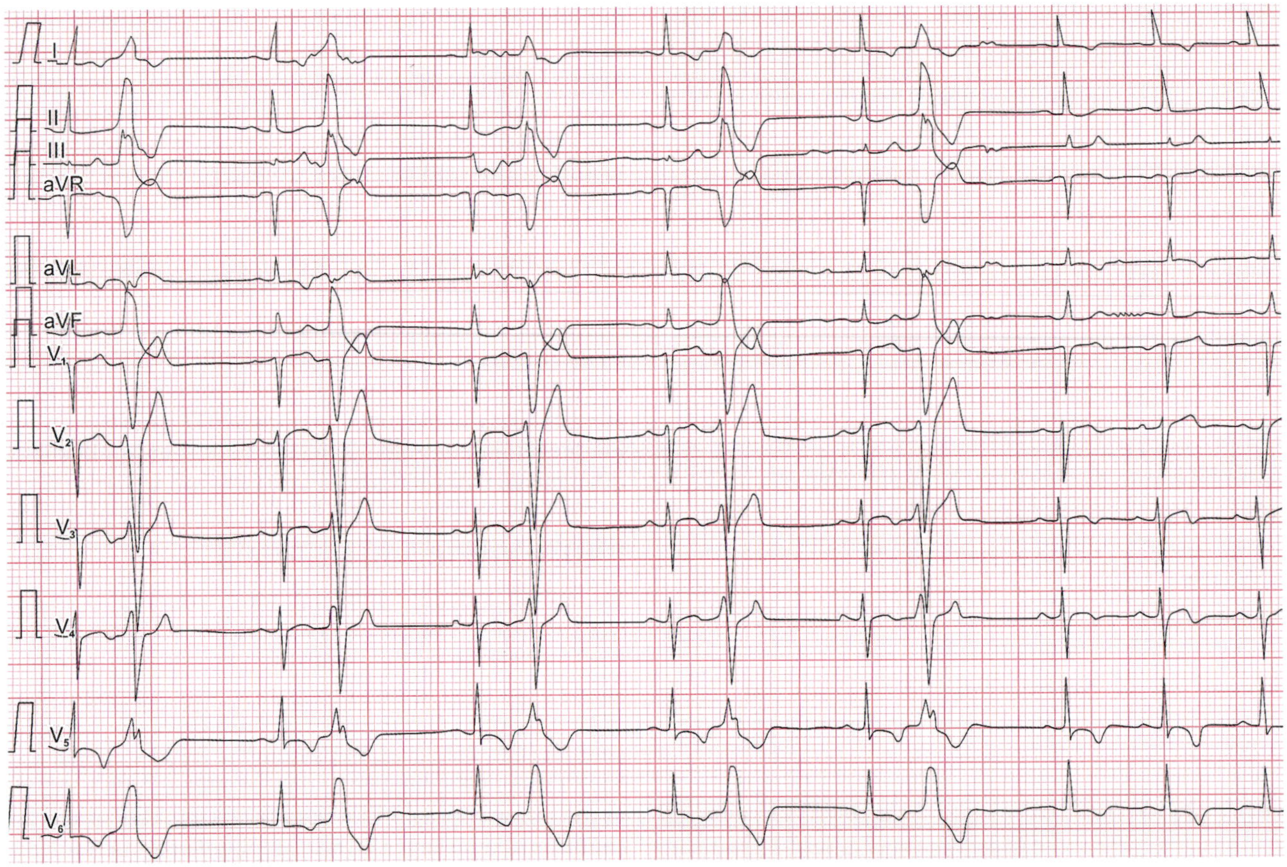

FIG. 2: ECG shows a PVC originating from RVOT.

TABLE 4: Numerous ECG prediction algorithms for differentiating sites of OT PVC.[13]

Site	ECG criteria	
Septal vs. free wall RVOT	PVC QRS duration/QRS duration of the preceding sinus beat	If > 1.9, it suggests free wall RVOT origin
RVOT vs. LVOT	Earliest onset or first peak/nadir in V_2	RVOT
	R-wave duration index (RWDI) and R/S amplitude	If RWDI < 0.5 and R/S wave amplitude < 0.3, it suggests RVOT
	V_3 R-wave deflection interval and V_1 R-wave amplitude	If V_3 R-wave deflection interval is > 80 ms and V_1 R-wave amplitude > 0.3, predicts LVOT origin
	V_2 transition ratio	Value > 0.6, predicts LVOT origin
	TZ index	Value < 0 predicts LVOT origin
	V_2S/V_3R index	Value ≤ 1.5, predicts LVOT origin
	V_4/V_8 index	Value > 2.28, predicts LVOT origin
	V_3R/V_7 index	Value ≥ 0.85, predicts LVOT origin

LV Summit Origin

Currently, only one article has described the differences in the ECG characteristics among PVCs originating from the LV summit, and intramural and endocardial LVOT. First, the maximal amplitude of the R wave in the inferior leads is the highest in the inaccessible area PVCs, second in the GCV PVCs, and lowest in the accessible area PVCs. Second, an RBBB pattern always occurs in the accessible area PVCs and is dominant in the GCV PVCs but rare in the inaccessible area PVCs. Third, a very early precordial transition of the PVCs (earlier than in lead V_1) is dominant in the accessible area PVCs and GCV PVCs, whereas it never occurs in

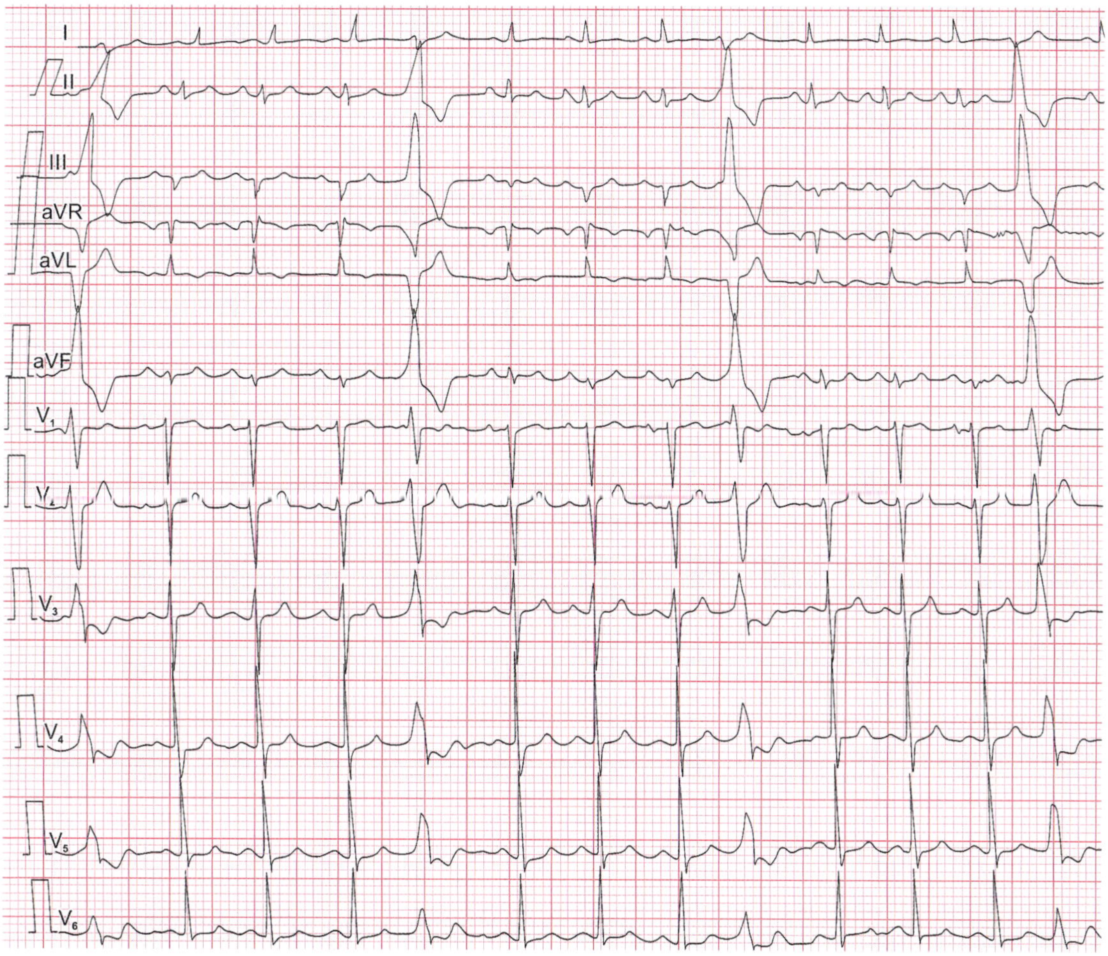

FIG. 3: ECG shows a PVC originating from LVOT.

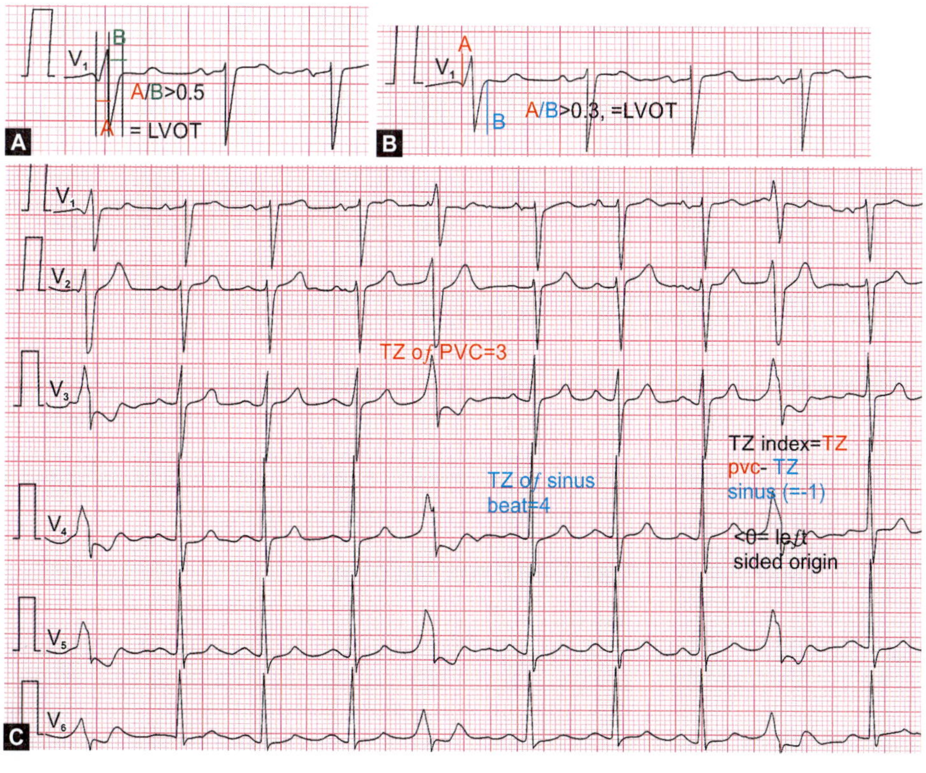

FIGS. 4A TO C: *Continued*

Continued

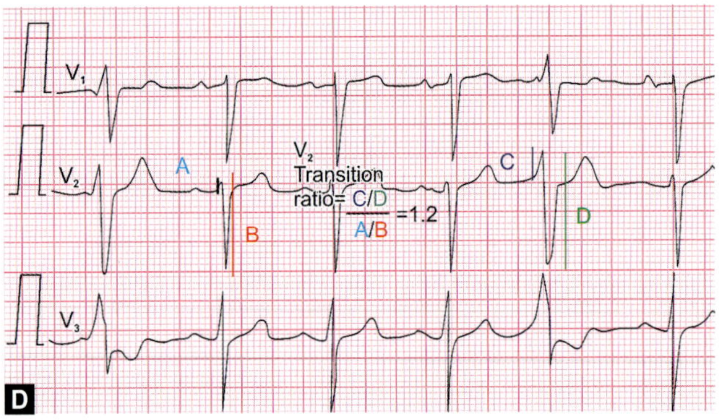

FIGS. 4A TO D: Various ECG prediction algorithms which favor LVOT origin of PVC. (A) R-wave duration index > 0.5, is suggestive of LVOT origin. (B) R/S Amplitude Index > 0.3, is suggestive of LVOT origin. (C) Transition zone index < 0, is suggestive of left-sided origin. (D) V_2 transition ratio ≥ 0.6, is suggestive of LVOT origin.

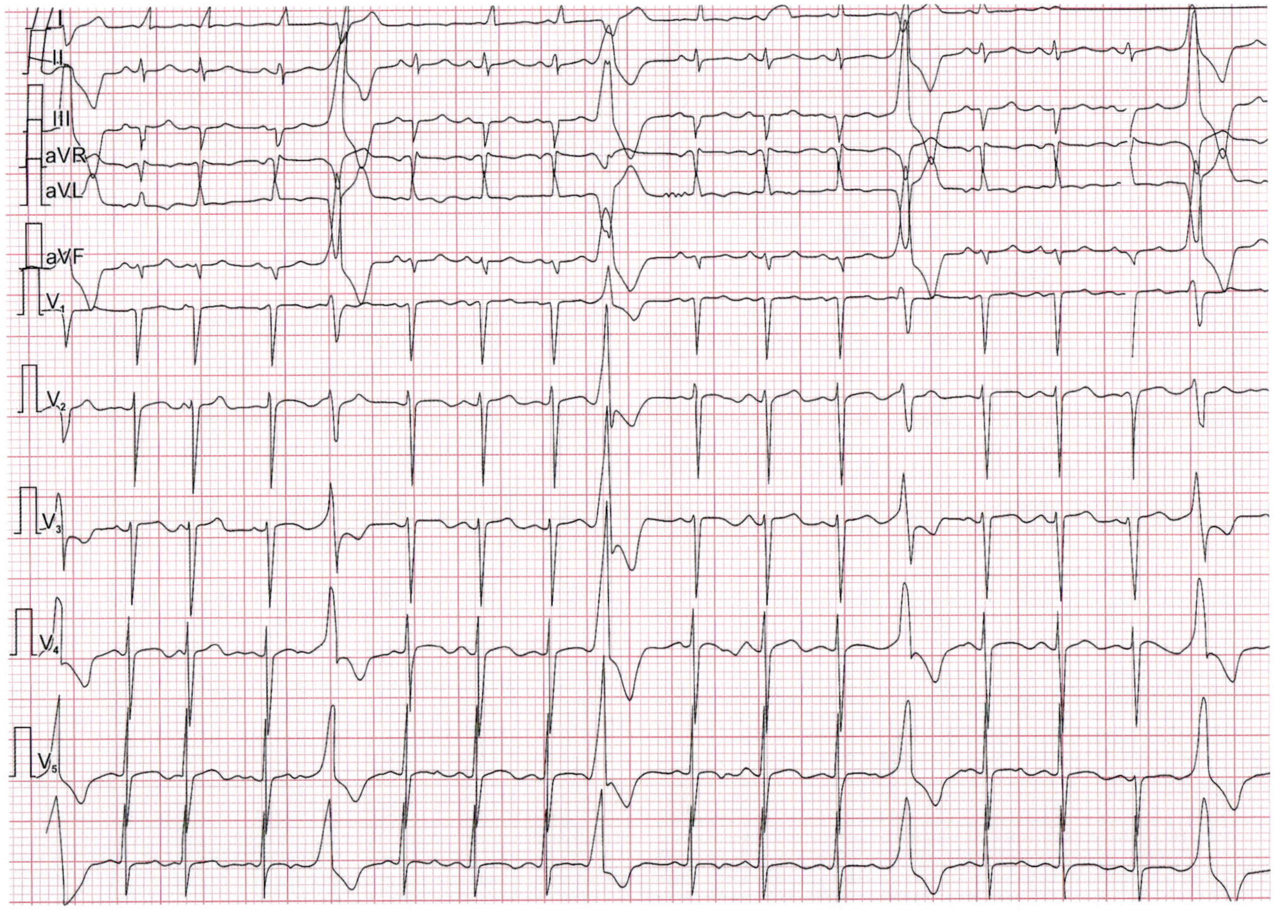

FIG. 5: An ECG with wide QRS, pseudo-delta wave and a deep S wave in lead 1, suggesting a possible origin from LV summit.

the inaccessible area PVCs. Fourth, the QRS duration is significantly longer in the accessible area PVCs and GCV PVCs than in the inaccessible area PVCs. Fifth, the III/II R-wave and aVL/aVR S-wave amplitude ratios are significantly higher in the accessible area PVCs than in the GCV PVCs and inaccessible area PVCs. When PVCs are considered to originate from the LV summit, an RBBB pattern, transition zone earlier than lead V_1, aVL/aVR ratio >1.1, and presence of S waves in lead V_6 suggest with a high accuracy that PVCs should originate from a GCV site and the accessible area.[13,14]

This is an ECG of a 45-year-old male; presented to us with chronic dyspnea. His 24-hour holter study revealed high PVC burden and his echocardiography showed the presence of LV dysfunction with EF-35%. He was taken up for RFA and ablation done in LV summit region **(Fig. 5)**.

Cardiac Crux Origins

The crux of the heart refers to the epicardial region near the junction of the AV sulcus and the posterior interventricular groove, but the term apical crux has been also used to describe the epicardium surrounding the more apical aspect of the interventricular groove. Basal crux PVCs have an LBBB pattern with left superior axis, early transition (lead V_2), and a QS pattern in inferior leads, usually with maximum deflection index > 0.55.

Premature ventricular contractions from the apical crux have also a superior axis and QS in inferior leads but usually exhibit an RBBB pattern and a deep S wave in V_6.[15] These ECG characteristics are similar to those associated with maximally pre-excited posteroseptal accessory pathways, because the latter insert into the same area of the LV as the origins of crux PVCs. The activation from the crux epicardially propagates to the ventricular apex first where it enters the Purkinje network in the endocardium. Thereafter, it propagates rapidly throughout the ventricle, resulting in a major negative deflection of the QRS in lead V_6. The MDI is always greater than 0.55.[1,13,15]

This is an ECG of a young patient presented with this basal crux VT **(Fig. 6)**.

Para-Hisian Region

The term para-Hisian PVC is used to describe PVCs that exhibit earliest activation in close proximity to a His electrogram (within 10 mm). The ECG shows an LBBB pattern, typically with V_2 to V_3 transition and R wave in I and aVL (vs. negative aVL in the RVOT), narrow QRS duration, and lead II more positive than III, which can even be negative (inferior lead discordance).[16]

This is an ECG of elderly male, who presented with palpitations and ECG revealed the presence of para-Hisian PVC **(Fig. 7)**.

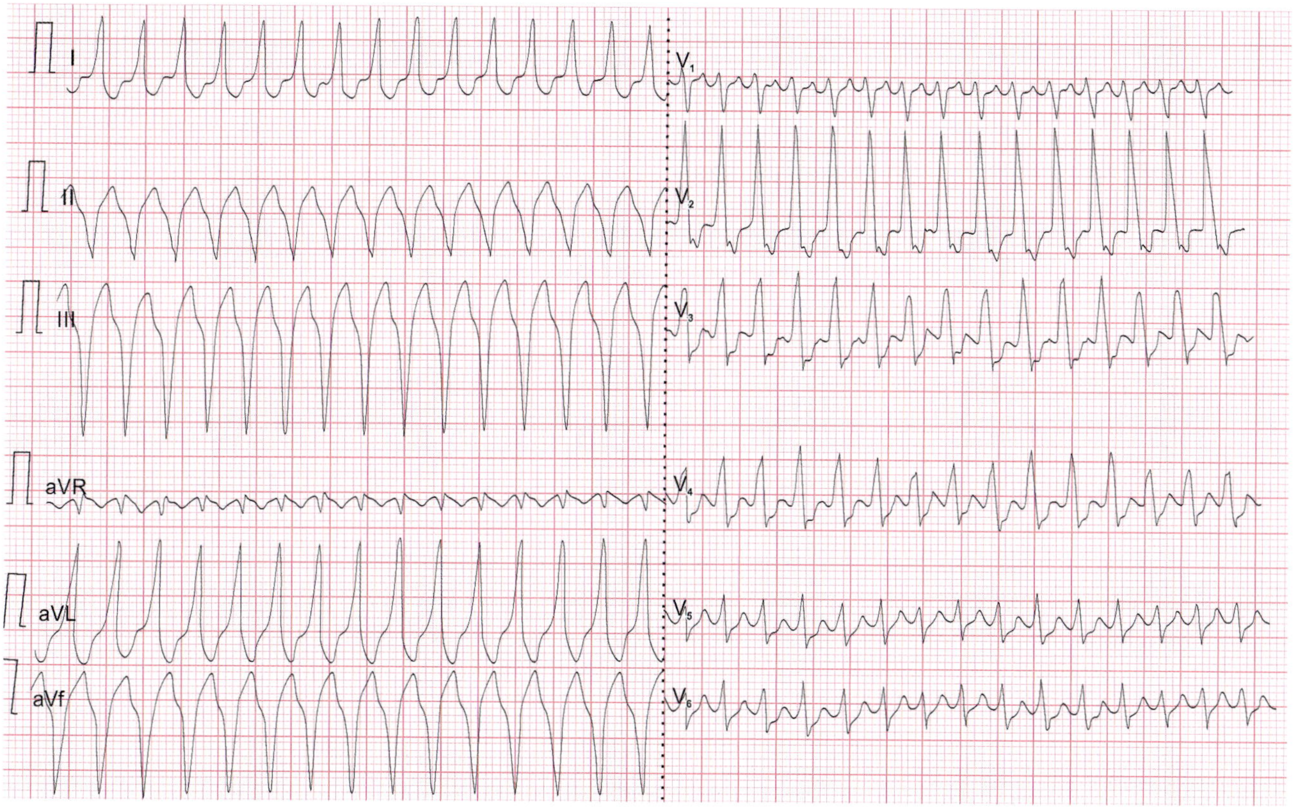

FIG. 6: An ECG with crux origin ventricular tachycardia.

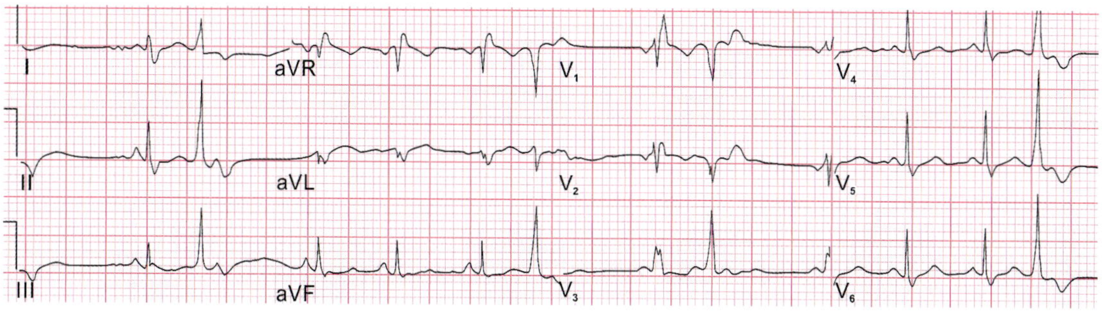

FIG. 7: A narrow QRS PVC with aVR, aVL discordance, and transition in V_3, suggesting para-Hisian origin.

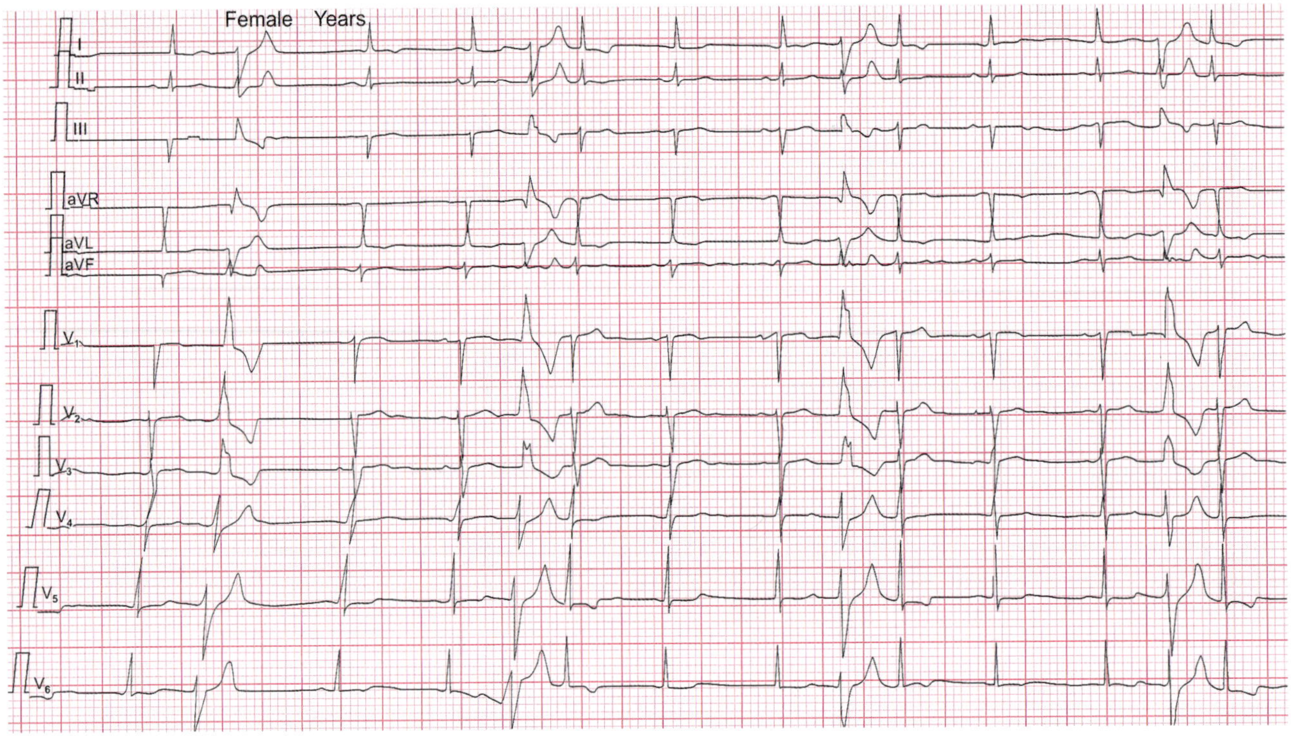

FIG. 8: An ECG with RBBB morphology PVC with precordial transition in V_4, suggesting originating from anterolateral papillary muscle.

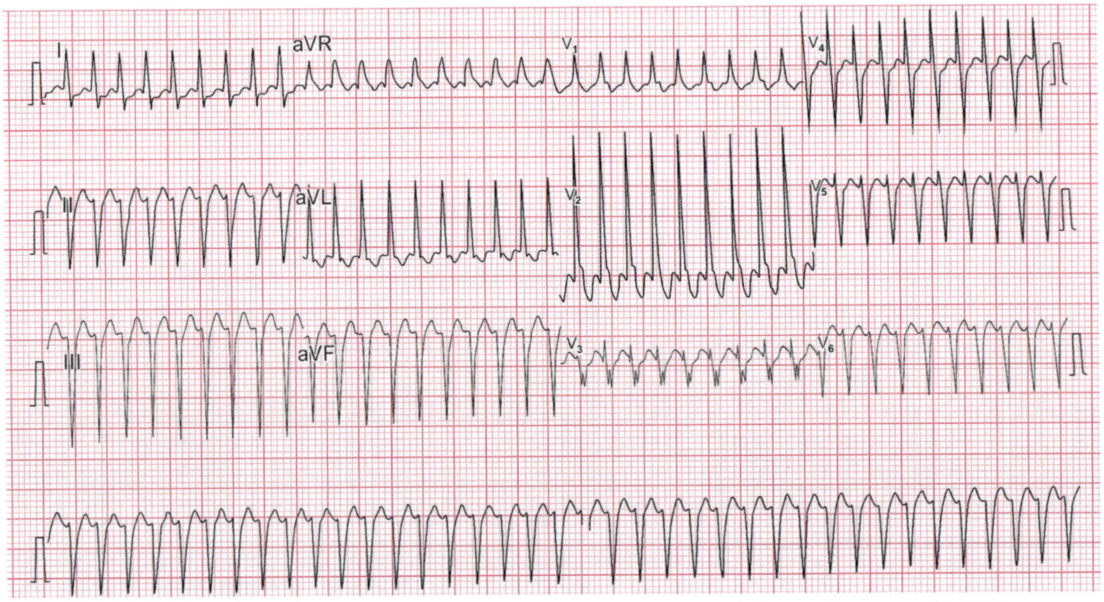

FIG. 9: An ECG with narrow QRS, typical RBBB morphology in V_1, suggesting fascicular ventricular tachycardia.

Papillary Muscle Origin

The posteromedial and anterolateral papillary muscles of the LV are a source of PVCs in both structurally normal and abnormal hearts. PVCs from the posteromedial papillary muscle exhibit an RBBB morphology, left or right superior axis, and precordial transition usually between leads V_3 and V_5.[17] Those from the anterolateral papillary muscle demonstrate an RBBB morphology, right inferior axis, transition between leads V_3 and V_5, and sometimes inferior lead discordance, with negative QRS polarity in lead II and positive QRS polarity in lead III.[17,18]

The ECG here shows frequent PVCs originating from anterolateral papillary muscle **(Fig. 8)**.

LV Purkinje System

Premature ventricular contractions from the LV Purkinje system represent about 4% of idiopathic PVCs and are the most common triggers for idiopathic VF in different series. Unlike LV fascicular VT, which is a re-entrant arrhythmia, the mechanism of fascicular PVCs is believed to be abnormal automaticity or triggered activity. The ECG is characteristic, showing a relatively narrow QRS duration (<130 ms), rsR′ pattern in V_1 resembling a typical RBBB and an initial Q wave in lead I. Those originating from the left posterior fascicle have a left superior axis and those from the left anterior fascicle have a right inferior axis.[18,19]

This is an ECG of a young patient presenting with left posterior fascicular tachycardia **(Fig. 9)**.

CONCLUSION

Ablation outcomes can be improved if the OTVA origin can be predetermined before CA. Differentiating LVOT and RVOT VA can be predicted with a variable accuracy using the ECG algorithms before CA. A combined model using the TZ index and V2S/V3R is the most accurate, but its clinical utility may be limited. Promising novel techniques altering the ECG configuration have been developed and can also be used to predict OTVA with high accuracy.

ONLINE REFERENCES

Please scan the QR code provided at the end of the table of contents for References of this chapter.

CHAPTER

203

Management of Refractory Ventricular Tachycardia

Satya Sahitya Mandava, Parag Barwad

ABSTRACT

Ventricular tachycardia (VT) is characterized by three or more ventricular premature complexes with a rate of over 100 beats/min. Refractory VT, also known as "VT storm" or "electrical storm," can occur after AICD therapy, with episodes following another within 5 minutes.

Keywords: Ventricular tachycardia, refractory, AICD, therapy, episodes

INTRODUCTION

Ventricular tachycardia (VT) is defined as ventricular premature complexes, three or more in number, with a rate of >100 beats/min. Three or more episodes of such sustained VT in 24 hours requiring treatment are defined as refractory VT. This situation is also called "VT storm" or "electrical storm." Other situations which are considered synonymous with refractory VT in the literature are as follows:

- VT, which fails to terminate after appropriate AICD therapy
- VT, in which one episode follows another within 5 minutes
- VT, which is ongoing and slower than the AICD programmed termination rate

EPIDEMIOLOGY OF VENTRICULAR TACHYCARDIA

Although the exact incidence of refractory VT cannot be determined, it remains the predominant cause of SCD and constitutes about a quarter of all deaths in the world. Most of the time, the VT burden is calculated from the ICD interrogation data; hence, there needs to be a consistent methodology to estimate the burden of VT. However, the association between the burden of VT and its relation to SCD has been established convincingly by various previous observational and interventional studies.

A study evaluating the association of cardiac arrhythmias and SCD in intensive care settings showed VT constituted 25% of all arrhythmias. Among 1,067 patients with VT, 29% had ischemic heart disease, and about 40% had no structural heart disease.[1] Of all patients hospitalized with acute myocardial infarction (AMI), 5–10% may have ventricular fibrillation (VF) or sustained VT before hospital presentation, and another 5% will have VF or sustained VT after hospital arrival, most within 48 hours of admission.[2] Among nonischemic heart disease, a plethora of conditions is known to present with VTs. These are:

- *Degenerative disease*: Dilated cardiomyopathy (DCM) and arrhythmogenic right ventricular cardiomyopathy (ARVC)
- *Inflammatory disease*: Acute myocarditis, chronic myocarditis, and cardiac sarcoidosis
- *Hypertrophic disease*: Hypertrophic cardiomyopathy (HCM) and cardiac amyloidosis
- Congestive heart disease
- Post-surgery (tetralogy of Fallot, postvalvular surgeries)
- Mitral valve prolapse
- Neuromuscular disease (myotonic dystrophy)

Ventricular tachycardia secondary to nonacute coronary syndrome (non-ACS) conditions are usually monomorphic, but poly- and pleomorphic VT are also well described in them. VTs occurring in structurally normal hearts may be monomorphic (idiopathic VT) or polymorphic (cardiac channelopathy, medication-induced long QT syndrome

(LQTS), Brugada syndrome, catecholaminergic VT). Many times, ES or refractory VT is precipitated by acute myocardial ischemia, electrolyte disturbances (e.g., hypokalemia, hyperkalemia, and hypomagnesemia), worsening heart failure (HF), sepsis, and poor compliance with antiarrhythmic medications. It often presents as a medical emergency. It may present with recurrent ICD therapies, recurrent syncope in patients without ICD, or with dizziness, chest pain, and features of HF and is associated with increased mortality. A meta-analysis showed a 2.5- to 3-fold increase in mortality after a VT storm.[3]

This chapter will discuss the sequential management of refractory VT with relevance to their etiologies in the ICU/CCU/emergency room setting. The initial hemodynamic stabilization should be followed by a multimodality approach, which may include pharmacological treatment, device programming, neuraxial modulation, deep sedation, and catheter ablation (CA). **Flowchart 1** shows managing of the VT storm.

ELECTRICAL CARDIOVERSION

Electrical cardioversion is the first line of therapy in the case of VTs, which are hemodynamically unstable and the second line after antiarrhythmic drugs in the case of VT, which are relatively hemodynamically stable. In the case of VT with no hemodynamic compromise, the DC cardioversion is synchronized to the R wave. It needs to be performed asynchronously when the VT is polymorphic, and there is significant hemodynamic compromise. DC cardioversion is usually performed with 150–200 J in biphasic defibrillators, and sedation with a short-acting agent should preferably be given before energy delivery in a conscious patient. Antiarrhythmic drugs such as amiodarone should be considered if VT is not terminating with two or three DC cardioversions. Lidocaine may also be used if amiodarone is not available.[5] For shock-refractory VT/VF, there are two other defibrillation strategies other than the standard approach, where the defibrillation pads are placed one along the sternum and the other at the back. These two strategies are double sequential external defibrillation (DSED; rapid sequential shocks from two defibrillators) and vector change (VC) defibrillation (switching defibrillation pads to an anteroposterior position). The DOSE VF study compared DSED and VC with a standard defibrillation approach in out-of-hospital cardiac arrest patients in a RCT. In this study, survival to hospital discharge was more common in DSED and VC than compared to the standard strategy.[6]

Patients with implanted ICD with VT storm present with recurrent ICD shocks. These recurrent shocks are associated with increased mortality and morbidity. Also, they are associated with anxiety, depression, and PTSD. When encountering such a situation, one must immediately do a device interrogation to determine if the therapies delivered

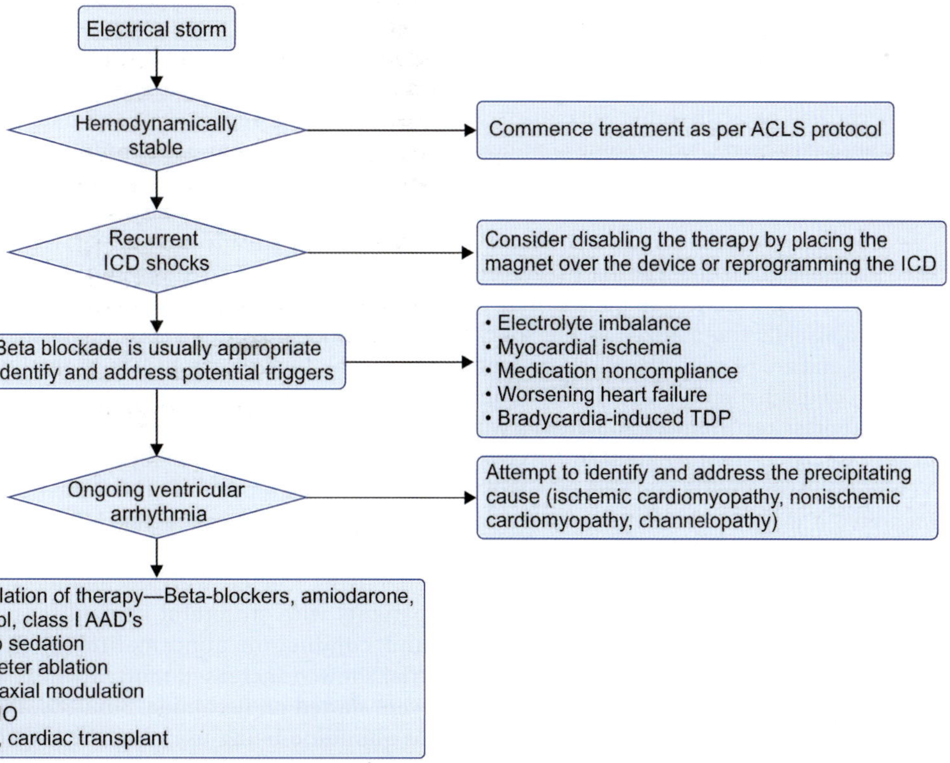

FLOWCHART 1: Management of refractory VT.[4]

were for appropriate indication. In case of incessant VT, the ICD can be turned off by placing a magnet over it or by turning off ICD detection. In the meantime, the patient can be evaluated for reversible causes and considered for sedation. An attempt at terminating the VT with measures such as ATP, pharmacological cardioversion, or else neuromodulation techniques can be tried.

PHARMACOLOGICAL MANAGEMENT

Amiodarone

Amiodarone was initially introduced as an antianginal medication, but its antiarrhythmic properties were soon recognized. It is now a first-line agent broadly used for VT due to various underlying etiologies. The loading dose of amiodarone is 5 mg/kg, followed by an infusion rate of 1 mg/min for the first 6 hours and 0.5 mg/min for the next 8 hours. Amiodarone is a useful drug even in the early postinfarction period and in the presence of HF and hypotension, as it has very little negative ionotropic support. It has been seen to be useful in other causes of VT, such as acute and chronic myocarditis and scar-related VT. The effectiveness of amiodarone has been shown in multiple studies. In a study of 273 patients with incessant VT refractory to intravenous (IV) lidocaine, procainamide, and bretylium, there was a 40% response rate to IV amiodarone.[7] In another multicentric study of 412 ICD patients randomized to beta-blocker (BB), BB plus amiodarone, and sotalol for 1 year, amiodarone plus BB significantly reduced the risk of shock compared with BB alone and sotalol.[8] Sotalol also showed a trend toward a decrease in recurrent episodes. Amiodarone can be used as first-line therapy, but it should be used under the supervision of cardiac or arrhythmia specialists as sometimes the VT cause may be related to some channelopathies where the prolonged QT interval may get exacerbated by the effect of amiodarone and can lead to refractory VT or VF.

Beta-blockers have a significant role in VT storms. VT storm is a hyperadrenergic state. The patient may be physically and psychologically traumatized as the shocks come without warning and are painful. The VT storm tends to exacerbate because of this hyperadrenergic effect. Thus, BBs can effectively suppress recurrent VF in patients with recent MI, with an associated improvement in survival.[9] The ACC 2017 Ventricular Arrhythmias and Sudden Cardiac Death guidelines give a class IIa recommendation for BBs in patients presenting with VF secondary to ischemia and in incessant VTs resistant to repeated shocks and antiarrhythmic medications.

Regarding the choice of BB, nonspecific agents such as propranolol are preferred over metoprolol. The clinical superiority of propranolol can be explained by the downregulation of the B1 receptor and upregulation of the B2 receptor in the setting of HF. In a study by Chatzidou et al., 60 ICD patients presenting with VT storm were randomized to receive propranolol versus metoprolol and an amiodarone infusion for 48 hours. Patients under propranolol therapy, compared to metoprolol-treated individuals, presented 2.67 times decreased incidence of ventricular arrhythmic events (tachycardia or fibrillation) and 2.34 times decreased rate of ICD discharges. Time to arrhythmia termination and length of hospital stay were significantly shorter in the propranolol group.[10] Meta-analysis of studies using beta-blockade for the management of cardiac arrest caused by refractory VF or pulseless VT showed its use may lead to increased rates of return of spontaneous circulation, survival to discharge, and survival with a favorable neurologic outcome. The agents used were esmolol, propranolol, and left stellate ganglion block (SGB).[11]

Amiodarone is more effective than lidocaine in terminating incessant VT with improved survival at 24 hours.[12] In this study comparing the two medications, VT termination was achieved in 78% of the patients with amiodarone compared to 27% of the patients with lidocaine. Lidocaine is effective in terminating VAs associated with myocardial ischemia but less effective in terminating ventricular arrhythmia (VA) associated with healed myocardial infarction (MI). For patients with recurrent, stable VT not in the setting of an AMI, IV procainamide is superior to lidocaine for terminating the arrhythmia. Procainamide successfully terminated VT in 79% of the cases in this study.[13] The PROCAMIO was a multicenter, prospective, randomized study that compares the safety and efficacy of IV procainamide and amiodarone in the acute treatment of wide QRS complex monomorphic tachycardias (presumably VT), which are hemodynamically well tolerated. Occurrence of major adverse cardiac events was more common in the amiodarone group, and VT termination was higher in the procainamide group. Similar findings were seen in patients with structural heart disease.[14] The potassium-blocking properties of procainamide may prolong the QT interval. In patients with already prolonged QT, it may lead to torsades de pointes (Tdp) and thus should be used with caution. The ACC 2017 Ventricular Arrhythmias and Sudden Cardiac Death guidelines give a class IIa indication for amiodarone and sotalol for recurrent VTs in nonischemic cardiomyopathy (NICM) and a class I indication for recurrent VTs in ischemic cardiomyopathy (ICM) despite optimal ICD programming and BB therapy.

There are reports of other antiarrhythmic medications also being used for refractory VT. In a study of 94 patients with VT storm refractory to multiple AADs, 72% were effectively treated with flecainide. This study included patients with structural heart disease, low baseline EF, and conduction abnormalities.[15] However, the CAST trial showed increased mortality in post-MI patients who were started on flecainide. Similarly, there is a case report of quinidine being useful in the case of VT refractory to multiple AADs.[16]

Magnesium is also important in terminating VT by suppressing early and late after-depolarization and automaticity. It is particularly effective in marked hypokalemia-induced VT and medication-induced Tdp.

Ranolazine

Ranolazine is an antianginal drug approved for use in chronic stable angina. It has an antiarrhythmic effect on the ventricles and atria. The principal mechanism in ventricles is the inhibition of the late INa channels, and in atria, it is via use-dependent inhibition of peak INa and IKr. It can suppress arrhythmias associated with ischemia, ACS, reperfusion, HF, and prolonged QT. It can suppress atrial tachycardias and atrial fibrillation. In animal studies, ranolazine has suppressed drug-induced Tdp and Tdp in experimental models of LQTS. It caused a marked increase in the threshold for induction of repetitive ventricular extrasystole and VF without increasing the defibrillation threshold. In the experimental ischemia-reperfusion model, it caused a reduction in ventricular premature beats, VT, and VF. In comparison to the vast experimental data, clinical studies are limited. In a study of 12 patients with refractory ICD shocks despite antiarrhythmic drugs, ranolazine caused a reduction in VT and ICD shocks in 11 patients.[17] In the MERLIN-TIMI 36 trial, 6,560 patients hospitalized with a non-ST-elevation ACS were randomized to ranolazine or placebo in addition to standard therapy, and 1 week ECG recording was done. Ranolazine caused a reduction in the incidence of VT lasting ≥8 beats (5.3% in ranolazine vs. 8.3% in the placebo group, $p < 0.001$).[18] In the RAID trial, 1,012 high-risk ICD patients were randomly recruited for ranolazine versus placebo. It showed that treatment with ranolazine did not significantly reduce the incidence of the first VT or VF or death.[19] In a multivariate analysis of the RAID trial, ranolazine was noted to be effective in reducing VT burden in CRT-treated patients, those without AF, and those not on concomitant AADs. In patients already on AADs or those with AF, adding ranolazine did not affect VT burden.[20]

In LQTS type 3, ranolazine, mexiletine, and flecainide shorten the QTc and have been used to reduce recurrent arrhythmias. Similarly, in cases of CPVT with recurrent sustained VTs, adding flecainide, propafenone, and verapamil is effective. Quinidine and isoproterenol infusion can be used in case of recurrent sustained VTs in Brugada syndrome and short QT syndrome.

In patients already on AADs and having VT storm, proarrhythmic because of AADs and their interactions should be considered.

SEDATION

Endotracheal intubation and deep sedation have shown promising results in terminating refractory VT. Rapid sequence induction is used for intubation, followed by IV infusion of midazolam or propofol and opioids to maintain deep sedation. It serves to tide over the VT storm period before definitive treatments such as CA, sympathectomy, medical treatment, revascularization, etc. Caution must be taken in administering sedative drugs that have a myocardial depressant action in patients with significantly impaired LV function. In a study of 15 patients with VT storm (due to ischemia, cardiomyopathy, primary arrhythmia, and postvalve surgery), complete resolution of VT/VF was seen within minutes of administering deep sedation in 12 (80%) patients and partial resolution in 2 (13%) patients. One patient who required repeated deep sedation developed cecal necrosis.[21] In another retrospective study by Martins et al., 116 patients with VT storm were given deep sedation after nonresponse to multiple AADs. Acute response was seen in 47.5%. Pulmonary edema before deep sedation was seen as a predictor for nonresponse.[22]

CATHETER ABLATION

Catheter ablation has a significant role in patients with VT storms and has the most extensive data supporting its role. CA should be considered when initial pharmacotherapy fails. CA is beneficial in ICM and is less likely to achieve total success in NICM due to patchy areas of scarring, which may require epicardial ablation and endocardial ablation. Clinical guidelines give class I indication for CA in cases of ICM and class IIa indication for NICM.[23] CA has better outcomes in patients with monomorphic VT than with polymorphic VT. In patients with previous MI and an ICD who had arrhythmia while on AAD, it was seen that patients who received CA had lesser recurrence of VT and mortality compared to patients who received an escalation of AADs.[24] CA is efficacious in both acute and long-term suppression of VT storms. In a study of 50 patients who underwent CA for VT storm, it was suppressed in 84%. This study included patients with coronary artery disease, idiopathic cardiomyopathy, ARVC, and combined etiology.[25] Acute complete success was achieved in 61% of NICM patients with recurrent monomorphic VT. During a median follow-up of 23 months, 61% of the patients had no recurrence of VT. Among those who initially failed endocardial ablation, epicardial ablation was successful in 87% of the patients.[26] In a long-term follow-up study of 267 patients with ICM and NICM who underwent CA for VT storm, at 60 months follow-up, 48% NICM, and 54% ICM had VT-free survival.[27] CA can be effective in recurrent VT in postoperative conditions, PVCs-induced VF, and Brugada syndrome.[28-31]

AUTONOMIC NEUROMODULATION

The autonomic nervous system has a vital role in triggering arrhythmia. There is evidence suggesting the clustering of events with stressful situations despite the apparent stability of the myocardial substrate.[32] Thus, BB therapy and sedation have been recommended as the mainstay of therapy for a long time. However, when initial therapies are ineffective, more invasive neuromodulation has been seen to be effective.

Thoracic epidural anesthesia can be provided in acute settings as a bedside procedure. TEA provides complete sympathetic blockade by blocking segments C8-T4. They block the fibers proximal to both left and right SG and may be more efficient than LSGB. Its immediate onset of action can interrupt the vicious circle of recurrent shocks that lead to the elevation of catecholamine levels that potentiate further arrhythmias. The efficacy of TEA in refractory VA in humans has been documented in a few case series. The single largest case series, including 11 patients, showed a partial or complete response in >50% of the patients after TEA.[33] Bourke et al. reported a case series of modulation of neuroaxis in which eight patients had undergone TEA. Out of eight patients, six patients had >80% reduction in VT.[34]

Percutaneous SGB can be performed at the bedside under fluoroscopy or ultrasound guidance. The local anesthetic is injected into the region of the stellate ganglion. It provides sympathetic blockade for a more extended period (3–4 days) compared to pharmacotherapy. A systematic review of 35 published cases showed a significant (mean 16.5% vs. 23.1 events post-SGB; $p = 0.0002$) reduction of VA episodes and the need for defibrillation. It is efficacious irrespective of the etiology (ischemic vs. nonischemic), morphology (monomorphic vs. polymorphic), and LV dysfunction (preserved vs. decreased EF).[35] In a study comparing sympathetic blockade versus AAD in post-MI VT storm patients, 1-week mortality was lower in the additional sympathetic blockade group versus AAD group (22% vs. 82%; $p < 0.0001$).[9] In a systematic review of 38 cases by Meng et al. with SGB, there was a decrease in VA burden and the number of defibrillator shocks (10 ± 9.10 shocks/day vs. 0.05 ± 0.22 shocks/day; $p < 0.01$) and 80% survival to discharge.[36] In 2020, Fudim et al. reported bilateral SGB in 20 patients with refractory arrhythmia who had failed CA, sedation, AADs, and mechanical circulatory support. There was a drastic decrease in the number of VA episodes 24 hours before and after SGB (median 5.5 vs. 0) and the number of defibrillations.[37]

It has been observed that abnormal cardiac sympathetic afferent neurotransmission is associated with increased renal nerve activity and norepinephrine release. This norepinephrine spillover may contribute to autonomic dysregulation that leads to initiation and maintenance of VT. Thus, renal denervation was thought to have a role in managing VT. The largest multicentric case series reported by Ukena et al. consisted of 13 patients with CHF and VAs refractory to AADs and CA. 85% of the patients were free from VA at the end of 3 months.[38] In a second study, which included 10 patients with refractory VT, the mean episodes of VT/VF, ICD shocks, or ATPs were reduced to zero at the end of 6 months.[39] Bradfield et al. studied renal denervation as an adjunct to cardiac sympathetic denervation (CSD) in patients with VT refractory to CA. It was performed as a staged procedure and showed a significant decrease in all ICD therapies (shocks and ATPs) at the end of 6 months.[40] Renal nerve denervation, though looks promising, needs further study before being put to routine use.

Surgical CSD involves surgical resection of the stellate ganglion's lower half and the second through fourth thoracic ganglia. CSD has long been established as a treatment modality in CPVT and LQTS. In 147 LQTS patients undergoing LCSD for primary and secondary prevention, there was a significant decrease in the cardiac events (<91% post-LCSD; $p < 0.001$), and ICD shocks decreased by 95% ($p = 0.02$).[41] Similarly, among 63 CPVT patients undergoing LCSD for primary and secondary prevention, the cumulative event-free survival at 2 years was 81%. The primary cardiac events decreased from 100 to 32% ($p < 0.001$), and in those with ICD, the ICD shocks decreased by 93% ($p < 0.001$).[42] In a study by Vaseghi et al., 120 patients who underwent left or bilateral CSD were studied for a mean period of 1.5 years. At 1 year, 58% of patients were free of ICD shocks or sustained VT and freedom from ICD shocks, sustained VT, death, and orthotopic heart transplant was 50%. CSD reduced the number of ICD shocks by 88%. No differences were noted in terms of outcomes between ICM and NICM patients. Those patients who had undergone bilateral CSD had longer ICD shock-free, transplant-free survival compared to patients who underwent a left-only procedure ($p = 0.014$). At the end of the follow-up, 32% of the patients had come off AADs and received BBs for cardiomyopathy.[43] Another cohort of 65 patients that included patients with both ischemic and nonischemic heart disease who underwent CSD were followed up for a mean duration of 27 months. A complete response to CSD, as defined by >75% freedom from ICD or external defibrillation events, was achieved in 72.3% of patients. Freedom from the combined end point of death or ICD shocks was 51% at the end of 2 years.[44]

There has been one systematic review on cardiac sympathetic denervation in structural heart disease. It included 13 studies with 173 patients having cardiomyopathy due to ischemic and nonischemic (HCM, valvular, viral, and ARVC) causes. Patients undergoing both left or bilateral sympathectomy were included. Different case series showed freedom from events ranging between 58 and 100%. 1 year of event-free survival ranged between 58 and 63%.[45]

EXTRACORPOREAL MEMBRANE OXYGENATION

Extracorporeal membrane oxygenation (ECMO) acts as a bridge to more definitive therapies such as ablation and transplant. It improves myocardial perfusion and decreases LVEDP, thus helping restore and maintain sinus rhythm. In a study of 26 patients with intractable arrhythmias refractory to multiple AADs and causing cardiogenic shock who underwent VA-ECMO, stable sinus rhythm was restored in 61% after a median time of 3 hours. 13 patients (50%) died of multiorgan failure, and the remaining 50% could be discharged. Patients with alternating VT/VF episodes with sinus rhythm at the time of implantation had better survival than those with persistent VF.[46] In another study of 83 patients with treatment-refractory electrical storm, 45% were successfully weaned off, and 15% underwent successful CA while on ECMO.[47] Beyond hemodynamic support, ECMO decreases myocardial oxygen consumption, enables rapid weaning off ionopressors, and enables adequate levels of antiarrhythmic drugs.

CONCLUSION

Refractory VT is a life-threatening condition that increases short-term and long-term mortality and also has a significant effect on morbidity. It requires a prompt multimodal approach and one must always look for any correctable factors for the VT. While pharmacological ablation and CA have been the mainstay of treatment, new, emerging strategies such as deep sedation, neuromodulation, and hemodynamic support have shown promising results. All these therapies are complementary to each other and thus should be utilized for the best patient outcome.

ONLINE REFERENCES

Please scan the QR code provided at the end of the table of contents for References of this chapter.

CHAPTER 204

Novel Nonradiofrequency Ablation Modalities in the Management of Cardiac Arrhythmias: An Update

Oruganti Sai Satish, Purushotham Reddy Ramireddy Gari

ABSTRACT

Radiofrequency ablation (RFA) has been the most successful and most used modality of ablation for various arrhythmias. But, it has its own drawbacks creating a need for alternative ablation modalities. Much research has been going on in the field of ablation using alternative sources of power for ablation including cryoablation, photoablation, and electroporation. These new non-RFA ablation modalities have been able to overcome the drawbacks of RFA and are proven to be equally effective.

Keywords: RF, cryoablation, photoablation, electroporation, PFA, acoustic ablation, ethanol ablation, autonomic neuromodulation

INTRODUCTION

Radiofrequency catheter ablation (RFA) is the preferred modality for ablation of various arrhythmias to date. But, there is an unmet need for newer modalities that can target functionally critical and conventionally inaccessible areas with reliable effectiveness. The field of ablation is growing beyond well-established RF technology with several alternative energy sources and delivery modes proposed, some of which are proven to be safe and effective with minimal associated risks and rapid recovery times.

CHALLENGES WITH RADIOFREQUENCY ABLATION

The efficacy relies on precise catheter positioning, adequate catheter-tissue contact, and the energy levels applied. Collateral damage is frequent, which can lead to cardiac tamponade, thromboembolism, pulmonary vein (PV) stenosis, phrenic nerve and esophageal injury, and mitral valve trauma.[1] "Steam up" can result from overheating the target site with RF energy and can lead to myocardial perforation.[1,2] Coronary blood flow during the RFA procedure can cause a heat sink effect preventing uniform tissue heating or lesion formation. At times, RF can damage coronaries by causing intimal hyperplasia, shrinkage of collagen fibers, and coagulation.[2,3]

CURRENT ABLATION MODALITIES

Multiple ablation modalities are available using different energy sources and delivery modes. They can be classified into thermal, nonthermal energy sources, and nonenergy-dependent modalities such as chemical ablation and denervation **(Table 1)**.

TABLE 1: Different types of ablation modalities for cardiac arrhythmias.

Energy source-based ablation				
Thermal energy	**Nonthermal energy**	**Mixed**	**Chemical ablation**	**Other**
Radiofrequency ablation (RFA)	Electroporation (pulse field ablation)	Acoustic (ultrasound) mechanical + thermal	Ethanol	Autonomic neuromodulation
Cryoablation				
Photoablation (laser)				

CRYOABLATION

Biophysics

Cryoablation is based on the "Joule–Thomson effect," which states that if a gas is compressed at high pressure and then expands suddenly at low pressure, it expands utilizing the heat energy, thereby decreasing the temperature.[2] In cryoablation catheters, liquid nitrous oxide is delivered under constant pressure from console to tip where the balloon acts as an expansion chamber, where the liquefied nitrous oxide expands, absorbing heat from surrounding tissue, and cools the surface. This results in tissue freezing and ice formation. Extracellular ice formation occurs at temperatures of 0 to –20°C, leading to hypertonicity and osmotic gradient leading to cell shrinkage. The effects are reversible, if rewarming is achieved within 30–60 seconds. If not, it leads to cell death. Rapid cooling of tissue surface to below –40°C leads to both intra- and extracellular freezing. Intracellular freezing leads to irreversible organelle damage and cell death. The disruption of membranous organelles is enhanced by cellular thawing. So, repeated freeze–thaw cycles can extend the cellular injury.

Clinical Advantages of Cryoablation

Reversible lesions can be created with slow cryoablation (over 240 seconds) at –30°C, which can help in cryomapping, where functional assessment of efficacy and safety of ablation site can be done before permanent ablation.[2,4] This advantage is of importance while ablating close to critical structures such as atrioventricular (AV) node or His bundle. Cryo lesions are less thrombogenic compared to RFA. Cryoablation results in well-demarcated lesions and does not cause collagen denaturation or contracture like RFA and is less likely to cause coronary stenosis or perforation.[5] The cryoadherence effect (attachment of catheter tip to target tissues by formed ice) helps in the formation of very focal lesion and avoids catheter instability during sudden changes in heart rate during ablation. The hypothermic effect desensitizes the nerves, so the procedure is pain-free.

Clinical Applications

Atrioventricular Nodal Reentrant Tachycardia

Although RFA has a high success rate and low risk, in unselected atrioventricular nodal reentrant tachycardia (AVNRT) cases, cryoablation of slow pathway is especially useful in patients with difficult anatomy, failed prior RFA, in children, and in patients who cannot even tolerate the small risk of AV node blockade.[6]

Accessory Pathways

Ablation of accessory pathways (APs) in anteroseptal and paraseptal areas are at high risk of permanent AV block when done with RFA, where cryoablation is highly safe and successful. Cryoablation can also be done in specific cases of epicardial left-sided APs within the coronary sinus (CS), safely. Limited steerability, maneuverability, and catheter stiffness are its disadvantages.[7]

Atrial Fibrillation: Pulmonary Vein Isolation

By using a cryoablation balloon which evenly distributes the cryoenergy, PV isolation can be done safely and effectively with results comparable to RFA. Cryoenergy is expected to be safer and the incidence of PV stenosis and thromboembolic events is expected to be reduced compared to RFA.[8] Phrenic nerve injury is more common with first generation (13%) and second generation cryoballoons (3%) compared to RFA.[9]

Recently, the POLARx (Boston Scientific) cryoballoon was approved for clinical use, which has greater compliance and operates at a lower ablation pressure. It can increase the balloon diameter, useful in PVs with larger diameters.[10]

The ultra-low temperature cryoablation (ULTC, Adagio medical) system employs a single diagnostic and therapeutic flexible linear catheter, which can achieve multiple configurations by preformed stylets facilitating pulmonary venous isolation as well as linear bi-atrial ablation lesions. The ULTC system maintains and circulates liquid nitrogen at its near-critical phase within a closed-loop system, achieving ultra-low temperatures (–185°C) and creating a rapid and deeper myocardial lesion.[10,11]

Ventricular Tachycardia

Cryoablation can be used in epicardial ablation of ventricular tachycardia (VT). The cryoadhesion effect along with deep lesion formation gives an advantage in targeting papillary muscle and moderator band VTs.[12]

PHOTOABLATION (LASER ENERGY)

Biophysics

Laser produces a narrow frequency range beam at a specific wavelength, which can be directed for specific duration and intensity, and as it penetrates the tissue, energy is absorbed and scattered. Tissue injury is created by the thermal effect. Lesion size depends on the extent of light diffusion and heat transport. Three laser systems are used: Argon laser (wavelength 500 nm), neodymium:yttrium aluminum garnet (Nd:YAG wavelength 1,060–2,000 nm), and diode laser (700–1,500 nm).[2]

Clinical Applications

Pulmonary Vein Isolation

The most recent generation of laser ablation balloon is a nonsteerable, compliant balloon (HeartLight, CardiFocus, Marlborough, MA, USA). The balloon is filled with contrast and deuterium oxide (D_2O) for cooling effect and is positioned at PV antrum and monitored through imaging for monitoring intrusion of blood into space between the balloon and tissue. Lesions are deployed in a point-by-point manner in a circumferential, contiguous, and overlapping manner around PV.[2] In paroxysmal atrial fibrillation (AF), laser appears to be as safe and effective as RFA. Recently visually guided laser balloon ablation has been developed, which uses titrable laser energy for PV isolation. First-generation VGLB has shown good isolation rates and long-term freedom from AF was 78.8% for paroxysmal AF and 65.3% for persistent AF.[13,14]

Ventricular Tachycardia

Laser can give unidirectional emission without producing tissue edema, avoids collateral damage, and the lesion depth can be titrated with wavelength. These properties make it useful in ablation of VTs near critical structures like para-Hisian area, coronaries, and phrenic nerve.[15] Laser ablation can achieve transmurality at a given thickness in a safe and efficient way. So, subepicardial surfaces can be targeted from endocardium alone (e.g., postcardiac surgery with inaccessible pericardial space). Lastly, as there will not be any tissue edema produced during laser ablation, the durability of the lesion is more predictable. Other energy sources may produce reversible injury mimicking acute success but conduction may recover over time.[12]

ACOUSTIC ABLATION (ULTRASOUND ENERGY)

Biophysics

Acoustic waves can generate thermal and mechanical effects. The amount of energy transmitted depends on the intensity of the wave and absorption coefficient of tissue. Ultrasound ablation does not require tissue contact, in contrast to RFA. Ultrasound energy decreases inversely with radius, where RF electrical conduction decreases proportional to the square of the distance ($1/r^2$). Because of this feature, ultrasound energy can create deeper and transmural lesions.[2]

Clinical Applications

Pulmonary Vein Isolation

A novel noncontact system for PV isolation has been developed—the low-intensity collimated ultrasound system (LICU; VytronUS, Inc, Sunnyvale, CA, USA) which combines automated three-dimensional high-resolution, ultrasound-guided anatomic mapping, and robotic ablation. It creates transmural lesions around PVs. A recent human trial (VALUE trial) has shown it to be effective and safe but needed touch-up RFA in 5.8–22.7% of cases. Freedom from AF recurrence was 79.6–92.3%.[16]

Ventricular Tachycardia

The surface and coronary sparing effects of acoustic ablation make it an interesting option for VT ablation at sites otherwise at risk of coronary injury or covered by thick epicardial fat (e.g., LV summit). Attempts are going on to utilize acoustic ablation to minimize periprocedural morbidity and risk of complications of VT ablation while ablating VT source.[12]

ELECTROPORATION (PULSE FIELD ABLATION)

Biophysics

Electroporation is a form of low-energy DC catheter ablation. Electroporation can be reversible or irreversible. Reversible electroporation (RE) is used for temporary pore formation on cell membranes for drug delivery. Irreversible electroporation (IRE) causes permanent damage and cell death used in ablation. The extent and targeting can be controlled by parameters such as pulse amplitude, frequency, pulse shape, number of pulses, and duration.[1,17] Stankevic et al. reported that pulse shape is a major factor for determining electropermeabilization, and asymmetric waveforms have significantly lower IRE thresholds compared to equivalent symmetrical waveforms in vitro studies.[18]

Nanosecond pulsed electric fields (nsPEFs) have been shown to improve the controllability of pore size, limit solute movement, overall reducing the osmotic imbalance, and improving cell targeting with PEF exposure. ns-PEFs can induce a uniform activation of the myocardium by forming a consistent electric field distribution.[1,19]

Advantages of Pulse Field Ablation

Recently, different types of catheters for pulse field ablation (PFA) have been developed **(Figs. 1A to D)**. In first human trials IMPULSE and PEFCAT, using the FARAPULSE endocardial ablation system, the tissue-specific nature of PFA was shown. There were no reports of esophageal or phrenic nerve injury **(Fig. 2)**. They also showed that the incidence of PV stenosis was virtually eliminated. IRE procedures require significantly less time, energy, and number of applications of energy in comparison to RF or cryoablation.[20]

Safety

Irreversible electroporation has some specific risks of electrolysis when untuned current is passed through body fluids, instigating gas formation. These gaseous microemboli could result in myocardial infarction (MI) or cerebral ischemic events. There can be an overall decrease in the resting cell membrane potential of the myocardium leading to ST- and T-wave changes on ECG. Some cases of lethal and nonlethal arrhythmias were found in animal studies.[21]

Thus, its use requires meticulous monitoring of blood pressure, ECG, and electrolytes. It has been concluded that an application of IRE-PEFs directly to cardiac tissue both endo- and epicardially in preclinical and clinical studies is safe when timed with the R-wave during sinus rhythm.[22]

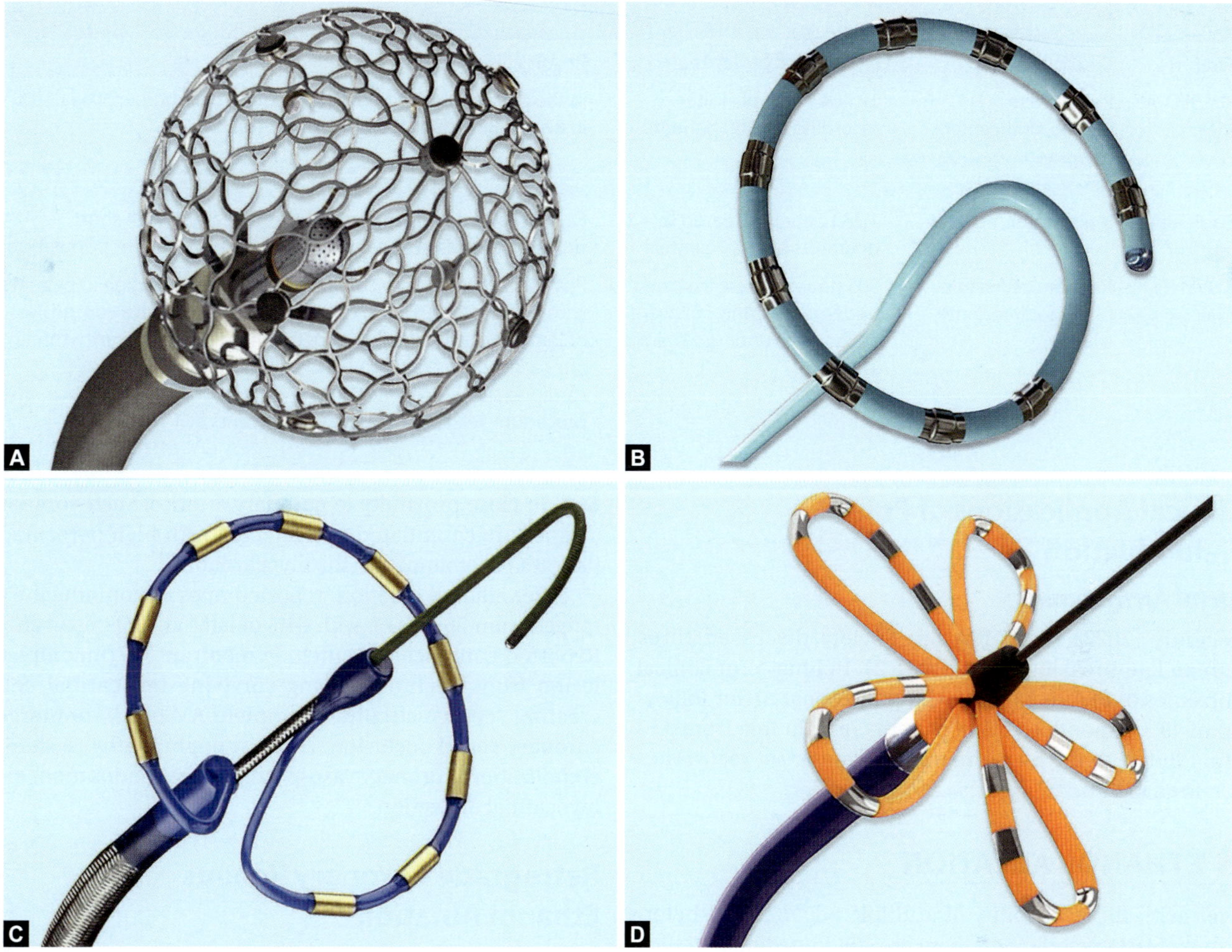

FIGS. 1A TO D: Different pulse field ablation catheters. (A) Sphere-9 (Medtronic), (B) Varipulse (Biosense Webster), (C) PulseSelect (Medtronic), and (D) Farapulse (Boston Scientific).

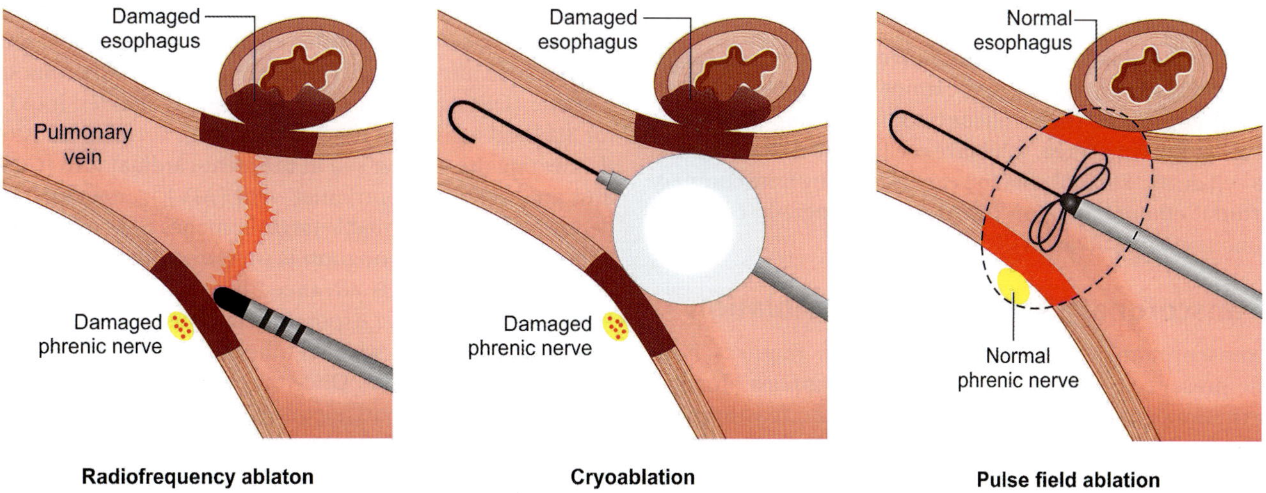

FIG. 2: Chances of phrenic nerve and esophageal damage with RFA and cryoablation, but very less with PFA.

TABLE 2: Recent late-breaking trials in PFA.

Trial	Trial type	Number of patients	Results
PULSED-AF trial[23]	Prospective, global, multicenter, nonrandomized, paired single-arm trial	12,264 hours of Holter recordings in 300 patients	In the paroxysmal and persistent cohorts, AF burden was <10% in 87 and 82% of patients, respectively
EU-PORIA registry[24]	Multicenter registry	1,233 patients treated by 42 operators across 7 centers	Favorable single procedure success rate along with short procedure times in a real-world all-comer AF patient population
ADVENT trial[25]	Randomized single-blind noninferiority trial	305 patients were assigned to undergo PFA, and 302 were assigned to undergo thermal ablation	PFA was noninferior to conventional thermal ablation in patients with paroxysmal AF with respect to freedom from a composite of initial procedural failure, documented atrial tachyarrhythmia after a 3-month blanking period, antiarrhythmic drug use, cardioversion, or repeat ablation and with respect to device- and procedure-related serious adverse events at 1 year

Clinical Applications of Pulse Field Ablation

Atrial Arrhythmias

Recently (2023) Heart Rhythm Society discussed three human late-breaking trials **(Table 2)**. In long-term clinical outcomes of PFA in patients with paroxysmal AF for follow-up of 49 ± 7 months, 73% of patients remain free from AF/atrial flutter at the 5-year mark, and late onset recurrence occurred in 11%.[23-25]

ETHANOL ABLATION

Even with the availability of multiple advanced catheter-based ablation modalities, there are still impediments, such as proximity to coronary vessels, and possible damage to phrenic nerve. This is particularly true for LV summit VTs. It lies underneath the left main coronary artery bifurcation. Catheter ablation is challenging in this region, given the difficulty of accessing this area via transseptal, retroaortic, and epicardial approaches.[26]

Ethanol ablation is an alternative treatment option for intramural arrhythmias that cannot be targeted with the usual approach. High concentration of ethanol, when it reaches the target area, solubilizes cell membranes and leads to cell death. Ethanol ablation can be done by transcoronary arterial ethanol ablation (TCAEA) or retrograde coronary venous ethanol ablation (RCVEA) routes.[27]

Transcoronary Arterial Ethanol Ablation

Transcoronary arterial ethanol ablation requires both the presence of an arterial branch that supplies blood to arrhythmogenic ventricular tissue and the feasibility of selective cannulation of an angioplasty balloon. Intramural mapping over guidewires or small 2Fr linear mapping catheters can identify substrates deep within the myocardial wall, in close proximity to coronary arteries. Such coronary arteries are cannulated and injected with high percentage (96–98%) of ethanol into the myocardium.[27]

After ethanol ablation, reported rates of noninducibility ranged from 56 to 84% with 64% of later any VT recurrence. Reported complications include reentrant VT (incomplete lesion from ethanol, leaving surviving myocardial cells creating reentry circuits), complete AV block, nontarget coronary vessel occlusion, contrast nephropathy, systemic embolization, coronary vasospasm, arterial perforation, and myocardial dissection.[27]

Retrograde Coronary Venous Ethanol Ablation

This approach is advantageous compared to the transarterial route: Ethanol backflow is diluted by retrograde flow into the CS reducing the risk of collateral myocardial damage. Complications related to arterial cannulation, such as vessel dissection and perforation, are avoided.

Initially, the 3D mapping should be done to identify the source of PVC or VT. After identification of endocardial earliest activation site, CS is cannulated, and a multipolar catheter (DECANAV® Biosense Webster) is inserted into CS for 3D local activation time or pace-map correlation. After delineating the earliest site in the great cardinal vein (GCV) and anterior interventricular vein (AIV), venograms are performed to locate suitable target branches close to that site. Balloon occlusion venogram is preferred. Then preloaded angioplasty balloon is advanced over guide wire into CS leaving the tip of wire exposed. This is used as a unipolar electrode connected with an alligator clip to the input of the recording amplifier. Once the signals from the wire in cannulated vein support adequacy, the wire is removed, the balloon inflated, and contrast is injected into the targeted venule to determine the size and extent of myocardial straining.[27,28]

An international registry of long-term efficacy of RCVEA was completed, showing acute success of 98% and 77% had no recurrent arrhythmias on 1-year follow-up with only two venous dissections leading to pericardial effusion.[29]

For adequate response, there should be no collateral vessels back to CS, circumventing the myocardium. Successful ablation is confirmed by an intracardiac echocardiogram showing increased echogenicity and myocardial staining.[30,31]

Advanced Techniques for Ethanol Ablation

One limitation of ethanol ablation is collateral flow and technical challenges cannulating intramural veins in complex venous anatomies. Advanced techniques using multivein multiballoon approach have proven to be of use. Key techniques use multiple balloons to (1) block collateral dissipation of alcohol within a target vein with both balloons inflated in the same vein; (2) occlude a second intramural vein with a second balloon and deliver multivein venous ethanol ablation (VEA); (3) use collaterals to reach a target that is not otherwise accessible via direct intramural vein cannulation; (4) block flow into the CS while delivering VEA antegradely via collateral cannulation; (5) serve as a mechanical block to facilitate intramural vein cannulation; and (6) the use of ethanol's sclerosing effects to reduce distal flow and restrict flow to the target area.

Double Balloon for Distal Protection

For the therapeutic effect of VEA, adequate myocardial reach is necessary, not just venous exposure to ethanol. In cases of large intramural veins (most commonly first septal veins), signals compatible with the site of origin of VA were recorded in a limited portion of the vein, making it necessary to avoid delivering ethanol beyond that portion to avoid unintended damage. After VEA via the proximal balloon, myocardial staining was restricted to the interballoon portion of the vein.[30,31]

Multiple Vein Venous Ethanol Ablation—Cross Fire Approach

When multiple veins drain the tissue targeted by VEA via one vein, ethanol may escape the arrhythmia site of origin and be shunted away toward the CS through a second vein. If the vein-to-vein communication is postcapillary, then ethanol may eliminate such communication by sclerosing the capillaries, in which case, repeated injections serve the purpose of target tissue ablation after the initial injection blocks postcapillary vein-to-vein communication. By targeting the same region with ethanol injection from two different vantage points, ethanol is more efficiently delivered to the tissue without shunting from vein to vein.[30]

AUTONOMOUS NERVOUS SYSTEM MODULATION

Antiadrenergic Neuromodulation

In ischemic heart disease, due to postinfarct remodeling, sympathetic hypersensitivity and nerve sprouting develop. The heterogeneous decrease in action potential duration and increase in spatial dispersion of repolarization following sympathetic activation predisposes to ventricular arrhythmias (VAs). Similarly, sympathetic arousal is also a described trigger for arrhythmias in catecholaminergic polymorphic VT (CPVT), and certain subtypes of long QT syndrome (LQTS). In such patients, cardiac sympathetic denervation has shown to be effective in reducing VT episodes.[12]

Methods of Antiadrenergic Neuromodulation

- Renal sympathetic denervation
- Spinal cord stimulation
- Surgical cardiac sympathetic denervation
- Percutaneous pharmacological stellate ganglion blockade

Vagal Stimulation

In patients with previous MI, vagal tone maintains ventricular electrical stability. Vagal nerve stimulation suppresses ganglionated plexi activity of both adrenergic and cholinergic components and the stellate ganglion activity. A beneficial impact on ventricular remodeling and anti-inflammatory effect may also contribute to arrhythmia suppression.[12]

Modes of Vagal Nerve Stimulation

- *Low-level vagus nerve stimulation*: A small surgical procedure done to a right cervical segment of the vagus nerve with a neurostimulator positioned to stimulate the vagus nerve. Other noninvasive handheld devices for self-administration achieving vagus nerve stimulation via skin have been approved.[32]
- *Auricular branch vagus nerve stimulation*: Transcutaneous stimulation via ear clip attached to tragus in patients with MI showed decreased VA events within 24 hours.[33]
- *Baroreflex activation therapy*: Surgically implanted carotid sinus lead implanted subcutaneously in infraclavicular chest wall pocket activates baroreceptors. Animal infarct model studies have shown reduced incidence of VTs and are successful in heart failure patients for arrhythmia prevention.[34,35]

STEREOTACTIC ABLATIVE RADIOTHERAPY

Stereotactic ablative radiotherapy (SABR) uses a 3D coordinate system by a planning computerized tomography (CT) scan to prevent damage to surrounding tissues. The same principle is applied to deliver a potent ablative energy to critical target areas for VAs, minimizing the risk of collateral damage, in patients too unstable for conventional ablations and patients with electrical storms. Photons are the most commonly used energy for this purpose.[12,36,37]

Even though first in human case reports showed a reduction in VT burden, long-term data showed the risk of VT recurrence, rare but life-threatening complications such as heart failure, gastropericardial fistula, pericardial effusions, and pneumonitis.[38] Several prospective controlled trials are undergoing in SABR to improve safety and long-term efficacy.

CONCLUSION

Novel non-RFA modalities in the management of cardiac arrhythmias are energy-based, chemical-based, and neuromodulation. Cryoablation and PFA are less thrombogenic and lesions can be created without damage to surrounding vital structures, of proven benefit in PV isolation. A novel ultrasound-based ablation system has also been of proven benefit in PV isolation. Ethanol ablation is particularly useful in LV summit VAs. Autonomic neuromodulation has been useful in post-MI arrhythmias and heart failure.

ONLINE REFERENCES

Please scan the QR code provided at the end of the table of contents for References of this chapter.

CHAPTER

205

Approach to a Patient with Syncope

Shivani Rao, Pradyumna Kumar Singh, Karthikeyan R

ABSTRACT

Syncope is a common complaint in the emergency department. It is often described as loss of consciousness for a brief period, with rapid and complete recovery. However, the cause and underlying mechanism may need extensive work-up, and priority should be given to recognizing patients at risk of unfavorable outcomes in busy setups. These patients should undergo expedited evaluation for the underlying mechanism and should receive mechanism-targeted therapy. This chapter focuses on how to approach a patient presenting with syncope and subsequent management.

Keywords: Syncope, vasovagal, arrhythmia, orthostatic intolerance

INTRODUCTION

Syncope is characterized by transient loss of consciousness (TLOC) caused by reduced blood flow to the brain. The condition typically has a sudden onset, is of brief duration and recovery is spontaneous and complete.[1] Additionally, it is often accompanied by a loss of muscle tone. Syncope is classified under the nontraumatic causes of TLOC. TLOC refers to a condition characterized by a genuine or perceived loss of consciousness, which can result from a wide range of underlying causes, each categorized according to its specific pathophysiological mechanisms. Global cerebral hypoperfusion is the underlying characteristic of syncope, and abnormal excessive brain activity is a qualifying criterion for epileptic seizures. The psychological process of conversion marks psychological TLOC. Syncope may be preceded by a short prodrome of dizziness, lightheadedness, faintness, weakness, or fatigue. However, these presyncopal symptoms may not always be present.

MAGNITUDE OF THE PROBLEM

Syncope has a lifetime cumulative incidence of 35% in the general population. Syncope accounts for 1% of hospital admissions and 3% of emergency department visits, with 20% of patients experiencing recurrence within a year.[2] Cardiac syncope is associated with the highest risk of mortality, approaching 50% over 5 years and 30% in the first year after diagnosis.[3] Syncope of noncardiac or unexplained origin in young adults carries an excellent prognosis. The risk of syncope recurrence increases with increasing age, presence of underlying cardiac ailment, and use of multiple drugs. Thus, it is crucial to identify patients at risk of adverse outcomes among nearly all patients who are most likely to have a benign condition.

CLASSIFICATION OF SYNCOPE

Based on the underlying mechanism of cerebral hypoperfusion, syncope has been classified into three groups—(1) reflex syncope, (2) cardiac syncope, and (3) orthostatic hypotension (OH) **(Box 1)**.

DIAGNOSTIC APPROACH

Determining the exact cause of syncope can be challenging. Syncope episodes are typically sporadic and infrequent; thus, it is challenging to examine the patient or obtain an electrocardiogram (ECG) during an episode. Therefore, the main objective in evaluating patients with syncope is to make an initial presumptive diagnosis of the underlying cause.

An effective syncope diagnostic strategy **(Flowchart 1)** involves the following four steps:

1. Distinguishing syncope from other types of TLOC
2. Assess prognosis to determine the risk level.

BOX 1 Classification of syncope.

Reflex (neutrally medicate) syncope:
- *Vasovagal*:
  - Orthostatic
  - Emotional: Triggers can be fear, pain, blood phobia, etc.
- *Situational*:
  - Cough and sneezing
  - Micturition
  - Postexertional
  - Postexercise
  - Other (e.g., laughing, brass instrument playing, and defecation)
- Carotid sinus syndrome

Syncope due to OH:
- *Drug-induced OH (most common cause of OH):*
  - For example, vasodilators, diuretics, and antihypertensives
- *Intravascular volume depletion*: Diarrhea and vomiting
- *Primary autonomic failure (neurogenic OH)*: Pure autonomic failure, neurodegenerative disorder such as MSA, Parkinson's disease, and dementia with Lewy bodies
- *Secondary autonomic failure (neurogenic OH)*:
  - Diabetes (most common), amyloidosis, autoimmune autonomic neuropathy, and paraneoplastic autonomic neuropathy
  - Spinal cord injuries

Cardiac syncope:
- Arrhythmia as primary cause
- *Bradycardia*:
  - Sinus node dysfunction (including bradycardia/tachycardia syndrome)
  - Atrioventricular conduction system disease
- *Tachycardia*:
  - Supraventricular
  - Ventricular
- *Structural cardiac*:
  - Acute aortic dissection
  - Severe pulmonary hypertension
  - Cardiac tamponade
  - Hypertrophic obstructive cardiomyopathy
  - Severe aortic stenosis
  - Congenital heart disease
  - Cardiac masses (atrial myxoma, tumors, etc.)
  - Massive pulmonary thromboembolism, pulmonary hypertension

(MSA: multiple system atrophy; OH: orthostatic hypotension)

3. Differentiating between cardiac and noncardiac causes of syncope and following the relevant diagnostic pathway
4. Recognizing "high-risk" indicates serious underlying health conditions presenting as syncope.

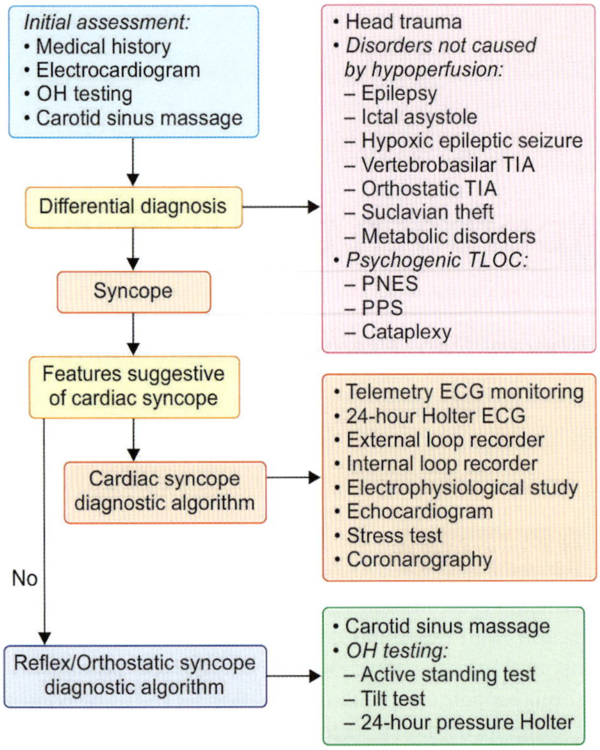

FLOWCHART 1: Diagnostic approach to syncope.

INITIAL EVALUATION

The patient's history and physical examination are crucial for evaluating TLOC and syncope. These components can help identify the cause in >25% of cases.[4]

History

When a patient presents with possible TLOC, history taking usually helps whether the event was actually a TLOC or not. Second, it allows the distinction between the major causes of TLOC. History is usually obtained from the patient and bystanders. The following points need to be evaluated in history **(Table 1)**.

Transient loss of consciousness is characterized by certain specific features—it is brief in duration, involves loss of or abnormal motor control, and is often followed by amnesia for the duration of the episode. History will guide the diagnosis of possible types/etiologies of syncope. These features might be able to discriminate between syncope types and help predict prognosis **(Box 2)**.

Once a patient is diagnosed, he/she should be assessed for high-risk features so that he/she can be advised for admission, further workup, or immediate intervention as deemed necessary. According to the ESC 2018 guidelines, the following are the high-risk features associated with syncope **(Boxes 3 and 4)**.[1]

TABLE 1: Points to be considered while taking history.

Before TLOC	During TLOC	After TLOC
• Age of onset of presumed syncope • Duration of episode • Frequency • *Predisposing factors*: Warm, crowded environment, and prolonged standing • *Precipitating event*: Severe pain, fear, and emotional stress • *Prodrome*: Nausea, vomiting, palpitations, cold, dizziness, blurring of vision, and duration of prodrome	• Eyewitness record • *How was the fall*? Abrupt rodlike suggestive of seizure or cloth-like suggestive of syncope • Any video recording • Lack of response • *Duration of LOC*: ○ 10–30 s syncope ○ >1 minute seizure ○ > 5 minutes probably psychogenic • Skin color during episode pale or cyanosed • Tongue bite and urinary incontinence • Abnormal body movements to be described	• Nausea and vomiting • Having chest pain and sweating • Mental confusion • Trauma • Focal neurological signs
Medical history		
Background: • Preexisting cardiac, metabolic, or neurological conditions • Family history of sudden cardiac death *Drugs*: • Diuretics, vasodilators, antiarrhythmic, antiarrhythmic, and antidepressants *Recurrent TLOC*: • Frequency of TLOC • Interval between previous and current episode		

(TLOC: transient loss of consciousness)

BOX 2 Clinical features that can suggest diagnosis during the initial evaluation.

Reflex syncope:
- Recurrent syncope before the age of 40 years
- After unpleasant sight, sound, smell, or pain
- Standing for long duration
- Being in crowded and/or hot places
- Pallor, sweating, and nausea/vomiting prior to event
- With head rotation or pressure on the carotid sinus (as in tumors, shaving, or wearing tight collars)
- No history of heart disease

Syncope due to OH:
- While or after standing for some time
- Standing after exertion
- Postprandial hypotension
- Recent history of start or change of antihypertensives or diuretics leading to hypotension
- Known case of autonomic neuropathy or parkinsonism

Cardiac syncope:
- Usually during exertion or sometimes during supine
- Abrupt-onset palpitation immediately followed by syncope
- Family history of unexplained SCD at a young age
- Typically, a history of structural heart disease or coronary disease

(SCD: sudden cardiac death)

BOX 3 High-risk features.

High-risk:
- *Major*:
  - Associated with chest discomfort, shortness of breath, abdominal pain, or headache
  - Syncope occurred when the patient was doing any activity (exertion) or when supine
  - Syncope occurs immediately after a palpitation episode
- *Minor (in presence of structural heart disease or coronary artery disease considered high-risk)*:
  - Short (<10 second) prodrome
  - Family history of sudden cardiac death at young age
  - Syncope while in the sitting position

Past medical history:

Low-risk:
- Long history (years) of recurrent syncope with low-risk features with the same characteristics of the current episode
- Absence of structural heart disease

High-risk:
- *Major*:
  - Features of severe cardiac disease, such as heart failure, low ejection fraction, and previous myocardial infarction

A normal ECG was considered low-risk, whereas several ECG changes were considered high-risk **(Table 2)**.

Physical Examination

The physical examination should involve measuring blood pressure and heart rate in the supine, sitting, and standing positions, as well as again 3–5 minutes after standing to assess for any abnormal changes in orthostatic regulation. The two abnormalities that should be sought are:

1. Early OH, defined as a 20-mm Hg drop in systolic or 10-mm Hg drop in diastolic BP within 3 minutes of standing.
2. *POTS*: An increase in heart rate of 30 beats/min or more during standing (or ≥40 beats/min in those 12–19 years of age),and absence of a >20-mm Hg reduction in systolic BP.

Cardiac examination may reveal structural or congenital heart disease.

Carotid Sinus Massage

Carotid sinus massage is the diagnostic maneuver of choice for carotid sinus hypersensitivity (CSH). CSH is an exaggerated reaction to stimulation of the carotid sinus baroreceptors, resulting in significant bradycardia and hypotension. It is of three types:

1. *Cardioinhibitory*: This is the major CSH variant. The predominant manifestation is marked bradycardia in either the sinus, atrioventricular block, or ventricular asystole >3 seconds. It is caused by vagal action at both the sinus and atrioventricular nodes. This response can be inhibited by anticholinergics, e.g., atropine.
2. *Vasodepressor*: It is the least common type with a decrease in vasomotor tone without significant changes in heart rate. This effect is not abolished by atropine.
3. *Mixed type*: This condition presents as bradycardia and hypotension.

Carotid sinus massage is performed with the patient in a supine position with the neck slightly extended. Then, the point of maximal carotid impulse is massaged for 5–10 seconds, and each carotid sinus is massaged consecutively with a gap of 1 minute between each massage. The presence of carotid bruit or TIA/stroke history within 3 months is a contraindication to performing carotid sinus massage. A massage can be considered positive if it receives any of the following three responses:

1. Asystole for more than 3 seconds (cardioinhibitory type).
2. Reduction in systolic blood pressure of >50 mm Hg irrespective of symptoms or >30 mm Hg with symptoms (vasodepressor type).
3. Both responses are observed (mixed type).

BOX 4 Physical examination.

High-risk:
- *Major:*
    - Systolic BP < 90 mm Hg without any predisposing condition
    - Heart rate < 40/min in the awake state in the absence of physical conditioning
    - Systolic murmur was not previously diagnosed
    - Evidence of gastrointestinal bleed

OTHER DIAGNOSTIC TESTS

Basic Autonomic Tests

- *Valsalva maneuver*:
    - The lack of blood pressure overshot and heart rate increase during the Valsalva maneuver are characteristic of autonomic failure or neurogenic OH, which usually occurs in primary or secondary autonomic failure.
    - A significant drop in blood pressure beyond what is typically expected during forced expiration, whereas the heart rate response remains normal, can occur in patients with situational syncope, such as during coughing, singing, or weightlifting.

TABLE 2: High-risk.

Major	Minor (high-risk only if history consistent with arrhythmic syncope)
• ACS • Mobitz's second- and third-degree AV block • AF with HR < 40 bpm (slow AF) • Sustained VT/VF • Nonsustained VT • Typical Brugada pattern • Bundle branch block, intraventricular conduction disturbance, ventricular hypertrophy, or Q waves consistent with ischemic heart disease or cardiomyopathy • Pacemaker or IC dysfunction • Prolonged QT, QTc > 450 ms in 12-lead ECGs indicate LQTS	• Mobitz I second-degree AV block and 1-degree AV block with markedly prolonged PR interval • Preexcitation • Asymptomatic inappropriate mild sinus bradycardia (40–50 bpm) • Paroxysmal SVT or atrial fibrillation • Short QTc interval (<340 ms) • Atypical Brugada patterns • Negative T waves in the right precordial leads and epsilon waves suggestive of ARVC

(ACS: acute coronary syndrome; AF: atrial fibrillation; ARVC: arrhythmogenic right ventricle cardiomyopathy; LQTS: long QT syndrome)

- *Deep breathing*:
  - Normally, in a healthy individual older than 50 years, heart rate variability during deep breathing is ≥15 beats/min, with the heart rate increasing during inspiration and decreasing during expiration.
  - Blunted heart rate variability is a marker of autonomic dysfunction, particularly in the parasympathetic system.
- *24-h ABPM and HBPM*:
  - Both tests are increasingly used for the diagnosis of hypertension.
  - Nocturnal "nondipping" or reverse dipping patterns are associated with autonomic dysfunction.
  - ABPM may also help prove postprandial, exercise-induced, and drug-induced hypotension.
  - ABPM and HBPM may help to record lower BP during syncope episodes.

Head-up Tilt Test

- Tilt-table test may provoke a vasovagal response by venous pooling, causing orthostatic distress. The test usually takes up to 20–45 minutes, with a tilt of about 60–70%. Sometimes, pharmacologic agents, such as intravenous proterenol and sublingual nitroglycerin, are needed to unmask a response. Although it increases the sensitivity of the test, it decreases the specificity of the test.
- There are three types of positive responses in the tilt-table test:
  i. Type 1 mixed where coexisting bradycardia and hypotension.
  ii. Type 2 cardioinhibitory condition presenting as persistent bradycardia or long pauses without significant hypotension; it can be either type 2A without asystole or type 2B with asystole.
  iii. Type 3 vasodepressor with only significant hypotension and no bradycardia.

Orthostatic Challenge

This test helps diagnose orthostatic intolerance and differentiate orthostatic intolerance **(Table 3)**. A sphygmomanometer is adequate for classical OH and delayed OH. However, Initial OH requires continuous beat-to-beat noninvasive BP monitoring.

Blood Investigations

Blood tests can sometimes aid in diagnosis. These measures may include a complete blood count to check for anemia, serum electrolytes such as potassium and magnesium

TABLE 3: Diagnostic features of different types of orthostatic hypotension (OH).

Syndrome	Diagnostic test	Time from upright position to abnormal BP response	Definition	The most frequently associated conditions
Initial OH	Beat-to-beat BP on active standing test (lying to standing)	0–15 seconds	BP decreases on standing >40 mm Hg for systolic and/or >20 mm Hg for diastolic within 15 seconds	Young, asthenic subjects; old age, drug-induced (alpha-blockers)
Classical OH	Active standings test, table-tilt test	<3 minutes	Sustained decrease in SBP ≥20 mm Hg, DBP ≥ 10 mm Hg, or sustained decrease in SBP < 90 mm Hg within 3 minutes of active standing or HUTT at 60°	Frail elderly patients, vasoactive drugs, and diuretics autonomic failure
Delayed OH	Tilt test active standing test	>3 minutes	Response is same as classical but occurs after 3 minutes	Frailty , incipient autonomic failure, drug induced (any vasoactive drugs and diuretics), and comorbidity
Orthostatic vasovagal syncope (VVS)	Tilt test	Prolonged standing	In VVS, the BP drop starts several minutes after standing up, BP drop rapidly accelerates till person faints or lies down. This is opposite of classical OH where BP fall starts immediately on standing, but rate of drop is slow	• Women • Chronic orthostatic intolerance
Postural orthostatic tachycardia syndrome	Active standing, table-tilt test	<10 minutes	HR increase > 30 bpm from baseline or >120 bpm within 10 minutes of standing	Young women with connective tissue disorders

to identify abnormalities that could lead to or worsen arrhythmias, and measurement of serum catecholamine levels in both the supine and upright positions when postural orthostatic tachycardia is suspected. Additionally, drug levels may be assessed if there is a concern that a medication or illicit drug could trigger arrhythmia.

ECG Monitoring

The diagnosis of arrhythmic syncope can be unanimously agreed upon when ECG and clinical symptoms are simultaneously correlated. This approach can reveal abnormalities that may predispose to syncope, such as previous infarctions, ventricular preexcitation (e.g., WPW syndrome), AV or bundle-branch blocks, abnormal QT intervals, incomplete right bundle-branch block with right precordial ST segment elevation (indicative of Brugada syndrome), epsilon waves, or right precordial T-wave inversion suggestive of ARVC or an arrhythmic event. If arrhythmias are not documented on ECG during the symptom episodes, this helps rule out arrhythmias as the cause of syncope.

Cardiac Monitoring

- *In hospital monitoring*: Usually performed in patients admitted in emergency cases with syncope due to ECG abnormalities.
- *Holter monitoring*: Most patients do not have daily symptoms, so if there is no episode, the patient can go undiagnosed or have symptoms attributed to a noncardiac cause. Holter monitoring has a higher yield in patients with daily single or multiple episodes. Thus, short-term Holter monitoring has a low diagnostic yield, and patients may need long-term recordings.
- *Event recorder*:
    - External loop recorder: Indicated when recurrent syncope(>1/month)
    - Internal loop recorders—indicated if:
        - Indeterminate syncope in high-risk patients
        - Low-risk patients with a high probability of recurrence within 36 months (≥3 syncope's in the previous 2 years)
        - Identify bradycardia in reflex syncope.

Echocardiography

Echocardiography helps identify structural heart disease (severe aortic stenosis, hypertrophic obstructive cardiomyopathy, massive pulmonary thromboembolism, cardiac tamponade, or aortic dissection) as the cause of syncope. However, additional testing, such as exercise stress ECHO, may be needed, and this is especially considered in patients with HCM who complain of syncope during exertion or changes in posture.

Electrophysiological Testing

Despite advancements in noninvasive techniques such as prolonged ECG monitoring, electrophysiological studies (EPS) remain valuable in certain scenarios. These include cases of asymptomatic sinus bradycardia in which sinus arrest is suspected, bifascicular block, and suspected tachycardias. Although the prognostic value of prolonged sinus node recovery time (SNRT) has not been well-defined, a study showed that in patients with asymptomatic sinus bradycardia, a corrected SNRT of ≥800 ms is associated with an eightfold increased risk of syncope.[5] Additionally, in patients with bifascicular block, a prolonged HV interval of ≥70 ms or the induction of second- or third-degree AV block through pacing or pharmacological challenge suggests a risk of imminent high-grade AV block.[6]

TREATMENT

The treatment principles are based on the identification of the underlying mechanism and risk stratification of further recurrence. Rivasi et al.[7] described the underlying mechanism as either a hypotensive phenotype or bradycardia phenotype. Thus, the efficacy of the therapy is largely determined by the dominant phenotype. In most cases, either one of the phenotypes is dominant, such as classical OH is a predominant hypotensive phenotype, whereas low adenosine paroxysmal idiopathic block is a predominant bradycardia phenotype.[8] However, in real-world scenarios, the final mechanism may be a mixed one but with varying contribution. For instance, in patients with delayed OH, there is an accompanying vasodepressor response, where pointing toward the predominant mechanism is difficult. Conversely, patients with long asystolic pauses may still have these changes during syncopal episodes despite adequate cardiac pacing.[9,10] In such conditions, patients may have an underlying vasodepressor reflex that may be unmasked by the tilt-table test.

Reflex Syncope

- *Educational and lifestyle modification*: Educational and lifestyle modifications are first-line syncope treatment approaches. This approach includes reassuring patients of the benign nature of their condition, educating them on recognizing warning signs, and advising them on the avoidance of known triggers. Patients should be taught techniques to avoid syncope, such as suppressing cough when it is a known trigger. The patient should lay horizontally in a safe place to prevent injury. Liberal salt intake (120 mmol/day) and maintaining hydration.[11] Despite the lack of controlled studies, education and lifestyle modification have been given class I recommendations because they have a marked effect on the recurrence of syncope.[1]

- *Discontinuation of hypotensive therapy*: Common drugs that cause hypotension are diuretics, antihypertensives (CCB, prazosin, hydralazine, ACEI, methyldopa, and labetalol), nitrates, MAO inhibitors, phenothiazines, and barbiturates. There is moderate evidence (class IIa recommendation) that discontinuation or reduction of the dose of these drugs with a target systolic BP of 140 mm Hg leads to a decrease in syncopal episodes.[1,12]
- *Physical counter-pressure maneuvers*: Squatting, arm tensing, leg crossing, and leg crossing with lower body muscle tensing are some forms of isometric exercise that help reduce recurrence.[13] Usually, these maneuvers can be performed only when the patient has a long enough prodromal period in which he or she can react.[14] These are effective in reducing the burden and recurrence of syncope in patients < 60 years age (class IIa recommendation).[1]
- *Tilt-table training*: In young patients with recurrent vasovagal symptoms triggered by orthostatic stress, prolonged periods of forced upright posture is occasionally prescribed to reduce syncope. However, this approach is generally shown to have limited effectiveness.[15,16]
- *Pharmacological therapy*: It is considered when patients experience recurrent syncope despite education, lifestyle modification, and counter-pressure techniques. Insufficient evidence from few clinical trials supports or refutes these drugs. These drugs, such as fludrocortisone (volume expanders) and midodrine alpha agonists (vaso/venoconstrictor), have a class IIb recommendation.[1]Although beta-blockers were once widely regarded as the primary treatment option, recent research has shown that metoprolol, propranolol, and nadolol are no more effective than a placebo.[17] Some new emerging therapies include theophylline in patients with recurrent onset syncope who have low circulating adenosine levels; reboxetine and sibutramine seem to attenuate vasovagal syncope.[18] Radiofrequency ablation of the vagal ganglia has been reported to abolish vagal activity during vasovagal syncope.[19]
- *Cardiac pacing* has a class IIa recommendation to reduce syncopal recurrence in patients aged > 40 years with documented asystole pause > 3 seconds or asymptotic pause > 6 seconds due to sinus arrest or AV blockade.[1]

Orthostatic Hypotension

Most management strategies for orthostatic intolerance involve reflex syncope. Educational and lifestyle modification (adequate hydration and increased salt intake), which are class I recommendation. All other measures stopping or reducing vasoactive drugs, counter-pressure measures, abdominal compression garments, head-up tilt sleeping, midodrine, and fludrocortisone are class IIa recommendations. Abdominal binders are used in older patients. Sleeping with the head elevated at >10°, known as head-up tilt sleeping, can help prevent nocturnal polyuria and reduce the risk of nocturnal hypertension.[20] Droxidopa improves orthostatic tolerance by increasing systolic standing BP.[21,22]

Cardiac Arrhythmia (Cardiac Syncope)

Cardiac pacing is indicated in:[1]

- Symptomatic sinus bradycardia due to sick sinus syndrome or intrinsic AV block.
- Intermittent/paroxysmal intrinsic third- or second-degree AV block, although symptoms and ECG are not correlated.
- Syncope, BBB, positive EPS, or ILR documented AV block.

Catheter ablation is indicated for syncope due to SVT or VT to prevent recurrence.

An ICD is indicated:[1]

- Syncope due to VT and EF ≤ 35%
- Syncope and previous MI who have EPS induced VT
- To prevent sudden cardiac death (in HCM, ARVC, LQTS, and Brugada syndrome).

Cardioneuroablation

Cardioneuroablation (CNA) is increasingly acknowledged for its success in treating vasovagal syncope. CNA involves precise targeting and cauterization of intrinsic epicardial ganglia within the heart. This procedure leads to parasympathetic denervation to a certain extent, leading to a decrease in vagal tone in cardiac fibers and a reduction in the tendency to develop bradyarrhythmias.[23] A meta-analysis conducted by Vandenberk et al. examined 465 patients aged 18–60 years who experienced severely symptomatic recurrent reflex syncope with either spontaneous or orthostatic challenge-induced asystole but did not have sinus or AV node dysfunction. This analysis included data from 14 studies.[24] According to these results, the freedom-from-syncope (FFS) rate after CNA was 91.9%, with a higher rate of FFS after left atrial and biatrial ablation than after right atrial ablation.[24] Despite these encouraging results, several issues have emerged regarding patient selection, the optimal ablation site, verification of ablation effectiveness, and long-term durability of the procedure. Consequently, additional clinical trials and real-world studies with a large participant pool and extended follow-up are required.[25,26]

CONCLUSION

Not all persons reporting to the emergency department or OPD with complaints of TLOC have syncope. Recognition of high-risk symptoms, signs, examination, and ECG findings may help in expedited workup for syncope and avoid extensive and futile workup for all patients. Once diagnosed, the predominant underlying mechanism must be evaluated to initiate targeted therapy. For hypotensive phenotypes, patient education, lifestyle modification, counter-pressure maneuvers, and occasional drugs may be beneficial. Cardiac pacing is indicated for cardioinhibitory response and symptomatic bradycardia. ICDs are indicated for VT and for the prevention of sudden cardiac death.

ONLINE REFERENCES

Please scan the QR code provided at the end of the table of contents for References of this chapter.

CHAPTER 206

Approach to Ischemic Ventricular Tachycardia

Muralidharan TR, Preetam Krishnamurthy, Abhilasha

ABSTRACT

Ventricular arrhythmia can often complicate ischemic heart disease and can have a plethora of presentations including benign VPC and accelerated idioventricular rhythm to malignant sustained monomorphic ventricular tachycardia (VT) or polymorphic VT and ventricular fibrillation. The pathophysiology of VT is often variable depending on the presentation and requires meticulous assessment of patient's clinical conditions to tailor the approach for the management of ventricular arrhythmia. Though various treatment options are available, early revascularization and beta blockers have shown the maximum benefit.

Keywords: Ventricular tachycardia, sudden cardiac arrest, acute coronary syndrome

INTRODUCTION

Coronary artery disease is the most common cause of clinically documented ventricular tachycardia (VT) or ventricular fibrillation (VF) (76–82% patients). There has been significant decrease in the incidence of ventricular arrhythmias (VAs) in the peri-infarct period and long-term post-MI in the past few decades, likely due to significant improvements in coronary revascularization strategies and pharmacotherapies that have 1-year mortality to >5%. However, sustained VT and VF remain the major cause of death in the first 30 days after MI, particularly in patients with left ventricular (LV) dysfunction or heart failure.[1]

Among acute coronary syndrome, incidence of ventricular arrhythmia is more in patients with ST elevation myocardial infarction (STEMI) compared to patients with non-ST elevation myocardial infarction (NSTEMI). In the setting of STEMI, sustained VA is more common in the first 24–48 hours. In contrast, in NSTEMI, events do not seem to be confined to the first 48 hours.[2]

PATHOPHYSIOLOGY

The main causes for ventricular arrhythmia in the setting of ischemic heart disease are active ischemia and chronic infarct—the pathophysiology of the arrhythmia in these settings is significantly different and warrants a different management approach.

Active Ischemia

Acute myocardial ischemia leads to intracellular acidosis and a decrease in ATP levels, which disrupts the function of the ATP-dependent Na^+-K^+ pump. This causes a net loss of K^+ from the myocytes, raising the extracellular K^+ concentration. As a result, the resting membrane potential of surviving Purkinje fibers becomes depolarized, leading to abnormal automaticity.

Intracellular acidification and the buildup of H^+ ions activate the Na^+-H^+ exchanger, leading to the expulsion of H^+ in exchange for Na^+ entry, resulting in an increased intracellular Na^+ concentration. This, in turn, triggers the Na^+-Ca^{2+} exchanger to operate in reverse mode, exchanging Na^+ for Ca^{2+} entry. The resulting intracellular Ca^{2+} overload in the ischemic myocardium leads to delayed afterdepolarizations and can trigger arrhythmias.

Membrane depolarization leads to the inactivation of Na^+ channels, reducing the fast Na^+ current and the action potential upstroke. This results in slowed conduction and changes in refractoriness.

BOX 1 Mechanisms of ventricular arrhythmia in active ischemia.

- *Abnormal automaticity:* Abnormal depolarization of Purkinje fibers
- *Triggered activity:* Increased intracellular calcium and delayed depolarization
- *Functional re-entry:* Heterogenous effect of ischemia on myocardial cells in ischemic and nonischemic zone

The effects of ischemia on myocardial cells are uneven. In the central ischemic zone and subepicardium, there is a more pronounced shortening of action potential duration and a greater reduction in upstroke velocity and amplitude compared to the border zone and subendocardium. Meanwhile, the surrounding healthy myocardium may exhibit increased conduction velocity (due to elevated catecholamine levels) and reduced refractoriness. This variability in action potential duration and refractoriness creates conditions for injury currents to flow between ischemic and nonischemic cells at the border zone. Additionally, ischemia disrupts gap junctions, causing cellular uncoupling, leading to slower, anisotropic conduction, and unidirectional conduction block, which promotes re-entry **(Box 1)**.

Based on experimental models, there are two phases noted during the active ischemia: Phase 1 (reversible ischemia) lasting from 2 to 30 minutes of ischemia and phase 2 (irreversible ischemia) extending from 1.5 to 72 hours of ischemia. In phase 1, during the initial 10 minutes (phase 1A), the ischemia produces reentry circuit secondary to heterogeneity of conduction and refractoriness in normal and ischemic tissues. These manifest as bursts of VT that rarely degenerate to VF. From 10 to 30 minutes (phase 1B), more often VT is caused by abnormal automaticity, and tendency to degenerate to VF is higher. Beyond 30 minutes, there is irreversible ischemia (phase 2). During this phase subendocardial Purkinje fibers are more resistant to ischemia and may survive, but with altered electrophysiological (EP) properties predisposing to arrhythmia generation. Reduced resting membrane potentials, Ca^{2+} overload, and heterogeneity of conduction and refractoriness at the infarct border zone can all lead to focal (abnormal automaticity and triggered activity) and reentrant arrhythmias.[3]

Healed Infarction

Sustained ventricular arrhythmia most often associated with post-myocardial infarction (MI) scar tissue is sustained monomorphic ventricular tachycardia (SMVT). Left ventricular (LV) remodeling starts almost immediately after an acute MI. Studies indicate that the EP substrate for monomorphic VT gradually develops during the subacute phase (within the first week) after an acute MI, and once established, remains stable into the chronic phase. These sites are primarily located in the border zone near areas of dense injury during both phases.[4]

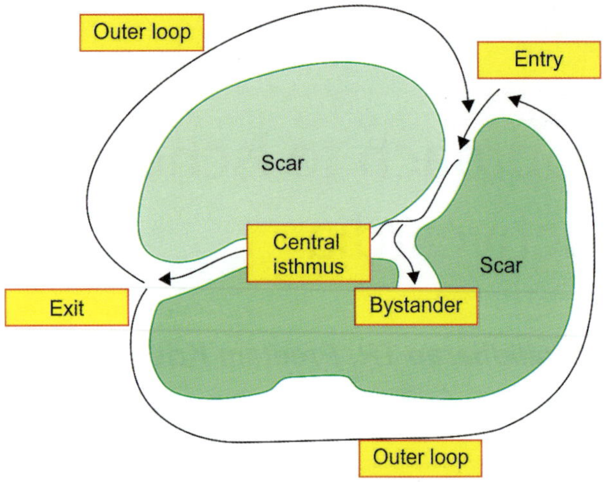

FIG. 1: Typical circuit in scar-related monomorphic ventricular tachycardia.

Variations in tissue composition and autonomic innervation in these regions can create zones of slow conduction and block, facilitating reentry. Within this arrhythmogenic substrate lies the common central pathway, or critical isthmus—a narrow tract of tissue with abnormal conduction properties that enables reentry to occur **(Fig. 1)**.

CLINICAL PRESENTATION

In patients with acute ischemia, sustained VAs often manifest as syncope or cardiac arrest. In chronic ischemic heart disease, VT can present with a wide range of symptoms, from mild issues like palpitations to more serious signs of hypoperfusion, such as lightheadedness, altered mental status, presyncope, and syncope. It may also worsen heart failure, trigger angina, or cause cardiovascular collapse. Patients with implantable cardiac defibrillators (ICDs) may experience shocks due to the arrhythmia. Incessant VT, even at slower rates, can lead to hemodynamic decline and heart failure. The hemodynamic effects of VT are influenced by factors such as ventricular rate and duration, the extent of LV dysfunction, ventricular dyssynchrony, and loss of atrioventricular (AV) synchrony.

EVALUATION

Identification of Type and Burden of Ventricular Arrhythmia

Using 12-lead ECG or ambulatory cardiac monitoring, the type of VT, burden, and clinical impact should be evaluated. ICD electrogram can provide information regarding the type of VT, VT morphology, and the tachycardia cycle length (TCL).

TABLE 1: Guidelines for invasive EP testing in patients with ischemic cardiomyopathy.[2]

Level of recommendation	Recommendations
IIa	For patients with ischemic cardiomyopathy presenting with syncope or other ventricular arrhythmia symptoms who do not meet indications for primary prevention ICD, an EP study can be useful in assessing the risk of sustained VT
III: No benefit	In patients who meet criteria for primary prevention ICD, EP study for the sole reason of inducing ventricular arrhythmia is not indicated

Source: Adapted from Al-Khatib et al. (2018).

BOX 2 General overview for management of ventricular arrhythmia.

Immediate treatment/suppression of the trigger:
- *Ischemia*: Urgent revascularization
- Correct metabolic abnormality

Maintenance of hemodynamics:
- Mechanical circulatory support
- Inotropes

Suppression of arrhythmia:
- Drug management
- Overdrive pacing
- Neuraxial modulation
- Ablation strategy

Identification of Triggers of Ventricular Arrhythmia

Possible reversible causes need to be evaluated. These include electrolyte imbalance, acute ischemia, hypoxia, heart failure, and drug effects. Patients will need early coronary evaluation and revascularization, especially in the setting of acute coronary syndrome. Even in patients with SMVT, where the likely pathogenesis is secondary to scar-related re-entry, revascularization will be required if ischemia is documented to improve patient outcomes.

Role of Electrophysiological Study

Invasive EP testing may be considered for post-MI patients who present with unexplained syncope, sustained palpitations, or wide complex tachycardia of unknown origin. It can also be used for risk stratification in patients with ischemic cardiomyopathy and nonsustained VT later after an MI. EP testing is not advised for patients with documented sustained VT unless catheter ablation is being considered **(Table 1)**.

MANAGEMENT

The main pillars of management in ventricular arrhythmia include identification of the trigger, suppression of arrhythmia, and maintenance of hemodynamics **(Box 2)**. A summary of the management is highlighted in **Flowchart 1**

Resuscitation and Revascularization

Urgent reperfusion **(Figs. 2A to D)** is the most important therapy, as acute ischemia triggers arrhythmias as described earlier.[6] Beta-blocker treatment is also recommended to prevent VA. Correction of electrolyte imbalances is strongly recommended.[7] In a hemodynamically unstable patient, appropriate cardiac support should be initiated to maintain the cardiac output. Ionotrope support, though it would help to maintain the hemodynamics in the short term, is highly proarrhythmic and must undergo judicious

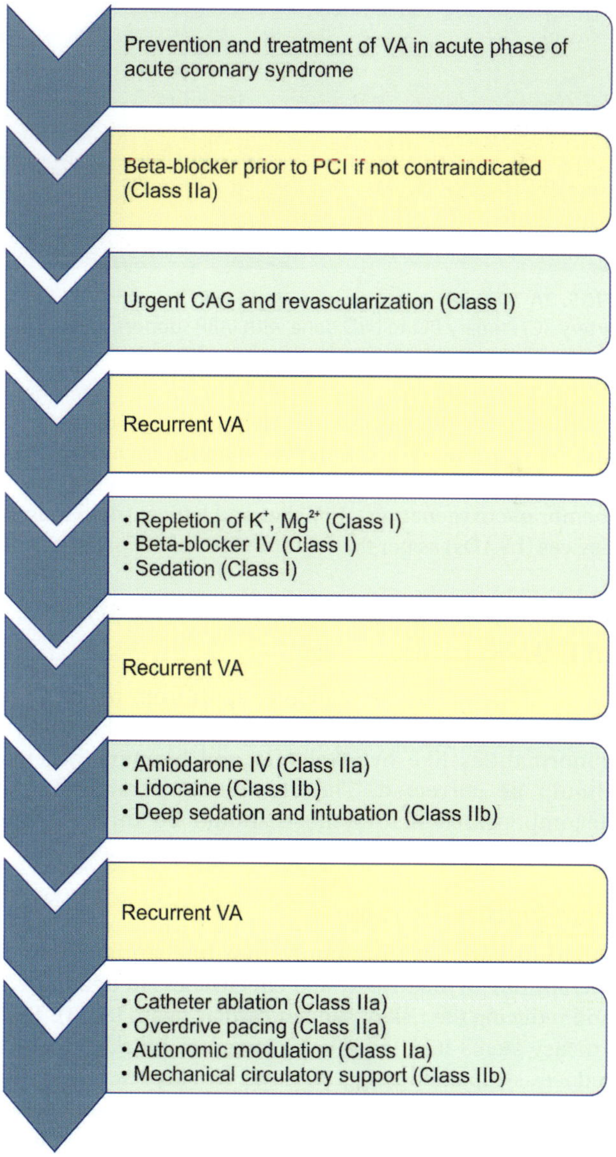

FLOWCHART 1: Approach to management of ventricular arrhythmia in the presence of acute ischemia.[5]

Source: Adapted from Zeppenfeld et al. (2022).

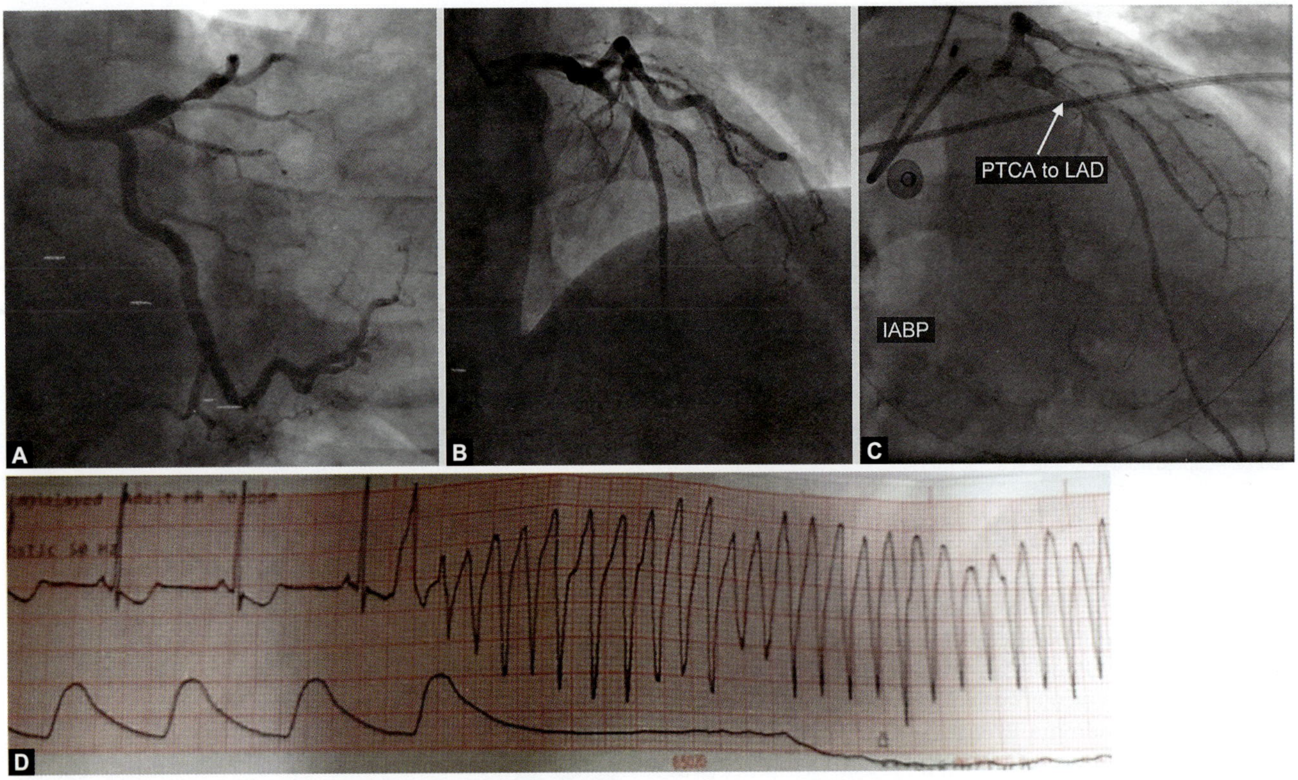

FIGS. 2A TO D: Revascularization strategy in ischemic VT. (A and B) Initial CAG showing 99% stenosis of the mid left anterior descending artery; (C) Primary PCI to LAD done with IABP support; and (D) presentation ECG—runs of polymorphic VT requiring ICD shock.

titration. Mechanical circulatory support may often be required to maintain the hemodynamics including IABP (intra-aortic balloon pump), ECMO (extracorporeal membrane oxygenation), Impella, and left ventricular assist devices (LVADs) as per the requirements of the patient.

Electrolyte Management and Initiation of GDMT

In the setting of acute ischemia, apart from revascularization, beta-blockade should be started. Electrolyte abnormalities like hypokalemia and hypomagnesemia should be corrected. The concomitant treatment for decompensated heart failure should be initiated and proarrhythmic medications should be discontinued.

Beta-blocker Therapy

Beta-blockers are commonly first-line antiarrhythmic therapy due to their safety and effectiveness in treating VAs and reducing the risk of sudden cardiac death (SCD). Their efficacy stems from adrenergic-receptor blockade, which reduces sympathetic triggers, slows the sinus rate, and may inhibit excess calcium release. Trial in STEMI patients found that early intravenous metoprolol before PCI lowered the incidence of acute-phase arrhythmias without increasing adverse events.[2,8]

Among beta-blockers, nonselective beta-blockers, like propranolol, have shown superiority over selective beta-blockers (metoprolol) in the setting of VT storm. The selective blockade of β_1 receptors may facilitate continuous sympathetic signal transductions through unblocked cardiac β_2 receptors, which is not cardiostimulatory, but may also increase the likelihood of VAs. Propranolol being lipid soluble also can cross the blood-brain barrier to act on the central nervous system to reduce sympathetic drive.[9]

Amiodarone and Sotalol

Amiodarone is a multichannel blocker including sodium, potassium, and calcium currents with additional beta-blockade. There is no clear benefit to use of amiodarone as primary prevention in patients with ischemic cardiomyopathy.[10,11] Intravenous amiodarone has a role in reducing recurrent VT/VF during resuscitation, which is predominantly attributed to its beta-blocking property.[12] The role of amiodarone in acute ischemia is not well established and lidocaine is preferred over amiodarone in patients presenting with cardiac arrest.[13]

Sotalol can suppress VAs but has notable proarrhythmic risks and has not been shown to improve survival. The SWORD trial found that d-sotalol increased mortality in heart failure patients. Unlike other antiarrhythmics, sotalol lowers the defibrillation threshold and may cause heart failure decompensation, so it is generally avoided in patients with an LVEF below 20%.[14]

Lidocaine and Mexiletine

Lidocaine and mexiletine are both class IB antiarrhythmic drugs that act as rapid sodium channel blockers, binding in a use-dependent manner. The key difference is that mexiletine has an 80% bioavailability, allowing for oral administration. Lidocaine's use in electrical storms is limited due to its lower efficacy in terminating scar-related VTs. However, during ischemic VT, altered membrane potential and reduced pH enhance lidocaine's effectiveness in terminating ventricular arrhythmias (VAs), making it recommended primarily for VA suppression in acute ischemia. Mexiletine reduces VA burden but shows a trend toward increased mortality and is typically used as an adjunct to amiodarone, helping to reduce appropriate therapies in ICD patients when amiodarone is ineffective. Both lidocaine and mexiletine have dose-dependent side effects mainly related to central nervous system accumulation, especially in heart failure patients, which can include tremors, seizures, and hallucinations. These side effects are generally reversible with dose reduction or discontinuation.[15,16]

Neuraxial Modulation

Stellate Ganglion Blockade

Stellate ganglion blockade is useful in patients with drug-refractory VA in electrical storms. It involves administration of local anesthesia percutaneously with or without imaging guidance. Left sympathetic ganglion blockade is the common practice, though bilateral ganglion blockade can also be administered in selected cases. Drugs that are commonly used include lidocaine, bupivacaine, ropivacaine, and mepivacaine. Stellate ganglion blockade has been shown to reduce VA and ICD shocks in patients presenting with electrical storm.[17]

Deep Sedation and General Anesthesia

Deep sedation with intubation is the most used method to reduce sympathetic excitation and avoid further arrhythmias and shocks while awaiting definitive treatment. Deep sedation with intubation can be initiated more rapidly. However, mechanical ventilation and deep sedation can cause hypotension in patients with already compromised cardiac function, limiting the depth of sedation achievable without depending on highly arrhythmogenic inotropes.

Thoracic Epidural Anesthesia

Thoracic epidural anesthesia (TEA), which involves infusing anesthetic agents like bupivacaine or opioids into the epidural space, achieves sympathetic block at the T1 to T4 levels **(Fig. 3)**. TEA offers rapid onset and can be adjusted for the desired effect. It has been shown to increase the VF threshold during acute myocardial ischemia, prolong ventricular repolarization and effective refractory periods, suppress sympathetic-induced repolarization heterogeneity, and reduce arrhythmia burden in VT storms.[18]

Renal Artery Denervation

Renal artery denervation (RDN) provides an alternative approach to targeting the sympathetic nervous system. Abnormal signaling from the heart is linked to increased renal nerve activity and noradrenaline release. RDN aims to

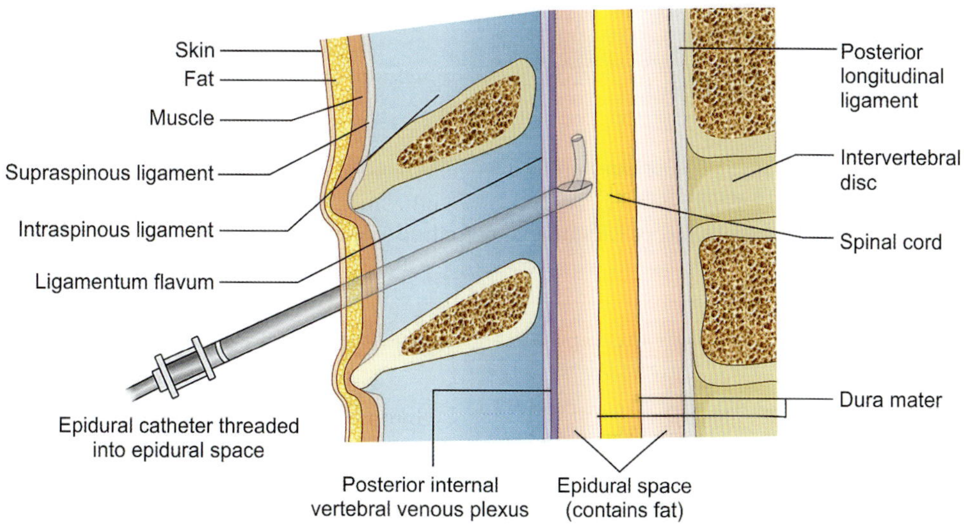

FIG. 3: Anatomy of thoracic epidural catheter placement for the management of ventricular tachycardia storm.

Source: Adapted from Do DH et al. (2017).

interrupt this process, lowering circulating catecholamines by targeting both efferent and afferent sympathetic pathways within the renal arteries. The procedure typically involves catheter insertion via transcutaneous access, creating spiral-shaped circumferential lesions through point-by-point radiofrequency ablation to destroy sympathetic fibers, usually requiring 5–6 lesions per artery. Small studies and meta-analyses suggest that RDN can effectively reduce VAs.[19]

Implantable Cardiac Defibrillator

Implantable cardiac defibrillator therapy significantly reduces mortality in patients with structural heart disease and a history of VT or VF, showing a 7% absolute reduction and a 25% relative reduction in all-cause mortality compared to amiodarone therapy, primarily due to a 50% decrease in arrhythmic deaths. ICD implantation is recommended for secondary prevention in patients with previous cardiac arrest or sustained VT, even if systolic function is normal or if they are undergoing successful catheter ablation or responding to antiarrhythmic therapy, as these methods do not sufficiently mitigate the risk of SCD. Additionally, ICDs are advised for patients with syncope and inducible sustained monomorphic VT, even if they do not meet primary prevention criteria. However, in patients with incessant VT or VF, ICD implantation should be postponed until adequate arrhythmia suppression is achieved through drug therapy or ablation to prevent frequent shocks **(Table 2)**.

Catheter Ablation

Catheter ablation can reduce VT recurrences and subsequent ICD interventions by over 75% in patients experiencing multiple ICD shocks. However, most post-MI VT patients have various types of monomorphic VTs, making it difficult to eliminate all VTs. Since the recurrence of an ablated VT or the emergence of a new VT can be life-threatening, RF ablation is rarely the sole therapy for VT. Instead, it is usually combined with ICD therapy in patients with coronary artery disease. The risk of death related to the ablation procedure ranges from 0 to 3%, while major complications occur in 3.6% to 10% of cases.

The various options of VT ablations are discussed in **Flowchart 2**.

Unstable VT can often be difficult to map **(Figs. 4A and B)**. Additional, mechanical circulatory support would be required if activation mapping is planned for unstable VT. High-definition catheters like HD grid catheter and penta-ray catheter enable fast mapping of activation

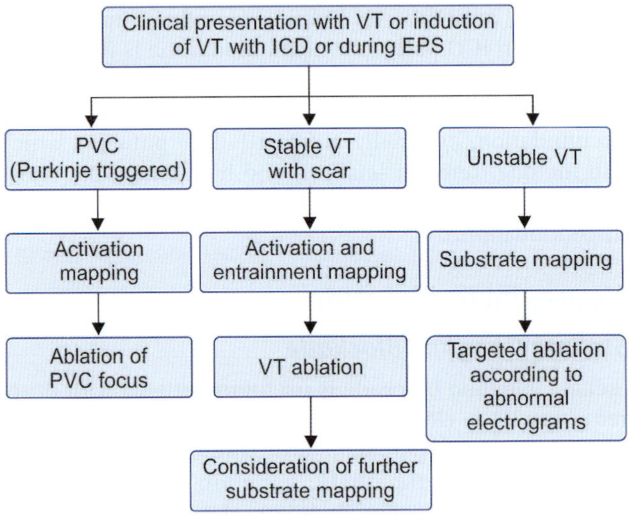

FLOWCHART 2: Approach to VT ablation in ischemic substrate.[20]
Source: Adapted from Shivkumar K et al. (2019).

TABLE 2: Indications for implantation of AICD.[2]

Level of recommendation	Recommendations
Secondary prevention	
I	SCA due to VT/VF or experiencing hemodynamically unstable VT or stable VT not due to reversible causes, an ICD is recommended
I	Unexplained syncope with inducible sustained monomorphic VT on electrophysiological study, an ICD is recommended
Primary prevention	
I	LVEF <35% at least 40 days post-MI and at least 90 days postrevascularization, and with NYHA class II or III HF despite GDMT, an ICD is recommended
I	LVEF <30% at least 40 days post-MI and at least 90 days postrevascularization, and with NYHA class I HF despite GDMT, an ICD is recommended
I	NSVT due to prior MI, LVEF of 40% or less, and inducible sustained VT or VF at electrophysiological study, an ICD is recommended
III: No benefit	An ICD is not indicated for NYHA Class IV patients with medication-refractory HF who are not candidates for cardiac transplantation, LVAD, or a CRT defibrillator

Source: Adapted from Al-Khatib et al. (2018).

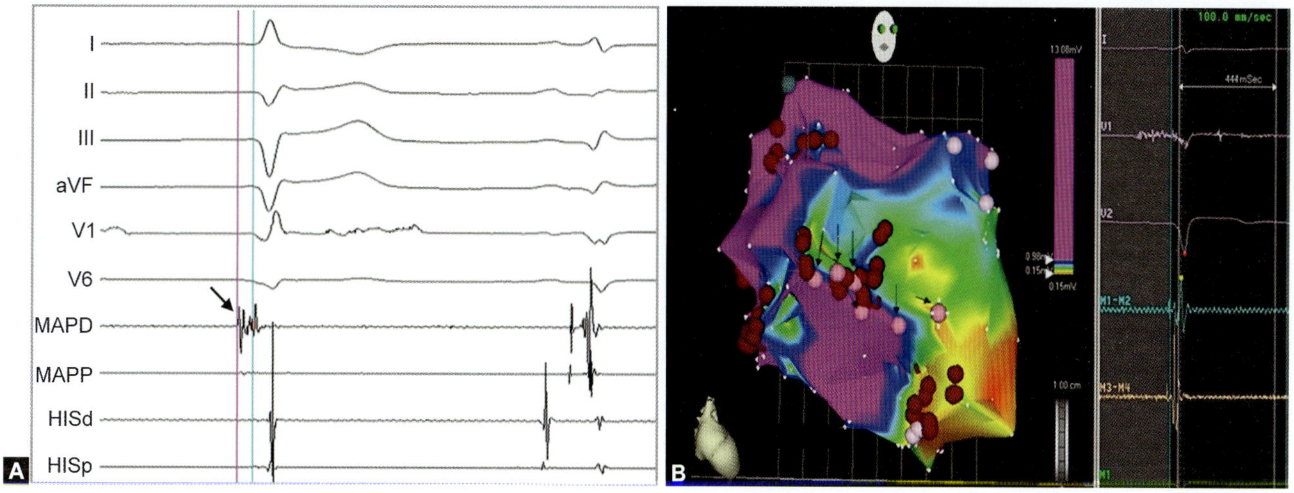

FIGS. 4A AND B: Purkinje fiber VPC initiating polymorphic VT. (A) Spontaneous VPC is preceded by sharp prepotential (black arrow), which is not seen in sinus rhythm; and (B) Targeted ablation of the sites with earliest activation.

Courtesy: C Narasimhan, AIG Hospital, Hyderabad, India.

sequence in patients with unstable VT and reduce the time for mapping. Without induction of VT, the electrograms can be assessed to identify possible substrate. These include identification of late potentials, fractionated electrograms, decremental evoked potentials, which can potentially identify the isthmus channel. Stable VT can be mapped by activation, entrainment, or substrate mapping. Pace-mapping in a scar VT often is not accurate and is usually not practiced.

Destination Therapy (LVAD) and Transplantation

In patients with refractory VT, not responding to medications, VT ablation, and other adjunctive therapy, it may be necessary to plan for LVAD as destination therapy. However, in patients with persistent VT in the presence of LVAD, there is a potential to develop RV dysfunction and biventricular assist devices may be needed. Heart transplantation should be planned in VT that is refractory to all the abovementioned management.

CONCLUSION

Ventricular arrhythmia complicating MI is a high-risk subset. The treatment involves a multidisciplinary approach requiring treatment modalities extending from pharmacotherapy, revascularization to catheter ablation that should be tailored as per the patient's requirements.

ONLINE REFERENCES

Please scan the QR code provided at the end of the table of contents for References of this chapter.

CHAPTER

207

Sudden Cardiac Death

Avishkar Agrawal, Mohsin Raj Mantoo, Sandeep Singh

ABSTRACT

Sudden cardiac death (SCD) is a global public health issue with genetic and environmental factors. Early diagnosis and prevention through diagnostic advancements and interventions like implantable cardioverter-defibrillator (ICD) are crucial. Understanding the pathophysiology of SCD and implementing effective management strategies, including immediate resuscitation and postresuscitation care, are essential for reducing incidence and improving patient outcomes.

Keywords: SCD, ICD, early diagnosis, pathophysiology

INTRODUCTION

Sudden cardiac death (SCD) is a global public health challenge and is a leading cause of death. It has multifaceted etiology, which includes genetic and environmental factors. Early diagnosis and prevention through diagnostic advancements and interventions like implantable cardioverter-defibrillator (ICD) are crucial. This chapter covers epidemiology, pathophysiology, clinical manifestations, and management strategies of SCD, with emphasis on research and clinical advancements.

DEFINITION

To understand the spectrum of SCD and its causes clearly, it is crucial to differentiate between two closely related terms:

1. *Sudden cardiac death:* Sudden natural death presumed to be of cardiac in origin, which can either occur within 1 hour of onset of symptoms in case of a witnessed event or within 24 hours of last being seen alive in an unwitnessed event. Although a heart disease may or may not have been previously diagnosed, the circumstances of the individual's death are unexpected.
2. *Sudden arrhythmic death (SAD):* Sudden unexplained death occurring in an individual older than 1 year with a negative pathological and toxicological assessment. To ascertain whether any death is sudden arrhythmic in origin, an autopsy is required.

EPIDEMIOLOGY

Sudden cardiac death is a leading cause of death globally, accounting for 15–20% of all fatalities. It surpasses the combined mortality rates from lung cancer, breast cancer, and AIDS, highlighting its crucial role in global health.[1] Historically, SCD prevalence in the adult population has been estimated to be between 0.05–0.2%, annually. Recent data from SCD registries across European Union countries confirm this range, suggesting a consistent trend in different regions.[2]

PATHOPHYSIOLOGY

Sudden cardiac death is a complex phenomenon caused by the interaction of a susceptible heart condition and an acute triggering event. Typical substrates include structural heart diseases (SHD) like coronary artery disease (CAD), cardiomyopathies, and inherited arrhythmogenic disorders. These conditions can lead to an electrophysiological unstable myocardium characterized by scarring, fibrosis, or ischemia, thereby increasing the risk of life-threatening arrhythmias.[3]

An acute event triggers a fatal arrhythmia in susceptible individuals. Triggers include acute myocardial ischemia, electrolyte imbalances, autonomic nervous system fluctuations, or external stimuli like physical exertion or emotional stress. For instance, in CAD patients, acute plaque rupture leading to MI can cause electrical instability in the affected region. This intricate interaction results in a terminal rhythm, manifesting as asystole, pulseless electrical activity (PEA), ventricular tachycardia (VT), or ventricular fibrillation (VF). Asystole is the most prevalent rhythm (50%), while PEA ranges from 19–23%. Once predominant, VT and VF have declined to <30% in recent decades.[4]

ETIOLOGY AND RISK FACTORS

The common risk factors predisposing to SCD are listed in **Table 1**. Traditionally, data from older studies, where autopsies were not routinely performed have shown that CAD accounted for 80% of all SCDs, followed by cardiomyopathies (15%) and valvular heart diseases (3%), while genetic arrhythmia syndromes contributed to approximately 2% of cases **(Fig. 1)**.[5]

TABLE 1: The common risk factors predisposing to sudden cardiac death (SCD).

Lifestyle factors	• Smoking • Obesity • Physical inactivity
Cardiac conditions	• Coronary artery disease • Cardiomyopathies • Congenital heart defects • Previous myocardial infarction • Heart failure • Arrhythmias (e.g., VT/VF)
Genetic factors	• Inherited arrhythmogenic disorders • Family history of SCD
Demographic factors	• Age (higher risk in older adults) • Gender (higher risk in males) • Race/ethnicity (higher prevalence in certain populations)
Other conditions	• Hypertension • Diabetes • Electrolyte imbalances

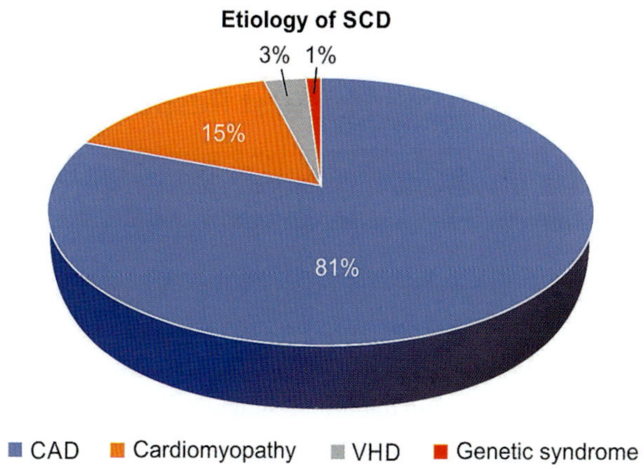

FIG. 1: Significant causes of sudden cardiac death (SCD).

However, contemporary series that performed autopsies in virtually all the cases provided a different perspective. In the POST-SCD study, 60% of SCDs were due to cardiac etiology, while 40% were due to noncardiac causes. Among cardiac causes, nearly 90% were SAD, which is the one preventable by current strategies of ICDs.[6]

The SCD due to noncardiac etiologies has a grim prognosis, with two-thirds dying before reaching the hospital. Of those who arrived, a staggering 90% were nonresuscitable at the hospital. Among the few resuscitable cases, most of the sudden deaths were arrhythmic in origin, with VT and VF being the most common rhythms, unlike asystole or PEA. This also highlights the fact that not all arrhythmic deaths are necessarily cardiac in origin.[7]

CLINICAL PRESENTATION

Sudden cardiac death is the first sign of underlying cardiovascular disease in half of the patients. Prodromal symptoms like chest pain or fatigue may precede SCD. Cardiac pumping failure leads to reduction in cerebral blood flow and loss of consciousness. Mechanical conditions like pericardial tamponade, aortic dissection, ventricular free wall rupture, or pulmonary embolism usually cause asystole or PEA. One-third of cases may have unclear symptoms.

Loss of cerebral circulation causes irreversible brain injury within 4–6 minutes, reducing chances of survival and having intact neurologic function. Anoxic brain injury and sepsis are common causes of death in out-of-hospital cardiac arrest (OHCA) survivors who attain hospitalization. Recurrent events are expected within the first 24–48 hours.

DIAGNOSTIC EVALUATION

Survivors of SCD are evaluated for reversible triggers, SHD, primary cardiac electrical disorders, genetic counseling and testing, and detailed neurologic assessment.

History

It is essential to obtain a history of cardiac diseases (e.g., CAD and heart failure), prodromal symptoms (e.g., angina), physical activity before the event, illicit substance or medication use that may predispose to arrhythmic events, or family history of cardiac disorders from patient's attendants or relatives, since patients may have retrograde amnesia postresuscitation.

Laboratory Tests

Routine laboratory tests, including electrolytes (potassium, magnesium, and calcium), arterial blood gas analysis, and toxicology screen (in selected patients) should be performed. Electrolyte and acid-base abnormalities can occur in SCA survivors due to profound hypoperfusion and anaerobic metabolism. Troponin levels are elevated in patients resuscitated from cardiac arrest, but these do not necessarily indicate an acute myocardial infarction.

Electrocardiogram

An electrocardiogram (ECG) provides essential clues regarding the underlying pathology.

- ST-segment elevation or new Q-waves indicate ST-segment elevation myocardial infarction, which may require urgent coronary revascularization.
- Nonspecific ST-T abnormalities like ST depression and T-wave inversions are common ECG findings, which are usually transient.
- Cardiac conduction abnormalities like atrioventricular conduction block or bundle branch block may suggest complete heart block as cause of SCA.
- Other ECG pointers that can be seen in specific etiologies are the coved ST segment of Brugada syndrome and the epsilon waves of arrhythmogenic cardiomyopathy.

Echocardiography

Echocardiography is the initial investigation for diagnosing an SHD. Regional wall motion abnormality suggests myocardial infarction, while a thinned-out dyskinetic segment suggests a ventricular aneurysm. SHDs that can cause SCD and can be diagnosed based on echocardiography include arrhythmogenic right ventricular dysplasia (ARVD) and hypertrophic cardiomyopathy (HCM). Echocardiography is crucial for diagnosing valvular heart diseases like severe aortic stenosis. Myocardial stunning can be induced by global hypoperfusion during cardiac arrest and resuscitation, so the assessment of left ventricular function should be repeated at least 48 hours after resuscitation.

Coronary Angiography

Since CAD is the most common cause of OHCA, coronary angiography is crucial in hospitalized survivors. Timing is vital in patients with ST-segment elevation on the ECG after resuscitation; an immediate invasive coronary angiography (ICA) and coronary revascularization are recommended.[8,9] Neurological status and overall survival probability should be considered before an invasive test, especially in patients who have received prolonged cardiopulmonary resuscitation (CPR). Patients with OHCA with VT/VF as initial rhythm and without ST-segment elevation in ECG should have a delayed ICA. Randomized clinical trials (TOMAHAWK and COACT trial) have not shown any superiority of immediate ICA in this setting.[10]

The ICA is crucial in detecting coronary anomalies in young patients with unexplained OHCA. However, it may not be necessary in patients without CAD risk factors and where other causes like HCM, ARVD, or Brugada syndrome are apparent on noninvasive investigations.

Cardiac Magnetic Resonance Imaging

Cardiac magnetic resonance imaging (CMR) is indicated in patients when the earlier-mentioned evaluation cannot establish SHD and is especially useful in cardiomyopathies and infiltrative disorders such as sarcoidosis.

Unexplained Cardiac Arrest

Patients with unexplained cardiac arrest (no SHD detected) may benefit from extended testing, including advanced cardiac imaging, exercise testing, drug provocation, and genetic testing.

Family Screening

Familial cardiomyopathies and channelopathies may affect multiple family members. First-degree relatives should be screened for risk using investigations like ECG, echocardiography, or provocation testing. Genetic testing is recommended only for pathogenic mutations detected in the index patient.

MANAGEMENT STRATEGIES

The management of cardiac arrest patients involves the initiation of early and uninterrupted CPR and life support until return of spontaneous circulation (ROSC) is achieved. Some salient aspects of the management of a case of cardiac arrest are discussed below:

Initial Assessment and Essential Basic Life Support

A quick assessment of voice response and confirmation of breathing, followed by palpation of carotid or femoral pulse is advised. On-site bystander CPR is recommended as it has shown a 2.5 times higher survival rate compared to those who received CPR after the arrival of medical team.[11]

The recommended basic life support (BLS) sequence is "CAB" (compression, airway, and breathing) with concepts of "minimally interrupted CPR" and the hypothesis that chest compressions are the most critical component of a successful CPR.

Early Defibrillation by First Responder

About 25% of OHCA patients have shockable rhythms (VT/VF) at presentation; therefore, early cardioversion/defibrillation is recommended to improve the survival.

Advanced Cardiovascular Life Support

Advanced cardiovascular life support (ACLS) is aimed to restore cardiac rhythm quickly, optimize ventilation, and support blood pressure to perfuse vital organs.

The CPR with intubation and rapid intravenous (IV) access are prioritized for bradyarrhythmia, asystole, and PEA. Reversible causes like hypokalemia, acidosis, tamponade, toxins, or pulmonary thromboembolism should be ruled out during resuscitation. Temporary transcutaneous pacing may be considered for bradycardia and heart blocks, though evidence of its usefulness is lacking.

Stabilization after Initial Return of Spontaneous Circulation

Optimization of ventilation, hemodynamics stabilization, and treatment of underlying etiologies should be undertaken. In patients with frequent ventricular ectopics or nonsustained VT (NSVT), intravenous antiarrhythmic agents like amiodarone or lignocaine should be given. Beta-blockers and IV magnesium sulfate are given for polymorphic VT. IV catecholamine is often required post-ROSC to augment cardiac contractility and peripheral vascular resistance. Isoproterenol or temporary pacing may be considered for persistent bradycardia or atrioventricular conduction blocks.

Temperature Control

During the initial 24 hours postarrest, active temperature management with a target to maintain normothermia (37.5°C) in postcardiac arrest patients is recommended. The HYPERION and TTM-2 studies showed no difference in mortality between targeted hypothermia (32°C) and normothermia (37.5°C). Systematic reviews also reported no improvement in survival or neurologic outcomes with a temperature target of 32–34°C compared to normothermia (37°C).[12]

PREVENTION

Primary Prevention

Primary prevention of SCD involves identifying and managing high-risk individuals to reduce the likelihood of fatal cardiac events. Premature ventricular contractions (PVCs) though usually benign, may have certain high-risk characteristics like frequency (>10 PVCs/h), short coupling interval (R on T phenomenon) or couplets which have shown to be independent predictors of mortality.[13,14] Additionally, numerous studies have shown that systolic heart failure with reduced left ventricular ejection fraction (LVEF) on two-dimensional (2D) transthoracic echocardiography is associated with a higher risk of SCD.[15] The prevention strategy involves two main approaches:

Pharmacological Interventions

The CAST trial showed increased mortality with antiarrhythmic drugs (AADs) (encainide and flecainide) when given for asymptomatic or minimally symptomatic ventricular arrhythmia after MI, though these drugs were effective in suppressing ventricular arrhythmia.[16] Both EMIAT and CAMIAT trials, which enrolled patients with ejection fractions <40%, failed to demonstrate a statistically significant overall mortality benefit with the use of amiodarone.[17,18] Despite the antiarrhythmic effects, the proarrhythmic effects and systemic toxicities counterbalanced the impact in reducing arrhythmic deaths or resuscitated VF **(Table 2)**.

Implantable Cardioverter-defibrillator

The role of ICD therapy in the prevention of SCD has been well-established, and ICD is widely utilized globally for this purpose. To comprehensively evaluate the effectiveness of ICD in preventing SCD, its role can be categorized into the following subgroups:

Role in Ischemic Cardiomyopathy

The role of ICD in preventing SCD in ischemic cardiomyopathy (ICMP) is more established than in other etiologies. Landmark trials such as MADIT and MUSTT showed that ICD reduced the risk of SCD as compared to AADs in patients with severe left ventricular systolic dysfunction and NSVT or inducible VT on electrophysiological (EP) study. Following these trials, ICD was approved for primary prevention in patients with LVEF <35%.[19,20] This was further substantiated by the MADIT-II trial, which demonstrated similar results in patients with ICMP with LVEF <35% without needing an EP study.[21] The current 2022 ACC guidelines give a class I recommendation for primary prevention ICD therapy in ICMP, at least 40 days after MI or 90 days after revasculari-

TABLE 2: Trials of antiarrhythmic agents in the setting of ventricular premature contractions (VPCs) or nonsustained ventricular tachycardia (NSVT) in post-MI patients.

Name	Inclusion criteria	Intervention versus control	Conclusions
CAST Trial (n = 1,498)	Patients with asymptomatic or mildly symptomatic ventricular arrhythmias post-MI	Class I antiarrhythmics (encainide, flecainide, and moricizine) versus placebo	Encainide and flecainide caused increased cardiovascular mortality with a relative risk of 2.5 (confidence interval 1.7–8.5; $p < 0.001$)
EMIAT Trial (n = 1,486)	Post-MI patients with left ventricular ejection fraction (LVEF) <40%	Amiodarone versus placebo	Amiodarone reduces arrhythmic deaths but does not improve overall survival in post-MI patients with low LVEF
CAMIAT Trial (n = 1,202)	Post-MI patients with NSVT and LVEF <40%	Amiodarone versus placebo	Similar to EMIAT, amiodarone reduces arrhythmic deaths but does not improve overall survival

zation (PCI/CABG) with LVEF <35%, and NYHA II–III symptoms with an expected meaningful survival of more than 1 year. ICD therapy is also recommended in NYHA I (asymptomatic) ICMP patients with severely reduced LVEF (<30%) despite guideline-directed medical treatment (GDMT).[22]

Role in Nonischemic Cardiomyopathy (NICMP)

Recent trials like DEFINITE and DANISH, challenge the utility of ICD in patients with nonischemic cardiomyopathy (NICMP). The DEFINITE trial showed that ICD reduced SCD in NICM patients but not the overall mortality.[23] The DANISH study showed that ICD reduced SCD incidence but did not significantly decrease the overall mortality, especially among those aged 68 and above.[23]

The SCD-HeFT trial, the most extensive study to assess the benefit of ICD therapy in patients with NICMP, demonstrated a significant 23% relative reduction in all-cause mortality with ICD therapy compared to optimal medical therapy alone.[24] Furthermore, the benefit was observed equally in patients with ICMP and NICMP.

The current guideline (2023) from the European Society of Cardiology (ESC) recommends (class IIa) ICD for symptomatic patients of NICMP with LVEF ≤35% despite more than 3 months of GDMT.[25] However, the AHA/ACC/HFSA guideline (2022) continues to give a class I recommendation to the primary prevention ICD therapy in NICMP patients with NYHA II or III symptoms and LVEF ≤35% despite GDMT.[22]

Timing of Implantable Cardioverter-defibrillator Implantation in Postmyocardial Infarction Patient

Although ICD implantation for SCD prevention is crucial, revascularization offers additional benefits and reduces the risk of SCD. The CABG-Patch trial found no significant mortality benefit with ICD therapy despite arrhythmic death reduction after MI.[26] Coronary revascularization improved outcomes, prompting deferring SCD risk stratification and reassessment. Coronary revascularization itself is an effective antiarrhythmic therapy. Two landmark trials studied patients in the immediate post-MI period. The DINAMIT trial, which investigated early ICD implantation (within 40 days) in patients with reduced LVEF (≤35%), failed to show a significant reduction in mortality compared to conventional therapy.[27] The IRIS trial, assessing ICD implantation in post-MI patients with LVEF ≤30% and NSVT, showed reduced arrhythmic events but not overall mortality.[28] ICD utilization in ICMP is recommended after 40 days of MI, 90 days of revascularization, or 90 days of treatment initiation and optimization in NICMP.[25]

Wearable Cardioverter Defibrillator

In high-risk patients who are ineligible for ICD therapy, such as within 40 days of a recent MI or 90 days of revascularization, or who declined ICD therapy, temporary increases in SCD risk occur during the waiting periods for ICD implantation. The VEST trial assessed the efficacy of wearable cardioverter-defibrillator (WCD) therapy in these patients.[29] The trial found no significant mortality difference between WCD users and usual care, suggesting limited survival benefits. However, WCDs were associated with higher appropriate shocks, indicating the potential to prevent SCD in high-risk individuals.

All major trials of ICD for primary prevention are summarized in **Table 3**.

Secondary Prevention

Three randomized clinical trials: AVID, CIDS, and CASH showed that ICD therapy reduced the incidence of sudden

TABLE 3: Trials of primary prevention implantable cardioverter-defibrillator (ICD) therapy in ischemic cardiomyopathy (ICMP) and nonischemic cardiomyopathy (NICMP).

Trial	Inclusion criteria	Results
ICMP		
MADIT (1996) $n = 196$	Prior MI LVEF ≤35% NYHA I/II/III NSVT on ECG monitoring Inducible VT during EPS	*Total mortality*: HR 0.46 (95% CI 0.26–0.82) compared with conventional medical therapy alone
MUSTT (1996) $n = 704$	Prior MI LVEF ≤40% NYHA I/II/III NSVT on ECG monitoring Inducible VT during EPS	*SCA or death from arrhythmia*: RR 0.24 (95% CI 0.13–0.45) for ICD versus no ICD
CABG-PATCH (1999) $n = 900$	<80 years old Scheduled for elective CABG LVEF <35% Abnormal SAECG	*Death from any cause*: HR 1.07 (95% CI 0.81–1.42) ICD versus control

Continued

Continued

Trial	Inclusion criteria	Results
MADIT-II (2002) $n = 1,232$	Prior MI LVEF ≤35% NYHA I/II/III	*Total mortality*: HR 0.65 (95% CI 0.51–0.93) compared with conventional medical therapy alone
DINAMIT (2003) $n = 674$	6–40 days post-MI LVEF ≤35% Impaired autonomic function	*Total mortality*: HR 1.08 (95% CI 0.76–1.55), ICD versus control
IRIS (2007) $n = 298$	5–31 days post-MI LVEF ≤40% and HR ≥90 BPM on first ECG or NSVT	*Total mortality*: HR 1.04 (95% CI 0.81–1.35) ICD versus control group
NICMP		
DEFNITE (2004) $n = 458$	LVEF ≤35% NYHA I/II/III PVCs or NSVT	*Total mortality*: HR 0.65 (95% CI 0.4–1.06) compared with conventional medical therapy alone
DANISH (2016) $n = 1,114$	LVEF ≤35% NYHA II/III (or IV if CRT is planned)	*Total mortality*: HR 0.87 (95% CI 0.68–1.12) compared with conventional HF therapy alone
SCD-HEFT (2005) $n = 2,521$ ICMP = 52% NICMP = 48%	HF for ≥3 months LVEF ≤35% NYHA II/III	*Total mortality*: HR 0.77 (95% CI 0.62–0.96) compared with conventional medical therapy alone

TABLE 4: Secondary prevention implantable cardioverter-defibrillator (ICD) therapy.

Name (N)	Inclusion criteria	Results
AVID (1016) 1997	VF or VT with syncope; VT with LVEF ≤40%	27% relative risk reduction in mortality with ICD compared to AADs in patients with LVEF ≤35%; no overall mortality benefit
CIDS (659) 2000	VF, resuscitated out-of-hospital cardiac arrest secondary to VF or VT; symptomatic VT with LVEF ≤35%; unwitnessed syncope with inducible VT	No significant difference in mortality between ICD and conventional therapy (although trend toward benefit in patients with LVEF ≤35%)
CASH (288) 2000	VF and VT	23% relative risk reduction in mortality with ICD compared to conventional therapy, but not statistically significant ($p = 0.081$)

death and total mortality compared to AAD therapy.[30-32] A meta-analysis of the three trials demonstrated a robust 50% relative risk reduction for arrhythmic death and 28% reduction for all-cause mortality with ICD therapy **(Table 4)**.[33]

Multiple analyses suggest that patients with impaired LV systolic function benefit most from ICD therapy, with no benefit if LVEF >35%. Despite these limitations, both ACC and ESC guidelines give class I recommendations for the use of ICD in secondary prevention for survivors of OHCA or hemodynamically significant VT, regardless of EF, after the identifiable and correctable transient causes of cardiac arrest have been ruled out.[22,25]

CONCLUSION

Sudden cardiac death remains a primary global health concern, with multifactorial etiology, including genetic and environmental factors. Advances in diagnostics and interventions, such as ICD are vital for prevention and management. Understanding the pathophysiology reveals that susceptible heart conditions combined with acute triggers often result in fatal arrhythmias. Prompt diagnostic evaluations and effective management strategies are crucial, including immediate resuscitation and appropriate postresuscitation care. Primary prevention through pharmacological interventions, ICD, and ongoing research is essential to further reduce SCD incidence and improve patient outcomes.

ONLINE REFERENCES

Please scan the QR code provided at the end of the table of contents for References of this chapter.

CHAPTER 208

Implantable Cardioverter Defibrillator Therapy: Critical Evaluation of Selection Criteria and Postimplant Care

Anish Bhargav, Raja J Selvaraj, Balachander Jayaraman

ABSTRACT

Sudden cardiac death is a leading cause of mortality in patients with left ventricular dysfunction. Implantable cardioverter defibrillator (ICD) is effective in patients at risk. These include patients with previous cardiac arrest or ventricular arrhythmias (secondary prevention) as well as patients without prior arrhythmias (primary prevention). In ischemic patients, the efficacy of ICD is without question. In patients with nonischemic cardiomyopathy, however, the evidence indicates lower mortality benefit as compared to patients with ischemic cardiomyopathy. Therefore, a nuanced approach is required in these patients, and other risk markers may be required. Apart from clinical assessment and echocardiography, cardiac MRI can guide selection of appropriate patients who are more likely to benefit from ICD implantation.

Keywords: Implantable cardioverter defibrillator, sudden cardiac death, primary prevention, secondary prevention, left ventricular dysfunction

INTRODUCTION

Sudden cardiac death (SCD) is a leading cause of mortality in patients with left ventricular (LV) dysfunction and accounts for 15–20% of global mortality.[1] Ventricular fibrillation (VF) is a common cause of SCD and is sometimes preceded by monomorphic or polymorphic ventricular tachycardia (VT). Implantable cardioverter defibrillator (ICD), first used in the 1980s, was designed to treat malignant ventricular arrhythmias and prevent arrhythmic sudden death.[2] Initially, ICD was offered to patients with VT for secondary prevention. This strategy was validated by the AVID (Antiarrhythmics versus Implantable Defibrillator) trial that showed significant reduction in mortality with ICD use compared with antiarrhythmic therapy.[3] Soon thereafter, studies were conducted to assess the utility of ICD for primary prevention. Most of the early studies were done in patients with ventricular dysfunction as a consequence of coronary artery disease (CAD) and ischemic cardiomyopathy (ICMP), in whom mortality reduction was consistently seen with the use of an ICD. This held true both in populations with specific risk markers, like in the MADIT (Multicenter Automatic Defibrillator Implantation Trial) and MUSTT (Multicenter Unsustained Tachycardia Trial) trials,[4,5] and in a population selected based on ejection fraction alone, like the MADIT II (Second Multicenter Automated Defibrillator Implantation Trial II) trial.[6]

The magnitude of benefit for primary prevention ICD in patients with nonischemic cardiomyopathy (NICMP) is more variable and with publication of the results of the DANISH trial, implantation of an ICD in these patients has become controversial. This is not surprising, however, because since the first use of ICD, the natural history of SCD has changed drastically with improvement in medical management and increased use of biventricular pacing in patients with heart failure (HF). These recent developments necessitated a closer scrutiny of the available evidence to further risk stratify and justify ICD implantation, especially for primary prevention indications in patients with NICMP.

IMPLANTABLE CARDIOVERTER DEFIBRILLATOR FOR SECONDARY PREVENTION

The most important step for successful ICD therapy is careful selection of appropriate patients. The term secondary prevention is used for the patients who have experienced a symptomatic life-threatening sustained VT or VF. While there are differences between guidelines for the primary prevention of SCD, they unanimously recommend ICD for secondary prevention of SCD.[7,8] The most important trial supporting this indication is the AVID trial that enrolled 1,016 patients with resuscitated VF arrest, sustained VT with syncope, or sustained hemodynamically unstable VT with a left ventricular ejection fraction (LVEF) ≤ 40% to receive either ICD implantation or class III antiarrhythmics, primarily amiodarone.[3] After 3 years of follow-up, there was a significant reduction in the primary end point of mortality in patients who received ICD, with a predominant benefit in those with reduced LVEF. Two other smaller RCTs were conducted in a similar group of patients, namely the Canadian Implantable Defibrillator Study (CIDS) and the Cardiac Arrest Study Hamburg (CASH).[9,10] Both the studies demonstrated a nonsignificant reduction in overall mortality in the ICD group. However, a meta-analysis of these three studies showed an absolute risk reduction in mortality of 3.5% per year with an effect that an ICD would have to be implanted in 29 patients to save 1 life per year of follow-up. This forms the foundation of secondary prevention ICD indications in current guidelines.

IMPLANTABLE CARDIOVERTER DEFIBRILLATOR FOR PRIMARY PREVENTION: ISCHEMIC CARDIOMYOPATHY

Identification of patients at a high risk of mortality and successful management with prophylactic ICD is a challenge. The MUSTT and MADIT were among the initial trials that helped establish the role of ICD in primary prevention.[4,5] The MUSTT trial included patients with CAD with LVEF ≤ 40% and asymptomatic nonsustained VT. In the patients with inducible VT at electrophysiology (EP) study, survival benefit was seen only in ICD recipients, while antiarrhythmic drugs did not reduce the risk of arrhythmic death. Similarly, the MADIT trial enrolled subjects with prior myocardial infarction (MI), LVEF ≤ 35%, nonsustained VT, and inducible VT at EP study not suppressible with intravenous procainamide. They were randomized to ICD (n = 95) or conventional drug therapy (n = 101): Amiodarone, digitalis, sotalol, disopyramide, mexiletine, procainamide, tocainide, and beta-blockers. In the ICD group, 15 patients (15.8%) died, whereas the conventional therapy group had 39 deaths (38.6%) with absolute risk reduction of 22.8% with the use of ICD so that 1 mortality is prevented if 4.4 patients are treated with ICD.

Reduced LVEF is the parameter most commonly associated with all-cause and cardiovascular mortality that indicates benefit with ICD. MADIT II and SCD-HeFT (Sudden Cardiac Death in Heart Failure Trial) were two landmark trials that established the efficacy of ICD therapy in patients with severely depressed LV systolic function.[6,11] The MADIT II trial included patients with a prior MI and a LVEF ≤ 30% who were randomized to receive an ICD (742 patients) or conventional medical therapy (490 patients). Interestingly, for the first time, inducible arrhythmia at EP study or NSVT was no longer a requirement for enrollment, thereby allowing the evaluation of a much broader population. Proportion of deaths in the defibrillator group and conventional therapy group was 14.2% and 19.8%, respectively, with an absolute risk reduction of 5.6% with the use of ICD with 17.8 patients requiring treatment with ICD to prevent 1 death over a period of 20 months. The SCD-HeFT trial was the largest study evaluating the role of primary prevention ICD and randomly assigned 2,521 patients with HF with ischemic or nonischemic substrate and LVEF ≤ 35% to the ICD arm (829 patients), amiodarone (845), or placebo (847). ICD therapy reduced the risk of mortality by 23%, whereas placebo and amiodarone groups were not associated with any decrease in the risk of death. There was no difference in benefit with regards to the etiology of HF, i.e., ischemic or nonischemic patients. The results of these two trials form the foundation of guidelines that recommend primary prevention ICD in patients with symptomatic HF (NYHA classes II–III) and LVEF ≤ 35% and asymptomatic patients with previous MI and LVEF < 30%.

IMPLANTABLE CARDIOVERTER DEFIBRILLATOR FOR PRIMARY PREVENTION: NONISCHEMIC CARDIOMYOPATHY

Nonischemic cardiomyopathy (NICMP) refers to patients without CAD in whom the ventricular dysfunction is due to varied causes. There are only a few studies in literature that focused exclusively on NICMP. The Cardiomyopathy Trial (CAT) followed 104 patients with idiopathic dilated cardiomyopathy and ejection fraction <30% after ICD implantation (50 patients) or medical management (54 patients).[12] At a mean follow-up of 5.5 years, total mortality was not different between the two groups. In the AMIOVIRT trial, 103 patients with NICMP and nonsustained VT were randomized to treatment with amiodarone or an ICD.[13] There was no difference in survival at 3 years of follow-up. Thus, the first studies of ICD in patients with NICMP showed that, at least with the small number of patients, no significant survival benefit of ICD could be demonstrated as compared to medical management.

This was followed by larger studies such as the Defibrillators in Nonischemic Cardiomyopathy Treatment Evaluation (DEFINITE) trial and SCD-Heft trial. The DEFINITE trial randomized 458 patients to ICD or medical therapy alone.[14] At 2 years, total mortality was higher in the medical management group (14.1% vs. 7.9%), but did not reach statistical significance. A significant reduction in risk of sudden death was, however, noted. In the SCD-HeFT trial, there was a significant mortality reduction with the use of ICDs in the overall study population.[11] About half the patients in this study had NICMP. While there was reduction in mortality with a hazard ratio of 0.73 in this group, this failed to reach statistical significance. Thus, these two large trials, while showing a trend toward mortality reduction with the use of ICDs in patients with NICMP, did not appear to have an adequate number of patients for this to achieve statistical significance. A pooled analysis of the primary prevention trials[15] showed a significant 31% reduction in all-cause mortality with the use of ICD compared to medical management alone and formed the basis on which this indication was added to the guidelines.

The DANISH study, published in 2016, was a large trial, specifically targeting patients with NICMP.[16] When 556 patients underwent implantation of an ICD and 560 patients were treated medically, at a mean follow-up of 67 months, total mortality was not different between the two groups (120 vs. 131 patients, respectively). Unlike the initial, smaller trials that were underpowered to detect a small benefit, the negative results in this large trial raised questions about the usefulness of ICD implantation in patients with NICMP. A closer look suggests that the difference in results compared to earlier trials was driven mainly by three factors—improvement in overall outcomes in these patients due to better medical management, increased use of CRT with attendant reduction in mortality, and an older patient population. Keeping in line with the results of DANISH trial, the 2021 ESC HF guidelines downgraded the indications for primary prevention ICD in symptomatic patients with NICMP from earlier class I (LOE: B) recommendation in the 2016 ESC HF guidelines to a class IIa (LOE: A) recommendation.[8] However, American Heart Association (AHA) guidelines still make no differentiation between ICMP and NICMP with both categories having a class I, LOE A recommendation for ICD implantation.[7]

Trials of CRT-P versus CRT-D for Nonischemic Cardiomyopathy

With the availability of CRT as an effective treatment option for patients with NICMP and a broad QRS, a decision has to be taken if a patient would be offered CRT alone (CRT-P) or a device that combines a defibrillator with CRT (CRT-D). Almost all patients with NICMP eligible for CRT-P implantation are also eligible for an ICD by guidelines. However, most of these patients have significant improvement in cardiac function after CRT placement and a few may even show complete normalization (super-responders). In such responders, the improvement in LV function is expected to be associated with a significant reduction in risk of sudden death, making the benefit from an ICD questionable. In the Comparison of Medical Therapy, Pacing, and Defibrillation in Heart failure (COMPANION) study, patients with both ICMP and NICMP showed a benefit with either CRT-P or CRT-D compared to medical management.[17] However, this trial was not powered to detect a difference between these devices. In the DANISH trial, 58% of patients in each group received a CRT in addition to ICD or medical management. In this subset of patients, there was no difference in outcomes suggesting lack of incremental benefit from adding a defibrillator in those receiving a CRT device. In two recently published retrospective analyses of registry data, one from the United States[18] and one from Europe,[19] no benefit was seen with CRT-D implantation over CRT-P implantation in patients with NICMP.

Taking a Decision

Today, in the post-DANISH era, how should the patient with NICMP be managed with regard to ICD use? In patients with NICMP, an EF < 35%, and HF (NYHA class II or III), the ACC/AHA and the European guidelines indicate ICD implantation as a class I indication and a class IIa indication, respectively. These recommendations have justification in the form of a meta-analysis[20] and a Cochrane review[21] which confirm mortality benefit with ICD implant in patients with NICMP even when data from DANISH are included.

However, a survey of cardiologists in various European centers found that the use of ICDs in this group of patients was less and had decreased after the publication of DANISH despite the guidelines, while use in ICMP was more prevalent.[22] This reflects the practice of most cardiologists who view the group of patients with NICMP as less likely to benefit from ICD as compared to patients with ICMP.

Combining the results of DANISH with earlier trials is a questionable strategy. The results of DANISH have to be viewed in isolation because they represent outcomes seen with contemporary management unlike the older studies. It can even be argued that there might be further improvement in outcomes after DANISH due to the introduction of newer therapies like angiotensin receptor inhibitor–neprilysin inhibitor combination (ARNI). Perhaps the message to learn from DANISH is that implantation of ICD in an unselected population with NICMP has little benefit. What is needed is a method to risk stratify these patients and identify a group who are more likely to benefit from ICDs.

Risk Stratification

This is an evolving field and the best approach is not known at present. We will present here only a brief overview of the approaches to risk stratification.

The simplest and first approach is to use clinical scores. There was a clear interaction with age in DANISH, suggesting that younger patients are likely to benefit more. Patients should also be evaluated for comorbidities as patients more likely to die of noncardiovascular causes or from HF benefit less from ICDs. In this regard, clinical scores like the Seattle Heart Failure Model[23] which provides survival estimates for patients with HF and the MADIT-ICD Benefit Score[24] which incorporated raw data from all the MADIT trials could be useful.

Electrocardiographic markers have been evaluated for risk stratification in addition to ejection fraction. However, markers like signal-averaged ECG (SAECG), T-wave alternans (TWA), and heart rate turbulence (HRT) have shown conflicting results in various studies and are not recommended for regular use at present.

Circulating biomarkers have been evaluated for risk stratification and have not performed well,[25] but proteomics-based approaches may perform better and are being studied. Similarly there is a possibility that genetic studies may identify specific mutations associated with a higher risk.

At present, the most promising approach appears to be cardiac magnetic resonance imaging (CMRI). Mid myocardial fibrosis identified by late gadolinium enhancement (LGE) using CMRI is a promising tool to identify patients at risk for sudden death.[26] In patients requiring CRT, midwall LGE also identified patients likely to benefit from CRT-D.[27] This is an area of active investigation.

POSTIMPLANT CARE

After ensuring proper selection and implantation of ICD, it is important to have disciplined postimplant care of the patient in order to have desired results from the procedure. It is clear at this point that apart from preoperative antibiotics, there is no role of IV or oral antibiotics thereafter and hence any antibiotic beyond the perioperative period is not recommended. Maintaining a proper environment of asepsis during the procedure along with preoperative IV antibiotics alone is enough to reduce the risk of infection. Once-daily dressing of the implant site for 3 days is usually enough to ensure proper healing. Restricting strenuous activity and lifting of the hands above the level of the shoulder for 4–6 weeks are required to ensure proper lead maturation without dislodgment.

The next important aspect of the care is programming of the device. Conservative programming with long delays between detection and therapy delivery reduces the risk of inappropriate and appropriate but unnecessary shocks and is hence recommended. Generally, for primary prevention, ICD is programmed to tachycardia treatment zone > 200 bpm. For secondary prevention, programming should be adapted according to the patient's specific needs.[8]

After discharge of the patient, an initial in-person follow-up is necessary to detect any complications such as infection, bleeding, and lead dislodgment. The first follow-up visit is usually recommended 2–12 weeks after implantation. Subsequently, in-person or remote monitoring is recommended every 3–6 months.[28] Remote monitoring increases follow-up adherence and provides earlier detection of actionable events without compromising safety. In devices approaching elective replacement, the frequency of remote transmissions should be increased to every 1–3 months.

CONCLUSION

In contemporary practice, ICD devices have evolved significantly from defibrillation-only devices to more advanced multichamber devices with enhanced features. The benefit of ICD is not uniform and proper risk stratification and patient selection are critical, especially in resource-limited countries with an increased risk of non-SCD deaths such as India. ICD remains important to reduce the risk of sudden death in patients with previous cardiac arrest or ventricular arrhythmias (secondary prevention). In ischemic patients with HF who meet the criteria for ICD therapy as primary prevention, treatment with ICD remains the cornerstone in SCD prevention. In patients with NICMP, the bulk of evidence indicates lower mortality benefit as compared to patients with ICMP. Therefore, ICD implantation in all these patients may not be warranted, despite the current guidelines. Selection of patients who are more likely to benefit from ICD implantation is essential. Apart from clinical assessment and echocardiography, CMRI appears to be promising in this regard.

ONLINE REFERENCES

Please scan the QR code provided at the end of the table of contents for References of this chapter.

SECTION 19

Cardiorenal Diabetes

Section Outline

CHAPTER

209

Top Ten Papers in Diabetes and Metabolic Disorders: 2023–2024

Ravi Vishnu Prasad

ABSTRACT

Cardiovascular diseases (CVDs) are the main cause of death among patients with type 2 diabetes mellitus (T2DM). A close link exists between T2DM and CVD, which is the most prevalent cause of morbidity and mortality in diabetic patients. Cardiovascular (CV) risk factors such as obesity, hypertension, and dyslipidemia are common in patients with T2DM, placing them at increased risk for cardiac events. In addition, many studies have found biological mechanisms associated with T2DM that independently increase the risk of CVD in diabetic patients. Therefore, targeting CV risk factors in patients with T2DM is critical to minimize the long-term CV complications of the disease. To effectively prevent the development of CVDs in T2DM, considerable effort has been made to explore novel preventive approaches, individualized glycemic control, and CV risk management together with recently developed glucose-lowering agents and lipid-lowering drugs. In this chapter, we are describing top ten works in diabetes and metabolic disease of the year 2023–2024.

Keywords: Diabetes, cardiovascular disease

INTRODUCTION

The year 2023–2024 witnessed major guidelines, trials, risk scores, new drugs, epidemiological studies, and research that make diabetic treatment and management easier than before. These are discussed in detail as follows below.

GUIDELINES FOR THE MANAGEMENT OF CARDIOVASCULAR DISEASE IN PATIENTS WITH DIABETES

This was published by European Society of Cardiology in 2023.[1]

This guideline focused on two major aspects:

1. Identification and evaluation of patients with cardiovascular disease (CVD) and type 2 diabetes mellitus (T2DM).
2. Diabetes and chronic kidney disease (CKD).

The T2DM patients are prone to develop increased risk of CVD as well as CKD, and both these comorbidities in a given patient have a major impact on the prognosis as well as treatment strategies. Therefore, we must give utmost importance to identifying patients with diabetes and CVD as well as patients with diabetes and CKD.[2]

- Due to high prevalence of undetected diabetes, it is recommended that all patients with CVD are screened for the presence of diabetes using fasting plasma glucose and HbA1c.
- Presence of CVD in diabetic patients is assessed by history and symptoms suggestive of atherosclerotic cardiovascular disease (ASCVD).
- Evaluation of heart failure (HF) symptoms and signs of HF is recommended at each clinical encounter in all patients with diabetes.
- Patients with diabetes should be regularly screened for the presence of CKD by assessing estimated glomerular filtration rate and urine albumin-to-creatinine ratios (UACR).
- It is recommended to categorize CV risk in patients with T2DM based on the presence of ASCVD or severe target organ damage, or in absence of ASCVD or severe target organ damage—based on the results of the dedicated T2DM CVD risk score, *SCORE2-Diabetes*.
- Glucose-lowering medications with proven benefit should be given preference over drugs without proven CV benefit or safety.
- It is recommended to switch drugs from glucose-lowering medications without proven benefit or safety to drugs with proven benefit.

- To reduce CV risk in patients with T2DM and ACSVD, it is recommended to treat with a GLP-1 receptor agonist and an SGLT-2 inhibitor with proven benefit, on top of standard of care and independent of glucose control or target HbA1c.
- In patients with HF, irrespective of ejection fraction, it is recommended that patients with T2DM are treated with an SGLT-2 inhibitor on top of standard of care to reduce HF-related endpoints such as HF hospitalization or CV death.
- Patients with T2DM and CKD should be treated with an SGLT-2 inhibitor and the nonsteroidal mineralocorticoid receptor antagonist finerenone to reduce both CV and kidney failure risk. In addition, these patients should receive a statin-based regimen, treatment with angiotensin-converting enzyme (ACE) inhibitors or angiotensin-II receptor blockers, and appropriate blood pressure control (≤130/80 mm Hg).

Overall, the management of CVD in patients with diabetes requires an interdisciplinary approach to implement evidence-based, person-centered strategies to reduce the burden of disease and improve the prognosis **(Fig. 1)**.

SCORE2-DIABETES RISK SCORE

Patients with T2DM have high risk of developing CVD. The SCORE2-Diabetes Working Group and the European Society of Cardiology Cardiovascular Risk Collaboration developed a T2DM-specific risk score (SCORE2-Diabetes) to estimate the 10-year risk of fatal and nonfatal CV events (MI and stroke)

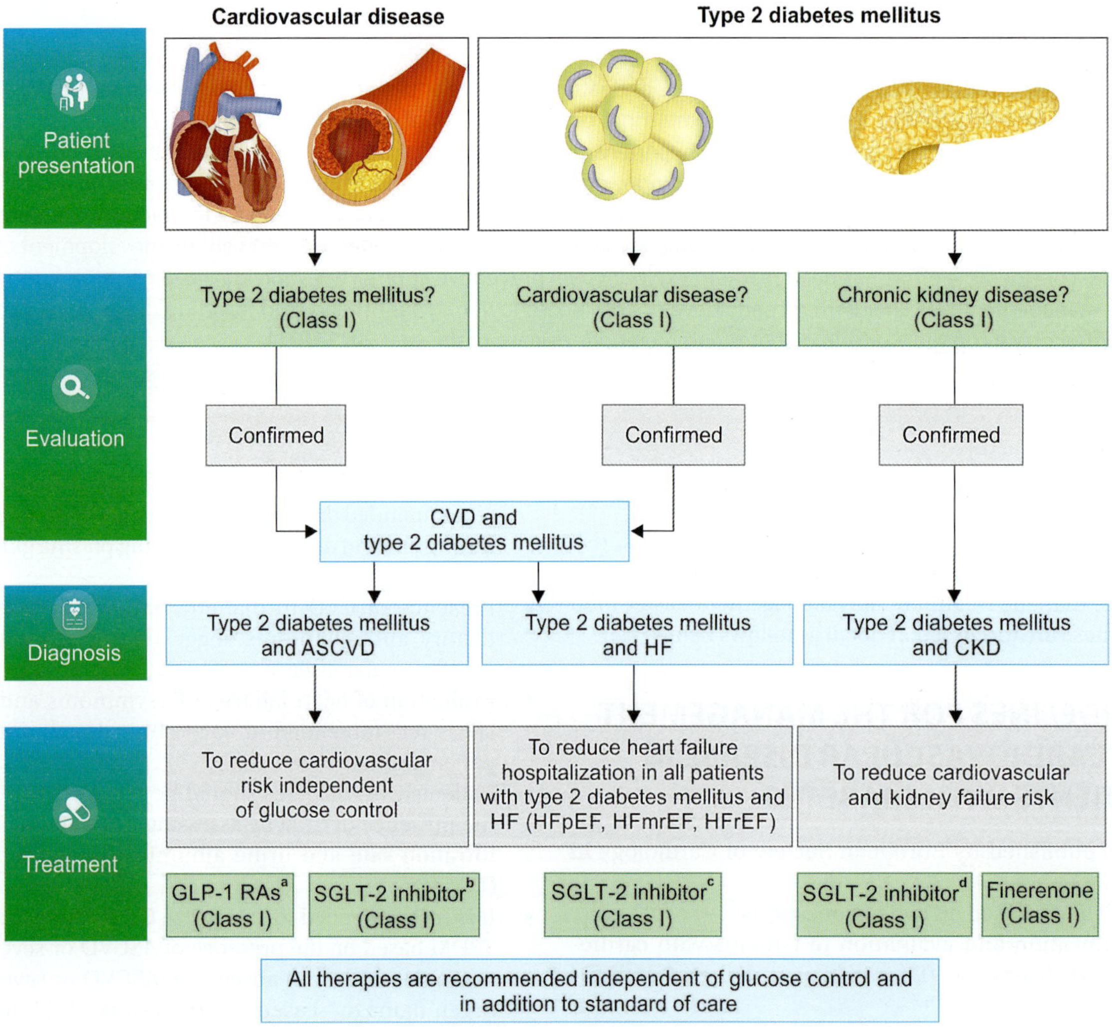

[a]*GLP-1 RAs with proven cardiovascular benefit:* Liraglutide, semaglutide sc, dulaglutide, and efpeglenatide.
[b]*SGLT-2 inhibitors with proven cardiovascular benefit:* Empagliflozin, canagliflozin, dapagliflozin, and sotagliflozin.
[c]Empagliflozin, dapagliflozin, and sotagliflozin in HFrEF; empagliflozin and dapagliflozin in HFpEF and HFmrEF.
[d]Canagliflozin, empagliflozin, and dapagliflozin.[1]

FIG. 1: Management of cardiovascular disease in patients with T2DM.

in Europe **(Fig. 2)**.[3] It involves information on conventional CVD risk factors (age, smoking status, systolic blood pressure, total cholesterol, and high-density lipoprotein-cholesterol) with diabetes-specific information (age at diabetes diagnosis, HbA1c, and estimated glomerular filtration rate) and is validated for patients aged ≥40–69 years without ASCVD or severe target organ damage. According to the results of SCORE2-Diabetes, patients are categorized into those at low (<5%), moderate (5 to <10%), high (10 to <20%), and very high risk (≥20%) **(Fig. 3)**.

CARDIOVASCULAR DISEASE AND RISK FACTORS IN SWEDISH STUDY

An important epidemiological study based on the Swedish cohort looked at trends for CV events and risk factors in 679,072 individuals with T2DM and 2,643,800 matched controls from 2001 to 2019.[4] Among individuals with T2DM, the analysis demonstrated a decrease in the incident rates per 10,000 person-years in 2019 as compared to 2001 for acute MI, cerebrovascular disease, and HF. Interestingly, around 2013, a plateau for the incidence of HF was observed with a trend that persisted until 2019. Overall, the CVD incidence in patients with T2DM was much higher compared to matched controls. The data also suggest that body mass index (BMI) alone explained >30% of HF risk in T2DM patients. This study demonstrates that the rates for ASCVD and HF are generally decreasing but over the last 10 years the incidence of HF in patients with T2DM has plateaued with no such effect in subjects without diabetes.

DAPAGLIFLOZIN, HEART FAILURE, AND PERIPHERAL ARTERY DISEASE

In more than 11,000 patients with HF enrolled in the DAPA-HF and DELIVER trials, the benefit of dapagliflozin,

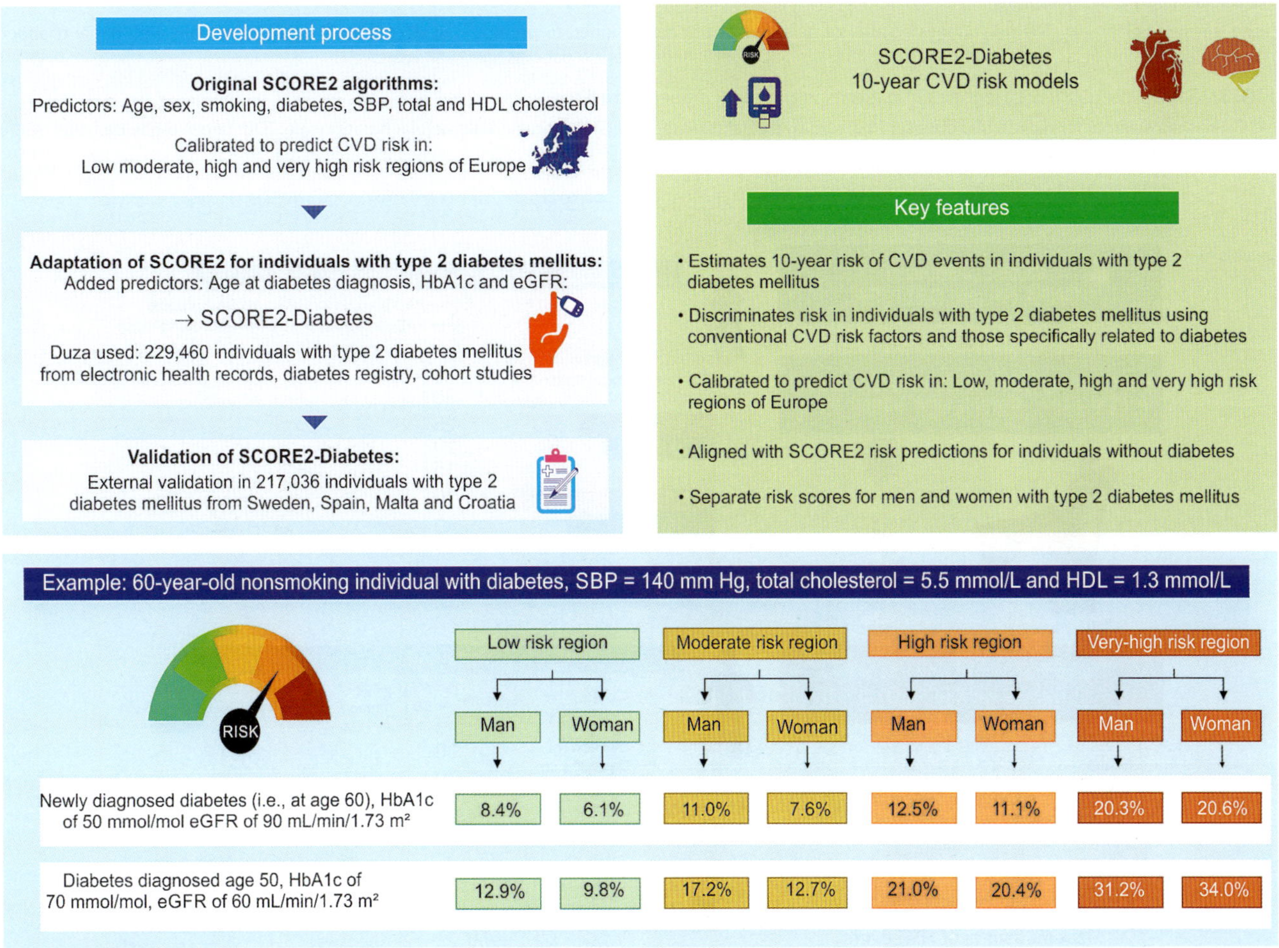

FIG. 2: SCORE2-Diabetes accurately estimates CVD risk in individuals with type 2 diabetes mellitus. It extends SCORE2, aligning CVD risk prediction for those with and without diabetes, while accounting for variation in risk across Europe. This facilitates the identification of individuals at high CVD risk.

(CVD: cardiovascular disease risk; eGFR: estimated glomerular filtration rate; SBP: systolic blood pressure)

compared with placebo, on the primary outcome and key secondary outcomes was consistent in patients with and without peripheral artery disease (PAD) **(Fig. 4)**. While amputations and other adverse events were more frequent in PAD patients, they were not more common with dapagliflozin, compared with placebo, irrespective of PAD status. In both trials, the primary outcome was the composite of worsening HF or CV death, and amputation was a prespecified safety outcome. This is an important finding because early SGLT-2 inhibitors trials generated uncertainty about the balance of benefits and risks of SGLT-2 inhibitors use in patients with PAD.[5]

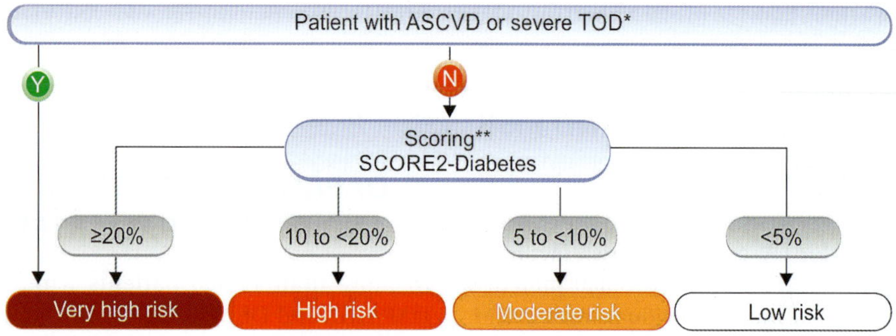

* Severe TOD is defined as eGFR <45 mL/min/1.73 m^2 irrespective of albuminuria; or eGFR 45–59 mL/min/1.73 m^2 and microalbuminuria (UACR 30–300 mg/g; stage A2); or proteinuria (UACR >300 mg/g; stage A3), or presence of microvascular disease in at least three different sites [e.g., microalbuminuria (stage A2) plus retinopathy plus neuropathy].

** The thresholds (10-year CVD risk) suggested are not definitive but rather designed to prompt joint decision-making conversations with patients about intensity of treatment, as well as additional interventions. SCORE2-Diabetes refers to patients aged ≥40 years.[1]

FIG. 3: Cardiovascular risk categories in patients with type 2 diabetes mellitus.

(ASCVD: atherosclerotic cardiovascular disease; CVD: cardiovascular disease risk; eGFR: estimated glomerular filtration rate; TOD: target-organ damage; UACR: urinary albumin-to-creatinine ratio).

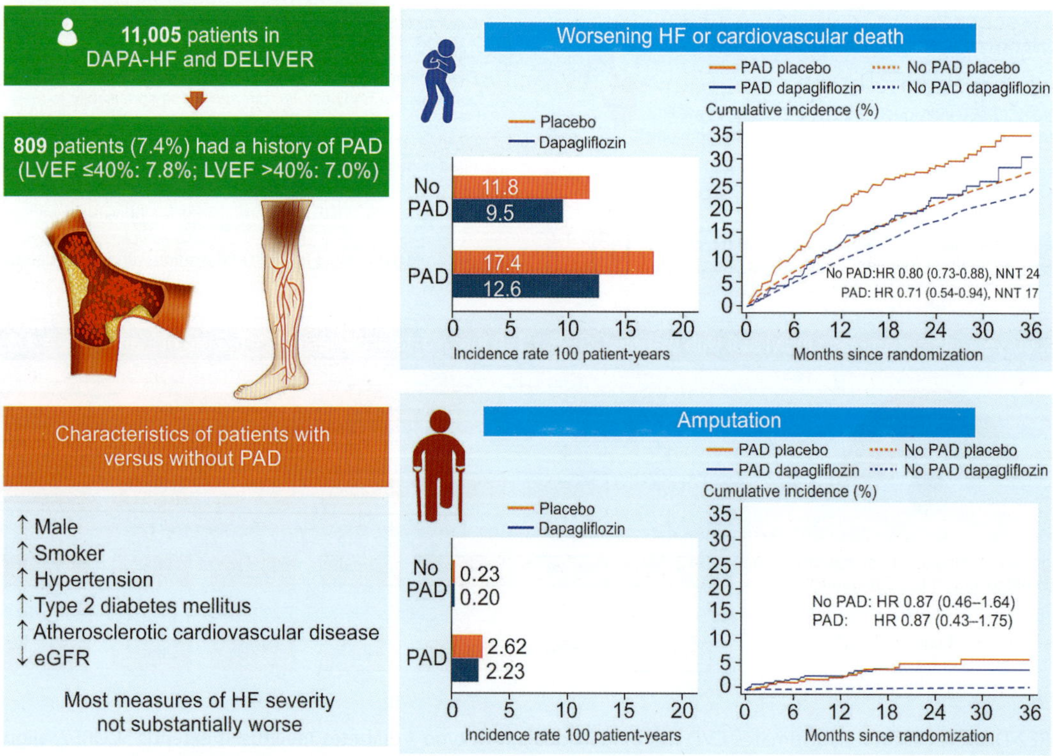

FIG. 4: Dapagliflozin, heart failure, peripheral artery disease, and amputation.[5]

RELATION OF SOCIAL ISOLATION, LONELINESS, AND CARDIOVASCULAR DISEASE IN DIABETES PATIENTS

Is there any association of loneliness or social isolation with CVD in diabetes and their relative importance compared to traditional risk factors? Loneliness, but not social isolation, was associated with a higher risk of CVD in diabetes, and ranked higher for predicting CVD than traditional lifestyle factors. The detrimental effect of loneliness on CVD risk was greater than additive (p for additive interaction = 0.005). Loneliness in diabetic patients is a potent and neglected risk factor for CVD. Wang et al. conducted population-based cohort study, which addressed the association of loneliness or social isolation with CVD in patients with diabetes and their relative importance compared to traditional risk factors[6] **(Fig. 5)**. A better understanding of the mechanisms driving the effect of loneliness on CVD risk in vulnerable population is highly needed. Nonetheless, these findings should prompt physicians to evaluate the role of psychosocial factors as biomarkers of CVD.

SEMAGLUTIDE IN PATIENTS WITH HEART FAILURE WITH PRESERVED EJECTION FRACTION AND OBESITY PHENOTYPE

The obesity phenotype of heart failure with preserved ejection fraction (HFpEF) is associated with reduced physical function and worse quality of life and represents an unmet treatment need. Therefore, it was postulated that semaglutide with its benefits on weight loss, inflammation, and cardiometabolic risk factors could be an attractive approach to treat obese people with HFpEF. *STEP-HFpEF* randomized 529 individuals with HFpEF and BMI ≥30 kg/m^2 to 2.4 mg semaglutide weekly versus placebo for 52 weeks.[8] Semaglutide significantly improved HF-related symptoms and physical limitation measured by the Kansas City Cardiomyopathy Questionnaire clinical summary score, exercise function measured by 6-minute walking distance, and reduced inflammation and body weight. These findings represent a significant advancement in the management of

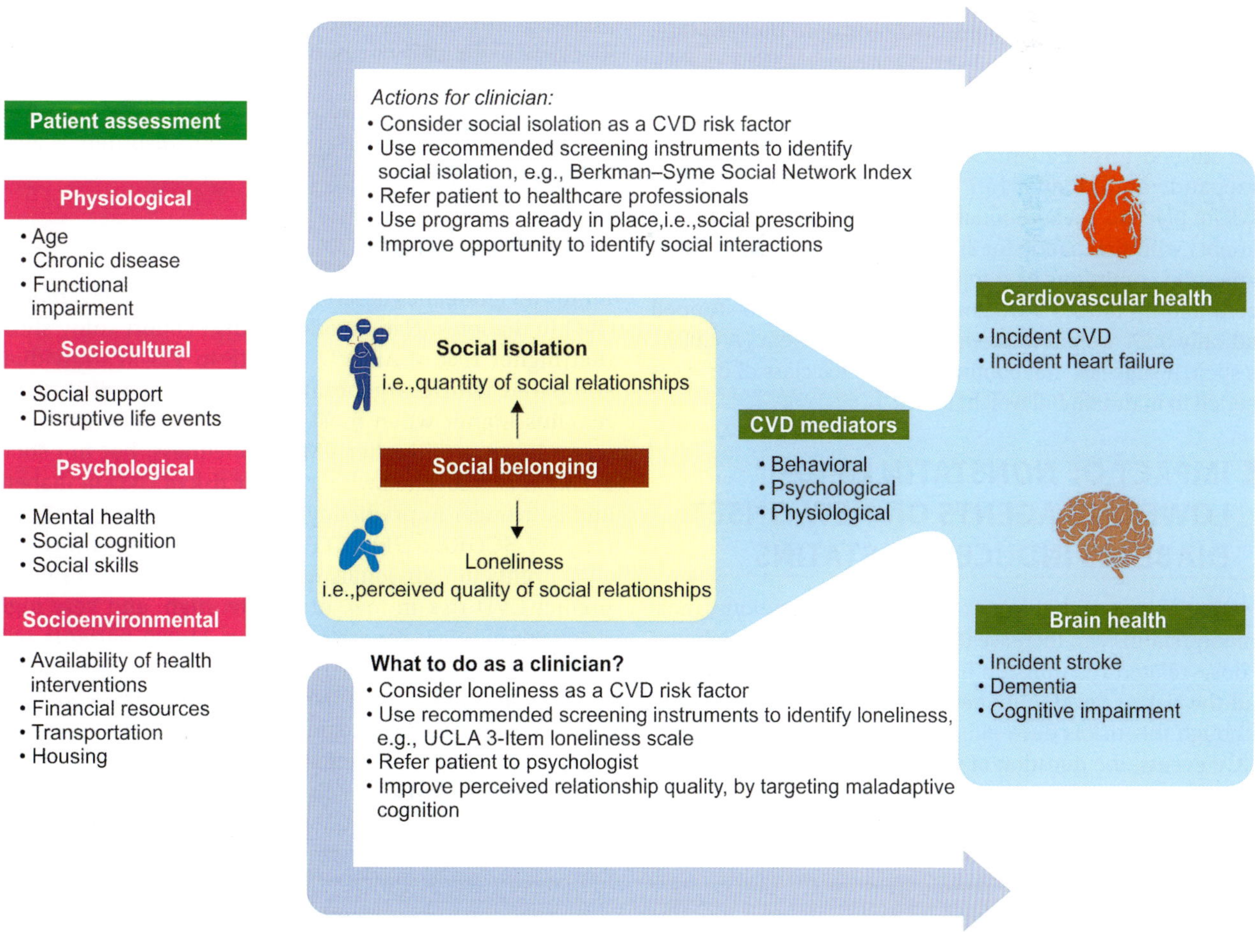

FIG. 5: Loneliness, social isolation, and cardiovascular diseases.[7]

the obesity phenotype of HFpEF. It is important to note that STEP-HFpEF was not powered for clinical events and whether semaglutide reduces "hard" outcomes in HF remains largely undefined. Nevertheless, this trial unmasks an important role for semaglutide in the HF treatment arena.

OBESITY, GLUCAGON-LIKE PEPTIDE-1 RECEPTOR AGONIST, AND CARDIOVASCULAR DISEASE

The *SELECT* trial studied patients with obesity, but not overt diabetes.[9] The trial randomized 17,604 patients who were overweight or had obesity (BMI ≥27 kg/m^2 and established ASCVD) but without diabetes to semaglutide 2.4 mg or placebo. The primary endpoint of CV events (cardiovascular death, MI, or stroke) was reduced by semaglutide by 20%, MI alone by 28%, and all-cause mortality by 19% over a mean follow-up period of 3.3 years. The expected gastrointestinal side effects were observed.

SURMOUNT SERIES

The *SURMOUNT* trials evaluated tirzepatide, i.e., a dual agonist, a glucose-dependent insulinotropic polypeptide, and glucagon-like peptide-1 receptor agonist (GLP-1 RA). The first trial in patients with obesity found an average 21% weight loss versus 3% for placebo.[10] The SURMOUNT-2 trial studied 1,514 patients with diabetes and obesity with tirzepatide and found a 15.7% reduction in weight versus 3.3% for placebo. An additional study, SURMOUNT-4, treated patients with tirzepatide for 36 weeks and then randomized patients to continuing or stopping. Those who continued the agent had up to 25.3% weight loss, but those who stopped had only 9.9% weight loss remaining after a year ($p < .001$). As such, it suggests that continuation of this class of drugs is needed to maintain full weight loss.[11]

IMPACT OF NONSTATIN LIPID-LOWERING AGENTS ON NEW-ONSET DIABETES INDUCED BY STATINS

Another aspect of diabetes is that some medications, most notably, statins can increase the risk of developing diabetes. A dose-related relationship has been seen between statins and the risk of developing new-onset diabetes (NOD), and although this risk is outweighed by a benefit on prevention of CV events, the question of whether other classes of lipid-lowering agents have the same risk is thus important.

The *CLEAR OUTCOMES* trial was a trial of nearly 14,000 patients with statin intolerance that found a benefit of a nonstatin agent bempedoic acid on CV outcomes.[12] An analysis by baseline glycemic status showed benefits on CV outcomes across those with diabetes, prediabetes, and normoglycemia. Importantly, bempedoic acid did not increase risk of NOD nor did it worsen HbA1c and was associated with modest weight reductions. As such, the efficacy and cardiometabolic safety profile of bempedoic acid make it a clinical option for those with and without diabetes. Similarly, no increase in NOD has recently been seen with ezetimibe as also with PCSK9 inhibitors, so use of any of the nonstatin lipid-lowering agents avoids the risk of NOD.[13]

SCAN ENZYME: NEW TARGET TO TREAT DIABETES

The researchers discovered a novel "carrier" enzyme [called SNO-CoA-assisted nitrosylase (SCAN)] that attaches nitric oxide to proteins, including the receptor for insulin action. They found that the SCAN enzyme was essential for normal insulin action, but also discovered heightened SCAN activity in diabetic patients and mice with diabetes. Mouse models without the SCAN enzyme appeared to be shielded from diabetes, suggesting that too much nitric oxide on proteins may be a cause of such diseases. Blocking this enzyme protects from diabetes, but the implications extend to many diseases likely caused by novel enzymes that add nitric oxide.[14]

A graphical summary of the year in cardiovascular medicine 2023—diabetes and metabolic disorders is given in **Figure 6**.

CONCLUSION

European guidelines described in detail the management of CVD in diabetes. Nationwide Swedish cohort study shows that higher risk of ASCVD and HF in T2DM individuals compared with the general population and risk for HF remains higher when most or all risk factors are within target because of higher BMIs. Loneliness, but not social isolation is associated with a higher risk of CVD in diabetes and is stronger in predicting CVD than traditional lifestyle factors. SCORE2-DIABETES estimates 10-year risk of CVD events in individuals with T2DM and is calibrated to predict CVD risk in low, moderate, high, and very high-risk regions of Europe. More than 11,000 patients with HF enrolled in the DAPA-HF and DELIVER trials showing the benefit and safety of dapagliozin in patients with and without PAD. In HFpEF, semaglutide improves HF-related symptoms, physical function and results in greater weight loss compared with placebo. The SELECT trial provides evidence of improved CV outcomes with GLP-1 RA in overweight patients with preexisting ASCVD but no history of diabetes. The SURMOUNT 2 and 4 trials with tirzepatide, a glucose-dependent insulinotropic polypeptide (GIP), and

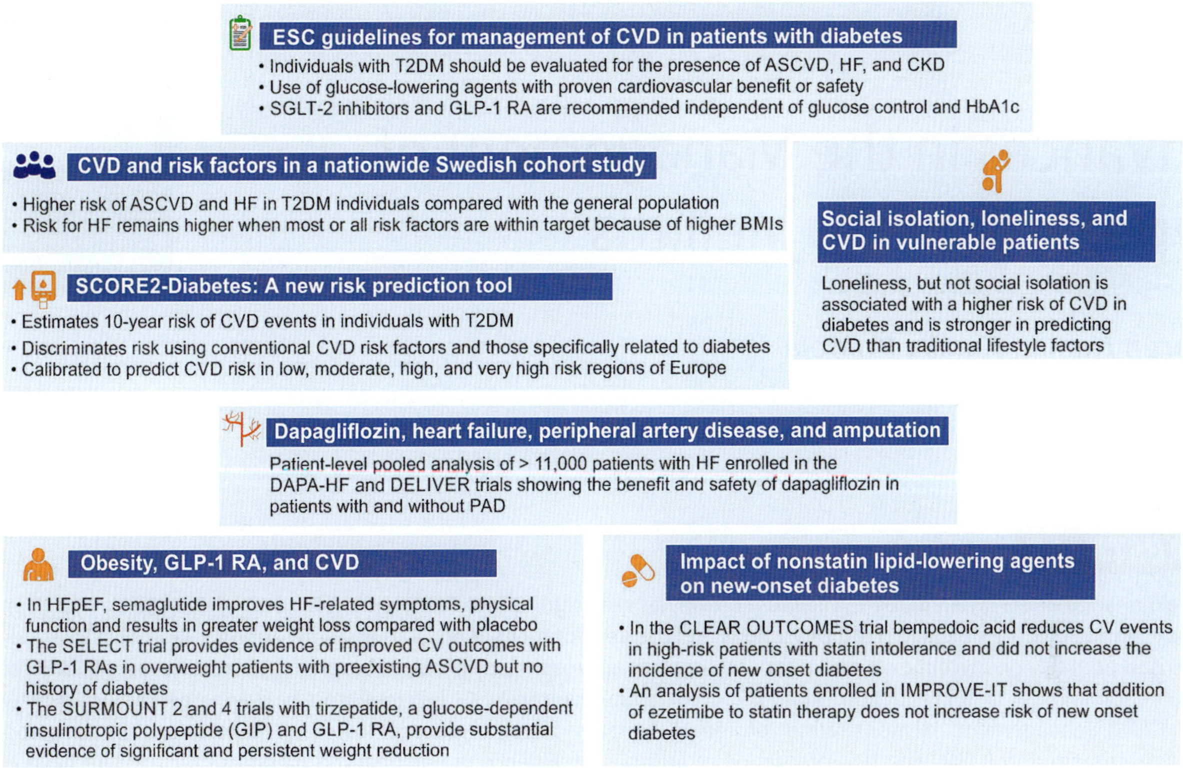

FIG. 6: Graphical summary. The year in cardiovascular medicine 2023: Diabetes and metabolic disorders.[1]

GLP-1 RA, provide substantial evidence of significant and persistent weight reduction. In the CLEAR OUTCOMES trial, bempedoic acid reduced CV events in high-risk patients with statin intolerance and did not increase the incidence of NOD. Addition of ezetimibe to statin therapy does not increase risk of NOD.

ONLINE REFERENCES

Please scan the QR code provided at the end of the table of contents for References of this chapter.

CHAPTER 210

Advances in the Management of Type 2 Diabetes Mellitus

Barun Kumar, Kanika Kukreja

ABSTRACT

The management of type 2 diabetes mellitus (T2DM) has seen significant advancements in recent years, driven by a deeper understanding of the disease's pathophysiology and the development of novel therapeutic agents. Traditional treatments focused primarily on glycemic control, but contemporary approaches emphasize comprehensive cardiovascular and renal protection and risk factor reduction. Sodium-glucose cotransporter-2 (SGLT-2) inhibitors have emerged as a cornerstone in T2DM management, demonstrating profound benefits beyond glucose lowering. Innovations in continuous glucose monitoring (CGM) and the integration of artificial intelligence in personalized diabetes mellitus care have also revolutionized patient management, enabled real-time data-driven adjustments, and improved glycemic outcomes. This chapter reviews the latest pharmacological therapies, technological advancements, and evidence-based guidelines that have collectively enhanced the management strategies for T2DM.

Keywords: Type 2 diabetes mellitus, SGLT-2 inhibitors, GLP-1 receptor agonists, continuous glucose monitoring, personalized medicine, advances, telemedicine

INTRODUCTION

Type 2 diabetes mellitus (T2DM) is characterized by insulin resistance and relative insulin deficiency, leading to hyperglycemia. It is a multifactorial disease influenced by genetic, environmental, and lifestyle factors. T2DM is associated with numerous complications, including cardiovascular disease, neuropathy, nephropathy, and retinopathy, significantly impacting patients' quality of life and posing a substantial burden on healthcare systems globally.[1] However, ongoing research and technological advancements have revolutionized the management of T2DM, offering new treatment modalities and strategies to improve patient outcomes. The management of T2DM has been revolutionized by recent advances in pharmacology and technology, including the development of drugs that improve insulin sensitivity or enhance insulin secretion. The ongoing research and technological advancements have revolutionized the management of T2DM, offering new treatment modalities and strategies to improve patient outcomes.

RECENT ADVANCEMENTS IN PHARMACOLOGICAL INTERVENTIONS

Pharmacotherapy remains a cornerstone in the management of T2DM. Recent years have seen the introduction of several novel classes of antidiabetic medications, expanding the therapeutic options available to clinicians and patients. These include:

- *SGLT-2 inhibitors:* Sodium-glucose cotransporter-2 (SGLT-2) inhibitors represent a breakthrough in T2DM management by promoting glycosuria and lowering blood glucose levels independent of insulin secretion. Additionally, SGLT-2 inhibitors have demonstrated cardiovascular and renal benefits, making them valuable agents in patients with T2DM and established cardiovascular disease or chronic kidney disease. SGLT-2 inhibitors, such as empagliflozin, dapagliflozin, and canagliflozin, have gained prominence. SGLT-2 inhibitors reduce the risk of MACE across a broad range of patients irrespective of ASCVD, diabetes mellitus, kidney function, or other major clinical characteristics at baseline.[2]

- *Glucagon-like peptide-1 (GLP-1) receptor agonists:* GLP-1 receptor agonists mimic the action of endogenous GLP-1, stimulating insulin secretion and inhibiting glucagon release in a glucose-dependent manner.[3] These agents not only improve glycemic control but also promote weight loss and have shown cardiovascular benefits. GLP-1 receptor agonists like semaglutide and dulaglutide have been highlighted for their dual benefits of glycemic control and weight loss. Oral formulations of semaglutide have also been introduced, offering a noninjectable option with a reasonable reduction in HbA1c and weight.[4]
- *DPP-4 inhibitors:* Dipeptidyl peptidase-4 (DPP-4) inhibitors (alogliptin, sitagliptin, saxagliptin, linagliptin) enhance endogenous GLP-1 activity by inhibiting its degradation, thereby improving glycemic control with a low risk of hypoglycemia and weight neutrality.[5]
- *Insulin analogs:* Advances in insulin therapy have led to the development of long-acting basal insulin analogs and rapid-acting insulin analogs, offering more flexibility and improved glycemic control compared to traditional insulins.

COMBINATION THERAPIES

Fixed-ratio combinations of GLP-1 receptor agonists and basal insulin (e.g., iGlarLixi and iDegLira[6]) have been developed to simplify treatment regimens and enhance efficacy.[7]

TECHNOLOGICAL ADVANCEMENTS

- *Continuous glucose monitoring (CGM):* Advances in CGM technology, such as the Freestyle Libre and Dexcom G6 systems, provide real-time glucose monitoring, leading to improved glycemic control and reduced hypoglycemic episodes **(Table 1)**.

  Real-time CGM (rtCGM) or intermittently scanned CGM (isCGM) should be offered for diabetes mellitus management in adults with diabetes mellitus on multiple daily injections (MDI) or continuous subcutaneous insulin infusion (CSII) who are capable of using the devices safely (either by themselves or with a caregiver). The choice of device should be made based on the individual's circumstances, preferences, and needs.[9]
- *Automated insulin delivery systems:* Hybrid closed-loop systems, often referred to as "artificial pancreas" systems, integrate CGM with insulin pumps to automate insulin delivery. The MiniMed 670G and Tandem tX2 with Control-IQ technology are examples of such systems.[10]

TABLE 1: Continuous glucose monitoring devices.[8]

Type of CGM	Description
rtCGM	CGM systems that measure and display glucose levels continuously
isCGM with and without alarms	CGM systems that measure glucose levels continuously but require scanning for visualization and storage of glucose values
Professional CGM	CGM devices are placed on the person with diabetes mellitus in the healthcare professional's office and worn for a discrete period of time (generally 7–14 days). Data may be blinded or visible to the person wearing the device. The data are used to assess glycemic patterns and trends. Unlike rtCGM and isCGM devices, these devices are clinic-based and not owned by a person with diabetes mellitus

TELEMEDICINE AND REMOTE PATIENT MONITORING

Telemedicine has emerged as a crucial tool in diabetes mellitus management, particularly useful in remote areas or for patients with limited access to traditional healthcare facilities. Telehealth platforms enable remote monitoring of glucose levels, which has been shown to improve HbA1c levels and patient satisfaction. Additionally, telemedicine facilitates the delivery of diabetes mellitus self-management education and supports the continuous monitoring of patients through devices like CGM systems. During the COVID-19 pandemic, telemedicine proved effective in managing diabetes mellitus by allowing continuous care while minimizing the risk of virus transmission. The integration of telemedicine into routine diabetes mellitus care can enhance access to healthcare services, reduce costs, and improve health outcomes for patients with diabetes mellitus. Telemedicine is efficacious, particularly for rural populations or those with limited physical access to health care for glycemic control as measured by HbA1c.[11]

STEM CELL THERAPY

The field of stem cell research has seen significant advancements, particularly in the differentiation of insulin-producing β cells from pluripotent stem cells (PSCs). This approach is considered more viable than using cells derived from human donors due to limitations such as donor scarcity and potential compatibility issues.

Techniques have been developed to induce embryonic stem cells and induced pluripotent stem cells (iPSCs) to differentiate into insulin-producing cells. These methods, known as the "five-stage differentiation protocol," have been refined over the years to enhance the efficiency and outcome of the differentiation process. iPSCs, created by reprogramming somatic cells, have shown potential as an autologous source for generating β cells. This technology, however, faces challenges such as genetic variability and low differentiation efficiency, which can affect the functionality of the derived β cells. Recent studies have utilized CRISPR-Cas9 genome editing to correct gene variants that cause diabetes mellitus, which has improved the differentiation and function of these cells. Moreover, advancements in in-vitro differentiation techniques have enabled the production of functional mature islet cells, which have been successfully used to reverse diabetes mellitus in animal models without causing tumors. Mesenchymal stem cells (MSCs), derived from various tissues like bone marrow, adipose tissue, and umbilical cord blood, have also been explored for their therapeutic potential in diabetes mellitus. Clinical trials using MSCs have shown promising results in improving blood glucose levels, enhancing insulin sensitivity, and supporting β cell function in diabetic models. These findings underscore the potential of stem cell therapy as a transformative approach for treating diabetes mellitus.[12]

PHARMACOGENOMICS-GUIDED TREATMENT APPROACHES

The integration of pharmacogenomics into clinical practice offers a pathway to personalized diabetology, where treatment plans are tailored based on an individual's genetic profile. This approach optimizes both pharmacokinetics and pharmacodynamics to achieve desired drug efficacy and minimize adverse effects. The falling costs of sequencing and genotyping technologies are making it feasible to implement pre-emptive genotyping, where actionable genotypes are embedded in medical records and used to guide prescribing decisions.[13]

Moreover, the development of clinical decision support tools that incorporate genotyping information can facilitate the use of genetic data at the point of prescribing, making it as easy to use as other clinical markers like body mass index or sex. This integration can help clinicians decide between treatment options when they are otherwise in equipoise, using genetic information to steer clinical decisions and improve patient outcomes.

As the technology and infrastructure continue to advance; it is likely that pharmacogenomic-guided treatments will become an integral part of diabetes mellitus management.[14]

LIFESTYLE INTERVENTIONS AND BEHAVIORAL MODIFICATIONS

Customized Lifestyle Plans

Recent guidelines emphasize a personalized approach to managing T2DM, which includes developing customized lifestyle plans that cater to individual patient needs. Clinicians are encouraged to collaborate with patients to establish personalized treatment goals that encompass glycemic control, weight management, and the prevention and treatment of comorbidities. This tailored approach helps in enhancing patient satisfaction, improving medication adherence, and ultimately, better health outcomes.

Mobile health applications are instrumental in facilitating behavior change to increase physical activity tailored to the patient's characteristics. These applications utilize data from activity trackers and genetic variants to provide personalized recommendations, which adapt over time to match the patient's evolving capabilities.[15]

Dietary Recommendations and Exercise

Diet and exercise are pivotal in the treatment of T2DM. A personalized meal plan focusing on complex carbohydrates, low glycemic index foods, and gut-healthy options helps in managing blood glucose levels effectively. Regular physical activity is equally important, with guidelines suggesting at least 2.5 hours per week of moderate to vigorous exercise to prevent the onset of T2DM in high-risk adults. Furthermore, intervention studies have demonstrated that moderate-intensity physical activity can significantly lower HbA1c levels, underscoring its role in improving insulin sensitivity and glycemic control.[16]

RECENTLY APPROVED DRUGS FOR TYPE 2 DIABETES MELLITUS

On May 13, 2022, the US Food and Drug Administration (FDA) approved tirzepatide (Mounjaro) for the treatment of T2DM. This medication is a first-in-class, dual incretin agonist, administered as a once-weekly injection. Tirzepatide uniquely impacts by decreasing blood sugar and promoting significant weight reduction, performing more effectively than existing treatments.

Tirzepatide functions by enhancing the body's response to incretin hormones, which are less effective in T2DM patients. It activates GLP-1 and GIP receptors, stimulating insulin release and inhibiting glucagon, thus controlling blood glucose levels. Additionally, it delays stomach emptying and suppresses appetite, contributing to weight loss.[17]

PIPELINE DRUGS

Sotagliflozin

Sotagliflozin is a dual inhibitor of SGLT-1 and SGLT-2. It works by blocking glucose absorption in the intestines and increasing urinary glucose excretion, leading to improved glycemic control in patients with T2DM.[18]

CONCLUSION

Recent advancements in the management of T2DM have transformed diabetes mellitus care, offering patients and healthcare providers a plethora of therapeutic options and strategies to optimize glycemic control, prevent complications, and improve quality of life. From novel pharmacological agents and lifestyle interventions to technological innovations and emerging therapies, the landscape of T2DM management continues to evolve, heralding hope for better outcomes and ultimately, a cure for this prevalent chronic disease. Continued research, innovation, and interdisciplinary collaboration are essential to realizing the full potential of these advancements and addressing the growing global burden of T2DM **(Box 1)**.

BOX 1 Summary of recent advances in the management of type 2 diabetes mellitus.

Pharmacological advancements:
- SGLT-2 inhibitors
- GLP-1 receptor agonists
- Insulin analogs
- Combination therapies

Technological advancements:
- Continuous glucose monitoring (CGM)
- Automated insulin delivery systems
- Telemedicine and remote patient monitoring

Individualized treatment:
- Pharmacogenomics-guided treatment approaches
- Lifestyle interventions and behavioral modifications

ONLINE REFERENCES

Please scan the QR code provided at the end of the table of contents for References of this chapter.

CHAPTER

211

Cardiovascular–kidney–metabolic Syndrome: Staging and Prevention

Umeshwar Pandey, Kumar Himanshu, Awadesh Kumar Sharma

ABSTRACT

Cardiovascular–kidney–metabolic (CKM) syndrome is an escalating health epidemic across the globe which leads to significant morbidity and mortality. In spite of the poor outcomes once the disease escalates, it is well recognized that it can be prevented and delayed by active screening and management. The American Heart Association recognizing the importance of CKM in future decades has come up with a presidential advisory regarding the stages and thereby the screening and management strategies. The traditional way of looking upon cardiac illness, chronic kidney disease, and obesity as separate entities has changed over the time to include a holistic approach and they are now recognized as different manifestations of the same pathology.

Keywords: Cardiovascular–kidney–metabolic syndrome, cardiorenal metabolic syndrome, epidemic, chronic kidney disease, obesity, staging, prevention

INTRODUCTION

Cardiovascular-kidney-metabolic (CKM) syndrome refers to a clinical syndrome characterized by dysfunctional obesity, renal dysfunction, and cardiac disease. Historically, the teaching has been clear about cardiorenal syndrome where disease in one organ leads to the other. Similarly, cardiac-metabolic disease is also widely appreciated where insulin resistance leads to cardiac disease.[1] But now there is enough evidence to understand that metabolic abnormalities lead to both cardiac and renal dysfunction which in turn propagates each other leading to worse outcomes. This holistic approach to a disorder which can have many presentations will lead to easy screening and management. It is also to be noted that while CKM does affect the heart and kidneys primarily, it also leads to other adverse health outcomes such as cancer, stroke, peripheral arterial disease, and atrial fibrillation.[2,3] While CKM is for obvious reasons more prevalent amongst the upper economic strata there is, however, significant heterogeneity amongst the population affected by it. There are people with metabolic risk factors without somatic obesity; at the same time there are others who just exhibit moderate kidney dysfunction without clinical cardiac disease for a long duration. Such subsets are often undiagnosed and lose out on the best preventive management strategies.[4] By defining CKM stages and including all manifestations this likelihood of missing these patients is significantly reduced. At the same time, it will also help us to prognosticate and treat them according to the stages of illness.

STAGING

The purpose of staging is to decide on the preventive or curative treatment to be offered to the patient. It also helps in deciding the various risk and prognosis **(Table 1)**.[1,4]

Stage 0

The purpose of defining this stage is to identify individuals who will be considered healthy and free of risk factors for CKM syndrome. Such individuals will be subjected to primordial prevention that is counseling them to adapt to a lifestyle that will prevent the development of CKM risk factors.

TABLE 1: The various stages of CKM syndrome.

Stages	Risk and prognosis
Stage 0	*No CKM risk factors*: No evidence of CKD/CVD, normal BMI, waist, normotensive, euglycemic, and normal lipids
Stage 1	*Excess/dysfunctional adiposity*: BMI > 23 kg/m^2, waist circumference > 80/90 cm in women/men: FBS 100–124 mg/dL or HbA1c 5.7–6.4%
Stage 2	*Metabolic risk factors and CKD*: Hypertriglyceridemia, hypertension, diabetes, and metabolic syndrome
Stage 3	*Subclinical CVD in CKM:* • Subclincal ASCVD-CT calcium score/angiography • Subclinical HF-elevated BNP, NT-proBNP, hs-troponin, or echocardiography
Stage 4	*Clinical CVD in CKM (CAD, HF, stroke, peripheral artery disease, and atrial fibrillation):* • 4A—no kidney failure • 4B—kidney failure present

(ASCVD: atherosclerotic cardiovascular disease; BMI: body mass index; BNP: brain natriuretic peptide; CKD: chronic kidney disease; CKM: cardiovascular-kidney-metabolic; CVD: cardiovascular disease: HF: heart failure)

Stage 1

This includes individuals who are found to have excess or dysfunctional adiposity. It is identified by the presence of any one or more of these three factors:

1. Excess weight, i.e., BMI > 25 kg/m^2
2. Waist circumference > 88 cm females, >102 cm males
3. Impaired glucose tolerance/prediabetes

They do not have the predefined metabolic risk factors. They also do not have any evidence of subclinical or clinical ASCVD nor do they have CKD.

Stage 2

Other than the presence of excess adiposity this group is defined by the presence of metabolic risk factors or moderate-high risk chronic kidney disease or both.

The metabolic risk factors are objectively identified by the presence of these risk factors:

- Hypertriglyceridemia > 135 mg/dL
- Hypertension (stage 1/2)
- Diabetes mellitus
- Metabolic syndrome

Stage 3

In addition to the features of stage 2, this stage is identified by the presence of subclinical heart failure or coronary artery disease. This requires targeted investigations in the form of cardiac biomarkers and coronary calcium scoring for heart failure and coronary artery disease, respectively. The importance of this stage lies in deciding when is the right time to screen for these diseases in a patient with risk factors. As we shall see later the protocol for screening addresses the issues partially. Those with an intermediate to high likelihood should be subjected to evaluation at yearly or 2 yearly intervals.

Stage 4

While this stage is the easiest to diagnose, it carries the worse prognosis and limited avenues for prevention. It is identified by the presence of clinical cardiovascular disease whose manifestations can be in the form of coronary artery disease, heart failure, stroke, peripheral artery disease, or atrial fibrillation. It is further subdivided into two stages based on the presence or absence of renal failure.

SCREENING

With the above described CKM staging, we can identify individuals at different stages of the syndrome. Early detection, especially in the subclinical phase is of prime importance so that the risk can be mitigated. As advised by the AHA two factors are to be screened.[4]

1. The first is the biological factors that include metabolic, kidney, and cardiac function which all of us are familiar with. The focus has to be start screening early including children. While western societies have already included screening children >3 years of age in view of rising childhood obesity even in India the affluent sections of the society do not appear to be different from western counterparts now. Hence a change in mindset to screen children and younger population is required.
2. The second interesting aspect which the AHA asked to screen is social determinants of health (SDOH) which we as physicians completely overlook. While there are many questionnaires available to screen for these factors which may be cumbersome, we as cardiologists must at least focus on addressing the diet, sedentary lifestyle, addictions such as smoking and alcohol, depression, and stressful lifestyle. The individual must understand that these factors do contribute as much as the biological ones in development of CKM.[3,4]

Screening Protocol

Early life, i.e., <21 years of age—start early at 3 years of age:

- Annual screening for weight, obesity, blood pressure measurement, and behavioral health
- Fasting lipid panel should be done once between 9 and 11 years of age and then again between 17 and 21 years of age.
- Checking for HbA1c and impaired glucose tolerance should start from 9 to 11 years of age and repeat it every 2–3 years.

Adult life, i.e., >21 years of age:

- Annual measurement of BMI, waist circumference, and components of metabolic syndrome (lipids and blood sugar measurement)

- Assessment of urinary albumin-creatinine ratio along with serum creatinine/cystatin C, annually for those with stage 2 CKM or higher
- Coronary artery calcium screening is reasonable in those with intermediate ASCVD risk score or stage CKM-2 and higher.
- Subclinical heart failure screening as per physicians' discretion as of now

MANAGEMENT

Stage 0: No Risk Factors

- Encouraging healthy lifestyle, addressing the social aspects of healthcare such as discouraging use of addictive drugs, alcohol, and excessive intake of fats and red meat.
- Spreading awareness to overcome sedentary lifestyle, to encourage 30–45 minutes of moderate intensity exercises for at least 4 days a week.
- Educating about the need of regular screening and understanding the various risk factors likely outcomes and ways to prevent them.

Stage 1: Excess/Dysfunctional Adiposity

- Discussion regarding weight loss using various lifestyle changes/other options
- Pharmacotherapy (BMI > 25 kg/m^2)
- Bariatric surgery (BMI > 30 kg/m^2 without comorbidities)
- Consider metformin if there is persistent or progressive impaired glucose intolerance despite lifestyle measures.

Stage 2: CKM Risk Factors

- *Hypertriglyceridemia*:
  - *Statin therapy* in those with intermediate/high ASCVD risk
  - If TG > 500 mg/dL—*fibrates*
  - If TG 135–499 mg/dL with diabetes or other risk factors—*eicosapentaenoic acid*
  - Lifestyle medications
- *Hypertension*:
  - Lifestyle modifications
  - To follow established guidelines to achieve target BP of <130/80 mm Hg
  - ACE inhibitors or ARBs to be preferred in those with established CKD or albuminuria.
- *Chronic kidney disease*:
  - With albuminuria, urinary ACR > 30 mg/g—ACEi or ARB to be used.
  - CKD with or without diabetes—SGLT-2 inhibitors
  - Diabetic kidney disease with persistent proteinuria despite ACEi/ARB—finerenone[2]
- *Diabetes*:
  - Lifestyle modifications
  - Moderate-to-high intensity statin therapy
  - Ezetimibe to be used for high-risk patients
  - In those with BMI > 35 kg/m^2 or HbA1c > 9%—GLP-1RA
  - In those with CKD-SGLT-2 inhibitors

Stage 3: CKM Syndrome at Risk for CVD

- Coronary artery calcium > 0—favors statin use
- Coronary artery calcium > 100—favors aspirin and statin use
- Subclinical heart failure—ACE/ARB + beta-blockers
- Subclinical heart failure with diabetes—add SGLT-2 inhibitor

Stage 4: CKM Syndrome with Existing CVD

Refer to **Flowchart 1**.

TREATMENT MODIFICATIONS FOR DIABETES

- *Patients with ASCVD*: To reduce MACE—use SGLT-2 inhibitors or GLP-1RA
- *Patients with HF*:
  - Avoid thiazolidinediones and DPP-4 inhibitors
  - SGLT inhibitors to be added to all
  - GLP-1RA to be added, e.g., HbA1c > 9% or high insulin requirement or BMI > 35 kg/m^2

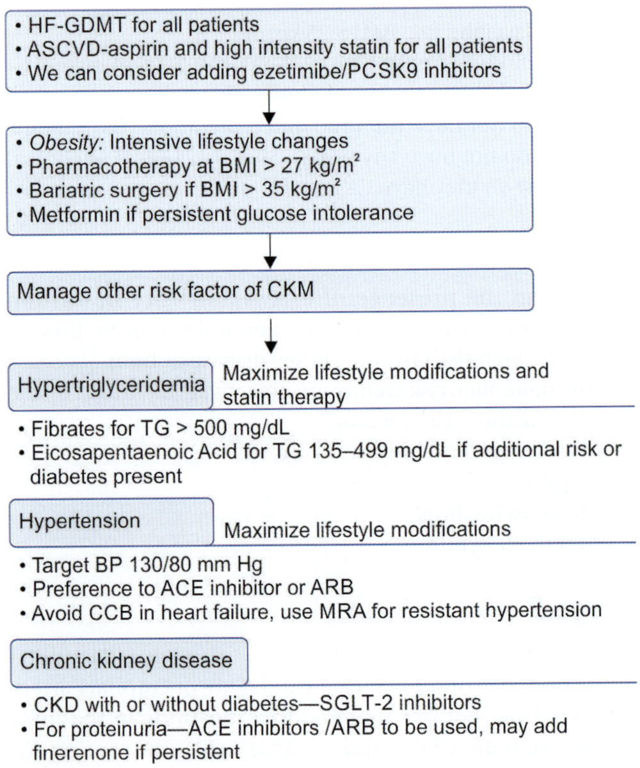

FLOWCHART 1: CKM syndrome with existing CVD, the flow chart describes a stepwise protocol to address the different aspects of treating CKM syndrome with existing CVD such as hypertriglyceridemia, diabetes, heart failure, etc.

- *Other factors*:
    - *Atrial fibrillation*: The use of anticoagulation for prevention of stroke is to be encouraged. While newer oral anticoagulants can be used in those with a normal or moderately reduced renal function, warfarin still continues to be the go to drug in cases of severe renal failure or on those undergoing dialysis. Obstructive sleep apnea also leads to fibrillation and is commonly found in those with CKM, hence addressing it is likely to be beneficial.[2]
    - *Stage 4b—Kidney failure*: The data to support use of most drugs is limited in renal failure. The use of ACE inhibitors or beta-blockers is encouraged but must be tailored to meet individual needs. There is limited data available regarding statins but their continuation seems reasonable. As CKD progresses pulmonary hypertension and advancement of heart failure is likely, hence treatment should be individualized to meet these needs.[3,4]
    - *Social factors*: The recent advisories have focused on the social aspects of health more than the previous ones. Merely relying on pharmacotherapy without addressing the social factors specially the sedentary and stressful lifestyle of the present times is inadequate. The physician should try to address the social aspects as far as possible.

CONCLUSION

As the living standards rise and the population starts ageing the number of people found suffering from CKM is going to rise. Treating it as a holistic entity and starting the screening early on will help us prevent morbidity and mortality. While specialized care will always have its niche a general consensus framing guidelines that can be used by even primary care physicians will help expand the reach of healthcare.

ONLINE REFERENCES

Please scan the QR code provided at the end of the table of contents for References of this chapter.

CHAPTER

212

Diabetic Cardiomyopathy

AK Pancholia

ABSTRACT

Development of myocardial dysfunction in diabetes mellitus in the absence of hypertension, atherosclerosis, or valvular defect is defined as diabetic cardiomyopathy (DCM). According to the UK Prospective Diabetes Study (UKPDS), there is a clear association between development of heart failure and increasing levels of glycated hemoglobin (HbA1c). Prevalence of DCM is on the rise globally as well as in India, which is why its proper diagnosis and treatment are so important. The primary pathological manifestations include myocardial hypertrophy, myocardial fibrosis, and widespread myocardial necrosis, which can progress to the development of heart failure. Appropriate therapy focusing on good glycemic control, associated diabetic dyslipidemia, and guideline-directed medical therapy for the control of heart failure reduces the risk of cardiovascular complications. In the future, we see new hope with therapies like stem cells and gene therapy targeting microRNA (miRNA) in DCM.

Keywords: Diabetic cardiomyopathy, diabetes mellitus, molecular mechanisms, risk factors, diagnosis, therapy

INTRODUCTION

Diabetic cardiomyopathy has been defined by the American College of Cardiology Foundation (ACCF), American College of Cardiology (ACC), and European Society of Cardiology (ESC) in collaboration with the European Association for the Study of Diabetes (EASD) as myocardial dysfunction without any associated coronary atherosclerosis and hypertension.[1,2] Therefore, all patients with diabetes mellitus without significant coronary artery disease, hypertension, and any valvular disease but having cardiac dysfunction are classified as patients with DCM.[3] However, it is challenging to define this disease correctly because most patients with type 2 diabetes mellitus (T2DM) have cardiovascular disease (CVD). The incidence of DCM proportionally increases with the onset of diabetes mellitus in the population.[4] Overall, the process of DCM formation is still an unsolved disease despite progress in clinical possibilities.[5]

PREVALENCE

Current data from small studies suggest that the prevalence of DCM is 1.1% in the general population and up to 17% in patients with diabetes mellitus, with morbidity and mortality approaching 31% over 10 years.[6,7]

PATHOGENETIC MECHANISMS OF DIABETIC CARDIOMYOPATHY

The exact pathophysiological mechanisms are still not very well known because of the complexity. The direct and indirect toxic effects of hyperglycemia on the myocardium lead to cardiac remodeling, diastolic and systolic dysfunction, and ultimately severe heart failure **(Flowchart 1)**.

ABNORMAL GLUCOSE METABOLISM AND INSULIN RESISTANCE

Persistent hyperglycemia causes reduction in glucose clearance and increase in gluconeogenesis, which are the initiating factors for DCM. Normally to sustain systolic and diastolic function glycolysis provides only 30–40% of the cardiomyocyte energy demands.[8] Glucose transporters 1 and 4 (GLUT1 and GLUT4) are responsible for glucose uptake. In

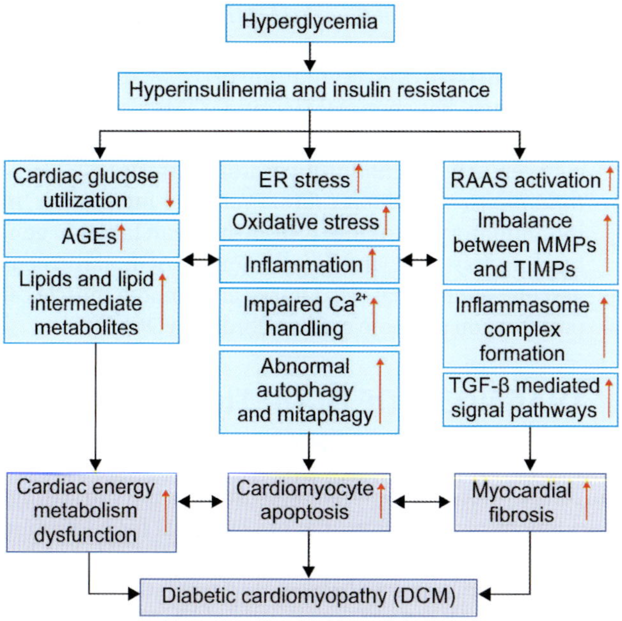

FLOWCHART 1: Pathogenetic mechanisms of DCM.

Source: Huo J-L, Feng Q, Pan S, et al. Diabetic cardiomyopathy: Early diagnostic biomarkers, pathogenetic mechanisms, and therapeutic interventions. Cell Death Discov. 2023;9:256.

DCM, there is a decrease in GLUT1 and GLUT4 in myocardial cells; hence, there is decreased glucose uptake and abnormal glucose metabolism.[9] Apart from that there is an increase in the formation of advanced glycation end products (AGEs) in myocardial cells, which cross-link with extracellular matrix (ECM) proteins, leading to increased cardiac fibrosis and thus causes diastolic dysfunction **(Fig. 1)**.[10] Impaired insulin utilization due to hyperinsulinism and cardiac insulin resistance leads to oxidation of nonesterified fatty acid, which is responsible for all myocardial energy metabolism.[11] This whole process results in the deposition of lipids and lipid intermediate metabolites, such as ceramide, diacylglycerol, and uncoupling protein-3, in cardiomyocytes and ultimately affects the energy supply of the myocardium, causing necrosis, fibrosis, remodeling, and ultimately dysfunction.[10] Chronic hyperglycemia also promotes the excessive release of reactive oxygen species (ROS) through the electron transport chain. ROS initiates an increase in AGEs and the protein kinase C (PKC),[12,13] which is responsible for stimulation of collagen expression and accumulation that leads to increased myocardial fibrosis and decreased cardiac muscle compliance.[14,15]

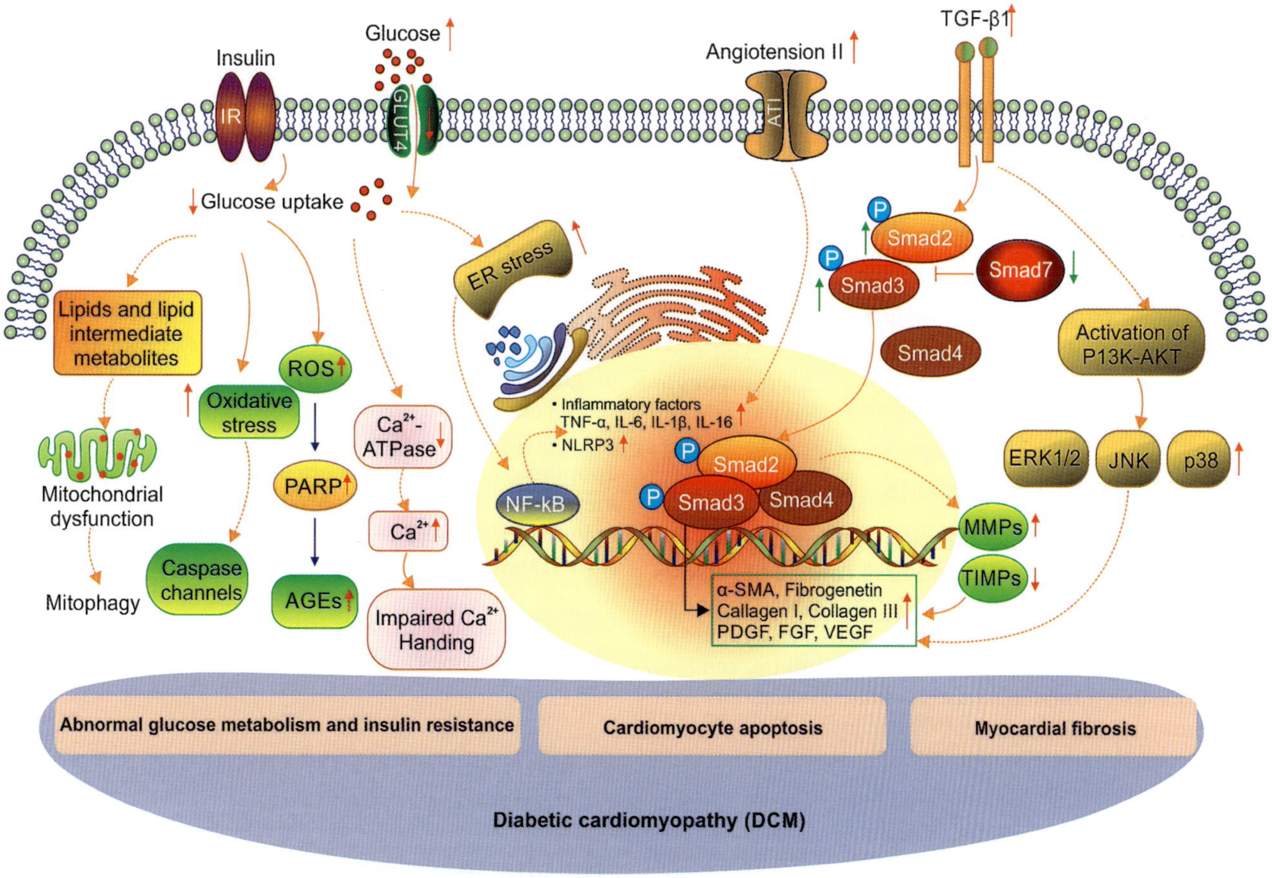

FIG. 1: Key pathogenetic mechanisms involved in DCM progression.

Source: Huo JL, Feng Q, Pan S, et al. Diabetic cardiomyopathy: Early diagnostic biomarkers, pathogenetic mechanisms, and therapeutic interventions. Cell Death Discov. 2023;9:256.

CARDIOMYOCYTE APOPTOSIS

In the early stage of DCM, abnormal apoptosis and cardiomyocyte injury may occur and are directly related to left ventricular hypertrophy and heart failure. In animal models, cardiomyocyte apoptosis is increased that leads to ventricular remodeling with reduction in cardiac systolic and diastolic function.[16-18] The factors which are responsible for abnormal cardiomyocyte apoptosis in DCM are as follows:

- Endoplasmic reticulum (ER) stress.[19-21]
- Oxidative stress in the myocardial endoplasmic reticulum[22-24]
- Activation of caspase-8 and caspase-9, which are responsible for the extrinsic and intrinsic apoptosis pathways in cardiomyocytes, and subsequently activate caspase-3, leading to neonatal rat cardiomyocyte apoptosis[25]
- Chronic inflammation responsible for not only inducing the production and release of nitric oxide (NO) in cardiomyocytes but also promoting the expression of proto-oncogenes, causing left ventricular diastolic dysfunction[26]
- Release of proinflammatory cytokines, including interleukin-1β (IL-1β), IL-6, IL-18, tumor necrosis factor-α (TNF-α), and transforming growth factor-β (1 TGF-β1), which leads to cardiomyocyte apoptosis, promoting the occurrence of diabetic cardiomyopathy[27]
- Increase in ROS in cardiomyocytes can also cause inflammation, cardiomyocyte apoptosis, and myocardial fibrosis.[28,29]
- Evidence has shown that excessive changes in or regulation of *NLRP3* inflammasome activity can promote the immunomodulatory response in DCM mice, whereas *NLRP3* gene silencing can improve diabetic cardiac remodeling and impair cardiac function **(Fig. 1)**.[30]
- Abnormal gene transduction of Ca^{2+}-ATPase in the cardiac sarcoplasmic reticulum with increased Ca^{2+} influx in cardiomyocyte causing cardiomyocyte apoptosis[21]

MYOCARDIAL FIBROSIS

Long-term hyperglycemia and severe insulin resistance are responsible for the proliferation of cardiac fibroblasts and thus development of cardiac fibrosis, which is one of the main histological manifestations of DCM. Myocardial fibrosis increases the stiffness of the myocardium, reduces cardiac diastolic function, causes systolic dysfunction, and finally induces sudden death.[31,32] For myocardial fibrosis and hypertrophy in DCM, the following multiple signaling pathways are involved:

- *Renin–angiotensin–aldosterone system (RAAS) activation:* RAAS activation is responsible for collagen deposition, cardiac fibrosis, and hypertrophy and thus responsible for the progression of diabetes mellitus to heart failure.[33]
- *Matrix metalloproteinases (MMPs):* MMPs and tissue inhibitors of metalloproteinases (TIMPs) are important antagonists in the regulation of ECM degradation. Imbalance between MMPs and TIMPs leads to an imbalance in the synthesis and degradation of ECM and collagen, thus promoting myocardial fibrosis
- *Inflammasome complex formation:* The increase in the inflammatory cytokine TNF-α, nuclear factor-κ-gene binding (NF-κB), and generation of AGE can trigger vascular endothelial cell damage and smooth muscle cell proliferation promote cardiac fibrosis in DCM.[34]

DIAGNOSIS OF DIABETIC CARDIOMYOPATHY

Currently, there are no biochemical indicators or distinct morphological alterations that are essential for confirming a diagnosis of DCM. In the early phase, it quite often lacks symptoms and is frequently correlated with other diabetic complications, making a definitive diagnosis very difficult. In the early prolonged subclinical period, significant histological and functional changes may occur, yet clinical symptoms remain absent. Thus, it is beneficial to make early diagnosis during the asymptomatic period. Identification of structural and functional changes in the left ventricle is important in the early diagnosis of DCM and ruling out other causes of HF. Both invasive and noninvasive methods can detect structural alteration, while echocardiography can identify functional changes. Other metabolic changes can be characterized by tools like magnetic resonance spectroscopy, positron emission tomography (PET), and single-photon emission computed tomography.[35,36] Biomarkers that can specifically detect DCM are still under investigation; however, in recent years, cardiac microRNAs (miRNAs) have emerged as crucial regulators in the development of DCM. These are potent diagnostic and prognostic biomarkers of DCM and play significant roles in regulating genes associated with the key pathophysiological pathways of DCM, such as hypertrophy, apoptosis, and fibrosis. There are some inflammatory and metabolic biomarkers that are linked to cardiac alterations in individuals with DM, such as mitral annular calcification (MAC) that can be picked up early by echocardiography in diabetic patients.[37] Diagnostic methods for DCM are shown in **Table 1** while possible diagnostic criteria for the two subtypes of diabetic cardiomyopathy are shown in **Box 1**.

MANAGEMENT OF DIABETIC CARDIOMYOPATHY

Nonpharmacological

Nonpharmacological treatment is given in **Box 2**.

TABLE 1: Diagnostic methods of DCM.

Method	Evaluation	Evaluated criterion
Echocardiography	Functional	Mitral inflow for diastolic function
	Structural	• Tissue Doppler imaging for diastolic and systolic function • In two-dimensional echocardiography LV hypertrophy
Cardiac PET	Metabolic and hemodynamic	Myocardial metabolic abnormality and disordered blood flow
Cardiac MRI	Functional	Late gadolinium enhancement for diastolic and systolic function
	Structural	Myocardial steatosis, LV hypertrophy
	Metabolic	Magnetic resonance spectroscopy for myocardial TG content and PCr/TP
Coronary angiography	Functional and hemodynamic	Mean PCWP and LVEDP for diastolic function, microvascular coronary artery disease
Serology	Functional	• mi-RNA for contractile function • BNP for diastolic and systolic function • Troponin for LV dysfunction
	Structural	MMPs and TIMPs for myocardial fibrosis
MAC biomarkers	Inflammatory and metabolic	Increase in TNF-alpha and HOMA-C peptide levels

Source: Radzioch E, Dąbeket B, Balcerczyk-Lis M, et al. Diabetic Cardiomyopathy—From Basics through Diagnosis to Treatment. Biomedicine. 2024;12(4):765.

BOX 1 Possible diagnostic criteria for the two subtypes of diabetic cardiomyopathy.

1. DMCMP Dilated/HFrEF phenotype:
- Presence of DM
- Exclusion of CAD, valvular or congenital heart disease
- Exclusion of hypertensive heart disease (= DBP < 90 mm Hg)
- Exclusion of viral myocarditis by endomyocardial biopsy
- LVEF < 50%; LVEDVI > 97 mL/m^2

2. DMCMP (Restrictive/HFpEF phenotype):
- Presence of DM
- Exclusion of CAD, valvular or congenital heart disease
- Exclusion of hypertensive heart disease (= DBP <90 mm Hg)
- Exclusion of infiltrative heart disease by endomyocardial biopsy
- LVEF > 50%; LVEDVI < 97 mL/m^2
- *E/E'* >15 or
  - 8 < *E/E'* < 15 + LAVI > 40 mL/m^2 or
  - 8 < *E/E'* < 15 + BNP > 200 pg/mL or
  - 8 < *E/E'* < 15 + atrial fibrillation or
  - 8 < *E/E'* < 15 + LVH (LVMI ♀ σ + >122 g/m^2; LVMI ♂ > 149 g/m^2)

Source: Modified from Seferović PM, Paulus WJ. Clinical diabetic cardiomyopathy: a two-faced disease with restrictive and dilated phenotypes. Eur Heart J. 2015;36:1718-27, 1727a-1727c.

BOX 2 Nonpharmacological treatment.

- Regular physical activity
- Proper weight maintenance
- Ceasing smoking
- Proper diet
- Bariatric surgery

Pharmacological Approaches

The latest treatment methods are now more individualized, targeting the different pathophysiological mechanisms for better treatment outcomes **(Flowchart 2)**.

EMERGING THERAPEUTIC MEDICATIONS

SGLT-2 Inhibitors

Promising results have been observed with SGLT-2 inhibitors in DCM in recent years.[38,39] These molecules have insulin-independent action and inhibit SGLT-2 receptors in the proximal renal tubules reducing glucose reabsorption and enhancing glucosuria, thus useful in reducing blood glucose.[39] Thus, the beneficial effect of SGLT-2 inhibitors in DCM is mainly because of its osmotic diuretic and natriuretic effects with reduction in pre- and afterload, leading to an improvement in cardiac output. The proposed mechanism of action in DCM is shown in **Figure 2**.

GLP-1 Receptor Agonists

GLP-1 RAs promote insulin secretion and reduce glucagon secretion, thus improving insulin resistance and reducing weight. They also slow gastric emptying and reduce food intake. GLP-1 RAs have antifibrotic effect by activating AMP-activated protein kinase (AMPK) pathway and hence improve LV diastolic function.[40] Cardiovascular benefit with reduction in CV mortality has been observed in the Cardiovascular Outcomes Assessment trial in patients with T2DM treated with liraglutide.[41]

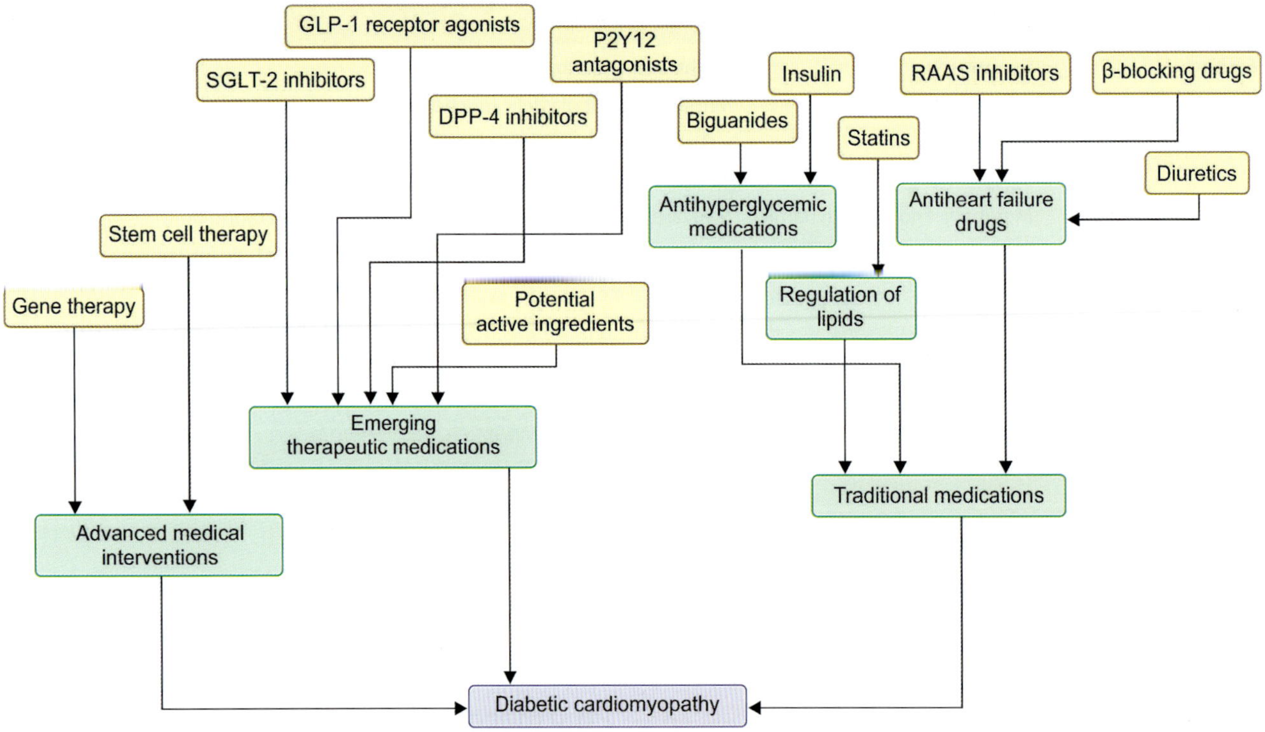

FLOWCHART 2: Pharmacological treatment of diabetic cardiomyopathy.

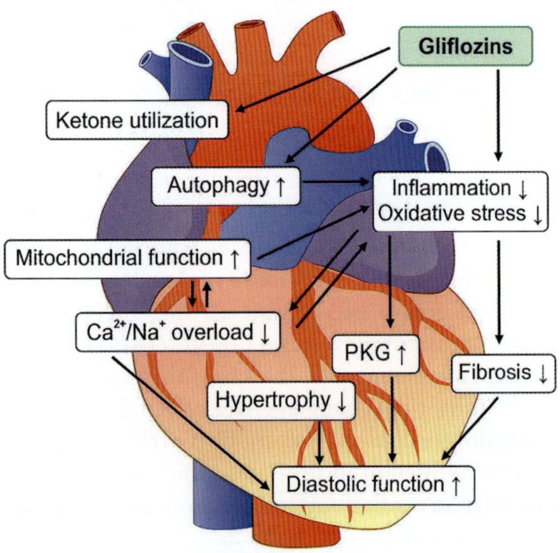

FIG. 2: Proposed myocardial mechanism of SGLT-2 inhibitors in DCM and HF.

Source: Pabel S, Hamdani N, Luedde M, et al. SGLT-2 Inhibitors and Their Mode of Action in Heart Failure-Has the Mystery Been Unravelled? Curr Heart Fail Rep. 2021;18:315-28.

DPP-4 Inhibitors

The hypoglycemic effect of DPP-4 inhibitors is mainly by increasing insulin secretion from beta cells and inhibiting glucagon through alpha cells.[42] Large prospective cardiovascular trials have confirmed that DPP-4 inhibitors are safe and have neutral effect on CV outcome.[43] Large clinical trials have also confirmed the safety of DPP-4 inhibitors as well as their benefits in improving outcomes of patients with diabetes mellitus complicated by heart failure.

Renin–Angiotensin–Aldosterone System Inhibitors

These are the first-line treatment for cardiovascular disease in patients with DM. They have anti-inflammatory and antifibrotic effects and thus are responsible for improving cardiovascular systolic and diastolic responses in patients with cardiovascular disease. The antiremodeling effect of RAAS inhibitors is useful in preventing DCM and also for the treatment of DCM.[44,45] Inhibiting cardiac-specific NF-κB signaling is another mechanism for their use in DCP.

β-blocking Drugs

β-blocking drugs are the frontline drugs for treating heart failure with reduced ejection fraction.[46] β-blocking drugs can reduce mortality in patients with HFrEF by reducing myocardial oxygen consumption, improving cardiac metabolism, and attenuating myocardial fibrosis. Various studies confirm that carvedilol reduces mortality in heart failure by improving myocardial hypertrophy, oxidative stress-induced cardiomyocyte apoptosis and myocardial fibrosis, ameliorating ventricular remodeling and cardiac dysfunction.

Mineralocorticoid Receptor Antagonist

Mineralocorticoid receptor antagonists have shown beneficial diuretic, anti-inflammatory, and antifibrotic effects, leading to reduction in morbidity and mortality in landmark trials.[47]

Gene Therapy

Recently, many studies have shown that miRNAs are aberrantly expressed in DCM; hence, these can be used as the pathogenesis of DCM and also the therapeutic target in the management of DCM.[48] Recently, *cmiR-21* gene demonstrates significant alterations in expression levels within the heart and circulation following myocardial injury, suggesting its close association with cardiac functional impairments, such as myocardial hypertrophy and fibrosis.[49] Experimental evidence demonstrates that inhibiting the activation of G protein-coupled estrogen receptor can suppress myocardial fibroblast proliferation in ovariectomized female rats with DM by reducing nitric oxide synthase activity and nitric oxide (NO) levels. At present, this therapy is not widely adopted in the management of DCM.

Stem Cell Therapy

Stem cell therapy might be promising in improving cardiac function, reducing myocardial damage, and improving the quality of life for patients.[50,51] They can show promising result, particularly mesenchymal stem cells, in cardiac regeneration and the treatment of cardiovascular diseases, including DCM.[52] The mesenchymal stem cells also have beneficial paracrine effects on the heart and vasculature, including antiapoptotic, anti-inflammatory, antifibrotic, and proangiogenic outcomes.

How Emerging Therapies are Compared with Existing Therapies?

Gene therapy and stem cell therapy are the emerging therapies and novel treatment approaches, which are developed based on existing therapies. They primarily target the pathological mechanisms and pathogenesis of DCM by either blocking or reversing these, thus leading to more pronounced treatment effects. Gene therapy targets the root cause of the disease, potentially achieving long-term and personalized treatment effects. Existing therapies are mainly focused on symptom relief to control disease progression, but they cannot enhance the recovery of diseased myocardium. For patients with DCM, the current existing therapies remain essential for the management but research is still going on for the new emerging intervention measures that will require clinical trials for their safety and efficacy.

CONCLUSION

In recent years, DCM has been considered as an independent disease. The primary aim to treat DCM has mainly been focused on effective control of glucose, blood pressure, lipids, and other risk factors as well as cardioprotection. The emerging therapeutic drugs like SGLT-2i and GLP-1 RA and gene and stem cell therapies have demonstrated unique advantages in treating DCM by delaying myocardial remodeling and reducing adverse reactions. Proper understanding of the basic pathophysiology of DCM will pave the way for discovering the effective gene-targeted therapies in future.

ONLINE REFERENCES

Please scan the QR code provided at the end of the table of contents for References of this chapter.

CHAPTER

213

Metabolic Ill Health: A New Therapeutic Target for Improving Outcome of Cardiometabolic Diseases

PC Manoria, Pankaj Manoria

ABSTRACT

Metabolic ill health is an emerging concept to encompass the conglomeration of cardiometabolic disease under one head. This is being done so that if a patient has one component of metabolic ill health, the other components of it can be screened, and a holistic approach can be provided for improving outcomes for patients suffering from metabolic ill health.

Keywords: Emerging concept, cardiometabolic, patients

INTRODUCTION

Metabolic ill health implies that the individual is prone to or has already developed obesity, type 2 diabetes (T2D), metabolic dysfunction associated with fatty liver disease (MAFLD), obstructive sleep apnea (OSA), polycystic ovarian syndrome (PCOS), atherosclerotic cardiovascular disease (ASCVD) such as coronary artery disease (CAD), stroke, and kidney disease **(Fig. 1)**. But the concept of metabolic ill health has not been widely percolated, so if a physician sees a patient with any of the above diseases, he tries to treat himself or tries to refer to the concerned specialist. But the correct approach is that if the patient has one of the manifestations of metabolic ill health, he must look at other components present in the same patient because they tend to conglomerate in the same patient.

Obesity is central to the pathogenesis of metabolic illness and is the root cause of cardiometabolic diseases. The global prevalence of obesity in 2022 was above one billion, whereas in India, the prevalence in 2023 was 224 million. Obesity, on the one hand, is a driver of diabetes, and on the other hand, it is also a driver of cardiovascular disease (CVD). If patients develop diabetes, it is also a driver of CVD. Therefore, cardiologists and diabetologists are very concerned about obesity. The adipocentric approach has therefore come to the forefront, even ahead of the glucocentric or cardiorenal approach. Any magnitude of weight loss is beneficial, but if the weight loss is >15%, it is a predictor of remission of diabetes, improves heart failure with preserved ejection fraction (HFpEF), and also decreases cardiovascular mortality. Lifestyle modification decreases the weight by 5–10%, but its compliance in the long run is difficult. The conventional drugs for obesity also decreased in weight by 5–10%. Endoscopic bariatric procedures decrease weight by about 15–20%, and bariatric surgery decreases weight by above 25% or so.

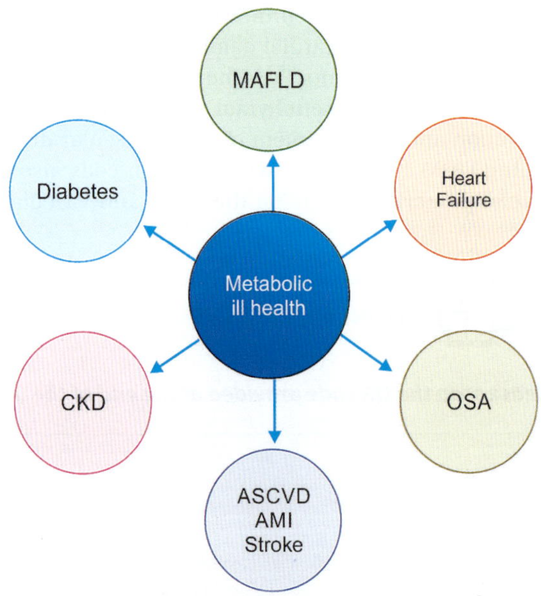

FIG. 1: Components of metabolic ill health.

(AMI: acute myocardial infarction; ASCVD: atherosclerotic cardiovascular disease; CKD: chronic kidney disease; MAFLD: metabolic dysfunction associated with fatty liver disease. OSA: obstructive sleep apnea)

DRUG REVOLUTION IN OBESITY

During the last couple of years, there has been a drug revolution in obesity. We have a single agonist, a double agonist, and triple agonist.

Single Agonist

Injectable semaglutide 2.4 mg (SC): This is a powerful drug for treating obesity and has shown a reduction in weight in the STEP trial by about 15–17%. Oral semaglutide 14 mg has shown a decrease in weight of about 5 kg across the pioneer program. Recently, higher oral doses of oral semaglutide 25 and 50 mg have shown incremental benefits. The 50 mg oral dose has shown a reduction in weight of 15%. Interestingly, injectable semaglutide has shown improvement in cardiovascular outcomes in nondiabetic obesity as well. However, injectable semaglutide is not yet available in India.

Dual Agonist

Dual agonist tirzepatide (GIP + GLP-1 RA) has shown a reduction in weight by 9.5–13 kg.[1] The reduction in HbA1C ranged from 2.07 to 2.59. CagriSema, which is a combination of semaglutide (2.4 mg) and cagrilintide (0.16–4.5 mg), has shown a reduction in weight of about 17%.

Triple Agonist

GIP + GLP-1+ GRA such as retatrutide in a phase II trial[2] has shown a reduction in weight up to 24.2% in a dose of 12 mg SC weekly.

Thus, monotherapy with a single agonist decreases weight by about 15–17%, dual agonists by 20–23%, and triple agonists by 24%, and therefore the gap between pharmacotherapy and bariatric surgery has narrowed down tremendously **(Fig. 2)**.

Weight loss promotes better glycemic control, impacts cardiometabolic risk factors, slows down disease progression, and helps in preventing diabetes microvascular complications.[3-7] If the weight loss is 5%, it starts impacting insulin sensitivity and beta-cell function. If the weight loss is 10–11%, the magnitude of the benefit is greater, the spectrum of benefits is wider, and it starts impacting gene expression and adipose tissue. If weight loss is about 15%, there is a greater benefit, and it also starts impacting inflammatory markers. The effect of weight loss on comorbidities is shown in **Figure 3**.

Obesity is also associated with increasing healthcare cost **(Table 1)**.[8]

Obesity should be treated upfront so that the development of diabetes can be minimized.

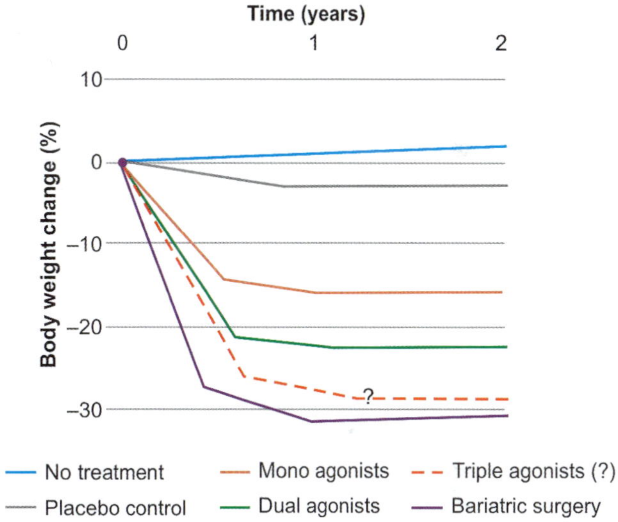

FIG. 2: Effect of drug revolution on change in body weight.

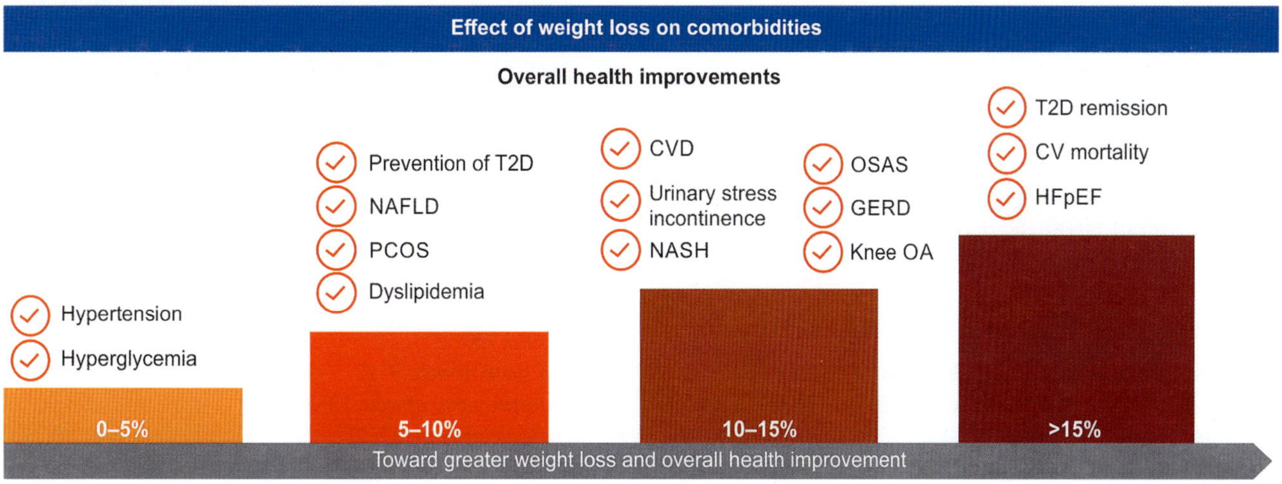

FIG. 3: Effect of weight on comorbidities.[3-7]

(GERD: gastroesophageal reflux disease; HFpEF: heart failure with preserved ejection fraction; NASH: nonalcoholic steatohepatitis; OSAS: obstructive sleep apnea syndrome)

TABLE 1: Costs for emergency room, inpatient, and outpatient services, plus pharmacy dispensing in overweight or obese.

Obesity	BMI	Increased healthcare costs
Overweight	BMI 25.0–29.9 kg/m^2	+ 11% cost
Obesity (Class I)	BMI 30.0–34.9 kg/m^2	+ 17% cost
Obesity (Class II)	BMI 35.0–39.9 kg/m^2	+ 29% cost
Obesity (Class III)	BMI ≥ 40 kg/m^2	+ 46% cost

METABOLIC DYSFUNCTION-ASSOCIATED FATTY LIVER DISEASE, METABOLIC DYSFUNCTION-ASSOCIATED STEATOHEPATITIS, AND METABOLIC DYSFUNCTION-ASSOCIATED STEATOTIC LIVER DISEASE

Nonalcoholic fatty liver disease (NAFLD) has been relabeled as metabolic dysfunction-associated fatty liver disease (MAFLD) and nonalcoholic steatohepatitis (NASH) has been designated as metabolic dysfunction-associated steatohepatitis (MASH). A new terminology of metabolic dysfunction-associated steatotic liver disease (MASLD) has been added. The normal amount of fat in the liver is 5%, when it exceeds 10%, it is termed MAFLD.

The most common cause of death in MAFLD is CVD and not liver disease. MAFLD is a gateway for the development of CVD. Most of these patients remain symptomatic till late in the course of the disease, and therefore it is also termed a silent killer. MAFLD is a global problem, and roughly 25–30% of the population is suffering from it. India falls into the high zone with a prevalence of greater than 30%. MAFLD is a systemic disease and is not merely a liver disease. It is associated with panoply of cardiometabolic diseases such as obesity, T2D, OSA, atherogenic dyslipidemia, hypertension, ASCVD, and PCOS. Diabetic MAFLD may progress to NASH and then to fibrosis. Diabetic patients have faster progression of fibrosis as compared to nondiabetic patients, which leads to compensated cirrhosis and finally decompensated cirrhosis. A small percentage of patients develop hepatocellular carcinoma.

Follow-up for Patients with NAFLD

If patients belong to a low-risk group, i.e., the Fibrosis-4 (FIB-4) < 1.3, liver stiffness measurement (LSM) < 8 kPa, or enhanced liver fibrosis (ELF) < 7.7, then this can be managed by a primary care physician with a focus on obesity management and CVD prevention. If the patient is at intermediate risk, i.e., FIB-4 1.3–2.67, LSM 8–12 kPa, or ELF 7.7–9.8, he should be referred to a hepatologist. If he has a high-risk FIB-4 > 2.67, LSM > 12 kPa, or ELF > 9.8, then he requires a multidisciplinary team to prevent cirrhosis and CVD.

Treatment

Lifestyle modification and a low-calorie diet are very important parts of treatment and should be strictly applied.

Drugs

- *Saroglitazar*: This is approved in India by DCGI. It is administered in doses of 4 mg per day for treatment of MASH and fibrosis F1 to F3. It also decreases blood glucose due to its dual PPαR action. It decreases triglycerides and decreases fibrosis. It is not effective if the patient has developed cirrhosis.
- *Vitamin E 400 mg* is given once daily in nondiabetic biopsy-proven NASH.
- *Pioglitazone*: This is administered in biopsy-proven NASH in diabetic as well as nondiabetic patients.
- *GLP-1 RA*: It decreases fat in the liver and histological resolution of MASH, but it is not effective when fibrosis has developed.

Resmetirom

This is a new drug approved by US FDA on March 24th, 2024. It is a liver-directed oral thyroid hormone receptor beta (THR-β) agonist therapy targeting the underlying cause of NASH. The drug was approved after the MAESTRO-NASH trial,[9] which showed positive results. It showed NASH resolution without worsening of fibrosis at week 52 ($p < 0.001$) and improvement in fibrosis by >1 stage with no worsening of NAFLD activity score ($p < 0.001$). The drug is administered in doses of 80 mg or 100 mg per day in a single dose. The drug is well tolerated. A small number of patients may develop diarrhea and nausea. The place lifestyle modification and various drugs are outlined in **Figure 4**.

OBSTRUCTIVE SLEEP APNEA

This is another component of metabolic ill health. OSA is diagnosed by polysomnography by apnea hypopnea index, i.e., AHI, which is calculated by dividing the number of apnea (pauses in breathing) + the number of hypopneas (periods of shallow breathing) events by the number of hours of sleep. The AHI limits per hour of sleep for adults are mentioned below:

- *Normal*: <5
- *Mild sleep apnea*: 5–15
- *Moderate sleep apnea*: 15–30
- *Severe sleep apnea*: ≥30

The OSA increases risk of recurrent heart attack, stroke, atrial fibrillation, and sudden cardiac death.

The OSA associated with a reduced mean nocturnal oxygen saturation < 93% and a lowest nocturnal oxygen

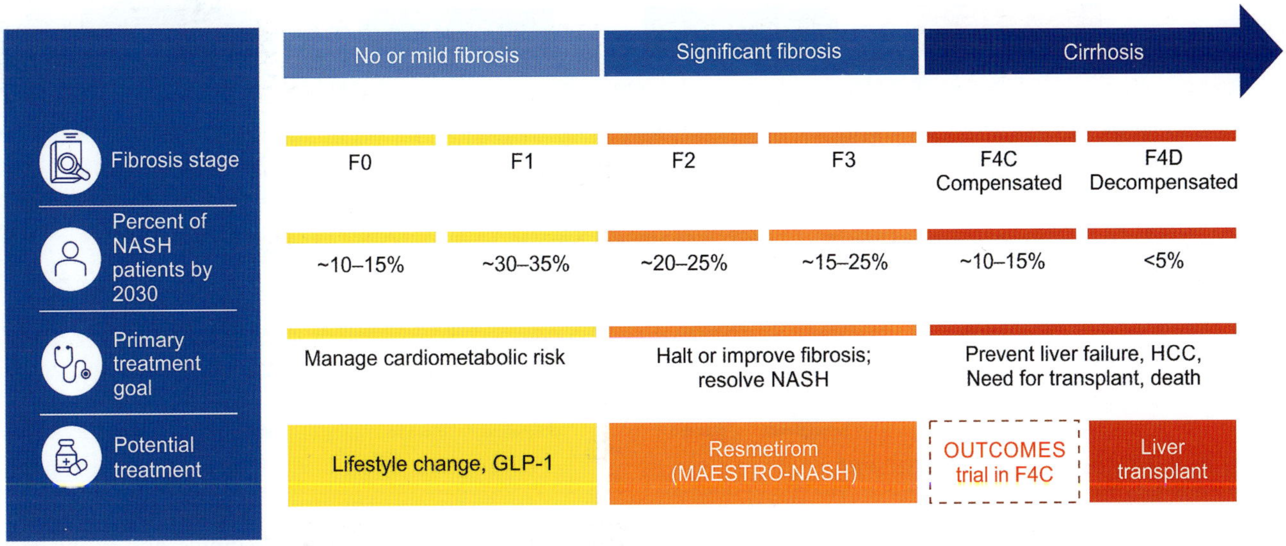

FIG. 4: Progression of MAFLD and its effect on therapies.

Source: Adapted from Estes C, Razavi H, Loomba R, Younossi Z, Sanyal AJ. Modeling the epidemic of nonalcoholic fatty liver disease demonstrates an exponential increase in burden of disease. Hepatology. 2018;67(1):123-33.

BOX 1 Concomitant diseases with OSA.

- Arterial Hypertension 30–60
- Drug-resistant hypertension 80–90%
- Coronary heart disease 30–60%
- Heart failure (HFrEF) 10–50%
- Heart failure (HFpEF) 20–60%
- Stroke 40–90%

saturation < 78% were independent risk factors for SCD (p = 0.0001). A circadian pattern of ventricular arrhythmia and a higher rate of SCD during sleep time (midnight to 6 AM) have been demonstrated. OSA is commonly with CVDs **(Box 1)**.

POLYCYSTIC OVARY SYNDROME

Its main features can include cysts in the ovaries, high levels of male hormones, and irregular periods.

HEART FAILURE

Heart failure is an important complication of diabetes. In diabetes, HFpEF is more common. SGLT-2i has a class one recommendation from HFpEF. Recently, injectable semaglutide 2.4 mg weekly has shown positive results in STEP-HFpEF trial and STEP-HFpEF DM trial. The drug is suitable for the obese phenotype of HFpEF. ARNI and MRAs have class 2B recommendations. Diuretics are, of course, used to decrease congestion in HFpEF. For HFrEF, besides diuretics, which are utilized to decrease congestion, the four foundational, i.e., SGLT-2i, beta-blockers ARNI, and MRAs, have kicked off a drug revolution in heart failure. For worsening heart failure, vericiguat is used.

CHRONIC KIDNEY DISEASE

Chronic kidney disease (CKD) is a progressive disease; there is no available treatment that can reverse it to normal. However, we have three guideline-recommended pillars of CKD that slow down the trajectory of CKD by slowing down the decline in eGFR and postpone dialysis by 10–15 years.

These include RAS blockers, SGLT-2i, and nonsteroidal MRAs, i.e., finerenone.[10] In the recent past, the FLOW trial[11] with injectable semaglutide 1 mg weekly has shown positive results, and in the future, this is lightly to become the fourth pillar of CKD management.

CORONARY ARTERY DISEASE

Diabetes is a leading cause of death in people with T2D. About 70% of diabetics die from acute myocardial infarction. CVD in India occurs a decade earlier and is two times more common than nondiabetics. The mere presence of diabetes cuts short the life span by 6 years, and if myocardial infarction gets superimposed, the life span is cut short by 12 years. Besides conventional therapies for the prevention of CAD of diabetes, GLP-1 receptor agonists have shown a reduction in ASCVD events both for primary and secondary prevention and are the standard of care for primary prevention for high-risk diabetics and for secondary prevention of diabetes **(Fig. 5)**.

Oral semaglutide 14 mg has shown good glycemic control and weight reduction in the PIONEER program, but the CV outcome is ongoing[12] to evaluate its cardiovascular effects.

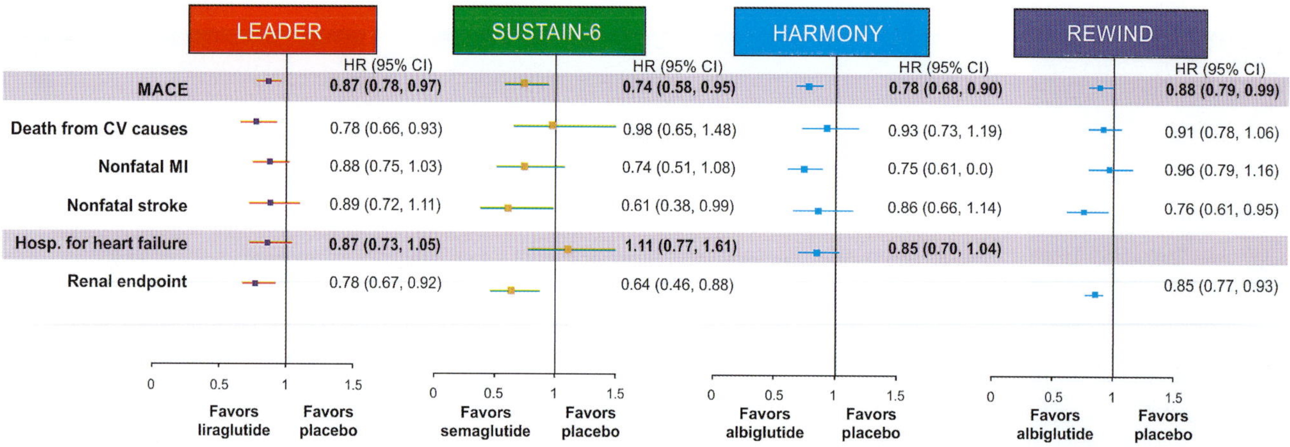

FIG. 5: Positive CV outcome trials with GLP-1 RA.

STROKE

People with diabetes are at a higher risk for both ischemic and hemorrhagic strokes. The risk of stroke is two to four times higher in individuals with diabetes compared to those without.

Diabetes accelerates atherosclerosis, leading to a greater likelihood of ischemic strokes. Hypertension is more common in diabetes, and these result in an increased incidence of hemorrhagic stroke. Diabetes, particularly in association with hypertension, also involves small arteries producing lacunar infarcts. After a stroke, diabetics are at higher risk of complications such as delayed recovery and poor functional outcomes. Lytic therapy is the standard of care for a large artery stroke if the patient is present within the window period. Endovascular therapy for extraction of the clot is also utilized in advanced centers. Besides this, good glycemic control, control of BP, lipids, and antiplatelet therapy are also useful. A dual pathway inhibitor, i.e., aspirin 100 mg plus rivaroxaban 2.5 mg twice daily, is also utilized to decrease the incidence of ischemic stroke in the future.

CONCLUSION

Cardiometabolic diseases due to metabolic ill health are rocking the entire universe and are the leading cause of cardiovascular morbidity and mortality. Obesity is central to the pathogenesis of metabolic ill health and its further consequences. Due to this obesity has come in forefront of therapeutics. If this can be minimized, most of the components of metabolic ill health will become a rarity. For those who have already developed metabolic ill health panoply of diagnostic and therapeutic strategy are available to improve their outcome.

ONLINE REFERENCES

Please scan the QR code provided at the end of the table of contents for References of this chapter.

CHAPTER

214

Antidiabetics and Cardiorenal Safety

Amit Aggarwal, MPS Chawla

ABSTRACT

Until 2008, antidiabetic drugs were exclusively approved on the basis of lowering of glycosylated hemoglobin (HbA1c), as trials with intensive glycemic control demonstrated lower rates of microvascular complications. After the 2008 controversy regarding the increased risk of cardiovascular events with the use of rosiglitazone, the United States Food and Drug Administration (USFDA) mandated trials to adequately assess the cardiovascular safety of newer diabetic drugs before approval. As a result, a multitude of large cardiovascular outcomes trials (CVOTs) for antidiabetics were published after 2008, leading to a paradigm shift in the management of type 2 diabetes mellitus (T2DM). For the first time, this led USFDA to approve label changes to drugs used in the management of diabetes for lower risk of major adverse cardiovascular events (MACE) and cardiovascular (CV) deaths.

Keywords: SGLT-2 inhibitors, GLP-1 receptor agonists, cardiovascular safety, renal safety, cardiovascular outcomes trials, antidiabetics

INTRODUCTION

The most famous trial that initiated the debate on cardiovascular (CV) safety of antidiabetics was a meta-analysis of 42 studies, in which it was determined that the odds-ratio for myocardial infarction (MI) in diabetics (mean HbA1c: 8.2% and mean age: 56 years) was 1.43, and for deaths due to CV causes was 1.64 in subjects taking rosiglitazone (minimum duration 24 weeks) in comparison with controls.[1] Responding to this controversy, the United States Food and Drug Administration (USFDA) published guidance for pharmaceutical industry recommending the inclusion of enough patients with high atherosclerotic cardiovascular disease (ASCVD) risk in order to adequately assess the CV risks of antidiabetics. The agency mandated that for novel drugs to demonstrate sufficient CV safety and win approval, a premarketing outcomes trial must show that the upper bound of two-sided 95% confidence interval of the estimated hazard ratio is <1.8 for composite three-point major adverse cardiovascular events (MACE) (CV death, nonfatal MI, and nonfatal stroke) or four-point MACE (CV death, nonfatal MI, nonfatal stroke, and hospitalization for unstable angina). For the approved drugs also, it is required that a postmarketing safety trial must demonstrate that the estimated risk ratio is <1.3 for the composite MACE outcomes. In order to achieve this, most enrolled patients must have established cardiovascular disease (CVD) or high ASCVD risk. Drug manufacturers adapted quickly to these new regulations and large number of cardiovascular outcomes trials (CVOTs) for antidiabetic drugs were published after 2008. These trials led to a shift in the primary objective of the management of diabetes from a mere reduction in HbA1c to focusing on associated comorbidities.

DRUGS THAT LOWER CARDIOVASCULAR OR RENAL DISEASE RISK

Metformin

Trials on CV outcomes of metformin preceded the FDA guidance, and as a result, there are no definitive CVOTs similar to those with sodium-glucose cotransporter-2 (SGLT-2) inhibitors, glucagon-like peptide-1 (GLP-1), and gastric-inhibitory polypeptide (GIP) receptor agonists, and dipeptidyl peptidase-4 (DPP-4) inhibitors. Current evidence on CV effects of metformin relies on numerous smaller studies that point toward CV benefits. A meta-analysis of 179 trials and 25 observational studies demonstrated lower CV mortality for metformin compared to sulfonylureas.[2] Andersson et al. in Danish retrospective national cohort study[3] demonstrated that patients with T2DM and heart failure (HF) had lower risk of mortality with metformin as compared to sulfonylureas and/or insulin.

Reducing with Metformin Vascular Adverse Lesions (REMOVAL)[4] was the largest and longest double-blinded randomized control study assessing metformin and observing the progression of atherosclerosis in patients with type 1 diabetes mellitus (T1DM). The primary outcome was the assessment of averaged mean far wall carotid intima-media thickness (cIMT), quantified annually for 3 years using repeated measures regression. Secondary outcomes were measurement of HbA1c, LDL cholesterol, estimated glomerular filtration rate (eGFR), incidental microalbuminuria, retinopathy, body weight, insulin dose, and endothelial function. The progression of mean cIMT was not significantly reduced with metformin, although the maximal cIMT was significantly reduced as a prespecified tertiary outcome. The overall data did not support the use of metformin to improve glycemic control in adults with long-standing T1DM but suggested a wider role in CV risk management.

Sodium-glucose Cotransporter-2 Inhibitors

The American Diabetes Association (ADA) 2019 Standards of Medical Care stated that in patients with established ASCVD, the evidence favoring SGLT-2 inhibitors is strongest with significant clinical benefits in individuals with HF. **Figure 1** shows the physiological mechanisms of SGLT-2 inhibitors and GLP-1 receptor agonists.

EMPA-REG OUTCOME,[5] a randomized double-blinded trial, evaluated the effect of empagliflozin on a composite of CV death, nonfatal MI, or nonfatal stroke. Even though designed for noninferiority, the study concluded that empagliflozin was superior as it reduced the relative risk of primary endpoints by 14% as compared to placebo. The CV death was reduced by 38% with empagliflozin, although it was only a secondary outcome and the reason why FDA-approved empagliflozin in 2016 "to reduce the risk of CV death in adult patients with T2DM and CVD". In addition, empagliflozin reduced the risk of HF in patients with or without HF at baseline, within a large range of HbA1c values. The American College of Cardiology/American Heart Association (ACC/AHA) 2019 Standards of Care recognized this potential of empagliflozin for primary prevention of HF.[6] The EMPA-KIDNEY[7] trial showed that empagliflozin reduced the risk of progression of kidney disease or CV deaths in

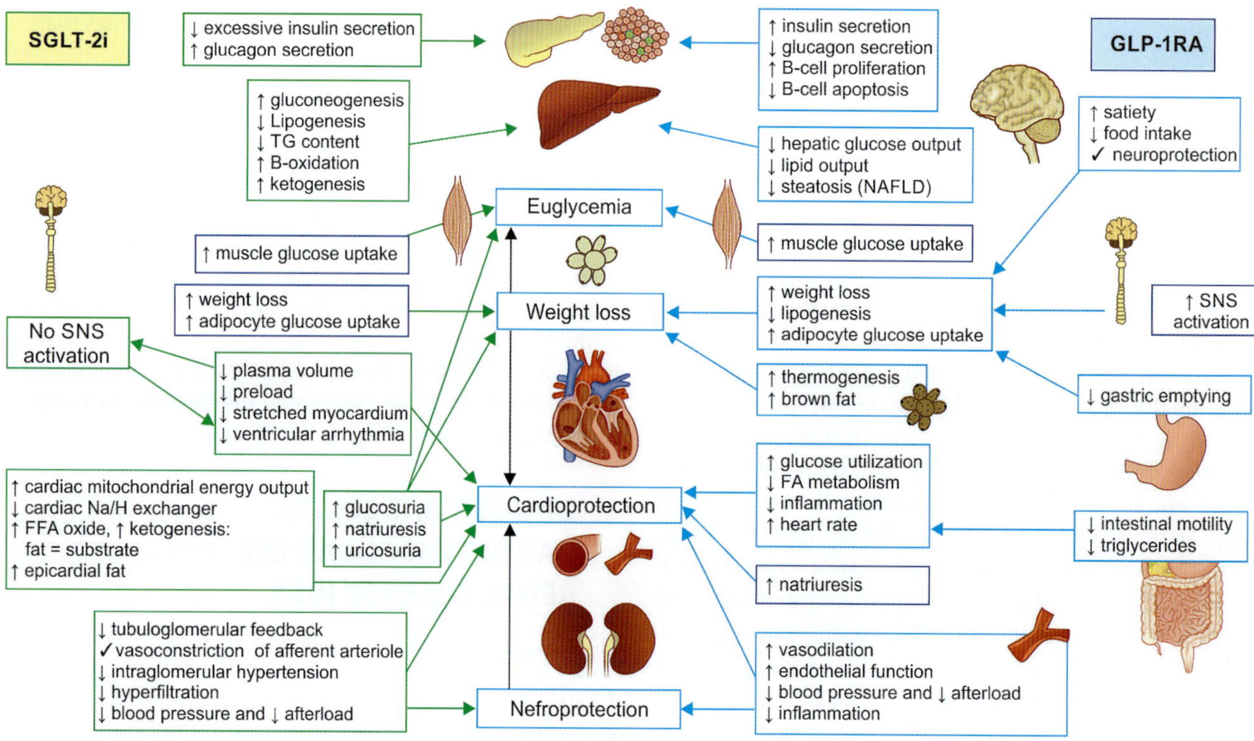

FIG. 1: Physiological mechanisms of SGLT-2 inhibitors and GLP-1 receptor agonists.

patients with chronic kidney disease (CKD), suggesting that SGLT-2 inhibitors should be part of standard of care to minimize progression of kidney function in CKD. This study not only used more uniformly defined composite renal endpoints such as new onset macroalbuminuria (urinary albumin-creatinine ratio, UACR > 300 mg/g) and doubling of serum creatinine with an eGFR ≤45 mL/min per 1.73 m^2, but also included initiation of renal replacement therapy (RRT) or death from renal causes.

EMPEROR-Reduced,[8] a double-blinded randomized trial, evaluated patients with New York Heart Association (NYHA) class II–IV HF and ejection fraction of ≤40%, receiving empagliflozin (10 mg once daily) or placebo, in addition to recommended therapy. The primary outcome was a composite of CV death or hospitalization for worsening HF. It was seen that among patients receiving recommended therapy for HF, those in the empagliflozin arm had a reduced risk of CV death or hospitalization for HF than those in the placebo group, regardless of the presence or absence of T2DM. It was also concluded that the annual rate of decline in the eGFR was slower with empagliflozin, indicating lower risk of major adverse renal events (MAREs).

In EMPEROR-Preserved,[9] patients with class II–IV HF and ejection fraction >40% were randomly assigned to receive either empagliflozin (10 mg once daily) or placebo, along with usual therapy. The primary outcome was similar to EMPEROR-Reduced. Empagliflozin reduced the composite risk of CV death or HF hospitalization in patients with HF and preserved ejection fraction by 21%, regardless of the presence or absence of diabetes. The lowered risk of composite primary outcome was mainly owing to a reduction in hospitalization for HF by 29%, with no significant reduction in CV deaths.

In DAPA-HF,[10] a phase-3 placebo-controlled randomized trial, patients with NYHA class II–IV HF and ejection fraction of 40% or less were randomly assigned to receive either dapagliflozin (10 mg once daily) or placebo, along with recommended therapy. The composite primary outcome was worsening of HF (hospitalization or an urgent visit resulting in intravenous therapy for HF) or CV death. Dapagliflozin was associated with reduction in the risk of composite outcome regardless of the presence or absence of diabetes.

DECLARE-TIMI 58[11] was the first SGLT-2 inhibitor CVOT to enroll a majority (59%) of primary prevention patients without CVD, and only 41% patients had established ASCVD. While dapagliflozin was noninferior to placebo in the primary outcome—three-point MACE, it did result in lower rates of hospitalization due to HF. Also, the progression of CKD occurred less often with dapagliflozin similar to DAPA-CKD.

CANVAS[12] evaluated CV effects of canagliflozin, and a reduction in the rate of three-point MACE from 31.5 to 26.9 participants per 1,000 patient-years was demonstrated. However, there were no significant findings for CV deaths or death by any cause.

CREDENCE[13] studied the renal effects of canagliflozin, the primary outcome being a composite of end-stage renal disease (ESRD), doubling of serum creatinine, and death from renal or cardiovascular cause. Compared to placebo group, the rates of the primary outcome were lower in the canagliflozin group. As per the guidelines, SGLT-2 inhibitors are not recommended in patients with eGFR <30 mL/min, but results from CREDENCE suggested that they are most beneficial in precisely these patients in order to reduce MAREs.

VERTIS CV[14] studied the safety of two different doses of ertugliflozin in adults with T2DM and ASCVD, with primary objective being noninferiority to placebo with respect to primary outcome of three-point MACE. A post hoc analysis of the cardiorenal outcomes, kidney functions, and other safety outcomes in adults older than 75 years in the trial was compared with participants below 75 years of age. Ertugliflozin was noninferior to placebo with respect to MACE and was the only SGLT-2 inhibitor CVOT to miss out on superiority. Reduction in the risk of hospitalization for HF, composite kidney outcome, and slower rate of decline of eGFR were also seen.

The CV efficacy of the dual SGLT-1 and 2 inhibitor, sotagliflozin, was studied in two large-scale randomized trials. In SCORED,[15] patients with T2DM and diabetic kidney disease were studied, and in SOLOIST-WHF,[16] patients with T2DM during or just after admission for decompensated HF were studied. Both trials demonstrated statistical superiority of sotagliflozin against placebo in the primary composite outcome of CV death/hospitalization for HF/urgent HF visit. In SCORED, sotagliflozin also reduced the risk for the secondary outcome of MACE.

Glucagon-like Peptide-1 Receptor Agonists

Glucagon-like peptide-1 receptor agonists (GLP-1RAs) enhance the incretin system by stimulating insulin secretion and suppressing glucagon release while reducing appetite and promoting weight loss. For patients with ASCVD, HF, or CKD; the ADA and European Association for Study of Diabetes (EASD) Standard of Care recommend the addition of SGLT-2 inhibitors or GLP-1RAs if HbA1c targets are not achieved through metformin or lifestyle intervention alone. GLP-1RAs are divided into short- and long-acting agents. Exenatide and lixisenatide are short-acting and have a more marked effect on postprandial glucose and gastric emptying but less on fasting glucose. Dulaglutide, liraglutide, and semaglutide are long-acting with greater effect on fasting glucose and less on gastric emptying.

The first GLP-1RA CVOT, ELIXA,[17] tested lixisenatide in 6,068 T2DM patients with recent acute coronary syndrome (ACS) and found no change in the primary composite four-point MACE outcome.

In LEADER,[18] involving 9,340 patients with a median follow-up of 3.8 years, liraglutide reduced the risk of MACE by 13% with concordant results for CV death, nonfatal MI, and stroke. In addition, the active therapy group had reduced all-cause mortality, but the risk of hospitalization for HF did not differ. Consequently, liraglutide was given a label indication for reducing MACE in T2DM patients with established CVD.

In EXSCEL trial,[19] once-weekly exenatide proved neutral for MACE in comparison to placebo, although adherence to the drug was lower than in other similar trials and likely reduced the statistical power to detect any benefit. All-cause mortality was also reduced in the active therapy arm in this study.

SUSTAIN-6[20] examined once-weekly subcutaneous semaglutide versus placebo in 3,297 patients and followed for a mean of 2.1 years. The risk of the primary MACE outcome decreased by 26% in semaglutide group, an effect driven predominantly by a 26% risk reduction for MI, 39% for stroke, but no apparent effect on CV death. Rates of new or worsening nephropathy were lower in the semaglutide group, but rates of retinopathy complications requiring intravitreal interventions were significantly higher.

In the first CVOT involving an oral GLP-1RA, PIONEER 6,[21] once-daily oral semaglutide was evaluated in an event-driven, randomized, double-blinded, placebo-controlled trial involving patients at high CV risk with age ≥50 years, and established CVD or CKD; or age ≥60 years with CV risk factors only. The primary outcome in a time-to-event analysis was the first occurrence of three-point MACE. In this study involving patients with T2DM, the CV risk profile of oral semaglutide was noninferior to placebo.

REWIND[22] studied dulaglutide with the longest follow-up duration of 5.5 years. This trial included higher proportion of females (47%), lower baseline HbA1c, and a higher proportion of primary prevention patients with no established CVD (69%). Dulaglutide was associated with 12% risk reduction of MACE and 24% risk reduction in nonfatal stroke. It extended the benefits of GLP-1RAs to primary prevention.

HARMONY OUTCOMES[23] showed that albiglutide significantly reduced MACE when added to standard care of patients with T2DM. The incidence rate of three-point MACE was 7% in the albiglutide group compared to 9% with placebo.

The results of the CVOTs for GLP-1RAs showed somewhat heterogeneous results. Only four of the trials (LEADER, SUSTAIN-6, REWIND, and HARMONY OUTCOMES) significantly reduced the risk of primary outcome MACE. Only REWIND suggested that GLP-1RAs may be applicable to primary prevention. ELIXA, HARMONY OUTCOMES, LEADER, SUSTAIN-6, and EXSCEL suggested that GLP-1RAs reduce CV events in individuals with established ASCVD.

Dual Gastric-inhibitory Polypeptide and Glucagon-like Peptide-1 Receptor Agonist

Tirzepatide, a dual GIP and GLP-1 receptor agonist has been shown to have cardioprotective effects. In the SURPASS-4 trial,[24] tirzepatide significantly decreased blood pressure, body weight, and HbA1c in patients with T2DM. Improvement in multiple cardiometabolic risk factors, like reduction in hepatic steatosis, new-onset macroalbuminuria, and lipid profile, across the spectrum range of HbA1c was also seen. The SURMOUNT-1 trial[25] demonstrated the efficacy of tirzepatide in reducing cardiometabolic risk factors in people with obesity without T2DM. The dual receptor agonism improved lipids, increased insulin secretion, reduced vascular inflammation, and promoted endothelial integrity. Tirzepatide shows promise as a comprehensive therapeutic option for managing CV risk factors in patients with T2DM and obesity.

DRUGS THAT DO NOT LOWER CARDIOVASCULAR OR RENAL DISEASE RISK

Dipeptidyl Peptidase-4 Inhibitors

Dipeptidyl peptidase -4 inhibitors counteract the degradation of plasma GLP-1 and GIP after meals, thereby stimulating the release of insulin and inhibiting that of glucagon. However, DPP-4 inhibitors elevate GLP-1 only by a modest amount, compared to when administering GLP-1 RAs directly. This might account for the greater beneficial effects on weight loss, fasting glucose levels, and HbA1c reduction with GLP-1RAs compared to DPP-4 inhibitors.

The EXAMINE trial[26] evaluated the safety of alogliptin in patients of T2DM with recent ACS. Alogliptin was found to be noninferior to placebo regarding the primary endpoint of three-point MACE. However, post hoc analysis showed an increased risk of hospitalization from HF compared to placebo.

TECOS trial[27] concluded that sitagliptin did not increase the risk of CV events compared to placebo with regards to four-point MACE, in patients with T2DM and established ASCVD. Unlike alogliptin, it did not result in an increased risk of hospitalization due to HF.

Saxagliptin did not increase or decrease the rate of ischemic events in the SAVOR-TIMI-53 trial.[28] However, there was an increase in the rates of hospitalization due to HF with saxagliptin.

The CARMELINA study[29] examined the safety of linagliptin. Linagliptin was noninferior with regards to the risk of MACE and notably included a patient population with high CV and renal risks.

CAROLINA[30] studied linagliptin versus glimepiride in patients with relatively early T2DM and risk factors for CV events or established ASCVD. The trial evaluated 6,042 patients, followed for a median of 6.3 years. The risk of developing the primary three-point MACE outcome was equivalent in the two treatment groups.

In CVOTs involving the DPP-4 inhibitors, no agent was associated with direct cardiovascular benefit. On the contrary, saxagliptin and alogliptin demonstrated an elevated risk for hospitalization due to HF. Consequently, the AHA and Heart Failure Society of America (HFSA) concluded that for patients with HF or at high risk of HF, the use of DPP-4 inhibitors is not justified.

Thiazolidinediones

Thiazolidinediones improve insulin sensitivity of target tissues through activation of the peroxisome proliferator-activated receptor gamma (PPAR-γ), leading to favorable effects on intermediate markers of CVD and CVD risk. This engendered interest in their effects on CVD morbidity and mortality.

The PROactive study[31] assessed the effect of pioglitazone in addition to other glucose-lowering drugs in 5,238 patients with T2DM who had evidence of macrovascular disease. The primary endpoint was the composite of all-cause mortality, non-fatal MI, stroke, ACS, endovascular or surgical intervention in the coronary or leg arteries, and amputation above the ankle. Treatment with pioglitazone yielded a significant 16% risk reduction for the prioritized secondary composite MACE compared to placebo after 34.5 months follow-up, although effect on the primary endpoint was statistically insignificant.

In follow-up reports from IRIS study,[32] using updated international definitions, pioglitazone reduced ACS by 29%, type 1 MI by 38%, and ischemic stroke by 28%.

The TOSCA-IT study[33] compared CV effects of pioglitazone to various sulfonylureas in 3,028 patients with T2DM not controlled on metformin monotherapy, in those without CVD. The incidence of CV events was similar in both the treatment arms.

Rosiglitazone was initially suspected of increasing MI risk which led to product label restrictions in the United States and withdrawal from elsewhere. However, a randomized open-label CVOT, RECORD[34] showed a neutral effect of rosiglitazone on CV outcomes in high-risk patients taking metformin and sulfonylureas. Rosiglitazone label was later updated to reflect this finding.

Thiazolidinediones increase the risk of peripheral edema, with an increased risk for new or worsening HF. The labels for these agents warn against their use in patients with HF, with contraindication in patients with NYHA class III–IV symptoms.

Sulfonylureas

Sulfonylureas are oral insulin secretagogues that stimulate insulin secretion by inhibiting adenosine triphosphate (ATP)—sensitive potassium channels of pancreatic beta-cells. They are known for their high glucose-lowering efficacy but are associated with significant weight gain, risk of hypoglycemia, and consequent stimulation of the adrenergic stress-response system. Although tolbutamide increased CV and all-cause mortality in an early randomized trial from 1960s [University Group Diabetes Program (UGDP)], no such adverse CV safety concerns emerged from subsequent trials.

The sulfonylurea receptor SUR2a is expressed in cardiomyocytes, and these drugs might interfere with cardiac ischemic preconditioning through blockade of K_{ATP}-channels. This theoretical effect possibly explains the increased MI case-fatality rate observed in the more intensively treated patients in the ACCORD trial.[35] Observations from the UKPDS[36] counter the likelihood of such an effect because an intensive glucose control policy with two different sulfonylureas, chlorpropamide and glibenclamide, yielded outcomes related to MI and CV deaths, similar to those with insulin, metformin, or medical nutritional therapy.

Due to these concerns, 3rd generation sulfonylureas, for example, glimepiride, were developed, which are relatively specific for pancreatic K_{ATP} channels. In the CAROLINA trial,[30] while glimepiride was associated with significantly more hypoglycemia than linagliptin, occurrence of MACE was equal between the two randomized groups. On the basis of extensive clinical experience and efficacy of glycemic control, sulfonylureas are popular second-line drugs after metformin, for the treatment of T2DM but without the CV and renal advantages of the newer drug classes.

Insulin

The often-presumed increased risk of HF caused by fluid retention with insulin treatment has not been translated into a consistent increase in the rate of mortality or hospitalization for HF. In addition, the Outcome Reduction with an Initial Glargine Intervention (ORIGIN) trial[37] showed that the addition of glargine or standard care versus omega-3 fatty acids or placebo in patients with CV risk factors plus impaired fasting glucose, impaired glucose tolerance, or new-onset T2DM, did not increase the risk of CV events with respect to three-point MACE or revascularization or hospitalization for HF. When used to target normal fasting plasma glucose levels below 95 mg/dL for more than 6 years, insulin glargine had a neutral effect on CV outcomes.

DEVOTE[38] randomized 7,637 patients with T2DM to either insulin degludec or glargine. Although, the incidence of primary three-point MACE outcome proved similar at 8.5% versus 9.3% with degludec and glargine, respectively, the glycemic variations and risk of hypoglycemia were less pronounced with insulin degludec. A meta-analysis of four trials (ACCORD,[35] ADVANCE,[39] VADT,[40] and UKPDS[36]) evaluating outcomes of tight glycemic control showed an overall 9% risk reduction in MACE in the intensive glucose-lowering arm compared to the standard arm, mainly owing to 15% reduction in incidence of MI.

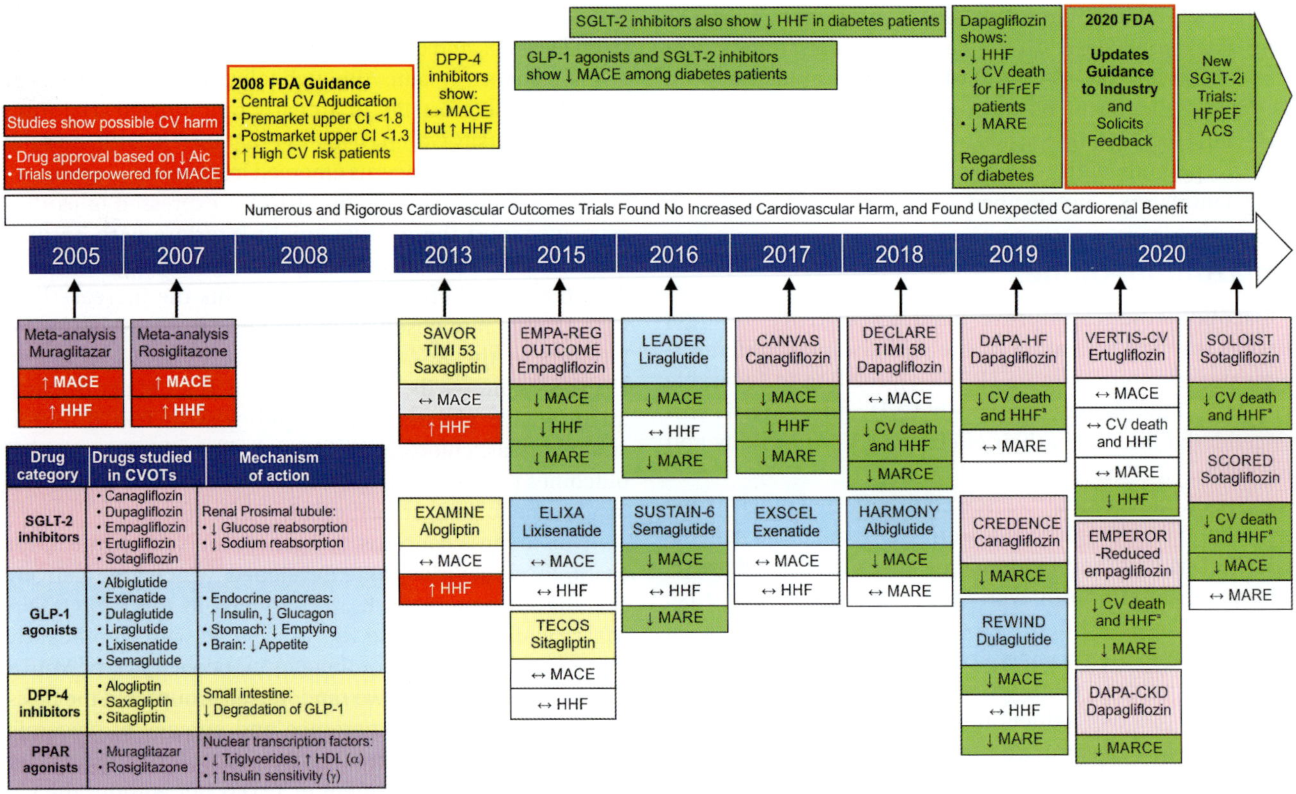

Drug category	Drugs studied in CVOTs	Mechanism of action
SGLT-2 inhibitors	• Canagliflozin • Dupagliflozin • Empagliflozin • Ertugliflozin • Sotagliflozin	Renal Prosimal tubule: • ↓ Glucose reabsorption • ↓ Sodium reabsorption
GLP-1 agonists	• Albiglutide • Exenatide • Dulaglutide • Liraglutide • Lixisenatide • Semaglutide	• Endocrine pancreas: ↑ Insulin, ↓ Glucagon • Stomach: ↓ Emptying • Brain: ↓ Appetite
DPP-4 inhibitors	• Alogliptin • Saxagliptin • Sitagliptin	Small intestine: ↓ Degradation of GLP-1
PPAR agonists	• Muraglitazar • Rosiglitazone	Nuclear transcription factors: • ↓ Triglycerides, ↑ HDL (α) • ↑ Insulin sensitivity (γ)

[a] Hospitalization for HF included as the part of primary end-point.

FIG. 2: Timeline of landmark CVOTs in diabetes drug development along with their results.
(↑: increased; ↓: decreased; <->: neutral; ACS: acute coronary syndrome; CI: confidence interval; CKD: chronic kidney disease; CVOT: cardiovascular outcome trial; DPP: dipeptidyl peptidase; FDA: US Food and Drug Administration; GLP: glucagon-like peptide; HDL: high-density lipoprotein; HFpEF: heart failure with preserved ejection fraction; HFrEF: heart failure with reduced ejection fraction; MACE: major adverse cardiovascular events; MARCE: major adverse renal and cardiovascular events; SGLT: sodium-glucose cotransporter)

CONCLUSION

Figure 2 summarizes the findings of most of the recent landmark CVOTs along with their timeline.

Intensive glucose control favorably affects microvascular disease risk, but its importance in CVD risk modification remains uncertain. Based on the accumulated data, the most recent guidelines from the ADA/EASD endorse a more individualized approach than previously recommended, with more liberal HbA1c targets for patients with shorter expected lifespans and significant comorbidities, including prevalent CVD. The landmark findings from SGLT-2 inhibitor and GLP-1RA trials demonstrated that the method that lowers glucose levels matters, particularly for those with established CVD. The benefits from SGLT-2 inhibitors on HF hospitalization and CKD progression appear to apply even in those without overt CVD. The MACE benefits of GLP-1RAs also appear to apply in patients with multiple risk factors but no established CVD.

The 2018 consensus report from the ADA/EASD advocates the use of either a GLP-1RA or an SGLT-2 inhibitor after metformin monotherapy in those with established ASCVD. In those patients where HF or CKD predominates the clinical profile, SGLT-2 inhibitors should be the preferred choice of therapy. Importantly, in the 2019 update to the ADA/EASD standards of care, the addition of these medications is now advised irrespective of the baseline HbA1c or HbA1c target. This shift from the previous HbA1c-centric approach of these organizations is noteworthy. From the cardiology community, both the ACC and the ESC advise the use of one of these drug categories in patients with T2DM and established ASCVD. In contrast, the ADA/EASD guidelines recommend these agents as first-line even in those not on metformin as summarized in **Flowchart 1**.

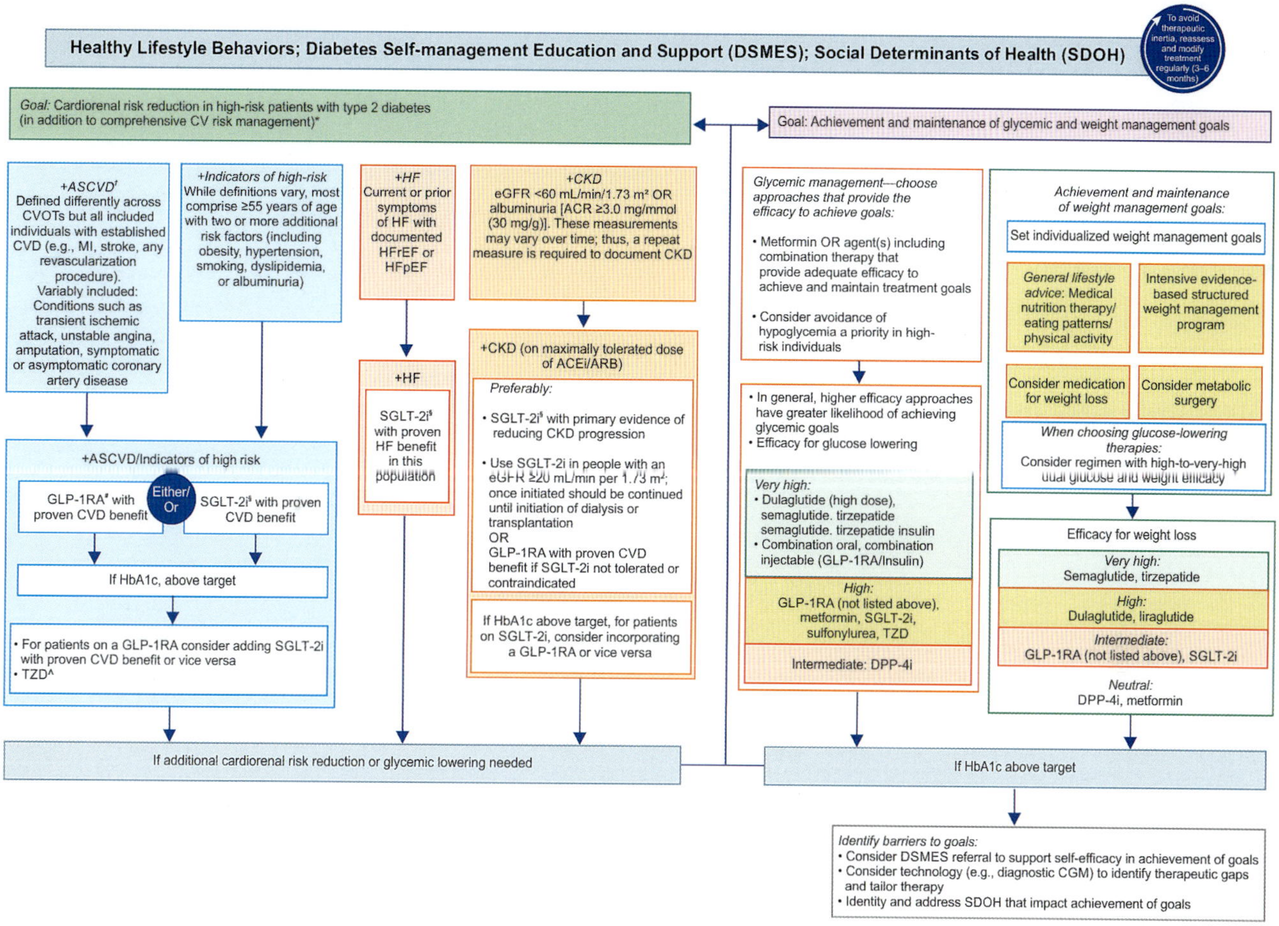

*In people with HF, CKD, established CVD or multiple risk factors for CVD, the decision to use a GLP-1RA or SGLT-2i with proven benefit should be independent of background use of metformin.

†A strong recommendation is warranted for people with CVD and a weaker recommendation for those with indicators of high CV risk. Moreover, a higher absolute risk reduction and thus lower numbers needed to treat are seen at higher levels of baseline risk and should be factored into the shared decision-making process. See text for details.

^Low-dose TZD may be better tolerated and similarly effective.

§For SGLT-2i, CV/renal outcomes trials demonstrate their efficacy in reducing the risk of composite MACE, CV death, all-cause mortality, MI, HHF, and renal outcomes in individuals with T2D with established/high risk of CVD.

#For GLP-1RA, CVOTs demonstrate their efficacy in reducing composite MACE, CV death, all-cause mortality, MI, stroke, and renal endpoints in individuals with T2D with established high risk of CVD.

FLOWCHART 1: Recommendations for the use of glucose-lowering medications in the management of type 2 diabetes mellitus.

ONLINE REFERENCES

Please scan the QR code provided at the end of the table of contents for References of this chapter.

SECTION 20

Emerging Drugs for Cardiovascular Disease

Section Outline

CHAPTER 215

Review of Thrombosis and Antithrombotic Trials of 2023–2024

Deepthi Kodati, Achukatla Kumar, Maddury Jyotsna

ABSTRACT

Even though "thrombosis" is a physiological process, it is the main culprit in many cardiovascular diseases. The field of antithrombotic therapy is continuously evolving with addition of new research and trials. The aim of this chapter is to concentrate on why there is a need in 2024 to talk about the advancement in antithrombotic therapy and what conclusion we can draw from the present-year published trials.

Keywords: Thrombosis, antithrombotic therapy, clinical trials

INTRODUCTION

Thrombosis is a physiological process of forming clots in vessels. However, it can turn into a very key pathophysiological mechanism in several diseases. It is well known that around one third of global deaths are due to cardiovascular diseases (most of these are due to thromboembolic events in coronary and cerebral vessels).

The stages in coagulation process are initiation, amplification, and propagation. In the initiation phase, a small quantity of thrombin, that is, factor IIa, will be generated. In the amplification phase, this thrombin in turn activates few platelets and some coagulation factor along factor XI (FXI) which in turn activates factors IX and X. In the propagation phase, the fibrin is generated from fibrinogen and forms the clot.

SIGNIFICANCE AND PRACTICAL CLINICAL ISSUES INVOLVED

Despite the growing understanding of the physiological process of thrombosis and several agents available to target individual pathways, there is still a lack of clarity in their optimal usage (different antiplatelet and anticoagulant drugs). No other area in clinical medicine offers such a confusion in the practice **(Fig. 1)**.

- There are several classes of drugs available targeting various pathways involved and the varying role played by each pathway in each particular disease scenario.
- Also, all drugs to prevent thrombus have a downside of risk for increased bleeding (*striking the perfect balance between thrombosis and hemostasis*—the Achilles heel of antithrombotic therapy).
- Treatment varies in the specific site of vasculature (arterial vs. venous) and specific organ involved.
- Availability of different agents among the same class of drugs, the local availability of individual drugs, their cost, varying pharmacokinetic profiles, drug-drug interactions, and presence of associated other chronic medical conditions (prior neurological, liver, or kidney diseases)
- The availability of specific reversable agents

The above-mentioned causes are some of the many factors responsible for the lack of clear consensus in the usage of these drugs and choosing the optimal agent for a particular patient. Hence, there are ongoing studies assessing these various agents in different clinical scenarios. Needless to say, studies with different drugs in varied spectrum of patient population are providing us with a lot of information albeit with some confusion (controversial results with different agents of the same class were noted too in the same subset of patients).

The aim of this chapter is to provide a short but clearer idea regarding the optimal usage of available antithrombotic drugs based on the latest trials available in this field (2023–2024) and hence simplify their clinical usage. A few recent trials which we thought offer better clarity in this regard are given in the following text.

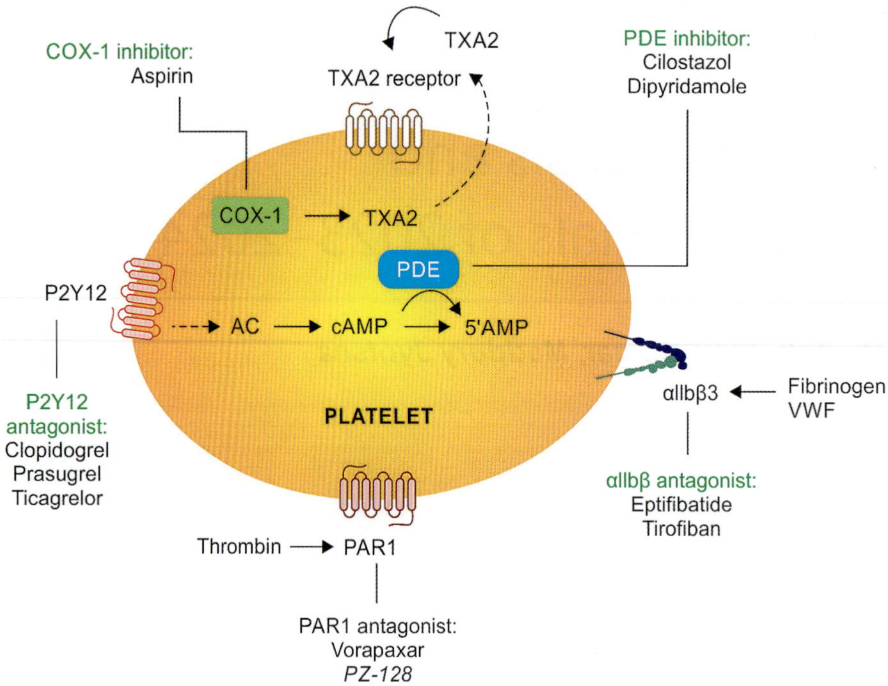

FIG. 1: Mechanism of action of different drugs to prevent or inhibit progression of thrombosis.

STUDIES OF 2023–2024

Bivalirudin Plus a High-dose Infusion versus Heparin Monotherapy in Patients with ST-segment Elevation Myocardial Infarction Undergoing Primary Percutaneous Coronary Intervention: A Randomized Trial—BRIGHT-4 Trial

BRIGHT-4 is an open-label, randomized controlled trial conducted at 87 clinical centers in 63 cities in China (6,016 patients; study period: 2019–2022). STEMI patients after primary angioplasty were grouped as either bivalirudin (B—bivalirudin plus a high-dose infusion after PCI in 3,009 patients) or only heparin (H—3,007 patients) group. GP IIb/IIIa inhibitor use was reserved for procedural thrombotic complications in both groups. The radial artery access was used in 5,593 (93.1%) of 6,008 patients. Primary endpoint was a composite of all-cause mortality or Bleeding Academic Research Consortium (BARC) type 3–5 bleeding at 30 days. Primary endpoint at 30 days was less with bivalirudin (92 events—3.06%) when compared to the heparin group (132 events—4.39%) with difference 1.33% [95% confidence interval (CI) 0.38–2.29%; hazard ratio (HR) 0.69, 95% CI 0.53–0.91; $p = 0.0070$], which is statistically significant. Similarly, all-cause mortality (B: 89 events, 2.96%, vs. H: 118 events, 3.92%; HR 0.75; 95% CI 0.57–0.99; $p = 0.0420$), BARC type 3–5 bleeding (B: 5 events, 0.17%, vs. H: 24 events, 0.80%; HR 0.21; 95% CI 0.08–0.54; $p = 0.0014$) **(Fig. 2)**, and stent

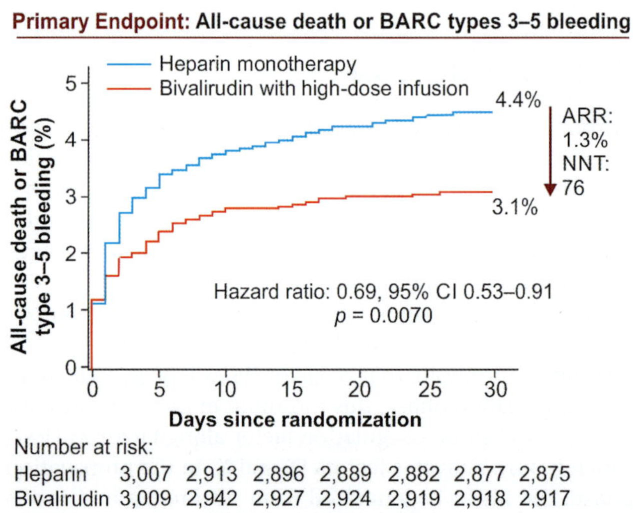

FIG. 2: All-cause death or bleeding in bivalirudin and heparin groups.

thrombosis (B: 11 patients, 0.37%, vs. H: 33 patients, 1.10%; $p = 0.0015$) were less with bivalirudin than with heparin. There were no significant differences in the 30-day rates of ischemia-driven target vessel revascularization, reinfarction, or stroke, between both the groups **(Fig. 2)**.[1]

Thus, this is a positive trial supporting use of bivalirudin in high-bleeding-risk (HBR) groups compared to a previous bivalirudin trial, and it also clarified the optimal regimen of administering bivalirudin.

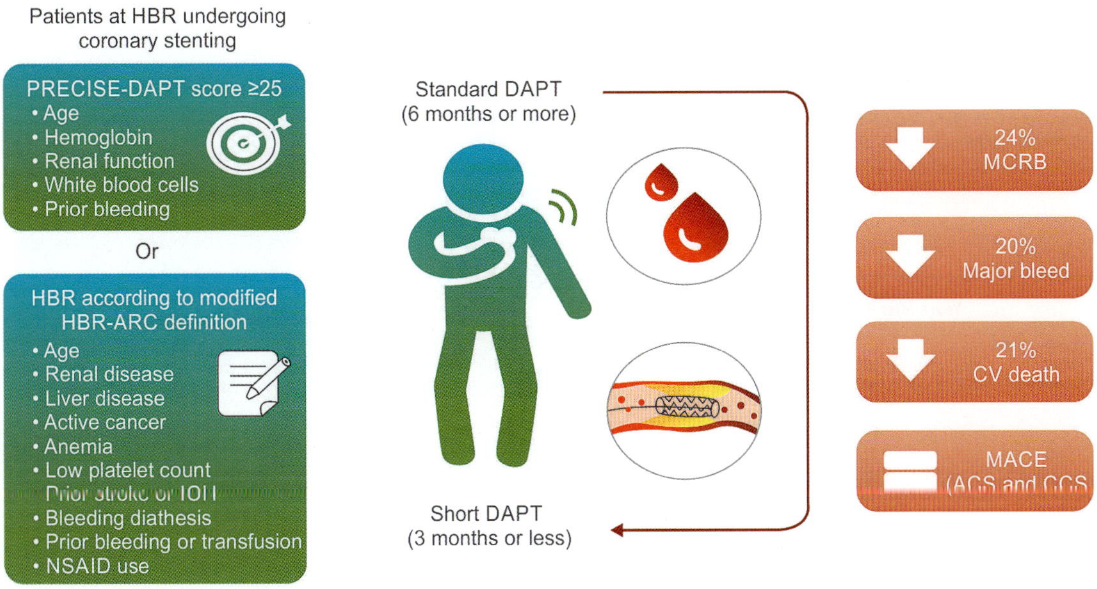

FIG. 3: Meta-analysis of 11 clinical trials.

Dual Antiplatelet Therapy Duration after Percutaneous Coronary Intervention in High Bleeding Risk: A Meta-analysis of Randomized Trials

This meta-analysis included 11 randomized clinical trials (900 patients) comparing abbreviated DAPT [ADTPT—very short (1 month) or short (3 months)] with standard (≥6 months) DAPT (SDAPT) in HBR patients without indication for oral anticoagulation **(Fig. 3)**.

Abbreviated DAPT reduced major or clinically relevant nonmajor bleeding [risk ratio (RR) 0.76, 95% CI 0.61–0.94, $I^2 = 28\%$], major bleeding (RR 0.80, 95% CI 0.64–0.99, $I^2 = 0\%$), and cardiovascular mortality (RR 0.79, 95% CI 0.65–0.95, $I^2 = 0\%$) compared with SDAPT. There was no difference in stent thrombosis, myocardial infarction, major adverse cardiovascular events, or all-cause mortality.

Thus, this meta-analysis support the use of shorter-duration DAPT in HBR patients.[2]

HOST-EXAM (Harmonizing Optimal Strategy for Treatment of Coronary Artery Stenosis–Extended Antiplatelet Monotherapy) Extended Study

This study is about 5,000 patients who were randomized to aspirin or clopidogrel monotherapy after initial SDAPT with a median follow-up of 5.8 years **(Figs. 4A to D)**. The event rates in both groups (aspirin group and clopidogrel group) are mentioned in **Table 1**.

Previously, the HOST-EXAM trial for 2-year follow-up had showed superiority of clopidogrel versus aspirin monotherapy in the prevention of the composite of readmission attributable to acute coronary syndrome (ACS), nonfatal myocardial infarction, major bleeding, and all-cause death. This benefit is persisting even in the extended-period follow-up at 5 years also.

Thus, this trial shows a clinical advantage of clopidogrel in that long-term clinical events are much lower with clopidogrel monotherapy compared to those with aspirin, thus making it the preferred choice of secondary prevention of CAD.[3]

Factor XI Inhibitor Trials

The major problem with till now known antithrombotic drugs is the bleeding. To decrease this incidence of bleeding, drugs like FXI inhibitors are studied (based on their differential effect in thrombosis vs. hemostasis, i.e., uncoupling thrombosis and hemostasis). It is not always that FXI inhibitors will be a strategy in all thrombotic conditions, as it depends on where FXI plays a major or a minor role in production of that thrombotic event. In orthopedic patients with atrial fibrillation (AF), Phase 2 trials with ASUNDEXIAN (FXI inhibitors) versus apixaban (the activated factor X inhibitor) showed a lower incidence of bleeding but no evidence of a therapeutic effect on stroke prevention. Only small Phase 2 positive trials in favor of FXI inhibitor versus enoxaparin are available in end-stage renal disease (ESRD), non-cardioembolic stroke, total knee arthroplasty (TKA), acute myocardial infarction, and AF **(Table 2)**.

The drugs available are abelacimab (MAA868), asundexian (BAY-2433334), milvexian (BMS-986177, JNJ-700-33093), osocimab (BAY-1213790), xisomab 3G3, IONIS-FXIRx (AB023), and IONIS-FXIRx (BAY-2306001, ISIS-416858, ISIS-404071). In **Table 2**, the drug details with trials are mentioned.[4]

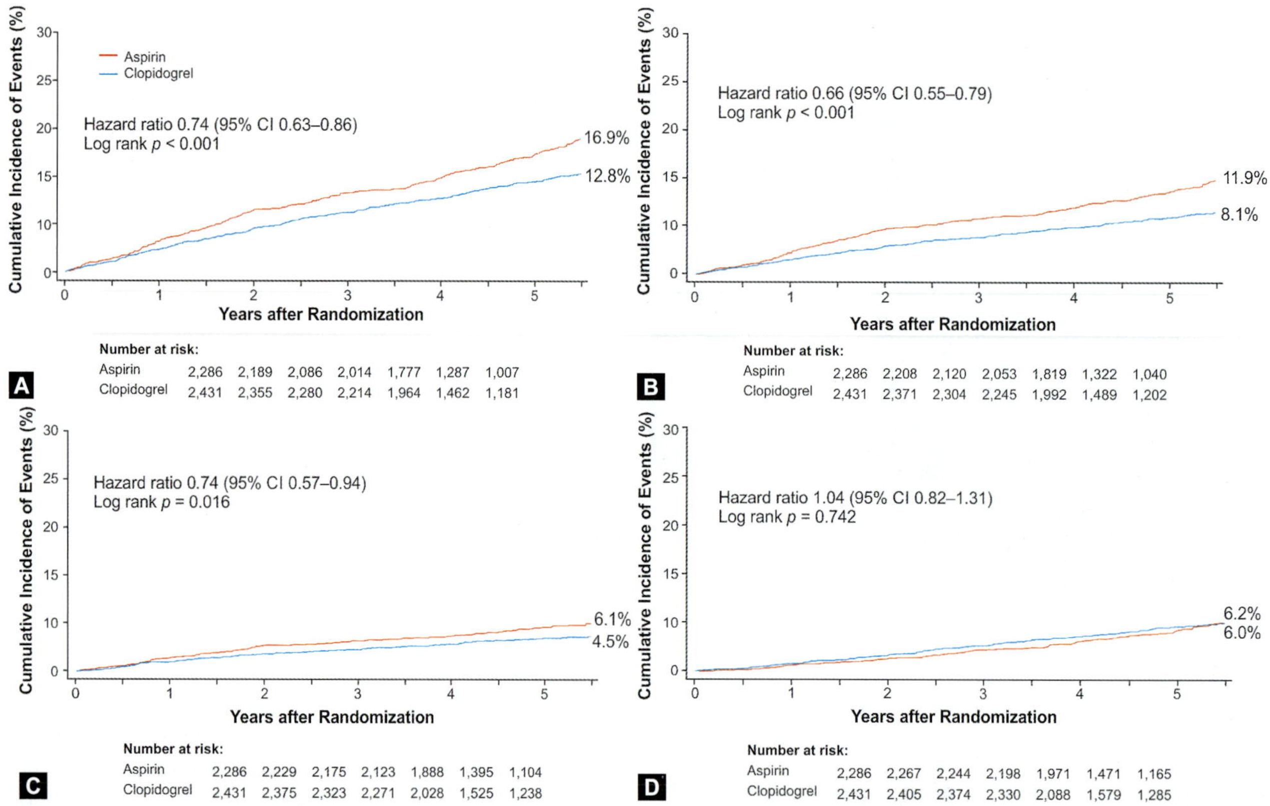

FIGS. 4A TO D: Cumulative incidence of the primary endpoint (A), secondary endpoints [(B) thrombotic and (C) bleeding], and all-cause death (D).

TABLE 1: Comparison of event rates in both groups.

Parameters during an extended follow-up of >5 years after randomization	Aspirin group (%)	Clopidogrel group (%)	Hazard ratio	*p*-Value
Primary endpoint (a composite of all-cause death, nonfatal myocardial infarction, stroke, readmission attributable to acute coronary syndrome, and Bleeding Academic Research Consortium type 3 or greater bleeding)	16.9	12.8	0.74 (95% CI 0.63–0.86)	< 0.001
Secondary thrombotic endpoint (cardiac death, nonfatal myocardial infarction, ischemic stroke, readmission attributable to acute coronary syndrome, and definite or probable stent thrombosis)	11.9	7.9	0.66 (95% CI 0.55–0.79)	< 0.001
Secondary bleeding endpoint (Bleeding Academic Research Consortium type 2 or greater bleeding)	6.1	4.5	0.74 (95% CI 0.57–0.94)	0.016
Incidence of all-cause death	6.0	6.2	1.04 (95% CI 0.82–1.31)	0.742

Apixaban and Valve Thrombosis after Transcatheter Aortic Valve Replacement: The ATLANTIS 4DCT Randomized Clinical Trial Substudy

After a successful TAVR procedure for severe aortic stenosis, follow-up is required for detection of hypo-attenuated leaflet thickening (HALT) which may lead to valve thrombosis and dysfunction [either reduced leaflet motion (RLM) or complete obstruction]. HALT can be suspected on echo, but CT confirms as it can differentiate thrombus from the other fibrotic tissue. The incidence of HALT may vary from 10% to 30% in different studies, and antithrombotic with antiplatelets may be useful in this situation. Previous GALILEO (Global Study Comparing a Rivaroxaban-Based Antithrombotic Strategy to an Antiplatelet-Based Strategy After Transcatheter Aortic Valve Replacement to Optimize Clinical Outcomes) suggested to use anticoagulants to prevent HALTs. There is no advantage of apixaban over standard therapy (S) for prevention of events; in fact, events were more in the apixaban (A) group. Composite events

TABLE 2: FXI inhibitor drugs and trials.

Parameters	Abelacimab	Milvexian	Xisomab 3G3	Asundexian	Osocimab	IONIS-FXIRx
Class	Monoclonal antibody	Small molecule	Monoclonal antibody	Small molecule	Monoclonal antibody	ASO
Mechanism of action	Inhibition of FXI and FXIa	Inhibition of FXIa	Inhibition of FXI activation by factor XIIa	Inhibition of FXIa	Inhibition of FXIa	Degradation of FXI mRNA
Route	Intravenous, subcutaneous	Oral	Intravenous	Oral	Intravenous	Subcutaneous
Doses tested in Phase II trials	30, 75, 150 mg	25, 50, 100, 200 mg twice daily; 25, 50, 200 mg once daily	0.25, 0.50 mg/kg	20, 50 mg	0.3. 0.6, 1.2, 1.8 mg/kg	200, 300 mg
Time to peak drug concentration	1 hour (intravenously), 7–21 days (subcutaneously)	3 hours	0.1–0.7 mg	1–4 hours	1–4 hours	6 hours
Time to aPTT prolongation	1 hour to 5 days depending on route	2–4 hours	10–30 minutes	4–8 hours	2 hours	3–12 weeks
Elimination	Phagocytic cells and RES	Hepatic (cytochrome P450) and renal (limited)	Phagocytic cells and RES	Metabolism and renal (limited)	Phagocytic cells and RES	Metabolism and renal (limited)
Half-life	20–30 days, depending on administrative route	11–18 hours	11–121 hours	14–21 hours	30–44 days	2 weeks
Drug–drug interactions	No	Cytochrome P450 3A4 inhibitors	No	No	No	No
Phase II studies ongoing	TKA	TKA, stroke	ESRD	• AF, stroke, AMI • PACIFIC-AF (the oral FXIa inhibitor BAY 2433334 and apixaban, in atrial fibrillation—*n* = 753)	• TKA • FOXTROT trial (factor XIa inhibition vs. enoxaparin and apixaban for the prevention of venous thromboembolism in patients undergoing total knee arthroplasty; *n* = 813)	• TKA, ESRD • FXI-ASO TKA trial (ISIS-FXIRx vs. enoxaparin in total knee arthroplasty; *n* = 300) • Bleeding was numerically lower with IONIS-FXIRx (3% with both doses vs. 8% with enoxaparin), but this difference did not reach statistical significance

(systemic embolism, myocardial infarction, any stroke, or death) at 1 year were 10.7% (*n* = 9 of 84) and 7.1% (*n* = 48 of 178) of the patients with and without subclinical valve thrombosis (grade 3 or 4 RLM or grade 3 or 4 HALT) at 90 days. So, the ATLANTIS main trial could not show the efficiency of apixaban.[5]

In the ATLANTIS 4DCT trial, after TAVI, 4DCT was done to find the incidence of subclinical obstructive thrombus on the implanted vale **(Fig. 5)**, its 1-year clinical outcome, and any difference with apixaban anticoagulation on the valve thrombosis.

The ATLANTIS 4DCT study is the largest evaluation of subclinical obstructive valve thrombosis in a TAVR randomized clinical trial. The primary endpoint of grade 3 or 4 RLM or grade 3 or 4 HALT occurred in 11.0% of the overall population, and grade 3 or 4 RLM occurred in 4.3% of patients [8.5% (antiplatelet therapy) vs. 1.1% (apixaban) in stratum 2 and 3.7% (VKAs) vs. 2.1% (apixaban) in stratum 1];

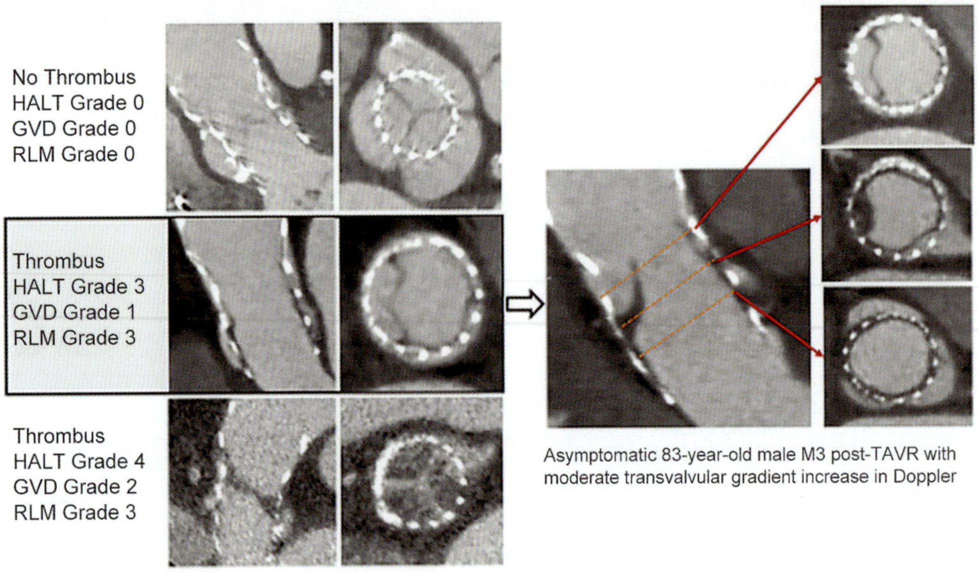

FIG. 5: Grades of valve thrombosis on 4DCT.
(GVD: global valvular dysfunction; HALT: hypoattenuated leaflet thickening; RLM: reduced leaflet motion; TAVR: transcatheter aortic valve replacement)

thrombi were detected in 22.2% of patients and significant global valve dysfunction (>50% opening limitation) in 2.9%.

Patients who had higher grades of HALTs of 4DCT had more ischemic events at 1 year. In this study, addition of 4DCT scanning in TAVR patients allowed to detect higher degradation of HALTs (>50%—incidence of 9.6%) at 90 days and these patients had more events subsequently in 1 year. The major drawback of this study is lack of power to draw conclusions. The ATLANTIS 4DCT study demonstrated that apixaban reduced valve thrombosis versus antiplatelet therapy at the cost of a nonsignificantly higher rate of thromboembolic and bleeding events. The important finding is that the benefit of apixaban was confined to the comparison with antiplatelet therapy and was consistent across the different imaging endpoints relating to both valvular dysfunction and thrombosis; no such benefit of apixaban was observed when compared with VKAs.

Apixaban for Stroke Prevention in Subclinical Atrial Fibrillation

It is well known that subclinical AF is also associated with a 2.5 times increased risk of stroke. However, there are clear clinical guidelines of benefit of oral anticoagulation in this scenario. This trial involved patients with AF detected on device monitoring, which lasted <24 hours only. If duration was >24 hours, they were excluded from trial and treated as per standard AF guidelines.

In a study of 4,012 patients with an average age of 76 and a mean CHA_2DS_2-VASc score of 3.9, 36.1% of whom were female, a 3.5-year follow-up revealed a lower incidence of stroke or systemic embolism in the apixaban (AP) group compared to the aspirin (AS) group (0.78% vs. 1.24% per patient-year, $p = 0.007$) **(Fig. 6)**. Even though the major bleeding is more in the apixaban group than in the aspirin group (1.71% vs. 0.94% per patient-year, $p = 0.001$), fatal bleed occurred less (5 patients vs. 8 patients) in the apixaban group.[6]

Thus, this trial concluded that apixaban lowered embolic event rate with a slight increase in bleeding.

Anticoagulation with Edoxaban in Patients with Atrial High-rate Episodes

Quite often, patients with devices are found to have atrial high-rate episodes (AHREs) on routine interrogation. These are nothing but native AF with a lower duration and frequency. However, the benefit of anticoagulation in this subset is uncertain. In this double-blind, double-dummy, randomized trial involving 2,536 patients [1,270 in the edoxaban (ED) group and 1,266 in the placebo (PL) group], with 37.4% being female, the study population consisted of individuals with AHREs and at least one additional stroke risk factor. The median duration of AHREs was 2.8 hours. The study was prematurely stopped due to safety concerns.

Among patients with AHREs detected by implantable devices, edoxaban did not significantly reduce the incidence of a composite of cardiovascular death, stroke, or systemic embolism as compared with placebo (3.2% vs. 4.0% per patient year, $p = 0.33$), but it led to a higher incidence of a composite of death or major bleeding (5.9% vs. 4.5% per patient-year, $p = 0.03$) **(Figs. 7A and B)**. The incidence of stroke was low in both groups (1%).

This trial shows us that the incidence of stroke was not further reduced by treatment with edoxaban, thus making it appropriate to withhold anticoagulant therapy in patients with AHREs (i.e., in patients with low arrythmia burden). However, this trial is underpowered to detect or rule out benefit of oral anticoagulation in AHREs. Further trials with other NOACs have to be considered.[7]

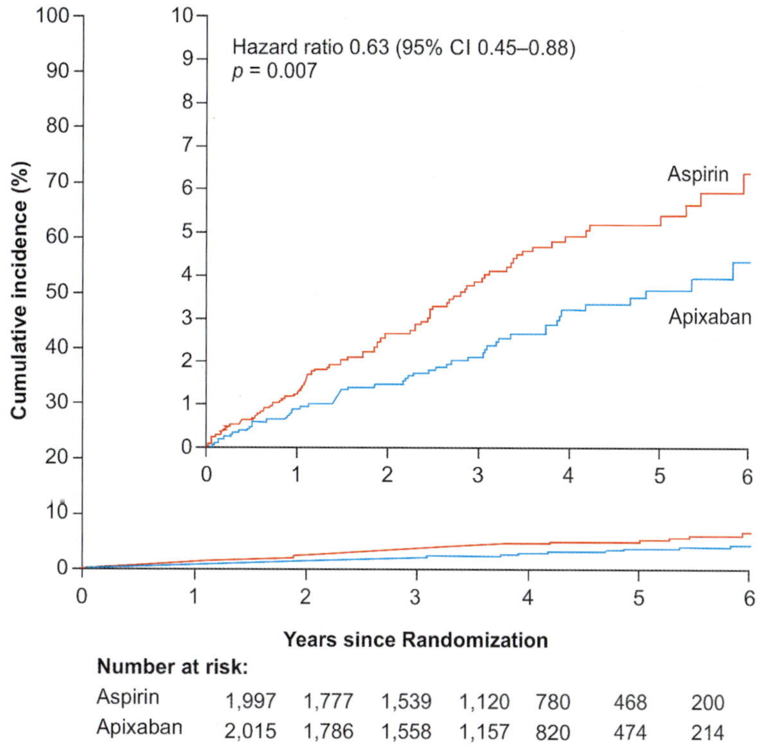

FIG. 6: Primary efficacy outcome of stroke or systemic embolism in two groups.

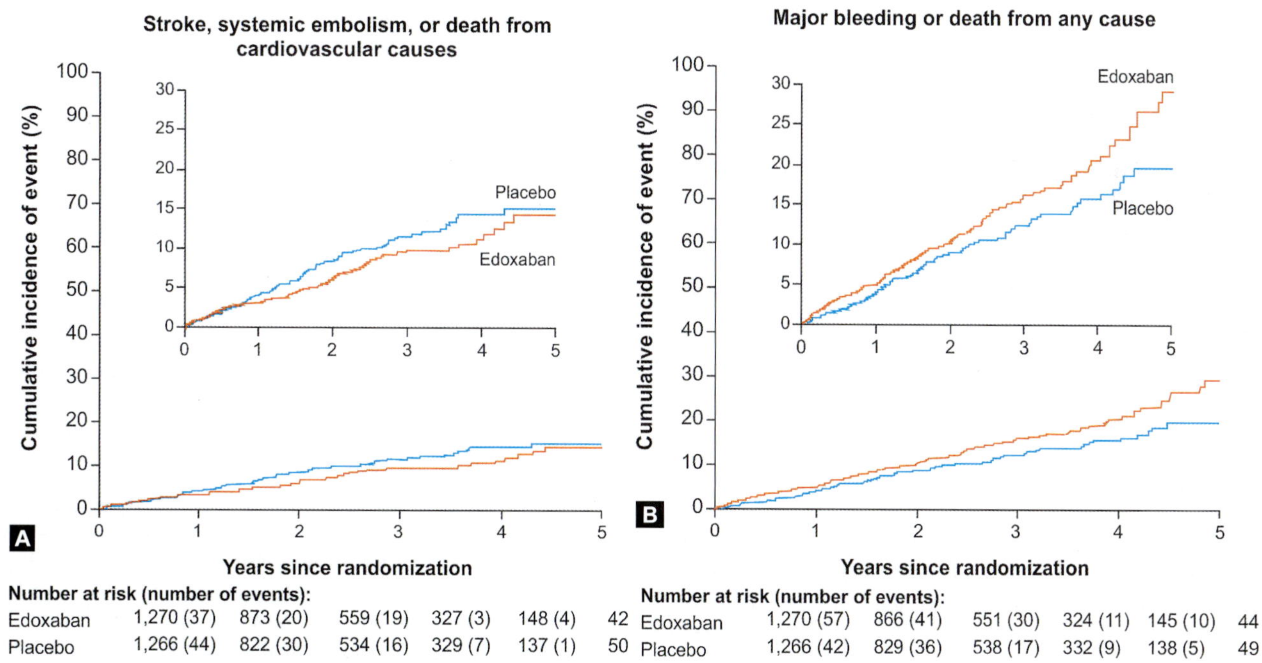

FIGS. 7A AND B: Primary efficacy and safety outcomes in the study group.

Stroke and Bleeding Risk in Atrial Fibrillation with CHA_2DS_2-VASc Risk Score of 1: The Norwegian AFNOR Study

Anticoagulation in intermediate-risk AF (nonsex CHA_2DS_2-VASc risk score of 1) which is a debatable topic was addressed in this trial in 118,762 patients. Mainly, it studied stroke and bleeding risk in AF patients with and without OAC treatment, and the risk of stroke in non-anticoagulated individuals with and without AF. Among AF patients, the ischemic stroke IR was 0.51%/patient-year in OAC users and 1.05%/patient-year in nonusers [aHR 0.47 (0.37–0.59)]. Intracranial hemorrhage IR was 0.28%/patient-year in OAC users and 0.19%/patient-year in nonusers [aHR 1.23

(0.88–1.72)]. Oral anticoagulant use was associated with an increased risk of major bleeding [aHR 1.37 (1.16–1.63)] but a lower risk of the combined outcome of ischemic stroke, major bleeding, and mortality [aHR 0.57 (0.51–0.63)]. Non-anticoagulated individuals with AF had a higher risk of ischemic stroke compared to non-AF individuals with the same risk profile.[8,9]

Thus, this trial concluded that in AF patients at an intermediate risk of stroke, OAC use was associated with lower embolic events including stroke. Non-anticoagulated AF patients had a higher risk of ischemic stroke compared to the general population without AF with the same risk profile.

Safety and Efficacy of Aspirin, Unfractionated Heparin, Both, or Neither during Endovascular Stroke Treatment (MR CLEAN-MED): An Open-Label, Multicenter, Randomized Controlled Trial

The effects and risks of antithrombotics for endovascular stroke treatment are unknown. This study aimed to study aspirin and unfractionated heparin, both or neither during endovascular stroke treatment to improve reperfusion and outcomes. This is an open-label, multicenter, randomized controlled trial from the Netherlands in 663 patients. Adult patients (i.e., ≥18 years) with ischemic stroke due to an intracranial large-vessel occlusion in the anterior circulation in whom endovascular treatment could be initiated within 6 hours of symptom onset were included with CT or MRI. Patients were randomly assigned (1:1) to receive either periprocedural intravenous aspirin (300 mg bolus) or no aspirin and randomly assigned (1:1:1) to receive moderate-dose unfractionated heparin (5,000 IU bolus followed by 1250 IU/h for 6 hours), low-dose unfractionated heparin (5,000 IU bolus followed by 500 IU/h for 6 hours), or no unfractionated heparin.

The risk of symptomatic intracranial hemorrhage was higher in patients allocated to receive aspirin (14% vs. 7%) as well as in patients allocated to receive unfractionated heparin (13% vs. 7%). Both aspirin and unfractionated heparin led to a nonsignificant shift toward worse modified Rankin Scale scores.[10]

Both periprocedural intravenous aspirin and unfractionated heparin during endovascular stroke treatment are associated with an increased risk of symptomatic intracranial hemorrhage, also without evidence for a beneficial effect on functional outcome.

Sustained Mechanical Aspiration Thrombectomy for High Thrombus Burden Coronary Vessel Occlusion: The Multicenter CHEETAH Study

It is well known that many cases of PCI in ACS subsets involve tackling high thrombus burden lesions. Needless to say, the final results in some of these are far from optimal—largely due to distal thrombus migration and embolization to distal bed with slow flow and no flow. Even on table, reinfarction and larger infarct size at follow-up are noted. To mitigate these complications, thrombus aspiration catheters prove advantageous (Thrombuster, Export, etc.). However, the routine use of these in a primary PCI setting did not prove to have an added advantage compared to routine strategy (6.9% vs. 7.0%; $p = 0.86$). Also, the varying results of trials on manual thrombus aspiration further led to their decreased usage. With the development continuing in thrombus aspiration using motorized engines, the interest in thrombus aspiration has been rekindled. The Indigo CAT RX Aspiration System (Penumbra Inc., Alameda, CA) differs from previously available coronary aspiration catheters in terms of soft distal tip, a larger aspiration port and lumen, and ability to provide continuous mechanical aspiration.

Primary composite endpoint of death, MI, and worsening heart failure was 3.60% [14/389 (95% CI 2.0–6.0%)]. The rate of stroke within 30 days was 0.77%. Final rates of thrombus grade 0, TIMI flow 3, and myocardial blush grade 3 were 99.50%, 97.50%, and 99.75%, respectively. No device-related serious adverse events occurred.[11]

Thus, it was concluded that this is a safe and effective option when used before stenting in cases with high thrombus burden.

As pregnancy, prosthetic valves, and antithrombotic management are out of the scope of this chapter since no new studies have been conducted in 2023–2024, for completion sake, we added the recommendation table in the **Appendix**. Interested readers can refer that.

CONCLUSION

Use of antithrombotic drugs continues to be a confusing aspect in certain clinical subsets. This chapter focuses on such scenarios.

- Bivalirudin bolus and continued infusion after primary PCI (unlike only the bolus given during procedure) appear to have beneficial effects on bleeding without an increase in thrombotic events.
- Careful assessment of bleeding and thrombotic risk in individual cases can help us to shorten the DAPT duration and thus the overall complications. Also, the results of HOST-EXAM are convincing to prefer clopidogrel as the agent of choice for secondary prevention of CAD after the initial DAPT duration is completed.
- FXI inhibitors appear to be very promising in tackling the Achilles heel of antithrombotic drugs, i.e., uncoupling hemostasis and thrombosis, thus playing an important role in preventing excessive bleeds while retaining optimal antithrombotic efficacy. But they still seem to have a long way to go before being implemented in clinical practice.
- NOACs, especially apixaban, after TAVI appear to minimize the CT-detected HALT and therefore are very

encouraging in enhancing the long-term outcomes of post-TAVI patients.

- Use of anticoagulation in lower-risk AF (CHA_2DS_2-VASc score ≤ 1) is not clear. However, data on apixaban usage in these subsets was associated with lower embolic events, especially stroke. However, this beneficial effect was not noted with other agents. Further trials on this subset need to be done before making any change in the guideline of management.
- In endovascular management of stroke, IV aspirin and heparin were found not to be beneficial.
- In device-detected asymptomatic AHREs, the routine use of oral anticoagulation was not warranted, unless there is another indication.
- CAT Rx aspiration catheter is a useful armamentarium in high thrombus burden cases, where routine stenting is likely to have lower TIMI flow, and a high incidence of no reflow may be noted otherwise. However, cost seems to be a major concern in its widespread usage. Dedicated trials in pulmonary bed and peripheral vasculature thrombus cases are needed.

ONLINE REFERENCES

Please scan the QR code provided at the end of the table of contents for References of this chapter.

Appendix

Recommendations for Anticoagulation for Pregnant Women with Mechanical Prosthetic Heart Valves

Recommendations	Class	Level
Pregnant women with mechanical prostheses should receive therapeutic anticoagulation with frequent monitoring during pregnancy	1	B-NR
Women with mechanical heart valves who cannot maintain therapeutic anticoagulation with frequent monitoring should be counseled against pregnancy	1	B-NR
Women with mechanical heart valves and their providers should use shared decision-making to choose an anticoagulation strategy for pregnancy; women should be informed that VKA during pregnancy is associated with the lowest likelihood of maternal complications but the highest likelihood of miscarriage, fetal death, and congenital abnormalities, particularly if taken during the first trimester and if the warfarin dose exceeds 5 mg/day	1	B-NR
Pregnant women with mechanical prostheses who are on warfarin should switch to twice-daily LMWH (with a target anti-Xa level of 0.8–1.2 U/mL at 4–6 hours after dose) or intravenous unfractionated heparin (UFH) [with an activated thromboplastin time (aPTT) 2 times control] at least 36 hours before planned delivery	1	C-LD
Pregnant women with mechanical prostheses who are on LMWH should switch to UFH (with an aPTT 2 times control) at least 36 hours before planned delivery	1	C-LD
Pregnant women with valve prostheses should stop UFH at least 6 hours before planned vaginal delivery	1	C-LD
If labor begins or urgent delivery is required in a woman therapeutically anticoagulated with a VKA, cesarean section should be performed after reversal of anticoagulation	1	C-LD

(NR: nonrandomized; LD: limited data)

In pregnant females with mechanical prosthesis, the increased risk of thrombosis should be counseled to the family. There is no need to switch from vitamin K antagonists (VKAs) to parenteral anticoagulation (except warfarin dose > 5 mg and nicoumalone dose > 3 mg). When LMWH (low-molecular-weight heparin) are planned to be given, they should be adjusted as per anti-Xa levels.

CHAPTER

216

Antiplatelet Agents in STEMI: Which, How, and When

Akhilesh Kumar, Suman Bhandari

ABSTRACT

Antiplatelet agents play a crucial role in the management of patients undergoing percutaneous coronary intervention (PCI) by mitigating the risk of thrombotic complications during and after the procedure. Administering these agents prior to PCI, particularly dual antiplatelet therapy (DAPT) with aspirin and a P2Y12 inhibitor such as clopidogrel, prasugrel, or ticagrelor, significantly enhances procedural success and reduces major adverse cardiovascular events. Recent advancements have demonstrated that newer P2Y12 inhibitors provide greater efficacy in preventing thrombosis compared to older agents, though they may be associated with an increased risk of bleeding. Therefore, selecting the appropriate antiplatelet regimen and timing is essential for optimizing patient outcomes, requiring careful consideration of individual risk profiles to balance the benefits of reduced thrombotic risk against potential bleeding hazards.

Keywords: Antiplatelet agent, thrombosis, PCI, ACS, zalunfiban, selatogrel, primary PCI

INTRODUCTION

ST-elevation myocardial infarction (STEMI) is a dynamic event in which platelet activation is a key step in the process leading up to thrombus formation. Early platelet inhibition facilitates epicardial reperfusion, reduces thrombotic burden, improves microcirculatory function, and reduces ischemic complications such as stent thrombosis (ST).[1] A rapid onset of action (especially in STEMI setting where both the duration of the period of platelet-rich dynamic thrombus formation and the reperfusion benefit are time dependent) and more effective platelet inhibition seem key elements in improving thrombotic outcomes. Antiplatelet therapy for patients undergoing primary PCI should include aspirin and a P2Y12 inhibitor.

ANTIPLATELET DRUGS

The commonly used antiplatelet drugs include aspirin, P2Y12 inhibitor (clopidogrel, and prasugrel, ticagrelor, and cangrelor), and glycoprotein IIb/IIIa inhibitor (GPI). Each agent has a distinct site of action **(Fig. 1)**.[2]

Aspirin works by irreversibly inhibiting cyclooxygenase-1 (COX-1), which prevents the formation of thromboxane A2, a key promoter of platelet aggregation.

P2Y12 inhibitors, such as clopidogrel, ticagrelor, and prasugrel, block the P2Y12 receptor on platelets, thereby reducing platelet activation and aggregation.

Cangrelor is the first and only IV, direct P2Y12 inhibitor, characterized by rapid onset and offset of action. It has been evaluated during PCI for CCS and ACS in clinical trials against clopidogrel, both with administration before (CHAMPION PCI) and after (CHAMPION PLATFORM and CHAMPION PHOENIX) PCI.[3-5]

The GPI prevents platelet aggregation by blocking the final pathway triggered separately by each of the different platelet activators, namely the binding of fibrinogen and vWF to activated GPIIb/IIIa receptors on the platelet surface. Three agents are currently approved for use—(1) the chimeric monoclonal antibody Fab fragment, (2) abciximab, and (3) the small-molecular GPI, eptifibatide, and tirofiban.

STEMI: PREHOSPITAL MANAGEMENT

The biggest delays and challenges in reducing the time to reperfusion are mostly seen in the prehospital setting. This consists of the time from the onset of symptoms to first medical contact (FMC) termed "patient delay".[1]

To minimize the patient delay there are two novel drugs as a subcutaneous injection; (1) selatogrel (P2Y12 inhibitor)

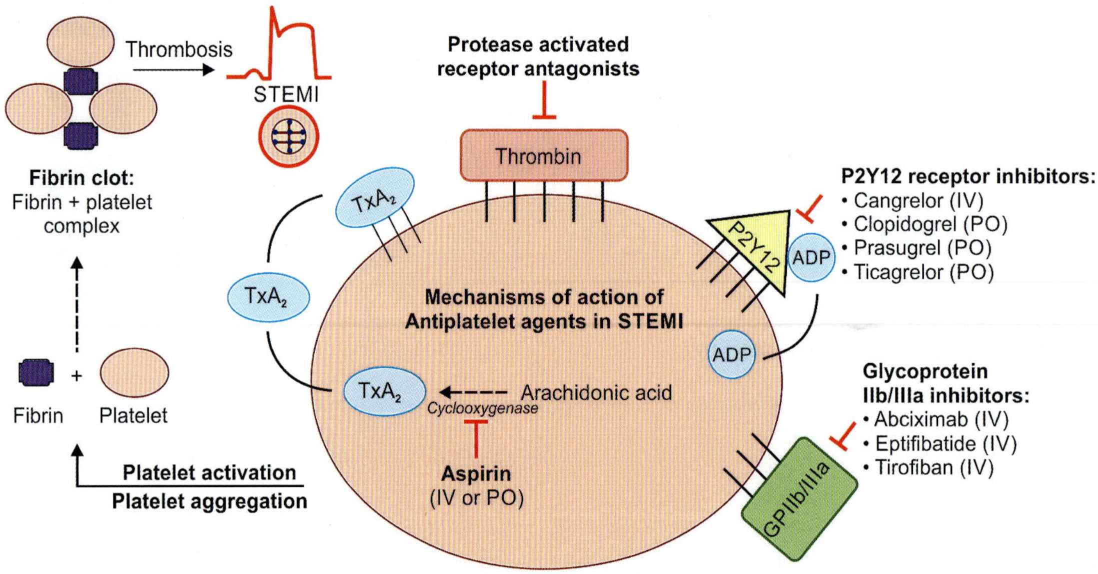

FIG. 1: Mechanism of action of antiplatelet agents in ST elevation myocardial infarction.

TABLE 1: Trials of selatogrel and zalunfiban.

Drug	Study	Population	No. of patients	Objective	Findings	Study
Selatogrel	Phase II: prospective, multinational, double-blind, randomized	ACS	29 STEMI	To compare administration of selatogrel 8 or 16 mg in terms of platelet aggregation: Response to treatment defined as P2Y12 reaction units < 100 evaluated at 30 minutes	The proportion of responders 30 minutes postdose was 91 and 96% with 8 and 16 mg, respectively	Sinnaeve et al.[7]
	SOS-AMI trial[8]	ACS	14,000	Multicenter, double-blind, randomized, placebo-controlled, parallel-group study to evaluate the efficacy and safety of self-administered subcutaneous selatogrel for prevention of all-cause death and treatment of AMI in subjects with a recent history of AMI		Ongoing, ClinicalTrials.gov Identifier: NCT04957719
Zalunfiban	Phase II, open-label trial	STEMI	24	To assess the PK/PD properties and safety	A single subcutaneous dose of RUC-4 at 0.075, 0.090, and 0.110 mg/kg showed dose-response high-grade inhibition of platelet function within 15 minutes	CEL-02 trial[9]
	CELEBRATE trial,[10] Phase III	STEMI with symptom onset < 4 hours		CELEBRATE trial is being conducted to determine whether a single prehospital subcutaneous injection of zalunfiban in addition to standard-of-care in patients with STEMI results in improved clinical outcome		Ongoing, ClinicalTrials.gov Identifier: NCT04825743

and (2) zalunfiban (GPI) are under trial. **Table 1** summarizes the ongoing trials.

Selatogrel

Selatogrel (ACT-246475) is a potent and reversible P2Y12 receptor antagonist developed for subcutaneous self-administration by patients with suspected acute myocardial infarction.[6]

After single-dose emergency treatment with selatogrel, patients are switched to long-term treatment with oral P2Y12 receptor antagonists. Selatogrel shows rapid onset and offset of inhibition of platelet aggregation to overcome the critical initial time after acute myocardial infarction. Long-term benefit is provided by oral P2Y12 receptor antagonists such as clopidogrel, prasugrel, and ticagrelor. Clinical studies in healthy subjects and phase 2 studies provided extensive information on the pharmacokinetics and pharmacodynamics of selatogrel.[7]

The ongoing global clinical phase 3 study, Selatogrel Outcome Study in Suspected Acute Myocardial Infarction (SOS-AMI)[8] evaluates the efficacy and safety of selatogrel in patients with AMI.

Subcutaneous GPI

Zalunfiban (RUC-4) differs from current GPIIb/IIIa drugs by its subcutaneous route of administration and its capacity to lock the receptor in its inactive state.[11]

The CELEBRATE trial, phase 3 prospective, blinded, randomized, placebo controlled, international study (NCT04825743) is assessing the safety and efficacy of a single subcutaneous injection of zalunfiban in patients with STEMI in the management of STEMI at FMC, a major unmet need in prehospital care that could potentially improve patient outcomes prehospital setting, with the trial due to end in 2024.[10]

The simple mode of administration of RUC-4, possibly by an autoinjector, makes it a promising candidate for the management of STEMI at FMC.

STEMI: PRE-PCI MANAGEMENT

In patients undergoing PCI, the association of aspirin plus a P2Y12 inhibitor, a strategy known as dual antiplatelet therapy (DAPT) has represented the cornerstone of treatment for patients undergoing PCI.

Dose regimen of antiplatelet drugs in ACS as per ESC 2023[12] recommendation is summarized in **Table 2**.

TABLE 2: Dose regimen of antiplatelet drugs in acute coronary syndrome patients: ESC 2023.[12]

Drug	Dose regimen
Aspirin	LD of 150–300 mg orally or 75–250 mg IV, followed by oral MD of 75–100 mg OD
P2Y12 receptor inhibitors (oral or IV)	
Clopidogrel	LD of 300–600 mg orally, followed by an MD of 75 mg OD
Prasugrel	• LD of 60 mg orally, followed by an MD of 10 mg OD • If weight ≤ 60 kg or weight > 75 kg, an MD of 5 mg OD is recommended • Prior stroke is a contraindication for prasugrel
Ticagrelor	LD of 180 mg orally, followed by an MD of 90 mg bid
Cangrelor	Bolus of 30 µg/kg IV followed by 4 µg/kg/min infusion for at least 2 hours or the duration of the procedure (whichever is longer)

Antiplatelet therapy reduces thrombotic-related periprocedural myocardial damage associated with blood vessel wall trauma such as dissections or plaque ruptures, embolization or side branch occlusions. In addition, it decreases the risk of ST, which is more frequent in the acute or subacute phase of PCI **(Fig. 2)**.[13]

STEMI: WHICH P2Y12 INHIBITOR

Based on the results of the PLATO[14] and TRITON-TIMI 38[15] studies, DAPT including aspirin and a potent P2Y12 receptor inhibitor (*prasugrel or ticagrelor*) is recommended as the default DAPT strategy for ACS patients.

Prasugrel should be considered in preference to ticagrelor for ACS patients who proceed to PCI. ISAR-REACT 5 trial[16] is the largest head-to-head comparison of 1-year DAPT with prasugrel versus DAPT with ticagrelor in patients with ACS planned for invasive evaluation, >80% of whom underwent PCI. A treatment strategy with prasugrel significantly reduced the composite endpoint of death, MI, or stroke without any increase in bleeding complications.

Clopidogrel, which is characterized by less effective and more variable platelet inhibition, should only be used when prasugrel or ticagrelor are contraindicated/not available, or in some patients considered otherwise at high bleeding risk (e.g., ≥1 major or ≥2 minor ARC-HBR criteria—discussed later). In addition, the use of clopidogrel may be considered in older patients (e.g., ≥70 years).[17-20]

Cangrelor may be considered on a case-by-case basis in P2Y12 receptor inhibitor-naïve ACS patients undergoing PCI, including in patients for whom it may not be feasible to give oral drugs in the setting of emergent PCI (e.g., cardiogenic shock patients and/or patients on mechanical ventilation). **Table 3** summarizes ESC recommendations.

STEMI: HOW: CRUSHED VERSUS WHOLE

Clopidogrel

Ines Khochtali et al.[21] compared the antiplatelet effect of crushed clopidogrel versus whole tablet in diabetic patients presenting with an ACS. No greater platelet inhibition by VerifyNow P2Y12 was achieved by crushed clopidogrel at 24-hour postloading dose compared with whole tablets in diabetic patients.

Ticagrelor

MOJITO study[22] was a prospective, randomized, four-center study, which evaluated the role of equal doses (180 mg) of crushed versus integral ticagrelor tablets in STEMI patients undergoing primary PCI. High on-treatment platelet reactivity was found in 35 and 63% of patients in the crushed and integral tablets groups, respectively.

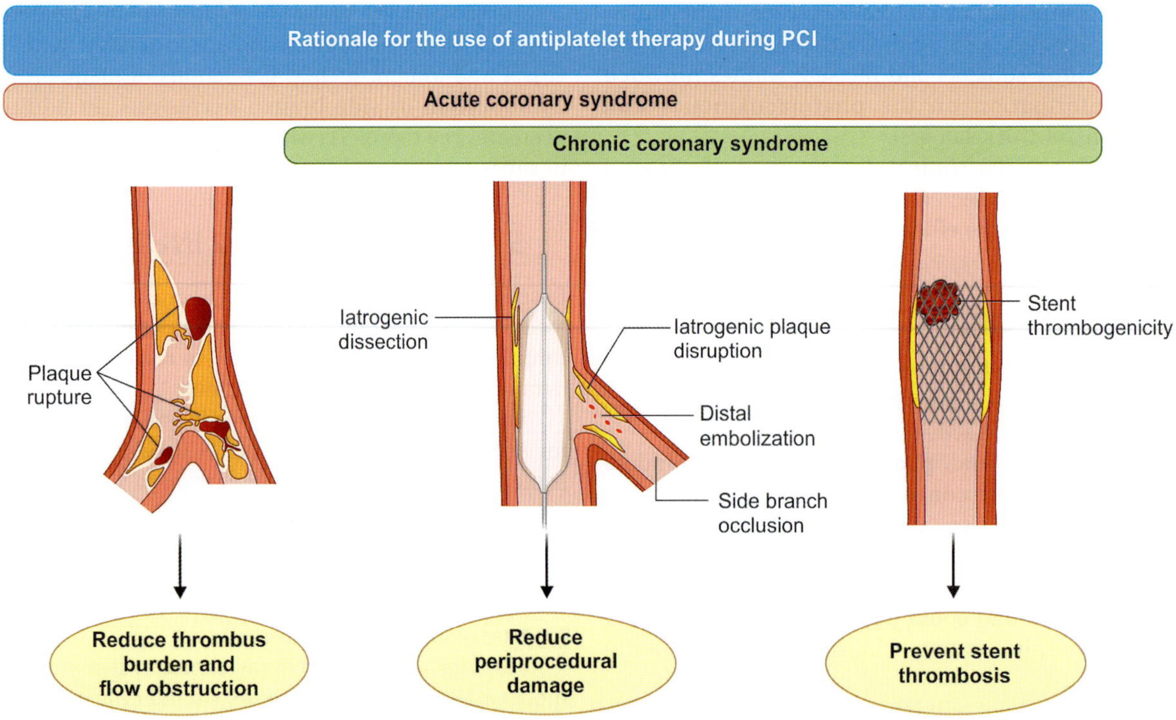

FIG. 2: Rationale for the use of antiplatelet therapy during percutaneous coronary intervention (PCI). In patients undergoing PCI in the setting of chronic coronary syndrome (CCS), antiplatelet therapy reduces the occurrence of intraprocedural or very early stent thrombosis (right), periprocedural damage caused by iatrogenic dissections, plaque disruption, distal embolization or side branch occlusion (middle). During acute coronary syndrome, antiplatelet therapy also plays a role in reducing thrombus burden and flow obstruction (left).

TABLE 3: ESC 2023 STEMI guidelines.[12]

Aspirin is recommended for all patients without contraindications	I	A
Prasugrel is recommended in P2Y12 receptor inhibitor-naïve patients proceeding to PCI	I	B
Ticagrelor is recommended irrespective of the treatment strategy	I	B
Clopidogrel is recommended when prasugrel or ticagrelor is not available, cannot be tolerated, or is contraindicated	I	C
In P2Y12 receptor inhibitor-naïve patients undergoing PCI, cangrelor may be considered	IIb	A

The LIQUID study[23] examined the pharmacokinetic and pharmacodynamic interactions of crushed versus oral ticagrelor administered in the semi-upright sitting position, in 20 patients with STEMI undergoing primary PCI. A more potent antiplatelet activity was apparent during the first hour postloading in the crushed ticagrelor group, which was attributed to the more rapid absorption and plasma exposure than with standard administration.

Prasugrel

The pharmacokinetic and pharmacodynamic profiles of crushed versus whole prasugrel tablets in 50 STEMI patients undergoing primary PCI were described in the CRUSH study.[24] The 60 mg LD of crushed prasugrel provided reduced platelet reactivity as early as 30 minutes after drug administration.

In COMPARE CRUSH trial,[25] STEMI patients being considered for primary PCI were randomized in a 1:1 fashion to either crushed or integral tablets of 60 mg prasugrel in the ambulance. Patients were followed for 48 hours. Crushed prasugrel did not improve TIMI 3 flow at first angiography or complete ST-segment resolution at 1-hour post-PCI compared with integral prasugrel. Platelet reactivity was lower in the crushed prasugrel arm, but this did not translate into lower ST events or need for less frequent bailout GPI.

Conclusion

Based on the afore mentioned studies, crushed ticagrelor or prasugrel instead of whole tablet administration may be a preferable treatment option in patients presenting with STEMI. Although crushing P2Y12A inhibitors (prasugrel and ticagrelor) prior to administration increases bioavailability and inhibits platelets faster, the clinical impact is unknown (all trials were underpowered for clinical events). However, to date, there has been no harm of crushing these drugs, so it makes sense to perform high risk PCI procedures with adequate antiplatelet drugs on board.

STEMI: WHEN

Pre-treatment refers to a strategy in which an antiplatelet drug, usually a P2Y12 receptor inhibitor, is given before coronary angiography and, therefore, before the coronary anatomy is known.

The optimal timing of the loading dose of a P2Y12 inhibitor in STEMI undergoing primary PCI remains controversial. The arguments for pretreatment in the ambulance or emergency department include the theoretical benefit of earlier onset of antiplatelet action in the prothrombotic setting of STEMI, while the arguments for drug administration in the cardiac catheterization laboratory include the potential for less procedural bleeding, reducing delays in patients who require urgent cardiac surgery, and avoiding the administration of large doses of platelet inhibitors to patients with STEMI mimics such as pericarditis, intracerebral hemorrhage, aortic dissection, or other STEMI mimics.

Clopidogrel

Use of clopidogrel as pretreatment for STEMI was evaluated in the PCI-CLARITY trial.[26] The trial demonstrated efficacy of clopidogrel; however, it is important to note that the median number of days from initiation of clopidogrel to PCI was 3 days, which does not mimic current clinical practice in which majority of the patients undergo primary PCI within 90–120 minutes.

Ticagrelor

Use of ticagrelor as a pretreatment strategy in STEMI was evaluated ATLANTIC trial.[27] In this trial, patients were randomized to receive a ticagrelor loading dose either during transfer to a PPCI center or immediately before angiography. But the trial failed to meet its primary endpoint of ST-segment resolution before PCI as well as restoration of TIMI 3 flow in the infarct-related artery. Rates of major and minor bleeding events were identical in both treatment arms.

Prasugrel

Use of prasugrel as a pretreatment strategy in patients with STEMI has not been evaluated in clinical trials.

GP IIb/IIIa Inhibitor

Upstream IV administration of GPI in the precatheterization setting in the STEMI population was determined in conjunction with aspirin in an era prior to the widespread use of oral P2Y12 inhibitors as well as prior to the use of stents.[28]

TABLE 4: ESC 2023 pretreatment guidelines.

Recommendation	Class	Level
Pretreatment with a P2Y12 inhibitor may be considered in patients undergoing a primary PCI strategy	IIb	B
Pretreatment with a GP IIb/IIIa receptor antagonist is not recommended	III	A
Pretreatment with a P2Y12 inhibitor may be considered in NSTE-ACS patients who are not expected to undergo an early invasive strategy (<24 hours) and do not have HBR	IIb	C
Routine pretreatment with a P2Y12 receptor inhibitor in NSTE-ACS patients in whom coronary anatomy is not known and early invasive management (<24 hours) is planned is not recommended	III	A

In the FINESSE,[29] AGIR-2,[30] and ON-TIME 2[31] trials, there was no statistically significant difference with the upstream administration of GPI in STEMI population. Based on the mixed data from these trials as well as evolution in the treatment of STEMI with oral antiplatelet agents, as well as primary PCI; as per the ESC 2023 guidelines, the upstream approach of GPI administration in the STEMI population is given a class III, LOE A recommendation.

Conclusion

In summary, pretreatment in STEMI with P2Y12 inhibitors does not have robust clinical trial evidence; however, due to minimal risk, administration of these agents upon diagnosis of STEMI is endorsed by the current ESC 2023 guidelines (class IIB, **Table 4**).

STEMI: IV ANTIPLATELET DURING PCI

Peri-interventional GPI (eptifibatide and tirofiban) should be considered for bailout if there is evidence of no-reflow or a thrombotic complication during PCI. Another potential use for GPI is in the setting of high-risk PCI in patients who have not been pretreated with P2Y12 receptor inhibitors.

Due to its proven efficacy of cangrelor in preventing intraprocedural and postprocedural ST in P2Y12 receptor inhibitor-naïve patients, cangrelor may be considered on a case-by-case basis in P2Y12 receptor inhibitor-naïve ACS patients undergoing PCI, including in patients for whom it may not be feasible to give oral drugs in the setting of emergent PCI (e.g., CS patients and/or patients on mechanical ventilation).

CONCLUSION

Dual antiplatelet therapy composed of ASA and a P2Y12 receptor inhibitor remains a mainstay of ACS therapy. The ESC guidelines recommend the use of potent P2Y12 inhibitors prasugrel or ticagrelor over clopidogrel in all ACS patients, unless contraindicated. Clopidogrel is reserved for situations when prasugrel or ticagrelor is not available, cannot be tolerated, or is contraindicated.

As a growing number of novel medications are introduced, there could be a paradigm shift in how antiplatelet medications are administered to patients with ACS. Nevertheless, studies have successfully proven the favorable effects of antiplatelet treatment on ACS patients, with remarkable safety and efficacy, provided that the prescribed medication and dose have been customized individually, following a meticulous evaluation of the patient's risk of bleeding.

ONLINE REFERENCES

Please scan the QR code provided at the end of the table of contents for References of this chapter.

What are Future and Novel Antithrombotic Drugs in Acute Coronary Syndrome and Percutaneous Coronary Intervention: Are there Still Unmet Needs

CHAPTER 217

Archit Dahiya, Harsh Wardhan

ABSTRACT

Antithrombotic therapy is crucial in managing acute coronary syndrome (ACS) patients to prevent adverse events. Two main categories of antithrombotic drugs are anticoagulants and antiplatelet drugs. Time is crucial in managing occlusive coronary thrombosis, and the management landscape is rapidly evolving with the development of novel antithrombotic agents. Current drugs have deficiencies, prompting researchers to develop new categories with varying pharmacokinetic and pharmacodynamic characteristics.

Keywords: Antithrombotic therapy, ACS, anticoagulants, antiplatelet drugs, researchers

INTRODUCTION

To reduce the effect of adverse ischemic events in acute coronary syndrome (ACS) patients, effective antithrombotic therapy is of utmost importance. Anticoagulants and antiplatelet drugs are the two categories of antithrombotic drugs available to us. Anticoagulants function by reducing clotting, resulting in less fibrin formation and helping to prevent the development and spread of clots.

The most important aspect in the management of occlusive coronary thrombosis is "time." The treatment should start as soon as possible to avoid irreversible damage to the heart. The ACS management landscape is rapidly evolving, especially with the development of novel antithrombotic agents **(Table 1)**. Antithrombotic therapy is an important pillar in the management of patients with ACS, proven to positively modify the outcome of such a highly vulnerable patient population. The currently used antithrombotic drugs in ACS patients have many deficiencies, and these have pushed researchers for the development of several categories of antithrombotic drugs with various pharmacokinetic and pharmacodynamic characteristics, leading to rapid changes in guideline recommendations for their indications in ACS management.

STANDARD ANTITHROMBOTIC DRUGS

The 2023 European Society of Cardiology (ESC) Guidelines recommend timely aspirin treatment, a cyclooxygenase (COX) inhibitor, for all patients with a diagnosis of ACS once contraindications for antithrombotic therapy have been ruled out.[1]

In ACS, a P2Y12 inhibitor is recommended with ticagrelor and prasugrel being the preferred agents.[2,3] Also, as per the ISAR-REACT 5 trial, prasugrel might be considered preferable to ticagrelor in patients with ACS proceeding to percutaneous coronary intervention (PCI) (Class IIa, B).[4]

In STEMI patients, the delayed onset and attenuated antiplatelet effects of oral P2Y12 receptor inhibitors are mainly due to impaired drug absorption resulting in decreased drug availability. As a result, strategies were developed to increase the bioavailability of orally administered drugs and to achieve a more immediate and fast antiplatelet effect. One technique is to take crushed or to chew the P2Y12 inhibitor (prasugrel or ticagrelor) as it may decrease the time for optimal platelet inhibition but fails to completely provide adequate results. There is prolonged contact of the drug with the saliva leading to more enzyme action and probably enhanced oral transmucosal absorption of the drug when chewed in the mouth.[5] Another technique was to implement higher loading doses of P2Y12 inhibitors (ticagrelor and prasugrel) to achieve faster and adequate platelet inhibition. However, it was seen that these higher loading doses have failed to accelerate or enhance platelet inhibition.[6]

Parenteral anticoagulation is an important cornerstone in the management of patients with ACS. In patients undergoing PCI, an unfractionated heparin bolus of 70–100 U/kg

TABLE 1: Antithrombotic drugs.

Drugs	Mechanism of action
Antiplatelet	
Aspirin	Thromboxane A2 inhibitor
Clopidogrel and prasugrel	Irreversible P2Y12 receptor inhibitor
Ticagrelor	Reversible P2Y12 receptor inhibitor
Cilostazol	Phosphodiesterase inhibitor
Tirofiban, eptifibatide, and abciximab	Intravenous glycoprotein IIb/IIIa receptor antagonist
Zalunfiban	Subcutaneous glycoprotein IIb/IIIa receptor antagonist
Cangrelor	Intravenous reversible P2Y12 receptor inhibitor
Selatogrel	Subcutaneous P2Y12 receptor inhibitor
Anticoagulant	
Unfractionated heparin	Antithrombin activation
Low-molecular-weight heparin	Antithrombin activation
Bivalirudin	Reversible and direct thrombin inhibitor
Fondaparinux	Antithrombin-mediated selective inhibition of Factor Xa
Rivaroxaban	Factor Xa inhibitor
Asundexian	Factor FXIa inhibitor

should be administered as the default therapy, followed by a titrated dosage in the cath lab to achieve a sufficient activated clotting time (ACT).

Enoxaparin (low-molecular-weight heparin) (ATOLL trial) may also be considered as an alternative to unfractionated heparin in STEMI and also in NSTEMI patients with early invasive strategies.[7]

NOVEL ANTITHROMBOTIC DRUGS

The initial success of classical antithrombotic drugs has come at the price of higher bleeding risk. However, recently newer research has shown potential differences between thrombosis and hemostasis, thus resulting in the possibility of developing newer antithrombotic drugs that do not significantly increase bleeding risk.

Bivalirudin

Bivalirudin is a reversible and direct thrombin inhibitor that can be used as an alternative to unfractionated heparin. This indication is based on the findings of the BRIGHT-4 trial, which randomized 6,016 patients with STEMI undergoing primary PCI to bivalirudin plus a high-dose infusion after PCI or unfractionated heparin. There was a significant reduction in the primary endpoints (all-cause mortality or major bleeding) at one month as well as a significant reduction in stent thrombosis in this study.[8] However, as per the HORIZONS trial, a significant increase in the incidence of stent thrombosis was seen during the first 24 hours after primary PCI for STEMI. Currently, it is mainly indicated for patients with heparin-induced thrombocytopenia (HIT) and patients with increased bleeding risk during primary PCI.

Fondaparinux

Fondaparinux acts by selectively binding to antithrombin and leads to rapid and irreversible inhibition of factor Xa. It can be used in patients with NSTEMI without an indication of early PCI. In the OASIS-5 trial, where fondaparinux was compared with enoxaparin, while the primary combined outcome of death, myocardial infarction (MI), and refractory ischemia at day 9 was similar, a significantly lower bleeding risk was observed in the fondaparinux group.[9] It is administered as a single subcutaneous dose of 2.5 mg/day. However, it is not recommended during primary PCI as per ESC guidelines.

Glycoprotein IIB/IIIA Receptor Antagonist

Regarding parenteral antiplatelet drugs, glycoprotein IIb/IIIa receptor antagonist is recommended only as a bailout drug for complex cases with high thrombotic burden and not for routine treatment. Eptifibatide, abciximab, and tirofiban belong to this group of drugs. They act by targeting the final common pathway by competing with fibrinogen and von Willebrand factor (vWF) to bind to activated GPI receptors on the surface of the platelets and thus prevent platelet aggregation. A recent study showed a beneficial effect of routine glycoprotein IIb/IIIa receptor antagonist use in STEMI patients who received morphine, as morphine use is associated with diminished absorption of oral P2Y12 receptor inhibitors and delayed onset of action of such agents.[10] However, currently these are not generally recommended in NSTEMI patients.

These drugs are given as a bolus dose and are followed by continuous infusion according to the patient's weight to achieve 80–90% platelet inhibition.

There is an unmet need for alternative agents for achieving early patency of the infarct-related artery within a limited time window and also to bridge the initial gap in platelet inhibition to preserve left ventricular function and reduce the infarction's expansion.

Nonvitamin K Antagonist Oral Anticoagulant

In the H-REPLACE trial, short-term oral rivaroxaban was compared with parenteral enoxaparin as an alternative in the acute phase of ACS. Two doses of oral rivaroxaban (2.5 mg twice daily or 5 mg twice daily) were compared with each other and also to subcutaneous enoxaparin (1 mg/kg) twice daily. The primary efficacy outcome in this trial was a composite of death from cardiac causes, MI, stroke, or revascularization during a 6-month follow-up period. 5 mg twice daily dose of rivaroxaban was found to be noninferior to enoxaparin with respect to major cardiovascular events and ISTH (International Society on Thrombosis and Haemostasis) bleeding events.[11] Due to the relatively low number of events and the short follow-up period of 6 months, this H-REPLACE trial had limited statistical power for comparing the long-term effects of rivaroxaban compared with enoxaparin.

When ACS treatment in an atrial fibrillation patient is needed, 1 week of triple antithrombotic therapy (aspirin, clopidogrel, and 20 mg rivaroxaban) followed by dual antithrombotic therapy using rivaroxaban and a single oral antiplatelet agent (preferably clopidogrel) for up to 12 months has been recommended.[1] In high-bleeding risk patients, 15 mg of rivaroxaban can be used in place of 20 mg.

As per the COMPASS trial, in patients with chronic coronary syndromes and/or peripheral artery disease (PAD), a combination of rivaroxaban 2.5 mg twice daily and aspirin once daily compared with aspirin once daily, reduced the risk of cardiovascular events but at an increased risk of major bleeding and has recently been approved by the US Food and Drug Administration (FDA) agency for these patients.[12]

Cangrelor

Cangrelor is the only intravenous P2Y12 inhibitor available and can be used in place of clopidogrel. Cangrelor is administered as a bolus dose followed by infusion. It has rapid and strong antiplatelet action. It is a short-acting drug and its effect lasts up to 30–60 minutes after termination of infusion. It induces reversible inhibition like ticagrelor. It acts directly on the P2Y12 receptor without requiring metabolic conversion in the liver. Optimal antiplatelet effect with cangrelor is achieved within minutes of intravenous cangrelor injection, whereas clopidogrel reaches maximum platelet inhibition after 4–6 hours of oral administration. Cangrelor is thus able to bridge the gap for optimal platelet inhibition. However, a pooled meta-analysis from the three CHAMPION trials failed to show any significant difference with cangrelor with regard to all-cause mortality or MI. However, cangrelor significantly reduced the risk of ischemia-driven revascularization and stent thrombosis.[13] Cangrelor does not need dose adjustment in patients with kidney or liver impairment.

The Champion Phoenix trial compared cangrelor to clopidogrel standard of care therapy in subjects who require PCIs. It showed reductions in ischemic events and overall efficacy with cangrelor. In the initial 2 hours, cangrelor significantly decreased the primary composite endpoints (death, MI, ischemia-driven revascularization, or stent thrombosis) compared with clopidogrel (4.1% vs. 5.4%; $p = 0.002$). Also, the most common events in the initial 2 hours were MI, stent thrombosis, ischemia-driven revascularization, and death. The risk of moderate to severe bleeding in the initial 2 hours between the cangrelor and clopidogrel groups was similar and also infrequent. After 2 hours and up to 48 hours, no significant difference was seen in the primary composite endpoint.[14]

Cangrelor may only be considered on a case-by-case basis in selected P2Y12-receptor-naïve patients undergoing PCI including hemodynamically unstable patients who cannot take oral medication.[15]

Zalunfiban

Zalunfiban is a type of glycoprotein IIb/IIIa receptor antagonist, but it differs from current glycoprotein IIb/IIIa receptor antagonists as it is administered subcutaneously and also it locks the glycoprotein IIb/IIIa receptors, which are present on the surface of the platelets in their inactive form.[16,17] Zalunfiban has a half-life of about 2 hours and reaches maximal efficacy within 15 minutes. After administration, it acts fast and causes a high grade of platelet aggregation inhibition. To assess the efficacy and safety of a single subcutaneous injection of zalunfiban in STEMI patients, a phase 3 trial (CELEBRATE) is ongoing and is estimated to be completed in the second half of 2024. In this trial, patients with STEMI planned for primary PCI will be given a single subcutaneous injection of either zalunfiban dose 1 (0.110 mg/kg), zalunfiban dose 2 (0.130 mg/kg) or placebo, and the injection will be given in the ambulance before being shifted to the hospital.[18]

Selatogrel

Selatogrel is a subcutaneous highly selective nonthienopyridine antagonist of the P2Y12 receptor and is under phase 3 trials to assess the clinical efficacy and safety of selatogrel 16 mg when self-administered above the standard of care upon the occurrence of symptoms suggestive of AMI.[19] It acts rapidly and has a short duration of action. Minor bleeding and dyspnea are the most commonly reported adverse effects of this drug.

Asundexian

Asundexian is one of the newer anticoagulants and acts by inhibiting Factor FXIa. It has already finished phase 2 trials (PACIFIC-AMI) to assess the efficacy and safety of oral asundexian when given along with oral DAPT in patients following an acute MI.[20] It concluded that lower ischemic events occurred when three doses of 50 mg asundexian were given in addition to DAPT to patients with recent acute MI and without a significant increase in bleeding risk.

CONCLUSION

As antithrombotic agents are the most important pillar in the management of ACS and during PCI, there has been a constant search for ideal antithrombotic agents with high efficacy, low bleeding risk, ease of administration, and fast onset of action. Whereas drugs such as ticagrelor and prasugrel have become the standard of care, rivaroxaban and cangrelor are finding a place in the management of a selective group of patients. Drugs such as zalunfiban, selatogrel, and asundexian are undergoing clinical trials and may become available in the near future, adding to the armamentarium of drugs to effectively manage ACS and PCI patients.

ONLINE REFERENCES

Please scan the QR code provided at the end of the table of contents for References of this chapter.

CHAPTER

218

Emerging Promising Drugs for Cardiovascular Disease

Safal, Mayank Shami

ABSTRACT

Cardiology is one of the most rapidly growing fields of modern medicine. It is a unique branch where medical and interventional therapy complement each other to optimize patient outcomes. In this chapter, we discuss some of the latest drugs that have either recently been added to the cardiologist's armamentarium or are likely to be added in the near future and have the potential to change patient outcomes significantly. The categories covered include antihypertensives, hypolipidemic agents, heart failure therapy, amyloidosis, and hypertrophic cardiomyopathy. Few established drugs that have the potential to be repurposed for newer cardiac indications, like semaglutide and colchicine, have also been discussed briefly.

Keywords: Newer drug therapy, emerging treatment, recent advances

INTRODUCTION

While substantial progress has been made with respect to the management of cardiovascular diseases (CVD) over the past few decades, there is still a lot of uncovered ground that needs to be covered. This chapter explores some of the most promising emerging drugs in cardiology, focusing on their mechanisms of action, clinical trial results, current status, and potential impact on patient care.

NEWER ANTIHYPERTENSIVE DRUGS

Aprocitentan

On March 19, 2024, the US Food and Drug Administration (FDA) approved aprocitentan (Tryvio) for treating patients with resistant hypertension. Aprocitentan (ACT-132577) is the first endothelin receptor antagonist to receive approval as an antihypertensive, specifically for resistant hypertension.

Mechanism of Action

Aprocitentan is an endothelin receptor antagonist that targets both endothelin-1 (ET-1) receptors, namely ET-A and ET-B receptors, which play a crucial role in regulating vascular tone and blood pressure. ET-1 is a potent vasoconstrictor peptide produced by endothelial cells. It acts through two types of receptors: ET-A, primarily located on vascular smooth muscle cells, and ET-B, which is found on both endothelial cells and smooth muscle cells. By blocking ET-A and ET-B receptors, aprocitentan reduces the vasoconstrictive effects of ET-1, in turn leading to vasodilation, decreased vascular resistance, and ultimately a reduction in blood pressure.[1]

Clinical Trial

PRECISION was a multicenter, blinded, randomized, parallel-group, phase 3 study done in centers across Europe, North America, Asia, and Australia. Patients with sitting systolic blood pressure (SBP) of ≥140 mm Hg despite three antihypertensive drugs (including a diuretic) were eligible to participate. In the first part of the study, 730 patients were randomized to receive aprocitentan 12.5 mg, aprocitentan 25 mg, or placebo for 4 weeks in a 1:1:1 ratio. This was followed by a 32-week single (patient)-blind period in which all patients received aprocitentan 25 mg. After this, there was a 12-week double-blind withdrawal part, in which patients were re-randomized to receive aprocitentan 25 mg or placebo in a 1:1 ratio. The study showed a significant reduction in office SBP as well as 24-hour ambulatory SBP with both 12.5 mg and 25 mg doses. Fluid retention/

mild-to-moderate edema led to drug discontinuation in seven patients. A significant antiproteinuric effect was also observed at both doses of aprocitentan, which is relevant and truly promising in terms of the reduction of target organ damage.[2]

Indication and Dosage

Aprocitentan has a half-life of ~44 hours and steady-state conditions are reached after 8 days.[1] While both 12.5 and 25 mg once daily doses were studied in the PRECISION trial, US FDA approval has been received for the 12.5 mg daily dose. As per the official FDA prescribing information, aprocitentan is indicated "for the treatment of hypertension in combination with other antihypertensive drugs, to lower blood pressure in adult patients who are not adequately controlled on other drugs."[3] Apart from fluid retention, other known side effects include a fall in hemoglobin, reduction in sperm count, and hepatotoxicity. The drug is contraindicated in pregnancy.

Zilebesiran

Zilebesiran is an investigational RNA interference therapeutic agent that inhibits hepatic angiotensinogen synthesis. RNA interference is a natural cellular process of gene silencing that has emerged as a highly promising drug development target. Synthetic small interfering ribonucleic acid (siRNA) are used to silence the target messenger RNA (mRNA)—thus halting the synthesis of the target protein—in this case, angiotensinogen. This action of halting protein synthesis is upstream of conventional drug targets like receptor blockade and has a long-lasting effect, thereby requiring infrequent dosing.

In a phase 1 study, dose-dependent decreases in serum angiotensinogen levels and 24-hour ambulatory blood pressure were found to be sustained for up to 24 weeks after a single subcutaneous dose of zilebesiran of 200 mg or more; mild injection-site reactions were observed. KARDIA-1, a phase 2 randomized double-blind study in adults with mild-to-moderate hypertension, also showed that treatment with zilebesiran across a range of doses at 3- or 6-month intervals significantly reduced 24-hour mean ambulatory SBP at 3 months. A number of phase 2 studies are ongoing with this drug, and it holds great hope for the near future.[4,5]

NEWER HYPOLIPIDEMIC DRUGS

Proprotein convertase subtilisin/kexin type 9 (PCSK9) monoclonal antibodies, including evolocumab and alirocumab, are now established therapies for CV risk reduction in patients at very high risk of future CV events when LDL targets are not achieved with maximum tolerated statins + ezetimibe.[4] Unfortunately, despite compelling evidence of CV risk reduction, their penetration in routine clinical practice in our country is still low, partly due to cost issues and in part due to physician inertia. However, discussing them as an "emerging" therapy would not be correct; hence we shall focus on newer hypolipidemic agents other than PCSK9 monoclonal antibodies in this chapter.

Inclisiran

Mechanism of Action

Inclisiran is a long-acting, synthetic siRNA that silences translation of PCSK9 mRNA by binding to RNA-induced silencing complex; this inhibits hepatic translation of PCSK9 protein, resulting in up-regulation of LDL receptor density on hepatocytes. Thus, inclisiran is also a "PCSK9 inhibitor"—although at an intracellular level.

Clinical Trials/Evidence

In a pooled patient-level analysis of 3,660 patients in phase 3 trials of inclisiran (ORION-9, ORION-10, and ORION-11), the drug showed approximately 51% reduction in LDL-cholesterol at day 510. Although there are no head-to-head comparisons of evolocumab or alirocumab with inclisiran, on comparing similarly designed trials, LDL-C-lowering response to inclisiran appears to be around 10% less than the PCSK9 monoclonal antibodies. Nevertheless, the twice-yearly dosing (after the first two doses) is a significant attraction aspect of this drug. Although LDL-C reduction as well as safety and tolerability have been established, the cardiovascular outcome trials with inclisiran (ORION-4 and VICTORION-2P) are still ongoing.[6,7]

Indications and Dosage

Inclisiran is currently approved by the US FDA "as an adjunct to diet and statin therapy for the treatment of adults with primary hyperlipidemia, including heterozygous familial hypercholesterolemia (HeFH), to reduce low-density lipoprotein cholesterol (LDL-C)."[8]

Inclisiran is administered as a subcutaneous injection in the abdomen or thigh. The standard dosing regimen starts with a dose of 284 mg, repeated at 3 months and then every 6 months. It is generally well-tolerated, with minor injection site reaction being the most common side effect. Arthralgia and bronchitis have also been described with increased frequency vis-à-vis placebo in individuals receiving inclisiran.[8]

Angiopoietin-like Protein 3 Inhibitors

Evinacumab

Mechanism of Action

Angiopoietin-like protein 3 (ANGPTL3) inhibits lipoprotein lipase and endothelial lipase, enzymes crucial for the breakdown of triglycerides and LDL-C. Evinacumab is a fully human monoclonal antibody that inhibits ANGPTL3, thereby activating both lipoprotein lipase and endothelial lipase. This prevents hepatic secretion of triglyceride-rich lipoproteins, in turn reducing triglycerides and total cholesterol. Notably, as the action of evinacumab is independent of the LDL receptor, the drug is expected to be successful even in homozygous familial hypercholesterolemia (HoFH) patients with absent or defective LDL receptors.

Clinical Trial/Evidence

The ELIPSE HoFH (Evinacumab Lipid Studies in Patients with Homozygous Familial Hypercholesterolemia) trial was a double-blind, placebo-controlled, phase 3 trial in which 65 patients with HoFH on stable lipid-lowering therapy with LDL-C ≥70 mg/dL were randomly assigned in a 2:1 ratio to receive an intravenous infusion of evinacumab every 4 weeks or placebo. There was a 47.1% relative reduction from baseline in LDL-C in patients treated with evinacumab, vis-à-vis an increase of 1.9% in the placebo group.[9]

Indications and Dosage

In 2021, evinacumab received US FDA approval as an adjunct to other LDL-C lowering therapies for the treatment of adult and pediatric patients, aged 12 years and older, with HoFH. The recommended dose is 15 mg/kg administered by intravenous infusion over 60 minutes once monthly (every 4 weeks). Serious hypersensitivity reactions can occur and have to be watched for; pregnancy must be avoided till at least 5 months after the last dose.

Other ANGPTL3 Inhibitors and Similar Agents

Vupanorsen is an *N*-acetyl galactosamine-conjugated therapy targeting the delivery of antisense oligonucleotides to hepatocytes to prevent upstream production of ANGPTL3. In a phase 2, double-blind, placebo-controlled trial of 105 patients with hypertriglyceridemia (>150 mg/dL), type 2 diabetes, and hepatic steatosis, the drug was associated with a 53% reduction in triglycerides. Additionally, there was a significant reduction in Apo-CIII, remnant cholesterol, total cholesterol, and HDL cholesterol, but no significant change in LDL-C.[10]

Phase 2b trial with *zodasiran*, a siRNA-based therapy targeting expression of *ANGPTL3* in the liver, has also shown a marked reduction in triglyceride levels on targeting this pathway. Significant reduction in triglyceride levels has also been seen with *plozasiran*, a hepatocyte-targeted *APOC3* siRNA, in patients with mixed hyperlipidemia. However, worsening glycemic control might be a concern with both zodasiran and plozasiran.[11,12]

Bempedoic Acid

Bempedoic acid received US FDA approval in 2020 as an adjunct to diet and maximally tolerated statin therapy for the treatment of adults with HeFH or established atherosclerotic CVD who require additional lowering of LDL-C.

Mechanism of Action

Bempedoic acid inhibits ATP-citrate lyase, an enzyme upstream of HMG-CoA reductase in the cholesterol synthesis pathway. This inhibition leads to reduced hepatic cholesterol synthesis and increased LDL receptor expression, an effect that is similar to that of statins. However, being a prodrug that is activated in the liver and not in the skeletal muscle, its potential for muscle-related side effects is much lower than statins.

Clinical Trial/Evidence

A number of trials have shown that bempedoic acid can lower LDL-C levels by approximately 17–28% and can be particularly effective in patients who are intolerant to statins or require additional LDL-C reduction. The CLEAR-Outcomes was a double-blind, randomized, placebo-controlled trial involving patients who were unable or unwilling to take statins owing to unacceptable adverse effects ("statin-intolerant" patients) and had, or were at high risk for, CVD. About 13,970 patients were randomized to placebo or 180 mg of bempedoic acid daily. After a median follow-up of 40.6 months, the therapy group had 21.1% reduction in LDL as well as a significantly lower incidence of major adverse cardiovascular events.[13]

Indications and Dosage

Bempedoic acid is given at a dose of 180 mg once daily. It is typically prescribed when patients are not able to achieve their LDL-C goals with maximally tolerated statin therapy and/or other lipid-lowering therapies, or in patients who are statin intolerant. The drug is well-tolerated, with common adverse effects including musculoskeletal pain and gastrointestinal symptoms. Its adverse effect frequency is more favorable compared to statins, particularly regarding muscle-related side effects.

NEWER HEART FAILURE DRUGS

Vericiguat

In 2021, vericiguat—a soluble guanylate cyclase (sGC) stimulator—received US FDA approval for use in a select group of HFrEF patients who had experienced recent worsening of heart failure.

Mechanism of Action

Vericiguat enhances the cyclic guanosine monophosphate (GMP) pathway by directly stimulating sGC through a binding site independent of nitric oxide; it also sensitizes sGC to endogenous nitric oxide by stabilizing nitric oxide binding to the binding site. Increased production of cGMP leads to vasodilation and reduced vascular resistance. This helps to decrease the heart's workload and improve cardiac output. As the mechanism of action is distinct from any component of the "four pillars" of HFrEF therapy, this drug has a niche use as an add-on to established HFrEF therapies.

Clinical Trial/Evidence

The VICTORIA trial was a phase 3, randomized, double-blind, placebo-controlled trial. It enrolled 5,050 patients with chronic heart failure, LVEF < 45% within 12 months before randomization, and an elevated natriuretic peptide level within 30 days before randomization. Each enrolled patient had at least one episode of "recent worsening of heart failure"—defined as hospitalization within 6 months preceding randomization or need for intravenous diuretic therapy within 3 months preceding randomization. The primary outcome was a composite of death from cardiovascular causes or first hospitalization for heart failure; this occurred in 897 patients (35.5%) in the vericiguat group and 972 patients (38.5%) in the placebo group [hazard ratio (HR) 0.90; 95% CI 0.82–0.98; $p = 0.02$].[14]

The phase III study VICTOR study is currently ongoing to assess vericiguat efficacy and safety in chronic HFrEF patients who have not had a recent worsening heart failure event.

Indications and Dosage

Based on the results of the VICTORIA trial, vericiguat has an IIb recommendation for use in selected HFrEF patients who are already on guideline-directed medical therapy and have a recent worsening of heart failure.[15] The recommended starting dose is 2.5 mg once daily, which may be doubled every 2 weeks to achieve a target dose of 10 mg daily. The drug is reasonably well tolerated but symptomatic hypotension and a fall in hemoglobin may occur. Vericiguat is contraindicated in pregnancy and in patients taking other sGC stimulators or phosphodiesterase-5 inhibitors.

Finerenone

Finerenone is a novel nonsteroidal mineralocorticoid receptor antagonist (MRA) that has emerged as a promising therapeutic option in the management of diabetic kidney disease and heart failure.

Mechanism of Action

Finerenone works by selectively antagonizing the mineralocorticoid receptor (MR), a key player in regulating electrolyte balance and blood pressure. Unlike traditional steroidal MRAs such as spironolactone and eplerenone, finerenone offers a more targeted approach, which can help mitigate some of the adverse effects associated with long-term steroidal MRAs. By blocking MR, finerenone reduces inflammatory and fibrotic processes in the kidneys and heart. Its action helps decrease the progression of CKD and improve outcomes in patients with HF by reducing fluid overload and vascular resistance.

Clinical Trial/Evidence

The FIDELIO-DKD trial in patients with diabetic kidney disease demonstrated a statistically significant reduction of 18% in the primary endpoint (composite of kidney failure, a sustained decrease of ≥40% in the eGFR from baseline over a period of ≥4 weeks, or death from renal causes) with finerenone, over a median follow-up of 2.6 years. Although finerenone was associated with a lower occurrence of the key secondary endpoint [a composite of CV death, nonfatal myocardial infarction (MI), nonfatal stroke, and hospitalization for HF], there was no reduction in heart failure hospitalization per se. Patients with HFrEF and NYHA classes II–IV were excluded from this trial.[16]

In the FIGARO-DKD trial, the primary outcome was a composite of death from CV causes, nonfatal MI, nonfatal stroke, or hospitalization for HF. It included 7,437 adults with T2DM and CKD treated with a renin–angiotensin system inhibitor at maximum tolerated dose. At a median follow-up of 3.4 years, the rate of primary outcome was significantly lower in the treatment arm compared with placebo (HR 0.87; 95% CI 0.76–0.98; $p = 0.03$). The benefit was driven by a numerically small, but statistically significant, lower incidence of HF hospitalization seen with finerenone.[17] A prespecified individual patient-level, pooled analysis of 13,026 patients with diabetic kidney disease (taken from both FIDELIO-DKD and FIGARO-DKD trials), also showed a reduction in the composite CV outcome, as well as in HF hospitalizations alone, with finerenone versus placebo. With this background, the ESC in 2023 gave a class I indication for the use of finerenone in patients with T2DM and CKD to reduce the risk of heart failure hospitalization.[18,19]

The recently published FINEARTS-HF trial affirmed the role of finerenone as one of the few therapies beneficial in HFmrEF and HFpEF. In this international, double-blind trial, patients with heart failure and LVEF of 40% or greater were randomized in a 1:1 ratio, to receive finerenone or placebo, in addition to usual therapy. The primary outcome was a composite of total worsening heart failure events ("event" defined as a first or recurrent unplanned hospitalization or urgent visit for heart failure) and death from cardiovascular causes. Over a median follow-up of 32 months, 1,083 primary-outcome events occurred in 624 patients in the finerenone group, and 1,283 primary-outcome events occurred in 719 patients in the placebo group ($p = 0.007$). The total number of worsening heart failure events was 842 in the finerenone group and 1,024 in the placebo group ($p = 0.006$). It is to be emphasized that this trial was done in a heart failure population, and diabetes or CKD were not essential inclusion criteria; all patients were in NYHA classes II–IV, 48% had eGFR < 60 mL/min/1.73 m^2, mean LVEF was 53%, and 48% patients were diabetic.[20]

Indications and Dosage

Finerenone is administered orally, typically starting at a dose of 20 mg once daily if eGFR is ≥60 mL/min/1.73 m^2.

For patients with eGFR between 25 and 60, the starting dose is 10 mg once daily. The drug should not be initiated if eGFR is <25 mL/min/1.73 m^2 or if serum potassium exceeds 5 mEq/L. Current FDA approval for finerenone is to reduce the risk of sustained eGFR decline, end-stage kidney disease, cardiovascular death, nonfatal MI, and hospitalization for heart failure in adult patients with CKD associated with type 2 diabetes. However, approval for use in HFmrEF and HFpEF can be expected in the near future.

Semaglutide

The glucagon-like peptide-1 (GLP-1) agonist semaglutide, a well-known antidiabetic and antiobesity agent, has shown promise in a number of cardiovascular outcome trials to reduce cardiovascular adverse events and heart failure symptoms. Based on the results of the SELECT trial, semaglutide received US FDA approval in 2024 for use in the nondiabetic population—to reduce the risk of major adverse cardiovascular events (cardiovascular death, nonfatal MI, or nonfatal stroke) in obese or overweight adults with established CVD. Additionally, recent studies have explored the impact of semaglutide on obese patients with HFpEF and found significant improvement in quality-of-life scores irrespective of diabetic status.[21,22]

In adults, semaglutide is started at 0.25 mg once a week subcutaneously and gradually escalated by week 17 to the target dose of 2.4 mg weekly. The drug is contraindicated in patients with a family history of medullary carcinoma thyroid. Diabetics need to be monitored for hypoglycemia as well as diabetic retinopathy complications. Acute pancreatitis and acute gallbladder disease have also been reported.

MISCELLANEOUS DRUGS

Acoramidis

Tafamidis, the currently approved treatment for transthyretin amyloidosis, stabilizes transthyretin tetramers (TTR), thereby reducing their dissociation into unstable monomers and subsequent deposition as amyloid fibrils in the myocardium. It has shown benefits in slowing disease progression but is not effective for all patients and does not reverse the condition. A more potent TTR stabilizing agent may improve outcomes further. A rare mutation *(T119M)* in the gene encoding TTR results in a variant with better stabilization of the tetramer than wild-type TTR; acoramidis is designed to mimic the action of this T119M variant and provide more effective TTR stabilization (over 90% stabilization as measured ex vivo).

The clinical efficacy of acoramidis was tested in the ATTRibute-CM trial, a phase III, multinational, double-blind, placebo-controlled study. About 632 patients with transthyretin amyloid cardiomyopathy were randomized in a 2:1 ratio to receive acoramidis hydrochloride at a dose of 800 mg twice daily or matching placebo for 30 months. Acoramidis administration was associated with significantly better outcomes (win ratio of 1.8).[23] FDA approval for this drug is currently pending.

Aficamten

Mavacamten, an allosteric, selective, and reversible inhibitor of cardiac myosin ATPase, received FDA approval in 2022 for the treatment of adults with symptomatic NYHA II–III hypertrophic obstructive cardiomyopathy (HOCM) to improve functional capacity and symptoms. Aficamten, another reversible cardiac myosin inhibitor, is designed to have a shallow dose-response relationship (small reductions in LVEF as the dose is increased, resulting in a wide therapeutic window) and a plasma half-life that allows for personalized dose adjustments as often as every 2 weeks—features that are likely to give the drug an advantage over mavacamten.

The SEQUOIA-HCM was a phase 3, double-blind randomized trial of 282 patients with symptomatic obstructive HCM. Patients were randomized to receive aficamten (starting dose, 5 mg; maximum dose, 20 mg) or placebo for 24 weeks, with dose adjustment based on echocardiography results. The primary endpoint was a change in peak oxygen uptake from baseline to week 24. At 24 weeks, the mean change in peak oxygen uptake was 1.8 mL/kg/min (95% CI 1.2–2.3) in the aficamten group and 0.0 mL/kg/min (95% CI –0.5 to 0.5) in the placebo group ($p < 0.001$). The incidence of adverse events was similar between the groups.[24] Aficamten is yet to receive regulatory approval for clinical use.

Colchicine for Coronary Syndromes

Colchicine, a well-known anti-inflammatory drug traditionally used for gout, has recently gained attention for its potential role in reducing cardiovascular events, particularly after MI.

Colchicine inhibits microtubule formation and reduces the activation and recruitment of neutrophils. This leads to a reduction in inflammatory mediators like interleukin-1β, which are involved in the inflammatory response following MI. By dampening this inflammation, colchicine may help to stabilize atherosclerotic plaques and prevent further cardiovascular events. Colchicine also suppresses NLRP3 inflammasome present in myeloid cells, including monocytes, neutrophils, and eosinophils or its downstream inflammatory cytokine activation. Highly mature inflammatory cytokines IL-1β and IL-18 produced from NLRP3 lead to the progression of atherosclerotic plaques and even shedding of plaques.

The COLCOT trial was a randomized, double-blind trial involving 4,745 patients recruited within 30 days after MI. Colchicine at a dose of 0.5 mg daily led to a significantly lower risk of ischemic cardiovascular events than placebo.

TABLE 1: Salient features of a few newer therapeutic agents in cardiology.

Drug	Class	MOA	Dosage	Status	Trial
Aprocitentan	Antihypertensive	ET-A and ET-B receptor	12.5 mg OD	US FDA approved March 2024	PRECISION
Zilebesiran	Antihypertensive	siRNA targeting angiotensinogen synthesis	200 mg or more	Phase 2 trials	KARDIA
Evinacumab	Hypolipidemic	ANGPTL3 inhibition	15 mg/kg every 4 weeks IV infusion	US FDA approved 2021 for HoFH	ELIPSE HoFH trial
Bempedoic acid	Hypolipidemic	ATP citrate lyase inhibition	180 mg OD	US FDA approved 2020	CLEAR outcomes
Inclisiran	Hypolipidemic	siRNA targeting PCSK9 synthesis	284 mg; repeat after 3 months followed by (f/b) 6 monthly	US FDA approved 2021	ORION
Zodasiran	Hypolipidemic	siRNA targeting ANGPTL3 synthesis	50–200 mg on day 1 f/b at 12 weeks	Phase 2b trial	ARCHES-2
Vericiguat	Heart failure therapy	Soluble guanylate cyclase stimulator	2.5 mg OD as starting dose to 10 mg OD	US FDA approved for worsening HF	VICTORIA published; VICTOR ongoing
Finerenone	Heart failure therapy	Nonsteroidal MRA	10 mg OD to maximum 40 mg OD	US FDA approved for diabetic kidney disease currently	FINEARTS-HF
Semaglutide	Heart failure therapy	GLP1-agonist	2.4 mg subcutaneous once weekly (target dose)	Approved for CV risk reduction in obese with CVD	SELECT; STEP-HFpEF; STEP-HFpEF DM
Acoramidis	Amyloidosis	TTR tetramer stabilization	800 mg twice daily	Approval pending	ATTRibute-CM
Aficamten	HOCM	Cardiac myosin inhibitor	5–20 mg daily	Approval pending	SEQUOIA-HCM
Colchicine for coronary syndromes	Coronary	Anti-inflammatory	0.5 mg OD	Class IIb recommendation in ACC/ESC guidelines	COLCOT; LoDoCo2

The LoDoCo2 (Low-Dose Colchicine 2) trial extended the findings of COLCOT by investigating the effects of colchicine in 5,522 patients with chronic coronary syndrome. Here also, the risk of cardiovascular events was significantly lower among those who received 0.5 mg colchicine once daily than among those who received placebo.[25,26]

The ACC/AHA 2023 and ESC 2023 guidelines give a class IIb recommendation for the use of colchicine in chronic coronary syndrome and after MI, respectively. Given the narrow therapeutic window and poor tolerability of this drug, a decision needs to be individualized after considering the residual risk of patients despite standard therapy **(Table 1)**.

CONCLUSION

We have come a long way since the GISSI trial for streptokinase—when the tested agent alone could reduce mortality by 18%. Most drugs being studied now are tested against an already solid background therapy, and incremental benefit is frequently small in magnitude. Nevertheless, there remains a sizeable population of patients in genuine need of that small incremental benefit—and as clinicians, it should be our constant endeavor that these newer therapies cross the last mile and finally reach the subset of patients they are most likely to benefit.

ONLINE REFERENCES

Please scan the QR code provided at the end of the table of contents for References of this chapter.

CHAPTER 219

Glucagon-like Peptide-1 Analogs in Cardiometabolic Disorders: State of the Art

Arijit Kumar Ghosh, Shinjan Patra

ABSTRACT

Cardiometabolic syndrome is a clinical entity associated with an increased risk of atherosclerotic cardiovascular disease (ASCVD) or death, even after controlling for its component risk factors. Glucagon-like peptide-1 receptor agonists (GLP-1 RAs) have pleiotropic effects and comprehensive metabolic improvement, and the benefits go beyond weight loss and extend across the cardiovascular–kidney–metabolic (CKM) syndrome. GLP-1RAs offer a multitude of pleiotropic effects and that is why comprehensive metabolic improvements can be seen in this drug's usage. The basic limitation in our country remains its mode of administration (all injectable except oral semaglutide) and cost.

Keywords: Glucagon-like peptide-1 (GLP-1 analogs), cardiometabolic disorders, cardiovascular–kidney–metabolic syndrome, cardiovascular outcome trial (CVOT)

INTRODUCTION

Cardiometabolic syndrome refers to a constellation of metabolic abnormalities and is a clinical entity associated with an increased risk of atherosclerotic cardiovascular disease (ASCVD) or death, even after controlling for its component risk factors.[1] Cardiometabolic disorders are a group of common preventable conditions including ASCVD, stroke, diabetes, insulin resistance, kidney disease, and nonalcoholic fatty liver disease. There is a global increase in the number of people who experience one or more of these conditions during their lifetime. The impact of cardiometabolic disease is far-reaching and approximately 31% of the global deaths are associated with cardiometabolic disease.

Glucagon-like peptide-1 receptor agonists (GLP-1RAs) are incretin analogs. They reduce glucose levels after meals and promote weight loss by reducing appetite and delaying gastric emptying.[2,3] GLP-1RAs appear to have substantial additional benefits beyond weight loss. Several studies have demonstrated that GLP-1RAs have pleiotropic effects and comprehensive metabolic improvement, and the benefits go beyond weight loss and extend across the cardiovascular-kidney–metabolic (CKM) syndrome.

Glucagon-like peptide-1 is a 30 amino acid peptide, produced by intestinal L-cells by processing from the proglucagon gene.[4] GLP-1 was discovered from the genetic sequence of glucagon in 1983 by Bell et al.[5] The first GLP-1RA (GLP-1 receptor agonist) with useful therapeutic activity was inspired by identifying exendin-4. This was isolated from the saliva of the venomous lizard Gila monster.[6] It was found to be a part of physiological incretins by Kreymann et al.[7] and secreted as a part of a response to oral glucose intake. Glucose and fat in the intestinal lumen can directly stimulate the GLP-1 secretion.[8]

Glucagon-like peptide-1 analogs can be broadly classified as exendin-based therapies (exenatide, exenatide once weekly), dipeptidyl peptidase-4 (DPP-4)-resistant analogs (lixisenatide, albiglutide), and analogs of human GLP-1 (liraglutide, taspoglutide).

Exenatide was the first GLP-1RA to be approved for type 2 diabetes mellitus (T2DM) patients in 2005. Following its approval, subsequent GLP-1RAs such as dulaglutide, albiglutide, liraglutide, semaglutide, and tirzepatide (dual

GLP-1 and GIP agonist) have been trialed and are currently approved for T2DM. Semaglutide became the first oral GLP-1RA to be approved for usage in T2DM.[9] Currently, commercially available analogs are exenatide (Bydureon, Byetta), lixisenatide (Adlyxin), liraglutide (Victoza, Saxenda), dulaglutide (Trulicity), tirzepatide (Mounjaro), and semaglutide (Ozempic, Rybelsus).

STRUCTURE, DISTRIBUTION, AND PHYSIOLOGICAL FUNCTIONS OF GLUCAGON-LIKE PEPTIDE-1

Glucagon-like peptide-1's primary structure begins with histidine and ends with glycine. It exerts its action through its receptors in specific nuclei of the pancreas, gastrointestinal tract, kidney, heart, bone, central nervous system, etc. Its presence has been confirmed in liver and adipose tissues also.[10] GLP-1 lowers glucose by stimulating the release of insulin and inhibiting glucagon.[11] Its glucose-dependent actions make this a perfect choice of drug in patients with higher risks of hypoglycemia.[12] Endogenous GLP-1 has a short half-life of 1–2 minutes and is degraded by the enzyme DPP-4. The short half-life of endogenous GLP-1 has prompted the development of GLP-1RA as an important treatment for T2DM.[13]

Glucagon-like peptide-1 stimulates the proliferation and regeneration of islet β-cells and inhibits their apoptosis in the pancreas. It reduces gastric emptying in the gastrointestinal tract and increases renal blood flow and glomerular filtration rate in the kidney.[14] After binding to its specific receptors in the cardiac system, it enhances cardiac contractility and directs myocardial functions.[15] It promotes bone marrow mesenchymal stem cell osteoblast differentiation and inhibits its differentiation into fat cells, thereby promoting bone formation.[16] Its main action on the central nervous system is satiety regulation and energy homeostasis. It induces satiety and that is how the patient's appetite is reduced significantly.

Glucagon-like peptide-1 induces hepatic gluconeogenesis, glycogen synthesis, and glycolysis by acting on the liver.[17] It reduces liver fat content through signal transduction of the AMP-activated protein kinase (AMPK)/mammalian target of the rapamycin (mTOR) pathway. It has been shown to reduce hepatic steatosis in vivo and in vitro by enhancing autophagy and lipid degradation through the GLP-1R-transcription factor EB (TFEB)-mediated autophagy lysosomal pathway.[18] GLP-1 stimulates systemic energy metabolism by regulating adipocyte development, accelerating plasma clearance of glucose and triacylglycerol-derived fatty acids, and improving insulin signaling along with thermogenesis in brown adipose tissues.[19] The cardiometabolic actions of the GLP-1 are quite diverse considering it has receptors in virtually all important major organs of the body. In this chapter, we will try to discuss the role of GLP-1RA in cardiovascular (CV) systems and will discuss its metabolic functions in terms of reducing plasma glucose, dyslipidemia, body fat and body weight, and liver steatosis.

CARDIOVASCULAR EFFECT OF THE GLUCAGON-LIKE PEPTIDE-1 RECEPTOR AGONISTS

Cardiovascular Outcome Trials

This class of drug has garnered attention not only for its excellent antidiabetic actions but also for its potential benefit on the CV system. Cardiovascular outcome trial (CVOT) is required by regulatory agencies to ensure that these drugs do not increase CV risk. All GLP-1RAs have undergone extensive CVOTs. These randomized controlled trials were designed meticulously among high CV risk T2DM patients and mostly the outcomes were 3-point major adverse cardiovascular events (MACE) (nonfatal stroke, nonfatal acute coronary syndrome, and death due to CV cause).[20] The accumulated evidence from all CVOTs has confirmed not only their safety but also their immense positive pleiotropic CV effects.[21]

The LEADER (Liraglutide Effect and Action in Diabetes: Evaluation of Cardiovascular Outcome Results) trial demonstrated the CV benefits of liraglutide in high-risk patients with T2DM. It reduced the risk of MACE by 13% in more than 9,000 patients with close to 4 years of follow-up.[22] Semaglutide was tested in the SUSTAIN-6 (Trial to Evaluate Cardiovascular and Other Long-term Outcomes with Semaglutide in Subjects with Type 2 Diabetes) trial and reduced the risk of MACE by 26% mostly by reducing the rate of nonfatal stroke (39%).[22] Similar results were seen in the REWIND study where dulaglutide reduced the risk of nonfatal strokes, and resultantly MACE significantly reduced in dulaglutide compared to placebo.[23] Albiglutide significantly reduced MACE compared to placebo in the HARMONY rewind trial where the maximum benefit was observed in myocardial infarction in contrast to the reduction in stroke events in the previously two discussed trials.[24] The AMPLITUDE-O trial, done for another once-weekly GLP-1RA efpeglenatide, which included 4,076 high-risk patients (established ASCVD and kidney disease), not only reduced MACE but also prevented the worsening kidney function.[25] GLP-1RAs have established their secondary preventive role in ASCVD.

In the ELIXA and the EXSCEL trials (once-daily lixisenatide and once-weekly exenatide, respectively), GLP-1RAs were proven noninferior to placebo in reducing MACE in contrast to previous findings of obvious superiority.[26,27] The only oral-approved GLP-1RA semaglutide has been tested in the PIONEER-6 trial and showed CV noninferiority to placebo.[28] CV benefit along with renoprotective actions of oral semaglutide is currently under investigation in the SOUL study where the primary and secondary outcomes for noninferiority had been achieved and soon will be published.[29] Dose-dependent CV benefit was observed in dulaglutide (1.5–4.5 mg weekly) and efpeglenatide where other CVOTs used maximum tolerated doses of the respective GLP-1RAs.

Mechanism in Brief for the Cardiovascular Benefit

Adequate glycemic control is the first major step in reducing CV risk burden in patients with T2DM, and GLP-1RAs' glycemic efficacies have been proven beyond doubt. Intensive glucose management, as demonstrated in landmark clinical trials, the United Kingdom Prospective Diabetes Study (UKPDS), has been related to the reduced risk of CV events.[30] Maintaining a stable glycemic level was the key to reduced CV events in patients with GLP-1RA. These drugs reduce body weight by previously mentioned mechanisms and by reducing insulin resistance, the CV risks decreased by many folds.[31] Moderate reductions in LDL cholesterol, total cholesterol, and triglycerides are seen with the usage of GLP-1RAs.[32] These drugs promote myocardial glucose uptake and utilization, reduce oxidative stress, inhibit cardiomyocyte apoptosis, and prevent adverse cardiac remodeling.[15] GLP-1RA causes vasodilation by producing endothelial nitric oxide (NO) and by modulation of the renin–angiotensin–aldosterone system (RAAS).[33] Natriuresis is enhanced by GLP-1RAs and it helps in reducing blood pressure status.[34] The anti-inflammatory and antiatherogenic effects of the GLP-1RAs prevent atherosclerotic plaque formation and its progression.[35]

Glucagon-like Peptide-1 Receptor Agonists and Heart Diseases (Heart Failure and Major Cardiovascular Events)

In current times, GLP-1RAs are expected to impart potential benefits in heart failure management. However, there are not many clinical trials available compared to SGLT-2 inhibitors where the benefit in heart failure extended to HFpEF. FIGHT and LIVE trials were conducted on liraglutide [300 patients with acute heart failure and reduced ejection fraction (<40%) and 241 patients of chronic heart failure with reduced left ventricular ejection fraction (LVEF ≤ 45%), respectively] which did not show any benefit compared to the placebo group.[36,37] The STEP-HFpEF (Semaglutide in Patients with Heart Failure with Preserved Ejection Fraction and Obesity) trial used semaglutide 2.4 mg once-weekly injections for efficacy in patients with preserved LVEF (LVEF ≥ 45%) and obesity [body mass index (BMI) ≥ 30 kg/m^2]. A total of 529 patients participated in the trial, and the results showed that in patients with HFpEF and obesity, semaglutide treatment reduced symptoms and physical limitations, improved exercise function, and reduced body weight.[38] The significant weight loss led to improvement in the 6-minute walk distance when compared to placebo. Interestingly, this benefit was observed in patients without diabetes.[38] These results have now been replicated in the T2DM population.[39]

Most of the CVOTs have demonstrated noninferiority in hospitalizations due to heart failure compared to placebo. No benefit in risk of HF hospitalization was observed with oral semaglutide. However, a meta-analysis encompassing eight CVOTs established promising trends regarding heart failure outcomes in terms of reduced rate of heart failure-related events.[40]

Cardiovascular outcome trial has given us immense opportunity to know about the CV safety and benefit data of GLP-1RAs over the years. Currently in our clinical practice, oral semaglutide and injectable liraglutide are the most prescribed GLP-1RAs in patients with T2DM and obesity with CV disease. GLP-1RA's pleiotropic actions and multisystemic actions make it a wonderful drug for cardiac ailments in patients with T2DM.

Semaglutide was recently studied in a multicenter, double-blind, randomized, placebo-controlled, event-driven superiority CV outcomes trial called SELECT (Semaglutide and Cardiovascular Outcomes in Obesity without Diabetes).[41] The SELECT trial demonstrated that weekly semaglutide was more effective than placebo in reducing MACE in patients who have preexisting ASCVD and are overweight or obese, but do not have diabetes.[41] Moreover, patients who were treated with once-weekly subcutaneous semaglutide showed a significant decrease in key secondary endpoints of all-cause mortality, hospitalization due to heart failure, and a composite nephropathy endpoint.[41]

A small step forward in the approach to exploring the benefits of these incretin-based therapies is being implemented in a study called SURMOUNT-MMO (A Study of Tirzepatide on the Reduction of Morbidity and Mortality in Adults With Obesity).[42] The primary outcome of the study is time to the first occurrence of any event of a broad combined outcome. This combined outcome consists of all-cause death, nonfatal myocardial infarction, nonfatal stroke, coronary revascularization, or heart failure events.[42]

GLUCAGON-LIKE PEPTIDE-1 RECEPTOR AGONISTS AND KIDNEY DISEASE

Two meta-analyses of several CVOTs explored whether the benefits of GLP-1RA extend beyond MACE in patients with T2DM.[40,43] This included a composite kidney outcome comprising the development of macroalbuminuria, doubling of serum creatinine, or at least a 40% decline in estimated glomerular filtration rate (eGFR), kidney replacement therapy, or death due to kidney disease. Both meta-analyses had over 50,000 patients and showed a significant 21% and 17% reduction in the composite kidney outcome, respectively.[40,43] Recently, it was announced that the FLOW trial of semaglutide in patients with T2DM and chronic kidney disease would be stopped early for the benefit of important renal outcomes.[44]

GLYCEMIC BENEFITS IN GLUCAGON-LIKE PEPTIDE-1 RECEPTOR AGONISTS

Starting from the approval of exenatide as a twice-weekly injection in 2005, many GLP-1RAs have evolved and gained prominence. Currently, worldwide dulaglutide, semaglutide, and tirzepatide are the most commonly prescribed GLP-1RAs.[45] As per ADA recommendations, the combination of basal insulin and GLP-1RA demonstrates potent glucose-lowering effects while minimizing weight gain and reducing the risk of hypoglycemia compared to intensified insulin regimens.[46] ADA currently approves GLP-1RAs in patients with T2DM who are not adequately controlled with diet and exercise. This drug can be used as the second choice antidiabetic drug in T2DM patients with increased CV risk or prior CV events after metformin. The glycemic efficacies between various GLP-1RAs have also been studied. The LEAD-6 trial compared liraglutide 1.8 mg once a day with exenatide 10 μg twice a day and demonstrated greater HbA1c reduction and fewer adverse effects with liraglutide, including hypoglycemia.[47] When dulaglutide's initiation in patients was compared to exenatide once weekly and liraglutide, dulaglutide had higher compliance and lower discontinuation rates within 6 months.[48] Liraglutide and dulaglutide were found similar in terms of HbA1c reduction.[49] Semaglutide has shown better HbA1c reduction compared to dulaglutide. Superior reduction of HbA1c and greater weight loss were seen with tirzepatide than with semaglutide 1 mg once weekly over 40 weeks in people with T2DM.[50] Higher doses of semaglutide (2 mg once weekly) and dulaglutide (up to 4.5 mg once weekly) have subsequently been approved for T2DM due to their superior benefit. The glycemic benefits of GLP-1RAs are glucose-independent, and HbA1c reduction is in the range of 0.5–0.8%.

OBESITY BENEFITS IN GLUCAGON-LIKE PEPTIDE-1 RECEPTOR AGONISTS

The initial weight-loss trends observed in GLP1-RAs in T2DM patients encouraged the practitioners and clinicians to trial such drugs for antiobesity management. Liraglutide 3 mg once daily was the first GLP-1RA approved (in 2014) for weight loss in people with overweight and comorbidities or people with BMI > 30 kg/m^2. The combined central and peripheral actions of GLP-1RA promote satiety, decrease hunger, and ultimately reduce food intake. Decreasing gastric motility along with nausea plays a minor role in this regard. When liraglutide was used in varying doses in obesity patients and compared to placebo and orlistat, the mean weight loss with liraglutide 3.0 mg was 7.2 kg, compared with 2.8 kg with placebo and 4.1 kg with orlistat. This 20-week-long trial of liraglutide till the maximum dose of 3 mg established its sheer efficacy along with reducing obesity-related risk factors.[51] 3 mg once-daily doses of liraglutide were found to be more effective compared to the 1.8 mg dosage used in T2DM. The weight-loss potential of liraglutide was found to be in the range of 5–10% body weight.[52]

Semaglutide has been studied extensively for weight loss. STEP-1 to STEP-7 trials have been done to investigate the weight-loss potential of injectable semaglutide in 2.4 mg once-weekly doses. It caused a greater reduction in waist circumference (MD –8.28 cm; 95% CI –9.51 to –7.04; p = 0.00001), BMI (MD –3.71 kg/m^2; 95% CI –4.33 to –3.09; p = 0.00001), and weight loss of 5, 10, 15, and 20% with a greater proportion of participants when compared to placebo.[53] The body weight reduction was observed to be in the range of 10–15% in injectable semaglutide 2.4 mg once-weekly dose.[54] Subsequently, it has been approved for obesity with or without diabetes. From a weight-loss perspective, tirzepatide needs special mention, as a dual GIP and GLP-1RA. From SURPASS 1 to SURPASS 7, this drug has been compared to placebo and semaglutide; dulaglutide; insulin degludec and glargine; and metformin. The tirzepatide group achieved an average weight loss from 5 to 15 kg in those trials.[6] At the SURMOUNT-1 trial tirzepatide was compared to placebo and at week 72, the mean percent change in weight was 15.0% with weekly doses of 5 mg tirzepatide, 19.5% with doses of 10 mg, 20.9% with doses of 15 mg, and 3.1% with placebo.[55] It has been subsequently approved for T2DM with obesity. The weight-loss potential of tirzepatide is enormous and we can expect this drug's use in our country soon.

GLUCAGON-LIKE PEPTIDE-1 RECEPTOR AGONISTS IN LIPID METABOLISM

Studies have indicated that GLP-1 in hepatocytes may mediate the outflow of intracellular cholesterol to apo AI through the ABCA1 (ATP binding cassette transporter pathway). Exendin-4 is mediated by Ca^{2+}/calmodulin (CaM)-dependent protein kinase pathway which increases liver ABCA1 expression and reduces cholesterol accumulation.[56] Other basic science studies have shown that GLP-1 may mediate cholesterol outflow in hepatocytes through the LXRα-ABCA1 (liver X receptors) pathway, consequently avoiding large amounts of cholesterol accumulation.[10] It also increases mRNA and protein expression levels of AP2 and PPARγ in a dose-dependent manner during pre-3T3-L1 adipocyte differentiation and thereby modulates adipocyte differentiation. GLP-1 increases the expression of thermogenic genes for browning phenotype maintenance and improves the expression of UCP1, mitochondrial biosynthesis, and thermogenic markers. All such mechanisms contribute immensely to weight loss and favorable lipid profile with the use of GLP-1RA. It reduces the LDL, total cholesterol, and triglycerides and increases HDL.[6]

GLUCAGON-LIKE PEPTIDE-1 RECEPTOR AGONISTS AND METABOLIC DYSFUNCTION-ASSOCIATED STEATOTIC LIVER DISEASE

Diabetes, obesity, and metabolic dysfunction-associated liver disease are a common association. This class of drug has been shown to positively impact hepatic gluconeogenesis, glycogen synthesis, and glycolysis.[57] It reduces hyperlipidemia, liver fibrosis, and inflammation and imparts favorable outcomes on metabolic dysfunction-associated steatotic liver disease (MASLD). This drug's significant weight-loss properties have made way for an exciting option for MASLD. In obese patients with MASLD, a reduction in body weight of 7–10% improves liver enzymes together with the histological grade of the disease.[58] The improvements in the liver injury biomarkers are also seen with the use of GLP-1RAs. Armstrong et al. conducted a meta-analysis of 4,442 patients with T2DM where liraglutide was proven to significantly lower ALT levels in patients with elevated baseline values in 1.8 mg/day doses.[59] Vanderheiden et al., Petit et al., and Yan et al. have demonstrated hepatic and subcutaneous fat reduction of up to 44% in patients with T2DM with liraglutide usage and obesity examined by MRI.[60] Liraglutide significantly improves hepatic steatosis and hepatocyte ballooning and was found to be associated with 4.5 times chances of resolution of MASLD.[61] Other hepatic steatosis markers APRI (AST-to-platelet count ratio index), NFS (NAFLD fibrosis score), and the FIB-4 (fibrosis index based on 4 factors) or from the assessment of liver stiffness measurement (LSM) all improved with the usage of liraglutide.[62] Post hoc analysis of two large trials on the effect of semaglutide on body weight and CV outcomes revealed significantly reduced ALT levels in patients with T2DM. After 72 weeks of treatment with semaglutide (0.4 mg/day dosage), histological resolution of NASH without progression of fibrosis was observed in 59% of patients compared to 17% in the placebo group.[63] The progression to liver fibrosis is also halted with the use of GLP-1 analogs as they reduce the expression of three out of five collagen genes.[55] The delayed progression to liver fibrosis has been observed with liraglutide; however, no such evidences exist with semaglutide as of now. Finally, with the convincing evidence of steatosis reduction, the chances of hepatocellular carcinoma are also thought to be reduced; however, larger clinical trials need to be conducted for confirmation.

SAFETY PROFILE

The safety profile of such GLP-1RAs has been evaluated in several clinical studies and meta-analyses. Mild-to-moderate gastrointestinal side effects were observed in all studies.[21] Once-daily exenatide was found to have the lowest risk of vomiting, while albiglutide had the highest risk for diarrhea. Nausea, abdominal pain, and dyspepsia were the other common side effects observed with GLP-1RA.

SUMMARY

Table 1 shows a summary of the GLP-1RA's cardiometabolic functions.

TABLE 1: Summary of the GLP-1RAs cardiometabolic functions.

System	Mechanism of benefit	Outcomes
Cardiovascular systems	• Adequate glycemic control • Promote myocardial glucose uptake and utilization • Inhibit cardiomyocyte apoptosis • Prevent adverse cardiac remodeling • Natriuresis	• MACE reduction (10–20%) • Hospitalization for heart failure reduction
Antihyperglycemic	• Stimulating the release of insulin and inhibiting glucagon • Proliferation and regeneration of islet β-cells and inhibits their apoptosis	HbA1c reduction of 0.5–0.8%
Obesity	• Promote satiety, decrease hunger, and ultimately reduce food intake • Decreasing gastric motility along with nausea	Weight loss in the range of 5–20%
Diabetic dyslipidemia	• Mediate the outflow of intracellular cholesterol to ApoA-I through the ABCA1 pathway • Cholesterol outflow in hepatocytes through the LXRα-ABCA1 (liver X receptors) pathway • Increases mRNA and protein expression levels of AP2 and PPAR-γ in a dose-dependent manner and modulates adipocyte differentiation	Reducing LDL, triglyceride, and increasing HDL
MASLD (Metabolic dysfunction-associated steatotic liver disease)	• Reduce hepatic gluconeogenesis and glycolysis • Increase glycogen synthesis • Weight loss	• Reducing hepatic fat content • Reduces hepatic ballooning

CONCLUSION

Glucagon-like peptide-1 receptor agonist is the best possible armamentarium in our fight to treat T2DM with metabolic syndrome and CV diseases. Plenty of clinical trials have demonstrated clear benefits in reducing cardiovascular risk, heart failure hospitalizations, improving lipid profiles, and reducing liver steatosis parameters. All such benefits are achieved in T2DM patients with obesity with impressive glycemic control and minimal gastrointestinal side effects. GLP-1RA offers a multitude of pleiotropic effects and that is why comprehensive metabolic improvements can be seen in this drug's usage. The basic limitation in our country remains its mode of administration (all injectable except oral semaglutide) and cost. As we navigate the evolving landscape of cardiometabolic disease management, it becomes imperative to think broadly about the calculation of cost-effectiveness to include broader individual and societal impact on key outcomes across the CKM continuum, such as kidney function and quality of life in conditions like HFpEF. With further clinical trials and clinician's experience, the usage of such drugs will increase tremendously in the coming times in India.

ONLINE REFERENCES

Please scan the QR code provided at the end of the table of contents for References of this chapter.

CHAPTER 220

Mitochondria-based Therapies in the Cardiovascular System

Ashwani Mehta, Kavita Tyagi

ABSTRACT

Cardiovascular diseases (CVDs) are a leading cause of global mortality, with mitochondrial dysfunction playing a significant role in their pathogenesis. Mitochondria are essential for adenosine triphosphate (ATP) production in cardiomyocytes, and their dysfunction leads to imbalances in reactive oxygen species (ROS), contributing to conditions like heart failure and atherosclerosis. Recent advancements in mitochondria-targeted therapies and nanoparticle-based drug delivery systems show promise in improving treatment efficacy and specificity. This chapter highlights the potential of these novel therapies in addressing mitochondrial dysfunction in CVDs and discusses future research directions and challenges.

Keywords: Mitochondria-targeted therapies, mitochondrial dysfunction, reactive oxygen species (ROS), nanoparticle-based drug delivery, cardioprotective effects

INTRODUCTION

Cardiovascular diseases (CVDs) represent a significant public health challenge globally, accounting for nearly one third of all deaths worldwide. The development of many CVDs is increasingly linked to mitochondrial dysfunction. In a healthy individual, the heart's continuous contraction requires a substantial amount of energy, primarily in the form of adenosine triphosphate (ATP). Cardiomyocytes are densely packed with mitochondria, which occupy approximately 30% of the cell volume. These mitochondria collectively produce about 6 kg of ATP daily through oxidative phosphorylation via the electron transport chain (ETC). This energy production process naturally generates reactive oxygen species (ROS) as by-products, which are neutralized by the mitochondria's own antioxidant systems. Beyond their role in energy production, mitochondria are crucial for calcium homeostasis, macromolecule synthesis, and intracellular signaling.[1]

Mitochondria can mitigate deleterious effects by regulating mitochondrial homeostasis. Recent years have seen growing interest in mitochondria-targeted therapies for CVDs. Numerous studies have demonstrated that many clinical drugs, such as β-blockers and angiotensin-converting enzyme inhibitors/angiotensin II receptor blockers, possess mitochondrial protective properties. Additionally, a growing number of cardiac mitochondrial targets have exhibited cardioprotective effects in both experimental and clinical settings. This trend offers potential directions for future experimental and clinical research.[2]

MITOCHONDRIA AS A THERAPEUTIC TARGET FOR NEW DRUGS

Mitochondrial dysfunction is increasingly recognized as a hallmark of various cardiovascular disorders. For instance, impaired ATP availability in the failing heart may reflect changes in fuel utilization and energy buffering. Excessive production of ROS can cause oxidative damage, particularly when endogenous antioxidants are depleted, contributing to heart failure and dysfunction of vascular endothelial cells, leading to conditions such as hypertension and atherosclerosis.[3]

Mitochondria also play a critical role in determining cell fate, particularly evident in ischemia–reperfusion (I/R) injury following myocardial infarction (MI). During ischemia, the lack of ATP production through oxidative phosphorylation results in energy depletion and ionic dysregulation, leading to changes in pH and elevated levels of calcium and succinate. Revascularization oxidizes succinate, generating a significant burst of ROS through reverse electron transport at complex I. This process is a potent trigger for the formation of the mitochondrial permeability transition pore (mPTP), which dissipates the mitochondrial membrane potential and leads to proinflammatory necrotic cell death.[3] Targeting complex I inhibition during early reperfusion and inhibiting the mPTP are potential therapeutic strategies for mitigating I/R injury. The mPTP is also a therapeutic target in heart failure, where elevated ROS and calcium levels, along with ATP depletion, increase the likelihood of pore opening. This condition contributes to the loss of cardiomyocytes, replacement fibrosis, and activation of inflammatory cells.[4]

ROLE OF NANOPARTICLES IN TARGETING MITOCHONDRIA

Mitochondria-targeted nanomedicines have primarily been investigated for cancer treatment, with varying outcomes for cell survival. The challenges of uptake and targeting are similar, involving delivery to hypoxic or poorly perfused tissues. Effective tumor delivery is facilitated by the enhanced permeability and retention (EPR) effect, wherein fenestrated blood vessels allow for extravasation, thus overcoming the endothelial barrier.[5] The EPR effect is also present in CVDs, particularly following acute injury (e.g., post-MI), and to a lesser extent in chronic heart failure.[6] Active targeting can be achieved by conjugating nanoparticles (NPs) with DNA, peptides, or antibodies that recognize specific molecular targets. These targets could include markers that are unique to or overexpressed in the injured tissue or cells, providing disease specificity.[7]

For mitochondrial targeting, NPs can be functionalized using techniques such as conjugation with triphenylphosphonium (TPP+), Szeto–Schiller (SS) peptides, or fusogenic lipid moieties. For example, MITO-Porter, a liposome-based nanocarrier functionalized with an octa-arginine peptide, can deliver cargos into the mitochondrial matrix via membrane fusion, including CoQ10 in cultured fibroblasts,[8] and is under investigation for mitochondrial gene delivery.

Liposomes have been widely studied for drug delivery due to their potential for subcellular delivery, controlled drug release, excellent biocompatibility, and targeting efficacy. NP-based drug delivery systems offer significant advantages by modifying the biodistribution of therapeutic molecules through targeted delivery, controlled release, and customization to the specific molecular properties of diseased tissues. This can enhance drug potency at the target site, thereby improving efficacy with fewer off-target effects. Several liposomal NP drugs have been clinically approved by the US FDA, including the COVID-19 mRNA vaccines. Polymeric NPs, such as those made from polylactic/glycolic acid (PLGA), also represent a promising approach, offering good biocompatibility along with higher stability and better-controlled release than liposomes.[9,10] For example, PLGA NPs have been studied as carriers for cyclosporine A (CsA), where they were found to be cardioprotective by inhibiting mPTP opening in a murine I/R injury model in vivo.[11]

ADDITIONAL MITOCHONDRIA-TARGETED THERAPEUTICS

Further exploration into mitochondria-targeted therapeutics has revealed several promising compounds. Some of them are listed below:

- *SS peptides*: SS-31, for instance, has shown potential in modulating mitochondrial function. These peptides selectively target cardiolipin, a phospholipid crucial for maintaining mitochondrial inner membrane integrity and function. By binding to cardiolipin, SS-31 has been demonstrated to preserve mitochondrial structure and function, reduce ROS production, and improve cellular bioenergetics in various preclinical models of cardiac injury and metabolic diseases.[12]
- *Bendavia (elamipretide)*: A derivative of SS-31, Bendavia has shown promise in clinical trials aimed at treating primary mitochondrial myopathy and heart failure with preserved ejection fraction (HFpEF). Although early results were mixed, ongoing trials with optimized dosing regimens and extended treatment periods are underway to better understand its therapeutic potential.[13]
- *MitoTEMPOL*: This mitochondria-targeted version of the general antioxidant TEMPOL specifically localizes to mitochondria, offering targeted ROS scavenging capabilities. Preclinical studies suggest that MitoTEMPOL can mitigate oxidative stress-induced damage in cardiac cells, highlighting its potential for treating conditions like MI and chronic heart failure.[14]
- *MitoSENS therapies*: These involve the expression of engineered mitochondrial genes to replace defective endogenous genes, an emerging approach in mitochondrial medicine. This gene therapy strategy aims to correct mitochondrial dysfunction at its genetic root, providing a potential treatment avenue for mitochondrial diseases and secondary mitochondrial dysfunction observed in CVDs.[9,15]

CHALLENGES AND FUTURE DIRECTIONS

Despite the promising results of mitochondria-targeted therapies in preclinical studies, several challenges remain in translating these findings into clinical practice. One major hurdle is the efficient and selective delivery of therapeutics to mitochondria within the context of complex human physiology. While conjugation with lipophilic cations like TPP+ has shown some success, ongoing research into alternative delivery mechanisms, such as NPs and mitochondria-penetrating peptides, aims to enhance targeting precision and drug uptake.

Another challenge lies in the variable response observed in clinical trials, which may be attributed to differences in disease etiology, patient demographics, and the inherent complexity of mitochondrial biology. Therefore, personalized medicine approaches, where treatments are tailored based on individual mitochondrial genetic profiles and metabolic states, could enhance therapeutic efficacy and patient outcomes.[16]

CONCLUSION

Targeting mitochondrial dysfunction represents a promising strategy for the treatment of CVDs. Continued research and clinical trials are essential to fully understand the therapeutic potential and limitations of mitochondria-targeted drugs. As our understanding of mitochondrial biology and pathophysiology deepens, new and more effective therapeutic strategies are likely to emerge, offering hope for improved management of CVDs and associated mitochondrial dysfunction.

Currently, the application of mitochondria-targeted nanomedicines for CVD remains at the preclinical proof-of-principle stage. While the foundational framework exists, significant work is needed to optimize circulation times and uptake across multiple membranes while avoiding phagocytic and lysosomal capture. For I/R injury, rapid uptake is crucial, presenting an additional challenge, whereas long-term safety and clearance pathways must be considered for chronic diseases such as heart failure. Progress in this field will require multidisciplinary expertise bridging materials science, chemistry, pharmacology, and cardiovascular medicine.

The ultimate goal is a new generation of targeted therapeutics that can rejuvenate borderline therapies by improving efficacy through targeted accumulation at the site of injury. Mitochondria targeted nanomedicines also hold potential for novel applications, such as regulating mitophagy for mitochondrial quality control, modulating mitochondrial calcium, and delivering genetic material such as mitochondrial microRNAs.

ONLINE REFERENCES

Please scan the QR code provided at the end of the table of contents for References of this chapter.

CHAPTER

221

Different Response to Same Drug: Effect of Pharmacogenomics on Statin Efficacy

S Ramesh, SR Sharath Shanmugam

ABSTRACT

Statins, also known as 3-hydroxy-3-methylglutaryl coenzyme A (HMG-CoA) reductase inhibitors, have established themselves as the cornerstone in the treatment of coronary artery disease. Since discovery of lovastatin in 1980, statins are widely prescribed and used worldwide for several decades. Statins are effective in lowering plasma LDL, thereby reducing cardiovascular events risk, and improving health outcomes in individuals with cardiovascular disease. Generally, statins are considered very effective and safe, with side effects mainly related to muscles (such as myalgia) or transient increase in liver enzymes, which are usually mild. Serious adverse effects like myopathy and rhabdomyolysis are very rare and often occur when statins are combined with other medications like fenofibrate or drugs that affect their pharmacokinetics. Since the introduction of lovastatin in 1980, various statins with different pharmacokinetic properties and varying potencies have been developed.

Trials have shown that there is considerable variation in individual response in terms of efficacy of statin and also in genetic predisposition to possible adverse effects. Plasma concentrations of statins can also vary among patients receiving the similar dose. A recent study revealed up to a 40-fold variability in plasma concentration of atorvastatin and rosuvastatin in patients taking the same dose.[1] Advances in knowledge of the pharmacogenomics of statin, both beneficial and harmful, have led to the identification of several genes that may influence the pharmacokinetic and pharmacodynamic aspects of statin response. Till now, over 40 genes have been found to affect statin efficacy and safety, thereby reflecting the complexity of cholesterol homeostasis and the varying pharmacological profiles of individual statins. Some genetic variants have been associated with more severe side effects, leading to reduced medication adherence.

Keywords: Statin, transporter, genes, genetic variants

COMMON GENETIC VARIANTS THAT AFFECT THE PHARMACOKINETICS OF STATINS

The statins available in the market differ in their physicochemical properties and pharmacokinetics, including uptake, transport, metabolism, and excretion. This variability is determined by genetic variation in genes encoding major importers, exporters, and drug-metabolizing enzymes. These genetic variants can also lead to considerable differences in pharmacokinetic properties such as systemic exposure (AUC) and half-life. Even though most statins share common mechanisms for drug transporters, substrate affinities for each specific transporter for statin may vary. Similarly, the differences in drug-metabolizing enzymes among statins can be particularly important when combining statins with other medications, which may affect statin metabolism, thereby increasing side effects of statin.

Here, we will discuss several candidate genes for which substantial experimental evidence supports their role in influencing statin pharmacokinetics. Recent reviews have summarized the minor allele frequencies for many of these genes.

SLCO1B1

SLCO1B1 gene is commonly implicated to affect the pharmacokinetics of statin. It encodes the OATP1B1 importer. OATP1B1 is predominantly expressed in the liver on the basolateral side of the sinusoidal membrane. Two variants (*rs4149056 and rs2306283*) of *SLCO1B1* have been extensively studied, both in isolation and as part of *SLCO1B1* haplotypes. The *SLCO1B1* 521T>C variant (*rs4149056*), present in the coding region of the transporter, results in a V174A substitution in a putative transmembrane region of the protein. Many functional studies suggest that the SLCO1B1-V174A protein may have reduced cell surface expression, potentially leading to decreased hepatic statin uptake. Individuals homozygous for the CC variant have shown higher systemic exposure (AUC) for statins, including simvastatin (40 mg), atorvastatin (20 mg), rosuvastatin (10 mg), and pitavastatin (2 mg). Especially, the off-target effects are more pronounced for simvastatin, with this SNP linked to a significant risk of simvastatin-induced myopathy at higher doses.[2,3] For example, the cumulative incidence of myopathy was 18% in patients expressing the CC variant compared to 0.6% in TT carriers in a cohort on simvastatin 80 mg/day. Often, the 521T>C variant has also been associated with reduced medication adherence due to side effects. There is variation in occurrence of this SNP in different ethnic groups; it is reported to be 14–23% in individuals of European ancestry and 10–15% in those of Southeast Asian ancestry.[3,4] Due to the strong evidence linking the 521T>C variant to simvastatin-induced myopathy, genetic-based dosing is recommended for this statin. The Clinical Pharmacogenetics Implementation Consortium (CPIC) recommends that patients homozygous or heterozygous for the 521C allele to be prescribed with an alternative statin or have their simvastatin dose restricted to 20 mg/day. These recommendations have been endorsed by the FDA, and genetic testing for this SNP is being increasingly used in the Western countries for high-risk individuals.

ABCG2

ABCG2 is a member of the ABC cassette transporter gene family, encoding the ABCG2 protein, a G-subfamily ABC half-transporter. *ABCG2* is expressed in various organs, including the intestine, liver, kidney, and blood–brain barrier. Primarily known for its role in multidrug resistance, this export pump is also involved in transport of many drugs, metabolites, and endogenous substrates, including most statins. Enhanced activity of this transporter usually results in reduced absorption and increased excretion of its substrates.

The 421C>A variant, located in the coding region of the *ABCG2* gene (*rs2231142*) has notable effect on pharmacokinetics of statins. This SNP results in a Q141K substitution in an intracellular domain of the protein, leading to reduced export capacity in the enterocyte and enterohepatic circulation, thereby increasing plasma statin concentrations and systemic exposure. The homozygous 421AA variant has been linked to increased AUC and Cmax for most prescribed statins (except pravastatin and pitavastatin). The prevalence of this variant is highest among individuals of Southeast Asian ancestry, with approximately one in three people expressing at least one copy. In one of the studies, this genetic variant (421A) was found to enhance LDL-cholesterol-lowering capacity. Patients homozygous for this 421A variant had an average 7% greater reduction in LDL-cholesterol levels compared to those homozygous for the 421C variant when taking 10 mg/day of rosuvastatin. This single genetic variant accounted for 5.4% of inter-individual variation in statin response in the above study. Additionally, the *ABCG2* variant also has been linked to a significantly greater risk of adverse drug reactions after taking fluvastatin in patients with renal dysfunction, highlighting the importance of screening for genetic variants in more vulnerable patient populations.[5,6]

ABCB1

ABCB1, also known as *MDR1*, is a member of the ABC transporter gene family and encodes the ABCB1 protein, also known as p-glycoprotein (P-gp). Like *ABCG2*, P-gp is widely expressed on physiological barriers such as the intestine, liver, and blood–brain barrier. Three SNPs that have strong linkage to disequilibrium and account for two common haplotypes (*rs1128503, rs2032582, and rs1045642*), have been extensively investigated for their effect on statin pharmacokinetics and efficacy.[7-9] The effects of these variants may be statin-specific. Some of the studies reported no significant effects of the three SNPs on pharmacokinetics of fluvastatin, pravastatin, lovastatin, or rosuvastatin, but have been observed to have higher AUCs for simvastatin and atorvastatin. Although the physiological consequences of this SNP in vivo are not fully clarified, observations suggest that synonymous SNPs may have more significant consequences than previously thought of. Reductions in LDL cholesterol after pravastatin treatment ranged from 23% for GG carriers to 17% for T/A homozygotes. In another study by Thompson et al., there was a difference in LDL-lowering efficiency in homozygote carriers of *rs2032582*,[10] but only for low-dose atorvastatin and not for other statins. The effects of this SNP on *ABCB1* transporter function remain grossly undetermined, making the phenotypic impact of these observations inconclusive.

CYP Enzymes

Drug metabolism has an important role in variation in medicine response of many molecules including statins. Genetic polymorphisms in selected *CYP* genes may have significant effect on hepatic metabolism of specific statins, impacting clinical response and risk of adverse effects.

CYP2C9

Fluvastatin is metabolized by several CYPs, but *CYP2C9* is crucial for its hepatic clearance. Genetic polymorphisms in *CYP2C9* have been linked to significant changes in fluvastatin pharmacokinetics.[11,12] In a study by Kirchheiner et al., carriers of the *CYP2C9*3/*3* genotype (rs1057910) had a threefold higher AUC of the active enantiomer of fluvastatin compared to *CYP2C9*1/*1* carriers. Also in a recent study, patients with a reduced-function *CYP2C9* genotype (*CYP2C9*1/*3*) experienced greater reductions in LDL-C and total cholesterol compared to those with a fully functional *CYP2C9* gene. CYP2C9 also plays a small role in pitavastatin metabolism, but this is not clinically significant. While rosuvastatin is a substrate for *CYP2C9* and *CYP2C19*, clinical studies have not shown any significant associations between *CYP2C* genetic mutations and changes in rosuvastatin pharmacokinetics, response, or tolerability.

CYP3A4

Atorvastatin, simvastatin, and lovastatin are substrates for *CYP3A4*. Small number of studies have examined *CYP3A4* polymorphisms, these studies suggest that *CYP3A4*22* (*rs35599367*) is associated with low hepatic CYP3A4 expression, affecting statin pharmacokinetics.[13,14] A study on atorvastatin showed no significant impact of *CYP3A5* genotype on atorvastatin pharmacokinetics. However, a small study by Kivistö et al., indicated that lovastatin, simvastatin, and atorvastatin were less effective in *CYP3A5* "expressors" (*CYP3A5*1* allele) compared to "non-expressors" (*CYP3A5*3* allele).

Gene–Gene Interactions

While evaluating the risk of dose-related side effects for statins, it may be prudent to consider genetic determinants of drug response alongside other factors affecting its metabolism. In a case report, a patient with atorvastatin-induced rhabdomyolysis and acute renal failure had carried SNPs in *SLCO1B1* and *ABCB1*, predisposing them to a higher risk of side effects. This was compounded by a *CYP2C19* gene mutation affecting the metabolism of concomitant therapy (pantoprazole), which, at high concentrations, could inhibit *CYP3A4*-mediated atorvastatin metabolism. This scenario underscores the importance of considering both genotypic and phenotypic factors in understanding variability in response.

Summary

Genetic variants in importers, exporters, and CYP enzymes can significantly affect statin pharmacokinetics, although the extent of impact varies with individual statins. The *SLCO1B1* 521T>C variant has the strongest evidence for its role in statin pharmacokinetics and side effects and is already partially implemented in clinical practice. Variants in the *ABCG2* gene have consistently been linked to statin efficacy and side effects, making them potential candidates for screening. For CYP enzymes, more studies are needed before any specific variants can be recommended for inclusion in clinical practice.

GENETIC MARKERS AFFECTING PHARMACODYNAMICS OF STATINS

Pharmacodynamics of Statins

Statins primarily work by inhibiting HMG-CoA reductase (*HMGCR*), leading to reduced cholesterol synthesis in the liver and consequently increased expression of LDL receptors (LDLR), which enhances LDL clearance from the bloodstream. Despite their general efficacy, responses to statins can vary significantly among individuals. This variability can be influenced by genetic differences that affect the drug's pharmacodynamics, i.e., the effects and mechanisms of action of statins. The following are key genetic markers that have been shown or proposed to influence statin efficacy.

HMG-CoA Reductase and Related Genes

- *HMGCR (rs3846662):* Variants in the *HMGCR* gene can influence statin response. The SNP rs3846662 has been associated with altered splicing of exon 13, resulting in a truncated, nonfunctional protein isoform. This isoform, known as Δ13 or *HMGCRV1*, is thought to impair statin binding and reduce the drug's effectiveness. However, evidence is mixed, with some studies confirming the association and others not finding a significant impact.
- *HNRNPA1 (rs1920045):* This gene encodes a protein involved in splicing regulation. Variants in *HNRNPA1* have been linked to reduced response to statins, possibly through their effects on *HMGCR* splicing and subsequent protein functionality. The rs1920045 SNP was associated with statin efficacy in multiple trials, highlighting its potential role in determining statin efficacy.
- *HMGCR haplotypes:* Specific haplotypes in the *HMGCR* gene (e.g., H2 and H7) have been linked to baseline LDL-C levels and response to simvastatin. The prevalence of these haplotypes varies among different racial populations, which might contribute to observed differences in statin response across ethnic groups.

LDL Receptor (LDLR) and Related Genes

- *LDLR (rs688):* This synonymous SNP in exon 12 of *LDLR* affects exon 12 splicing efficiency, leading to two isoforms of *LDLR*. The *LDLR* (–12) isoform has altered localization and function compared to the *LDLR* (+12) isoform, which may impact LDL clearance and statin efficacy. This variant has been associated with differences in basal LDL cholesterol levels and statin response.
- *PCSK9:* This gene encodes an enzyme that regulates *LDLR* degradation. Variants in *PCSK9* can significantly impact statin response. For instance, the rare insertion mutant *c43-44insCTG* (L10) was associated with reduced

LDL cholesterol levels, possibly due to decreased *PCSK9* function and enhanced *LDLR* stability.

- *IDOL:* The E3-ubiquitin ligase IDOL, a negative regulator of *LDLR* stability, has recently been identified as a potential marker for statin response. Variants in *IDOL* might affect *LDLR* degradation, and thereby influence statin efficacy.

Apolipoproteins (APOE, APOC1, and APOC2)

Apolipoprotein E (*APOE*) is crucial for lipoprotein metabolism. The *APOE* gene has three common alleles (ε2, ε3, ε4). Variants such as *rs7412* and *rs429358* influence the *APOE* isoform, which affects statin response. Individuals with the ε2 allele tend to have greater LDL reduction on statin therapy compared to those with the ε4 allele.

Lipoprotein(a)

LPA (rs10455872 and rs3798220): LPA encodes for lipoprotein (a), an atherogenic lipoprotein. Variants like *rs10455872* are associated with statin response, with evidence suggesting that these SNPs can influence LDL lowering and cardiovascular risk. Another SNP, *rs3798220*, was found to affect simvastatin efficacy but not pravastatin, highlighting the need for further research into the role of LPA variants in statin response.

CONCLUSION

Several candidate genes have been found to influence the efficacy and safety of statin therapy. Among these, *SLCO1B1* has been particularly notable, with gene-based dosing recommendations for simvastatin implemented in some countries. However, whether genetic testing will become a standard practice to guide individualized statin therapy remains uncertain. An economic review by Sorich et al., suggested that it might be more cost-effective to avoid statin types and doses with a high risk of serious side effects rather than implementing routine genetic screening.

Moreover, patients at highest risk for statin-induced myopathy are often older individuals receiving multiple medications, increasing their risk for drug–drug interactions. While these patients would benefit most from personalized treatment, genetic screening alone may not be sufficient. Currently, statin efficacy can be effectively gauged through routine blood tests to measure lipid profiles. Although the pharmacodynamics of all statins are similar, their pharmacokinetic properties differ significantly. Therefore, genetic screening would need to be tailored to specific statins, requiring prescribing physicians to be educated accordingly. Therefore, the value of pharmacogenomic research extends beyond merely identifying genes for personalized medicine; it also holds promise for developing novel treatment strategies in the future.

ONLINE REFERENCES

Please scan the QR code provided at the end of the table of contents for References of this chapter.

SECTION 21

Preventive Cardiology

Section Outline

CHAPTER

222

Prevention of Coronary Artery Disease

Hem Chandra Kalita, Anupam Srivastava

ABSTRACT

Coronary artery disease (CAD) remains a foremost cause of cardiovascular afflictions across the globe, underscoring the imperative for vigilant prevention. Preventive healthcare advocates for the adoption of a heart-healthy regimen, encompassing a balanced diet, regular exercise, weight management, and the cessation of smoking. It further addresses individuals with preexisting risk factors by melding lifestyle modifications with appropriate medications to mitigate the likelihood of CAD. This chapter elucidates the CAD risk score and delineates the guidelines for primordial, primary, secondary, and tertiary prevention of CAD. Through the integration of these measures, we may substantially reduce the prevalence of CAD, thereby enhancing cardiovascular well-being and extending longevity.

Keywords: Atherosclerosis, coronary artery disease, modifiable risk factors, atherosclerotic cardiovascular disease (ASCVD) risk score

INTRODUCTION

Coronary artery disease (CAD) is a major cause of death globally, resulting in over 18 million fatalities annually, accounting for 32% of all deaths worldwide.[1] The ischemic heart disease deaths in India constituted around 13.9% of total deaths in 2021.[2] CAD encompasses a spectrum of conditions, from asymptomatic atherosclerosis to sudden cardiac death and stable angina to acute coronary syndromes (ACS), such as unstable angina, non-ST-elevation myocardial infarction (NSTEMI), and ST-elevation myocardial infarction (STEMI).

The risk factors for CAD are categorized into two categories—modifiable and nonmodifiable. Nonmodifiable risks include age, gender, ethnicity, and family history of CAD. Modifiable risk factors for CAD include hypertension, dyslipidemia, diabetes, obesity, smoking, alcohol, infections, sedentary lifestyle, increased C-reactive protein (CRP), hyperhomocysteinemia, chronic inflammatory diseases, environmental, air pollution, and AGE (advanced glycation end products)-RAGE (receptor for AGE) stress. These contribute to an increase in reactive oxygen species (ROS) within the blood and tissues through various mechanisms. This subsequently elevates levels of inflammatory cytokines and adhesion molecules, which play a crucial role in the development of atherosclerosis.

Prevention of CAD is divided into the following sections: Primordial, primary, secondary, and tertiary. Primordial prevention entails taking proactive steps to prevent the creation and reinforcement of environmental, economic, social, and behavioral factors, as well as cultural habits that are known to elevate the risk of CAD. Primary prevention is aimed at individuals who have risk factors but show no clinical signs of CAD, focusing on preventing the disease's onset. Secondary prevention is for individuals who have already been diagnosed with CAD and aims to reduce the development of complications. Tertiary prevention aims to reduce the impact of CAD by enhancing quality of life, reducing disability, delaying complications, and restoring cardiac function.

This chapter covers strategies for all levels of prevention that aim to prevent, reverse, and slowdown CAD progression. These measures can improve patients' quality of life and reduce healthcare expenses.

PREVENTION OF CORONARY ARTERY DISEASE

Primordial Prevention

To achieve the lowest possible risk for CAD and prevent the greatest number of incidents, it is crucial not only to manage individuals with existing risk factors using evidence-based strategies but also to prevent the initial development of these risk factors, a principle known as primordial prevention.

Young adults who adhere to five key healthy lifestyle practices—such as a Dietary Approaches to Stop Hypertension (DASH)-style diet, regular physical activity, a normal body mass index (BMI), nonsmoking, and minimal alcohol consumption—have roughly a 60% likelihood of maintaining optimal risk factor levels into midlife. In comparison, those who follow none or just one of these healthy practices have only about a 2% chance of achieving the same outcome.[3] Individuals with all risk factors at optimal levels and those who do not smoke have a lifetime risk of major atherosclerotic cardiovascular (CV) events of ≤8%. In contrast, those with one risk factor at suboptimal levels have a lifetime risk of about 30%, and those with two or more elevated risk factors face a lifetime risk of up to 70%.[4]

To determine the effectiveness of primordial prevention strategies in our country, it is crucial to conduct specific projects such as *The Special Turku Coronary Risk Factor Intervention Project* (STRIP study),[5] which took place in Turkey from 1990 to 2010, aimed to prevent atherosclerosis and coronary heart disease through dietary interventions starting in infancy and extending into early adulthood. Results showed that adults in the early intervention group had improved CV health, including lower smoking rates and more favorable blood pressure (BP) and cholesterol levels, compared to those who did not receive the intervention. The positive outcomes continued to be observed in the adults even after the intervention had ceased. Implementing a similar study in India would be highly beneficial for assessing the effectiveness of primordial prevention in reducing the overall burden of CAD.

The American Heart Association's (AHA's) *Healthy for Good program*,[6] along with its wellness toolkit, offers straightforward guidance for improving health and controlling risk factors for patients and clinicians. Meanwhile, *Voices for Healthy Kids*[7] supplies resources and information to assist community and advocacy efforts focused on bettering children's health in both school settings and daily life.

Primary Prevention

Cardiac Risk Assessment for Primary Prevention

Identifying heart health risks is the initial step in formulating a primary prevention strategy for individual patients. Various tools have been developed to aid this assessment, including the Framingham CVD risk score, the Reynolds risk score, and the QRISK3 assessment **(Tables 1 to 3)**.[8] These tools estimate the future risk of a cardiac event. The American College of Cardiology (ACC) and the AHA recommend using the atherosclerotic cardiovascular disease (ASCVD) risk estimator for this purpose **(Table 4)**. This tool calculates a 10-year risk of a first CV event using patient-specific data such as gender, age, race, cholesterol levels, BP, diabetes status, and tobacco use.

The ASCVD risk score helps determine the appropriate intensity of preventive measures and optimizing benefits

TABLE 1: Framingham risk score.[8]

Risk factors—men				Points assigned	
Age (20–79 years)				–9 to +13	
Total cholesterol (<160 to >280 mg/dL)				0 to +11	
Tobacco use (yes or no, by age)				0 to +8	
High-density lipoprotein (HDL) (>60 to <40 mg/dL)				–1 to +2	
Systolic blood pressure (<120 to >160 mm Hg)				0 to +3	
Risk factors—women				**Points assigned**	
Age (20–79 years)				–7 to +16	
Total cholesterol (<160 to >280 mg/dL)				0 to +13	
Tobacco use (yes or no, by age)				0 to +9	
HDL (>60 to <40 mg/dL)				–1 to +2	
Systolic blood pressure (<120 to >160 mm Hg)				0 to +6	
Risk score (RS) and corresponding 10-year risk (%)					
RS	*%*	*RS*	*%*	*RS*	*%*
<9	<1			21	14
9–12	1	17	5	22	17
13–14	2	18	6	23	22
15	3	19	8	24	27
16	4	20	11	25+	>30

TABLE 2: Reynolds risk score.[8]

Risk factors assessed	Data to be entered
Age and sex	–
Smoking status	–
Systolic blood pressure (in mm Hg)	–
Total cholesterol (mg/dL)	–
High-density lipoprotein (HDL) (mg/dL)	–
HbA1c (if diabetic)	–
High sensitivity CRP (mg/L)	–
Family history coronary artery disease (CAD) < 60 years old	–
10-year CVD risk	–

TABLE 3: QRISK3 score.[8]

Risk factors assessed	Data (input) to be given
Age	–
Sex	–
Ethnicity	–
Smoking status	–
Diabetes	–
Chronic kidney disease	–
Atrial fibrillation	–
Systolic blood pressure	–
BMI	–
Migraines	–
Rheumatoid arthritis	–
Severe mental illness	–
Use of atypical antipsychotic	–
Routine steroid use	–
Erectile dysfunction	–
Cholesterol/HDL ratio	–
hsCRP	–
Family history CAD < 60 years old	–
Calculate risk	

(BMI: body mass index; CAD: coronary artery disease; HDL: high-density lipoprotein)

TABLE 4: ASCVD risk estimator.[14]

Risk factors assessed	Patient profile to be entered
Age	
Sex	
Ethnicity	
Blood pressure	
Total cholesterol	
HDL	
LDL	
Diabetes	
Smoking status	
Hypertension treatment status	
Statin therapy	
Aspirin therapy	
Calculate risk	
ASCVD risk assessment	
Low risk	<5%
Borderline risk	5–7.4%
Intermediate risk	7.5–19.9%
High risk	>20%

(ASCVD: atherosclerotic cardiovascular disease; HDL: high-density lipoprotein; LDL: low-density lipoprotein)

while minimizing side effects and potential harms. Based on the estimated risk, individuals are categorized as low, borderline, intermediate, or high risk.[8] This categorization informs whether to initiate lifestyle modifications or pharmacological interventions to manage modifiable risk factors. The ASCVD tool is designed for adults aged 40–75 years; based on the cohort, it was validated in 2013.[9] Nevertheless, it has been observed that this tool might overestimate risk in Asian populations, particularly among Chinese and South Asians, and might underestimate risk in individuals with conditions that involve increased inflammation, such as HIV,[10] autoimmune diseases,[9] and radiation exposure.[11]

While the ASCVD risk estimator has its limitations, it remains a useful tool for engaging patients in conversations about their risk profiles. However, in 2024, the AHA introduced PREVENT (Predicting Risk of CVD Events),[12] a new CV risk predictor **(Table 5)** using data from 46 cohorts. It includes BMI, GFR, glycosylated hemoglobin, and urinary albumin-to-creatinine ratio, highlighting the role of metabolic and renal factors. Unlike earlier models, PREVENT omits race and offers 10-year CV risk estimates for those aged 30–79 years and 30-year estimates for those aged 30–59 years. The patient's data will be input into various sections of the calculator, which will then estimate the risk separately for CV disease (CVD), ASCVD, and heart failure. Researchers

TABLE 5: PREVENT calculator (American Heart Association).[12]

Risk factors	Input to be entered	
Sex		
Age	In years	
Total cholesterol	mg/dL	
HDL cholesterol	mg/dL	
Systolic BP	mm Hg	
BMI		
eGFR		
Diabetes	Yes	No
Currently smoking	Yes	No
Antihypertensive medication	Yes	No
Lipid-lowering medication	Yes	No
UACR	Yes	No
HbA1c	Yes	No
Zip code (for estimating social deprivation index)	Yes	No
Calculate risk		
• Risk of CVD • Risk of ASCVD • Risk of heart failure		

(ASCVD: atherosclerotic cardiovascular disease; BMI: body mass index; CVD: cardiovascular disease; HbA1c: glycated hemoglobin; HDL: high-density lipoprotein; UACR: urinary albumin creatinine ratio)

found that 17 million people eligible for statins under the 2013 model would not qualify under PREVENT.[12] Clinicians should consistently incorporate the ASCVD or PREVENT calculation into a holistic risk assessment process.

The following recommendations for primary prevention are based on guidelines from the AHA (2019) and ESC (2021):

- Implementing a team-based care approach is a proven strategy for the prevention of CVD. Clinicians should assess the social determinants of health that influence individuals to guide treatment decisions effectively. RCTs and systematic reviews with meta-analyses demonstrated a greater reduction of ASCVD risk with team-based care than with usual care in patients with hypertension, diabetes, and hyperlipidemia.
- Adults aged 40–75 years undergoing evaluations for CVD prevention should receive a 10-year ASCVD risk assessment. For individuals aged 20–39 years, it is advisable to evaluate traditional ASCVD risk factors every 4–6 years.[13,14] Before initiating pharmacological treatments such as antihypertensives, statins, or aspirin, it is crucial to have a risk discussion between the clinician and the patient. Additionally, considering other risk-enhancing factors and using coronary artery calcium scanning can aid in making well-informed decisions about preventive strategies for certain individuals.
- A healthy diet **(Box 1)** is recommended for all adults, emphasizing the consumption of vegetables, fruits, nuts, whole grains, lean sources of protein (more plant based), and fish, while reducing the intake of transfats, red and processed meats, refined carbohydrates, and sweetened beverages. In a multicenter randomized trial conducted in 2018 by the PREDIMED (*Prevencion con Dieta Mediterranea*) study group,[15] which involved individuals at high CV risk, those who followed a Mediterranean diet supplemented with extra-virgin olive oil or nuts experienced a lower incidence of major CV events compared to those who adhered to a reduced-fat diet.[15] For adults who are overweight or obese, counseling and calorie restriction are advised to support weight loss and maintenance. The Adventist Health Study 2 cohort comparison showed that consuming animal protein was linked to a 61% higher mortality rate while substituting meat with nuts and seeds was associated with a 40% decrease in mortality rate.[16]
- Reducing dietary sodium was shown to decrease BP by an average of 5.8 mm Hg in hypertensive patients and 1.9 mm Hg in normotensive patients, as well as lower the risk of CV events in both the DASH trial[17] and the Trials of Hypertension Prevention (TOHP).[17,18] Data from the National Health and Nutrition Examination Surveys (NHANES)[19] indicate that consuming >2,000 mg of sodium per day, along with a high intake of red meat (over 14 g/day), sugar-sweetened beverages, and processed red meat, was linked to an increased risk of CV death. Additionally, "each 7 g/day increase in total fiber intake is associated with a 9% reduction in the risk of CAD [relative risk (RR) 0.91]."[20]
- Adults should engage in at least 150 minutes of moderate-intensity physical activity (3–5.9 MET) or 75 minutes of vigorous-intensity exercise (>6 MET) each week as advised by the *Physical Activity Guidelines Advisory Committee, Washington DC (2008)* **(Box 2)**.[21] People who are overweight or obese should focus on losing weight to lower BP, improve cholesterol levels, and reduce the risk of type 2 diabetes, which can lead to a better metabolic profile. Although various diets can aid in weight loss, it is crucial to adhere to a calorie-restricted diet that supports CV health for long-term effectiveness.
- For adults with type 2 diabetes mellitus, lifestyle changes, including better dietary habits, smoking cessation, meeting exercise recommendations, and maintaining an HbA1c target < 7.0% are critical. Meta-analyses of the UKPDS,[22] ADVANCE, ACCORD,[23] and VADT studies, including 27,049 participants, have demonstrated that lowering HbA1c reduces MACE, driven by a reduction in myocardial infarction (MI). Metformin shall be the first-line therapy and if additional ASCVD risks are present, it will be a good choice to initiate SGLT-2 inhibitors or a glucagon-like peptide-1 receptor (GLP-1R) agonist to improve glycemic control and reduce CVD **(Box 3)**.
- Smoking represents a significant modifiable risk factor for CAD and is responsible for approximately 20% of global CAD-related deaths.[24] Smoking just one cigarette per day increases the risk of developing CAD by 40–50%.[25] Specifically, heavy smokers—those with 20 or more pack-years of smoking—who cease smoking experience a 39% reduction in CAD risk within 5 years compared to those who continue smoking.[26] Tobacco use should be

BOX 1 Dietary recommendations.[8]

- Emphasize intake of vegetables, fruits, legumes, nuts, whole grains, and fish
- Replace saturated fat with monosaturated fat and poly-unsaturated fat
- Avoid transfats
- Reduce cholesterol and sodium intake
- Minimize the intake of sweetened beverages, refined carbohydrates, and processed meats

BOX 2 Exercise recommendations.[8]

- Adults should be routinely encouraged to maintain a physically active lifestyle
- Each week adults should perform 150 minutes of moderate-intensity exercise, or 75 minutes of high-intensity exercise, or a combination of the two
- Any amount of physical activity in those unable to meet the recommended amount is still beneficial
- Decrease sedentary factor

BOX 3 Diabetes mellitus recommendations.[8]

- Each week adults should perform 150 minutes of moderate-intensity exercise, or 75 minutes of high-intensity exercise, to improve glycemic control and achieve weight loss
- At the time of diagnosis, initiate lifestyle therapies as well as metformin as first-line therapy
- For those with additional ASCVD risk factors who require further glucose lowering therapy, it is reasonable to initiate SGLT2 inhibitor or GLP-1R agonist as a first line

(ASCVD: atherosclerotic cardiovascular disease; GLP-1R: glucagon-like peptide-1 receptor; SGLT-2: sodium glucose cotransporter-2)

BOX 4 Pharmacotherapy for smoking cessation.[8]

Stable cardiovascular disease

- *First line*: Varenicline or combination nicotine replacement therapy
- *Second line*: Bupropion or single nicotine replacement product
- *Third line*: Nortriptyline

Acute coronary syndrome

- *First line*: Nicotine patch or combination nicotine replacement therapy in the hospital, a combination nicotine replacement therapy or varenicline at discharge
- *Second line*: Single nicotine replacement therapy product
- *Third line*: Bupropion

evaluated at every healthcare visit and individuals who use tobacco should receive assistance such as nicotine replacement therapy, varenicline, and bupropion, as well as individual or telephone counseling **(Box 4)**. Exposure to second-hand smoke is recognized as a cause of CAD in nonsmokers and it can lead to immediate negative health effects. No level of second-hand smoke exposure is considered safe. Even short-term exposure to second-hand smoke has the potential to trigger a MI.

- The cardioprotective effects of light to moderate alcohol consumption might primarily result from confounding lifestyle factors. Genetic analyses indicate a causal link between alcohol intake and CVD, though the risk increases exponentially with higher levels of consumption.[27]
- Aspirin use is not recommended in individuals with low/moderate CV risk due to the increased risk of major bleeding. Contemporary primary prevention trials such as ASCEND (2018),[28] ASPREE (2018),[29] and ARRIVE (2018)[30] reported no or little benefit in patients without ASCVD and a consistent increase in bleeding.
- According to 2019 ESC/EAS dyslipidemia guidelines, statin therapy is the recommended first-line treatment for primary prevention of ASCVD in patients with high low-density lipoprotein cholesterol (LDL-C) levels (≥190 mg/dL), adults aged 40–75 years with diabetes mellitus and those identified as being at sufficient ASCVD risk after a thorough discussion with their clinician.[31] In patients aged 75 years and younger, the effectiveness of statins for primary prevention is well supported by numerous randomized trials which have demonstrated a 20–30% reduction in the RR of major vascular events.[32] New meta-analyses from the contemporary JUPITER[32] and HOPE-3 randomized trials in 2017 showed that the use of rosuvastatin significantly lowered the risk for a composite outcome of nonfatal MI, nonfatal stroke, or CV death by 26%, compared with placebo, in subjects >70 years of age initially free of ASCVD.[32]

  For primary prevention in patients at very high risk who do not have familial hypercholesterolemia (FH), if the LDL-C target is not met with the maximum tolerated dose of a statin and ezetimibe, adding a proprotein convertase subtilisin/kexin type 9 (PCSK9) inhibitor to the treatment regimen may be considered.[33,34]

  While elevated fasting triglycerides (TG) above 1.7 mmol/L (150 mg/dL) are associated with an increased risk of CAD, medications to lower TG levels are generally considered only for high-risk patients when TG levels exceed 2.3 mmol/L (200 mg/dL) and cannot be managed through lifestyle changes. Available pharmacological options for managing TG include statins, fibrates, PCSK9 inhibitors, and n-3 polyunsaturated fatty acids (PUFAs), with icosapent ethyl being particularly effective at doses of 2–4 g/day.[35]
- In managing hypertension, it has been suggested that physical activity can contribute to weight loss, which may reduce inflammation and decrease vascular resistance. This reduction is thought to be associated with lower oxidative stress, reduced sympathetic activity, decreased vascular sensitivity to adrenergic and endothelin-receptor stimulation, diminished renin–angiotensin system (RAS) activity, and a thinning of the intima-media layer.[36] For all adults with hypertension, nonpharmacological interventions are advised first. If not controlled, the addition of medications should be done to achieve a target BP of <130/80 mm Hg **(Box 5)**.

Secondary Prevention

Secondary prevention targets those with established CAD to prevent disease progression and reduce further risk. The goals are to slow the advancement of CAD, reverse its progression, and lower the likelihood of recurring events or mortality.

Key measures of secondary prevention include:

- Regular physical activity is a key element in the secondary prevention of CAD as it enhances exercise capacity, manages comorbid risk factors, and boosts overall quality of life. Studies confirm that exercise-based cardiac rehabilitation lowers both all-cause and cardiac-specific mortality compared to routine care. The recommended target for patients is 30–60 minutes of moderate-intensity

BOX 5 Hypertension recommendations.[8]

- Adults with hypertension adopt nonpharmacological interventions including weight loss, a heart-healthy dietary pattern, sodium reduction, potassium supplementation, increased physical activity, and limited alcohol intake
- In patients with a 10-year ASCVD risk score of 10% or higher, or with hypertension and diabetes, and with BP of 130/80 mm Hg or higher, BP-lowering medications should be initiated
- In adults with hypertension and CKD, diabetes, or 10-year ASCVD risk score of 10% or higher, a target BP < 130/80 mm Hg should be used
- In patients with a 10-year ASCVD risk score of 10% or lower, BP-lowering medicines should be initiated at BP > 140/90 mm Hg
- In adults without additional ASCVD risk factors, targeting a BP of 130/80 mm Hg may be reasonable

(ASCVD: atherosclerotic cardiovascular disease; BP: blood pressure; CKD: chronic kidney disease)

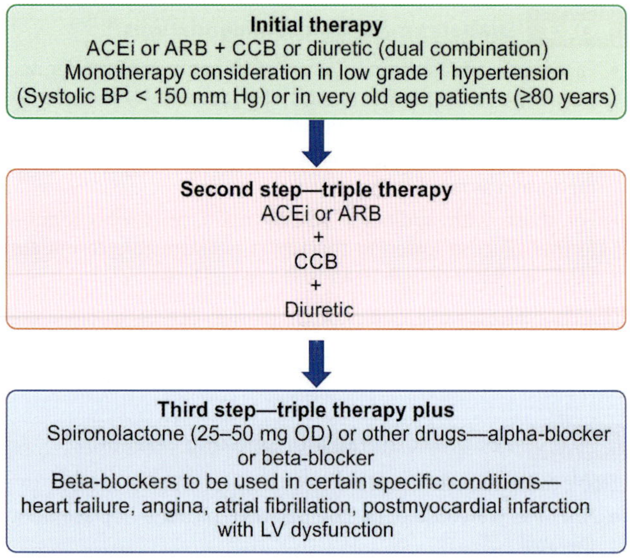

FLOWCHART 1: ESC 2023 based hypertension core drug management plan.[42]

[ACE: angiotensin-converting enzyme; ARB: angiotensin receptor blocker; BP: blood pressure; CCB: calcium channel blocker; OD: omni die (once a day)]

exercise, such as brisk walking or cycling, on most days of the week. After an ACS or revascularization procedure, exercise-based cardiac rehabilitation can be initiated. Before patients embark on a more rigorous exercise regimen, physicians need to assess their CV health by taking a detailed physical activity history or conducting an exercise test **(Box 1)**.[37]

- *Weight management*: Reduce BMI to 18.5–24.9 kg/m^2 and target waist circumference <40 inches for men and <35 inches for women.
- *Lipid management*: A consistent 2 mg/dL reduction in LDL-C through statin therapy is associated with a 1% decrease in the risk of major coronary events, coronary revascularization, and stroke.[38] Use of statins, ezetimibe, and PCSK9 inhibitors to lower LDL-C and manage TG levels with fibrates or omega-3 fatty acids. The target for LDL-C under the age of 70 years is <55 mg/dL for very high risk and <70 mg/dL for the high-risk group patients with multiple events.[39] If the maximum tolerated dose of a statin does not achieve the desired goals, adding ezetimibe is advised (IMPROVE-IT TRIAL).[40] Fibrate or a high dose of omega-3 fatty acid should be used if the TG level is 500 mg/dL or non-HDL-C level is 100 mg/dL.
- *Hypertension*: Treat with antihypertensive medications and maintain BP below 130/80 mm Hg.[41] It is advised to increase the use of single-pill combination therapies to improve adherence to BP treatments. A straightforward drug treatment plan should be employed for most patients, utilizing combinations of a RAS blocker with either a calcium channel blocker (CCB) or a thiazide/thiazide-like diuretic, or all three. Beta-blockers can also be prescribed when indicated by clinical guidelines **(Flowchart 1)**.
- *Antiplatelet therapy*: For antithrombotic therapy following an ACS, the typical regimen is dual-antiplatelet therapy (DAPT) for 12 months, ideally with prasugrel or ticagrelor in addition to aspirin.[42] The debate continues over whether prasugrel offers superior benefits compared to ticagrelor. A 6-month course of DAPT is generally regarded as inadequate after ACS, although it might be suitable for patients with a high risk of bleeding. In the case of patients with chronic coronary syndromes (CCS) undergoing elective percutaneous coronary intervention (PCI), DAPT is usually prescribed for 6 months.[43] For those at very high risk of bleeding, a shorter period of 1–3 months might be considered. While clopidogrel is commonly used as the P2Y12 inhibitor, prasugrel and ticagrelor may be employed for more complex situations. Extending DAPT beyond 12 months may be considered for patients who tolerate the therapy well and exhibit a high ischemic risk, whether following ACS or CCS. In stable CAD patients, adding low-dose rivaroxaban (2.5 mg twice daily) to aspirin can improve CV outcomes, though it increases the risk of major bleeding compared to aspirin alone.

  According to the AHA CCS Guidelines 2023, for long-term secondary prevention, adding a second antithrombotic agent (either a P2Y12 inhibitor or low-dose rivaroxaban) to aspirin is recommended for patients at high ischemic risk without a high bleeding risk. This strategy may also be appropriate for those at moderate ischemic risk, provided there is not a high risk of bleeding, though the benefits are less definitive.[43]
- *Diabetes management*: Achieving optimal blood glucose levels is crucial, typically using antidiabetic medications. The recommended HbA1c target is below 7%. Specific glucose targets are fasting levels between 72 and 126 mg/dL and 2 hours post-meal < 180 mg/dL.[44] Managing

hypertension and elevated serum cholesterol is also advised while monitoring for any diabetes-related end-organ damage. SGLT-2 inhibitors (evidenced by six CV outcome trials)[45-50] and GLP-1R agonists (GLP-1RAs)[51-59] are two drug classes that have shown CV benefits, which seem to be independent of both glycemic control and, where studied, prior use of metformin **(Box 3)**.

- *Smoking cessation*: Support efforts and medications to quit smoking as described for primary prevention **(Box 4)**.
- *AGE–RAGE stress*: To mitigate AGE-RAGE stress, it is important to lower levels of AGES and increase soluble RAGE (S-RAGE) levels. Avoiding cigarette smoking and engaging in regular moderate exercise can reduce AGE levels. Prevention of AGE formation can be supported by consuming acidic foods such as lemon juice and vinegar, along with linolenic acid, flaxseed, and vitamins C, D, and E. To elevate S-RAGE levels, statins, ACE inhibitors, and rosiglitazone[60] may be beneficial, along with the potential exogenous administration of S-RAGE if available.
- *Oxidative stress*: Plant-based antioxidants play a role in preventing atherosclerosis. Vitamins E and C together have been shown to slow the progression of hypercholesterolemic atherosclerosis. Other antioxidants, such as probucol, garlic, and flaxseed lignan complex, may also help reduce oxidative stress. However, supplements as drugs did not show benefits as evidenced by the HOPE trial.[61]
- *CRP*: Several medications are known to lower serum CRP levels, including aspirin, clopidogrel, statins, β-adrenoreceptor blockers, ACE inhibitors, ARB's (such as candesartan), rosiglitazone, and vitamins-E[62] and C. Observational studies have suggested that vitamins A and E might be inversely related to the risk of ASCVD. However, intervention trials have not supported these results. Additionally, supplementation with B vitamins (B6, folic acid, and B12), as well as vitamins C and D, has not demonstrated any beneficial effects.[63,64]
- *Others*: Recently, air pollution (especially airborne particulate matter), environmental exposure, and climate change have been shown to increase CAD risk. Hence, policies directed to reduce the impact of the above factors should be implemented globally.

Tertiary Prevention of Coronary Artery Disease

Tertiary prevention is focused on individuals who already have CAD. Its primary goal is to enhance the quality of life for these patients by reducing disability, preventing, or managing complications and restoring cardiac function. Achieving these goals involves treating CAD and undergoing rehabilitation. The treatment team typically includes a family physician, cardiologist, cardiac surgeon, exercise specialist, physiotherapist, dietitian, and nurses. The strategies used in tertiary prevention often overlap with those used in secondary prevention. Treatment options in tertiary prevention may involve procedures such as PCI, coronary artery bypass grafting (CABG), pacemakers, defibrillators, and ventricular assist devices. Efforts should also be directed toward promoting neovascularization in ischemic heart tissue. Various approaches have been explored to encourage this neovascularization.

CONCLUSION

Coronary artery disease leads to substantial morbidity and mortality for millions of patients in India and globally. Consequently, effective management and prevention of CV risks at various levels can significantly enhance their health and quality of life.

ONLINE REFERENCES

Please scan the QR code provided at the end of the table of contents for References of this chapter.

CHAPTER 223

Management of Inflammation in Cardiovascular Disease

SR Sharath Shanmugam, S Murugarajan, MS Ravi

ABSTRACT

Inflammatory heart disease encompasses group of diseases that occur following an injury to myocardium, pericardium, and endocardium secondary to infectious or noninfectious insult. Variety of immune cells can infiltrate and cause tissue destruction.[1] Inflammatory heart disease can occur in any age group and usually, spontaneous recovery occurs but in few subsets of patients, persistent damage can occur, which may lead to chronic damage to the heart. Myocarditis can have varied presentations from asymptomatic heart failure (HF) to cardiogenic shock and sudden cardiac death. Diagnosis is usually challenging due to its complex presentation. Pericarditis can be self-limiting but persistent inflammation can lead to chronic constrictive pericarditis. Endocarditis can occur as part of systemic autoimmune diseases like systemic lupus erythematosus (SLE) and rheumatoid arthritis in addition to infectious etiology.[2] Endocarditis can lead to valvulitis and congestive HF. Electrocardiogram, echocardiography, cardiac biomarker, cardiac MRI, and cardiac nuclear scan (PET scan) are the investigations that will be useful for inflammatory heart disease. Autoimmune panels may be required in few subsets of patients. Patients are managed with guideline-directed HF treatment. Patients are treated with immunosuppressive drugs.

Keywords: Inflammation in CVD, myocarditis, pericarditis, endocarditis

INTRODUCTION

Inflammatory heart disease (IHD) is a group of diseases that includes pericarditis, myocarditis, and endocarditis. Males are more commonly affected than females; IHD can be seen in any age group. While the disease can be self-limiting leading to full recovery, individuals can develop chronic disease, suggesting that identification of primary triggers is critical for successful therapies. In addition to this complexity, IHD can be triggered by a variety of infectious and noninfectious causes that can also occur as secondary events to primary insults.[3]

PATHOGENESIS

The pathogenesis given here is common for immune-mediated injury.

Following an injury (infectious or noninfectious) to pericardium, myocardium, or endocardium, a variety of innate immune cells like neutrophils, macrophages, dendritic cells including γδ T cells, ILCs, and NK-T cells can infiltrate and take part in tissue destruction.[4]

The inflammatory damage can also lead to the release of cardiac antigens such as cardiac myosin, actin, cTnI, ANT, BAR, BCKD, SERCA2a, laminin, muscarinic receptor (MR), and heat shock proteins (HSP). The newly released antigens can trigger autoimmune responses by activating T cells and B cells in the draining lymph nodes, which can in turn infiltrate the heart and aggravate inflammation **(Fig. 1)**.[5]

MYOCARDITIS

Myocarditis is an inflammatory disease of the heart that involves myocyte and interstitial and vascular elements of the heart. Myocarditis usually occurs as a consequence of infections, exposure to toxic substances, and immune system activation. It has a wide clinical presentation ranging from asymptomatic to fulminant HF. It is also a relatively common cause of sudden cardiac death (SCD) in young people (from 6–10% in autopsy-based series). Pathologically, myocarditis can be classified as eosinophilic, lymphocytic, giant cells, or granulomatous (based on the cell types infiltrating).[6] Exact prevalence is unknown due to heterogeneity in clinical presentation and complexity in diagnosis but roughly

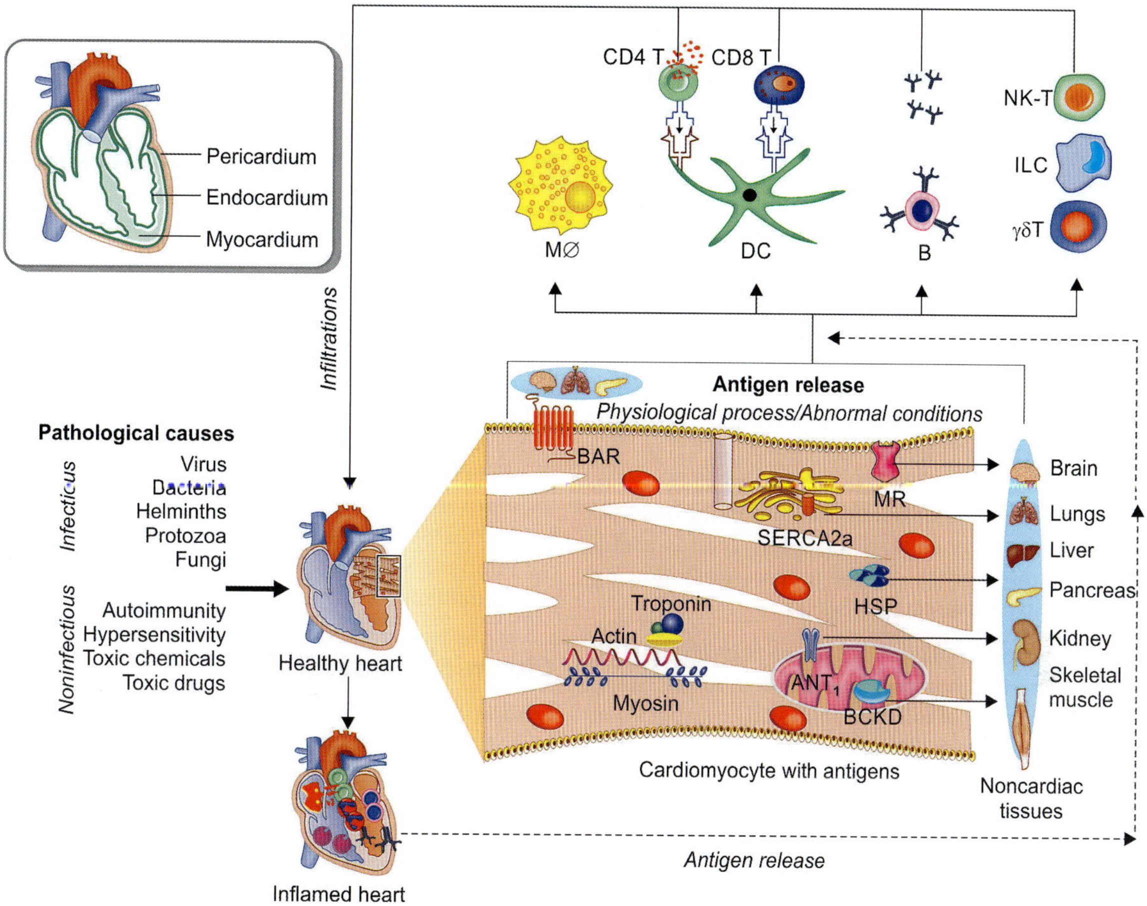

FIG. 1: Proposed mechanisms of inflammatory heart disease.[8,9]

estimated to be 20–40 cases per 100,000 people based on hospital-based discharge study.

Clinically, myocarditis is classified into acute (<1-month symptom onset), subacute (1–3 month symptom onset), and chronic myocarditis (>3-month symptom onset).

Acute myocarditis (AM) usually presents with chest pain (most common), dyspnea, fatigue, palpitation, and syncope. Some patients may have prodromal symptoms like sore throat, fever, gastrointestinal disorder, or respiratory tract infections. In history, focus on recent exposure to drugs (e.g., antibiotics and clozapine) or toxic substances (e.g., cocaine or amphetamine) or to infectious agents (e.g., ingestion of raw meat suggesting helminthic infections, travels to areas where viruses associated with AM, such as dengue, are endemic). Recent retrospective study showed that 26.6% of AM will have eventful presentations like LV dysfunction, arrhythmias, cardiogenic shock, whereas 73.4% have uneventful presentation with chest pain and ST segment changes.[7]

An ECG abnormality will be seen in 85% of AM with predominant ST-segment elevation mimicking STEMI. It usually involves inferolateral leads. Bradycardia, tachycardia, ventricular arrhythmias, and widened QRS (QRS >120 ms) points to high-risk myocarditis.

Second-degree or complete AV block is uncommon in preserved LV function except in cardiac sarcoidosis and Lyme carditis.

Laboratory investigations include CRP, ESR, and biomarkers such as troponin and CK-MB. The correlation between biomarkers level and severity of cardiac function is weak. Peripheral eosinophilia is seen in eosinophilic myocarditis. Viral PCR for influenza and SARS-2 may point to the etiology in few cases. Serological tests for HIV and *Borrelia burgdorferi* antibodies may provide etiological clues. ANA and autoimmune panel will point toward autoimmune myocarditis.

Imaging

Echocardiography: LVEF is a powerful prognosticator on admission. AM usually will have normal dimensions, normal thickness, mild segmental hypokinesia, pericardial effusion, and increased myocardial echogenicity with low ejection fraction. LVEF may improve during the course of illness either spontaneously or with treatment.

Cardiac MRI (CMRI): It is the most important noninvasive tool indicated in all patients suspected to have AM. It should be performed ideally 2–3 weeks after symptom onset to rule out or rule in myocardial inflammation reliably. Original Lake Louise Criteria have three hallmarks of CMRI biomarkers for myocardial inflammation: (1) Hyperemia (intense signal in early gadolinium enhancement images), (2) tissue edema (increased signal intensity in T2-weighted images), and (3) necrosis/fibrosis based on late gadolinium enhancement (LGE) images. Two out of three criteria positive will have 86% specificity and 74% sensitivity. Updated criteria include native T1 images and T2 weighted images to improve sensitivity and specificity. CMRI cannot identify the specific cause for inflammation and cannot subtype myocardial inflammation histopathologically. Regional distribution can give some clue to etiology such as basal septal involvement suggests cardiac sarcoidosis. Persistent LGE suggests unfavorable prognosis in follow-up CMRI study **(Fig. 2)**.

Role of PET in myocarditis is limited to diagnosing cardiac sarcoidosis and other systemic autoimmune diseases with multiorgan involvement. ^{18}F-FDG PET scan is useful to diagnose and monitor the disease progression following immunotherapy in cardiac sarcoidosis.

Role of endomyocardial biopsy (EMB) in myocarditis: It is an invasive procedure and has lesser yield based on the site of sampling and presence of inflammation with complication rate 1–2% at expert center and 8.9% at low-volume center. To improve the diagnostic yield Marburg criteria is used, based on the presence of >14 mononuclear leukocytes/mm^2 on bioptic samples, with the presence of >7 T lymphocytes per mm^2.

Current Indications for EMB:

- AM presenting with severe HF or cardiogenic shock (i.e., fulminant myocarditis)
- AM complicated by severe myocardial dysfunction, acute HF, ventricular arrhythmias, or high-degree atrioventricular block
- AM or [suspected chronic inflammatory cardiomyopathy (infl-CMP)] associated with peripheral eosinophilia
- AM or chronic infl-CMP with persistent release of biomarkers of myocardial necrosis, particularly if associated with a suspected/known autoimmune disorder or ventricular arrhythmias or high-degree atrioventricular block
- Myocarditis in the setting of immune checkpoint inhibitor, where appropriate diagnosis has implications for patients receiving additional chemotherapy.

Chronic Myocarditis

Chronic myocarditis represents the evolution of >1 episode of AM that was diagnosed or missed leading to chronic myocardial damage resulting in HF. This can be dilated

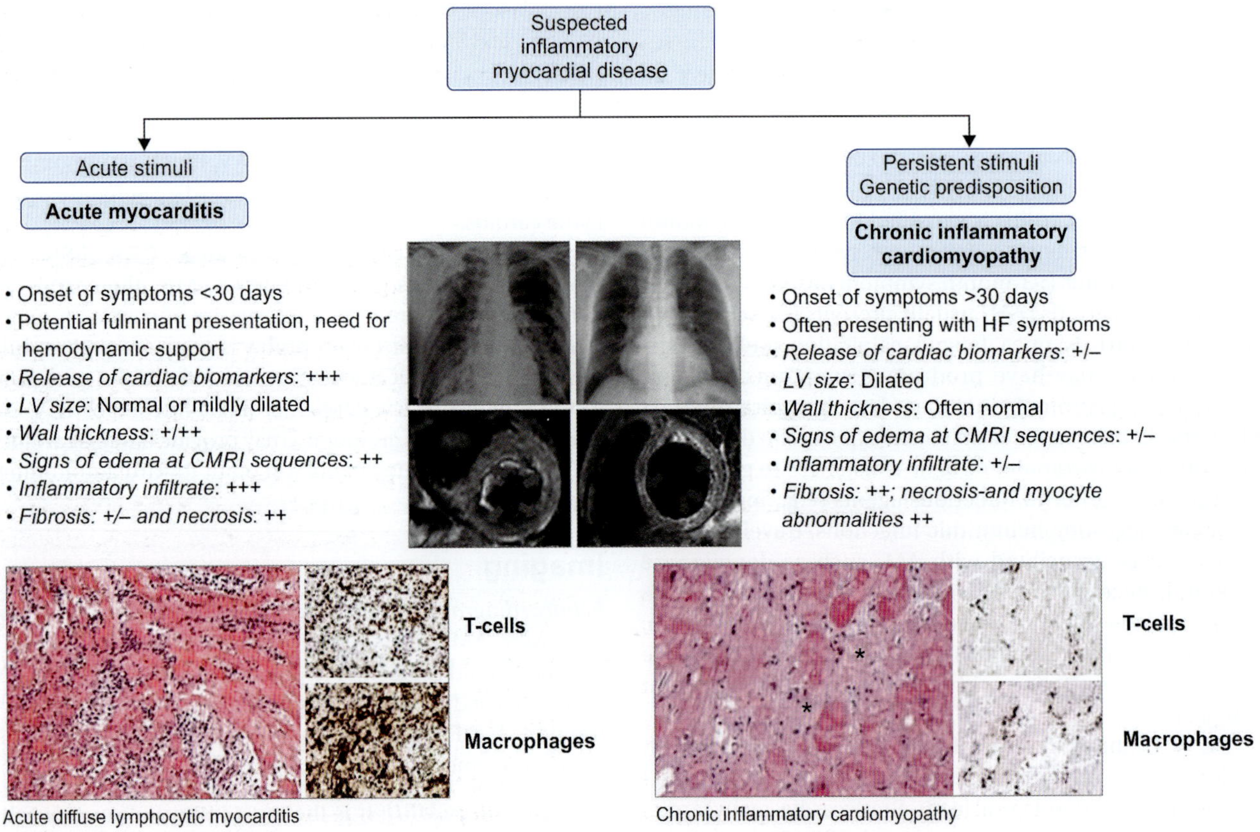

FIG. 2: Characteristic features of lymphocytic acute myocarditis and chronic inflammatory cardiomyopathy.

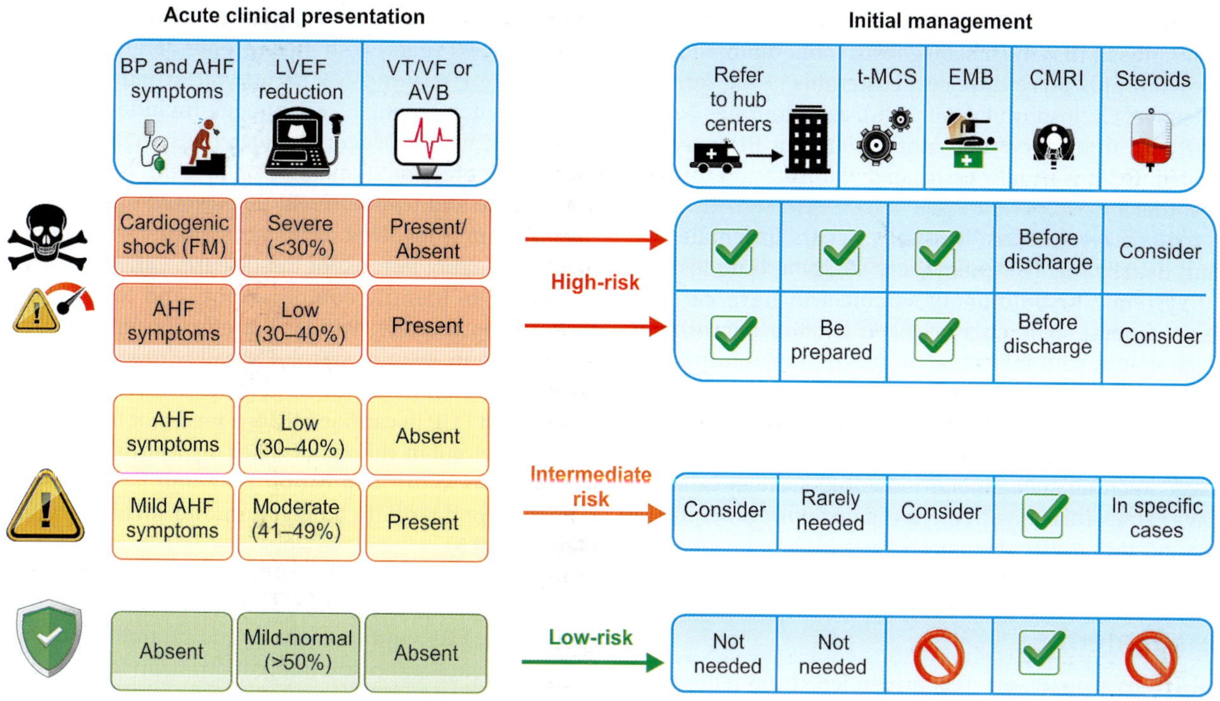

FIG. 3: Proposed risk-based approach to acute myocarditis.

cardiomyopathy phenotype or nondilated hypokinetic phenotype. Usually, these patients will have LV systolic dysfunction with normal wall thickness. Subtle clues such as low voltage, fragmented QRS, minor conduction disturbance, ST-T abnormalities, persistent troponin elevation, failure to respond to standard HF treatment should arouse the suspicion of chronic myocarditis **(Fig. 3)**.

Salient Features of Different Forms of Myocarditis

- *Lymphocytic myocarditis*: Viral-mediated and immune-mediated myocarditis will cause lymphocytic myocarditis. Viral-mediated myocarditis can be viral-induced or viral-triggered myocarditis, e.g., viral-induced include enterovirus (coxsackie) that affects infants and children. Respiratory viruses (influenza or corona) will trigger the immune-mediated damage due to molecular mimicry. So, if the virus is replicating and damaging myocardium, it is reasonable to use antiviral drugs or interferon-beta, which will enhance native immunity.[10] If the virus is not replicating or it simply a bystander then immunosuppression will be useful based on AHA scientific statement. Immune-mediated lymphocytic myocarditis could be a part of systemic autoimmune diseases like SLE, dermatomyositis, and inflammatory bowel disease.
- *Immune checkpoint inhibitors associated myocarditis*: Immune checkpoint inhibitors have revolutionized the cancer chemotherapy but their use is associated with myocarditis within 1 month of exposure. High-dose intravenous corticosteroids associated with withdrawal of ICI are considered the first-line therapy, Alemtuzumab (anti-CD52 antibody), antithymocyte globulin (anti-CD3 anti-body), and abatacept (a CTLA-4 agonist) have been proposed as second-line therapy.
- *Eosinophilic myocarditis (EM)*: It is usually due to hypersensitivity reactions secondary to chemicals (clonazipine), systemic condition (Churg–Strauss syndrome and EGPA) or idiopathic (HES) or parasitic infection (*Toxocara*). EM usually occurs in middle-aged individuals; equal in both sexes. Patients may have skin rash, asthma, eosinophilia, and LV dysfunction. Typically, they have intracardiac thrombosis at the LV apex (HES) and LV dysfunction. EM have subendocardial LGE pattern in contrast to other forms of myocarditis where they have subepicardial LGE. Steroids are usually effective. Along with steroids, cyclophosphamide, azathioprine, and methotrexate will be useful in systemic eosinophilic conditions. Albendazole and steroids are useful in *Toxocara*-mediated myocarditis. Imatinib is utilized in myeloproliferative variants of HES.
- *Giant-cell myocarditis (GCM)*: It is a rapidly progressive necrotizing myocarditis caused due to infiltration of cytotoxic T cells, macrophages, giant cells, and eosinophils with poor prognosis, and has an occurrence of 1% of all cases of myocarditis and 8% of FM (fulminant myocarditis). Usually, it occurs in 43–53 years of age, presenting with severe LV dysfunction with arrhythmias. Apart from mechanical circulatory support (MCS),

immunosuppressive therapy should be initiated promptly. EMB is the first diagnostic tool. Antithymocyte globulin plus pulse dose corticosteroids (1 mg/kg) are effective. Cyclosporine (100 ng/L), azathioprine (1 mg/kg), and mycophenolate mofetil 500 mg BD may be added. GCM is usually associated with IBD and thyroid disorder.

- *Sarcoidic myocarditis*: It usually occurs in female sex and usually involves pulmonary and lymph nodes. 5% of systemic or pulmonary sarcoid will have cardiac involvement. It is characterized by non-necrotizing granulomas with infiltration of macrophages forming a multinucleate giant cell or epithelioid cell. Conduction abnormalities, ventricular arrhythmias, and HF are the common presentations. The ventricular septum and basal free wall are commonly involved. Cardiac imaging plus extracardiac involvement of sarcoidosis is helpful in diagnosing cardiac sarcoidosis. Steroids are the first-line therapy.

Management

Usual HF treatments are recommended in patients with chronic infl-CMP or AM with reduced LVEF and stable hemodynamics. β-blockers are often used after an AM also in patients with uncomplicated presentation. For SCD prevention, general guidelines are followed for chronic myocarditis. For AM, risk stratification should be done based on family history of SCD, arrhythmogenic cardiomyopathy, presence of LGE scar on CMRI, ventricular tachycardia on VT presentation, and various factors like EMB being compatible with GCM or cardiac sarcoidosis should be taken into account. No major trials have been conducted in this group of diseases due to heterogenous presentation and delayed diagnosis, but few small studies favor the usage of steroids and immunosuppression in selected subtypes of myocarditis.

Patient complicated by refractory HF or cardiogenic shock need inotropic support or MCS. AM is usually a reversible condition and temporary devices like IABP, VA ECMO are needed. Theoretically, centrifugal pump or intra-aortic axial pump should give better results than VA ECMO, but studies show no significant difference in the circulatory support. If there is no weaning from MCS within 2–3 weeks, then consider long-term LV-assisted device or urgent heart transplantation.

PERICARDITIS

Pericardium is the outer covering layer of heart consisting of outer fibrous membranous sac and inner serous layer. Two out of four criteria must be followed to diagnose pericarditis: (1) Chest pain, (2) pericardial rub, (3) ECG changes, and (4) new or worsening pericardial effusion. Symptoms include sharp chest pain with rapid onset, radiating to trapezius ridge, aggravated by cough and breathing, relieved by sitting and leaning forward. Pericarditis can occur in all age groups (20–50 years) with male preponderance. Estimated prevalence is around 5% among chest pain admissions in emergency room. ECG changes include PR segment depression with ST-segment elevation specifically, but PR segment depression alone may be present. Biomarkers are nonspecific and troponin will be elevated only if adjacent myocardium is involved. Echocardiography will be the only needed imaging in most of the disease. Echo is helpful for diagnosis, to identify complications, and to monitor the response to therapy. Pericardial effusion may be graded as trivial (only seen in systole), small (<10 mm), moderate (10–20 mm), large (21–25 mm), and very large (>25 mm). Presence of LGE in cardiac MRI is a predictor for recurrence. CMRI is helpful in ruling out other myocardial pathologies. CT scan has short acquisition time and is very useful in detecting pericardial calcification and localized effusion **(Figs. 4 and 5)**.

Infectious triggers include bacteria (*Staphylococcus, Streptococcus, Haemophilus,* and *Mycobacterium*), viruses (echovirus, EBV, and coxsackie), and mutation in immune response genes will result in Mediterranean fever and TNF-receptor associated periodic syndrome.

Autoimmune pericarditis can occur in SLE, rheumatoid arthritis, and Sjögren syndrome. Serum Carcinoembryonic antigen cell adhesion molecule 1 and MHC class I chain-related protein A can be used as biomarkers and prognostic markers, respectively. Pericardial fluid may contain markers like IL-6, IL-8, and INF-γ.

The disease is self-limiting in most patients (70–90%) and responds well to anti-inflammatory medications like aspirin or nonsteroidal anti-inflammatory drugs with colchicine, corticosteroids, and anakinra (IL-1 receptor antagonist) **(Table 1)**.

ENDOCARDITIS

Endocarditis can be due to infectious or noninfectious-mediated immune activation. Endocarditis can be seen in patients with RA, SLE, and rheumatic fever, in which both joints and cardiovascular systems could be affected. Antibodies crossreact with cardiac proteins like cardiac myosin, laminin and other cytoskeleton proteins. Damage to endocardium can result in valvulitis and endothelial scarring and ultimately lead to congestive HF.

Endocarditic lesions, primarily called vegetation, consist of microorganisms, inflammatory cells, platelets, and fibrin. Infective organisms like *S. aureus*, *Streptococcus* species, *Enterococcus*, HACEK organisms, and *Candida* species all can cause vegetations. Vegetations are common in IV drug abusers, HIV, diabetes, cancer patients. Management consists of antifailure medications, appropriate antibiotics, and immunosuppression based on the subtype of endocarditis and anticoagulation for APLA syndrome.

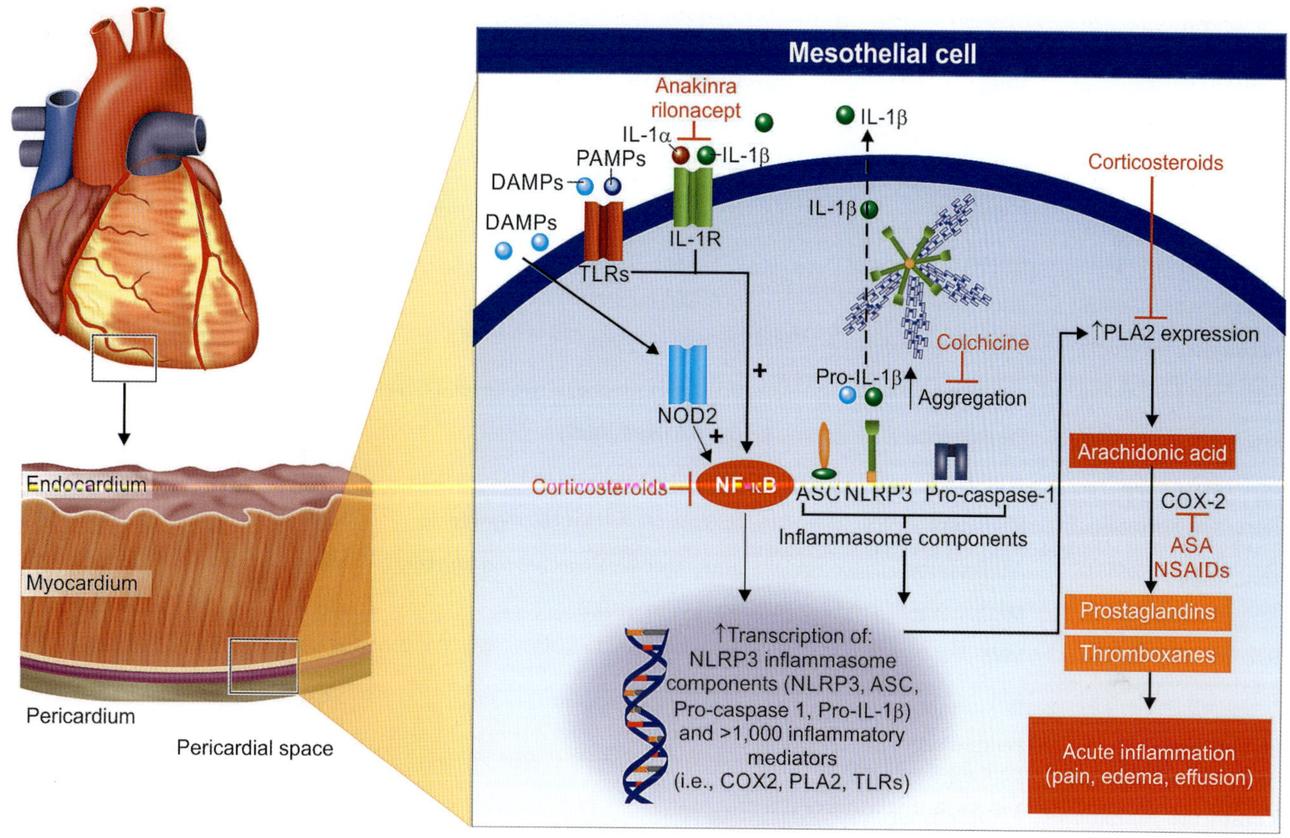

FIG. 4: Pathophysiology of acute pericarditis.

Source: Chiabrando JG, Bonaventura A, Vecchié A, et al. Management of acute and recurrent pericarditis: JACC State-of-the-Art Review. J Am Coll Cardiol. 2020;75(1):76-92.

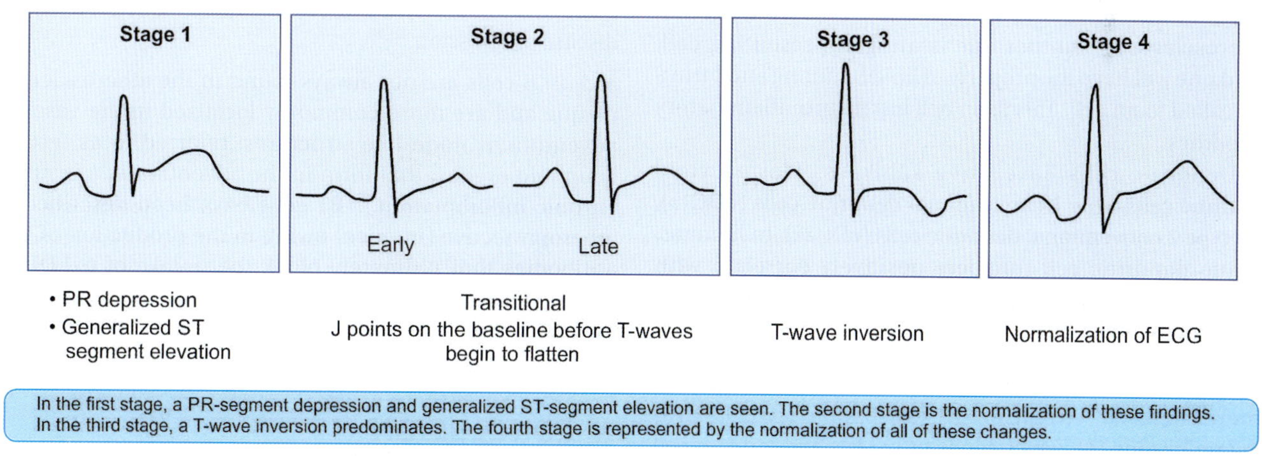

FIG. 5: Electrocardiogram (ECG) changes of pericarditis.

Role of Inflammation in Atherosclerosis

Immune cells involved in atherosclerosis are monocytes, dendritic cells, and macrophages.

Monocytes are divided into classical monocytes (CD14 + CD16–) and nonclassical monocytes (CD14– CD16+). In atherosclerosis, classical monocytes are recruited into the plaque.[11-13]

Increase in classical monocytes into the blood pool is associated with increased severity of atherosclerosis. Moreover, the conventional atherosclerotic risk factors will drive the hematopoietic system toward classical monocyte production.

Macrophages are of three types in human atherosclerotic plaque. One is proinflammatory, which expresses high

TABLE 1: Treatment of pericarditis and their complications.

Stage of pericarditis	Drug	Dose	Duration
Acute pericarditis	Aspirin	750–1,000 mg Q8hrly	1–2 weeks
Acute pericarditis	Ibuprofen	600–800 mg Q8hrly	1–2 weeks
Acute pericarditis	Colchicine	0.5–1.2 mg in one or two divided doses	3 months
Recurrent pericarditis	Aspirin	750–1,000 mg Q8hrly	Weeks–months
Recurrent pericarditis	Ibuprofen	600–800 mg Q8hrly	Weeks–months
Recurrent pericarditis	Indomethacin	25–50 mg Q8hrly	Weeks–months
Recurrent pericarditis	Colchicine	0.5–1.2 mg in one or two divided doses	At least 6 months
Recurrent pericarditis	Prednisolone	0.2–0.5 mg/kg/daily	Months
Recurrent pericarditis	Anakinra	1–2 mg/kg/daily up to 100 mg/daily	Months
Recurrent pericarditis	Rilonacept	320 mg once, then 160 mg weekly	Months
Recurrent pericarditis	Azathioprine	1 mg/kg/daily up to 2–3 mg/kg/daily	Months
Recurrent pericarditis	Methotrexate	10–15 mg weekly	Months
Recurrent pericarditis	MMF	2,000 mg daily	Months
Recurrent pericarditis	IVIg	400–500 mg/kg/day	5 days
Tamponade	Pericardiocentesis pericardial window		
Constrictive pericarditis	Active inflammation	Yes	Anti-inflammatory as first-line/ pericardiectomy for refractory cases
Constrictive pericarditis	Active inflammation	No	Pericardiectomy

levels of IL-1β, a well-recognized immune target in atherosclerosis. Another one is antigen presenting cell. Third one will have the property of lipid handling and form a cell called foam cell. This foam cell has no proinflammatory properties.

Dendritic cells have three subtypes: Plasmacytoid dendritic cells, type 1 conventional dendritic cells (cDC1s), and type 2 conventional dendritic cells (cDC2s). In humans, plaque dendritic cell numbers positively correlate with plaque vulnerability. Dendritic cells express CCL17s that have proatherogenic role.[14-16]

Neutrophils: Neutrophils are involved in all stages of atherosclerosis.[17] Neutrophil extracellular traps (NETs) contain histone H4, which binds to VSMCs and induces cell lysis, resulting in plaque destabilization. Moreover, NETs induce plaque erosion and platelet aggregation, leading to thrombosis **(Fig. 6)**.

T cells are important in atherosclerosis formation and progression. CD4 T-helper cells are proatherogenic and activated CD4 cells promote atherogenesis. Treg cells called regulatory T cells are antiatherogenic and help in disease regression via IL-10 and TGF-β secretion. Immune dysregulation and imbalance in immune activation lead to disease progression.[18-20]

B cells: B cells are not always found in the atherosclerotic plaque and are more commonly localized in the vascular adventitia or node-like structures, referred to as tertiary lymphoid organs, that form in the adventitia as a result of chronic inflammation.[21] B1 cells have been described as atheroprotective (in mice) owing to the production of IgM antibodies that ultimately block the uptake of oxLDL by macrophages in atherosclerotic lesions. By contrast, B2 cells have been shown overall to be proatherogenic **(Table 2** and **Fig. 7)**.

CONCLUSION

Immune-mediated injury is the key pathway in IHD pathogenesis and disease progression. Latest research work has found the role of inflammation in atherosclerosis progression and HF disease progression. Elevated plasma CRP, IL-6, and TNF levels are linked to adverse cardiovascular events. Various immune targets have been under investigation for immune modulation and altering the disease progression. Promising immunotherapies are in the future pipeline.

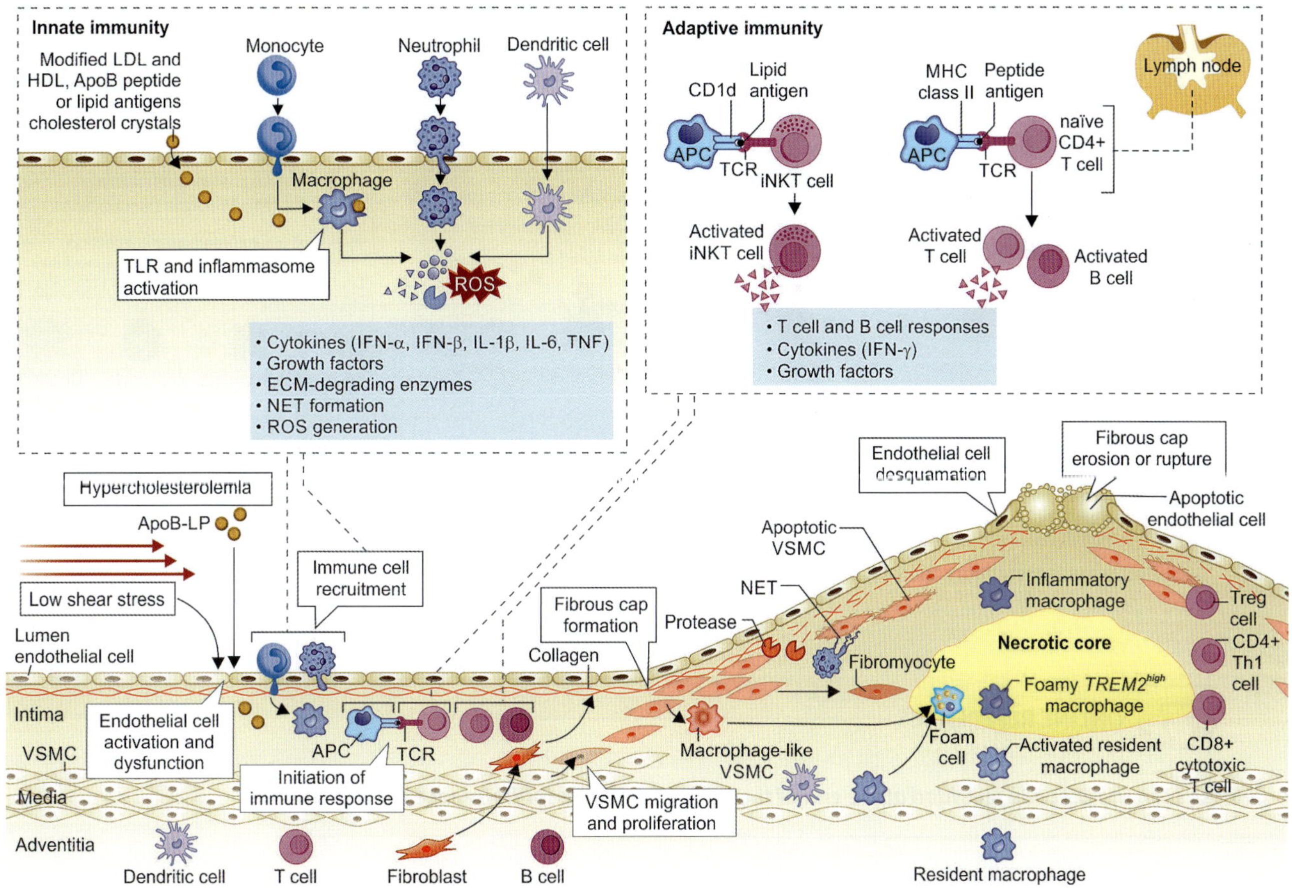

FIG. 6: Role of inflammation in atherosclerosis.[22-24]

TABLE 2: Immunotherapies effective trials in CVD.

Trial (year)	Agent	Drug target	Trial design	Patient cohort	Primary endpoint	Main outcomes
CANTOS (2017)	Canakinumab	Inhibition of IL-1B pathway	Randomized, double-blind, placebo-controlled	10,061 patients with previous MI and elevated plasma CRP levels	Nonfatal MI, nonfatal stroke, or death from cardiovascular causes	The 150 mg dose of canakinumab reduced CV events compared with placebo independent of lipid level interactions
COLCOT (2019)	Colchicine	Broad cellular effects, including inhibition of tubulin polymerization, inhibition of inflamma-some assembly, and IL-1 release	Randomized, double-blind, placebo-controlled	4,475 patients with MI within 30 days before enrolment	Death from CV causes, resuscitated cardiac arrest, MI, stroke, or hospitalization for angina leading to coronary revascularization	Colchicine decreased the risk of the composite endpoint compared with placebo
LoDoCo2 (2020)	Colchicine	Broad cellular effects, including inhibition of tubulin polymerization, inhibition of inflamma-some assembly, and IL-1 release	Randomized, double-blind, placebo-controlled	5,522 patients with chronic coronary artery disease	Death from CV causes, resuscitated cardiac arrest, MI, stroke, or ischemia-driven coronary revascularization	Colchine decreased the risk of the composite endpoint compared with placebo

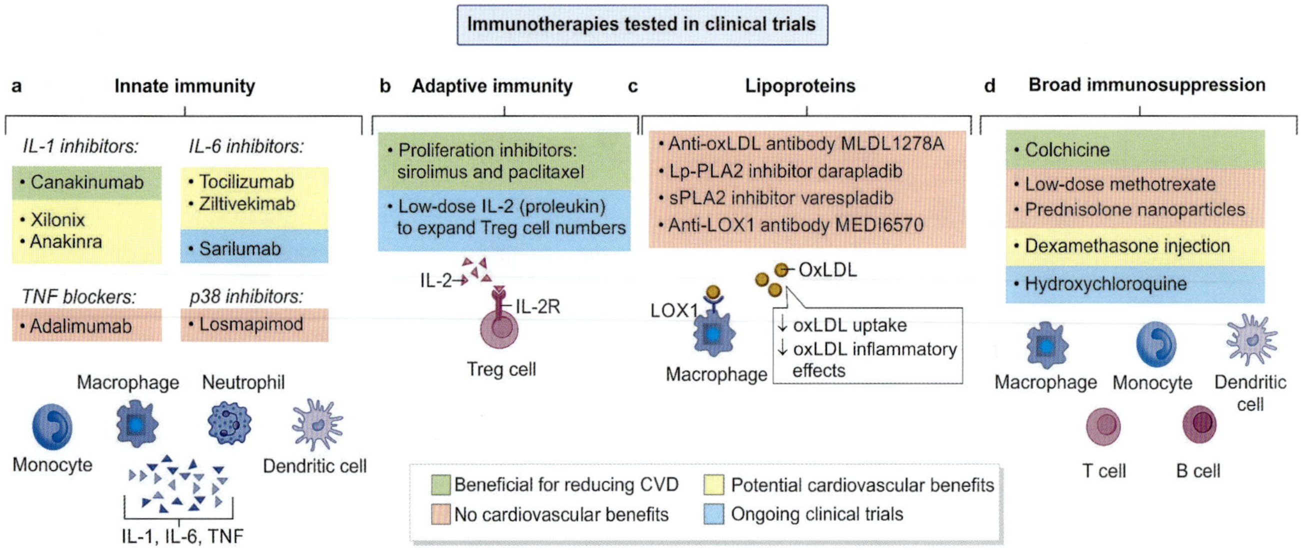

FIG. 7: Immunotherapies tested for atherosclerosis.[16,25-30]

ONLINE REFERENCES

Please scan the QR code provided at the end of the table of contents for References of this chapter.

CHAPTER

224

Geriatric Preventive Cardiology

Aftab Khan, Navanil Biswas, Debayan Sarkar

ABSTRACT

Aging is the most powerful nonmodifiable risk factor for cardiovascular disease (CVD). Older adults with CVD have to contend with various challenges unique to their age group like frailty, multimorbidity, polypharmacy, impairment of cognitive function, and lack of social support. This complicates management and often denies them optimum guideline-based treatment. *Thus, four key domains that must be addressed while dealing with this geriatric population are the (1) medical domain, (2) mind and emotional domain, (3) functional domain, and (4) social domain*. This has been incorporated in five essential principles of geriatric cardiology. Prevention and treatment goals mirror those of the general populace with some special considerations. The *"what matters"* principle is an important construct, providing importance to the priorities of this age group. It is becoming increasingly necessary to integrate fundamental cardiovascular care concepts with relevant geriatric principles to tailor comprehensive patient-centered approaches that will allow us to optimize outcomes in elderly patients.

Keywords: Aging, geriatrics, preventive cardiology, geriatric cardiology

"A man is as old as his arteries".

—Thomas Sydenham

INTRODUCTION

Elderly patients with cardiovascular disease (CVD) have to deal with problems across different health domains. This usually occurs due to age-related physiological changes which negatively impact their cardiovascular health and treatment. Due to advances in healthcare and living standards, coupled with globalization, life expectancy is on the rise, leading to a dramatic increase in the elderly populace. *It is likely that by the year 2034, the number of older adults (aged >65 years) will outnumber the youth (aged < 18 years).*[1] This drastic change in the demographic pattern of the world population will lead to a higher prevalence of both clinical and subclinical CVD. This becomes more important when we realize that age, besides being a non-modifiable risk factor for CVD, is also directly related to a number of important CVD conditions including hypertension, heart failure, coronary artery disease, cerebrovascular disease, peripheral artery disease, valvular disease, and arrhythmia to mention a few.[2] This proves the increasing clinical relevance that geriatric cardiology assumes in the modern world. A systemic approach, combining disciples from various medical fields is the need of the hour, to deal with this challenging clinical subset.

GERIATRIC CARDIOLOGY: WHAT IS IT?

Geriatric cardiology refers to the "merging the management of CVD while focusing on the healthcare of the elderly, thus infusing cardiovascular medicine with geriatric principles in order to provide holistic, individualized, and patient-centered care to older people with or at risk of CVD".[3] *It essentially deals with persons with CVD aged 65 years or above*. Among them, special care is needed to deal with the most vulnerable, *the oldest old, i.e., those above 80 years*. Geriatric cardiology thus is a collaborative and multidisciplinary approach, which combines the expertise of not only cardiologists and geriatricians, but also primary care clinicians, advanced healthcare providers, nurses, pharmacists, dieticians, physiotherapists, and social workers to effectively address and manage the complex needs of this elderly populace.

CHALLENGES IN THE FIELD OF GERIATRIC CARDIOLOGY

Geriatric cardiology is still in its adolescence, when compared to other disciplines of cardiology like pediatric cardiology, heart failure, interventions, and imaging. But like other fields, the challenges to overcome are many and need to be understood and appreciated to effectively prevent the development and progression of CVD in the elderly. Some of these challenges are enumerated here:[1]

- *Research*: There is restricted enrolment of this population in major trials, for both drugs and devices, leading to a paucity of data while dealing with this vulnerable subgroup. There is also a lack of research into *"geroscience"* where the mechanisms of cardiovascular aging still remain to be elucidated.
- *Clinical care*: There is a significant lack of geriatric constructs when it comes to the care of the elderly with CVD. The use of *poly pills, competing drugs prescribed for different comorbidities, and aggressive approach* while dealing with this vulnerable group all negatively impact their cardiovascular health. An "all-size-fits-all" approach does not work in this field where treatment needs to be individualized based on patient profile and healthcare goals.
- *Education*: Paucity of data leads to paucity of knowledge. Increased awareness and education of physicians, pharmacists, and nurses about geriatric principles of care is warranted. Better and wide circulation of elderly focused guidelines will help in this regard.
- *Public policy*: Better reimbursement models and elderly focused insurance policies will help providers in ensuring optimal multidisciplinary patient-centered care to complex elderly patients. Also, ensuring that drugs and devices have been adequately tested in this elderly population and proper notification of unexpected adverse events will allow more mainstream use of them in the elderly.

PHYSIOLOGICAL CHANGES ASSOCIATED WITH AGING

A myriad of physiological changes occur within multiple organ systems with aging. In the cardiovascular system, the changes can be classified into *structural changes* (like atherosclerosis, endothelial dysfunction, increase in vascular stiffness, increase in left ventricular wall thickness, diastolic dysfunction) and *functional changes* (like decreased functional capacity, exercise intolerance, increased risk of heart failure, increased risk of arrhythmia and other conduction disorders).[4] In fact, aging and inflammatory processes are so intimately entwined that they have been together named as *"inflammaging"*.[5] Other aging-related changes that occur in other systems but directly or indirectly affect the cardiovascular system are described in **Figure 1**. Thus, these age-related biological changes coupled with the increasing incidence of complex conditions across multiple organ systems in the aging population make geriatric cardiology, especially preventive geriatric cardiology, not a preferred approach, but a necessary approach.

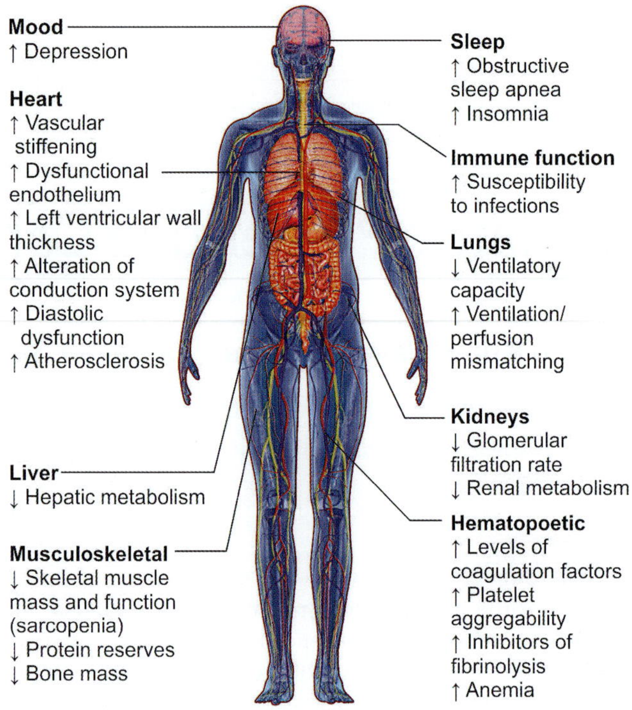

FIG. 1: Age-related changes across different organ systems affecting CV health.

ESSENTIAL PRINCIPLES IN GERIATRIC CARDIOLOGY

After knowing the "what" and the "why", let us come to the "how"? How can we incorporate the principles of geriatric cardiology into the routine care of older adults? What are the principles to apply that will help us to treat this elderly population better, and be useful for both primary and secondary prevention? *This has been lucidly described by Goyal et al.*[1] *and summarized into five essential principles* **(Box 1)**, which are described in the following text.

Recognition and Consideration of the Impact of Multimorbidity

Multimorbidity is Defined as Coexistence of Two or More Chronic Conditions

The prevalence of multimorbidity increases with advancing age because of both age-related changes and the cumulative

BOX 1 Five essential principles of care for the geriatric population.

1. Recognition and consideration of the impact of multimorbidity
2. Evaluation and integration of cognition into the decision-making process
3. Evaluation of integration of the three physical functioning domains into management
4. Incorporation of socioenvironmental factors while considering management decisions
5. Ensuring that the care plan is aligned with the patient's priorities and health goals

effects of CVD and other diseases. For treating such adults with multimorbidity, *it is important to consider the overall treatment burden, life expectancy, and the risk of death from both CVD and non-CVD conditions.* Also, as the severity and the number of these disease conditions increase, management plans of these complex disease states lead to increased burden for both the patient and his family, ultimately impairing quality of life.

Polypharmacy is defined as taking at least five medications and is another serious and common problem afflicting elderly persons. *A recent study observed that >50% of elderly hospitalized for heart failure had been prescribed 10 or more medications at discharge.*[6] That is a seriously high pill burden. The combined effects of multimorbidity, polypharmacy, and age-related degenerative changes, especially involving the renal and the hepatic systems that influence both pharmacokinetics and pharmacodynamics, put the elderly population at a very-high-risk of adverse drug reactions. More significantly, with an increasing number of chronic conditions and their medications, there remains a high chance of *"therapeutic competition"* whereby a drug prescribed for one condition may adversely affect and exacerbate another condition.

Managing polypharmacy is essential, and to do this is by ensuring effective and safe prescribing and deprescribing. Medications in this age group should only be prescribed when they demonstrate a favorable risk-benefit outcome and are aligned with the patient's health goals. *Tools that have been developed to help us in this regard are the Beers criteria (for drugs of concern) and the STOPP/START (Screening Tool of Older Persons' Prescriptions/Screening Tool to Alert to Right Treatment) criterion.*[7]

Evaluation and Integration of Cognition into Decision-making Process

Aging results in various anatomical and functional changes in the brain, leading to worsened cognition and subsequent dementia. *This might lead to limitations in self-care behavior and may even be misconstrued as noncompliance, even though the lack of engagement was unintentional and not by choice.* Cognitive impairment, depending on its severity, is related to reduced life expectancy. *The tools available for screening for dementia are the Mini-Cog and the AD8,* which can be applied in just 3 minutes.

The *Patient Health Questionnaire and the Geriatric Depression Scale* are the validated tools for screening for *depression*, another CVD risk factor, that increases with age and affects both quality of life and cardiovascular health. *Delirium*, a common problem in old age, especially in hospitalized patients, can be screened via the validated *"Confusion Assessment Method"*. *Referral for evaluation of these neuro-cognitive functions and their effective management, both behavioral and pharmacological, have shown to have positive outcomes in treating elderly with CVD.*[8]

Evaluation of Integration of the Three Physical Functioning Domains into Management

Physical function affecting cardiovascular health can be adequately represented by three domains—disability, frailty, and falls. *Disability* can be assessed by *the ability to perform activities of daily living (ADLs). This has been defined by Katz,*[9] *as including bathing, toileting, continence, feeding, transferring, and dressing.* Inability to perform even one ADL has been shown to be associated with almost halving of life expectancy, as well as decreased independence and reduced quality of life.

Frailty is defined as *"a clinical syndrome of increased vulnerability resulting from age-associated declines in reserve and function across multiple physiological systems such that the ability to cope with everyday acute stress is compromised"*.[10] Frailty has been observed to affect up to half of the adults with coronary artery disease, heart failure, and severe aortic stenosis. It has also been demonstrated that a bi-directional association exists between frailty and CVD, where frailty can lead to CVD and CVD can lead to frailty. *Frailty can be assessed and graded by the FRAIL (Fatigue, Resistance, Ambulation, Illness, Loss of weight) Scale, Frailty Index, Timed Up and Go test, and the Short Physical Performance Battery (SPPB) test.*

Falls is another important factor affecting CV health in the elderly. A number of factors can be responsible for falls including hypotension, reduced autonomic reflex, decreased baroreceptor sensitivity, impaired fluid hemostasis, electrolyte imbalance, hearing and vision impairment, neurological disorders, and cognitive dysfunction. *For assessment, a one-question inquiry of any history of falls in the past 6 months is often adequate. Other screening tools include the John Hopkins Fall Risk Assessment Tool, Hendrich II Fall Risk Model, and Fall Risk Questionnaire.*

Referral of these patients to tailored exercise programs has been seen to increase strength, balance, and aerobic endurance resulting in improvement in ADLs and reduction in frailty and falls. Thus, physical rehabilitation therapy has been proven to improve all three physical domains.[11]

Incorporation of Socioenvironmental Factors while Considering Management Decisions

Social isolation and loneliness are two important social constructs plaguing this age group. *Social isolation* can be defined as the physical lack of social support, while *loneliness* is defined as the emotional perception associated with the absence of intimate connections. The death of a spouse or a loved one results in a decline in social interactions ultimately leading to lower life satisfaction, a sense of belonging, and a reduction in self-esteem. Retirement and the resultant reduction in income coupled with the limited availability of health insurance for the elderly also becomes a barrier to their appropriate and optimum treatment.

Various services required by older adults like vision and hearing aids, dental needs, and the costs of long-term hospitalizations or stay at care homes are expensive and require significant out-of-pocket expenditure. Clinicians involved in treating the elderly must be aware of such social vulnerabilities. *Inquiring about social support and using tools like the UCLAS Loneliness Scale should be applied to all elderly patients.* Development of novel technologies, such as *remote monitoring or teleconsultation, referred to as "gerontechnology"*, will significantly reduce transportation problems and allow better care for these vulnerable populace.[12]

Ensuring that the Care Plan is Aligned with the Patient Priorities and Health Goals

One of the most important concepts in geriatric cardiology is the *"what matters" concept.* This concept is essential for clinicians to address effectively the complexities of managing CVD in order to increase the likelihood of assisting the patients to achieve their care goals with the help of shared decision-making. *It refers to aligning the treatment plan with the patient's individual healthcare goals.* This is especially important, as such patients receive care from multiple clinicians, leading to different treatment strategies that might compete with one another, and even deviate from what the patient actually desires. For example, the logistical challenges of repeated commuting to and from medical appointments may come at the cost of spending time with their loved ones, likewise, paying for their poly-medications might even come at the cost of other basic necessities like food and clothing. Though most interventions both prolong life and improve its quality, some can only achieve one at the expense of the other.

It is also important to recognize that a patient's healthcare goals might change with time depending on their social and economic environment at that time. *The Patient Priorities Care Toolkit is a recently developed resource that can assist clinicians in assessing and addressing "what matters" to the patient and tailor treatment to the patient's healthcare goals.*[13] This signals a shift from a disease-centric approach to a more holistic patient-centered approach to deal with the complex management of the elderly with CVD.

DISCUSSIONS ON A FEW CLASSICAL CARDIOVASCULAR RISK FACTORS IN ELDERLY PATIENTS

According to the latest ESC guidelines for Cardiovascular prevention,[14] a new and modified scoring system, *the SCORE2-OP (Systematic Coronary Risk Evaluation-Older Persons)*, has been proposed for classifying the cardiovascular risk in those >70 years. This is a landmark shift in the management of such people as it signifies a dedicated risk score for the elderly, instead of just extrapolating data from the general population. *Accordingly, this risk score reclassifies older patients as being at very-high-risk (>15%), high risk (7.5–15%), and low-to-moderate risk (<7.5%) of CV death as well as nonfatal CV events at 5–10 years separately.* Recommendations have also been made on controlling the common classical CVRF, some of which are briefly described in the following text.

Dyslipidemia

Cardiovascular risk recommendations in this regard *mirror the general population with a goal of >50% reduction in LDL-C levels to reach <55 mg/dL in very-high-risk and <70 mg/dL in high-risk elderly people.* Regarding pharmacotherapy, statins are the first choice followed by ezetimibe and PCSK9. Special considerations regarding statin-induced myopathy must be kept in mind while prescribing these drugs to such patients.

Hypertension

Treating hypertension in this cohort is complex, *as usually hypertension is more severe, more resistant to treatment, and carries a higher risk of postural hypotension.* The *SPRINT trial*[15] (Systolic Blood Pressure Intervention Trial), which included a subgroup of elderly patients (>75 years), showed that more intensive treatment was associated with reductions in CV morbidity and mortality.

Accordingly, the recommended cutoff to initiate blood pressure treatment is >140 mm Hg in those > 75 years and >160 mm Hg in those >80 years. The ideal treatment goal should be 130–139 mm Hg and not below 130/70 mm Hg due to the possible deleterious effect of the J-curve of hypertension. Some more recommendations are outlined in **Box 2**.[16]

Diabetes

Like hypertension, the adverse effects of hypoglycemia should be kept in mind while prescribing drugs in this populace. Also, the presence of comorbidities and frailty should guide the physician in selecting lenient treatment targets. *SGLT-2 inhibitors and GLP-1 agonists have been proven to have CV benefits and should be the first line treatment.* Diabetic control recommendations are summarized in **Box 3**.[17]

Obesity and Diet

Weight loss in elderly patients is important, as it leads to improved quality of life, functional capacity, and long-term prognosis. Personalizing diet recommendations, tailoring caloric intake to a patient's activity and energy expenditure, and keeping in mind the risks of sarcopenia and malnutrition in frail patients are required. The target body mass index in patients > 60 years of age may be >25.

BOX 2 Recommendations regarding treatment of hypertension in the elderly.

- Monotherapy is recommended in patients >80 years or frail patients
- Drugs should be started at lower doses and uptitrated according to BP
- Postural hypotension should be avoided
- ACE inhibitor (angiotensin-converting enzyme inhibitor) are the drugs of choice
- Caution of use and if possible avoidance of diuretics and alpha-blockers due to their side effects
- Monitoring of renal function, especially after initiation of RAAS inhibitors
- Frequent monitoring, to increase tolerance, adherence to treatment, and reduction in adverse events

BOX 3 Recommendations regarding treating diabetes in the elderly.

- Treatment should be tailored to the individual based on frailty, comorbidities, CV risk, and renal function
- Drugs like SGLT-2i and GLP-RA with proven cardiovascular benefits should be preferred
- Severe hyperglycemia should be avoided, as it might lead to life-threatening complications
- Insulin regimens should be simplified to reduce the risk of hypoglycemia
- It is to be noted that hypoglycemia might occur even in the presence of high HbA1c
- Screening for diabetes-related microvascular and macro-vascular complications should constitute an essential part
- Less stringent diabetic targets (HbA1c < 8) might be considered in the very elderly and frail patients

TABLE 1: Recommendations for physical exercise in the elderly.

Type	Intensity	Frequency	Duration
Aerobic/Endurance	Moderate	>5 days/week	>30 minutes/ session
Strength/Force	Moderate	2 days/week	1–2 sets
Flexibility/Balance	Moderate	>5 days/week	>10 minutes/ session

Physical Exercise

Physical exercise is not a risk factor per se, but an important adjunct in the treatment and prevention of CVD. In the normal population, physical exercise has been shown to reduce CV morbidity and mortality and also improve the quality of life in elderly patients. *Structured physical exercise and cardiac rehabilitation have been given a Class IA recommendation in all CVD patients.*[14] Other benefits of exercise include reduction in the prevalence of anxiety, depression, obesity, osteoporosis, and cancer, counteracting functional limitation, improving pain control, increasing muscle power, leading to reduction in the risk of falls, and allowing improved functional independence. In fact, it is one of the pillars of promoting the reversal of frailty in nonagenarians in its initial stages.

The Borg scale or adapted scales may be used to tailor exercise regimens based on individual baseline functional capacity, frailty, comorbidities, and treatments received. The recommended exercise modalities in the elderly populace are summarized in **Table 1**.[18]

CONCLUSION

Prevention and management of CVD in the elderly is a complex and multidisciplinary effort, which comes with its own set of obstacles and challenges. Keeping the five essential principles in mind while treating such patients will go a long way in providing optimum and all-comprehensive holistic, patient-centered individualistic care to these vulnerable groups of patients. Though recent times have seen substantiative advances being made in the field of geriatric cardiology, much still remains to be done in the realms of research, education, clinical care, and health policy.

ONLINE REFERENCES

Please scan the QR code provided at the end of the table of contents for References of this chapter.

CHAPTER

225

Vegetarian and Vegan Diets: Benefits and Drawbacks

Asha Moorthy, Supraja Moorthy, Prashant Moorthy

ABSTRACT

Plant-based diets have gained considerable attention due to their health benefits and environmental impact, characterized by the exclusion of meat and the potential omission of other animal products such as dairy and eggs. These diets focus on plant-based foods such as leafy greens, vegetables, mushrooms, grains, legumes, fruits, and nuts. The diets are classified into veganism, lacto-ovo vegetarianism, pescetarianism, and flexitarianism, each differing in the inclusion of animal-derived products.

Health benefits associated with plant-based diets are well documented, including reduced risks of obesity, type 2 diabetes mellitus, coronary heart disease, and other noncommunicable diseases. These benefits are attributed to the high intake of dietary fibers, antioxidants, phytochemicals, and omega-3 fatty acids found abundantly in plant foods. Plant-based diets positively impact cardiometabolic risk factors by lowering LDL cholesterol, improving glucose metabolism, and supporting healthy body weight.

However, concerns persist regarding potential nutritional deficiencies in strict vegan diets, especially for omega-3 fatty acids, vitamin B12, calcium, iron, and zinc. Addressing these concerns requires careful dietary planning, supplementation, and consumption of fortified foods to ensure adequate nutrient intake.

In conclusion, plant-based diets offer substantial health advantages, particularly in reducing cardiovascular risk factors and promoting overall well-being.

Keywords: Vegetarian, vegan, cardiovascular disease, coronary heart disease, cardiometabolic risk factors, nutrient deficiency

INTRODUCTION

Plant-based diets have become increasingly popular for their beneficial effects on human health and the environment.[1] These diets commonly eliminate all types of meat, including fish, and may additionally exclude other animal-derived products such as eggs and dairy. These diets primarily consist of plant-based foods, such as leafy greens, root vegetables, mushrooms, grains, legumes, fruits, and nuts.[2]

Plant-based diets are mainly classified as vegan, lacto-vegetarian, lacto-ovo vegetarian, and ovo-vegetarian.[2] Other plant-based diets, such as semi-vegetarian, pescetarian, and flexitarian, vary in their consumption levels of meat and/or fish and can be classified as distinct types within the broader spectrum of plant-based diets.[2-4] All vegetarian diets (VDs) prohibit the consumption of meat, including chicken, pork, lamb, beef, venison, and other related meat products.[5] The different types of VDs based on the inclusion of animal products or dairy intake have been given in **Table 1**.

Plant-based diets generally provide health benefits. The Academy of Nutrition and Dietetics recognizes that a balanced VD is nutritionally adequate and supports human growth and development.[6] VDs have been linked to reduced risks of various health conditions such as obesity, type 2 diabetes mellitus (T2DM), coronary heart disease (CHD), and other noncommunicable diseases (NCDs).[6] This recommendation aligns with existing evidence suggesting that decreasing the consumption of red meat and processed meat may lower the risk of several NCDs.[3] Moreover, the health effects of plant-based foods vary considerably.[5] VDs that incorporate hydrogenated oils, high-fructose corn syrup, artificial sweeteners, sucrose,

TABLE 1: Categorization of different types of plant-based diets.

Diet type	Meat	Dairy	Fish	Eggs	Honey
Vegan[2,3]	×	×	×	×	×
Lacto-vegetarian[2-4]	×	✓	×	×	✓
Lacto-ovo vegetarian[2-4]	×	✓	×	✓	✓
Ovo-vegetarian[2-4]	×	×	×	✓	✓
Pesco-vegetarian/ Pescatarian[2-4]	×	×	✓	×	✓
Semi-vegetarian (flexitarian)[2,3]	✓	✓	✓	✓	✓

refined flour, salt, and preservatives have been linked to increased risk of morbidity and mortality.[5] Plant-based diets, such as vegan diets, may result in possible deficiencies in crucial micronutrients such as iron and vitamin B12.[3]

Cardiovascular diseases (CVDs) such as CHD, stroke, and peripheral vascular disease are the most common NCDs globally. The root cause of CVD is atherosclerosis. Atherosclerosis progression can be slowed down by managing the risk factors, thereby reducing CVD risk. The key risk factors include high blood pressure (BP), dyslipidemia, obesity, T2DM, and behavioral factors such as unhealthy diet, smoking, and lack of physical activity.[7]

The importance of a balanced diet in preventing CVD is widely acknowledged. Research indicates that consuming certain nutrients and some types of food, or following a specific diet can effectively contribute to CVD prevention.[7]

This chapter summarizes the effects of vegetarian and vegan diets on CVD, its risk factors, and associated clinical outcomes. Thus, it highlights the overall beneficial effects of these diets in promoting cardiovascular (CV) health.

BENEFITS OF VEGETARIAN AND VEGAN DIETS FOR CARDIOVASCULAR HEALTH

The VD offers a wide array of beneficial components such as fiber, phytosterols, flavonoids, carotenoids, various other phytochemicals, antioxidants, and omega-3 fatty acids.[4] Vegetarian or vegan diets, when carefully planned and balanced, have distinct mechanisms that could potentially decrease the likelihood of CHD.[5]

Effect on Cardiometabolic Risk Factors

Lipid-lowering Effect and Cardiovascular Diseases Risk

There is a clear understanding that the quality, rather than the quantity, of dietary fats significantly influences dyslipidemia and CVD management. Saturated fatty acids (SAFA) are prevalent in animal-derived fats such as butter, fatty meats, full-fat dairy, palm oil, and coconut oil. Conversely, plant-based fats such as vegetable oils are rich in unsaturated fatty acids, including monounsaturated fatty acids (MUFA) such as oleic acid and polyunsaturated fatty acids (PUFA).[7] Substituting SAFA with unsaturated fatty acids in the diet reduces low-density lipoprotein cholesterol (LDL-C) levels without impacting high-density lipoprotein cholesterol (HDL-C) and triglycerides (TGs). The reduction in LDL-C levels is more pronounced when SAFA is substituted with PUFA compared to MUFA.[7] Substituting 5% of energy intake from SAFA with an equivalent amount from PUFA, MUFA, or carbohydrates from whole grains has been linked to a 25%, 15%, and 9% reduced risk of CHD, respectively.[5]

Dietary fibers and phytosterols decrease the absorption of cholesterol and bile acids in the small intestine, leading to greater uptake of LDL by the liver.[5] Seeds and nuts are rich sources of PUFA, soluble and insoluble fibers, and sterols, which are recognized for their cholesterol-lowering properties.[5]

Evidence from randomized clinical trials (RCTs) supports that incorporating a diet abundant in nuts, dietary fibers, and margarine enriched with plant sterol esters can lower plasma LDL-C by 13%.[5] Furthermore, increasing daily dietary fiber intake by an additional 7–10 g/day was associated with a 9% decrease in CVD mortality and a 9–11% decrease in CHD mortality.[7] Observational studies have also demonstrated that increased consumption of dietary fiber and diets rich in fiber not only reduces the risk of CVD but also T2DM and obesity, both of which are risk factors for CVD.[7]

For individuals adhering to vegetarian or vegan diets, the phytosterol intake can rise by as much as 600 mg/day. In a meta-analysis including 124 clinical studies, it was found that the intake of phytosterol significantly reduces LDL-C levels from 6 to 12% when consuming 0.6–3.3 g/day, while having no impact on HDL-C levels.[7] Another meta-analysis indicated that phytosterols decrease atherogenic apolipoproteins, such as Apo-B and Apo-E, while increasing antiatherogenic apolipoproteins, such as Apo-AI and Apo-CII.[7]

Phytosterols have shown efficacy in reducing LDL-C levels in both healthy individuals and those with various health conditions, including familial hypercholesterolemia, T2DM, and metabolic syndrome.[7] Consuming 2 g/day of phytosterols reduces absorption of cholesterol by 30–40%, resulting in a subsequent 10% decrease in circulating LDL-C levels.[7]

Studies have indicated a significant decrease in TG levels linked to phytosterol intake, particularly evident in individuals with higher baseline TG concentrations.[7]

The benefits of different dietary components on lipid profile have been summarized in **Figure 1**.

Lower Blood Pressure and Cardiovascular Diseases Risk

Observational studies suggest that individuals on vegetarian and vegan diets generally have lower BP levels compared to those who follow Western diets. Vegetarians have been

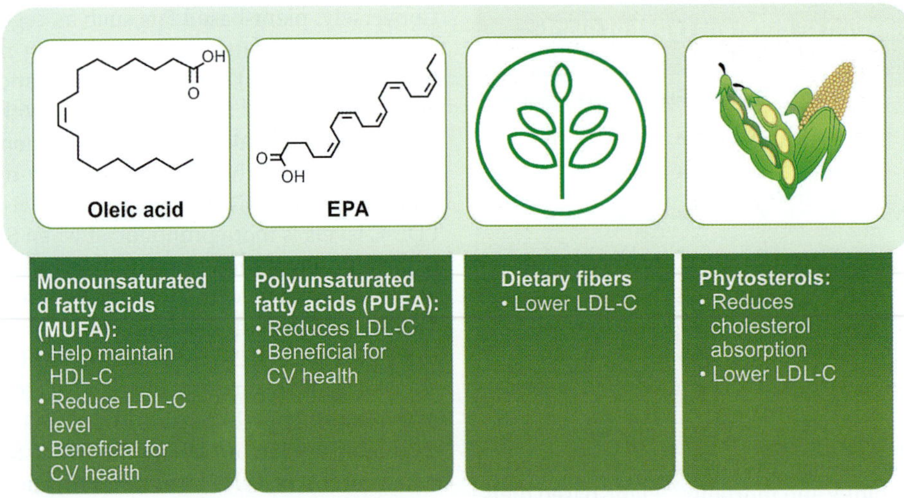

FIG. 1: Dietary components and their effect on lipid profile.
(LDL-C: low-density lipoprotein cholesterol; HDL-C: high-density lipoprotein cholesterol; CV: cardiovascular)

reported to have lower BP and a decreased prevalence of hypertension compared to omnivores, regardless of their body weight and sodium intake. Evidence from multiple observational studies suggests that consuming red meat and poultry is linked to a higher risk of hypertension, irrespective of intake levels of vegetables, whole grains, and fruits.[5]

Glucose-lowering Effects

High-fiber diets cause stomach expansion, slow down stomach emptying, and help stabilize blood sugar levels after meals. Short-chain fatty acids, produced on the breakdown of oligosaccharides and starch found in minimally processed plant foods, promote satiety by slowing down stomach emptying through incretins such as peptide-YY and glucagon-like peptide-1. Clinical trials demonstrate that these mechanisms result in reduced body weight and blood glucose levels.[5]

Diets based on whole-food vegan and vegetarian principles could lead to a decrease in bioavailable calories. Implementing calorie restriction while ensuring adequate nutrition has been widely recognized for its substantial improvement in glucose tolerance, insulin sensitivity, and other cardiometabolic outcomes in human subjects.[5]

Healthy, minimally processed VDs offer multiple benefits that contribute to improved insulin sensitivity and lowered blood glucose levels. These diets achieve these effects through several mechanisms. Firstly, they have a low glycemic index/load, which helps to stabilize blood sugar levels after meals. Additionally, they typically contain lower amounts of protein, specifically sulfur and branched-chain amino acids. These branched-chain amino acids are associated with an increased risk of developing prediabetes and T2DM. So, a diet lower in proteins like these amino acids would reduce the risk of T2DM.[5]

Anti-inflammatory Effects

Extensive prospective studies indicate that diets with higher inflammation potential are significantly associated with increased systemic and vascular inflammation, less favorable lipid profiles, and ultimately higher rates of CHD and stroke. Conversely, diets that have lower inflammatory potential include foods rich in dietary antioxidants.[5]

Vegetarian diets rich in legumes, seeds, nuts, vegetables, whole grains, and fruits are abundant sources of antioxidants. These antioxidants include vitamins such as vitamins C and E; beta-carotene; plant compounds, including tannins, phenols, alkaloids, and flavonoids; and minerals such as selenium. Increased intake of dietary antioxidants might reduce the likelihood of atherosclerotic plaques by promoting adaptive changes in enzymes and receptors involved in stress response. These changes help prevent lipoprotein oxidation, endothelial dysfunction, and immune system activation.[5]

EVIDENCE ON BENEFICIAL EFFECTS OF VEGETARIAN AND VEGAN DIETS

Based on the evidence, there are no RCTs specifically evaluating the effect of VDs on the incidence of CHD events.[5]

Effect of Vegetarian and Vegan Diets on Cardiometabolic Parameters

Numerous RCTs have investigated the impacts of various types of VDs on cardiometabolic risk factors.[5]

Recent evidence indicates that both Mediterranean and vegan diets are linked to weight loss and improvement in cardiometabolic risk factors. However, until recently, there had been no randomized trials comparing their relative effectiveness. In a recent study by Barnard et al., a low-fat vegan diet resulted in improved insulin sensitivity, body weight, and lipid levels compared to baseline and a Mediterranean diet. BP decreased on both diets, with a slightly greater reduction observed on the Mediterranean diet **(Table 2)**.[8]

Recent findings suggest that a vegan diet may provide CV benefits compared to an omnivorous diet by improving overall diet quality. Landry et al. demonstrated through an RCT that adopting a healthy vegan diet resulted in superior improvements in cardiometabolic outcomes compared to a healthy omnivorous diet **(Table 2)**.[9]

Koch et al. assessed the effect of vegetarian and vegan diets on total cholesterol, LDL-C, TGs, and Apo-B levels. Both diets were linked to a reduction in total cholesterol, LDL-C, and Apo-B levels **(Table 2)**. These effects were consistent across different types of studies and characteristics of participants. Hence, plant-based diets can decrease the accumulation of atherogenic lipoproteins, potentially reducing the risk of CVD.[10]

In another study by Crosby et al., participants on a low-fat vegan diet raised their consumption of plant-based foods while reducing the intake of animal products, nuts, seeds, and added fats in comparison to their usual diets. Higher legume intake was strongly correlated with weight loss. The AHEI-2010 score, which indicated the quality of the diet, improved on the low-fat vegan diet, indicating improved weight management and metabolic health outcomes **(Table 2)**. This indicates that consuming low-fat plant-based foods and reducing consumption of high-fat and animal-based foods can effectively lead to weight reduction and enhance overall diet quality and metabolic health.[11]

Argyridou et al. also demonstrated that adopting a vegan diet is a beneficial approach for enhancing glucose tolerance and lowering plasma TMAO levels in individuals with dysglycemia or obesity **(Table 2)**.[12]

In their randomized crossover study, Djekic et al. investigated the impact of a VD compared to an isocaloric meat diet (MD) on individuals diagnosed with ischemic heart disease (IHD) who were receiving optimal medical treatment. Over 4 weeks, participants following the VD experienced notable reductions in oxidized LDL-C, LDL-C, total cholesterol, and body mass index compared to those on the MD **(Table 2)**. These improvements in cardiometabolic risk factors were attributed to changes in the composition of gut microbiota, specifically with increased levels of genera from families such as Ruminococcaceae and Barnesiellaceae among VD participants. Moreover, people following the VD had lower amounts of specific gut bacteria and plasma metabolites related to metabolic disorders such as CVD. At the same time, they showed higher levels of gut bacteria and blood substances associated with reduced risks of heart and metabolic problems compared to those following the MD.[13,14]

Effect of Vegetarian and Vegan Diets on Inflammatory Markers

Emerging evidence indicates that low-grade inflammation is associated with an elevated risk of developing various chronic diseases. Increased levels of inflammatory markers such as high-sensitivity C-reactive protein (hs-CRP), tumor necrosis factor-alpha (TNF-α), and interleukin 6 (IL-6) have been linked to the pathogenesis of numerous chronic conditions including T2DM and CVD.[15]

Adopting vegetarian or vegan diets may mitigate inflammatory processes and reduce circulating levels of inflammatory biomarkers. These dietary choices offer anti-inflammatory properties that could potentially lower the risk of chronic diseases involving inflammation.[15]

Craddock et al. indicated that adopting vegetarian dietary patterns correlated with reduced levels of serum CRP, fibrinogen, and total leukocytes **(Table 3)**. However, future investigations should prioritize large-scale trials to explore disparities in inflammation and immune function between vegetarian and nonvegetarian populations.[16] Similarly, Menzel et al. also reported significant associations between reduced CRP levels and vegan or VDs **(Table 3)**. However, their study also mentioned that additional research is warranted, given that most inflammatory biomarkers have only been studied in isolated instances so far.[15]

DRAWBACKS OF VEGETARIAN AND VEGAN DIETS

A well-planned VD can fulfill all nutritional requirements. However, the interpretation of vegetarianism varies, and deficiencies in nutrients may occur depending on the variety and amount of food consumed. Nutrient deficiencies that may arise due to a VD, particularly a vegan diet, include omega-3 fatty acids; minerals such as iron, calcium, and zinc; vitamins D and B12; and protein.

Protein

Concerns about protein deficiency in vegetarians persist, but adequate protein intake (0.8 g/kg body weight per day) can be achieved through a solely plant-based diet. However, it is crucial to conduct a thorough nutritional assessment to ensure sufficient consumption of essential amino acids. For example, diets rich in cereals, nuts, and corn but lacking in legumes may lead to a deficiency in lysine, which can be easily addressed by increasing the intake of beans, peas, or lentils.[4]

Vitamin B12

Vitamin B12 plays a vital role in human health by supporting DNA synthesis, myelin production, hemoglobin formation,

TABLE 2: Studies supporting the beneficial effects of vegetarian and vegan diets on cardiometabolic parameters.

Author	Participants	Design	Methods	Main outcomes
Barnard et al.[8]	62 overweight adults	Randomized crossover trial	• Compared Mediterranean versus vegan diets for 16 weeks each with a 4-week washout • *Measured*: Body weight, plasma lipids, blood pressure, body composition, insulin sensitivity	• *Vegan diet*: ○ Significant weight loss (6.0 kg; $p < 0.001$) ○ Insulin sensitivity (OGIS +35.8 mL/min/m^2; $p = 0.003$) ○ Reduced total cholesterol (−18.7 mg/dL; $p = 0.001$) ○ LDL-C (−15.3 mg/dL; $p = 0.001$) • *Mediterranean diet*: No significant weight loss; slight reduction in blood pressure
Landry et al.[9]	44 twins (22 pairs)	Population-based randomized clinical trial	• Compared vegan versus omnivorous diets for 8 weeks. Provided meals initially; participants prepared their meals later • *Measured*: LDL-C, cardiometabolic factors (fasting insulin, body weight, plasma lipids, and glucose), TMAO, and vitamin B12	• *Vegan diet (mean change)*: ○ Reduced LDL-C: −13.9 mg/dL ($p = 0.02$) ○ Insulin: −2.9 μIU/mL ($p = 0.03$) ○ Body weight: −1.9 kg ($p = 0.01$) ○ No significant changes in other cardiometabolic parameters, TMAO, and vitamin B12 • *Omnivorous diet*: No significant changes
Koch et al.[10]		Meta-analysis	• Analyzed 30 trials comparing vegetarian/vegan versus omnivorous diets on blood lipids	• *Plant-based diets (mean difference)*: ○ Reduced total cholesterol: −0.34 mmol/L ($p = 1 \times 10^{-9}$) ○ LDL-C: −0.30 mmol/L ($p = 4 \times 10^{-8}$) ○ Apo lipoprotein B: −12.92 mg/dL ($p = 0.01$)
Crosby et al.[11]	219 healthy adults	Randomized clinical trial	• Assessed changes in food groups, nutrient intake, and diet quality (AHEI-2010) on a low-fat vegan diet versus control (usual diet) • Measured: Food group intake, nutrient intake, AHEI-2010, body weight, body composition, insulin sensitivity	• In the vegan group, body weight, fat mass, and visceral fat volume decreased, unlike in the control group • *Treatment effects of vegan diet*: ○ Body weight: −5.9 kg ($p < 0.001$) ○ Fat mass: −4.1 kg ($p < 0.001$) ○ Visceral fat volume: −238.3 cm^3 ($p < 0.001$) ○ Insulin resistance (HOMA-IR) decreased (treatment effect: −1.2; $p = 0.008$) ○ Insulin sensitivity improved significantly (treatment effect: +0.87; $p < 0.001$) following the vegan diet • *Strong correlation between weight loss and the following*: ○ Increased intake of legumes ($r = -0.38$; $p < 0.0001$) ○ Decreased intake of total meat, fish, and poultry ($r = +0.43$; $p < 0.0001$) ○ AHEI-2010 score ○ Increased by 6.0 points in the intervention group ($p < 0.001$) ○ No significant change in the control group

Continued

Continued

Author	Participants	Design	Methods	Main outcomes
				• *Correlation of AHEI-2010 scores with weight and insulin sensitivity*: ○ An increase in AHEI-2010 score correlated with lower body weight ($r = +0.14$; $p = 0.04$) ○ Higher AHEI-2010 score associated with reduced fat mass ($r = -0.14$; $p = 0.03$) ○ Improved insulin resistance (HOMA-IR) linked to an increase in the AHEI-2010 score ($r = -0.17$; $p = 0.02$)
Argyridou et al.[12]	23 participants	Interventional prospective trial	• Examined effects of an 8-week vegan diet on glucose tolerance and plasma TMAO levels in individuals with dysglycemia/obesity	*Vegan diet*: • Reduced plasma TMAO levels (week 1: 5.66 µmol/L, week 8: 6.38 µmol/L) • Improved glucose tolerance (week 1: 7.14 mmol/L, week 8: 7.34 mmol/L)
Djekic et al.[13]	Subjects with ischemic heart disease	Randomized crossover trial	• Compared isocaloric vegan versus meat diets for 4-week periods with washout • Measured: Oxidized LDL-C, total cholesterol, LDL-C, body weight, BMI, blood pressure	*Vegan diet*: Lower the levels of the following— • Oxidized LDL-C (−2.73 U/L; $p = 0.02$) • Total cholesterol (−5.03 mg/dL; $p = 0.01$) • LDL-C (−3.87 mg/dL; $p = 0.02$) • Body weight (−0.67 kg; $p = 0.003$) • BMI (−0.21 kg/m^2; $p = 0.009$) • No significant differences in other parameters

(AHEI-2010: Alternative Healthy Eating Index 2010; BMI: body mass index; LDL-C: low-density lipoprotein cholesterol; TMAO: trimethylamine N-oxide)

TABLE 3: Studies supporting beneficial effects of vegetarian and vegan diets on inflammatory biomarkers.

Author	Study design	Population	Methods	Main outcomes
Menzel et al.[15]	Systematic review and meta-analysis	General population, patients with impaired kidney function	• Conducted literature search in PubMed and EMBASE up to April 2020 • Included 21 cross-sectional studies • Assessed mean differences in various inflammatory biomarkers between vegans, vegetarians, and omnivores	• A vegan diet significantly lowers CRP levels compared to omnivorous diets (MD −0.54 mg/L, $p < 0.0001$) • Vegetarians show a weaker reduction in CRP levels (MD −0.25 mg/L, $p = 0.05$) • No notable effects were observed for other inflammatory biomarkers
Craddock et al.[16]	Systematic review and meta-analysis	General population	• Searched PubMed, Medline, and Cochrane databases for relevant studies • Included 30 observational and 10 interventional studies • Conducted random effects meta-analyses	The vegetarian diet was associated with lower levels (expressed as WMD) of the following markers compared to nonvegetarian diets: • *CRP*: −0.61 mg/L ($p = 0.0001$) • *Fibrinogen*: −0.22 g/L ($p = 0.02$) • *Total leukocyte*: $-0.62 \times 10^3/\mu L$ ($p = 0.02$)

(CRP: C-reactive protein; MD: mean difference; WMD: weighted mean difference)

and the conversion of amino acids and fatty acids into energy, as well as maintaining nervous system function.[17]

Vegans encounter significant challenges related to vitamin B12 deficiency, as it is predominantly present in animal-derived foods. A high prevalence of vitamin B12 deficiency is observed in populations such as those in Hong Kong and India, particularly among vegans who do not consume adequate fortified foods or supplements.[4]

The absence of animal products in vegan diets can lead to serious deficiencies, potentially causing conditions such as megaloblastic anemia and neurological disorders. Symptoms may include numbness, tingling sensations, difficulty walking, memory impairment, and depression. Since vitamin B12 is exclusively found in animal products, vegans must depend on supplementation or fortified plant-based alternatives such as plant milk, cereals, and nutritional yeast. Hence, vitamin B12 levels should be regularly monitored in vegans and supplementation should be considered to maintain optimal health.[4,17]

Vitamin D and Calcium

Several studies suggest that vegans frequently do not intake sufficient levels of calcium and vitamin D, largely because they do not consume dairy products and face challenges related to the bioavailability of calcium in plant-based diets.[18]

Insufficient calcium intake can hinder the attainment of peak bone mass and may accelerate bone loss as well, possibly resulting in conditions such as osteopenia or osteoporosis. Symptoms associated with low serum calcium levels include tingling and numbness in the extremities, muscle cramps, reduced appetite, lethargy, seizures, and irregular cardiac rhythms.[4]

Vitamin D insufficiency further compounds calcium deficiency by impairing intestinal absorption. Recent studies indicate a higher likelihood of hip fractures in vegetarians, vegans, and individuals who eat fish compared to those who consume meat. Vegans also exhibit higher rates of overall fractures, leg fractures, and fractures in other major sites. These increased fracture risks may be attributed to significantly reduced dietary protein intake, lower calcium intake, and lower BMI in vegans.[18]

Other Minerals and Micronutrients

Vegans need to consume higher amounts of iron compared to other dietary patterns, as the plant-based foods they primarily consume contain nonheme iron, which has lower bioavailability. This is due to the presence of phytic acid in nuts, whole grains, and legumes, which inhibits iron absorption. Additionally, vegans often experience a zinc deficiency. Animal products such as dairy, meat, and eggs are rich sources of zinc, whereas nuts, seeds, and whole grains, also high in zinc, may have reduced bioavailability due to their phytate content, which limits absorption in the gut. Insufficient zinc intake among vegans has been associated with mental health concerns such as depression, as well as conditions such as dermatitis, diarrhea, and alopecia, which are more commonly observed in this population. Selenium insufficiency has also been noted in vegetarians.[18]

CONCLUSION

Diets rich in minimally processed plant foods, such as VDs, have been linked to lower risks of developing chronic diseases such as CVD, diabetes, and hypertension. These diets result in the improvement of certain cardiometabolic markers such as LDL-C, fasting glucose, and HbA1c and reduce body weight in individuals with diabetes or those at high risk of CVD. Clinical trials also support the protective effects of VDs against conditions such as diabetes, high cholesterol, high BP, and overweight.

As VDs gain popularity globally due to various factors, it is essential to determine which dietary compositions yield optimal health benefits and identify components that may have adverse effects on health. Further RCTs are needed to establish whether the advantages of nutritious plant-based diets are universally applicable. Additionally, these studies should assess the impact of less stringent plant-based diets, which may include limited amounts of animal products like those in pescatarian or traditional Mediterranean diets, on diverse health outcomes. This includes evaluating their role in preventing conditions such as hemorrhagic stroke and bone fractures. Moreover, there is a need for mechanistic studies to deepen our understanding of the biological mechanisms that connect dietary factors to chronic diseases in healthy plant-based dietary patterns.

ACKNOWLEDGMENT

We are thankful to Ms Heena Bhojwani for her Academic Assistance.

ONLINE REFERENCES

Please scan the QR code provided at the end of the table of contents for References of this chapter.

CHAPTER

226

Beneficial Cardiovascular Plants

Shridhar Dwivedi, Deepti Chopra

ABSTRACT

Cardiovascular diseases (CVDs) have emerged as a major killer globally. Conventional medications commonly available for treatment of various cardiovascular ailments have been noted to have adverse effects and are expensive too. Herbal medicines have been used to treat diseases since the beginning of civilization, are safer, are less costly, and can be an alternative approach for treatment of CVDs. The present chapter examines the available scientific information regarding beneficial cardiovascular plants with therapeutic potentials against CVDs.

Keywords: Cardiovascular diseases, traditional medicine, medicinal plants

INTRODUCTION

Cardiovascular diseases (CVDs), particularly coronary artery disease (CAD), have become a growing health problem and are the leading cause of death and disability in both developed countries and developing nations. Despite the widespread prescription of cardiovascular drugs and the availability of prevention information, this disease continues to devastate societies globally. Herbal remedies have long been used to treat a variety of ailments; they play a significant role in improving the progression of these conditions. More than 80% of people in Asian and African countries depend on traditional medicine for their primary health needs.[1] Several medicinal plants have been described as beneficial for cardiac ailments, including *Allium sativum* (garlic), *Commiphora mukul* (guggul), *Curcuma longa* (turmeric), *Eugenia jambolana* (jamun), *Terminalia arjuna* (arjuna), etc. In this chapter, we will discuss the plants that have shown promising results in treating CVDs.

AEGLE MARMELOS (BAEL)

Aegle marmelos, commonly known as *Bael,* belongs to the family Rutaceae, and contains several active constituents including marmelosin, marmelide, luvangetin, auraptene, psoralen, and tannin. *Bael* has shown significant potential in reversing cardiac cell damage and improving membrane permeability. The fruit extract exerts antioxidant activity. Further, the extract scavenges hydroxyl radical and nitric oxide (NO) radical. The increased plasma levels of ascorbic acid in treated rats further indicate its beneficial role in preventing myocardial infarction.[2] The methanolic extract has been shown to reduce blood sugar in alloxan-induced diabetic rats. Additionally, there was a significant decrease in lipid peroxidation and conjugated diene and hydroperoxide levels in serum as well as in the liver. Further, superoxide dismutase, catalase, and glutathione peroxidase activities were found to be increased.[3] Studies have shown the protective effect of aqueous extract on the histopathology of the pancreas in streptozotocin-induced diabetic rats. The fruit extract-treated groups showed improved functional state of the pancreatic cells and partially reversed the damage caused by streptozotocin.[4]

ALLIUM SATIVUM (GARLIC)

Allicin (allyl 2-propenethiosulfinate or diallyl thiosulfinate) is the principal bioactive compound present in garlic; other sulfur-containing compounds present in garlic include allyl methyl thiosulfonate, 1-propenyl allyl thiosulfonate, and γ-L-glutamyl-*S*-allyl-L-cysteine. Allicin is produced when alliinase enzyme, present in garlic, is activated and acts on alliin (present in intact garlic). The sulfur compounds in garlic are known to have hypolipidemic and hypercholesterolemic effects. The principal sulfur compound in garlic oil, diallyl disulfide, is known to decrease plasma and liver tissue lipid levels by inhibiting enzymes such as acetyl-CoA carboxylase, and HMG-CoA reductase subsequently reduce fatty acid and cholesterol synthesis. Garlic also increases the excretion of cholesterol.[5] Various animal studies have shown that garlic significantly attenuated serum LDL levels, VLDL, cholesterol levels, and increased HDL levels. Further, human studies have also shown that garlic significantly lowered LDL-C and other plasma lipid levels in adults with moderate hypercholesterolemia.[6-8]

Adverse effects of garlic include heartburn, nausea, vomiting, allergic reactions, bloating, headache, dizziness, and profuse sweating. In studies, garlic has been shown to have additive effects with anticoagulants or platelet aggregation inhibitors leading to hemorrhage.[5]

COMMIPHORA MUKUL (GUGGUL)

Commiphora mukul **(Fig. 1)**, commonly known as *Guggul*, has shown significant cardioprotective potential. Ojha et al. conducted a study demonstrating its efficacy against isoprenaline-induced myocardial necrosis in rats. Pretreatment with *guggul* resulted in a significant increase in myocardial antioxidants while reducing MDA levels. Furthermore, it prevented the leakage of LDH and CK-MB from the heart. Histopathological examinations revealed a reduction in necrosis, edema, and inflammation following *guggul* pretreatment. The potential beneficial effects can be attributed to its antioxidant and antiperoxidative activities.[9]

Guggulsterone isolated from *guggul* has been identified as the bioactive constituent responsible for *guggul*'s therapeutic effects. It acts as an antagonist at the farnesoid X receptor (FXR), which is a key regulator for cholesterol and bile acid homeostasis. The FXR antagonism has been proposed as a mechanism for its hypolipidemic effect. Further, another proposed mechanism for hypolipidemic effect is upregulation of the bile salt export pump, by guggulsterone. This is responsible for removing cholesterol metabolites and bile acids from the liver. This upregulation promotes cholesterol metabolism into bile acids.[10]

The hypolipidemic effect of guggulipid and guggulsterone has been consistently demonstrated in various animal studies. Guggulsterone has shown to significantly reduce serum cholesterol and triglycerides, LDL, and very low-density lipoprotein levels. Additionally, guggulsterone treatment was found to increase lipolytic enzyme activity and receptor-mediated catabolism of LDL. Various clinical studies have also demonstrated hypolipidemic activity of *guggul*. Short-term use of either *guggul* or guggulipid has been shown to be generally safe with no significant side effects observed on renal and liver functions, hematological parameters, and electrolytes.[10] The pioneering studies done by Satyavati et al. in 1988 have proved its utility in clinical cases of dyslipidemia long back. However, its clinical use has been overshadowed by statins. Guggulipid received regulatory approval in India in 1987 for use as a lipid-lowering drug, and it is available in the United States as a dietary supplement. Guggulipid is marketed in the United States to maintain normal levels of serum cholesterol, and as part of multiherbal supplements for "heart health," weight loss, and arthritis. In a recent study conducted by Szapary et al., its effect on LDL cholesterol is less than encouraging. One of the plausible reasons for such discouraging result could be use of Western diet/junk diet or nonvegetarian items by the study group subjects. It is surmised that the drug may be reexplored in cases of statin intolerance and/or statin resistance.[11]

CRATAEGUS OXYACANTHA (HAWTHORN)

Crataegus oxyacantha **(Fig. 2)**, commonly known as hawthorn, is a well-regarded herb in the management of hypertension. Hawthorn has been used for its beneficial

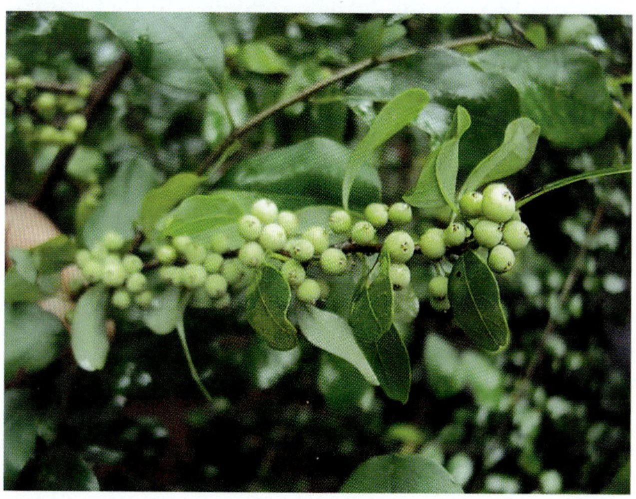

FIG. 1: *Commiphora mukul.*

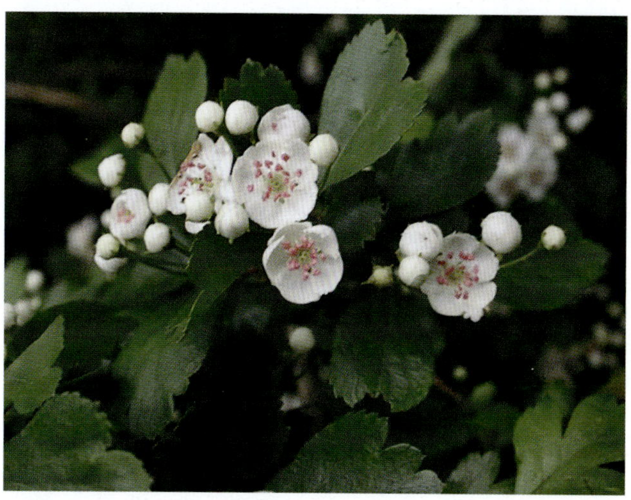

FIG. 2: *Crataegus oxyacantha.*

effects for various CVDs, such as angina, hypertension, hyperlipidemia, ischemia/reperfusion injury, arrhythmia, and class II congestive heart failure. Its mechanism of action involves the modulation of endothelial nitric oxide synthase (eNOS), which plays a crucial role in vasorelaxation. Hawthorn extracts have been shown to enhance the production of NO in endothelial cells, leading to vasodilation and reduced vascular resistance. This vasorelaxation effect helps in lowering blood pressure and improving overall cardiovascular function. Additionally, hawthorn is noted for its antioxidant properties, which further support its cardiovascular benefits by reducing oxidative stress. These effects make hawthorn a valuable herb for managing hypertension and supporting cardiovascular health.[12]

CURCUMA LONGA (TURMERIC)

Turmeric, derived from the rhizome of the *C. longa* plant belonging to the Zingiberaceae family, has long been revered for its medicinal properties. Curcumin, the active component of turmeric, offers various cardiovascular benefits through its antioxidant, anti-inflammatory, and antihypertensive properties.[13] Evidence from literature demonstrated that hydrogen peroxide-induced premature senescence in endothelial cells is attenuated by pretreatment with curcumin. This is accompanied by a decrease in reactive oxygen species production, increased eNOS activation, and enhanced NO production. Curcumin counteracts these effects by upregulating sirtuin 1 (SIRT1) and NRF2 and downregulating the p53/p21 pathway.[13-15] Studies have shown that turmeric extract reduces oxidative stress and attenuates atherosclerosis development and also has shown to reduce the size of atherosclerotic lesions.[16,17] There is a protective role of curcumin in myocardial infarction and remodeling. In isoproterenol-treated rats, curcumin has shown to attenuate the morphological changes in the heart. Protective effect of curcumin in obesity-induced adipose tissue dysfunction has been demonstrated. Curcumin has shown to improve fatty acid oxidation, impair lipogenesis, attenuate differentiation into mature adipocytes, and induce apoptosis in these cells. Furthermore, curcumin increases adiponectin levels while decreasing leptin, reducing inflammation.[13] Hajleh et al. conducted a randomized controlled trial and found that turmeric concentrate intake can reduce BP and improve antioxidant and anti-inflammatory status and arterial compliance. Turmeric may also improve exercise performance and ameliorate oxidative stress. It also has antihypertensive effects due to its antioxidant and anti-inflammatory properties, Ca^{2+} ion interference, α2-adrenergic receptor stimulation, and renin-angiotensin system inhibition.[18-20]

Despite these benefits, some adverse effects of turmeric have been reported. Few of the adverse effects reported in different studies are abdominal pain, nausea, dyspepsia, constipation, hot flashes, and mild diarrhea.[21-24]

EMBLICA OFFICINALIS (AMLA)

Emblica officinalis (**Fig. 3**), commonly known as *amla*, belongs to the Euphorbiaceae family, and is a fruit rich in tannins, alkaloids, phenols, amino acids, carbohydrates, vitamins, flavonoids, and organic acids. *Amla* has shown to improve vascular endothelial function and protect against myocardial ischemia/reperfusion injury as well as doxorubicin and isoproterenol cardiotoxicity.[25,26] In various animal and human studies, *amla* has demonstrated diverse activities including antihyperglycemic, hypoglycemic, anti-inflammatory, antihyperlipidemic, antihypertensive, and antioxidant activities. These properties make it a valuable medicinal plant for managing cardiovascular health.[26,27] Experimental studies have shown that the extract possesses antiplatelet activity, which may increase the risk of bleeding when taken with medications such as aspirin, warfarin, heparin, clopidogrel, ibuprofen, or naproxen. The fruit extract also lowers blood sugar levels, necessitating caution when used with hypoglycemic drugs. *Amla* is a rich source of tannins, which may interfere with intestinal absorption of iron, and its high ascorbic acid content can potentially trigger gastric hyperacidity and constipation.[25]

EUGENIA JAMBOLANA (JAMUN)

Eugenia jambolana, commonly known as *jamun*, belongs to the family Myrtaceae and has been widely used in traditional medicine to treat diabetes. Achrekar et al. first reported that the water extract of fruit pulp exhibited hypoglycemic activity and was found to be more potent in reducing fasting blood glucose compared to the ethanolic fruit pulp extract. The seeds of *jamun* are well documented for their antihyperglycemic activity. In streptozotocin-induced diabetic rats, a purified active compound obtained from aqueous extract has resulted in significant improvement in

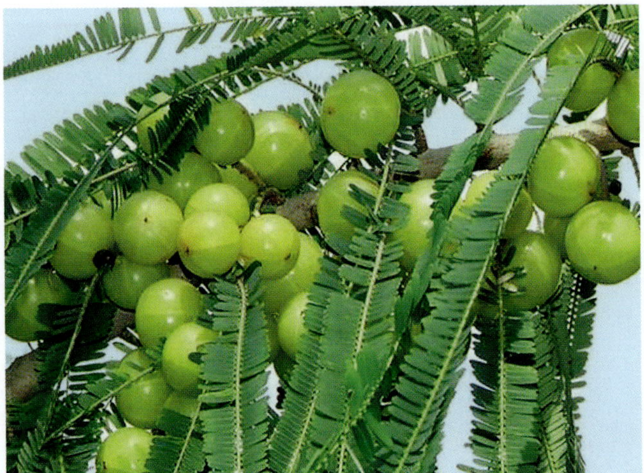

FIG. 3: *Emblica officinalis.*

blood glucose, serum lipid profile, apolipoproteins (apoA1 and apoB100), and endothelial dysfunction parameters.[28]

Shukla et al. evaluated the hydroalcoholic extract of the fruit pulp for its effects on isoproterenol-induced myocardial damage in rats. The study showed pretreatment with extract provided cardioprotective activity by decreasing levels of malondialdehyde, cardiac markers, and markers of inflammation. Further, it also increased levels of superoxide dismutase and reduced glutathione.[29] A study on patients diagnosed with prediabetics showed that *E. jambolana* seed powder significantly improved total cholesterol and LDL levels.[30]

MOMORDICA CHARANTIA (BITTER GOURD)

Momordica charantia, commonly called bitter gourd or balsam pear, belongs to the Cucurbitaceae family. The phytochemical constituents include alkaloids, flavonoids, cardiac glycosides, saponins, steroids, terpenoids, tannins, and anthraquinones, which are of significant biochemical and cardiovascular relevance.[31,32] Consumption of extract has been shown to favorably alter blood lipid profiles in obese rats, while increasing systemic insulin levels. This ultimately results in decreased serum glucose levels in treated animals. The potential mechanism of action of seed extract is modulation of peroxisome proliferator-activated receptor gamma (PPAR-γ) gene expression.[33] Studies have demonstrated that *M. charantia* polysaccharides augment the production of the cytoprotective heat shock protein heme oxygenase-1. This protein has been demonstrated to mitigate major symptoms of streptozotocin-induced diabetes and diabetic nephropathy in a rat model.[34] Extremely bitter *karela* have been noted to cause severe gastritis associated with gastrointestinal bleeding which could be fatal.

PUNICA GRANATUM (POMEGRANATE)

Punica granatum belongs to the family Punicaceae; it possesses many bioactive compounds such as ellagic acid, cinnamic acid, genistein, linoleic acid, anthocyanin, gallic acid, catechin, quercetin, rutin, kaempferol, cyanidin, punicalin, delphinidin, punicalagin, ellagitannins, anthocyanins, urolithins, flavonoids, alkaloids, and tannins. These compounds exhibit free radical scavenging properties in the myocardium.[35-37] Niewiadomska et al. demonstrated the cardioprotective potential of dietary polyphenols found in pomegranate peels in an animal model of metabolic syndrome.[35] Gupta et al. studied the peel extract against isoproterenol-induced myocardial infarction. The results showed that the treated groups showed reduced serum marker enzymes of MI, increased myocardial tissue superoxide dismutase activity, reduced glutathione and nitrite levels, and decreased lipid peroxidation.[38] Santoz et al. investigated the effects of the extract on damage associated with hypertension and aging in animal model. The results showed that the levels of superoxide anion were found to be significantly lower in animals pretreated with extract. Further, peel extract consumption conferred protection against hypertension in animal models.[39]

PTEROCARPUS MARSUPIUM (VIJAYSAR)

Pterocarpus marsupium **(Fig. 4)** has been used in Ayurveda to treat various diseases. The bark, seed, and heartwood have been particularly beneficial in decreasing hyperglycemia in pharmacological trials. The methanolic heartwood extract was found to have high phenolic and flavonoid content. It contains antidiabetic saturated and unsaturated fatty acids, alcohols, and sterols such as myristic acid, succinic acid, isoeugenol, linolic acid, and citronellal.[40] The sterol isoeugenol found in the heartwood extract has been reported to activate AMP-activated protein kinase and improve glucose uptake in rat myotubes. Further, esters of succinic acid which is present in the extract are potent insulin secretagogues, and their prolonged use has shown to improve pancreatic beta-cell functioning.[41] The presence of quercetin in the extract enhances its antidiabetic potential by increasing antioxidant enzyme activity. Experimental data from studies revealed that the ethanolic extract reduced blood glucose, increased serum insulin levels, and showed marked antidyslipidemic effects. The potential reason for its effects is attributed to the high content of phenolic compounds, tannins, and flavonoids present in extract.[40,42] The aqueous extract of heartwood also shows cardiotonic effect in a dose-dependent manner.[43]

TERMINALIA ARJUNA (ARJUNA)

Terminalia arjuna **(Fig. 5)**, commonly known as *arjuna*, belongs to the Combretaceae family. Both experimental and clinical studies suggest that this plant possesses

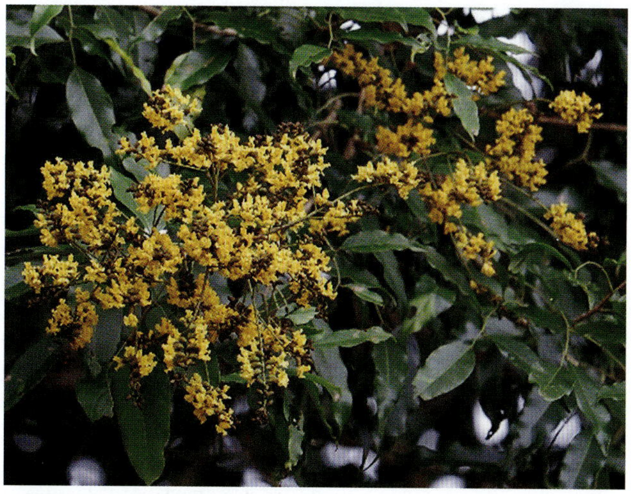

FIG. 4: *Pterocarpus marsupium.*

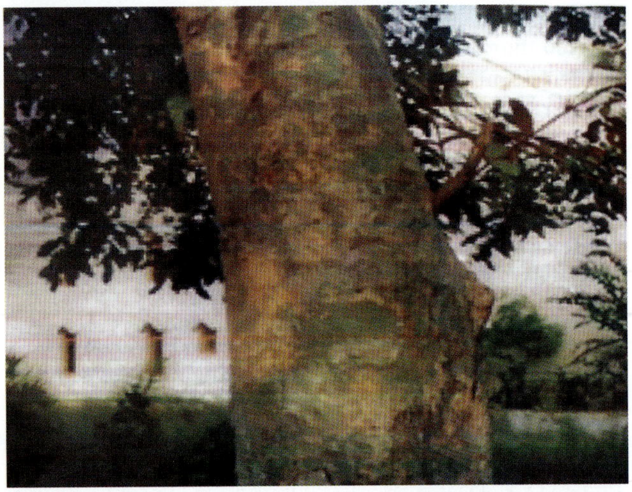

FIG. 5: *Terminalia arjuna.*

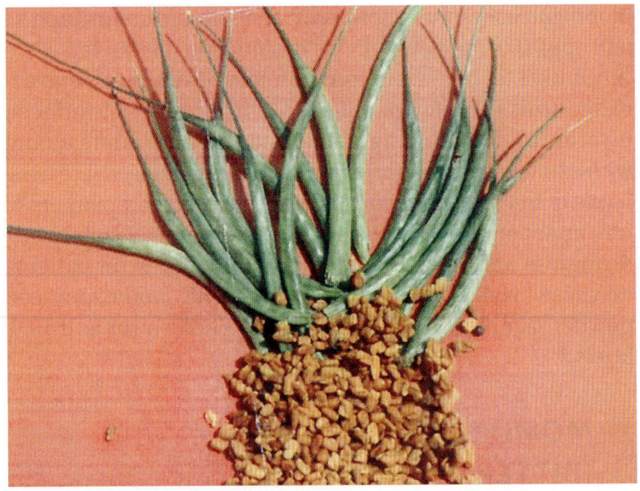

FIG. 6: *Trigonella foenum-graecum.*

anti-ischemic, antioxidant, hypolipidemic, and antiatherogenic activities. The plant contains a variety of phytoconstituents including triterpenoids, β-sitosterol, flavonoids, and glycosides. Experimental studies have shown a dose-dependent decrease in blood pressure in animals. The hypotensive effect may be mediated by cholinergic mechanisms, adrenergic β2-receptor agonistic action, and/or direct action on heart muscle. *Arjuna* bark extract has also shown protective effects against doxorubicin-induced cardiotoxicity. Studies have demonstrated that *arjuna* protects the heart against myocardial changes induced by chronic β-adrenoceptor stimulation.[44] Praveen et al. studied the protective effect of bark extract on left ventricular and baroreflex function in rat model of chronic heart failure. Both prophylactic and therapeutic treatment with *arjuna* improved cardiac functions and baroreflex sensitivity. Further, *arjuna* extract also attenuated the hypertrophy and fibrosis of the left ventricle, reduced serum oxidative stress, and lowered serum TNF-α levels.[45] In clinical studies, *arjuna* has been demonstrated to be effective in patients with angina and hypertension, and shown to improve lipid profile.[44]

TRIGONELLA FOENUM-GRAECUM (FENUGREEK)

Trigonella foenum-graecum (**Fig. 6**), commonly known as fenugreek, is a medicinal herb from the Fabaceae family that has been used in traditional medicine for its numerous therapeutic benefits. Fenugreek is particularly known for its ability to reduce total cholesterol and low-density lipoprotein cholesterol levels.[46] The seeds of fenugreek contain 4-hydroxyisoleucine (an unusual amino acid), which enhances cell glucose uptake by increasing GLUT-4 to plasma membrane in skeletal muscle cells.[47] Additionally, administration of fenugreek seed polyphenolic extract has shown to improve insulin sensitivity by enhancing the phosphorylation of tyrosine kinase and improving insulin signaling.[48] Fenugreek's antihyperlipidemic properties are also significant. It contains diosgenin, which can alter intracellular calcium concentration, regulate membrane binding proteins, increase lipid transportation into cells, and decrease tissue fatty acids. Diosgenin has shown to decrease body weight gain, blood glucose, insulin, and insulin resistance, and also it modulated lipid profile in animal models.[49] The polysaccharide components in fenugreek seeds are fermented by the intestinal bacteria to yield short-chain fatty acids, which inhibit the absorption of cholesterol and enhance its excretion.[46] Ramesh et al. investigated the effect of fenugreek seeds on alloxan-induced diabetic rats. The extract lowered the total cholesterol and serum triglycerides. Histopathological analysis of the pancreas showed that treatment with fenugreek extract restored the extensive damage to the islets of Langerhans and reduced dimensions of the islets that were found in alloxan-induced diabetic rats.[50] Clinical studies have shown that seed powder improved lipid metabolism in newly diagnosed type II diabetic patients with no adverse effects.[51]

WITHANIA SOMNIFERA (*ASHWAGANDHA*)

Withania somnifera has structural similarity to digoxin, and exhibits significant cardioprotective effects. Treatment with *ashwagandha* has been shown to increase heart rate and contractility, decrease preload, and enhance antioxidant enzyme activity while inhibiting lipid peroxidation. Additionally, it demonstrates antiapoptotic properties also. Evidence from literature demonstrated that *ashwagandha* improved myocardial energy substrate utilization and cardiac function, and reduced infarct size in ischemia-reperfusion models. *Withania* and its withanolides exhibit potent anti-inflammatory effects by inhibiting proinflammatory transcription factors. The plant also has hypolipidemic and antiatherogenic properties, including delayed plasma recalcification time, and enhanced lipoprotein lipase enzyme release. In terms of antidiabetic activity, *ashwagandha* favorably alters blood and urine glucose levels, glycated hemoglobin, and liver enzymes in diabetic rats.[52,53]

ZINGIBER OFFICINALE (GINGER)

Zingiber officinale, commonly known as ginger, has several cardioprotective effects, attributed to its cardiotonic, antihypertensive, antihyperlipidemic, and antiplatelet properties. The oleoresin from ginger rhizomes contains bioactive compounds such as gingerols, shogaols, diarylheptanoids, phenylbutenoids, flavonoids, diterpenoids, and sesquiterpenoids. These compounds have shown to reduce inflammation, improve dyslipidemia, and lower blood pressure.[54,55] In hypertensive animals, ginger has demonstrated a dose-dependent hypotensive effect. It has been shown to cause vasodilation in animal models following induced vasoconstriction and exhibits calcium channel-blocking activity. Ginger extract has also been found to increase the levels of apolipoprotein A-1 and lecithin-cholesterol acyltransferase mRNA in the liver, which is related to the formation of high-density lipoprotein.[54,56] Ginger can reduce levels of plasma total cholesterol, triglycerides, and very low-density lipoprotein cholesterol in high-fat diet rats. This effect is linked to higher liver expression of peroxisome proliferator-activated receptors, which are involved in lipid metabolism and regulation.[57]

CONCLUSION

The present chapter highlights the therapeutic potential of various plants in treating CVDs through their diverse mechanisms of action, including antioxidant, anti-inflammatory, hypolipidemic, and antihypertensive effects. These observations support the need for extensive in-depth studies investigating for active drug molecules from medicinal plants such as *T. arjuna* (*arjuna*), *A. sativum* (garlic), *C. mukul* (*guggul*), *C. longa* (turmeric), and *E. jambolana* (*jamun*). It is worthwhile to remember that use of these herbal drugs also mandates maintaining a healthy lifestyle to get the best relief out of them.

ONLINE REFERENCES

Please scan the QR code provided at the end of the table of contents for References of this chapter.

Index

Page numbers followed by *b* refer to box, *f* refer to figure, *fc* refer to flowchart, and *t* refer to table.

A

B

G

H

I

J

K

L

N

Q

R

T

W

X

Y

Z